To Fred Enslell
in recognition of six
good months in the
tradition of the Guild.

Feb 10/78

General Pathology

J. B. Walter *T.D.*, M.D., M.R.C.P., F.R.C.Path.

Department of Pathology, Banting Institute, University of Toronto, and Departments of Medicine and Pathology, Toronto General Hospital, Toronto, Canada.

M. S. Israel M.B., M.R.C.P., M.R.C.Path., D.C.P.

Department of Pathology, Institute of Basic Medical Sciences, Royal College of Surgeons of England, and Lewisham Group Laboratory, London.

General Pathology · 4th Edition

J. B. WALTER & M. S. ISRAEL

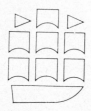

CHURCHILL LIVINGSTONE   EDINBURGH AND LONDON 1974

CHURCHILL LIVINGSTONE
Medical Division of Longman Group Limited

Represented in the United States of America by Longman Inc.,
New York, and by associated companies, branches and
representatives throughout the world

© Longman Group Limited 1974

ISBN 0 443 01120 6

Reprinted 1975

Library of Congress Catalog Card Number 73–84620

Printed in Great Britain by Hazell Watson & Viney Ltd.,
Aylesbury, Bucks

Preface to the Fourth Edition

For over a hundred years pathology has been one of the keystones of medicine, and as an academic subject it has been taught as part of the medical curriculum to prepare the student for the more nebulous clinical programme that completes his training. Unfortunately the practice of pathology has come to be relegated to the full-time pathologist and clinical medicine to the specialised clinician. This separation of pathological practice from the direct care of the patient is quite artificial, and has in any case never been absolute. Recently this cleavage has been bridged, and the process is being accelerated by the advances that have taken place during the last two decades in clinical pathology, namely cytology, biochemistry, haematology, and microbiology. Even the isolation of histopathology, surely the last bastion of the non-clinical medical pathologist, has eroded before the advancing techniques of needle biopsy and the various types of endoscopy. Diseases even of previously inaccessible organs like the kidneys and the central nervous system can now be adequately investigated during life and their progress mapped with precision. The necropsy has ceased to be the final event of revelation, but has rather assumed the role of an epilogue to a drama already well documented. Nevertheless, the epilogue quite frequently provides engaging and disquieting twists to the story—but it is no longer the major part of the record of the tale itself.

Pathology is the scientific study of disease: it follows the morbid process from its inception to its termination and it investigates the lesions produced. Wherever possible it uses accurate measurement, for the scientific method demands reproducible data. Thus, the size of a cancer cell, its content of DNA, its characteristics in tissue culture, and the life span of the patient in whom it is found can all be measured; all these considerations fall within the scope of pathology. The subject is therefore the concern of clinicians no less than pathologists, a fact well attested by the many valuable contributions made to pathology by clinicians and to clinical medicine by pathologists. The medical graduate who restricts his practice either to the bedside or to the laboratory can be sure of having only an incomplete and unbalanced understanding of medicine.

The fourth edition of General Pathology is our continued effort to provide an account of the fundamental processes of pathology in relationship to medical practice. A full understanding of the subject involves the disciplines of morbid anatomy, biochemistry, haematology, microbiology, physiology, and clinical medicine; all these aspects of disease process are dealt with in this book, and in particular we have tried to give a careful description of the basic pathological processes, for both these and the terms which are commonly used to describe them are a constant source of difficulty to the beginner. We do not aim at giving a comprehensive account of recent advances; many fine books and reviews are available for such information.

In the three years which have elapsed since the last edition, there have been no dramatic advances in medicine, but there has been steady progress in many areas so that a complete revision has been necessary. The section on immunology has undergone the greatest change, and in particular the pathogenesis of cell-mediated responses has become further clarified. The properdin system and the alternate pathway for the activation of complement are now known to be important, and the immunological mechanisms are better understood in relationship to immune-complex disease and other forms of hypersensitivity and autoimmunity. A new section has been added on the principles of fixation and staining of tissues, and some modification has been necessary in the section on the mediators of acute inflammation—particularly the role of the prostaglandins. The ravages of research have yet again struck amyloid, the nature of which is now thought to be closely related to the immunoglobulins.

Amongst the numerous topics which have either been expanded or introduced for the first time are the following: scanning electron microscopy, demonstration of the Y chromosome in the interphase nucleus, cytoplasmic DNA, genetic polymorphism, the Lesch-Nyhan syndrome, cyclic AMP, the avoidance and methods of treatment of genetic defects, myxomatous change of heart valves, the biosynthesis of collagen, selective chemotaxis in acute inflammation particularly in relation to the eosinophil, the pathogenesis of granulomata, the use of silicones and silastics, candidiasis, antiviral agents of clinical importance, the virus haemorrhagic fevers, the hepatitis associated antigen, vaginal adenocarcinoma induced by stilboestrol, the classification of lymphomata, immune aspects of carcinogenesis, the role of the oncogenic RNA viruses and the importance of their DNA polymerase, the clinical detection of venous thrombosis, the importance of micro-emboli in the pathogenesis of disease, alpha-1 antitrypsin deficiency, the importance of 2:3-diphosphoglycerate in red cells, and finally the importance of the isoenzymes of lactic dehydrogenase and alkaline phosphatase. Some unsatisfactory figures have been removed and a number of new ones added. Inevitably this has involved some increase in size, and the new, more modern format has been introduced to accommodate this and present the material in a more pleasing way.

The references at the end of each chapter have been scrutinised, augmented, and updated, so that the reader can gain easy entry to the preceding literature. In doing this, we have sometimes omitted references which, although of fundamental and original nature, can readily be found in the later literature.

J.B.W.,
Toronto, Canada.

M.S.I.,
London, England.

Acknowledgements

The great majority of the specimens illustrated are from the Wellcome Museum of Pathology, and we are grateful to the President and the Council of the Royal College of Surgeons of England for permission to reproduce them. In accordance with their wishes each is acknowledged at the end of the caption and their catalogue number is indicated. We are grateful to Mrs. Marie Crookston for her continued help with Chapter 52. In the case of published work we wish to thank the authors, editors, and publishers who have allowed us to reproduce their material. The references are given after each figure. We owe special gratitude to those who have given us unpublished material, or have allowed us to modify their original published work: Abell, M. R., 16.10; Bernhard, W., 22.5; Bithell, T. C., 51.3; Bloom, H. J. G., 26.14; Brewer, D. B., 4.8; Bywaters, E. G. L., 16.6, 16.7; Clark, Jr., J. W., 27.15, 27.16, 27.17; Cohen, A. S., 44.3, 44.4, 44.5; Comroe, J. H., 41.3, 41.4; Crick, F. H. C., 2.10; Crowle, A. J., 1.4; Cullen, J. B., 21.5, 26.33; Curry, R. H., 41.2; David, J. R., 14.2; Davidson, J. N., 2.13; Dawson, I. M. P., 11.9; Demshar, H. P., 38.3, 38.4; Director of Archaeological Museum, Florence, 15.1; Dixon, F. J., 12.14, 14.1; Dunphy, J. E., 9.9; Eastoe, J. E., 1.5, 1.6; Egan, R. L. 47.3, 47.4; Eisen, H. N., 12.8; Epstein, M. A., 2.5, 2.16, 2.19, 22.4; Flewett, T. H., 23.1, 23.3, 23.4; Gahan, P. B., 1.8; Hale, A. J., 1.1; Hansson, O., 23.2; Harrison, C. V., 16.9; Heptinstall, R. H., 16.8; Horne, R. W., 22.1, 22.2, 22.3; Kavanau, J. L., 2.6; Kawerau, E., 1.3; Kemp, N. H., 2.8, 2.9, 3.7, 3.10; Latner, A. L., 4.11; le Beux, Y., 2.2, 2.7; Levene, C. I., 5.1; Lewin, P. K. and Conen, P. E., 3.8; Miyai, K., 2.14, 2.15, 2.18, 2.20, 4.5, 4.6, 4.7; Miles, A. A., 6.5; Najarian, J. S., 15.2; Neely, J. and Davies, J. D., 11.10; Nirenberg, M. W. and Warner, J. R., 2.11; Nopajaroonsri, C., Luk, S. C., and Simon, G. T., 1.2; Palade, G. E., 42.1; Reese, A. J. M., 1.7; Schulz, H., 41.1; Sheward, J. D., 46.2; Simon, G. T., 42.2; Stewart, P. D., 30.7; Thompson, J. S. and Thompson, M. W., 2.12; Thomson, A. D., 21.3, 26.28; Turk, J. L., 12.10, 12.11, 12.12, 12.13; Waldenström, J., 45.1, 45.2; Wintrobe, M. M., 49.2, 51.3; Wood, P., 40.1.

Contents

Chapter

Chapter 1. Introduction

Pathology, the scientific study of disease processes, has its roots deeply implanted in medical history. The earliest observers, from Celsus (about 30 B.C.–A.D. 38) to Morgagni in the eighteenth century, based their work upon the naked-eye appearances of diseased individuals and organs. Only as the technique of microscopy improved was the Germanic School of Pathology, headed by Virchow (1821–1905), able to investigate changes at a cellular level.

In France, Pasteur, using the microscope, laid the foundation of the science of bacteriology, while later on the German dye industry enabled Koch, Ehrlich, and Domagk to extend this knowledge and open the era of chemotherapy. Advances in pathology thus have been closely related to advances in technology. This in no way belittles the efforts of inspired experimenters like Jenner, who in England pioneered the way to active immunisation.

Nowadays technological advances are occurring so rapidly that no doctor can hope to have a working knowledge of all the methods that are available. Nevertheless, it is by utilising all these complex techniques that problems are fully investigated. The student of medicine should therefore have some understanding of the techniques which are available, and the type of problem which they might be able to solve. In this way investigators conversant with many different disciplines are brought together to their mutual benefit.

TECHNIQUES AVAILABLE IN PATHOLOGY

MICRODISSECTION

Apparatus is available for dissecting cells. In this way the nucleus can be removed, and the effect of this on the deprived cell observed[1] (p. 11). Micropipettes can be inserted into the capillaries, and microelectrodes placed in single nerve cells or fibres.[2] More recently, microbeams of ultraviolet light, or Laser rays (*Light Amplification by Stimulated Emission of Radiation*), have been used to produce damage in a particular part of a cell.[3]

The micromanipulation of embryos can produce some interesting results. Thus the developing eggs from two pregnant mice of different strains can be removed and made to adhere to each other *in vitro*. If reimplanted into a pseudopregnant female, the combined embryo can develop into one animal called an allophrenic mouse. In this the two cell types form clones* of varying numbers in different organs. When hair colour is involved, roughly equal numbers of melanocytes of both genotypes are produced, and the animal has a series of transverse bands of alternating colours. It has been suggested that even in the normal animal mutations could lead to the production of clones of different genetic constitution. Furthermore, even if all the cells of an individual have the same genotype, some could exhibit a separate phenotype due to suppression of certain genes. Perhaps some type of clonal segregation can account for the irregular and patchy distribution of the lesions seen in some human diseases.[4]

MICROSCOPY

The Light Microscope[5]

The light microscope has two disadvantages:

(*a*) Its *resolution* is limited by the wavelength of light. The ability to distinguish between two adjacent points is called the resolving power. In theory resolution should be possible up to a distance of half the wavelength of the light used, but in practice using green light the resolving power of the microscope is about 250 μm.† Thus, only the largest viruses (the poxviruses) can be seen with a good optical microscope. The shorter the wavelength of the light used the better is the resolution, and with ultraviolet light it can be improved two to three times. It is important to distinguish between *visibility* and *resolution*. Particles as small as 75 μm may be visible, but no detailed structure can be resolved. A simple analogy illustrates this difference. If an open book is placed at a distance from the eyes, the writing can easily be distinguished as such, i.e. it is visible, but it may be quite impossible to recognise individual letters because their details cannot be resolved.

(*b*) Living tissue is transparent, and the homogeneity in optical density of its components hides its detailed structure. Staining techniques must therefore be used to see cellular details, but these must almost invariably be performed on dead fixed tissue. It is possible to stain cells by

---

* A clone is a group of cells of like hereditary constitution which has been produced asexually from a single cell. The word is derived from the Greek *klon* meaning a cutting used for propagation.

† 1 mm = 1 000 μm, 1 μm = 1 000 nm, 1 nm = 10 Å (Ångström unit). The present tendency is to dispense with Ångström units and use nanometres instead.

supravital techniques, e.g. the mitochondria of living leucocytes can be stained by Janus green, but even this damages them rapidly so that the cells soon lose their motility and begin to die.

Three techniques have been developed to overcome these difficulties in examining living cells.

Dark-ground illumination[5] relies upon the fact that objects placed in a beam of light may be seen by the rays which they reflect in much the same way that dust particles are rendered visible by a shaft of sunlight. The method finds particular application in the demonstration of organisms which cannot be readily stained, e.g. *Treponema pallidum*.

Phase contrast[5, 6] microscopy takes advantage of the different refractive indices of various parts of the cell. These differences are converted into differences in optical density. In this way living cells can be examined; mitochondria, at one time thought to be artefacts, have been shown to occur in the normal cell.

Interference[6] microscopy works on a different principle. It produces a picture of the cell in which its different components appear in different colours. The interference microscope has one further advantage: the actual amount of a chemical substance in a cell can be measured.

Examination of Fixed Tissues[7, 8]

Paraffin section technique. This is the most commonly used routine method of examination. Tissue is fixed, dehydrated in graded alcohols, cleared in xylol, chloroform, or other solvent which is miscible with both alcohol and wax, and finally embedded in paraffin wax.

Fixation. Fixation is a complex process which involves killing the cells rapidly and inhibiting the enzymatic processes of autolysis. Macromolecules are stabilised and aggregated, proteins are denatured, and some active groups, e.g.—NH_3^+ of protein and —PO_4^{---} of nucleic acid are exposed. The cell's membranes are altered in such a way that stains can penetrate into the cell and its organelles.

Formaldehyde, as a 10 per-cent aqueous solution of formalin, is the most useful, cheap, and commonly-used fixative. It penetrates tissue with ease and will therefore fix large specimens. It reacts by forming bridges between adjacent —NH_2 groups in the side-chains of proteins and in phospholipids. Only substances which are rendered insoluble, such as proteins, or which become attached to insoluble substances, such as nucleic acids, can be made visible by subsequent staining. Small soluble molecules, such as Na^+, glucose, and urea, cannot be localised with any degree of precision by present-day methods.

Frozen section technique. The paraffin-wax technique removes certain chemicals, e.g. fat, and alters others, e.g. enzymes. To meet this difficulty the cryostat has been developed: in essence this is a microtome with which sections are cut at —30°C. This is achieved by having the microtome enclosed in a refrigerator. The sections of frozen fresh material thus obtained are so little damaged

that they are suitable for histochemical study. They may also be stained with haematoxylin and eosin, and the method can be used for quick examination of tissue. Some hospitals employ the method for the routine examination of surgical material, but the sections, although adequate for diagnosis, are nevertheless of poor quality.

STAINING TECHNIQUES FOR DEMONSTRATING CELL STRUCTURE[9, 10]

Although many of the staining methods of histopathology have been developed empirically, some general principles can be discerned. There are three types of staining method:

Solution of lipid-soluble dyes in the liquid lipid of cells or tissue.

Staining of tissue by chemical union of coloured or chromogenic substances to reactive loci.

Coloration of added reagents by reactive loci (commonly enzymic) of tissue.

Each of these will be considered in more detail.

Lipid Soluble Dyes

An alcoholic solution of a lipid-soluble dye, such as Sudan III or Oil Red O, when applied to a frozen tissue section, will rapidly pass into cellular lipid droplets and thereby colour them. Similarly osmium tetroxide will dissolve in liquid lipid; it is then reduced by ethylenic double bonds to black lower oxides. Osmium tetroxide also acts as a fixative, and in this role finds particular application in electron microscopy (see p. 4).

Staining of Tissue by Chemical Union of Coloured or Chromogenic Substances to Reactive Loci of Cells

The attachment by chemical union depends on one of three mechanisms:

(*a*) electrostatic attraction of dye to oppositely charged tissue loci;

(*b*) precipitation of charged colloids on to oppositely charged tissue loci;

(*c*) covalent union to reactive sites.

(*a*) **Electrostatic attraction of dyes to oppositely-charged tissue loci.** *Acidophilic (positively-charged) tissue loci.* The principal cationic loci are the —NH_3^+ groups of basic amino acids. These can be demonstrated by anionic dyes such as eosin, picric acid, and acid fuchsin. If careful, controlled techniques are used, combinations of these dyes will stain cytoplasm and connective tissue selectively. Thus in Van Gieson's stain, picric acid stains cytoplasm and muscle yellow, while collagen takes up the red acid fuchsin.

Basophilic (negatively-charged) tissue loci. These include the —PO_4^{---} groups of nucleic acids, —SO_4^{--} of polysaccharides, and the —COO^- of uronic and amino acids. The union of cationic dyes with the last group is tenuous and, in practice, the dyes stain nucleic acids, polysaccharides, and some acidic lipids. Important members of this group are methylene blue, Azur A (formed by the oxidation of methylene blue), pyronin, and methyl green. As with the anionic stains, combinations of dyes can produce differential staining. Thus in Leishman's stain DNA is stained violet by Azur A, RNA of cytoplasm and nucleoli is coloured blue by methylene blue, while cytoplasmic protein including haemoglobin is tinted red by eosin (p. 583). The most useful cationic dye is derived from haematoxylin, a dye extracted from a tree. By oxidation haematein is produced, and this when mordanted with Al^{+++}, Cr^{+++}, or Fe^{+++} forms a useful deep purple, positively-charged dye, commonly referred to as "haematoxylin" and used in combination with eosin.

(*b*) **Precipitation of charged colloids on oppositely charged tissue loci.** A good example of this method is Hale's colloidal iron stain. Positively-charged colloidal iron is precipitated and bound to sulphate esters and uronic acids of polysaccharides. The bound ferric ions are converted to Prussian blue by the addition of potassium ferrocyanide.

(*c*) **Covalent union of coloured or chromogenic substances to reactive tissue loci.** Reactive loci in the cell can be demonstrated by combining them covalently with coloured compounds. Two examples will be considered.

Periodic Acid-Schiff (PAS) reaction. This stain is not specific, but nevertheless useful. When periodic acid is applied to a section, many carbohydrate components are oxidised to aldehydes. Aldehydes produce a red colour with Schiff's reagent (a solution of basic fuchsin decolorised by sulphurous acid). Therefore, if Schiff's reagent is applied to the treated section, the parts containing carbohydrate are stained red. The periodic acid-Schiff reaction is useful for the demonstration of glycogen, ground substance, and epithelial mucus. Glycogen can be differentiated from the others by pretreating the section with diastase, which removes it.

Feulgen stain. Tissue is treated with hydrochloric acid followed by Schiff's reagent. The reaction depends upon the hydrolysis by hydrochloric acid of the purine-deoxyribose linkages in the DNA molecule. The pentose-phosphoric acid complex which is released has a free aldehyde group, which can be detected by Schiff's reagent. Nuclei and chromosomes are therefore coloured magenta. The method is specific for DNA.

Coloration of added reagents by reactive loci of tissue. Some reactive loci, commonly enzymatic, can convert added reagents into coloured or opaque material. If this material is precipitated, the reaction product is located at, or very close to, the original locus. Several examples of this technique will be described:

(*a*) *Enzymatic localisation.* The demonstration of an enzyme is well illustrated by the method used for alkaline phosphatase. The section is placed in a solution of the substrate β-glycerophosphate in the presence of calcium.

The enzyme splits off phosphate, and this forms calcium phosphate which is invisible. Addition of cobalt nitrate converts it into cobalt phosphate, and ammonium sulphide changes this to black cobalt sulphide.

Although the amount and situation of the black sulphide is indicative of the amount and site of the phosphatase originally present, it is evident that errors can creep in at each of the stages: glycerophosphate → calcium phosphate → cobalt phosphate → cobalt sulphide. The X-ray microscope demonstrates these stages very well.[11, 12] This instrument takes radiographs of sections using X-rays generated at 5 to 10kV. The rays are absorbed by elements of high atomic number, and as in the conventional full-size radiographs show up deposits of calcium. Fig. 1.1 shows how the original calcium phosphate is localised, whilst there has been considerable diffusion by the time the last step is reached. The X-ray microscope can, of course, be used on unstained tissues to show deposits of calcium as well as other structures.

Histochemical techniques may also be applied to the study of cells by electron microscopy (see Fig. 2.5, p. 15).

(*b*) *Perls's Prussian-blue reaction for haemosiderin.* Acid is applied to the tissue to release Fe^{+++} from haemosiderin. Next, potassium ferrocyanide is applied; this reacts with the Fe^{+++} to form blue ferric ferrocyanide.

(*c*) *Reduction of silver nitrate to metallic silver.* Some loci, such as those present on melanin granules and in the cells of Kultschitzky, which are termed *argentaffin*, can reduce silver nitrate to metallic silver, and are thereby blackened.

Argyrophilic loci bind silver but do not reduce it. Subsequent treatment of the tissue with a reducing agent leads to the precipitation of metallic silver. This silver impregnation method is useful for demonstrating reticulin fibres and spirochaetes.

(*d*) *Metachromasia.* Some tissue components have the property of taking up certain dyes and so altering the dye's structure, usually by polymerisation, that the colour is changed. This is called metachromatic staining, and is a property exhibited by the granules of mast cells and by some acid mucopolysaccharides (p. 59). Dyes of the thiazine group are commonly used, and toluidine blue is the best known. It stains most tissues blue, while metachromatic material is coloured purple or even red.

The Electron Microscope[6, 13, 34]

The electron microscope resembles the ordinary microscope except that a stream of electrons is used instead of light, and electromagnetic fields instead of glass lenses. Its resolving power is 0·6–0·7 nm.* By its use viruses can be seen with ease, and our knowledge of detailed cell and tissue structure has increased enormously (see Chapter 2). The electron microscope of current design has, however, three disadvantages.

* For comparison the diameter of a globular protein of molecular weight 80 000 is 6 nm, glucose is 0·5 nm, and water 0·28 nm.

1. Only very small pieces of tissue can be examined; 1–2 mm blocks are usual.

2. The tissue must be examined in a vacuum—living cells cannot therefore be used.

3. Tissue must be fixed immediately, preferably *in vivo*, if artefacts are to be avoided. This must be borne in mind if it is proposed to examine human surgical material.

The most widely used fixative is osmium tetroxide; this also acts as a stain by virtue of the increased electron scattering power of the tissue after impregnation with osmium. It was at one time thought that it stained lipid structures, but this is no longer believed. Another good fixative is potassium permanganate; it shows up phospholipid well, and is therefore useful for the demonstration of the cell membranes. Contrast can be increased by "staining" the sections with salts of heavy metals; alkaline lead hydroxide and uranyl acetate are the ones most often used.

Other fixatives, especially glutaraldehyde, have proved useful in the application of histochemical methods to electron microscopy.[14] Whereas in light microscopy the final reaction product of a histochemical stain is coloured, in electron microscopy it contains a heavy metal and is therefore electron-dense (see Fig. 2.5). Another approach is to conjugate ferritin with protein; in this way intracellular antigens and antibodies may be localised[15] (see p. 152).

Methacrylate was the first embedding medium to gain popularity, but this plastic tends to disintegrate in the electron beam and artefacts are produced. It has therefore been replaced by more stable plastics, e.g. araldite and epon, and pictures of much higher quality can now be obtained. Two other developments of electron microscopy are of note:

Replication. A surface can be examined by making a replica of it, e.g. with a carbon film, and then examining the replica with the electron microscope. This technique has provided valuable information about the plasma membrane.

Negative staining. The method consists of embedding the particles to be examined in a layer of electron-dense material, e.g. containing sodium phosphotungstate or a uranium salt, so that the objects stand out against a dense

Figure 1.1

(*a*) Historadiograph of rat kidney after incubation of the section with β-glycerophosphate in the presence of calcium chloride. The deposits of calcium phosphate indicate the site of alkaline phosphatase activity. (*b*) Section treated as (*a*) above, but the calcium phosphate has been converted into cobalt phosphate by the action of cobalt nitrate. (*c*) Final treatment with ammonium sulphide converts the cobalt phosphate into cobalt sulphide. The historadiograph shows that there has been considerable diffusion, and that the distribution of the radio-opaque material no longer corresponds accurately to that of the alkaline phosphatase. Cobalt sulphide is black, and is visible under the light microscope. However, it is evident that a radiograph at stage (*a*) gives a clearer indication of the actual distribution of the enzyme. ×150. *(From photograph supplied by Dr. A. J. Hale. Published previously in Hale, A. J. (1961), J. biophys biochem. Cytol.,* **11,** *488)*

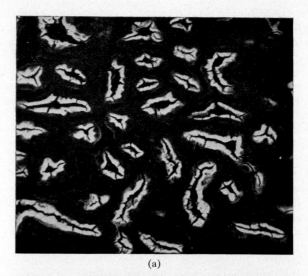

(a)

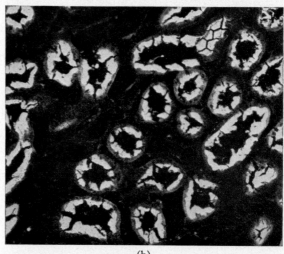

(b)

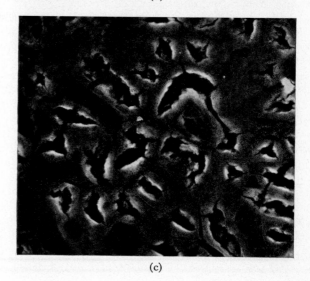

(c)

background. Viruses and amyloid fibres have been usefully studied by this technique (Figs. 22.1 and 2 and 44.4 and 5).

Instruments with a high accelerator voltage are now available, and by their use it has been possible to photograph living bacteria.[16] Although useful in metallurgy, their contribution to biological knowledge has so far been small.

Scanning electron microscope. This instrument works on a different principle from the conventional transmission electron microscope: a very fine beam of electrons is focused to a point and made to scan the surface of the specimen. The secondary electrons scattered from the surface are collected and amplified. The current so generated is used to modulate the brightness of a television tube which is scanned in synchronicity with the electron beam scanning the object. The method is useful for examining the surfaces of objects, and the pictures so obtained have a remarkable three-dimensional effect (Fig. 1.2). Micro-organisms, red cells, and intestinal epithelium have been studied with advantage.

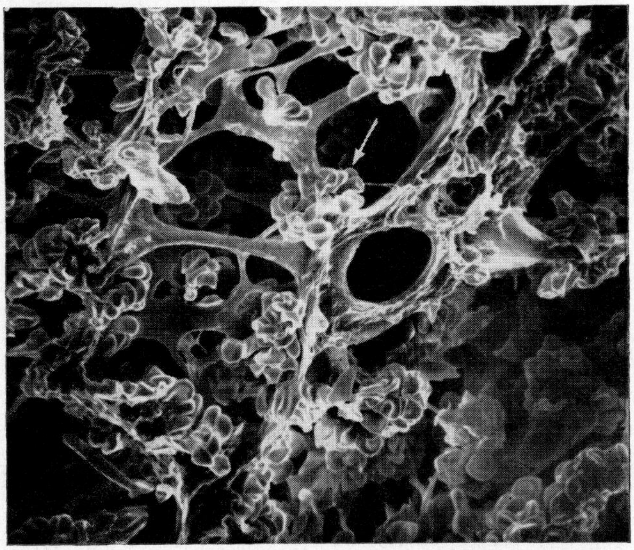

Figure 1.2
Scanning electron micrograph showing the sinuses of a haemolymph node of a rat. Trabeculae are seen crossing the sinuses, and in this mesh-work there are macrophages surrounded by red cells which are being phagocytosed. The sinus-lining cells cannot be discerned, but the groups of red cells forming a rosette around each macrophage are clearly seen and one of them is indicated by an arrow. *(Photograph supplied by Drs. C. Nopajaroonsri, S. C. Luk and G. T. Simon)*

THE ULTRACENTRIFUGE[17]

The tremendous centrifugal force that can be applied by this machine is utilised to separate mixtures of large molecular chemicals. The present-day instrument can develop a centrifugal field sufficient to spin down particles as small as 1 nm. The velocity with which sedimentation occurs can be measured, and the ratio:

$$\frac{\text{Sedimentation velocity}}{\text{Centrifugal field}}$$

is called the Sedimentation Constant. It is measured in Svedberg units (S).

The ultracentrifuge has been used to separate mixtures of proteins; it was in this way that the macroglobulins were identified (see p. 549).

The various components of cells can also be separated and examined by physical and chemical means. If cells are disrupted either physically or by ultrasonic vibration, the cell membranes, nuclei, mitochondria, and ribosomes can be isolated in a fairly pure state after centrifugation.[18] By analysing these fractions the results of histochemistry may be correlated with those of the well-established procedures of chemistry. The many enzyme systems of mitochondria have been investigated in this way. The granules in cloudy swelling have been isolated and identified as altered mitochondria (see p. 50).

CHEMICAL AND PHYSICAL ANALYSIS OF SUBSTANCES OF BIOLOGICAL INTEREST

It is beyond the scope of this book to deal with this subject. It is sufficient to note that methods are available which have led to the complete analysis of substances as complex as the insulin molecule (51 amino-acid residues), the enzyme ribonuclease[19] (124 amino-acid residues), and more recently immunoglobulin. X-ray diffraction techniques[17] have revealed the complex folded structure of a large molecule like myoglobin. Modern methods of rapid analysis have been introduced into clinical practice in many instances (see Fig. 1.3 and legend).

The techniques of immunology have been of great value in the identification and assay of proteins.[20] The radioimmunoassay method has been adapted to measure the blood levels of certain peptide hormones, e.g. insulin, glucagon, and ACTH, which are present in picograms or nanograms per ml.* The method depends upon the ability of unlabelled hormone to inhibit, by simple competition, the binding of labelled hormone (e.g. with ^{131}I or ^{125}I) by specific antibody. The hormone content of an unknown sample is determined by comparing the degree to which it inhibits the binding of labelled antigen with the inhibition produced by a series of standard solutions containing known amounts of hormone. The reagents required are therefore pure hormone, labelled hormone, and specific antibody. The amount of labelled hormone bound to antibody is determined after separating it from the free labelled hormone. This separation is done by electrophoresis or by chemical means.

* 1 milligram — 1 000 micrograms (μg). 1 microgram — 1 000 nanograms (ng). 1 nanogram — 1 000 picograms (pg).

Figure 1.3
Continuous blood sugar recording obtained by the use of an autoanalyser. The graph reads from right to left. Standard solutions of glucose (10, 25, 50, 100, 150, 200 mg/ml, etc.) were first fed into the instrument to obtain the calibration spikes shown on the right. Next, continuous sampling of blood was obtained by means of a small catheter inserted into an arm vein. At the point indicated by the arrow 20 g of glucose was administered intravenously, and the blood sugar level rose from 80 mg/100 ml to 195 mg/100 ml. The form of the curve showing the subsequent return to normal is within normal limits. The instruments can be adapted to measure other blood constituents either as a continuous recording or for a large number of separate specimens. *(Photograph of a recording provided by Dr. E. Kawerau)*

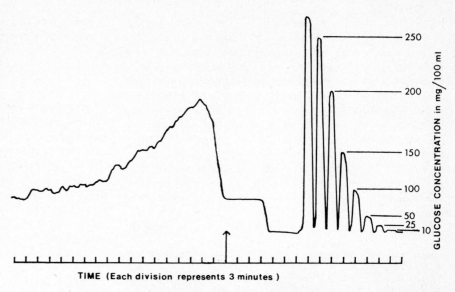

TIME (Each division represents 3 minutes)

Two other methods have found particular application in pathology:

Electrophoresis[6]

If a mixture of proteins is placed in an electric field at a known pH, individual proteins move at particular rates dependent to a great extent upon their size and charge. The test is conveniently performed on filter paper, and after passing an electric current for a suitable time the paper is dried, and the separated proteins are stained with a simple dye, e.g. light green. Electrophoresis is now commonly performed in other media, e.g. starch gel and cellulose acetate strip, the choice depending upon the nature of the substances being investigated. Fig. 45.1 shows a typical electrophoretic separation of the plasma proteins. Combined with the agar-diffusion technique electrophoresis has proved invaluable in separating protein mixtures (see Fig. 1.4 and legend).

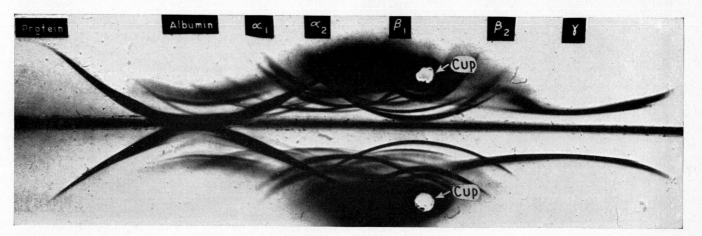

Figure 1.4
Immuno-electrophoresis of serum. This method entails the separation of the protein components by electrophoresis in an agar gel, and then demonstrating each fraction by means of a precipitin reaction using an antibody.

Serum is placed in the two cups in a sheet of agar gel at a pH of 8·2. At this pH albumin (isoelectric point 4·7) has a strong negative charge, and γ-globulin (isoelectric point 7·2) has a weak negative charge. Application of an electric field results in a tendency for the proteins to move towards the anode. Their actual movement, however, is determined not only by their molecular size and charge but also by a flow of water towards the cathode due to the phenomenon of electro-osmosis. This is due to a negative charge on the agar itself, and as the agar is fixed, its tendency to move towards the anode actually results in a movement of water to the cathode. The weakly charged γ-globulins are thus actually carried towards the cathode.

The separated plasma components are demonstrated by placing antiserum to whole plasma down the central strip. From there the antibodies diffuse to form precipitin lines with each separated serum protein. A stain, thiazine red R, has been used.

(Photograph by courtesy of Dr. A. J. Crowle. See Crowle, A. J. (1961), Immunodiffusion, New York and London: Academic Press)

Chromatography[21, 22]

Chromatography is an important technique for separating pure substances from mixtures. The chromatographic system consists of two immiscible phases, a *stationary phase* which is fixed and granular, and a *moving phase* which flows through the interstices of the stationary phase. The moving phase is fluid (liquid or gas), and its movement is effected by gravity, applied pressure, or capillarity. The stationary phase is usually a finely divided insoluble solid.

Chromatographic separation depends on the fact that different substances follow the moving solvent at different rates. All these substances must be soluble in the moving phase, but some become distributed on the surface (adsorption) or throughout the interior (partition) of the particles of the stationary phase (Fig. 1.5). Those substances whose

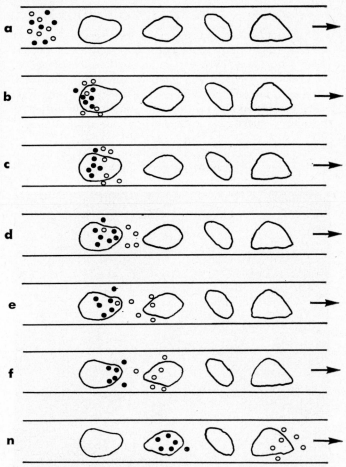

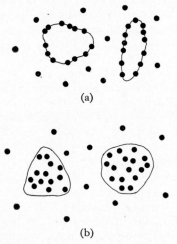

Figure 1.5
Distribution of a substance between moving and stationary phases (*a*) adsorption and (*b*) partition mechanisms. *(Eastoe, J. E. (1964), Ann. roy. Coll. Surg. Engl., **35**, 234)*

Figure 1.6
Mechanism of chromatographic separation as a result of differences in the distribution of two substances between moving and stationary phases. (The distribution of the black molecules favours the stationary phase with the result that they move through the system more slowly than the white molecules.) *(Eastoe, J. E. (1964), Ann. roy. Coll. Surg. Engl., **35**, 234)*

distribution favours the moving phase pass more rapidly through the chromatogram than those which favour the stationary phase. If the column is sufficiently long, a complete separation of substances between successive bands of pure solvent can be achieved as is seen in Fig. 1.6.

There are three main types of chromatography: (*a*) *column chromatography*, in which liquid passes down through powdered solid packed in a glass tube; (*b*) *paper chromatography*,[17] in which an organic solvent moves by capillary action through the pores of filter paper, the fibres of which contain a little water; (*c*) *thin-layer chromatography*, which resembles (*b*) except that the stationary phase is made to adhere to a glass plate, up which the solvent moves by capillarity.

Chromatography has found its greatest use in the separation of amino acids in solution. From a clinical point of view the most important type is paper chromatography. It

is invaluable for identifying amino acids and sugars in urine. Each moves at a specific rate along the paper depending on the solvent, so that the ratio

$$\frac{\text{Distance travelled by component}}{\text{Distance travelled by solvent}}$$

or the R_f value, is a constant for each component under the conditions of the test. After allowing the solvent to move a certain distance the paper is dried, and the area occupied by the component is "developed" by spraying the paper with a chemical that reacts with that component, e.g. ninhydrin turns purple with amino acids. If a series of known substances are run in parallel with the unknown components, their R_f values can be compared. In this way an unknown component can be identified.

FLUORESCENT TRACING TECHNIQUES[17, 23]

The ability of certain compounds to convert the energy of ultraviolet light into visible light can be utilised in various ways. Flourescent dyes, e.g. auramine, have been used to stain tubercle bacilli, which are then easily visible under the ultraviolet microscope. Fluorescein, if injected intravenously, is excreted into the bile, and beautiful illustrations of the biliary ducts can be obtained in the living animal[24] (Fig. 1.7).

Fluorescein and lissamine rhodamine B may be used in another way: they can by chemical means be incorporated

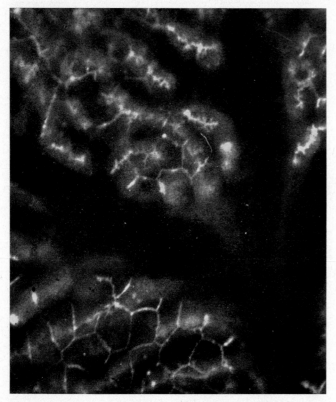

Figure 1.7
Photomicrograph of the surface of the liver illuminated by incident ultraviolet light. The rat has been injected intravenously with a solution of sodium fluorescein 5 mins. previously. The liver cells and bile canaliculi fluoresce brilliantly. The large centrilobular veins appear dark. ×520. *(Photograph supplied by Dr. A. J. M. Reese)*

into protein molecules. This is of great use as a tool in immunology, since antibodies so labelled have an unaltered specificity. They may then be used to localise antigens which have already been introduced. In this way it has been demonstrated that injected pneumococcal polysaccharide remains in the tissues long after its administration. Sections from such an animal are treated with fluorescein-antibody conjugate, washed, and examined under ultra-

violet light. The site of the polysaccharide antigen is revealed by the fluorescence of the attached antibody. Another method, the sandwich technique, is sometimes employed to identify an antigen in the tissues. Unlabelled immunoglobulin antibody is applied to the section, and the site of its attachment is revealed by a second labelled anti-immunoglobulin (Coombs's reagent). These techniques, pioneered by Coons at Harvard, have also been of great use in investigating the site of antibody production and deposition (see p. 152).

RADIOACTIVE ISOTOPES

The radioactive isotopes are treated by living cells in the same way as the normal elements. Their radiation can be detected by suitable counters, and they may usefully be employed as labels in a wide range of fields. Clinically, thyroid function can be investigated by estimating the distribution of an administered dose of radioactive iodine in the plasma and over the thyroid gland. Radioactive chromium can be attached to the red cells, and their length of survival estimated (see Chapter 49). The clearance of a small quantity of injected radioactive sodium from the skin has been used to measure blood flow.[25] In the experimental animal many compounds can be tagged and their metabolism followed, e.g. albumin.

Autoradiography[26]

The isotopes can also be used at a microscopic level. By placing a section of tissue on a photographic film, subsequent photographic development will reveal the site of isotope localisation as a series of black grains. As an example of the value of this it is found that tritiated thymidine given to a cell is incorporated into its nucleus. This may therefore be used as an indicator of DNA synthesis (see Fig. 1.8).

PHOTOGRAPHY

Apart from the value for record purposes photography plays an important role in many other fields. It is essential in ultraviolet, electron, and x-ray microscopy. The ultrafast films now available have made high-speed cine photomicrography possible, and blood flow can be examined from films shot at 7 600 frames per second[27] (the "normal" is 24 per sec.). Time-lapse cine photography, on the other hand, has made it possible to "speed up" the movement of living cells grown in tissue culture.[28] This technique, as yet but little used, has provided interesting information on the behaviour of phagocytes, lymphocytes, and tumour cells.

TISSUE CULTURE[6, 29]

Tissues of various types can be cultured outside the body with comparative ease. The usual surface employed

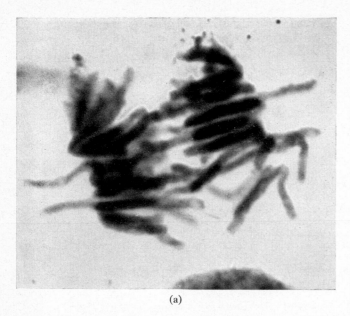

(a)

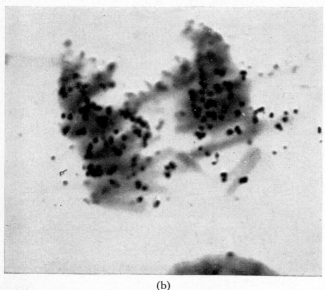

(b)

Figure 1.8
DNA localisation. Autoradiograph of a Feulgen-stained anaphase figure in a squash preparation of the root tip of *Allium cepa* fed with tritiated thymidine.
(*a*) Photographed at the level of the section to show the chromosomes.
(*b*) The same cell photographed at the level of the photographic emulsion. The labelled thymidine has been taken up by the cell and incorporated into the DNA. Note how the silver dots correspond to the chromosomes. ×3 200. *(Photographs supplied by Dr. P. B. Gahan)*

is glass or plastic, and the tissues can be grown in test-tubes, medicine-flat bottles, flasks, or simply on the surface of a cover-slip inverted over a slide with a hollow depression.

There are two types of tissue culture: (*a*) *cell culture*, in which the cells of an organ or tumour are allowed to grow out. The organ is first cut up into small fragments which are then digested with trypsin at 37°C until there is complete disintegration. The cells derived from the tissue are centrifuged, suspended in a liquid growth medium that usually contains serum and a balanced salt solution, and allowed to sediment in a container; they rapidly become attached to the surface, and within a few days multiplication is sufficient to cause it to be covered with a monolayer of confluent cells. Another method consists of attaching a tissue fragment, or explant, to the glass surface, adding a growth medium, and then waiting for an outgrowth of cells from it. Cell culture is an extremely important technique for cultivating viruses, and is described in Chapter 22. Its use in cancer research has proved disappointing except in the study of tumours of nervous tissue, where the cells growing out sometimes differentiate into specific elements, e.g. astrocytes or ganglion cells, thus allowing the tumour to be more easily classified. (*b*) *Organ culture*, in which a fragment of tissue is grown on a grid so that there is no cellular outgrowth, but the organ is kept as normal histologically as is possible. Limb buds, eye rudiments, and bones have been studied while growing in an artificial medium, and their differentiation observed. The effect of Vitamin A on the skin of chick embryos has been investigated in this way (see p. 307).

The culture of human cells has yielded much information.[30] Some normal human cells, e.g. fibroblasts, can be sustained in tissue culture for about fifty generations. Serially propagated mammalian cells do not normally carry out the specific functions of the organ from which they were isolated. However, enzyme studies on human cell cultures have shed some light on the genetic enzyme defects seen in some diseases (see p. 36).

Another interesting aspect of cell culture is the technique of making two somatic cells fuse to form a common cell. Sometimes the stimulus of a virus infection has been used, and the mononuclear hybrid cell may be capable of proliferation. For example, hybrid cells between a human cell line and a mouse cell line have been obtained.[31] Another method of combining DNA from two cells is based on the finding that certain DNA viruses, such as polyoma and S.V. 40, can add new genes to cells in culture when these are infected.[32] The viral DNA can become incorporated in the host's DNA and reproduce with the host-cell chromosomes. Sometimes the descendants of these infected cells can be stimulated to synthesise infectious virus particles again, and, in the case of the polyoma virus infecting mouse cells, the infected virus particles contain mouse genes.[33]

Tissue culture has played a useful part in adding to our knowledge of cellular metabolism, but its use is greatly limited by the fact that the cells are surviving in a completely abnormal environment; the vascular arrangement of the living body is replaced by a synthetic fluid medium which bathes the tissue.

It is certain from this bewilderingly large number of specialised techniques at our disposal that many of the intimate secrets of cellular physiology are now being revealed. Nevertheless, it is still as true as ever that the most important investigation into the nature of disease is based on a careful investigation of the patient himself.

REFERENCES

1. GOLDSTEIN, L. (1964). In *Cytology and Cell Physiology*, 3rd edn, p. 559. Edited by G. H. Bourne. New York and London: Academic Press.
2. SALMOIRAGHI, G. C. and BLOOM, F. E. (1964). *Science*, **144,** 493.
3. Occasional Survey (1964). *Lancet*, i, 1099.
4. MINTZ, B. (1969). In *The Clinical Delineation of Birth Defects, Birth Defects: Original Article Series*, vol. 5, no. 1, p. 11. New York: The National Foundation.
5. SWAIN, R. H. A. (1965). In *Medical Microbiology*, 11th edn, p. 605. Edited by R. Cruickshank. Edinburgh: Livingstone.
6. ATKINS, H. J. B. (1959). (Ed.) *Tools of Biological Research.* Oxford: Blackwell.
7. HAM, A. W. (1969). In *Histology*, 6th edn, p. 9. Philadelphia and London: Lippincott.
8. McMANUS, J. F. A. and MOWRY, R. W. (1960). *Staining Methods: Histologic and Histochemical.* New York: Hoeber.
9. PEARSE, A. G. E. (1968 and 1970). *Histochemistry, Theoretical and Applied*, 3rd edn, vols 1 and 2. London: Churchill.
10. DIXON, K. (1970). In *An Introduction to the Biology of the Skin*, p. 35. Edited by R. H. Champion, T. Gillman, A. J. Rook and R. T. Sims. Oxford: Blackwell Scientific Publications.
11. ENGSTRÖM, A. V. and FINEAN, J. B. (1967). In *Biological Ultrastructure*, 2nd edn, p. 9. New York: Academic Press.
12. TSALTAS, T. T. (1967). In *Methods and Achievements in Experimental Pathology*, vol. 2, p. 30. Chicago: Year Book Medical Publishers.
13. PEASE, D. C. (1964). *Histological Techniques for Electron Microscopy*, 2nd edn. New York and London: Academic Press.
14. MÖLBERT, E. R. G. (1967). In *Methods and Achievements in Experimental Pathology*, vol. 2, p. 1, *loc. cit.*
15. SINGER, S. J. (1959). *Nature*, **183,** 1523.
16. DUPOUY, G., PERRIER, R. and DURRIEU, L. (1960). *Comptes rendus hebdomadaires des séances de l'Académie des sciences (Paris)*, **251,** 2836.
17. ATKINS, H. J. B. (1960). (Ed.) *Tools of Biological Research*, 2nd series. Oxford: Blackwell.
18. SCHNEIDER, W. C. and KUFF, E. L. (1964). In *Cytology and Cell Physiology*, 3rd edn, p. 19, *loc. cit.*
19. STEIN, W. H. and MOORE, S. (1961). *Scientific American*, **204,** no. 2, 81.
20. LANDON, J. (1968). In *Recent Advances in Endocrinology*, p. 240. Edited by V. H. T. James. London: Churchill.
21. EASTOE, J. E., READING, H. W. and SLOANE-STANLEY, G. H. (1964). *Annals of the Royal College of Surgeons of England*, **35,** 234.
22. GORDON, A. H. and EASTOE, J. E. (1964). *Practical Chromatographic Techniques.* London: George Newnes.
23. NAIRN, R. C. (1969). *Fluorescent Protein Tracing*, 3rd edn. Edinburgh: Livingstone.
24. REESE, A. J. M. and RIMINGTON, C. (1964). *British Journal of Experimental Pathology*, **45,** 30.
25. BUCHANAN, T. J., WALLS, E. W. and WILLIAMS, E. S. (1954). *Clinical Science*, **13,** 333.
26. ATKINS, H. J. B. (1961). (Ed.) *Tools of Biological Research*, 3rd series. Oxford: Blakwell.
27. BLOCH, E. H. (1962). *American Journal of Anatomy*, **110,** 125.
28. PULVERTAFT, R. J. V. (1959). In *Modern Trends in Pathology*, p. 19. Edited by D. H. Collins. London: Butterworths.
29. PAUL, J. (1970). *Cell and Tissue Culture*, 4th edn. Edinburgh: Livingstone.
30. KROOTH, R. S. (1969). *Medical Clinics of North America*, **53,** 795.
31. WEISS, M. C. and GREEN, H. (1967). *Proceedings of the National Academy of Sciences of the United States of America*, **58,** 1104.
32. WESTPHAL, H. and DULBECCO, R. (1968). *Proceedings of the National Academy of Sciences of the United States of America*, **59,** 1158.
33. WINOCOUR, E. (1968). *Virology*, **34,** 571.
34. WEAKLEY, B. S. (1972). *A Beginner's Handbook in Biological Electron Microscopy.* Edinburgh and London: Churchill Livingstone.

Chapter 2. The Normal Cell

The importance of the cell as the basic building unit of the body has been recognised since the microscope was first applied to the analysis of biological material. This is scarcely surprising, because simpler forms of life like the amoeba consist entirely of one cell. Just over a hundred years ago Virchow published his text-book on "Cellular Pathology", and since then our concept of many diseases has been centred on abnormalities in cellular behaviour or appearance. No attempt will be made to describe in detail the various types of cells which are present in the body. Such descriptions are available in standard text-books of histology.

The majority of cells in the human body are not disposed separately, but are grouped together to form tissues. Traditionally two types of cells are distinguished—those of the epithelia and those of the connective tissue.

Epithelial cells cover surfaces, e.g. skin, or line cavities, e.g. the mouth, and in these situations they are essentially protective in function. Covering epithelium may also perform a secretory function: the respiratory epithelium, for instance, secretes mucus.

In addition to covering extensive surfaces, the secretory type of epithelial cell may be arranged to form glands. These may be simple, like the mucous glands of the colon, or more elaborate, like those of the breast and pancreas. In the endocrine glands secretion is absorbed directly into the blood stream, and in some situations, e.g. pituitary, no tubular or acinar spaces are present. A feature common to all epithelial cells is that they are closely contiguous to one another. This is evident on light microscopy, and even under the electron microscope these cells appear to be separated by only a thin layer of low electron density which is about 15 nm in width.

Connective tissue cells are the other cell type present in the body. These are usually widely separated from each other by a zone containing much ground substance, and in which there are embedded collagen fibres. This type of connective tissue, typified by tendon, bone, cartilage, and fibrous tissue, is primarily supportive in function. Other connective tissue cells have been endowed with a specialised cytoplasm either for contraction (muscle fibres) or conduction (nerve cells).

This classification of cells into "epithelial" and "connective tissue" is not as simple as is sometimes assumed. The flattened "endothelial" cells which line blood and lymph vessels are usually considered to be connective tissue, although they are, in fact, performing a covering function. The same may be said of the mesothelial cells lining the pleura and peritoneum, and those of the synovium.

Under abnormal conditions such cells may assume an "epithelial" appearance. Squamous metaplasia has been described in the pleura, and some pleural and synovial tumours have a frankly adenocarcinomatous appearance. It must be accepted that the distinction between epithelial and connective tissue cells is not as rigid as used to be supposed.

This is not merely of academic interest. Its implications are obvious when it is remembered that the common basis for the classification of tumours is their tissue of origin (see p. 313).

STRUCTURE OF CELLS

Although the different cells of the body possess striking features which readily distinguish them one from another, all are built upon a similar basic plan. This is to be expected, because in spite of their diversity of structure and function, each is in fact remarkably independent. Each receives a supply of oxygen and foodstuff from the blood stream, with which it must produce its own structural components and secretions and from which it must release energy required for mechanical, chemical, or electrical work. Each possesses an outer limiting membrane and within its protoplasm there is another limiting membrane which encloses the nuclear material. Most cells possess a single nucleus which is centrally placed. The basal nuclei of some columnar epithelial cells and the eccentric nucleus of the plasma cell are obvious exceptions. Cells with more than one nucleus are called *giant* or *multinucleate cells*. Osteoclasts and megakaryocytes are examples of such cells found normally in the body. To these may be added the syncytiotrophoblast of the placenta. Striated muscle fibres may be regarded as multinucleate cells with specialised cytoplasm. Giant cells are not infrequently found in pathological lesions: these are listed in Table 2.1 (see also pp. 128 and 341).

The nucleus forms an essential part of all living mammalian cells. The technique of microdissection has shown that after removal of the nucleus, respiratory activity may continue for two or three days, but the cell dies inevitably soon afterwards. Introduction of a nucleus may, however, ensure its continued life. Under some circumstances an

Figure 2.1
Diagrammatic representation of a hypothetical
composite cell, with some organelles shown around
it at a higher magnification. The free surface of
the cell has projecting microvilli, which on the left
are arranged regularly to form a brush border. In
the centre, the villi are irregular, and micropinocytotic vacuole formation is depicted. On the
right cilia are shown. The cell adjoins its neighbours with some interdigitation of their plasma
membranes; one junctional complex is shown.
The nucleus contains one nucleolus, and is surrounded by a double-layered membrane. Between
the nucleus and the free border is the cell centre, or
centrosome, surrounded by sacs of the Golgi
apparatus. There are two centrioles lying at right
angles to each other. The base of the cell rests on a
basement membrane which at high magnification
has three components; the plasma membrane, like
other membranes in the cell, has a trilaminar
structure. Ribosomes are scattered free in the cell
cytoplasm, and are also attached to the rough
endoplasmic reticulum and the outer nuclear
envelope. *(Drawn by Margot Mackay, Department
of Art as Applied to Medicine, University of
Toronto)*

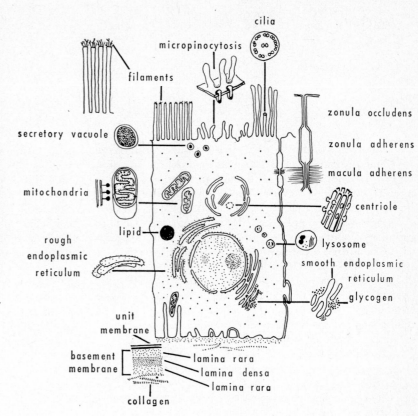

TABLE 2.1   Types of giant cell

Damaged striated muscle fibres

1. Regenerating sarcolemmal cells in damaged voluntary muscle.
2. Aschoff giant cell in heart muscle (? fused myocardial macro-phage).

Tumour giant cells

1. Giant-cell tumours, e.g. of bone, poorly differentiated astro-cytoma (glioblastoma multiforme), choriocarcinoma, Hodgkin's disease (Sternberg-Reed cell), etc.
2. Giant-cell variants of many tumours, e.g. carcinoma of lung and kidney.

Fused cells due to virus infection

1. Epithelial giant cells, e.g. in herpesvirus infections.
2. Connective tissue, e.g. Warthin-Finkeldey giant cells of measles.

Fused macrophages

See Table 11.1.

enucleated cell can continue to grow and differentiate for
many months. The messenger RNA already in the cytoplasm is responsible for this.[1] In man the only non-nucleate
cells are platelets and erythrocytes; both have a limited
existence and neither is capable of reproduction. The
extranuclear protoplasm, or cytoplasm, contains a number

of bodies: some of these can be seen with the light microscope, but others are recognisable only by means of the
electron microscope. The most conspicuous structures are
the mitochondria, the endoplasmic reticulum and its
associated ribosomes, lysosomes, and a variety of granules
or vacuoles which are present in many specialised cells, e.g.
eosinophils (Figs. 2.1. and 2.2).

The increasing complexity which the electron microscope reveals has brought morphology more into line with
function. The numerous complicated biochemical reactions
which are known to occur in the cell could hardly be recon-
ciled with a cytoplasm devoid of structure.

THE CELL MEMBRANE[2, 3]

The *cell* or *plasma membrane* is an extremely important
structure, for it forms the interface between the cell
cytoplasm and the interstitial tissue fluids or in lower forms
of life, the exterior. Its functions may be listed: movement;
cell recognition; cell growth; adhesion; transfer function.

Cell Movement[4]

The amoeboid movement and phagocytic activity of
white cells are well known, but apart from this, an examination of living cells by phase contrast microscopy reveals the
cell surface to be in constant movement. The undulating
surface of the macrophage is particularly characteristic.

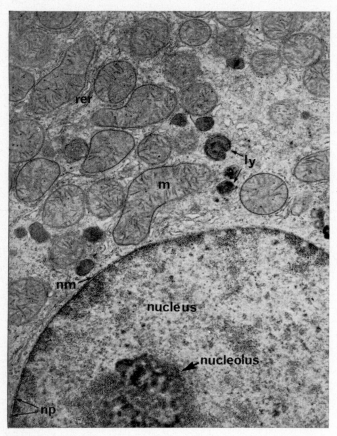

Figure 2.2
Rat liver cell showing the main features of a cell as revealed by electron microscopy. The nucleus is bounded by the nuclear membrane (nm) in which there is a nuclear pore (np). A nucleolus is present in the part of the nucleus which is included. In the cytoplasm there are mitochondria (m) with cristae, lysosomes (ly), and rough endoplasmic reticulum (rer). The tissue was fixed in osmic acid and embedded in epon-araldite mixture. ×17 300. *(Photograph supplied by Dr. Y. le Beux)*

Folds of the membrane have been observed to entrap a droplet of fluid by a process known as *pinocytosis*.[5]

Cell Recognition

The membranes of the cell, including the plasma membrane, are associated with the antigens by which the body is able to recognise its own cells and tolerate them. Cells from another individual are regarded as aliens, and are attacked.

Cell Growth

The phenomenon of contact inhibition (see p. 110) is a function of the cell surface. Some procedures, e.g. treatment with proteolytic enzymes, appear to alter the cell membrane and also remove components involved in the control of the cell growth. Malignant transformation may so alter the cell surface that it abolishes the control of cell

growth. This seems to be due to the exposure of previously hidden receptor sites; it is of interest that viruses can produce the same effect.[6]

Cell Adhesion

The cell membrane is concerned with adhesiveness, which is a factor that induces cells of like constitution to stick together. If the cells of an embryo are separated from each other and are then allowed to come together again, they aggregate to form organs and tissues. At first sight this would seem to indicate that differentiated cells have specific surface sites for recognition and adhesion. However, an alternative hypothesis is that differential adhesion is determined by the quantity and distribution of the sites of adhesion available. Groups of cells therefore strive to attain an arrangement that is thermodynamically most favourable.[7] This affinity which cells have for their own kind must be an important mechanism in the development and maintenance of the architecture of multicellular animals. But not all cells behave in this manner. The cells of the blood do not normally exhibit adhesiveness, nor to any great extent do cancer cells, for they are able to infiltrate freely into the surrounding tissues.

Transfer Function

All substances which enter or leave the cell protoplasm must cross the cell membrane, and the properties of this membrane are responsible for the peculiar chemical composition of the cytoplasm.

Small ions like Na^+ and K^+, as well as water, appear to cross the membrane with relative ease, while others are held back. Molecular size and electrical charge play a part. Chemicals soluble in organic solvents enter cells much more readily than do those which are water soluble. The absorption of some substances is related to enzymatic activity occurring at or near the cell surface. How chemicals cross the membrane and the factors which regulate their passage can be understood only in relationship to the structure of the membrane itself, for as in other realms of pathology, structure and function are interdependent.

Membrane structure in relation to function. Electron microscopy has shown an intact membrane some 7·5 nm in width, which at high magnification of suitably prepared material can be resolved into two electron-dense laminae with an intervening clear space. This trilaminar structure is known as a *unit membrane*, and it appears to have no pores such as have been postulated to explain the observed permeability of the cell membrane.[8]

In *micropinocytosis* small invaginations of the cell membrane, the *caveolae intracellulares*, become nipped off to form vesicles. In this way small quantities of fluid may be imbibed by a process which resembles pinocytosis but on a small scale. The formation of micropinocytotic vesicles on one surface of a cell and their discharge from another surface is one postulated mechanism whereby substances may cross a cellular barrier, e.g. blood-vessel endothelium. The process is known as *cytopempsis*.[9]

Substances may therefore enter the cell by diffusion across the cell membrane or by the processes of phagocytosis, pinocytosis, or micropinocytosis. In the latter event the vacuole is still membrane bound, and its contents are not in the cytoplasmic ground substance. The fusion of the vacuole with a primary lysosome containing hydrolytic enzymes results in the formation of a *phagosome*, and digestion of its contents may result in their being released into the ground substance of the cell.

Studies on the rate of diffusion of small molecules across the cell membrane led Pappenheimer to conclude that it

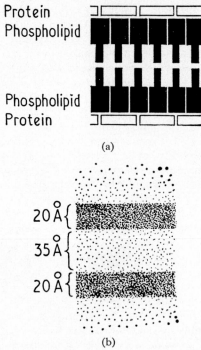

(a)

(b)

Figure 2.3
The unit membrane is composed of two electron-dense laminae separated by a third clear zone (*b*). The chemical structure shown in (*a*) is compatible with this appearance.

contained small pores.[8] No such static pores have been seen, but it is conceivable that the formation of a micropinocytotic vesicle and subsequent diffusion of its contents or fusion with other membranes in the cytoplasm of the cell constitute the equivalent *functional pore*.

It is generally accepted that the cell membrane is made up of a lipid–protein combination but the details of its construction are not known. Davson and Danielli introduced the concept of a bimolecular lipid leaflet with two layers of lipid molecules having their polar (hydrophilic) ends turned outwards, and being covered by protein (Fig. 2.3*a*). This concept of a lamellar structure fits well with the observed electron microscope appearance of an approxi-

mately 7·5 nm thick trilaminated membrane (Fig. 2.3*b*). Analysis of the protein component of cell membranes has indicated that about 25 per cent of the protein is present as α-helix and there is no β-structure.[*] Calculations based on this and of the polar residues available indicate that the Davson and Danielli model is not a stable configuration. An alternative view is that the membrane consists of globular subunits, or micelles, and Lenard and Singer have proposed a model depicted in Fig. 2.4. It will be seen that

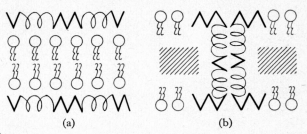

(a)   (b)

Figure 2. 4
Two diagrams to illustrate the possible structure of the cell membrane. (*a*) A modification of the Davson-Danielli-Robertson unit membrane. The outer layers are depicted as composed of protein, either helical, or random coil which is shown as straight lines forming W or M. The lipid molecules are in the centre of the membrane with their polar heads, shown as circles, pointing outwards. (*b*) The membrane as suggested by Lenard and Singer. The central cross-hatched areas is assumed to be occupied by relatively non-polar constituents (hydrophobic amino-acid residues or lipids) and single polypeptide chains are drawn to traverse the entire membrane. (*After Lenard, J. and Singer, S. J.* (1966), Proc. N.Y. Acad. Sci. **56**, 1824)

some lipid hydrophilic head groups are exposed on the surface and that protein with α-helix and non-structured configuration extends from one surface of the membrane to the other, thereby forming tube-like structures. It is possible that these form pores through which small water-soluble molecules can pass. When one observes living cells, the activity of the membrane is striking. It is by no means a static structure, and is continually changing shape. Change indicates the performance of work, and the presence of ATPase at the cell surface (Fig. 2.5) supports the concept that energy is released at the cell membrane. A model which allows for this is that proposed by Kavanau.[10] The membrane is pictured as having pillars of lipid covered by protein

* The *primary structure* of the protein is the order in which the individual amino acids are linked on the peptide chain. Orderly folding of this chain, such as the formation of a right-handed α-helix, is referred to as *secondary structure*. The peptide chains can also be held by adjacent chains to form sheet-like structures, β structures, or no structures at all (a random coil). Proteins whose major secondary structure is in the alpha form are elastic: keratin is a good example. Proteins that have extensive β structure, such as fibrin are not readily extensible, since the polypeptide chains are already fully extended. *Tertiary structure* is the result of the interaction between active groups lying in the side chains of the amino acids. Disulphide bonds are the most important linkages involved. *Quaternary structure* is the association of individual monomers to form dimers, trimers, tetramers, etc.

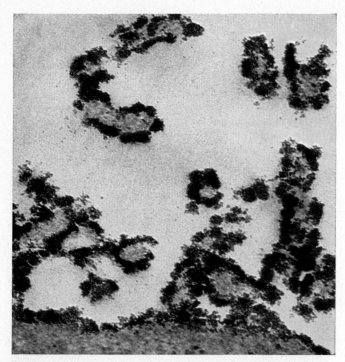

Figure 2.5
Detail of the plasma membrane of a HeLa cell with much surface activity in the form of profuse filamentous microvilli. After staining for enzymes splitting adenosine triphosphate, dense reaction-product has been deposited with close precision at the cell membrane, indicating that the enzymes are localised there, presumably for the supply of energy requirements. × 55 000. *(Electron micrograph provided by Dr. M. A. Epstein and Dr. S. J. Holt)*

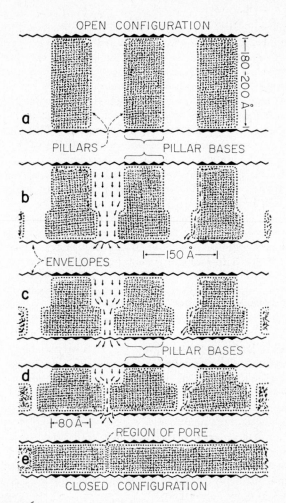

Figure 2.6
A diagrammatic cross-sectional representation of the plasma membrane. The protein envelope is depicted as zig-zag lines and between them are pillars of lipid, each with a base (heavy zig-zag lines). The pillars are widely separated when the membrane is in the open position (*a*). As the pillars collapse (*b, c, d*), fluid in the pores is pumped in the direction of the arrows. In the closed position some of the pores may remain (*e* left-hand end), or else fusion of the pillars takes place and the membrane structure is then very similar to that depicted in Fig. 2.3. *(From Kavanau, J. L.* (1963), Nature (Lond.) **198,** 525)

(Fig. 2.6). Between the bases of the lipid pillars are pores, which are large in the open and small in the closed configuration. This concept of cell membrane structure allows for ready change in membrane shape and in its permeability. The amoeboid movement of the polymorphs and the changed permeability of the plasma membrane of a neurone when an impulse passes are more readily explained than by the static structure depicted in Fig. 2.3. The technique of surface replication electron microscopy has indicated that this structure of cell membrane may indeed exist.[11]

It should be noted that the membrane in the closed configuration clearly approximates to the structure of Davson and Danielli. The "normal" appearance of the membrane as seen in routine electron microscopy may indeed be an artefact if the membrane readily adopts the closed configuration when subjected to fixation.

An interesting feature of the red-cell envelope is the ability with which influenza viruses attach themselves to it. The relationship between the two is quantitative, and it seems probable that viruses attach themselves to specific areas on the cell surface. These hypothetical areas which are presumably dependent upon particular chemical groupings are known as *cell* or *surface receptors*. It is likely that many

substances, e.g. drugs, toxins, etc., act in a similar manner by becoming fixed on to specific receptors. If the receptor units of the membrane are capable of rotation, a substance attached to an external receptor could enter the cell quite readily.

This mechanism would require the expenditure of energy, and could form the basis for active transport across the cell membranes.[12] Selective amino-acid transport is important in the gut and the renal tubules. In the case of amino acids one transport mechanism may serve a single amino acid, for instance defective cystine transport in the kidneys results in hypercystinaemia, and a selective failure to absorb tryptophane in the gut causes the blue diaper syndrome. Sometimes a single mechanism involves a group of amino acids; thus there is a failure to reabsorb cystine, lysine, ornithine, and arginine in the kidney in the classical type of cystinuria. An interesting application of the receptor concept is the supposition that many hormones react with a specific receptor on their target cells. The interaction between the two activates an enzyme, adenyl cyclase, which in the presence of magnesium ions, converts ATP to adenosine 3′,5′-cyclic monophosphate (cyclic AMP). This substance triggers a sequence of events specific for that cell, and leads to the response associated with the action of the hormone. Thus cyclic AMP has been termed a second messenger in hormonal action.[13]

In summary, the plasma membrane is a complex lipo-protein structure. It can consume energy and change its shape in response to stimuli. It contains protein molecules which are heterogeneous, some being responsible for the receptor sites, others for antigenicity, enzyme activity, etc.

Projections from the Cell Surface

Cilia, e.g. of respiratory epithelium, and flagella, e.g. of spermatozoa, are easily recognisable under the light microscope. Electron microscopy also reveals a very characteristic structure.[14] Cilia contain nine peripherally-placed electron-dense filaments which under higher magnification can be resolved into double structures like a figure-of-eight. These ciliary filaments terminate in the basal plate opposing which there is another plate*; this is part of the ciliary body, a hollow cylindrical structure with nine peripherally-arranged double rods. This ciliary body resembles the structure of the centriole. In the centre of each cilium there is a pair of single filaments. Flagella resemble cilia, but in addition have an outer spiral wrap.

The electron microscope has revealed projections, or *microvilli*, on cells which are not readily visible by light microscopy (see Fig. 2.5).

The function of the microvilli is probably related to absorption; certainly the well-marked villus formation in the renal tubules and small intestine appears to subserve this function. It forms the "brush border" seen by light microscopy.

Relationship of Cells to Each Other

Epithelial cells are generally closely applied to each other, but even then there is a clear area of about 15 nm between their adjacent cell membranes. This is probably due to a covering of mucopolysaccharide which may well prove to be an important component of the external cell membrane itself. The free surface of epithelial cells is also covered by an additional coat which on high-resolution electron microscopy can be seen to be filamentous. The degree of indentation of one cell into another varies according to the tissue.

The *junctional complex* is illustrated in Fig. 2.1. It should

* The precise manner in which the cilia terminate in the ciliary body varies in different species.

be noted that the *zonula occludens*, or tight zone, is a belt which surrounds the cells near their free edges. Adjacent cells are in very close contact, and the electrical resistance between them is very low. The underlying *zonula adherens* is also in the form of a belt in contrast to the *macula adherens*, or *desmosome*, which is button-shaped. Desmosomes can occur elsewhere along the lateral surface unconnected with this complex.

In connective tissue the space between individual cells is considerably greater, and it usually contains fibres, e.g. collagen and elastic, as well as ground substance.

THE CELL NUCLEUS

The Nuclear Membrane or Envelope

The nucleus is bounded by the nuclear membrane which under the electron microscope can be resolved into two laminae, each about 7·5 nm in width, and separated from each other by a space 40–70 nm wide (Fig. 2.7). The outer

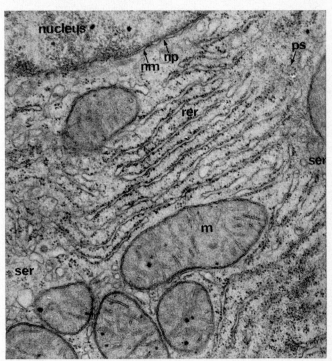

Figure 2.7
Rat liver cell. The double-layered nuclear membrane (nm) and nuclear pores (np) are well shown. The endoplasmic reticulum has two components, rough (rer) with its attached ribosomes forming parallel arrays, and smooth (ser) seen lower down in the section without ribosomes. Note the group of ribosomes (ps) apparently lying free in the cytoplasm; this probably corresponds to a polysome. The mitochondria (m) are bounded by a double membrane, the inner component of which is folded on itself to produce the cristae. The dense aggregates in the cytoplasm are composed of glycogen. The tissue was fixed in osmic acid and embedded in epon-araldite mixture. Lead hydroxide stain. ×41 250. *(Photograph supplied by Dr. Y. le Beux)*

lamina is studded with ribosomes, and is continuous with the endoplasmic reticulum from which it is produced at the completion of mitosis. The inner lamina is reinforced on its internal aspect by a layer of filamentous material called the "fibrous lamina". The two layers of the nuclear envelope are continuous with each other around the edges of the nuclear pores, which appear as circular holes 50 nm in diameter. Whether there is free communication between the nucleus and cytoplasm through these pores is undecided. High-resolution electron micrographs indicate that there is a membrane across each pore.

Nuclei are generally circular or oval in shape, but they may show indentations. Irregular folding of the nuclear membrane is seen in the actively dividing cells of regeneration and neoplasia, but is not uncommon in the normal cell.

The principal components of the nucleus are the chromatin, the nucleolus, and the nuclear sap, or nuclear matrix, in which they are suspended.

Chromatin

Chromatin is the acidic substance in the nucleus which takes up basophilic dyes like haematoxylin, and methylene blue in the Romanowsky technique. In the interphase nucleus, some chromatin (*heterochromatin*) appears as areas of deep staining and is thought to represent those regions of the chromosomes which remain condensed and relatively inert metabolically. The remainder of the nucleus is lightly stained, and the dispersed chromatin material (*euchromatin*) is in an active form. It follows that the actual morphology of the nucleus varies considerably from one cell to another, and that an assessment of function can be made from nuclear structure. In active cells, e.g. neurones, the nucleus is vesicular and very little heterochromatin is present. Heterochromatin is more abundant in epithelial cells, and gives the nucleus a stippled appearance. In inactive cells, e.g. lymphocytes and late normoblasts, the heterochromatin occupies much of the nucleus which therefore appears deeply basophilic. In the mature plasma cell the heterochromatin is disposed close to the nuclear membrane in clumps to produce the cart-wheeled, or clock-faced, appearance so typical of this cell.

Sex chromatin, or x-chromatin. A feature which has assumed great importance recently is a mass of heterochromatin, first noted by Barr in the nerve cells of the cat.[15] He observed a chromatin dot near the nucleolus in the female but not in the male. This is therefore called the *sex chromatin*, or *Barr body*. Further observations have shown a similar body in the human subject. It is best demonstrated in squamous epithelial cells of skin[16] or scrapings of the buccal mucosa, where the sex chromatin appears as a demilune on the nuclear membrane (Fig. 2.8). Most cells in the normal female are "chromatin-positive", while in the normal male they are negative.

An important site for the investigation of sex chromatin is the neutrophil leucocyte in the peripheral blood.[17, 18] In

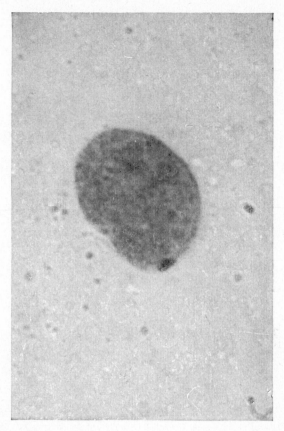

Figure 2.8
The Barr body. Nucleus of a cell from female buccal mucosal smear showing the sex chromatin mass on the nuclear membrane. Stained by orcein acetic. *(Photograph supplied by Dr. Nigel H. Kemp)*

this situation it is disposed as a drumstick attached to the side of the nucleus (Fig. 2.9). About 3 per cent of leucocytes in females exhibit drumsticks.[19]

The value of "sexing" somatic skin and mucosal cells is described in Chapter 3, and it is sufficient to note here that the number of Barr bodies present in a diploid cell is one less than the number of X chromosomes.[19] Hence the cells of a normal male have no Barr body while those of the female possess one.

Y-chromatin. The chromatin of the Y chromosome can now be seen in the interphase nucleus by staining with quinacrine and examining the cell under ultraviolet light (see p. 37).

Deoxyribonucleic Acid

The acid nature of chromatin led to it being regarded as a combination of protein (a histone in mammalian cells) with nucleic acid, two types of which exist. *Deoxyribonucleic acid* (DNA) occurs mainly in the nucleus, and is believed to be the essential constituent of genetic material.

DNA is a polymer of molecular weight around $6\text{--}10 \times 10^6$

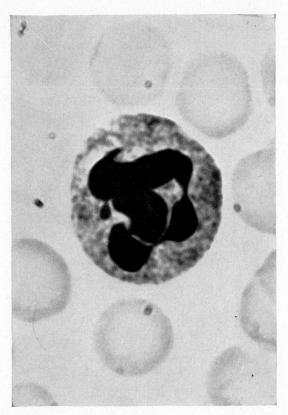

Figure 2.9
Polymorphonuclear neutrophil leucocyte from a normal female subject showing the drumstick appendage to the nucleus. The film has been stained by a Romanowsky technique. ×3 000. *(Picture supplied by Dr. Nigel H. Kemp)*

composed of a long chain of monounits, or nucleotides (Base—Sugar—Phosphate). The deoxyribose molecules are linked together by a phosphate: a base is attached to each sugar. The common bases are either purines (adenine and guanine) or pyrimidines (thymine and cytosine). As a result of x-ray diffraction studies Watson and Crick have proposed a structure which fits in remarkably well with our concept of DNA as a self-reduplicating genetic material. They proposed that the molecule is composed of two polynucleotide chains spiralled round a common axis (see Fig. 2.10). The bases are directed inwards towards the axis, and the two chains are linked by hydrogen bonds between a purine and a pyrimidine. They showed that only adenine could pair with thymine, and guanine with cytosine. DNA has a coat of protein, and this combination thus closely resembles in structure that of the simpler viruses.

Role of the Nucleic Acids as Genetic Material[20, 21]

It is believed that DNA in the nucleus contains genetic information which is passed *via* RNA into the cytoplasm where it is utilised in the manufacture of proteins (often enzymes) of exact composition.

The order of the bases in DNA constitutes the genetic code, a sequence of three bases corresponding to a single amino acid. A type of RNA (*messenger RNA*, or mRNA) is made in the nucleus in the presence of DNA-dependent RNA polymerase, or transcriptase, for the process is called *transcription*, and the mRNA is modelled on one of the polynucleotide chains of DNA which acts as a template. The base sequence of the RNA is thus complementary to that of DNA, i.e. cytosine corresponds with guanine, etc. This mRNA passes into the cytoplasm and becomes associated with a group of ribosomes[22] (a *polysome*). Here protein synthesis occurs. Each triplet of the RNA base

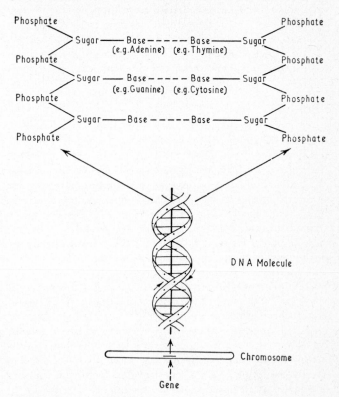

Figure 2.10
Suggested chemical structure of DNA. The two polynucleotide chains are united by their bases, the order of which constitutes the genetic code. *(After Watson, J. D. and Crick, F. H. C. (1963), Nature (Lond.) 171, 737)*

order is responsible for one amino acid.* As the ribosomes "read along" the RNA molecule, successive amino acids are added to an ever-increasing polypeptide chain. In this way a protein of exact composition is built up; secondary

* With 4 bases, 64 triplets are possible, but as only about 20 amino acids have to be coded, some duplication occurs. The code is therefore said to be degenerate. Thus UUU and UUC both correspond to phenylalanine. The actual order of the three bases in each triplet is not known. It is thought that the code is universal, i.e. the same for all organisms. The code is written in terms of the order of bases in mRNA.

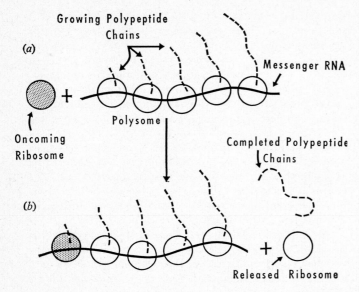

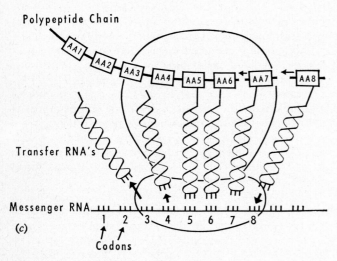

Figure 2.11
Schematic model of protein synthesis. In (*a*) and (*b*) a long single-stranded molecule of messenger RNA (mRNA) is seen associated with a group of ribosomes to form a polysome. As each ribosome moves along the mRNA, an ever-growing polypeptide chain is produced. In (*c*) a single ribosome is depicted as a combination of two particles of unequal size. The sequence of bases of the mRNA forms triplets, or codons, which for the sake of clarity are drawn as groups of three upright lines. Each molecule of transfer RNA (tRNA) is composed of a long thread bent on itself to form a helical structure. At one end of the molecule there is a particular amino acid (AA1, AA2, etc.), and at the other end, where it is bent on itself, there are three unpaired bases which form an anti-codon. Each codon of the mRNA is "recognised" by a corresponding anticodon of a tRNA. In this way specific amino acids are added to the polypeptide chain in a specific linear sequence determined by the mRNA which is itself modelled on the nuclear DNA. *(Drawn by the Department of Art as applied to Medicine, University of Toronto: after Warner, J. R. and Soeiro, R. (1967), New Engl. J. Med.* **276**, *613; and Nirenberg, M. W. (1965), in* The Living Cell, *San Francisco and London: Freeman)*

and tertiary structure are presumably a consequence of this. The actual addition of each amino acid is effected by another type of RNA (*transfer RNA*, or tRNA), a separate form of which exists for each of the amino acids. The process is complex and is described as *translation*, for the code of the DNA finally appears legible in the form of a polypeptide chain (Fig. 2.11).

Thus the genetic code of DNA consists of triplets, or *codons*, which determine the insertion of particular amino acids in the peptide chain. The sequence of the codons is colinear with the sequence of amino acids. The codons responsible for a whole peptide chain form a group called a *cistron*. It is believed that a number of cistrons are grouped together to form a larger unit, the *operon*,[23] which is described below. The actual code has been investigated by various means. Synthetic polyribonucleotides have been prepared and can act as mRNA in cell-free preparations containing ribosomes, suitable substrates, and a source of energy. Thus a polynucleotide containing uridine only (poly U) leads to the formation of phenylalanine. Hence the code for this amino acid is UUU.

Although it is well established that the encoded message of DNA is passed on to RNA, it is also known that the reverse can occur. Several RNA tumour viruses contain a polymerase activity which can lead to the formation of specific nuclear DNA (p. 385).

Relationship of DNA to Genes

It is apparent that DNA provides the chemical basis for the inheritance of characteristics which are described as genes (Chapter 3). The nucleotide sequence of a length of DNA comprises a gene whose message is first transcribed into mRNA and then translated into a polypeptide chain of specific amino-acid sequence.

Control of gene action. It is evident that each nucleated cell of the body contains the necessary information for the manufacture of every protein of which the body is composed. That they do not do so all the time is evidence that there is some very adequate control mechanism. Thus erythroid cells manufacture haemoglobin, plasma cells immunoglobulin, etc.

The degree of permanence with which genetic information is repressed when cells differentiate has been the subject of much speculation. A fertile adult frog can develop from the implantation of an intestinal-cell nucleus of an adult frog into an enucleate ovum.[24, 25] It would seem that in this instance none of the DNA in the differentiated cell is irreversibly repressed. If this is true, it is not surprising that under abnormal circumstances cells produce substances which are alien to their accustomed products. This occurs in metaplasia and neoplasia. An excellent example is the secretion by certain cancer cells of hormones which normally are produced only in the very specialised cells of the endocrine glands. The production of α_1-feto-globulin by some hepatomata is another example (p. 393).

The control of gene action is poorly understood, but is being actively investigated at the present time. Some genes lead to the production of proteins which are enzymes, or which are used in the metabolism of the cell. These are termed *structural genes*. In certain bacteria it has been found that a group of genes are closely linked, and either function together or are completely repressed, i.e. no mRNA is produced. The mechanism of control is also under genetic influence, and Fig. 2.12 illustrates a scheme of this based on

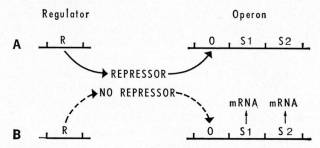

Figure 2.12
The regulator-operator hypothesis. A. The regulator gene (R) forms a repressor substance which acts through the cytoplasm to repress the operator gene (O). When O is thus inhibited, the structural genes (S1 and S2) in its operon cannot form mRNA. B. If the regulator gene cannot form repressor substance, or if the repressor does not reach the operator gene, the operator is *derepressed* and S1 and S2 are then able to produce mRNA. *(Diagram redrawn from Thompson, J. S and Thompson, M. W. (1966), Genetics in Medicine. Philadelphia and London: Saunders. The hypothesis is that of Jacob, F. and Monod, J. (1961), J. molec. Biol.* **3**, 318*)*

that proposed by Jacob and Monod.[26, 27] Each group of genes, or *operon*, is controlled by a closely associated gene called the *operator gene*. This itself is regulated by another gene, the *regulator gene*, which through its own mRNA leads to the production in the cytoplasm of a protein (*repressor substance*) which suppresses the operator gene. The regulator gene may itself be inhibited, and in that event the operator is derepressed and the genes of the operon are allowed to act; mRNA is produced and protein synthesis proceeds (Fig. 2.12). The model is derived from a study of bacteria which are haploid. In diploid organisms, such as man, more complex models have been proposed.[28] The complexity of the subject is apparent when it is appreciated that in every cell, every gene is under continuous control and so regulated that the requirements of the body are met. This applies not only during adult life but also during the complex processes of development. The ovum provides an excellent example of how protein synthesis can be inhibited, only to be switched on suddenly by the event of fertilisation.

Effect of antibiotics on nucleic acid metabolism. Certain antibiotics have a very specific action on nucleic-acid metabolism, which can be used therapeutically as well as in investigative work. Mitomycin C, which has antitumour and antibacterial activity, inhibits DNA synthesis, while RNA and protein synthesis are unaffected. Actinomycin D, on the other hand, inhibits DNA-dependent RNA polymerase activity by binding to DNA, and mRNA production is therefore stopped by its action. Streptomycin and puromycin block the transfer of amino acids from tRNA to the polypeptide chain, while chloramphenicol, which also inhibits protein synthesis, probably acts by preventing mRNA from binding to the ribosomes.

Replication of DNA. The DNA molecule has been observed to uncoil, and it is believed that each half can act as a template for the manufacture of another half. The enzyme concerned is called DNA polymerase. In this way the exact order of the bases is faithfully copied during cell division.

The amount of DNA is constant in all resting cells (the 2 c amount), whereas there is only half this amount in the germ cells (c). Prior to mitosis the cell builds up DNA until it contains the 4 c amount; division then occurs, and the 2 c quantity is restored. A histogram of the amount of DNA in the nuclei therefore provides a measure of the mitotic activity of a tissue. In tumour tissue cells may be found with even greater amounts of DNA; this is known as polyploidy, and accounts for the giant nuclei sometimes seen in neoplasms. Polyploid cells may also be found in normal tissues, e.g. liver (Fig. 2.13).

It can also be seen that by measuring the amount of DNA in a tissue, an estimate can be made of the number of cells present. Likewise the amount of DNA which appears on a surface can be used to estimate the number of cells which are exfoliated. Thus it has been calculated that from 20 to 50 million cells are shed from the human small intestine each minute.[29]

DNA is thus the material responsible for the appearance of chromatin of the cell nucleus. It is basophilic and stains dark blue with H. and E. Methyl green stains it green, and this is a selective reaction. Feulgen's method (p. 3) is also specific for DNA. It can furthermore be recognised by being depolymerised by specific enzymes (deoxyribonucleases), after which the stains mentioned above are all negative. It has a characteristic absorption of ultraviolet light of 260 nm wavelength, and can in this way be estimated quantitatively, since the amount of light absorbed is proportional to the amount of DNA present. (RNA has the same optical properties, and must be distinguished by some other form of separation.)

Nucleoli

The nucleus frequently contains one or more round bodies known as nucleoli. There may be a surrounding condensation of chromatin to form the *nucleolus-associated heterochromatin*. The nucleoli contain *granules* 15 nm in diameter, and *fibrils* which are 5 nm in diameter and of variable length. Together these are concentrated to form an electron-dense network (fibrillo-granular meshwork, or

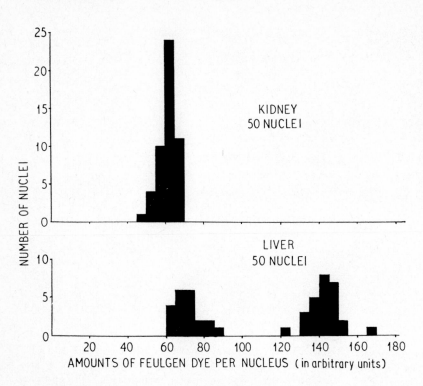

Figure 2.13
Histogram to show the DNA content of isolated rat kidney and liver nuclei as determined by quantitative microspectrophotometry after Feulgen staining. The upper diagram shows that kidney nuclei contain a constant amount of DNA (the 2c amount) which corresponds to the normal complement of chromosomes (the diploid or 2n number). In liver the second peak is largely due to the presence of tetraploid nuclei (i.e. nuclei with double chromosome complement). The cells about to undergo mitosis also contribute to this peak. *(From data of R. Y. Thomson published in Davidson, J. N. (1960), The Biochemistry of the Nucleic Acids, 4th edn. London : Methuen)*

nucleolonema) which encloses spaces of low electron opacity called the *pars amorpha* (Fig. 2.14). The nucleolus appears to be the site of RNA formation, and it is thought that the fibrillar component is the precursor of the granules. The latter closely resemble the ribosomes of the cytoplasm, but whether they migrate into the cytoplasm is not clear. Although the precise role of the nucleoli in RNA metabolism is not known, their presence in a cell is related to activity. Thus cells which are active metabolically, e.g. neurones, regenerating cells, and malignant cells, often have large and sometimes numerous nucleoli with a prominent granular component (Fig. 2.15).

Ribonucleic acid. RNA occurs in the cell in various forms. Its basic structure is similar to that of DNA in that it consists of a polynucleotide chain. However, uridine is present instead of thymine. mRNA, previously described, is single-stranded and has a short life, while tRNA is double-stranded (Fig. 2.11). RNA is the principal component of the ribosomes (p. 25) as well as the granular and fibrillar components of the nucleoli. RNA can be recognised by the action of specific enzymes (ribonucleases) which break it down, and also by its selective red staining with pyronin. Methyl green and pyronin are generally used together: the nucleus stains green and the cytoplasm and nucleoli red.

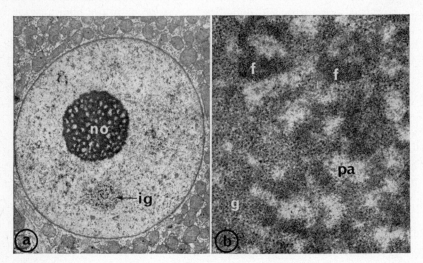

Figure 2.14
Nucleolar structure of the hepatocyte. (*a*) This shows the nucleus of a rat hepatocyte of an animal given ethionine. The nucleolus (no) is large, deeply staining, and shows the nucleolonema as a dense network enclosing spaces of low opacity called the pars amorpha. ig—interchromatin granules. Uranyl acetate. ×7 500. (*b*) A higher magnification of a nucleolus similar to that shown in (*a*). The fibrillar (f) and granular (g) components are seen, and together surround clear spaces—the pars amorpha (pa). Lead hydroxide. ×45 000. *(Photographs supplied by Dr. Katsumi Miyai)*

Figure 2.15
Nucleolar structure in a malignant cell. (*a*) This
shows the nucleus of a hepatoma cell. The
tumour was induced in a rat by the administration
of ethionine. The nucleolus is enlarged and irregular in size, and has an abundant granular component (g). The fibrillar zones (f) of the nucleolus
are distinct and form a twisted rope-like pattern.
Chromatin is inconspicuous. Lead hydroxide.
×6 300. (*b*) A higher power of a nucleolus similar
to that shown in (*a*). The abundant granular component is obvious. Lead hydroxide. ×43 750.
(*Photographs supplied by Dr. Katsumi Miyai*)

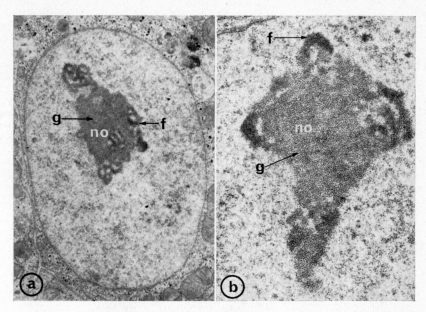

The Cytoplasm

Chemical composition.[30] The cytoplasm is composed
largely of water. There is also about 8 per cent of protein.
The contents differ from the extracellular fluid in several
important respects. There is a high concentration of potassium, magnesium, and phosphate which contrasts with the
sodium, chloride, and bicarbonate found in the extracellular
fluids. The osmotic pressure within the cells has in the past
been assumed to be two to three times greater than the
surrounding extracellular fluid, but this is denied nowadays.

The current view is that the osmotic pressure of the
contents of the cell (exerted principally by protein, potassium, magnesium, and phosphate) is equal to that of the
extracellular fluid (exerted by sodium, chloride, and bicarbonate). The electrolytes can move freely across the cell
membrane, but the protein is retained within the cell.
Sodium would continuously enter the cells because of its
concentration gradient, but there exists a "sodium pump"
which actively excludes it. In this way the intracellular
sodium concentration is maintained at a low level, and
other ions, e.g. potassium, are retained to support the
osmotic pressure of the cell contents. Water is extruded
pari passu with sodium, and does not enter or leave the cell
without a corresponding electrolyte change.

The cell is in osmotic equilibrium with its environment,
but this is entirely dependent upon the continuance of the
sodium pump. This is thought to reside at the cell membrane;
the energy to operate it is derived from cell respiration *via*
ATP.

The enzymes concerned with cell respiration are mostly
situated in the mitochondria and when these organelles are
damaged the sodium pump fails (see p. 50).

Cytoplasmic DNA.[31, 32] The presence of DNA in the
cytoplasm is well established. Some is present in the

mitochondria and directs protein synthesis *via* specific
tRNA. In trypanosomes a mass of DNA at the end of a
giant mitochondrion forms the kinetoplast. DNA is also
present in the mitochondria of mammalian cells, and this
has given rise to the concept, popular but not necessarily
true, that mitochondria originally evolved from intracellular
symbionts. Likewise the chloroplasts of *Euglena* may be
symbiotic algae.

Other forms of cytoplasmic DNA are known. These may
act as infective agents, e.g. bacteriophage and resistance
transfer factor, and can replicate in the cytoplasm and act
as genetic material. These agents are known as *episomes*, or
plasmids. Their presence can alter the functions of a cell.
Thus the production of toxin by *C. diphtheriae* and
colicines by *Esch. coli*, the antibiotic sensitivity of bacteria,
and even the sex of certain moulds are determined by these
agents. They have been extensively studied in bacteria and
protozoa, and undoubtedly also occur in the higher forms
of life. One can speculate about their importance in explain-
ing some types of inheritance, certain aspects of the immune
response, and the development of tumours.

Formed Structures (or Organelles)

Mitochondria.[33, 34] Situated in the cytoplasm of nearly
all cells there are oval or rod-shaped bodies known as
mitochondria (Fig. 2.16). Described in the middle of the
nineteenth century and named mitochondria by Benda in
1898, they were thought at one time to be artefacts; however,
phase microscopy reveals their presence in the unstained
living cell. They are plentiful in actively metabolising cells,
but sparse in others. Under the electron microscope the
mitochondria are seen to have a smooth outer limiting membrane and an inner electron-dense membrane, which is
folded into incomplete septa, or cristae, which subdivide the

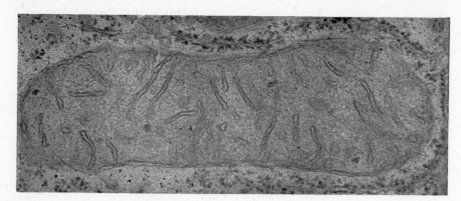

Figure 2.16
Liver cell mitochondrion. The organelle is surrounded by an outer membrane with a second, inner membrane close within it: the inner membrane is folded into shelf-like cristae which protrude into the interior. ×52 500. *(Photograph provided by Dr. M. A. Epstein)*

mitochondria into compartments. Both membranes can be resolved into double structures like the approximately 7·5 nm outer cell membrane. The cristae form plates which project into the mitochondrion, and in some cells form complete septa. High-resolution electron microscopy has revealed the presence of subunits 8–10 nm in diameter,

portant. They contain all the enzymes of the Krebs cycle, mostly in solution and of the terminal electron transport system (cytochrome system); the latter are membrane-bound. The Krebs cycle is a system whereby products of carbohydrate, fat, and protein metabolism are oxidised to produce energy. The latter is stored in the form of the high

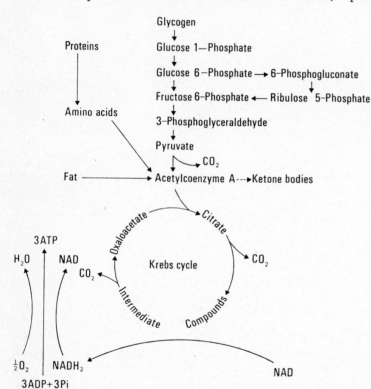

Figure 2.17
Outline of the metabolic pathways concerned in energy production. The whole process in the oxidation of glycogen to CO_2 and water can be considered as occurring in two phases. The first, or anaerobic, phase results in the formation of pyruvate, and is known as glycolysis. The second, or aerobic, phase is the Krebs cycle. Products of carbohydrate, fat, and protein metabolism are fed into the Krebs cycle *via* acetylcoenzyme A. Several enzymic reactions of the Krebs cycle involve the reduction of NAD to $NADH_2$. Reoxidation of $NADH_2$ by the cytochrome system is coupled with phosphorylation of ADP to ATP, viz.

$$NADH_2 + \tfrac{1}{2}O_2 + 3ADP + 3Pi \rightarrow NAD + H_2O + 3ATP.$$

The hexose monophosphate shunt, or pentose–phosphate pathway, leads to the formation of ribulose phosphate and is an alternative pathway in certain cells. It is an aerobic process, and in addition to its products re-entering the glycolytic sequence, sugars of 4–7 carbon atoms are formed and utilised in various synthetic processes. *Key:* NAD—Nicotinamide adenine dinucleotide. $NADH_2$—Dihydronicotinamide adenine dinucleotide. Pi—Inorganic phosphate. ADP—Adenosine diphosphate. ATP—Adenosine triphosphate.

which are attached to the inner membrane by narrow stalks (Fig. 2.1). Sometimes the inner membrane is folded to produce blind-ending tubules rather than plates. Mitochondria have been observed to divide by transverse fission, but there is considerable diversity of opinion as to whether they can also be formed from other cytoplasmic constituents.

The chemical composition of mitochondria is very im-

energy bonds of ATP, and is utilised whenever the cell performs any kind of work, whether mechanical, osmotic, or biosynthetic (Fig. 2.17). Mitochondria are therefore plentiful in actively metabolising cells, e.g. muscle. Furthermore, the complexity of their internal structure is a reflection of their activity; numerous cristae point to great activity. The mitochondria are thus intimately concerned with energy production, and are amongst the first structures to show the effects of the many adverse conditions which may affect the cell.

Lysosomes.[35, 36, 37] These are rounded, membrane-bound bodies which contain the lytic enzymes that are active at a low pH, i.e. acid phosphatase, esterases, deoxyribonuclease, and the proteolytic enzymes previously grouped under the term "cathepsins". They form the granules of the neutrophils, but in most cell types they cannot be seen by light microscopy. The lysosomes are thought to fuse with vacuoles containing ingested material and the *digestion vacuole*, or *phagosome*, so formed is a type of lysosome (*secondary lysosome*). Likewise portions of degenerate cytoplasm containing mitochondria, endoplasmic reticulum, etc., become membrane-bound and are digested by lysosomal enzymes. These are called *autophagocytic vacuoles*, or *cytolysomes*, and are to be found in normal cells as a result of wear and tear. Lipofuscin and other undigested

material may remain to form yet another type of lysosome. Various names have been applied—residual body, dense body, etc. (Figs. 2.18 and 2.19).

The concept of the lysosome is therefore in part biochemical and in part morphological. It is a membrane-bound structure containing lytic enzymes, and its morphology varies according to whether it is inactive (primary lysosome) or is actively engaged in digesting material, either of endogenous or exogenous origin.

The stability of the lysosomal membrane can be increased by the action of hydrocortisone, and this may be a factor in the protective action of this hormone against the effects produced by ultraviolet light[38] and bacterial endotoxin.[39] Vitamin A, on the other hand, has the reverse effect and causes the release of lysosomal enzymes. Thus, if administered to a rabbit there is softening of the cartilages so that the ears collapse.[40] A similar effect follows the

Figure 2.18
Various types of lysosome. (*a*) A lysosome (ly) in a normal parenchymal liver cell. Lead hydroxide. ×43 750. (*b*) Membrane-bound structures containing ferritin granules. These are sometimes called siderosomes (so). G—Golgi apparatus. Lead hydroxide. ×22 400. (*c*) A cytolysome (cly) in a normal rat hepatocyte containing small fragments of the rough-surfaced endoplasmic reticulum (er). Lead hydroxide. ×46 200. (*d*) A cytolysome (cly) containing structures which are probably degraded mitochondria. Lead hydroxide. ×17 900. (*Photographs supplied by Dr. Katsumi Miyai*)

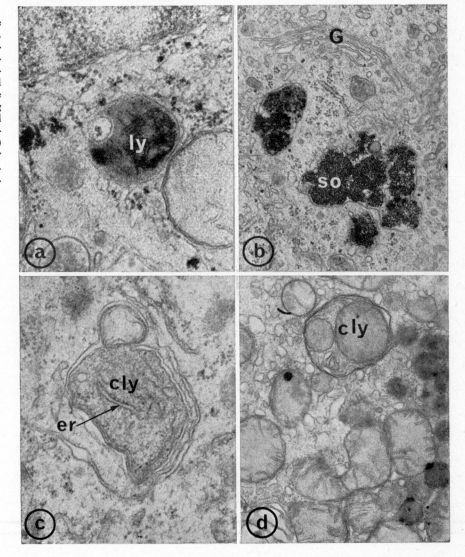

injection of the enzyme papain, for it has the same action on cartilage as does the released lysosomal enzymes.[41]

Lysosomal digestion plays a part in the removal of unwanted cells during embryonic development. For example there is a great increase in lysosomal enzyme activity in the tail during the metamorphosis of the tadpole *Xenopus laevis*.

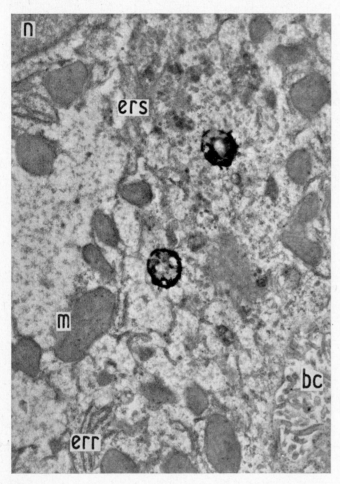

Figure 2.19
Rat liver cell. Survey of cytoplasm stained for acid phosphatase. The nucleus (n) lies in the top left corner and a bile canaliculus (bc) in the bottom right. The cytoplasm contains mitochondria (m) and both rough (err) and smooth (ers) endoplasmic reticulum. The specific localisation of heavy stain in two lysosomes indicates that these bodies are the storage site for the hydrolytic enzyme acid phosphatase. × 29 000. *(From S. J. Holt and R. M. Hicks (1961), J. biophys. biochem. Cytol. 11, 47)*

Interestingly enough, regression of the tail can be accelerated by administering vitamin A and retarded by hydrocortisone. In starvation the formation of cytolysomes is probably a factor in the mobilisation of cell constituents.

The enzyme defects that result in the abnormal accumulation of substances in the cells, e.g. glycogen-storage disease, can be regarded as lysosomal abnormalities (p. 36). The role of the lysosomes in cell degeneration and necrosis is described in Chapter 4.

The endoplasmic reticulum. Situated in the cytoplasm of all cells there are a series of membranes which include between them a complex series of intercommunicating tubes, vesicles, and cisterns. The secretion of some glandular cells, e.g. pancreas, appears between these membranes, and such cells show a well-developed endoplasmic reticulum, as the system of membranes is called. Situated on the endoplasmic reticulum there are granules about 15 nm in diameter and rich in RNA. These are the *ribosomes*, and they give the endoplasmic reticulum a rough appearance (Fig. 2.7). The rough endoplasmic reticulum is particularly well developed in cells engaged in the manufacture of protein for export, e.g. plasma cells. Ribosomes are also found lying free in the cytoplasm, either separately or in the form of polysomes. Again their function is related to protein synthesis, but here it is for use within the cell.

The endoplasmic reticulum and its associated ribosomal granules cannot be distinguished in the "paraffin" sections used in routine pathology. The RNA content, however, is distinguishable by its basophilia with haematoxylin and its red staining with pyronin. For this reason the cytoplasm of cells actively engaged in protein synthesis is blue or mauve in H. and E. sections. Plasma cells are an excellent example of this. The endoplasmic reticulum and its associated granules is also called the *ergastoplasm*.

Smooth endoplasmic reticulum. In some parts of the cell the endoplasmic reticulum also forms a complex lattice of tubules which has no attached ribosomes and therefore appears smooth. The smooth and rough elements of the endoplasmic reticulum are continuous with each other and also with the outer lamina of the nuclear membrane.

The smooth endoplasmic reticulum has been related to the following functions:

Drug metabolism.[42, 43] Following the administration of barbiturates and other toxins there is an increase in the smooth endoplasmic reticulum of the liver cells. This appears to be an adaptive response to ensure detoxification see Fig. 4.6.

Steroid and cholesterol metabolism[42, 44].

Carbohydrate metabolism.[42] In the liver glycogen synthesis occurs in close relationship to smooth endoplasmic reticulum (Fig. 2.20).

The Golgi apparatus. This consists of a series of flattened sacs and vesicles much smaller than those of the endoplasmic reticulum. They usually surround the *centrosome*, which is a clear area near the centre of the cell and which contains one or two *centrioles*. The Golgi apparatus is best developed in glandular cells, and is usually situated close to the nucleus on the side nearest the lumen. It has been suggested that secretion is formed in the endoplasmic reticulum, collects in the Golgi apparatus, and the vesicles so formed are then discharged on to the surface.

Microtubules and microfilaments. High-resolution

Figure 2.20
A perinuclear store of glycogen in a liver cell of a rat poisoned with ethionine. Glycogen (g) is mainly in the form of rosettes of particles, but occasional solitary particles are also present. Vesicular profiles of smooth endoplasmic reticulum are intermingled with glycogen particles. ly—lysosome, nu—nucleus. Lead hydroxide. ×30 800. *(Photograph supplied by Dr. Katsumi Miyai)*

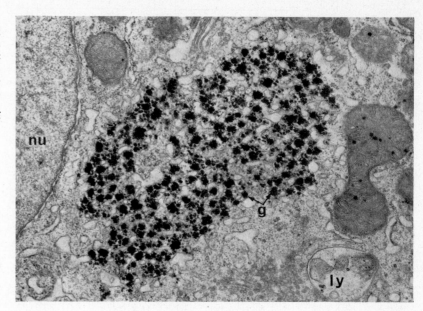

electron microscopy has revealed that most cells contain fibrillar material which is composed of either thin filaments or tubules. Their composition, structure, and function probably vary from one cell type to another and only a brief description will be given here.

Microtubules. These are tubular structures 20–27 nm in diameter. Their centres are composed of material of low electron density, and they therefore appear as hollow tubes. The outer dense wall is actually composed of approximately thirteen longitudinal filamentous subunits with a distance of 5·5–6 nm between them. In some cells, e.g. diatoms, the microtubules appear to give the cell rigidity, acting as a cyto-skeleton, and they may be responsible for the relatively fixed shape of some cells, e.g. blood platelets and podocytes. The transport of material within the cytoplasm is another suggested function. The filaments of the spindle at mitosis are composed of microtubules, and their formation is inhibited by colchicine.

Microfilaments. Most cells also contain long filaments about 5 nm in diameter. Bundles of these converging on the desmosomes (Fig. 2.1) are known as tonofibrils on light microscopy.

The centriole. The centriole is a cylindrical body about 150 nm long, which on transverse section shows nine electron-dense structures. The body divides into two immediately after mitosis, and is concerned with the orientation of the spindle in mitosis.

Cell Aging[45]

Although some cell clones can be cultivated indefinitely, there seems little doubt that normal diploid cells have a limited life in isolated tissue culture.[46] Established cell lines are usually malignant, e.g. HeLa cells. A clone of cells may exhibit aging, and the factors responsible are ill under-

stood. An immortal clone may be converted into a mortal one by suitably manipulating the environment, and the change may reside in either the cytoplasm or the nucleus.[47] Whether aging is the end-result of a programmed genetic sequence or whether it is due to the effects of random chemical damage is not known.[48]

CELL DIVISION—MITOSIS

The mechanism whereby somatic cells divide is a complicated process in which the nuclear material is reduplicated, and then carefully divided into two equal parts, which reform the nuclei of the two daughter cells (Fig. 2.21).

The nuclear material takes the form of long threads called *chromosomes*. Each somatic cell in man contains 46, comprising 22 pairs of autosomes and one pair of sex chromosomes (see p. 37).

During the period between mitosis (*interphase*) the chromosomes are present in the nucleus as long drawn-out threads. These are not visible as such using the light microscope, but in areas along the thread there is sufficient coiling for the condensation of material to render these areas recognisable as the heterochromatin of the nucleus. Each chromosome is thought to contain many DNA molecules rather than a single long one.

Following the synthesis of DNA there is a short period (G_2, or Gap 2) before the onset of mitosis. Each chromosome divides longitudinally into two *chromatids* which are held together by a *centromere*.

The strands show coiling along their whole length; in this way they become shorter and thicker and therefore visible. The cell has now entered into the first phase of mitosis—the *prophase*. Meanwhile in the centrosome the microtubules become arranged so as to form the spindle

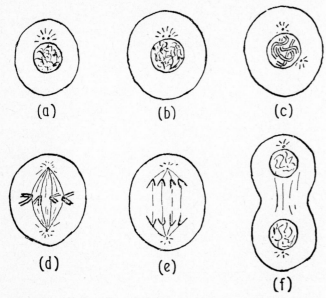

Figure 2.21
The stages of mitosis. (*a*) The resting cell. (*b*) Prior to mitosis the cell enlarges. There is a build-up of DNA and the nucleus now contains the 4c amount. (*c*) Prophase. The individual chromosomes become visible—for the sake of clarity only four are shown, but it should be remembered that the normal human cell contains 46 (the 2n number). Each chromosome has already split into two chromatids. (*d*) Metaphase. The chromosomes are arranged along the equatorial plate, and the spindle is fully formed. (*e*) Anaphase. The chromatids, now called chromosomes, move apart. (*f*) Telophase. The daughter nuclei reform and the cytoplasm divides to produce two new cells each with the 2c amount of DNA corresponding to the normal number of chromosomes (2n number).

fibres which converge on a dense body adjacent to the centrioles. The centrioles move away from each other to opposite poles of the cell, and in this way the *spindle* is formed. Its fibres are attached to the centromeres, and each centriole looks like a star, or *aster*.

Concurrently the nucleoli and nuclear membrane disappear. The cell is now in *metaphase* with the split chromosomes being arranged along a plane which bisects the cell (the "equatorial plate").

During the next phase (*anaphase*) the centromeres divide, and each set of chromatids (now called chromosomes) is pulled by the fibrils of the spindle to either pole of the cell.

The final stage (*telophase*) involves division of the cytoplasm of the cells, and the reconstitution of the nucleoli and nuclear membrane of each daughter cell. The cell now enters the G_1 period, which is terminated in due course by the onset of DNA synthesis prior to the next mitosis.

It can be readily understood how during mitosis each chromosome reduplicates itself exactly, and each daughter cell contains an identical quota of nuclear material. It is presumed that each DNA molecule (and genes) is also reduplicated exactly. Should an error occur during mitosis such that an abnormal gene is produced, the process is

called a *somatic mutation*. It is possible that cancer develops in this way.

MEIOSIS

In the testis the primitive spermatogonia on the basement membrane of the seminiferous tubules divide by mitosis to form *primary spermatocytes*. The next division is called meiosis, and is complex. Although each chromosome divides into two, the chromatids do not separate as in mitosis, but instead behave as a single structure. The double chromosomes line up on the equatorial plate to form 23 pairs. During this phase the pairs of chromosomes (actually four chromatids) may develop breaks and exchange homologous segments—a process known as *crossing over*. The chromosomes then separate and the cell divides. Each secondary spermatocyte contains 22 autosomes and one sex chromosome: each of these is still a double structure. It should be noted that as there is no fixed arrangement of the chromosomes on the spindle, each daughter cell contains a mixture of maternal and paternal chromosomes selected at random. Nevertheless, each cell possesses only one of each pair.

Each secondary spermatocyte divides once more, and it is at this stage that the chromatids actually separate. The two spermatids so formed thus contain 22 autosomes and one sex chromosome. This is the n, or haploid, number and the cells contain only half the normal amount of DNA. The meiotic division and the one that follows it are called the two *maturation divisions*. The spermatids do not divide further, but develop into spermatozoa (Fig. 2.22).

In the ovary the process is very similar, the oöcyte undergoing two maturation divisions, the first (meiosis) before and the second after ovulation. With each division, however, the cytoplasm is divided unequally between the daughter cells with the result that only one survives, and the other *polar body* dies. The sex chromosomes in the oöcyte are equal in size because both are X (Fig. 2.23).

It is interesting to note that in birds it is the male which is homozygous XX while the female is XY.

Thus each ovum and sperm contains 23 chromosomes, and with fertilisation the 2n, or diploid, number of 46 is restored. The pairs of chromosomes in the normal cell are important, because it is on them that the pairs of factors, or genes, are situated (see p. 30). It is noteworthy that only at meiosis do the chromosomes actually pair off.

Non-disjunction. At either of the two maturation divisions a pair of chromosomes may fail to separate, and both are drawn into one of the daughter cells. This is called non-disjunction. Thus, if the sex chromosomes are involved, abnormal secondary spermatocytes can be formed, one containing XY/XY and the other O. If the next division is normal, two types of spermatozoa are produced, one with no sex chromosome and the other with XY. If there is also non-disjunction at the second division, then gametes with XXYY, XYY, XXY, X, Y, or O can be produced. Such

Figure 2.22
Diagrammatic representation of spermatogenesis. Only the sex chromosomes are
shown. The primary spermatocytes are
depicted at the onset of meiosis with the
chromosomes already divided.

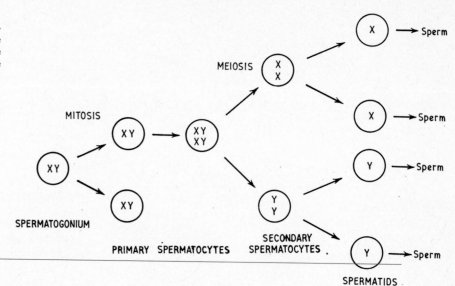

defects of gametogenesis can give rise to gross defects in the resulting offspring. When the autosomes are involved the zygote usually dies, or is produced as a macerated fetus.

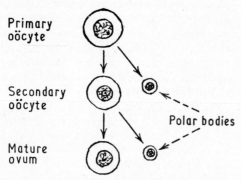

Figure 2.23
Diagrammatic representation of oögenesis.

Abnormalities in the sex chromosomes are, however, more often compatible with life.

It is evident that during the formation of the gametes there is ample opportunity for rearrangement of the genetic material. The extraordinary plasticity of the process of sexual reproduction is demonstrated by the fact that one human being is unlike any other. Errors may, however, occur. Faults in DNA synthesis result in *mutations*, while failure of the chromosomes to separate (*non-disjunction*) leads to an abnormal number of chromosomes. Breakage of chromosomes or chromatids is a common phenomenon, and although the broken ends may rejoin immediately, they may also join in other ways. These recombinations may be of importance in the evolutionary process. Sometimes parts of a chromosome are lost (*deletion*) or become attached to another chromosome (*translocation*). If two breaks occur in the same chromosome, the ends may join together to form a *ring chromosome*. Chromosome breaks can be induced by *ionising radiation, certain drugs*, and by *viruses*.[49] They are also more common in three rare syndromes:[50] ataxia telangiectasia (p. 172), Fanconi's anaemia (p. 608), and Bloom's syndrome.* Of interest is the observation that in all these conditions leukaemia or other types of malignancy are common in early life.

The next chapter deals with some of the effects of these errors.

---

* *Bloom's syndrome*[51] is characterised by low birth weight, stunted growth, and a sun-sensitive telangiectatic skin disorder affecting the cheeks and nose—called the butterfly area of the face and also affected in lupus erythematosus.

REFERENCES

 1. Annotation (1966). *Lancet*, ii, 1351.
 2. DALTON, A. J. and HAGUENAU, F. (1968). (Eds) *The Membranes*. New York and London: Academic Press.
 3. Various Authors (1968). *British Medical Bulletin*, **24**, 99–182.
 4. Various Authors (1961). Cell movement and cell contact. *Experimental Cell Research, Supplement* **8**.
 5. LEWIS, W. H. (1931). *Bulletin of the Johns Hopkins Hospital*, **49**, 17.
 6. Leading Article (1970). *Lancet*, ii, 1294.
 7. STEINBERG, M. S. (1964). In *Cellular Membranes in Development*, p. 321. Edited by M. Locke. New York: Academic Press.
 8. PAPPENHEIMER, J R. (1953). *Physiological Reviews*, **33**, 387.
 9. MOORE, D. H. and RUSKA, H. (1957). *Journal of Biophysical and Biochemical Cytology*, **3**, 457.
10. KAVANAU, J. L. (1963). *Nature*, **198**, 525.

11. KAVANAU, J. L. (1966). *Federation Proceedings. Federation of American Societies of Experimental Biology*, **25,** 1096.
12. SCRIVER, C. R. (1969). *Pediatrics,* **44,** 348.
13. Leading Article (1970). *Lancet,* ii, 1119.
14. SATIR, P. (1961). *Scientific American,* **204,** 108.
15. BARR, M. L. and BERTRAM, E. G. (1949). *Nature,* **163,** 676.
16. MOORE, K. L., GRAHAM, M. A. and BARR, M. L. (1953). *Surgery, Gynecology and Obstetrics,* **96,** 641.
17. DAVIDSON, W. M. and SMITH, D. R. (1954). *British Medical Journal,* ii, 6.
18. MITTWOCH, U. (1964). *Nature,* **201,** 317.
19. MITTWOCH, U. (1964). *Proceedings of the Royal Society of Medicine,* **57,** 643.
20. CRICK, F. H. C. (1967). *Proceedings of the Royal Society,* B, **167,** 331.
21. YČAS, M. (1969). *The Biological Code,* 360 pp. Amsterdam and London: North Holland Publishing Co.
22. RICH, A. (1963). *Scientific American,* **209,** 44.
23. STENT, G. S. (1964). *Science,* **144,** 816.
24. GURDON, J. B. (1962). *Journal of Embryology and Experimental Morphology,* **10,** 622.
25. GURDON, J. B. and UEHLINGER, V. (1966). *Nature,* **210,** 1240.
26. MONOD, J. and JACOB, F. (1961). *Cold Spring Harbor Symposia on Quantitative Biology,* **26,** 389.
27. JACOB, F. and MONOD, J. (1961). *Journal of Molecular Biology,* **3,** 318.
28. DREYFUS, J-C. (1969). *Progress in Medical Genetics,* **4,** 169.
29. CROFT, D. N. *et al.* (1968). *Lancet,* ii, 70.
30. CAMERON, G. R. and SPECTOR, W. G. (1961). *The Chemistry of the Injured Cell,* 147 pp. Springfield: Thomas.
31. PREER, J. R. (1971). Extrachromosomal inheritance: hereditary symbionts, mitochondria, chloroplasts. In *Annual Review of Genetics,* vol. 5, p. 361. Edited by H. L. Roman. Palo Alto: Annual Reviews Inc.
32. WOLSTENHOLME, G. E. W. and O'CONNOR, M. (1969). (Eds) *Bacterial Episomes and Plasmids, Ciba Foundation Symposium,* 268 pp. London: Churchill.
33. LEHNINGER, A. L. (1964). *The Mitichondrion,* 263 pp. New York and Amsterdam: W. A. Benjamin Inc.
34. PARSONS, D. F. (1965). *International Review of Experimental Pathology,* vol. 4, p. 1, ed. by G. W. Richter and M. A. Epstein. New York and London: Academic Press.
35. DE REUCK, A. V. S. and CAMERON, M. P. (1963). Edrs. *Lysosomes,* A Ciba Foundation Symposium, 446 pp. London: Churchill.
36. THOMAS, L. (1965). In *The Inflammatory Process,* p. 449, ed. by B. W. Zweifach, L. Grant and R. T. McCluskey. New York and London: Academic Press.
37. DINGLE, J. T. and FELL, H. B. (1969). Edrs. *Lysosomes,* vol. 1, 543 pp. and vol. 2, 668 pp. Amsterdam and London: North Holland Publishing Company.
38. WEISSMANN, G. and FELL, H. B. (1962). *Journal of Experimental Medicine,* **116,** 365.
39. WEISSMANN, G. and THOMAS, L. (1962). *Journal of Experimental Medicine,* **116,** 433.
40. THOMAS, L. *et al.* (1960). *Journal of Experimental Medicine,* **111,** 705.
41. FELL, H. R. and THOMAS, L. (1960). *Journal of Experimental Medicine,* **111,** 719.
42. JONES, A. L. and FAWCETT, D. W. (1966). *Journal of Histochemistry and Cytochemistry,* **14,** 215.
43. ORRENIUS, S. and ERICSSON, J. I. E. (1966). *Journal of Cellular Biology,* **28,** 181.
44. BLANCHETTE, E. J. (1966). *Journal of Cellular Biology,* **31,** 501 and 517.
45. ANNOTATION (1968). *Lancet,* **1,** 1240.
46. HAYFLICK, L. (1965). *Experimental Cell Research,* **37,** 614.
47. MUGGLETON, A. and DANIELLI, J. F. (1968). *Experimental Cell Research,* **49,** 116.
48. Leading Article (1967). *Lancet,* **2,** 502.
49. NICHOLS, W. W. (1966). *American Journal of Human Genetics,* **18,** 81.
50. GERMAN, J. (1969). *Birth Defects: Original Article Series,* vol. 5, No. 5, p. 117.
51. BLOOM, D. (1966). *Journal of Pediatrics,* **68,** 103.

Chapter 3.   The Cause of Disease

It is customary to regard pathology as the basis of both medicine and surgery. Certainly when the morbid anatomy and altered physiology of a patient are understood, the clinical picture falls into place, hence the popularity of the clinico-pathological conference. There is, however, a danger in regarding pathology in this light. Syndromes may be recognised, described, and named, but when once a condition acquires the distinction of becoming a "disease", further thought on the subject often tends to stop. It would perhaps be better to remember that the characteristics of each individual and each disease are the results of the interplay of two basic factors: inherited genetic constitution and environment.

The most characteristic feature of living matter, apart from its reproductive capacity, is the ability it has to adapt to changing circumstances and make good any damage that may be sustained. The mechanisms involved in the protective or reparative reactions are of fundamental importance; they are of a structural or chemical nature, and may be regarded as the units from which all pathological lesions are built. The fact that certain circumstances are sufficiently common for the body's reaction to them to be regarded as "diseases", does not detract from this concept.

Pathological processes frequently involve the body's normal responses to abnormal environmental influences. The major part of this book is, in fact, devoted to a consideration of the body's reaction to such noxious external influences as pathogenic organisms, trauma, and dietary deficiencies. Less frequently the body's response is abnormal, and in this chapter we shall first consider those abnormalities which are the result of innate errors.

THE GENETIC BASIS OF DISEASE

Mendel's laws of inheritance, which laid the foundations of the science of genetics, are of great importance in the understanding of many diseases.[1-4] It is postulated that a particular characteristic is determined by a pair of factors, or genes, each of which is situated at a specific site, or *locus*, on one of a pair of chromosomes. Such genes, forming a pair, are called *alleles* or *allelomorphs*. They may be alike (*homozygous*) or dissimilar (*heterozygous*). The genetic make-up of an individual is called the *genotype* and the effect which is produced is called the *phenotype*.

The simplest approach to the mode of inheritance of a particular characteristic, e.g. a disease, is to consider that genes may be either *dominant* or *recessive*. A dominant gene produces its effects whether combined with a similar dominant allele or a recessive one. Recessive genes, on the other hand, produce their effects only in the homozygous condition. This may be illustrated by reference to the inheritance of the Rhesus blood groups. "*D*" may be considered as dominant, and "*d*" as recessive*:

Genotype	Phenotype (*i.e. Blood group*)
D D	D
D d	D
d d	d

It is evident that if the phenotype is known, only in the case of Group d can the genotype be inferred. A person of Group D may be homozygous *DD* or heterozygous *Dd*. The actual genotype can be deduced only by investigating the whole family. The terms dominant and recessive are used in the context of a gene producing an obvious clinical effect. Heterozygotes for recessive genes can often be detected by biochemical tests (see p. 36).

Multiple alleles and co-dominance. In the above example the site, or locus, could be occupied by either *D* or *d*. In the inheritance of the ABO groups each locus may be occupied by one of three allelic genes, *O*, *A*, or *B*. *O* is recessive and *A* and *B* are co-dominant, i.e. both alleles are fully expressed in the heterozygote.*

Thus the possible genotypes are:

These correspond to the phenotypes:

AA, AO	AB	BO, BB	OO
A	AB	B	O

The presence of multiple alleles is common, e.g. in the inheritance of the transplantation antigens, haemoglobin, and the many variants of some of the plasma proteins and enzymes. The occurrence of two or more genetically different classes of individuals with respect of a single trait is known as *polymorphism*.[5]†

* It will be appreciated that the ABO and Rhesus blood groups are more complicated than this, see Chapter 52. Note that it is now conventional to depict genes in italics.

† The frequency of any one class should be greater than 1 per cent, since very rare traits can occur by mutation and their occurrence in a population does not constitute polymorphism in the sense in which this term is used. Polymorphism should be distinguished from *pleiotropism*, which means that a single aetiological factor, such as a defective gene, can produce multiple separate effects.

It is convenient at this point to describe the features of those diseases inherited as either dominant or recessive characteristics.

Diseases inherited as a dominant character are numerous, but none is common clinically. The skeletal system provides many of the best examples, e.g. diaphysial

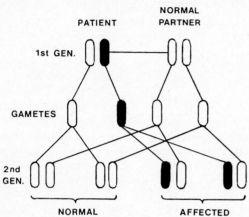

Figure 3.1
Diagram illustrating the transmission of a disease inherited as a dominant factor. One pair of chromosomes is shown for each individual, the black chromosome being the one carrying the defective gene. It will be seen that half the children of an affected patient are themselves diseased.

aclasis, achondroplasia, osteogenesis imperfecta, and cleidocranial dysostosis. Other important examples are polyposis coli, neurofibromatosis, Huntington's chorea, hereditary haemorrhagic telangiectasia, and some cases of cataract. The mode of inheritance is shown in Fig. 3.1.

The following features of a typical disease inherited as a dominant characteristic should be noted.

1. The disease appears in every generation of the family: i.e. one of the patient's parents should have the disease. The occasional instance of poor penetrance, e.g. in retinoblastoma, and the occurrence of a new mutant provide exceptions to this rule.

2. Unaffected members of the family need not usually fear transmitting the disease to their children. However, sometimes the disease becomes manifest only in adult life, when children have already been produced. This is the tragedy of Huntington's chorea.[6]

3. The affected members are usually heterozygous; therefore, if their breeding partner is normal, each of the offspring has a 50 per cent chance of being affected.

4. The disease is usually not severe enough to prevent reproduction, otherwise the affected genes would be rapidly lost from the community. In the few instances where the disease greatly diminishes the breeding potential of the sufferer, this loss is common and most cases are sporadic.

5. Some genes are lost in this way, but replacement is continuously occurring by mutation; new cases may therefore be found occasionally in previously unaffected families. An important factor in predisposing to such a mutation is an increased paternal age—this has been proved in acrocephalosyndactyly, Marfan's syndrome, and achondroplasia.[7]

6. Affected males and females occur in equal numbers.

Diseases inherited as a recessive character are frequently severe, and reduced the breeding chances of the sufferer. The mode of transmission is shown diagrammatically in Fig. 3.2.

The following features should be noted.

1. The birth of an abnormal child is usually the first indication of the condition.

2. As with other Mendelian characters the chances of further members of the family being affected or passing on

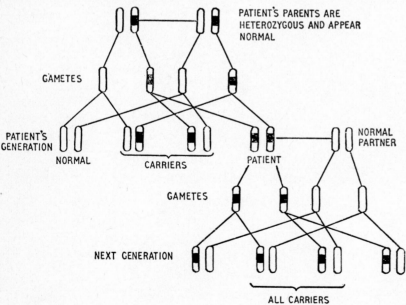

Figure 3.2
Diagram to illustrate the transmission of a disease inherited as a recessive factor. It will be seen that the patient's parents are both unaffected heterozygotes, and that all his children are likewise carriers.

the trait can be calculated: the family therefore is entitled to accurate counselling.[8] Thus the chances of the next child being affected are 1 in 4. Half the offspring will be carriers. If an affected individual mates with a "normal" partner, all the offspring will be carriers.

3. The seriousness of producing carriers should not be over-emphasised. It has been estimated that we all carry 1–3 harmful genes. The known carrier therefore differs from the rest of the population only in that he knows one of his genes!

4. The heterozygous carrier can often be detected because he exhibits minor stigmata of the condition, detectable either by clinical examination or biochemical investigation.

5. Since many members of one family are likely to have the same recessive genes, the dangers of close intermarriage are apparent.

Some of the best-known diseases inherited as recessive characters are retinitis pigmentosa, albinism, xeroderma pigmentosum, fibrocystic disease of the pancreas, and Werdnig-Hoffmann disease (the progressive spinal muscular atrophy of infancy).

Linkage of genes. The phenomenon of crossing over has revealed the location of some genes on a chromosome. The ABO genes and those responsible for the nail-patella syndrome* are always situated close together on one chromosome. This situation of genes at loci on the same chromosome is called *linkage*. When a gene is known to be situated on one of the sex chromosomes (almost invariably the X) the phenomenon is called *sex-linkage*. The only Y-linked characteristic so far described in man is hairy ears.[9]

* This comprises the tetrad: absence of patellae, deformed finger nails, dislocated radial heads, and bilateral iliac bone-spurs.[10]

Diseases inherited as a sex-linked recessive character (Fig. 3.3). The gene is located on the X chromosome; the female heterozygote is unaffected, since she is protected by the normal allele on the other X. In the male, however, the heterozygote is affected, since the Y does not carry the allele. Thus the disease affects males but is transmitted by the female. Father-to-son transmission never occurs. The disease may occur in the female, but this only follows the mating of an affected male with a female carrier—an unlikely event. Diseases inherited in this way are haemophilia, Christmas disease, red-green colour blindness, and often nephrogenic diabetes insipidus, congenital agammaglobulinaemia, and pseudohypertrophic muscular dystrophy. The complete list of conditions considered to be X-linked is well over fifty.[11]

Diseases inherited as a sex-linked dominant character. In this case affected females convey the gene to half their sons and daughters, whereas affected males transmit it only to their daughters; there can be no male-to-male transmission. Therefore there is an excess of female victims. Familial hypophosphataemia and haemolytic anaemia due to glucose 6-phosphate dehydrogenase deficiency are examples of diseases inherited thus. The locus for the Xg blood group is on the X chromosome. The two alleles are *Xg*[a] and *Xg*, and give rise to the phenotypes Xg(a+) and Xg(a−). *Xg*[a] is dominant.

Other Features of Gene Expression[12]

Not all human inherited disease can be explained in terms of simple dominant or recessive gene action. There are many complicating factors:

Penetrance and expressivity. It may happen that a trait, although dominant, occasionally misses a generation.

Figure 3.3
Mode of transmission of a disease like haemophilia, which is inherited as a sex-linked recessive Mendelian factor. The abnormal gene is situated on the X chromosome, and therefore produces its effect in the male but not in the female except in the rare event of her being homozygous. All the patient's daughters are carriers, but all his sons are normal.

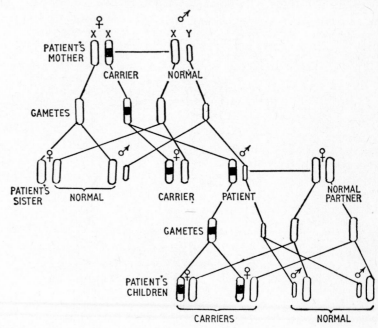

The trait is said to exhibit *reduced penetrance*. Another complication is seen in some families where a dominant gene produces a variable effect. Some individuals who possess it have a severe disease while others have a minor defect, or *forme fruste*, of the disease. In such instances the trait is said to exhibit *variable expressivity*. Penetrance and expressivity are closely related, and while penetrance is an all or none affair, expressivity is variable. Clearly when a gene produces a minor defect it is said to exhibit poor expressivity if the defect is detected, and poor penetrance if the defect is not detected.

Intermediate inheritance. When the heterozygote differs from either homozygote, the inheritance is described an intermediate. A good example is sickle-cell disease. The homozygote with the two sickle-cell genes has fully-developed sickle-cell anaemia, while the heterozygote carrying one defective gene and one normal allele has the mild sickle-cell trait—a state intermediate between the disease and the normal.

Sex limitation. A disease which is present only in one sex is said to be sex limited. Premature baldness may be an example, being inherited as a dominant autosomal factor, but manifest in the male and rarely in the female. Testicular feminisation may also be sex limited.

Interaction of several non-allelic genes. Genes situated at separate loci may interact in complex ways. A good example is that of the ABO, secretor, and Lewis blood-group systems.

Multifactorial, or polygenic, inheritance. Certain traits, e.g. intelligence and height, appear to be influenced by many genes, and the same may well apply to hypertension, diabetes mellitus, and other diseases where the line of division between disease and health is not clearly drawn. Environmental factors are almost certainly involved as well.

Genetic heterogeneity, or polymorphism.[13, 14] If variants of a single phenotype can be caused by different genes the trait is said to be genetically heterogeneous. Sometimes the diseases may be distinguished from each other on clinical grounds, for example the various types of muscular dystrophy,* and the defective genes are located at separate loci. In other instances the two conditions are almost indistinguishable, e.g. types of elliptocytosis and congenital deafness. The most direct proof that different genes are involved is where two individuals with similar defects inherited as autosomal recessive characters mate and produce a normal offspring.

Many examples of genetic polymorphism are known in respect of proteins and enzymes. Thus there are at least 150 variants of haemoglogin, 22 of glucose 6-phosphate de-

* The Duchenne type, which is inherited as a sex-linked recessive trait and affects males only, appears in early childhood, and progresses rapidly. The limb-girdle type is an autosomal recessive which appears at puberty and is less severe, while the facio-scapulo-humeral type is inherited a an autosomal dominant with variable expressivity which develops in the teens and progresses slowly.

hydrogenase, 3 of phenylketonuria, and three of galactosaemia. These variants could be due to defective genes at separate loci, but are usually due to the existence of multiple alleles at one locus. This raises interesting possibilities. In some patients, e.g. with galactosaemia, who are presumed to be homozygous, the phenotype is atypical. In these instances it is probable that the individual is in fact heterozygous for two abnormal alleles, in this instance the allele for the classical type of galactosaemia and that for the Duarte variant. Such a mechanism may provide the explanation for some instances of incomplete penetrance or expressivity of a particular gene. It might also explain why in some families the heterozygotes for a particular trait can be detected while in other families they are undetectable. This will occur if the test employed can detect the effects of one allele but not that of another.

Phenocopies. Characteristics can occur in the absence of the genes which are known to produce that particular effect in other families. The effects of genetic error may thus be mimicked by other factors, presumably acquired. These *phenocopies* are not inherited.

Finally it should be noted that some characteristics could be inherited from genetic material in the cytoplasm, or plasmagenes (p. 22). Such material need not be passed from one generation to the next in the precise way that mitosis determines the distribution of the nuclear genes. It is therefore no wonder that in human disease conditions are found which do not follow any simple Mendelian characteristic.

Mode of Gene Action[1]

It is now well established that the genetic material is composed of nucleoprotein, and that the DNA component is of prime importance in transfering information from each cell to its progeny and from one generation to the next. Its triplet code provides information whereby the cytoplasm is programmed for the manufacture of protein, and a defect in a part of the DNA molecule can result in the formation of an abnormal protein. Such a condition is called a *molecular disease*,[13] and several good examples are to be seen in the haemoglobinopathies.

In sickle-cell anaemia the red cells contain an abnormal haemoglobin (haemoglobin S) which precipitates at low oxygen tensions and leads to a sickle-shaped deformity of the cells. This is associated with their more rapid destruction in the body as well as their obstruction of small vessels with infarction locally.

The formation of the abnormal haemoglobin is determined by an abnormal gene. Cases of sickle-cell disease are homozygous, whilst those with the sickle-cell trait are heterozygous; their cells contain both normal and abnormal haemoglobin. The formation of normal haemoglobin is therefore determined by the normal allele. It has been found that the differences between the two haemoglobins lie in the globin moiety. In the abnormal form a valine residue replaces the normal glutamic acid residue at the sixth position in one of the two β-polypeptide chains of the molecule.

Many other abnormal haemoglobins have been described.[14] Usually the red cells containing them are more easily destroyed and anaemia results. One rare type, haemoglobin Zurich, predisposes to severe reactions from sulphonamides, while another, haemoglobin M, leads to hereditary methaemoglobinaemia. Thus an error of one codon can lead to widespread effects.

Sometimes genetic error results in the complete failure to form a protein, e.g. analbuminaemia. In many instances the protein formed as a result of gene action is an enzyme. The concept "one gene, one enzyme" is useful when one considers the conditions characterised by the presence of a defective enzyme. An example of this is the abnormal pseudocholinesterase which may be found in the plasma of certain individuals who in all other respects appear to be normal. These people are unduly susceptible to the action of short-acting muscle relaxant drugs, like suxamethonium, and this is of great importance to the anaesthetist.[15]

An ever-increasing number of conditions, usually inherited as Mendelian recessives, are being described in which there is a deficiency of a single enzyme. These are genetically determined biochemical lesions, or *inborn errors of metabolism*, a term coined by Sir Archibald Garrod over fifty years ago.[16] They are important, because they demonstrate how one simple biochemical error can affect many tissues and often produce severe disease. Furthermore, if they are diagnosed early enough, successful treatment may be instituted. The conditions are rare, but as noted by Harvey over 300 years ago, "nature is nowhere accustomed more openly to display her secret mysteries than in cases where she shows traces of her workings apart from the beaten path".*

It may be postulated that an abnormal allele can occupy the locus of a structural gene or of a gene that exercises control, such as an operator gene. When a structural gene is involved there can be one of several effects. The protein formed in the body, being of abnormal composition, may differ in chemical or physical properties. The many variants of haemoglobin are examples of this. In the case of enzymes, their specific activity may be lessened or their stability altered. It should be noted that it is technically difficult to distinguish between three possibilities:

(*a*) Less enzyme is produced and indeed there may be complete absence.

(*b*) A normal quantity of enzyme is produced but its specific activity is reduced or modified.

(*c*) The enzyme produced shows an increased lability and is rapidly catabolised.

Defective enzyme activity can therefore be due to several

mechanisms, and it is not surprising that apparently simple enzyme deficiency states such as glucose 6-phosphate dehydrogenase deficiency are in fact examples of complex genetic polymorphism.

A defective gene may also affect a control mechanism.[17] Thus a defective repressor gene might lead to excess formation of an enzyme. Acute intermittent porphyria may be an example of this, for there is an excess of δ-amino-laevulinic acid synthetase formation (p. 561). A defective operator gene might lead to a failure in the formation of several enzymes. *Hereditary orotic aciduria* has been cited as an example, for there is a deficiency of two enzymes responsible for the *sequential* steps in the conversion of orotic acid to uridine monophosphate. This is a precursor of RNA. The syndrome is characterised by retardation in infancy and a megaloblastic anaemia. Another example is sucrose intolerance, in which there is a deficiency of sucrase, maltase, and isomaltase in the gut.

It is sometimes stated that a particular germ-layer is affected, but in fact there is no known genetic error which affects one layer as a whole. One particular cell type may be affected; thus in albinism there is a failure of the melanocytes to form melanin. This affects the iris, retina, and skin, although these structures are not all formed at the same time embryologically. A genetic error therefore does not affect different processes merely because they are occurring at a particular stage of development.

Although a number of inherited diseases are explicable in chemical terms, the great majority are not. Presumably the obvious abnormalities, e.g. achondroplasia and polyposis coli, are far removed from the defective gene and its primary product. There is, however, every hope that these gaps in our knowledge will be spanned in due course, and ways will be found to foil such perverted developments.

Some Examples of Inborn Errors of Metabolism[1, 2, 12, 18]

Galactosaemia.[17] This is a condition in babies who fail to thrive, have large livers, and pass galactose, amino acids, and albumin in the urine. Mental retardation, cataract, and cirrhosis of the liver ultimately develop. The defect is due to absence of the enzyme galactose 1-phosphate uridyl transferase which is responsible for converting galactose 1-phosphate to glucose 1-phosphate (Fig. 3.4).

It follows that galactose (from the lactose of milk) cannot be utilised; it accumulates and is excreted in the urine. Galactose itself is not toxic, but galactose 1-phosphate probably interferes with some metabolic process (possibly involving phosphoglucomutase, which converts glucose 1-phosphate to glucose 6-phosphate), which is essential for the proper development of the brain, lens, liver, and kidney. The avoidance of galactose in the diet from an early age may prevent the baneful effects of this abnormality.

Alcaptonuria (or Alkaptonuria).[19] In this condition the urine contains large amounts of homogentisic acid, which

* "The Works of William Harvey, M.D.", translated by Robert Willis, p. 616, Sydenham Society, London, 1847. (Cited by Garrod, A. E., 1928, *Lancet*, **1**, 1055.)

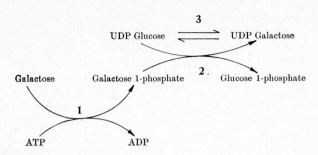

Figure 3.4
Metabolic pathway concerned in the conversion of galactose to glucose 1-phosphate.
Key: 1. Galactokinase. 2. Galactose 1-phosphate uridyl transferase. 3. UDP Galactose 4-epimerase. UDP—Uridine diphosphate. ATP—Adenosine triphosphate. ADP—Adenosine diphosphate.

causes it to darken on standing if the reaction is alkaline. Staining of the diapers may be the first sign of the disease. The condition is of little consequence except that as the patient grows older, his cartilages and ligaments become pigmented (ochronosis, p. 560). Osteoarthritis may develop, but the reason for this is not known. Alcaptonurics are unable to metabolise homogentisic acid, which is an intermediary in the metabolic breakdown pathway of tyrosine and phenylalanine. There are, however, alternative metabolic pathways, which probably explains why no serious lesion develops. Alcaptonuria was the first disorder in man found to be inherited as a Mendelian recessive characteristic, and the study of this condition led Garrod to formulate the concept of enzyme deficiency as a cause of disease.

Phenylketonuria.[20] Between 3 and 5 persons per 100 000 of the population exhibit this condition, which commences shortly after birth, and is characterised by retardation of mental development. Other neurological abnormalities, hypopigmentation of the skin, and sometimes eczema also occur.

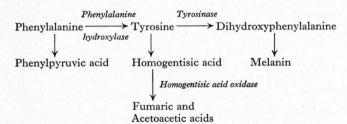

Figure 3.5
Some steps in the metabolism of phenylalanine. The absence of phenylalanine hydroxylase results in phenylketonuria, of homogentisic acid oxidase in alkaptonuria, and of tyrosinase in albinism (see p. 560).

In the classical form of the defect there is an absence of the hepatic enzyme phenylalanine hydroxylase, which normally converts into tyrosine that dietary phenylalanine not utilised in the synthesis of protein. Therefore the level of phenylalanine in the blood (normally up to 2 mg per 100 ml) and cerebrospinal fluid is high. The urine contains, in addition to phenylalanine, phenylpyruvic acid, which gives a green colour with ferric chloride solution. If the disease is detected early, certainly before the age of six months, and treated with a diet low in phenylalanine content, brain damage can be largely averted. The administration of tyrosine itself does not prevent the development of mental deterioration, so presumably phenylalanine or one of its derivatives is toxic. The condition is inherited as a Mendelian recessive; 1 per cent of the population are heterozygotes, and can be detected by the administration of a dose of phenylalanine, when the blood level rises. This does not occur in a normal individual.

Lesch-Nyhan syndrome.[21] This is inherited as a sex-linked recessive trait and is characterised by hyperuricaemia, gout, mental deficiency, and spastic paralysis with choreoathetosis. Its most remarkable characteristic is impulsive, uncontrollable self-mutilation of the fingers and lips. This bizarre behaviour may result in great tissue loss, and yet at autopsy no neurological structural abnormality can be found. These patients lack the enzyme hypoxanthine: guanine phosphoribosyltransferase used in the synthesis of nucleotides. In its absence there is an overproduction of uric acid. The enzyme defect can be demonstrated in cells cultured from the patients, and also in some individuals who suffer from gout only. The relationship between the enzyme defect and the other features of the Lesch-Nyhan syndrome is not understood. The disease is of great interest because of the association of a known biochemical lesion with a specific, aggressive, destructive type of behaviour, itself a gross caricature of the type of behaviour that afflicts man today.[21]

Glucose 6-phosphate dehydrogenase deficiency.[22] Patients lacking this enzyme in their red cells are liable to develop acute haemolytic crises if they take certain drugs, e.g. primaquin, sulphone, and sulphonamides. The defect is inherited as a sex-linked factor in negro Africans and their American descendants. Another type occurs in Greeks and Sardinians, and is responsible for haemolytic reactions to the bean *Vicia faba*, as well as to drugs.

At least 22 variants of glucose 6-phosphate dehydrogenase deficiency are now known. The enzyme is necessary for the conversion of glucose 6-phosphate to 6-phosphogluconate in the hexose monophosphate shunt (Fig. 2.17). On this depends the maintenance of glutathione in the reduced state in the red cell. For reasons which are not clearly understood, reduced glutathione is required for the maintenance of the integrity of the red-cell membrane particularly under the influence of certain drugs (see p. 585).

Pharmacogenetics.[15] The study of genetically determined variations in response to drugs is known as pharmacogenetics. Usually there is an increased sensitivity to a drug, and *suxamethonium sensitivity* has been described on p. 34. Another example is *isoniazid sensitivity*; certain individuals lack an isoniazid acetylating enzyme and maintain a high level of unaltered drug after the administration of a test dose. They are liable to develop toxic polyneuropathy. Hereditary resistance to a drug is rare, but cases are recorded of individuals resistant to coumarin.[23] Hereditary metabolic disorders which modify drug effects form a third group.

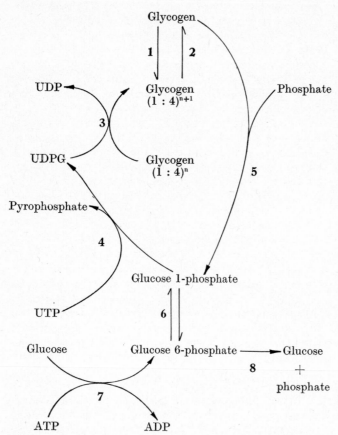

Figure 3.6
Metabolic pathways concerned in the formation and breakdown of glycogen. Straight chain growth of glycogen at the 1:4 linkage is effected by the transfer of one molecule of glucose by UDPG. Branching is achieved by linkage in the 1:6 position. Absence of the enzyme, glucose 6-phosphatase (8), is found in the common type of von Gierke's disease, and a normal type of glycogen is laid down in excess. Absence of other enzymes, e.g. the branching or debranching enzymes, leads to the formation of abnormal types of glycogen.
Key: 1. Amylo-1:6-glucosidase (debranching enzyme). 2. Amylo-1:4-1:6-transglucosidase (branching enzyme). 3. UDPG glycogen transglucosylase. 4. UDPG pyrophosphorylase. 5. Glycogen phosphorylase. 6. Phosphoglucomutase. 7. Hexokinase. 8. Glucose 6-phosphatase. ADP—Adenosine diphosphate. ATP—Adenosine triphosphate. UDP—Uridine diphosphate. UDPG—Uridine diphosphate glucose. UTP—Uridine triphosphate.

Glucose 6-phosphate dehydrogenase deficiency is a well-known example (p. 35).

Von Gierke's disease. The common form of glycogen-storage disease appears in infancy with liver enlargement, obesity, hypoglycaemia, and ketonuria. The condition is inherited as a recessive factor and is due to a deficiency of glucose 6-phosphatase. A normal type of glycogen is found to accumulate in the liver and renal tubules (Fig. 3.6).

Other rare types of glycogen-storage disease are associated with absence of the enzymes concerned in the building up or degradation of glycogen. In this way either a normal or an abnormal type of glycogen is laid down in the liver, heart, or skeletal muscle.

Lysosomal Enzyme Defects.[24] A considerable number of diseases are known in which there is a deficiency of one of the lysosomal enzymes. The corresponding substrate accumulates in the cell, emphasising the fact that lysosomes normally play a vital part in the removal of effete cytoplasmic components. Diseases which fall into this group are Type II glycogen-storage disease (Pompe), which is the most devastating of this group of disorders and is characterised by cardiomegaly culminating in death before the age of two years, metachromatic leucodystrophy, Gaucher's disease, Niemann-Pick disease, Tay-Sachs disease, and perhaps the mucopolysaccharidoses.

Many other inborn errors of metabolism are known, but they are rare and often restricted to particular families. Some are described elsewhere in this book: Wilson's disease, haemochromatosis, acatalasia, cystinuria, Crigler-Najjar syndrome.

Detection of Heterozygote Carriers[25–27]

In about two-thirds of the diseases inherited as recessive traits, the heterozygote carriers can be detected by a variety of tests.[25] In some there is a low level of a particular enzyme e.g. glucose 6-phosphate dehydrogenase, while in others a loading dose of the appropriate substrate, e.g. phenylalanine, reveals impaired tolerance. Another method is to examine cultured skin fibroblasts. In the Lesch-Nyhan syndrome there is lack of the enzyme which converts hypoxanthine and guanine to their respective ribonucleotides. In Pompe's disease the cells lack α-1, 4-glycosidase, and accumulate an excess of glycogen. In Hurler's syndrome the fibroblasts develop metachromasia as revealed by staining with toluidine blue. However, such a phenomenon is also seen in cystic fibrosis, Marfan's syndrome, and even in normal people. No doubt defects found in cultured cells are sometimes secondary events and cannot automatically be equated with events *in vitro*.

Diseases Associated with Genetic Errors[1]

There exist many examples of inherited characteristics which are associated with certain diseases. They are not, however, the obvious cause. The association of a particular disease with race, e.g. diabetes mellitus and Gaucher's disease in Jews, or with sex (goitres in women) is an example of this. Likewise, the ability to resist infection (innate immunity, p. 164) is an inherited characteristic, as is also the inherited liability to develop hypersensitivity (atopy, p. 179). The association of blood groups with disease has also been recognised; thus cancer of the stomach is more frequent in Group A subjects, while duodenal ulceration is more common in those of Group O.

We are quite ignorant of the mechanisms involved, but undoubtedly this type of association was noted by the great clinicians of the past, who often referred to a characteristic disease "diathesis".

Genetic Abnormality Associated with Gross Chromosomal Abnormalities[28, 29]

Advances in the technique of chromosome counting have played a leading part in the elucidation of certain congenital abnormalities. It has been found that colchicine holds up mitosis at the stage of metaphase by inhibiting spindle formation. If cells are grown in tissue culture and colchicine is added to the medium, there will be an accumulation of cells with nuclei showing arrested mitosis.[30] If these cells are placed in a hypotonic solution and squashed under a cover-slip, the individual chromosomes of the dividing cells can be clearly seen after using suitable stains, e.g. Feulgen or aceto-orcein.

Each chromosome has already divided into two chromatids, which are held together by a centromere. The method of preparation tends to separate the two chromatids except where they are held by the centromere. If this is near the middle, they appear X-shaped and are termed *metacentric*. If the centromere is off-centre the chromatid pair are *submeta-centric*, and when near the end the pair are V-shaped and are called *acrocentric*. Human acrocentric chromosomes, except

the Y, have small masses of chromatin attached by narrow stalks to their short arms. These masses are called *satellites*.

By using a photograph of a mitosis one can cut out the individual chromosomes and arrange them in pairs in order of length to form a *karyotype* (Fig. 3.7). An international system of nomenclature was put forward by the Denver Study Group,[31] and has subsequently been elaborated by conferences in London[32] and Chicago.[33] The pairs are numbered 1 to 22, leaving two extra chromosomes—a pair of Xs in females and an X and a Y in males (see Fig. 3.10). The human being therefore normally has 46 chromosomes. The term *autosome* is applied to any chromosome which is one of an equal pair. In man the only unequal pair is the XY of the male, but in practice an autosome has come to mean any chromosome other than X or Y, which are called *sex chromosomes*. As some of these chromosomes are of almost identical length and configuration, it is not easy to distinguish one from another. Seven groups are therefore defined: A (1–3), B (4–5), C (6–12 and the X chromosome), D (13–15), E (16–18), F (19–20), and G (21–22 and the Y chromosome).

Recently new staining techniques have been devised and these have revealed that each chromosome has a series of transverse bands. Each of the twenty-two chromosomes can now be positively identified, and minor racial and individual variations have been described. One method is the use of various modifications of Giemsa staining. The other is quinacrine staining and subsequent examination under ultraviolet light. A portion of the Y chromosome fluoresces so brilliantly that it can be seen even in the interphase

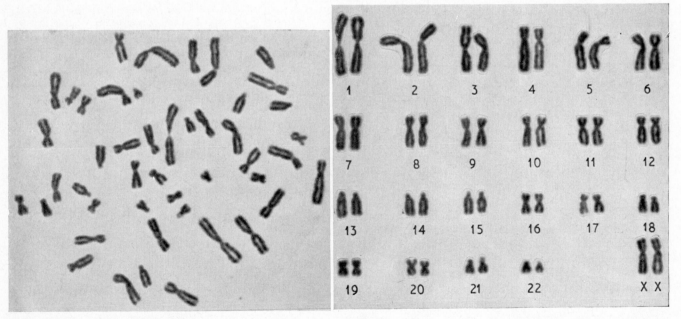

Figure 3.7
Normal human female. Above are shown the chromosomes of a somatic cell at metaphase, and below, these chromosomes are arranged as a karyotype. The latter demonstrates the 22 pairs of autosomes, numbered according to the Denver system of classification, and the two sex chromosomes XX of the female. *(Photograph supplied by Dr. Nigel H. Kemp)*

nucleus. This fluorescent Y body promises to be as useful as the Barr body in clinical medicine[34] (Fig. 3.8).

The present convention for recording a karyotype is as follows. First is given the total number of chromosomes and this is followed by the sex chromosomes, XX or XY in the case of normal individuals. Then a notation is made of any

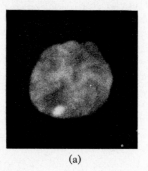 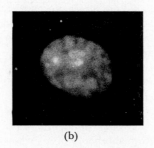
(a)   (b)

Figure 3.8
The fluorescent Y chromosome. Blood smears were air-dried, fixed in methanol, and after staining in 0·5 per cent quinacrine dihydrochloride (atebrine) and washing, were examined in ultra-violet light. The Y chromosome shows a characteristic point of fluorescence in the nuclei of the two cells shown. In (a) the blood was taken from a normal male, whilst in (b) the blood was from an individual with the karyotype 47/XYY. *(Photographs supplied by Dr. Peter K. Lewin. From Lewin, P. K. and Conen, P. E. (1971), Nature, **233**, 334)*

abnormalities. Additional chromosomes or deletions are shown as + or −, the affected chromosome or part of a chromosome being noted. The arms of a chromosome are recorded as p for short (petite) and q for long. Other abbreviations are: r = ring chromosome, s = satellite, t = translocation, and i = isochromosome. When mosaicism is present all cell types are given and are separated by a diagonal line.

There is no doubt that the Barr body, or X-chromatin, described on p. 17 is derived from a single X chromosome—the number of Barr bodies seen in the diploid nucleus is one less than the number of X chromosomes.[35–37]

Mary Lyon has put forward a hypothesis that one of the X chromosomes in each cell of a female fetus becomes inactive early in embryonic life.[38] This inactivation is random, so that about half the cells carry an active maternal chromosome and an inactive paternal one, and *vice versa*. This inactive chromosome replicates later than the other chromosomes during the mitotic cycle, and its descendants follow the same pattern. Since the two chromosomes may carry different sets of X-linked genes, there may be patchiness of a visible character transmitted thus, e.g. coat colour in an animal. Women heterozygous for glucose 6-phosphate dehydrogenase deficiency, an X-linked dominant character, possess two races of red cells,[39, 40] one normal and the other enzyme deficient, and it is these latter that undergo haemolysis. Two clones have also been isolated in women with other X-linked genetic abnormalities.[41] If the character is an

X-linked recessive, e.g. haemophilia, it is possible that some of the cells responsible for making AHG are inactive, but the defect is masked by those which are normal. The deficiency of AHG would escape notice except under the stress of a major procedure, such as extracorporeal circulation. This demonstrates once more how tenuous is the distinction between dominant and recessive.

This hypothesis of *lyonisation of the X chromosome* is now generally accepted, but there is evidence that part of the chromosome remains functional, p. 40.

Chromosomal Aberrations[2, 28, 42, 43]

Chromosomal aberrations may be of two types: (a) *an alteration in number*, either an addition or an absence of a chromosome. This is called *aneuploidy*, as the cells do not contain an exact multiple of the haploid number. In respect of autosomes, an additional chromosome produces *trisomy*, and the effect is always very severe with pronounced mental deficiency. An absence of an autosome is invariably lethal. Additional sex chromosomes, on the other hand, produce comparatively mild effects, and mental deficiency, though common, is by no means invariable. A single X chromosome is compatible with life and mental normality—it leads to ovarian dysgenesis. (b) *An alteration in structure*, i.e. deletion or translocation of part of a chromosome (see p. 28).

Both non-disjunction and loss of chromosomes may occur not only during meiosis, but also during the earliest mitotic divisions after fertilisation. The result of such post-fertilisation defects is *mosaicism*, the presence in one individual of cells which differ in their complement of chromosomes. The most important types of mosaicism are those involving the sex chromosomes, for, as already mentioned, changes implicating autosomes are usually lethal. If aberrations occur in later mitoses, a complex mosaic may result.

It should be noted that normal women are mosaics as regards the activity of their two X chromosomes, but this is not mosaicism as defined above.

SYNDROMES ASSOCIATED WITH
ABNORMALITIES OF THE SEX
CHROMOSOMES[43, 44]

Since many of the X and Y chromosomal abnormalities produce sexual abnormalities some of the features of sexual development should be noted. They may be considered under the following headings:

Anatomical Features
1. Chromosomal constitution, in respect of the sex chromosomes.
2. Structure of the gonads, as revealed by histology.
3. External genitalia.
4. Morphology of the Wolffian and Müllerian ducts.
5. Hormonal status, which is reflected in the secondary sexual characteristics, e.g. development of breast tissue and growth of beard.

Psychological Features

1. Sex of rearing, which is an indication of the sexual status of an individual as regarded by others. Usually this is based on the appearance of the external genitalia at birth.

2. Psychological sex, or the sex which the individual thinks himself to have. This includes sexuality in the sense of eroticism.

In the normal person, all features correspond to one sex. When the psychological features conflict with the anatomical ones, such disturbances as homosexuality and transvestism result. These will not be considered further. When there is conflict between the anatomical features, the condition is regarded as one of intersexuality. Some of the conditions will now be considered, but for details the reader should refer to specialised texts on this complex subject.

Hermaphroditism[45]

Individuals who possess anatomical features of both sexes are termed hermaphrodites. Three groups are commonly recognised, the basis of the classification being the morphology of the gonads.

Female pseudohermaphroditism. *Congenital adrenal hyperplasia.*[46] A defect in one of the enzymes necessary for the production of cortisol results in an oversecretion of ACTH by the pituitary and a corresponding hyperplasia of the adrenals. The common type is due to defective 21-hydroxylase, an enzyme involved in the synthesis of cortisol and aldosterone. An excess production of androgens results in the female fetus having ambiguous external genitalia at birth; later adrenal virilism develops and also a salt-losing state due in part to a failure in aldosterone secretion and in part to an overproduction of other hormones, e.g. progesterone, that antagonise aldosterone. In the male there is sexual pseudoprecosity, the testes being of normal size but the secondary sexual features being well developed.

In a less common type of adrenal hyperplasia, due to defective 11-hydroxylase, the overproduction of the mineralocorticoid deoxycorticosterone prevents a salt-losing state from developing but itself produces systemic hypertension. (See Fig. 3.9.)

Female pseudohermaphrodites may also be born to mothers who have an excess of androgens during pregnancy. Cases are recorded in which this was due to an arrhenoblastoma of the ovary or the administration of androgens for therapeutic purposes. All female pseudohermaphrodites have the chromosomal constitution 46,XX, and the gonads are ovaries.

True hermaphroditism. Both ovarian and testicular tissue is present, either combined as an ovotestis or in separate organs. The external genitalia are usually ambiguous. 46,XX is the usual chromosomal finding, but 46,XY and mosaics 46,XX/46,XY are known.

Male pseudohermaphroditism. The gonad or gonads present are testes but the genital ducts and external genitalia show deviation towards female type, e.g. a small vagina is usually present with or without a uterus. At puberty masculinisation occurs, and when the patient has been brought up as a girl this leads to investigation. This type of male pseudohermaphrodite is generally 46,XY when bilateral testes are present, and a mosaic of the type 45,X/46,XY when testicular development is unilateral.

There is another type of male pseudohermaphroditism which is inherited and in which the endocrine status is fully feminine; this is the remarkable condition of *testicular feminisation.* The individual is often of above average

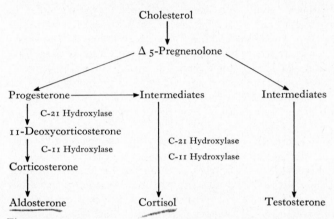

Figure 3.9
Diagram to illustrate the biosynthesis of the adrenal steroid hormones. Defective C-21 hydroxylase activity results in a failure in synthesis of aldosterone and cortisol. Overproduction of testosterone causes virilism in the female, an effect also seen when there is defective C-11 hydroxylase activity. An additional effect of this defect is the overproduction of 11-deoxycorticosterone. This counters the salt-losing state, but leads to systemic hypertension.

intelligence, and has a normal attractive female appearance with excellent breast development. The testes are situated in the inguinal region and their tenderness may cause the patient to seek medical advice. Amenorrhoea, sterility, or dyspareunia due to a short vagina are other common complaints. The chromosomes are usually normal, 46,XY. The pathogenesis of testicular feminisation is not clear. Assay of steroid hormones reveals that they are similar to those of a normal male. The embryonic testis appears to be competent in suppressing Müllerian duct development, but fails to stimulate the Wolffian ducts or the external genitalia. It seems likely that the defect lies in the unresponsiveness of these tissues to androgenic stimulation rather than to lack of hormones. Administration of androgens to the patients fails to produce masculinisation. The unopposed action of oestrogens is responsible for the breast development.

Klinefelter's Syndrome

In this syndrome, which occurs in about 1 in 500 births, there is an apparent male with gynaecomastia, small testes, poor facial hair growth, and a high-pitched voice. The limbs, especially the legs, are disproportionately long. The condition becomes apparent only at adolescence. In most cases examination of cells from skin or buccal scrapings reveals the unexpected presence of a Barr body. Chromosome counts show 47, the extra chromosome being an X. These individuals therefore have the constitution, 47,XXY. The condition usually arises by the fertilisation by a normal (Y) sperm of an XX ovum, but the fertilisation by an XY sperm of a normal (X) ovum can occur. In either event there has been non-disjunction in the abnormal gamete.

Some cases are more complicated, having a chromosomal composition of 48,XXXY, 49,XXXYY, 49,XXXXY, etc. Others exhibit mosaicism, e.g. 46,XY/47,XXY, 46,XX/47,XXY, and 46,XY/48,XXXY. 46,XX has been described (see p. 41). In general the greater the number of X chromosomes, the more likely is there to be mental retardation. The testes in Klinefelter's syndrome are atrophic, but there is very occasionally a limited degree of spermatogenesis. A few patients are said to be fertile, but some cases in which this has been claimed[47] have proved on subsequent analysis to be invalid.[48]

Chromatin-negative Klinefelter's syndrome. A substantial number of cases are chromatin-negative and appear to have the make-up 46,XY. Some may be mosaics in which the cell line XXY has remained undetected, but in others there appears to be primary failure in the formation or development of the germ cells (del Castillo syndrome). Another group may be phenocopies and due to testicular atrophy caused by inflammatory disease.

Ovarian Dysgenesis

This syndrome occurs in females and is characterised by two features:

1. The presence of hypoplastic ovaries, or *streak ovaries*, which contain ovarian stroma with rete ovarii and hilus cells but no germinal follicles. The patients are therefore sterile. The term ovarian agenesis has been used previously, but is inappropriate since the organs are abnormal rather than absent.

2. *Primary amenorrhoea* and *failure to develop secondary sex characteristics*, e.g. breast development. The internal and external genitalia are infantile.

Cases of ovarian dysgenesis may be females of normal stature, and the defect becomes evident with the failure to develop at adolescence. In other cases the individual is in addition of *short stature. Somatic abnormalities* are striking in the remaining cases. At birth there may be redundancy of the skin of the back of the neck and lymphatic oedema of the hands and feet. Webbing of the neck, a shield-like chest with widely spaced nipples, short fourth metacarpal bone, cubitus valgus, hypoplastic nails, multiple pigmented naevi, and coarctation of the aorta are all frequent. When two or more of these somatic anomalies are seen in a female of short stature and sexual infantilism due to streak ovaries, the eponym *Turner's syndrome* is applied.

Chromosomal abnormalities. The common defect is absence of one X chromosome giving the complement 45,X. Barr bodies are absent, and the incidence of colour blindness, a sex-linked recessive trait, is the same as in the normal male, i.e. about 8 per cent. Over twenty variants of ovarian dysgenesis have been found, and a few of these will be mentioned. Some are 46,XXp— in which one of the X chromosomes has deletion of the short arm; cells have a small Barr body. In 46,XXqi the abnormal isochromosome contains the two long arms of X; the Barr body is large. It therefore seems that *when an abnormal X is present it forms the sex chromatin during the process of lyonisation.* In 46,XXq— the abnormal X has deletion of its long arm. These individuals have streak ovaries but no somatic stigmata. Hence it appears that two normal X chromosomes are needed for the development of endodermal cells in the primitive ovary, so that a normal ovary with germ cells is formed. Absence of one short arm leads in addition to the somatic effects of Turner's syndrome.

Some cases of ovarian agenesis are transitional between the classical Turner's syndrome and the normal female. Some ovarian tissue may be present, and menstruation can occur. These patients are mosaics in which some cells have the normal XX, e.g. 45,X/46,XX, 45,X/47,XXX, and 45,X/46,XX/47,XXX. This emphasises the importance of examining chromosome preparations from various parts of the body in difficult cases.

Some cases of ovarian dysgenesis have male traits, e.g. 45,X/46,XYpi. In 46,XYqi the phenotype is female, but some testicular tissue may be found. It is evident that in the normal female XX, a component of the short arm of the "inactivated" X remains active; also the long arm of the Y chromosome probably has components in common with the short arm of the X, otherwise one would except the normal XY male to have the somatic anomalies of Turner's syndrome. A normal Y is necessary for normal male development. The study of these rare but fascinating cases of ovarian dysgenesis has, therefore, led to some understanding of the functions of the sex chromosomes.

The Turner phenotype. Short females have been encountered who have the somatic stigmata of Turner's syndrome but with normal sexual development and a 46,XX karyotype. A corresponding male variant (46,XY) is termed male Turner's syndrome.

Poly-X females. Many "super females", 47,XXX, have been described. The cells contain two Barr bodies. Cases have been described in which the patient is in all other respects normal, but in others there is secondary amenorrhoea and underdevelopment of the uterus, vagina, and external genitalia. Occasional instances of 48,XXXX and 49,XXXXX are recorded. Mental subnormality is common.

XYY syndrome.[49–51] The chromosomal constitution 47,XYY has been noted in males with normal sexual development. Some patients have been abnormally tall, and have exhibited an aggressive nature or have been mentally subnormal. XXXXY has been recorded.[52]

Summary of the Mechanism of Sexual Development

It is not possible to give a complete account of the factors which determine the normal development of sex. Abnormalities are common; indeed, aberrations of psychological sex constitute a major social problem, and one for which no adequate solution has been found. Even the factors which determine the development of the anatomical aspects of sex are not well understood, but nevertheless certain general features are evident.

The presence of a Y chromosome is generally regarded as essential for testicular differentiation, but several rare apparent exceptions to this rule are known. These are the 46,XX true hermaphrodites, the 46,XX Klinefelter's syndrome, and the very rare 46,XX male.[53] The explanation is not known. Perhaps an undetected chromosomal anomaly is present, e.g. translocation of a Y or a fragment of it to an X or other large chromosome, or XX/XY mosaics in which the XY cells are few in number or are in sites difficult to detect, such as in the testis itself.

Once the gonads have developed, further differentiation of the genital tubes and external genitalia is determined *in the male* by gonadal hormones. The testis produces two types of hormone: an androgenic steroid which stimulates the development of the Wolffian duct and the external genitalia, and a non-steroid, probably polypeptide, substance which suppresses the development of the Müllerian ducts. To a considerable extent this acts locally, for if testicular tissue is absent from one side, either as a result of an experimental procedure or in some cases of true hermaphroditism, the Müllerian duct of the same side develops to produce a uterine horn.

If an early embryo of either genetic sex is castrated, there is complete Müllerian duct differentiation, disappearance of the Wolffian duct, and development of female external genitalia.[54] This state of affairs is seen in ovarian dysgenesis.

Extragonadal hormones play some part in the differentiation of the genital ducts and external genitalia. These may be derived either from the mother or from the fetus itself, as in congenital adrenal hyperplasia.

SYNDROMES ASSOCIATED WITH ABNORMALITIES OF THE AUTOSOMES[55, 56]

Absence of one autosome (monosomy) is believed to be lethal to the developing embryo, and is therefore not found in post-embryonic life.[57] Occasionally there is deletion of part of a chromosome, but much more frequently non-disjunction causes one pair to become trisomic: for reasons which are not apparent, this additional chromosome causes severe damage.

Down's Syndrome (Mongolism)[58, 59]

The highly characteristic features of the "mongol" including the mental defect are associated with trisomy of one of the small acrocentric autosomes of group G; this is now defined as number 21. The condition occurs in about 1 in 600–700 live births, and is more common with increasing maternal age. The sex chromosomes are normal, therefore mongols can be of either sex; their chromosome number is 47 (Fig. 3.10).

In Down's syndrome the palm of the hand characteristically shows a simian crease and there are abnormalities of the dermal ridges of the fingers. Indeed, the study of these finger prints and palmar creases (dermatoglyphics) forms an important investigation in cases of chromosomal abnormality.[60, 61]

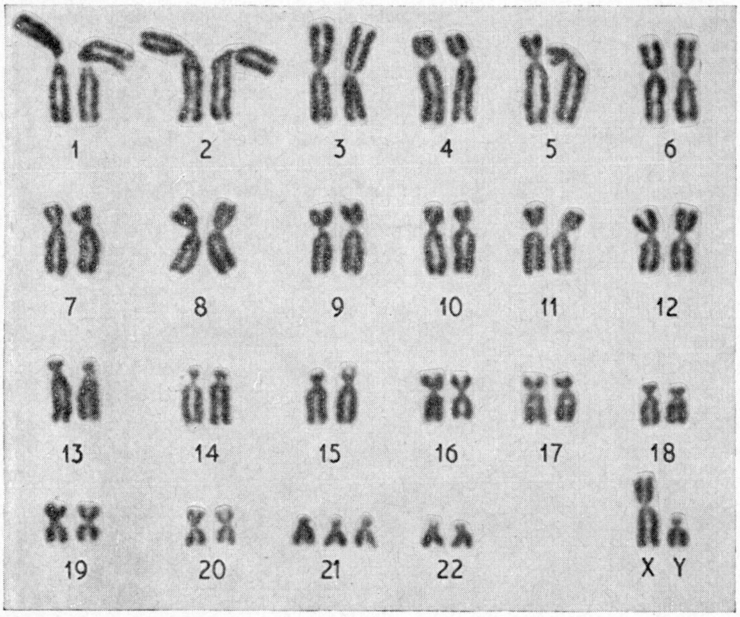

Figure 3.10
Karyotype of male patient with Down's syndrome. Note that there are 47 chromosomes due to trisomy of 21. Compare the sex chromosomes XY of the male with the XX of the normal female in Fig. 3.7. *(Photograph supplied by Dr. Nigel H. Kemp)*

Occasionally a mongol is found with 46 chromosomes. The constitution is: pairs (1–14), 15 alone, pairs (16–22)+XY+one odd big chromosome. This odd chromosome is thought to be a combination of 15 and 21. Thus the patient has in reality trisomy of 21, but the translocation has hidden it. In such cases one of the parents is found to have a similar translocation—45 chromosomes: pairs (1–14), 15, pairs (16–20), 21, pair 22, 15/21, XY. This is therfore called *translocation mongolism*.[62] It is important because further children are liable to be affected also, and the parents can be advised accordingly.

The D Trisomy Syndrome (Patau's Syndrome) 47,XY,D+ or 47,XX,D+[56]

Trisomy of one of the D chromosomes is associated with a variety of congenital defects, the most common of which are mental deficiency, cleft lip and palate, microphthalmia, polydactyly, and defects of the ear, heart, and urinary and genital tracts.

The E Trisomy Syndrome (Edwards's Syndrome) 47,XY,E+ or 47,XX,E+[56]

Multiple abnormalities occur in this syndrome. Affected infants usually die by the third month and few survive over one year. Low-set ears, micrognathia, heart disease, mental retardation, and failure to thrive are the common findings. As with Down's syndrome and the D syndrome, mosaics and translocation cases are also described.

The Cri du Chat Syndrome 46,XY,5p— or 46,XX,5p—[56]

The syndrome was named after the feeble mewing cry of the affected infants. Mental and growth retardation are combined with other defects. The chromosomal abnormality is a deletion of a portion of the short arm of one of the B chromosomes.

Many other chromosomal abnormalities have been described in association with developmental abnormalities, and no doubt other syndromes will be recognised. Ring chromosomes have been described in most of the syndromes noted above. They arise as a result of breaks in both the long and short arms of a chromosome; this is followed by the two ends joining together. The effects vary according to the chromosome affected and the amount of lost or added chromosomal material. The most severe chromosomal aberrations are found in aborted embryos.[63] Thus triploidy (69,XXY) and even tetraploidy (92,XXXX) are amongst the bizarre findings which have been reported. The incidence of these abnormalities has varied from 22 per cent[64] to 64 per cent[65] of spontaneous abortions in which cell cultures could be obtained. The earlier the abortion the more likely is a chromosomal abnormality to be found. About 30 per cent of zygotes are aborted spontaneously, and gross genetic errors are clearly a major cause.

CHROMOSOME ABNORMALITIES ARISING IN SOMATIC CELLS[56]

Although mosaics are described in many of the syndromes mentioned above, the abnormality presumably occurs at an early stage of development. The possibility that a similar event could occur later in life was suggested by the findings in some cases of chronic myeloid leukaemia. Some of the haematopoietic cells show a small chromosome which is 22 with a deleted long arm (46,XY,22q— or 46,XX,22q—). It is called the *Philadelphia* or *Ph' chromosome*.[66]

AVOIDANCE OF GENETIC DEFECTS[67]

Genetic counselling will dissuade some high-risk couples from procreation, but when once conception has occurred the only course open may be the induction of abortion. Amniocentesis can be employed for the prenatal detection of fetal abnormality. Fluid can be removed from the amniotic sac from the twelfth week onwards; about the sixteenth week is the optimal time. This gives the laboratory adequate time to examine the fluid and allows abortion to be performed before the twentieth week. In some societies legal technicalities make the performance of abortion more difficult after this time. The supernatant of the fluid obtained by amniocentesis can be examined biochemically and for the presence of virus. The cells can be examined for the presence of the X-chromatin and the Y-dot. They can also be cultured for biochemical investigation and chromosomal analysis.

TREATMENT OF GENETIC DEFECTS

The treatment of patients with genetic abnormalities is often very unsatisfactory, but there are some instances where expert attention can ameliorate the condition. These can be considered under eight headings:

1. *Administration of a missing protein*—e.g. immunoglobulin in agammaglobulinaemia.

2. *Avoidance of specific substances*—e.g. lactose in galactosaemia.

3. *Administration of missing metabolites*—e.g. cytidylic and uridylic acids in orotic aciduria.

4. *Avoidance of particular drugs*—e.g. primaquin.

5. *Adminstration of metabolic inhibitors*—e.g. allopurinol in gout.

6. *Administration of drugs to eliminate abnormally stored material*—e.g. penicillamine in Wilson's disease.

7. *Allografts*. The grafting of normal cells into individuals lacking specific enzymes or the ability to synthesise essential substances has been hindered by the unsolved problems inherent in grafting. Thus attempts to provide thymic or lymphoid cells in cases of immunological deficiency are in the experimental stage. Allografts of spleen cells in haemophiliac subjects have not been successful.

8. *Genetic engineering*. More complex means of treating genetic defects are now being investigated. Human fibro-

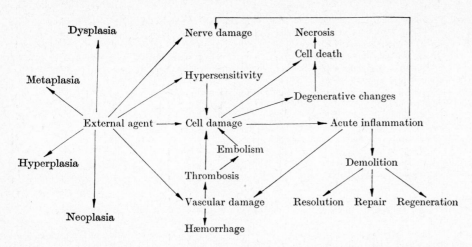

Figure 3.11
Diagram showing the main pathological processes of the body in response to an external agent.

blasts from patients with galactosaemia lack the enzyme α-D-galactose 1-phosphate uridyl transferase. A λ-bacteriophage which normally infests *Esch. coli* can carry the galactose operon. If the defective fibroblasts are infested with this phage, the enzyme activity of the cells is restored.[68, 69] Whether phages can ever be used as a vehicle for the introduction of selected genes into human cells *in vivo* is impossible to predict.

ACQUIRED DISEASE

ENVIRONMENTAL FACTORS CAUSING DISEASE

Much of human pathology is concerned with those diseases which are acquired in post-natal life as a result of the action of external factors. The effects of physical and chemical agents, living organisms, and dietary deficiencies are the common causes of these *acquired diseases*. It must not be forgotten, however, that the developing fetus is also sensitive to environmental influences—in some instances much more so than is the adult. Intrauterine events may produce defects which are present at birth (*congenital*) but which are not inherited, since no genetic mechanism is involved. The time of onset of a disease gives no indication as to whether the cause is environmental or genetic.

The cellular and tissue responses to external agents are summarised in Fig. 3.11. It can be seen that the types of reaction which can occur are strictly limited. Any pathological process is composed of a mixture of these basic units—the nature of the mixture being largely related to the cause. The remainder of this book is devoted to a description of these basic pathological processes and the common mixtures which are found.

GENERAL READING

ROBERTS, J. A. F. (1967). *An Introduction to Medical Genetics*, 4th edn, 290 pp. London: Oxford University Press.
VALENTINE, G. H. (1969). *The Chromosome Disorders*, 2nd edn, 172 pp. London: Heinemann.
LEVINE, H. (1971). *Clinical Cytogenetics*, 572 pp. Boston: Little Brown.

REFERENCES

1. Various Authors (1963). Symposium on genetics. *American Journal of Medicine*, **34**, 583–746.
2. Various Authors (1961). Human genetics, *British Medical Bulletin*, **17**, 177–259 and (1969). New aspects of human genetics, **25**, 1–114.
3. CANN, H. M. (1968). *Birth Defects, Original Article Series*, vol. 4, no. 6, p. 5.
4. CARTER, C. O. (1969). *Lancet*, i, 1014, 1041, 1087, 1139, 1203, 1252 and 1303.
5. TOWNES, P. L. (1969). *Medical Clinics of North America*, **53**, 886.
6. PLEYDELL, M. J. (1954). *British Medical Journal*, ii, 1121.
7. BLANK, C. E. (1960). *Annals of Human Genetics*, **24**, 151.
8. CARTER, C. O. (1969). *Medical Clinics of North America*, **53**, 991.
9. GATES, R. R. (1960). *Science*, **132**, 145.
10. RENWICK, J. H. and LAWLER, S. D. (1955). *Annals of Human Genetics*, **19**, 312.
11. McKUSICK, V. A. (1962). *Quarterly Review of Biology*, **37**, 69.
12. THOMPSON, J. S. and THOMPSON, M. W. (1966). *Genetics in Medicine*, 300 pp. Philadelphia and London: Saunders.
13. HARRIS, H (1968). *British Medical Journal*, ii, 135.
14. CHILDS, B. and KALOUSTIAN, V. M. D. (1968). *New England Journal of Medicine*, **279**, 1205 and 1267.
15. LA DU, B. N. (1969). *Medical Clinics of North America*, **53**, 839.
16. CHILDS, B. (1970). *New England Journal of Medicine*, **282**, 71.
17. HSIA, D. Y-Y. (1967). *Metabolism*, **16**, 419.

18. STANBURY, J. B., WYNGAARDEN, J. B. and FREDRICKSON, D. S. (1972). *The Metabolic Basis of Inherited Disease*, 3rd edn. New York, Toronto and London: McGraw-Hill.
19. O'BRIEN, W. M., LA DU, B. N. and BUNIM, J. J. (1963). *American Journal of Medicine*, **34**, 813.
20. CARPENTER, G. G., AUERBACH, V. H. and DiGEORGE, A. M. (1968). *Pediatric Clinics of North America*, **15**, 313.
21. Various Authors (1968). *Federal Proceedings. Federation of American Societies for Experimental Biology*, **27**, 1021.
22. PETERS, J. H. (1968). *Annual Review of Pharmacology*, **8**, 427.
23. O'REILLY, R. A., POOL, J. G. and AGGELER, P. M. (1968). *Annals of the New York Academy of Science*, **151**, 913.
24. Editorial (1970). *New England Journal of Medicine*, **282**, 337.
25. HSIA, D. Y-Y. (1968). *Birth Defects, Original Article Series*, vol. 4, no. 6, p. 75.
26. HSIA, D. Y-Y. (1969). *Medical Clinics of North America*, **53**, 857.
27. MELLMAN, W. J. and KOHN, G. (1970). *Medical Clinics of North America*, **54**, 701.
28. BARTALOS, M. and BARAMKI, T. A. (1967). *Medical Cytogenetics*, 419 pp. Baltimore: Williams and Wilkins.
29. Various Authors (1969). *Birth Defects, Original Article Series*, vol. 5, no. 5, p. 1.
30. FORD, C. E., JACOBS, P. A and LAJTHA, L. G. (1958). *Nature*, **181**, 1565.
31. Denver Report (1960). *Lancet*, i, 1063.
32. The London Conference on the Normal Human Karyotype (1964). *Annals of Human Genetics*, **27**, 295.
33. Chicago Conference: Standardisation in Human Genetics. *Birth Defects: Original Article Series*, II; 2 (1966). New York: The National Foundation.
34. Editorial (1971). *New England Journal of Medicine*, **285**, 1482.
35. OHNO, S., KAPLAN, W. D. and KINOSITA, R. (1959). *Experimental Cell Research*, **18**, 415.
36. GERMAN, J. L. (1962). *Transactions of New York Academy of Sciences*, **24**, 395.
37. MITTWOCH, U. (1964). *Proceedings of the Royal Society of Medicine*, **57**, 643.
38. LYON, M. F. (1966). *Advances in Teratology*, **1**, 25.
39. BEUTLER, E., YEH, M. and FAIRBANKS, V. F. (1962). *Proceedings of the National Academy of Sciences of the United States of America*, **48**, 9.
40. BEUTLER, E. and BALUDA, M. C. (1964). *Lancet*, i, 189.
41. KROOTH, R. S. (1969). *Medical Clinics of North America*, **53**, 795.
42. COURT-BROWN, W. M. (1962). In *The Scientific Basis of Medicine Annual Reviews*, p. 109. London: Athlone Press.
43. LENNOX, B. (1966). In *Recent Advances in Pathology*, 8th edn, p. 1. Edited by C. V. Harrison. London: Churchill.
44. MILLER, O. J. (1961). In *Recent Advances in Human Genetics*, p. 39. London: Churchill.
45. NEW, M. I. (1968). *Pediatric Clinics of North America*, **15**, 395.
46. BAULIEU, E. E., PEILLON, F. and MIGEON, C. J. (1967). In *The Adrenal Cortex*, p. 578. Edited by A. B. Eisenstein. London: Churchill.
47. LENNOX, B. (1963). *Lancet*, i, 611.
48. MILLER, O. J. (1964). *American Journal of Obstetrics and Gynecology*, **90**, 1078.
49. PRICE, W. H. *et al.* (1966). *Lancet*, i, 565.
50. Leading Article (1966). *Lancet*, i, 583.
51. COURT-BROWN, W. M., PRICE, W. H. and JACOBS, P. A. (1968). *British Medical Journal*, ii, 325.
52. ZALESKI, W. A. *et al.* (1966). *Canadian Medical Association Journal*, **94**, 1143.
53. DE LA CHAPPELLE, A. (1972). *American Journal of Human Genetics*, **24**, 71.
54. JOST, A. (1947). *Archives d'anatomie microscopique et de morpholgie expérimentale*, **36**, 271.
55. LEJEUNE, J. T. (1963). *Pediatrics*, **32**, 326.
56. CARR, D. H. (1969). *Progress in Medical Genetics*, **4**, 1.
57. Editorial (1967). *New England Journal of Medicine*, **277**, 825.
58. PENROSE, L. S. and SMITH, G. F. (1966). *Down's Anomaly*, 218 pp. London: Churchill.
59. PENROSE, L. S. (1966). *Advances in Teratology*, **1**, 9.
60. UCHIDA, I. A. and SOLTAN, H. C. (1963). *Pediatric Clinics of North America*, **10**, 409.
61. PENROSE, L. S. (1963). *Nature*, **197**, 933.
62. HAMERTON, J. L. and STEINBERG, A. G. (1962). *Lancet*, i, 1408.
63. INHORN, S. L. (1969). *Advances in Teratology*, **2**, 37.
64. CARR, D. H. (1965). *American Journal of Obstetrics and Gynecology*, **26**, 308.
65. SZULMAN, A. E. (1965). *New England Journal of Medicine*, **272**, 811.
66. Leading Article (1970). *British Medical Journal*, iii, 419.
67. NADLER, H. L. (1969). *Journal of Pediatrics*, **74**, 132.
68. Leading Article (1971). *Lancet*, ii, 965.
69. MERRIL, C. R., GEIER, M. R. and PETRICCIANI, J. C. (1971). *Nature*, **233**, 398.

Chapter 4.   Cell Response to Injury

The manner by which adverse conditions or poisons affect cells must now be examined. Most agents, it may be assumed, affect the cell by upsetting some important chemical reaction. A *biochemical lesion* is thus the first change and this in its turn may produce secondary results. Structural changes may take place within the cell, and if the damage is severe the cell may die; destructive enzymes are then liberated within the cell, and the process of *self-digestion*, or *autolysis*, occurs. When this happens after the death of the whole individual, the term *post-mortem change* is used. When, however, a group of cells dies in continuity with the living, similar changes occur and it is by them that cell death can itself be recognised: to this process the term *necrosis* is applied—it therefore means death of cells or tissue with structural evidence of this death.

BIOCHEMICAL LESIONS[1, 2]

The concept of a biochemical lesion was first put forward by Sir Rudolph Peters.[3, 4] It has been known for a long time that thiamine deficiency in pigeons leads to severe neurological complications. The birds develop opisthotonos and convulsions, but in spite of this evidence of a severe neurological lesion no abnormalities can be detected on histological examination of the brain. The situation is reminiscent of that seen in the Lesch-Nyhan syndrome.

When slices of brain tissue from thiamine-deficient birds are incubated in a Warburg apparatus, they show abnormally low oxygen consumption; if thiamine is added, the oxygen consumption rises to normal. Furthermore, if thiamine is injected intrathecally into a bird suffering from thiamine deficiency, it recovers from the neurological complications in about 30 minutes. Examination of the blood in thiamine-deficient birds reveals a raised pyruvate level, but this is not the cause of the symptoms since pyruvate itself is not toxic. The explanation of the symptoms is believed to be the hold-up in the activity of the Krebs cycle that occurs in the absence of the co-carboxylase thiamine pyrophosphate, which is one of the factors involved in the conversion of pyruvate to acetyl-coenzyme A. Pyruvate normally enters the Krebs cycle *via* acetyl-coenzyme A. A hold-up at this point results in an accumulation of pyruvate, which is thus an effect of the lesion rather than a cause of the symptoms. The impairment of glucose metabolism in the nerve cells is presumably the cause of the symptoms.

Thiamine deficiency thus provides an excellent example of a biochemical lesion due to a deficiency: a lesion which causes severe effects and even death, but which is not detectable by the current routine histological methods. Other similar examples may be mentioned.

Lewisite Poisoning[2, 4]

The trivalent arsenic compound lewisite was used as a poison gas in the 1914–18 war. It produces inflammation with blister formation when applied to the skin. As a systemic agent it also interferes with the action of pyruvate dehydrogenase by binding the enzyme. In this way a biochemical block is established, because pyruvate dehydrogenase plays an important part in the conversion of pyruvate to acetyl-coenzyme A.

$$\text{Protein}\!\!<^{SH}_{SH} + Cl_2AsCH = CHCl \rightarrow \text{Protein}\!\!<^{S}_{S}\!\!>AsCH = CHCl$$

$$\text{Enzyme} \quad + \text{Lewisite} \qquad \rightarrow \text{Inactivated enzyme}$$

$$\text{Protein}\!\!<^{S}_{S}\!\!>AsCH = CHCl + \begin{matrix} CH_2SH \\ | \\ CHSH \\ | \\ CH_2OH \end{matrix} \rightarrow \text{Protein}\!\!<^{SH}_{SH} + \begin{matrix} CH_2S \\ | \\ CHS \\ | \\ CH_2OH \end{matrix}\!\!>AsCH = CHCl$$

$$\text{Inactivated enzyme} \qquad + BAL \quad \rightarrow \text{Enzyme} \quad + BAL\text{-Lewisite compound}$$

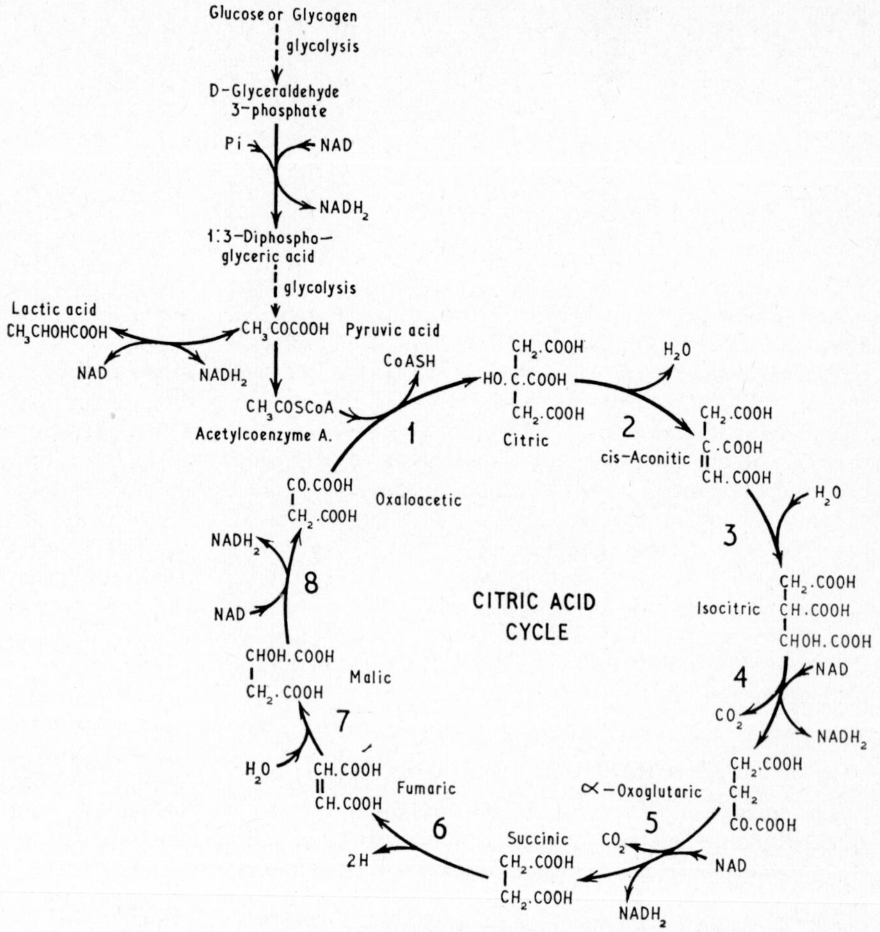

Figure 4.1
The Krebs cycle. Glucose is broken down predominantly by glycolysis, and enters the Krebs cycle as acetyl-coenzyme A. Under anaerobic conditions pyruvic acid is converted into lactic acid, whereby NAD is regenerated and allows glycolysis to continue. Under aerobic conditions the $NADH_2$ is oxidised by molecular oxygen, thus regenerating NAD, and the pyruvate is further metabolised *via* acetylcoenzyme A. The Krebs cycle is also known as the citric acid or tricarboxylic acid cycle.
Key: 1. Condensing enzyme. 2. and 3. Aconitase. 4. *Iso*-citric dehydrogenase. 5. α-oxoglutaric dehydrogenase. 6. Succinic dehydrogenase. 7. Fumarase. 8. Malic dehydrogenase. CoASH—Coenzyme A. $CH_2COSCoA$—Acetyl-coenzyme A. NAD—Nicotinamide adenine dinucleotide (previously called DPN). $NADH_2$—Dihydronicotinamide adenine dinucleotide ($DPNH_2$). Pi—Inorganic phosphate.

The compound British anti-lewisite (BAL) restores the activity of the enzyme.

Fluoroacetate Poisoning[4]

This substance was shown by Peters to block the Krebs cycle by a process described as *lethal synthesis*. It enters the cycle in place of ordinary acetate and is converted to fluoro-citrate. This cannot be further metabolised, and it blocks the Krebs cycle by interfering with the action of aconitase which is necessary for the conversion of citrate to *cis*-aconitate.

Bacterial Toxins

Diphtheria toxin is thought to inhibit the cytochromes.[2] Its exact mode of action is not understood, and it must be admitted that very little is known about bacterial actions in precise chemical terms.

Genetic Enzyme Defect

Another way in which a biochemical lesion may occur is by a specific enzyme deficiency dependent upon a genetic defect. This rare but important group of diseases is described in Chapter 3.

Some chemotherapeutic agents are used with the deliberate intention of producing a biochemical lesion in micro-organisms. This mechanism provides the basis for the action of sulphonamides and some antibiotics, e.g. rifamycin and its derivatives in bacterial and virus infections. Hopefully anti-cancer agents will also be found.

Finally, it has been suggested that some mental illnesses are the result of biochemical lesions. That this is possible is demonstrated by the dramatic effects of certain 5-HT antagonists, e.g. LSD.

Although only a few examples have been cited, this subject will certainly become increasingly important in the future. The routine methods of examining pathological material are inadequate for the detection of biochemical upsets. Other more refined methods will have to be employed for further advances to be made. For the present it may be postulated that chemical blocks or lesions may occur in the following ways:

1. The enzyme may be absent or abnormal through a genetic error.
2. The enzyme may be directly inhibited by a chemical agent.

3. There may be a deficiency of substrate for a variety of reasons—dietary deficiency, other biochemical lesions, etc.
4. Deficiency of co-enzyme.
5. Substrate competition by chemicals of similar nature to the natural substrate.

Whatever the mechanism causing the block, the effects can be brought about in three main ways:

1. The excess substrate which frequently accumulates may be toxic, or may cause some other biochemical lesion by affecting another enzyme system.

2. The inhibited reaction may be of vital importance to the cell.

3. Although the reaction itself may not be of great importance, the end-product may be an essential substance in some other important metabolic reaction.

CHANGES ASSOCIATED WITH ACCUMULATION OF WATER IN THE CELL[2, 5]

Cloudy Swelling

The changes of cloudy swelling are frequently to be found in parenchymatous cells, e.g. liver and kidney. The cells are swollen and the cytoplasm granular. These changes closely resemble those occurring in *post-mortem* autolysis,[6] but experimentally it has been shown that they can develop in the cells of the living animal when these are subjected to such adverse conditions as ischaemia, hypoxia, and the effects of a poison.

The organ whose cells show cloudy swelling is swollen, its cut surface bulges outwards, and it has a grey, parboiled appearance. The consistency is soft.

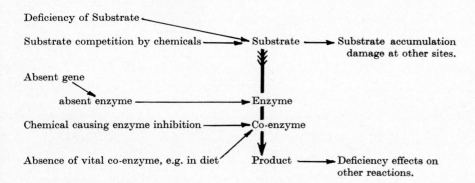

Figure 4.2
Some possible mechanisms which may be involved in the production of a biochemical lesion. The factors interfering with the basic reaction, substrate → product, are shown on the left and the effects are shown on the right.

The effects of a biochemical lesion vary considerably. The cell's metabolism may show gross abnormalities which may be exhibited as marked alteration in behaviour without any structural change; this has been considered above. The alterations in metabolism may, on the other hand, produce changes in the morphology of the cell. Such changes have been known for a long time as the *degenerations*, and great importance has been attached to them. The concepts of cellular degeneration were evolved during the last hundred years using the relatively crude methods available for cellular study. Three types of change have been described: these are firstly *cloudy swelling*, *vacuolar degeneration*, and *hydropic degeneration*. Secondly there is *fatty degeneration* and *fatty infiltration* which are related to each other. Finally there is a heterogeneous group in which eosinophilic material appears in the cell either as droplets or as ill-defined masses. This group is termed *hyaline degeneration* or *hyaline-droplet change*. These are depicted diagrammatically in Fig. 4.3. It must be appreciated that these are purely descriptive terms applied to the appearance of cells when viewed in the conventional manner by light microscopy of sections from paraffin-wax embedded tissue. Before considering the impact of biochemical and electron-microscopic studies the classical changes will first be examined.

Vacuolar Degeneration

The naked-eye appearance described as typical of cloudy swelling is sometimes associated with swollen cells containing vacuoles rather than granules. This is vacuolar degeneration, and its causes and distribution are similar to those of cloudy swelling.

Hydropic Degeneration

The cells show great swelling due to an accumulation of fluid (water-logging). The cytoplasm is pale and homogeneous. The condition is reversible, but this is the most severe form of this group of degenerations and may terminate in death of the cell. The balloon cells seen in the early epidermal lesions of some virus infections of the skin afford a good example of this. The hydropic epidermal cells soon undergo necrosis and produce the intraepidermal vesicle so characteristic of herpes simplex, varicella-zoster, vaccinia, and smallpox infections.

CHANGES ASSOCIATED WITH THE ACCUMULATION OF FAT

An accumulation of excess stainable neutral fat is a frequent finding in parenchymal cells. It is especially common

Figure 4.3
Diagram to illustrate the cellular changes which are generally described as the "degenerations". A damaged cell may exhibit progressive waterlogging, and pass through the stages of cloudy swelling, vacuolar degeneration, and hydropic degeneration. Alternatively, fat may accumulate, firstly as fine droplets, but later as the condition advances, a large globule is formed. Hyaline "degeneration" comprises several entities, and is here illustrated by hyaline droplet degeneration in a cell of the proximal convoluted tubule of the kidney.

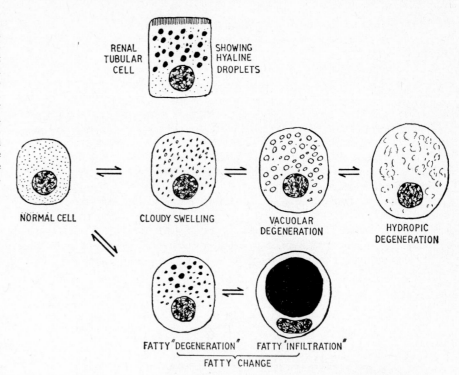

RENAL TUBULAR CELL — SHOWING HYALINE DROPLETS

NORMAL CELL ⇌ CLOUDY SWELLING ⇌ VACUOLAR DEGENERATION ⇌ HYDROPIC DEGENERATION

FATTY "DEGENERATION" ⇌ FATTY "INFILTRATION"
FATTY CHANGE

in the liver, and its causes include those which produce cloudy swelling. A fatty liver is enlarged, its cut surface bulges, and it is greasy to the touch. Its colour is pale, and in severe cases yellow. This is seen in alcoholism, cirrhosis, and in patchy distribution in the nutmeg liver of congestive heart failure. It is particularly well marked in cases of phosphorus poisoning. Fatty change is common in the convoluted tubules of the kidney, where it leads to pallor and swelling of the cortex. Accumulation of fat in the heart muscle cells is focal and may be sufficiently marked to produce yellow flecks visible on the endocardial surface (thrush-breast, or tabby cat, heart). Severe anaemia is the usual cause.

Microscopically the cells are swollen and contain small droplets composed of neutral fat (glyceryl triesters). This is the condition at one time known as "*fatty degeneration*" (Figs. 4.4 and 4.5). The fat was thought to be derived from hidden tissue fat by a process of unmasking, or *phanerosis*. In advanced cases the fat appears as one large globule pushing the nucleus to the side—an appearance described as "*fatty infiltration*", presumably because it was thought that adipose cells were infiltrating the organ (Fig. 4.4). This nomenclature is misleading and has been abandoned. It is now known that "fatty degeneration" is but an early stage in the development of "fatty infiltration", and that in both conditions the fat is brought to the cells from the fat depots. *Fatty change* is now used to include both conditions. It should not be confused with the accumulation of true fat cells in the tissues; this is common in the heart and pancreas of obese patients. Local deposits of fat are sometimes a feature of chronic inflammation (p. 134) and following

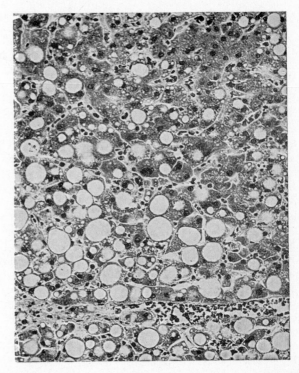

Figure 4.4
Fatty change of liver. Many of the liver cells are distended with fat globules to the extent that their nuclei are pushed to the cell wall. In other cells the fat is present as small droplets in the cytoplasm. The material was taken at the necropsy of an elderly woman who died of septicaemia. × 170.

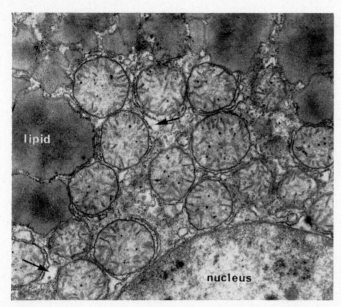

Figure 4.5
Fatty change in the liver. Electron micrograph of a rat liver cell, 4 hours following administration of ethionine. Accumulation of large lipid droplets is pronounced. The rough endoplasmic reticulum is disorganised and the two arrows point to dilated cisterns. Lead hydroxide. ×22 500. *(Photograph supplied by Dr. Katsumi Miyai)*

atrophy, e.g. lymph nodes and thymus. These conditions are sometimes called fatty infiltration, but confusion is most easily avoided if the term *adiposity* is used.

Hyaline degeneration and hyaline droplet change. These are described later (p. 52).

NATURE OF THE DEGENERATIVE CHANGES[5, 7]

It is often assumed that the cellular changes of cloudy swelling or hydropic degeneration are the same regardless of the organ affected, be it liver, kidney, or islet of Langerhans. Such is not the case. Using the electron microscope, it has been possible to probe more deeply into the nature of these changes. Whereas the light microscope can give a vague impression of intracellular events and detect the changes when they are severe enough to affect the cell as a whole, electron microscopy can reveal which parts of the cell are affected and indicate the sequence of events and metabolic changes which are occurring. The structure of the cell now appears more complex than did the anatomy of the whole body a hundred years ago. Just as "coma" ceased to be an intellectually satisfying ultimate diagnosis when specific conditions affecting the brain were recognised, so cloudy swelling is equally unsatisfactory now that organelles are known to exist. The first steps in the recognition of the cell's response to injury have been taken, and cellular pathology promises to become as complex as organ pathology. At this stage one must expect newly described lesions to prove as

useful—and at times as misleading—as were those used initially in organ pathology.

It is not easy to give a clear generalised account of the cell's response to injury, since relatively few cell-types have been investigated to any extent. Most work has been carried out on liver and kidney subjected to a variety of chemical poisons, e.g. carbon tetrachloride, ethionine, barbiturates, ethanol, etc. Some of the changes in the cell's components will be described:

Nuclear Changes

A variety of nuclear changes have been described in poisoned cells. One of the earliest is clumping of the chromatin adjacent to the nuclear membrane and around the nucleolus. The nucleoli show loss of their granular component, and the fibrillar material is sometimes dispersed into separate fragments. Nucleoli are therefore smaller but more numerous. The loss of granular material may indicate impaired synthesis of ribosomal material and mRNA. Reduced RNA synthesis is found in damaged cells,[8] and this is reflected in the cytoplasm as reduced protein synthesis. It should be stressed that by light microscopy nuclear changes are not obvious or characteristic in cells showing degeneration. Sometimes an increased number of nucleoli may be noted.

Cytoplasmic Changes

These may be considered under five headings:

Evidence of increased cell function. Cellular components may proliferate or reorganise in a manner which suggests a state of *hyperfunction*. In response to certain poisons the smooth endoplasmic reticulum becomes more abundant and forms complex whorls or gyrations (Fig. 4.6); this is regarded as an adaptive mechanism and indicates an attempt to increase the cell's ability to detoxify the substance. Likewise free ribosomes, rough endoplasmic reticulum, and the Golgi apparatus may proliferate; the number of lysosomes may increase, and mitochondria become more abundant, enlarge, and exhibit an increase in their internal complexity (Fig. 4.7). Evidently the cell's metabolism is increased, for protein synthesis, ATP production, and catabolic activity may all be stimulated as may sometimes glycogen synthesis.

Micropinocytotic activity may increase, and this results in the appearance of numerous vacuoles in the cytoplasm.

Evidence of decreased function. Cellular components may become less numerous and show evidence of *hypofunction*. In damaged liver cells the rough endoplasmic reticulum shows dilatation of its sacs and loss of attached ribosomes. Polysomes are reduced in number. These changes are particularly associated with hydropic degeneration, and indicate *impaired protein synthesis*.

Mitochondrial changes are frequent. These organelles may show swelling and a loss of cristae. An increase in calcium content and the formation of concentric laminated

Figure 4.6
Advanced proliferation of the smooth endoplasmic
reticulum (ser) in the periphery of a rat hepatocyte
following eithionine administration. The proliferated vesicles of the agranular reticulum are tightly
packed and well demarcated from the rough endoplasmic reticulum (rer), which can be identified
by the ribosomes studded on the membranes.
Mitochondria (m) are elongated. cm—cell membrane; lip—lipid droplet. Lead hydroxide.
×15 750. *(Photograph supplied by Dr Katsumi
Miyai)*

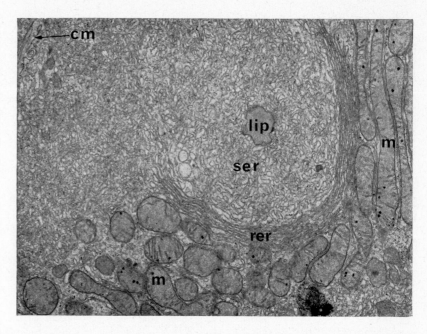

whorls in the matrix have also been described. Impaired
function results in reduced oxidative phosphorylation, and
ATP production is reduced. Since this substance forms the
main immediately available source of energy for cellular
metabolism, it is not surprising that many cell functions are

impaired. Thus ATP is required for the operation of the
mechanism, or pump, regulating the concentration of ions in
the cell. The sodium pump is impeded, and sodium and
water accumulate in the cell, which in this way becomes
progressively enlarged and waterlogged. The electrolytes
can pass freely across the cell membrane, but the proteins
within the cell cannot escape. When the sodium pump
breaks down, there is therefore a *tendency* for the cell to
become hypertonic. This is counteracted by the entry of
water into the cell which thereupon swells. The breakdown
of proteins into smaller molecules may further increase this
tendency to hypertonicity. This may not be the complete
explanation, but there is little doubt that changes in membrane permeability are an outstanding feature of cells undergoing degeneration.[7] Mitochondrial swelling is commonly
found in cells showing cloudy swelling.

Evidence of altered function. Changes may occur
which indicate that the cell has acquired a new function;
thus the endothelial cells of the glomerular tuft can become
actively phagocytic for fibrin, and cilia can develop in cells
which are not normally ciliated, e.g. those of the olfactory
mucosa.

Abnormal accumulation of substances in the cell.
Lipid is an example, and is described later.

Degenerative changes. Localised areas of the cell may
appear to become degenerate, and the term *focal cytoplasmic
degeneration* has been applied. Sometimes cytoplasmic components, e.g. endoplasmic reticulum and mitochondria, are
seen within vacuoles containing lysosomal enzymes. These
are called *autophagocytic vacuoles*, *autophagosomes*, or
cytolysomes, and an increase in their number is an indication
of cell injury.[9] Thus large numbers of autophagocytic
vacuoles are seen in the cells of an organ undergoing atrophy.

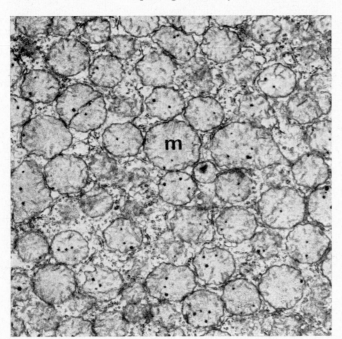

Figure 4.7
Marked proliferation of mitochondria (m) in a rat hepatocyte following the administration of ethionine. The mitochrondria are of
uniform size and shape, and other cytoplasmic organelles are inconspicuous. Lead hydroxide. ×15 600. *(Photograph supplied by
Dr. Katsumi Miyai)*

This may be due to progressive ischaemia or to a physiological cause, as in the breast following lactation or the secondary sex organs in old age.

Sometimes an area of cytoplasm degenerates and is actually cast off: damaged renal tubular cells can show loss of the brush border, which together with an area of the underlying cytoplasm is desquamated into the lumen. Such changes have been called necrosis of part of a cell.

It should be appreciated that these various changes indicating hyperfunction, hypofunction, altered function, and focal degeneration can all occur within a single cell either simultaneously or sequentially. A damaged cell is not an inactive cell, and its reaction to injury may end in recovery. Parts injured beyond recovery are lysed or extruded, and the remaining structures reform the lost components. The cell may return to normal but some alterations may persist. Thus the retention of an abnormal function is seen in metaplasia and perhaps also neoplasia. The reaction of damaged cells is a highly complex and varied affair, but so far as routine human pathology is concerned it is rarely possible to obtain tissue fresh enough to detect these intracellular events even if time and equipment were available.

Not all the changes described above occur under any single circumstance. Cells subjected to adverse conditions show a complex reaction: some changes may be regarded as degenerative, while others are adaptive. A liver cell showing cloudy swelling due to carbon tetrachloride poisoning would therefore not be expected to show the same changes as one infected with a virus, or a kidney cell damaged by hypoxia. The diversity of change is particularly well marked in cells showing hydropic change: the clarity and swelling of the β cells of the islets of Langerhans in diabetes mellitus is due to the accumulation of glycogen, while the apparent hydropic change in the kidney in hypokalaemia is due to an accumulation of fluid between the tubular cell and its basement membrane.[10]

Nature of Fatty Change[11, 12]

Electron microscopy has revealed that many normal cells contain small droplets of lipid, but these are not visible on light microscopy. An obvious exception to this is the adult fat cell. The excess fat which appears in damaged cells is generally considered to originate from outside the cell.[13] The evidence for this is as follows.

1. Both fine and large droplets are found in the cells of the same organ, and they can both be produced by the same agents.

2. If a normal animal is poisoned with phosphorus it develops acute hepatic damage with severe fatty change. If, however, the animal is starved so that its depot fat is severely depleted, poisoning causes cell damage without fatty change. The neutral fat droplets are evidently derived from the fat depots and not by a hypothetical process of phanerosis.

3. If cells grown in tissue culture are damaged, fat droplets accumulate when plasma is incorporated in the medium. If

no plasma is present, no fat appears. This is an excellent indication that the origin of the fat is from outside the cell.

4. The cells showing fatty change contain more fat than is normal; this would not be expected if phanerosis were the only mechanism involved.

5. Finally, if an animal is fed on a fat of different iodine value to its own, its fat depots accumulate the new type of fat. Poisoning of its liver then results in the appearance of droplets of this new type of fat.

Depot fat is composed mostly of neutral fat, and when it is mobilised it is transported in the blood as free fatty acid bound to albumin. This is removed by tissues and utilised for metabolic purposes. If the cells are damaged by hypoxia, poisoned, etc., their metabolic activity is impaired and the fat normally brought to them is inadequately utilised; it accumulates as droplets which are at first small, but later fuse into larger globules. It might be wondered why under some circumstances damaged cells show changes described as cloudy swelling, vacuolation, etc., but at other times there is fatty change. It must be admitted that often there is no adequate explanation. Many factors affect the susceptibility of cells to exogenous poisons. Thus, certain strains of mice are excessively sensitive to chloroform and develop bilateral renal cortical necrosis.[14] This in inherited as a sex-linked factor. Age is important; thus newborn animals are resistant to many liver-damaging compounds.[15]

Fatty change is particularly liable to occur in the liver, and is a reflection of the key position this organ occupies in fat metabolism. In addition to being able to manufacture fatty acids themselves, the liver cells remove free fatty acid from the blood stream and utilise it in the production of phospholipids. These are bound to protein, and passed back into the blood as lipoproteins by an active transport mechanism. If liver cells are damaged, protein synthesis is impaired; lipoprotein manufacture is impeded and the fat taken up by the liver is not exported. It accumulates and appears as droplets. This then is the explanation of fatty change in the liver under some circumstances.[16]

Fatty change in the liver due to an inadequate diet. The liver is also unable to metabolise fat unless there is an adequate supply of raw materials for the manufacture of lipoprotein. Substances which are necessary for this conversion are called lipotropic factors, and in particular *choline* is important. Without it, fatty acid cannot be converted to phospholipid and therefore fatty acid in the form of neutral fat accumulates. In experimental choline deficiency in the rat fatty change readily occurs in the liver, and if this is prolonged the damage leads to a type of cirrhosis.[17] The same effect is seen in starvation in man,[18] e.g. kwashiorkor, and the same mechanism is the most probable cause of the fatty liver of the chronic alcoholic. The fatty change in the liver seen in overfed animals is perhaps due to a relative deficiency of lipotropic substances.

The relationship between diet and liver disease is in fact complex. Total fasting does not lead to fat accumulation.

Ketones and fatty acids are utilised by the tissues as a source of energy, and gluconeogenesis almost ceases in the liver. Essential amino acids are therefore conserved. If small amounts of carbohydrate are given, this adaptation does not occur and the liver becomes fatty. An improper diet may be more damaging than one which simply lacks calories, a fact to be borne in mind when methods of reducing the weight of obese patients are devised. Thus the operation of small-bowel bypass effects a loss in weight, but sometimes leads to fatty liver, necrosis, and cirrhosis. It has therefore been abandoned.[19]

Although the concept of phanerosis (p. 48) has been largely discarded in relation to fatty change in the liver, it is probable that lipid droplets in other organs are sometimes formed by breakdown of cytoplasmic components. These have been described in the renal tubules in nephritis, and appear as vacuoles containing numerous internal vacuoles.

HYALINE DEGENERATION

Hyaline is a descriptive term applied to any homogeneous eosinophilic material. Literally the term means "glassy", and is commonly applied to changes in connective tissue (p. 65). Hyaline degeneration is also used to describe a change in cells when either the whole cell or part of it becomes eosinophilic and homogeneous. Many diverse conditions have been included. In the alcoholic patient the cells of the liver sometimes contain eosinophilic structures called Mallory bodies,

or alcoholic hyaline. The nature of this is not known, but the material consists of a meshwork of fibrils in an area where the rough endoplasmic reticulum has broken up. The giant mitochondria which are also found in the liver cells of the alcoholic are separate structures.

The droplets which appear in the proximal convoluted tubular cells of the kidney in the nephrotic syndrome are due to the excessive reabsorption of protein which has leaked through an abnormal glomerulus (Fig. 4.8). The condition is analogous to the effects of an intravenous sucrose injection, when droplets appear in the tubular cells.[20] Likewise, following the injection of mannitol and in diabetics with marked glycosuria these cells become greatly swollen and have a clear cytoplasm. In hyaline droplet "degeneration" of the kidney, there may be associated degenerative changes with the formation of large cytolysomes. Nevertheless, most of the droplets seen on light microscopy consist of reabsorbed protein and the condition is not really a degeneration.

ACCUMULATION OF ABNORMAL SUBSTANCES IN THE CELLS

The terms infiltration and degeneration have in the past been used indiscriminately in describing changes which may occur in cells. It is evident that cell function may be impaired by many agents, and the changes which ensue may be manifested either as altered function, altered appearance, or both. Sometimes the changes terminate in cell death, and at first sight it seems not unreasonable to use the term degeneration. However, the change is frequently associated with an abnormal accumulation within the cell, e.g. of water, fat, or

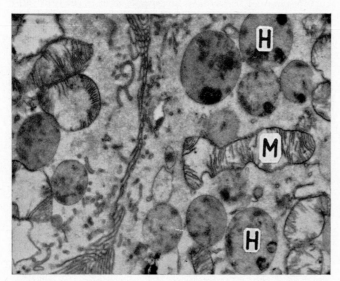

Figure 4.8
Hyaline droplet formation. This E.M. preparation shows part of the two adjacent proximal convoluted cells of a mouse kidney. The animal had been injected previously with egg-white. The foreign protein appears as droplets (H) which are distinct from the mito-**chon**dria (M). It is thought that the protein passes into the glomerular filtrate and then enters the tubular cells by a process of micropinocytosis. ×15 000. *(From Brewer, D. B. and Eguren, L. M. 1962), J. Path. Bact.,* **93**, 107–116)

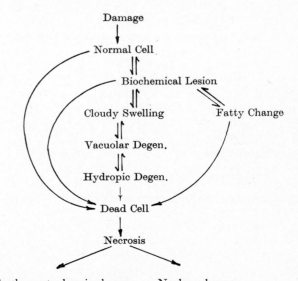

Further cytoplasmic changes   Nuclear changes

Figure 4.9
Diagram showing the stages whereby cell damage terminates in necrosis.

glycogen. When this is marked the term infiltration is sometimes used. Unfortunately the same term is also used to describe a condition where an abnormal substance is deposited in a tissue which is itself normal, e.g. glycogen in the heart and kidneys in diabetes mellitus, urates in gout, and amyloid. Depositions of other substances, e.g. calcium salts, haemosiderin, bile pigments, etc., are not generally termed infiltrations in classical accounts. Attempts to apply both terms to connective tissue have further complicated the situation. It is evident that the terms infiltration and degeneration served a useful purpose in the days of descriptive pathology, but that their continued use represents an attempt to impose unity where none exists. The terms cloudy swelling, hydropic degeneration, etc., are now used much less frequently than in previous periods. This is partly because the changes are so easily confused with those of *post-mortem* autolysis, and partly because changes which appear similar on light microscopy can be due to many diverse mechanisms, as revealed by biochemical analysis and electron microscopy. It is a mistake to regard these conditions as entities in themselves. If such terms are used at all they are better referred to as granular change, fatty change, hydropic change, etc., since these are convenient and indicate a particular appearance when the light microscope is used. It must not be thought that the terms represent anything more than a morphological description, and in the future it is to be hoped that each lesion will be described more precisely relating cause, biochemical lesion, and morphological changes.

CHANGES FOLLOWING CELL DEATH[21]

These differ according to whether or not the dead tissue remains an integral part of a living organism.

POST-MORTEM CHANGE

In the initial stages no alteration in cellular structure is visible: in this connexion it is important to remember that no changes will be found in the myocardium of patients dying suddenly of acute coronary insufficiency.

Evidence of cell damage will be seen only when the cause of cell death has itself produced recognisable injury, e.g. disruption of cellular structures by ice-crystal formation after freezing.

In the dying cell respiration ceases, glycolysis proceeds for a while, and there results a drop in pH due to the production of lactic acid. The synthetic activities of the cell stop, but the lytic destructive enzymes continue their work. These enzymes are mostly active at a low pH and include a wide range of proteases, lipases, esterases, deoxyribonuclease, ribonuclease, etc. The cell thus undergoes a process of *self-digestion*, or *autolysis*. The enzymes may be derived from lysosomes, and it has been suggested that disruption of these

bodies is an important factor in the causation of cell damage as well as in the autolysis which follows cell death. However, electron-microscopic studies of cells undergoing autolysis *in vitro* show that the changes (mitochondrial swelling, etc.) are diffuse, and not more advanced near the lysosomes.[22] Such evidence would suggest that lysosomal enzymes do not initiate the changes of necrosis.[22, 23]

Autolysis is rapid in certain tissues, and results in liquefaction, e.g. in the pancreas and gastric mucosa. In other tissues, e.g. fibrous tissue, autolysis is less rapid.

The microscopic changes that occur affect the whole cell. The cytoplasm becomes homogeneous and brightly eosinophilic; the early autolytic changes may resemble those seen in the degenerative lesions of living cells. Later on cellular and nuclear details become lost. It is important to note that these *post-mortem* changes can be distinguished from those occurring during life by the complete absence of any surrounding inflammatory response ("vital reaction"). This is particularly useful in the kidney, where it is often difficult to distinguish the changes of early necrosis from those of autolysis. The presence of oedema separating one tubule from another is good evidence that the degenerative changes existed before death.

Putrefaction in dead tissue occurs when there is invasion by protein-splitting, anaerobic, saprophytic organisms. This results in the formation of gas and a variety of foul-smelling substances which include ammonia, hydrogen sulphide, indol, skatol, and putrescent amines like putrescine and cadaverine. The tissue turns black or dark green as a result of the formation of iron sulphide from broken-down haemoglobin. The common putrefactive organisms are those clostridia normally present in the faeces, and therefore the process occurs earliest in the abdominal cavity.

CELL DEATH AND NECROSIS[21, 24]

The change in damaged cells which remain in continuity with the living varies according to the severity of the injury. The cells may be killed suddenly by direct physical or chemical trauma, and initially these show no changes other than those directly attributable to the agent concerned, e.g. disruption in electrical injuries, effects of freezing, burning, etc. Within a few hours, however, autolysis occurs, and the cells show the morphological changes (see below) by which cell death can be recognised: this is called *necrosis*,[25] which therefore means *circumscribed death of cells or tissues with structural evidence of this death*.

Cells less severely damaged, e.g. by poisons, may develop a biochemical lesion which may cause immediate death, or may first result in the degenerative and adaptive changes previously described. It will be recalled that these are mainly cytoplasmic, and in themselves do not indicate necrosis. Following cell death the nucleus also shows autolytic changes, and it is these which are to be regarded as pathognomonic of necrosis.

Nuclear Changes of Necrosis

The nucleus becomes smaller, while the chromatin loses its fine reticular pattern, becomes clumped, and stains darkly. This is called *pyknosis*. It is also characteristic of the late matured normoblast. The pyknotic nucleus either breaks up into fragments (*karyorrhexis*), or its outlines become indistinct as the nuclear material is digested (*karyolysis*).

Types of Necrosis

Coagulative necrosis. Necrotic material usually becomes firm and slightly swollen, a change well marked in 7–10 days old infarcts of the kidney and heart. It seems likely that the proteins are denatured.[26] This process involves an unfolding of the three-dimensional arrangement of the molecule without necessarily changing its primary structure. This causes the tissue to become opaque, as does an egg on boiling, to fluoresce with ultraviolet light (autofluorescence), and to become more reactive. Side-chains previously staturated become exposed and available for binding. This explains why dead tissue tends to calcify. It also explains why necrotic tissue binds dyes, e.g. eosin, more avidly than does normal tissue. Increased eosinophilic staining of heart muscle fibres and neurones is a useful indication of early necrosis before an inflammatory reaction develops.

Apart from the nuclear changes, another microscopic feature is noteworthy: the preservation of the general architecture of the tissue despite the death of its constituent cells. This is *structured necrosis*. In other examples of coagulative necrosis there is no residual structure—this is *structureless necrosis*, e.g. the caseous necrosis of tuberculosis.

Caseation is a particular type of coagulative necrosis in which the dead tissue has a firm, dry, cheesy consistency and contains much lipid material. Although this type of change may occur in other conditions, the term caseation is usually restricted to the necrosis of tuberculosis.

Colliquative necrosis. Necrosis with softening (colliquative necrosis) rarely occurs as a primary event except in the central nervous system. Here necrosis (usually due to infarction) always results in softening.

Liquefaction may occur in necrotic tissue as a result of secondary changes; this is seen in:

1. Suppuration, e.g. septic infarction.
2. Liquefaction of caseous material.

Necrosis in Special Sites

Necrosis of muscle. Striated muscle occasionally undergoes necrosis during acute fevers, e.g. typhoid and smallpox. The muscle fibres lose their striations, the nuclei disappear, and the whole appears as a brightly eosinophilic hyaline mass. The muscle, usually the rectus abdominis or the diaphragm, may rupture, and this leads to haemorrhage and pain. The condition is traditionally called "Zenker's degen-

eration", but is in fact a true necrosis. A similar change has been described in cardiac muscle in severe acute infections.

Fat necrosis. Necrosis may occur in the fat of the peritoneum following the liberation of lipases from an injured or inflamed pancreas. The neutral fat is split: glycerol is removed, while the fatty acid remains and gives the damaged cells a cloudy appearance. Macroscopic areas of necrosis appear as opaque white plaques. The lesions excite an inflammatory response, and may be removed within a week or two. Sometimes calcification ensues, and when extensive may lead to hypocalcaemia.

Traumatic fat necrosis is generally seen in the breast: the changes are similar to pancreatic fat necrosis, but the foreign-body giant-cell reaction is particularly marked (Fig. 4.10). Clinically it may resemble a scirrhous carcinoma.

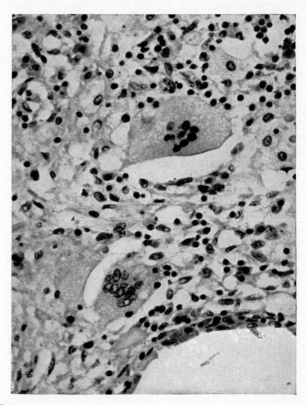

Figure 4.10
Traumatic fat necrosis of breast. The adipose tissue cells have an opaque, granular cytoplasm due to the breakdown of neutral fat and the production of fatty acid. Two large foreign-body giant cells with a foamy, fat-filled cytoplasm are present. × 330.

"Necrosis" of collagen. Whether it is permissible to describe the degenerative changes seen in collagen as necrosis is debatable. Certainly the associated fibrocytes undergo destruction. It is, however, difficult to define necrosis in an extracellular substance like collagen. This subject, necrobiosis, and "fibrinoid necrosis" are discussed in the next chapter.

DIAGNOSIS OF NECROSIS BY BIOCHEMICAL MEANS

Many soluble substances diffuse out of the cells following their death. These include potassium, protein breakdown products, and enzymes. The latter are absorbed into the blood-stream, and their presence can be utilised in diagnosis. Thus glutamate-oxaloacetate transaminase and other enzymes are released from infarcted heart muscle (p. 483). Similarly, the serum level of glutamate-pyruvate transaminase is useful in detecting liver necrosis.

Creatine phosphokinase is present in high concentration in skeletal muscle, and an increased blood level occurs after muscle damage, e.g. in polymyositis, alcoholic myopathy, malignant hyperpyrexia (p. 436), after severe exercise, and even following intramuscular injections. The highest levels are found in the muscular dystrophies. In the Duchenne variety (p. 33) such elevation is a constant feature, and its detection may be used to diagnose the disease even before clinical manifestations appear. An elevated level is also found in heterozygous carriers.[27]

Using column chromatography and starch-gel electrophoresis, it is possible to separate many enzymes into components called *isoenzymes*[28] (Fig. 4.11). The pattern of concentration of the various isoenzymes differs according to the tissue origin of the enzyme. This refinement in the study of

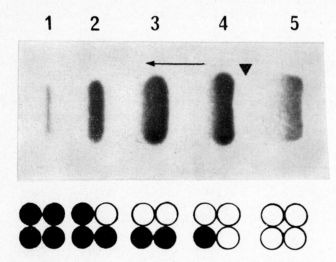

Figure 4.11
The lactate dehydrogenase activity of serum is shown as five component isoenzymes separated by electrophoresis. LDH 1 is the fastest component and has travelled farthest in the direction of the arrow towards the anode. In the lower part of the diagram each molecule is depicted as a tetramer made up of varying combinations of either H polypeptides (closed circles) or M polypeptides (open circles). The H and M chains are determined by separate genes. In the case of some other enzymes, the isoenzymes occur as a result of small variations in the structure of one or more polypeptides. *(After Latner, A. L. (1970). Journal of Clinical Pathology,* **24,** suppl. (Ass. Clin. Path.), **4,** 8*)*

G.P.—3

serum enzymes has been most rewarding in the diagnosis of myocardial infarction.

FURTHER CHANGES IN NECROTIC TISSUE

Acute inflammation. Necrotic tissue generally excites an acute inflammatory reaction in the surrounding tissue. This is well marked in infarction, and the infiltrating polymorphs by contributing their proteolytic enzymes to the dead tissue aid the process of autolysis. Similarly necrotic tumour excites an inflammatory response. Thus a melanoma of the choroid may be misdiagnosed as an inflammatory mass.

It is presumed that dead tissue releases some chemical which stimulates the inflammatory reaction, but no such substance has ever been satisfactorily identified. If a piece of liver is implanted free into the peritoneal cavity, it excites an acute inflammatory reaction and acquires the yellow-white appearance of coagulative necrosis. If it is now removed and reimplanted into another animal, very little reaction takes place. Boiled liver is similarly ignored. Presumably autolysing tissue exudes some chemical stimulus for the inflammatory reaction, but its nature remains obscure.[26] Activation of complement is probably important.

Repair and regeneration. Following autolysis and the inflammatory reaction, there ensues invasion by macrophages and granulation tissue. In this way the dead tissue is absorbed and replaced by scar tissue which may undergo dystrophic calcification. In some instances, e.g. necrosis of skin, regeneration of specialised tissue (in this case squamous epithelium) adds its contribution to the healing process.

Calcification. Some types of necrotic tissue appear to show limited autolysis; this is particularly true of caseation. Under these circumstances healing by repair appears to be hindered, and the necrotic tissue often undergoes calcification. Sometimes bone is formed.

Gangrene. This is an old descriptive clinical term applied to any black foul-smelling area which is in continuity with living tissue. In more precise terms it is *necrosis of tissue with superadded putrefaction*. The putrefactive organisms are usually the clostridia derived from the intestine or the soil (see Chapter 18). Necrosis of the gut is invariably followed by gangrene if the patient survives long enough. The necrosis may be ischaemic (mesenteric thrombosis, volvulus, etc.) or infective (e.g. acute appendicitis). Wounds infected with pathogenic saccharolytic clostridia are also contaminated by putrefactive clostridia—the result is gas-gangrene.

The putrefactive organisms which convert simple necrosis (with or without infection) to gangrene are not always clostridia. A variety of gangrenous lesions involving the skin and juxtacutaneous mucous membranes have been described: (*a*) *noma*,[29] a gangrenous lesion of the vulva or mouth (when it is alternatively called *cancrum oris*) occurring usually in malnourished children after an infectious disease such as measles. It is a slowly but relentlessly spreading

Figure 4.12
Sequelae of cell death.

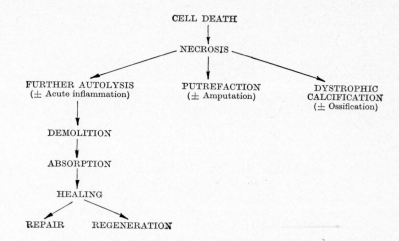

condition, and causes great tissue destruction. Death from inhalation pneumonia may occur. It is almost unknown in Britain, but is not uncommon in under-privileged communities; (*b*) *postoperative synergistic gangrene*, which implicates the anterior abdominal wall and thighs (see p. 221); (*c*) *Fournier's gangrene*,[30] a fulminating lesion of the scrotum, which is usually completely destroyed, so that the testes are left exposed; (*d*) *puerperal gangrene*.

The organisms concerned include anaerobic streptococci,[31, 32] and members of the family *Bacteroidaceae*.[33–35] This includes the genera *Bacteroides*, *Fusobacterium*, and *Necrobacterium*, a well-known member being *F. fusiforme* which is often found in the company of *Borrelia vincenti*. These bacteria are anaerobic and are cultured with considerable difficulty. They are Gram-negative bacilli, and are found as commensals in the mouth and intestine. Lesions caused by them are often called "fusospirochaetal gangrene", but it is doubtful whether *Borr. vincenti* plays any part in the disease process.[29] These gangrenous conditions are usually due to the combined effect of the above-mentioned organisms acting in debilitated tissues in association with *Strept. pyogenes*, staphylococci, and Gram-negative intestinal bacilli.

Gangrene of the lung. A putrid lung abscess is an occasional complication of dental extraction under general anaesthesia, when a piece of tooth is inhaled and lodges in a bronchus. Once again organisms belonging to the family *Bacteroidaceae* are responsible for the putrefaction.

Gangrene in the limbs. All the examples of gangrene so far mentioned are "wet". There is progressive tissue destruction, and unless effective treatment is instituted without delay, death results. A similar type of wet gangrene occurs in the limbs. It is usually due to vascular occlusion, and is not infrequently a complication of diabetes mellitus. Generally the legs are affected rather than the arms.

There is also described another type of gangrene, "dry gangrene". This is usually secondary to slow occlusive vascular disease. Commencing at the tips of the phalanges the tissues become desiccated and blackened.* There is no smell and no gas formation. The process is self-limiting, and the junction of dead with living tissue is sharp. Eventually the dead tissue is cast off by the process of spontaneous amputation. This lesion is in fact an infarct of a limb with minimal or no putrefactive changes. Tradition, however, dictates that it still be called gangrene. It is really an example of necrosis followed by mummification. All true gangrene is "wet".

Finally, it should be noted that gangrene is not massive necrosis, as is sometimes stated. Necrosis of the whole liver is not gangrene, nor is a gangrenous appendix large. It is the putrefaction of necrotic tissue, however caused, which constitutes the condition. It is this putrefaction which produces the smell and the blackening with iron sulphide which together are the pathognomonic features of gangrene.

It is evident from this account of cell structure and cell damage that many gaps exist in our knowledge. The advances in electron microscopy and cytochemistry are revealing wonderful details of cellular form and function. When these techniques are more widely applied to pathological material, it is to be expected that the changes occurring in damaged cells will be better understood.

---

* This blackening is probably due to the slow drying and oxidation of haemoglobin and myoglobin in the tissues.

REFERENCES

1. PETERS, R. A. (1963). *Biochemical Lesions and Lethal Synthesis*. Oxford: Pergamon Press.
2. CAMERON, G. R. and SPECTOR, W. G. (1961). *The Chemistry of the Injured Cell*. Springfield: Thomas.
3. GAVRILESCU, N. and PETERS, R. A. (1931). *Biochemical Journal*, **25**, 1397 and 2150.
4. PETERS, R. A. (1951). *Proceedings of the Royal Society*, B, **139**, 143.

5. TRUMP, B. F. and ERICSSON, J. L. E. (1965). In *The Inflammatory Process*, p. 35. Edited by B. W. Zweifach, L. Grant and R. T. McCluskey. New York and London: Academic Press.
6. TRUMP, B. F., GOLDBLATT, P. J. and STOWELL, R. E. (1965). *Laboratory Investigation*, **14,** 343.
7. MAGEE, P. N. (1966). *Laboratory Investigation*, **15,** 111.
8. VILLA-TREVINO, S., SHULL, K. H. and FARBER, E. (1966). *Journal of Biological Chemistry*, **241,** 4670.
9. SWIFT, H. and HRUBAN, Z. (1964). *Federation Proceedings. Federation of American Societies for Experimental Biology*, **23,** 1026.
10. BIAVA, C. G. *et al.* (1963). *Laboratory Investigation*, **12,** 443.
11. LOMBARDI, B. and RECKNAGEL, R. O. (1962). *American Journal of Pathology*, **40,** 571.
12. FARBER, E., LOMBARDI, B. and CASTILLO, A. E. (1963). *Laboratory Investigation*, **12,** 873.
13. DIBLE, J. H. and GERRARD, W. W. (1938). *Journal of Pathology and Bacteriology*, **46,** 77.
14. JUDAH, J. D. (1964). In *Cellular Injury, a Ciba Foundation Symposium*, p. 121. Edited by A. V. S. de Reuck and J. Knight. London: Churchill.
15. DAWKINS, M. J. R. (1964). In *Cellular Injury*, p. 106, *loc. cit.*
16. REES, K. R. (1964). In *Cellular Injury*, p. 53, *loc. cit.*
17. BEST, C. H., LUCAS, C. C. and RIDOUT, J. H. (1956). *British Medical Bulletin*, **12,** 9.
18. DIBLE, J. H. and LIBMAN, J. (1934). *Journal of Pathology and Bacteriology*, **38,** 269.
19. SNODGRASS, P. J. (1970). *New England Journal of Medicine*, **282,** 870.
20. TRUMP, B. F. and JANIGAN, D. T. (1962). *Laboratory Investigation*, **11,** 395.
21. KING, D. W. *et al.* (1959). *American Journal of Pathology*, **35,** 369, 575, 835 and 1067.
22. TRUMP, B. F., GOLDBLATT, P. J. and STOWELL, R. E. (1962). *Laboratory Investigation*, **11,** 986.
23. VAN LANCKER, J. L. and HOLTZER, R. L. (1963). *Laboratory Investigation*, **12,** 102.
24. DIXON, K. C. (1967). *Proceedings of the Royal Society of Medicine*, **60,** 271.
25. BESSIS, M. (1964). In *Cellular Injury*, p. 287, *loc. cit.*
26. MAJNO, G. (1964). In *Cellular Injury*, p. 87, *loc. cit.*
27. ROSALKI, S. B. (1970). *Journal of Clinical Pathology*, **24,** Supplement (Association of Clinical Pathologists) **4,** 60.
28. LATNER, A. L. (1970). *Journal of Clinical Pathology*, **24,** Supplement (Association of Clinical Pathologists), **4,** 8.
29. LINENBERG, W. B., SCHMITT, J. and HARPOLE, H. J. (1961). *Oral Surgery, Oral Medicine and Oral Pathology*, **14,** 1138.
30. KILBY, J. O. (1962). *British Journal of Surgery*, **49,** 619
31. MELENEY, F. L. (1931). *Annals of Surgery*, **94,** 961.
32. WEBB, H. E. *et al.* (1962). *Archives of Surgery*, **85,** 969.
33. OMATA, R. R. and BRAUNBERG, R. C. (1960). *Journal of Bacteriology*, **80,** 737.
34. BAIRD-PARKER, A. C. (1960). *Journal of General Microbiology*, **22,** 458.
35. MACDONALD, J. B. (1962). *Annals of the Royal College of Surgeons of England*, **31,** 361.

Chapter 5. Connective Tissue: Its Normal Structure and the Effects of Damage

The non-epithelial component of the body may be regarded as a gel of ground substance in which are embedded cells and fibres. It is one of the hallmarks of connective tissue that its component cells are widely separated from each other. They are responsible for the formation and perhaps the maintenance of the ground substance and the fibres, and it is these extracellular components which are responsible for giving each type of connective tissue its own special properties.

THE CELLS OF CONNECTIVE TISSUE

Fibroblasts. The major cellular component of the unspecialised connective tissue is the fibroblast, a cell of mesenchymal origin. The suffix "blast" is often used to denote the young plump cell of developing connective tissue as well as the thin spindle-shaped *fibrocyte* of mature collagenous tissue. Young fibroblasts are elongated or stellate in shape, and numerous processes project from the surface. There is an abundant cytoplasm which contains much rough endoplasmic reticulum as well as a prominent Golgi apparatus. When the cell is actively synthesising collagen, the cisterns of the endoplasmic reticulum contain material which is granular, but may also contain banded material which is probably collagen. The structure of the fibroblast is clearly that of a cell making protein for export.

In the mature fibrocyte the rough endoplasmic reticulum is less abundant. On light microscopy the cells appear to be inactive, with a small, densely staining nucleus and sparse cytoplasm compressed between surrounding collagen bundles.

Pericytes. Around blood vessels, but not lymphatics, there are cells which somewhat resemble fibroblasts except that they are surrounded by a basement membrane, as are smooth muscle cells. The pericyte is regarded by some as a primitive cell capable of differentiating along several lines—for instance into smooth muscle, cartilage, and bone.

Histiocytes. These cells are part of the reticulo-endothelial system, and are capable of exhibiting marked phagocytic activity—in which event they are called *macrophages*. Histiocytes have a vesicular nucleus and an abundant cytoplasm. This contains many ribosomes which are free rather than attached to endoplasmic reticulum. The cell outline is irregular due to the many short processes and in-vaginations which the plasma membrane exhibits. Lysosomes are abundant, and their internal structure is often complex because they contain fragments of cytoplasm, organelles, phagocytosed material, etc.

Eosinophil granulocytes. These cells are characterised by possessing cytoplasmic, membrane-bound granules which contain a central structure of crystalline appearance.

Mast cells. These cells have characteristic granules which contain heparin and histamine. Their actual structure varies from one species to another. The granules are not well preserved in some species unless alcohol is used as a fixative. In human tissue formalin is adequate, but the granules must be stained specially, e.g. with toluidine blue or Giemsa's stain, otherwise the cells may be mistaken for fibroblasts or histiocytes.

Mast cells form an important reservoir for histamine, and release this in response to certain chemical stimuli, e.g. compound 48/80, bee venom, basic peptides from polymorphs, C3a and C5a anaphylatoxins, and antigen when the cells have been sensitised by specific IgE antibody.

Plasma cells. A well-developed granular endoplasmic reticulum and Golgi apparatus are characteristic (p. 152). Plasma cells are particularly abundant in the lamina propria of the gastrointestinal tract, but a few are present in all loose connective tissue. A few *lymphocytes* are commonly present also.

THE GROUND SUBSTANCE

This material varies in consistency from an amorphous gel forming the solid translucent material of hyaline cartilage to the glairy fluid found in the synovial joint cavities. Its name is derived from the German *grundsubstanz*, which was regarded as the material from which the formed elements of the connective tissue were derived, as indicated in the French equivalent *substance fondamentale*.

It is in the molecular meshes of the ground substance that the *extracellular interstitial fluid* is contained. This constitutes about a third of the total body water, and lies between the blood vessels and the cells. It contains various electrolytes in a concentration similar to that of the plasma (see Chapter 34) and also small uncharged solute material, such as oxygen, CO_2, glucose, and urea, which is conveyed either for cellular metabolism or for excretion.

Ground substance itself contains *glycoproteins* as well as the soluble precursors of collagen fibrils and *mucoproteins*. Many of the characteristic properties of ground substance are attributed to these mucoproteins.

Glycoproteins[1] are proteins which contain a firmly bound moiety of carbohydrate. They stain red with the PAS method. Neither their site of formation nor their relationship with the glycoproteins of the blood is known.

The mucoproteins are loose combinations of protein with acid mucopolysaccharides. The latter have attracted much attention: they consist of polymers of hexose sugars, some of which possess amino groups, e.g. hexosamines like D-glucosamine and D-galactosamine. The amino groups are presumably responsible in part for the mucoid properties of the polymers. Meyer[2, 3] has subdivided the acid mucopolysaccharides as listed below. The alternative names in brackets are those proposed by Jeanloz.[4]

Non-sulphated group
> Hyaluronic acid
> Chondroitin

In these the acid grouping is due to a uronic acid, e.g. glucuronic acid.

Sulphated group
> Chondroitin sulphate A (chondroitin 4-sulphate)
> Chondroitin sulphate B (dermatan sulphate)
> Chondroitin sulphate C (chondroitin 6-sulphate)
> Heparitin sulphate (heparan sulphate)
> Keratosulphate (keratan sulphate)

The physical (e.g. optical) and presumably chemical properties of each connective tissue depend to a large extent upon the nature of the ground substance as well as upon the physical arrangement of the fibres themselves. For example, keratosulphate forms 50 per cent of the total acid mucopolysaccharide in the cornea, but is present only in small quantities in osteoid.

Formation of Acid Mucopolysaccharides

It is generally agreed that fibroblasts (and osteoblasts) form acid mucopolysaccharides.[5] Granules present in the fibroblasts of granulation tissue have the same staining properties as ground substance. Furthermore, in tissue cultures of pure osteoblasts or fibroblasts mucopolysaccharide is formed (mainly hyaluronic acid).[6] The evidence is therefore quite convincing. However, it is also claimed that *mast cells* liberate the substance of their granules to form the ground substance. Certainly these granules are metachromatic, and heparin or heparin-like anticoagulants have been demonstrated in ground substance. The case for the mast cell is, however, still not proven. It is important to note that tracer experiments using ^{35}S as a label have shown that the sulphur of ground substance is derived from inorganic sulphate, and not from sulphur-containing amino acids.[7]

Staining of Ground Substance

Its acidic nature renders it basophilic, i.e. blue in routine haematoxylin and eosin sections, as is seen in hyaline cartilage. The PAS method stains ground substance because of its high glycoprotein content (p. 3). The acid mucopolysaccharides themselves are PAS negative.

Staining properties of acid mucopolysaccharides.[8] A variety of staining techniques are in use but none can be regarded as very reliable for the identification of a particular mucopolysaccharide. Proper fixation of the tissue is important and aqueous formalin is unsatisfactory. Basic lead acetate solution, formalin-alcohol mixtures, and cetyl pyridium chloride-formalin are commonly used.

Thiazine dyes—Azur A and *Toluidine blue*. These dyes stain the mucopolysaccharides varying shades from purple to blue. They are therefore metachromatic stains (p. 3), but the precise results depend upon the pH employed. At one time it was thought that metachromasia was exhibited only by the sulphated compounds, but this is now known to be wrong. However, if the staining is performed at pH 2 or less only the sulphated mucopolysaccharides stain metachromatically.

Alcian blue. This is not a metachromatic stain. The substances are stained blue according to the pH used. A commonly employed method stains epithelial mucin as well as that of connective tissue.

Colloidal iron (Hale, Rinehart and Abul-Haj, and others). This method depends upon the affinity of mucopolysaccharides for ferric ions in colloidal form. The addition of potassium ferrocyanide leads to the formation of Prussian blue.

Enzymatic digestion. The alteration or elimination of staining after exposure of a section to a particular enzyme may be of assistance in identifying the substance responsible for the staining. Thus testicular hyaluronidase removes hyaluronic acid, chondroitin A, and C, while hyaluronidase of streptococcal origin removes only hyaluronic acid.

Role of Ground Substance in Disease

Remarkably little is known of the alterations that occur in ground substance under pathological conditions.

Reaction to injury. The mucopolysaccharides of ground substance appear to undergo depolymerisation, and consequently the ground substance itself becomes more watery.[9] Although in theory this might favour the spread of organisms, it might equally well enhance the penetrating power of the inflammatory exudate. If glucuronic acid is liberated, it could then form conjugates with toxins, thereby aiding the defence mechanism. The general loosening of the connective tissue in inflammation is well illustrated in the detachment of periosteum that occurs adjacent to a fracture (see p. 117).

The spreading factors, e.g. hyaluronidase of *Strept, pyogenes* and *Cl. welchii*, can be shown to depolymerise hyaluronic acid-containing ground substance, e.g. vitreous humour, *in vitro*. This also occurs *in vivo*, since it can be shown that dyes injected into the skin diffuse more readily when mixed with hyaluronidase. The enzyme is therefore used therapeutically for aiding the penetration of injections into the subcutaneous tissues, e.g. for parenteral fluid administration in babies. Whether hyaluronidase plays any part in the spread of infections is debatable (see p. 100).

Excessive accumulation of ground substance. The abnormal persistence of mucopolysaccharide in granulation tissue in scurvy, protein deficiency, and following cortisone administration is described in Chapter 9.

The amount of ground substance in connective tissue and its state of hydration are partly under hormonal control.[9] In *myxoedema* the increased accumulation of ground substance is responsible for the puffiness of the skin which gives the patient the characteristic appearance. It is probable that the exessive secretion of pituitary thyrotrophic hormone is responsible. In localised pretibial myxoedema of *hyperthyroidism*, LATS is incriminated (p. 297). Oestrogens and androgens also induce changes in connective tissue which are most marked in animals, e.g. the cock's comb and the sex skin of monkeys. Relaxin, secreted by the ovary, induces changes in the symphysis pubis in pregnancy.[10]

Under other less well-defined circumstances ground substance may accumulate in mature tissues, and appear as a basophilic material. The terms "mucoid" or myxomatous "degeneration" are generally applied to this condition, although its degenerative nature is neither always apparent nor provable. It is better to use the term *myxomatous change** to avoid this difficulty (see also p. 52).

Myxomatous change is seen in fibromatous tumours (myxofibroma, myxoma, myxosarcoma, etc.) and also in the connective-tissued stroma of epithelial tumours. In the giant intracanalicular fibro-adenoma of the breast (Brodie's tumour) the abundant myxomatous connective tissue is easily mistaken for a sarcoma.

---

* "Mucoid" is also applied to changes in epithelial tissues, e.g. "mucoid cancer", and is best avoided in relation to connective tissues.

Myxomatous change is also seen in the aorta in Erdheim's cystic medionecrosis, where it may form part of *Marfan's syndrome* (p. 64).

Myxomatous degeneration of the heart valves.[11, 12] Myxomatous degeneration of the valves may affect the cusps, annulus, or the chordae, and this by weakening the valves leads to incompetence. The valve leaflets are thin and diaphanous and may have a blue colour in this "floppy valve syndrome". It is the mitral valve which is most commonly affected, but aortic and rarely tricuspid involvement have also been reported. Intractable and progressive heart failure is the clinical manifestation of this condition, which is analogous to aortic cystic medionecrosis; moreover some cases have been associated with stigmata of Marfan's syndrome.[13]

Genetic defects of mucopolysaccharide metabolism.[14] There are at least six syndromes recognised in this group of diseases which may be called the *mucopolysaccharidoses*. The most common, and one of the most severe, is the *Hurler syndrome*, in which mucopolysaccharide is present in excess in connective-tissue cells as well as in certain epithelial cells, e.g. the liver. The disease becomes obvious in infancy or early childhood and results in gross skeletal deformities with dwarfism, hepatomegaly, mental defect, and corneal opacity. Involvement of the connective tissue of the heart valves leads to aortic and mitral lesions. Coronary-artery involvement leads to myocardial ischaemia. The grotesque appearance of the head is responsible for the alternative name by which the syndrome is commonly known—*gargoylism*.

The characteristics of the other syndromes is summarised in Table 5.1. All are inherited as autosomal recessive traits except the Hunter syndrome, which is an X-linked recessive. In all of them the affected cells are distended with mucopolysaccharide, but its precise composition is unknown, as indeed is the underlying defect in each syndrome. However, in each of them one or more acid mucopolysaccharides are excreted in the urine (Table 5.1); normally none is excreted. Two other laboratory tests are of value in diagnosis: (a) an

TABLE 5.1   The mucopolysaccharidoses

Syndrome	Clinical features	Compound in urine
I Hurler	Early onset, early death, mental deficiency, dwarfism, severe skeletal defects, corneal clouding	Chondroitin sulphate B Heparitin sulphate
II Hunter	As Hurler but less severe, skin lesions, no corneal clouding	Chondroitin sulphate B Heparitin sulphate
III Sanfilippo	Minor skeletal changes, severe mental retardation evident by school age	Heparitin sulphate
IV Morquio	Dwarfism with characteristic skeletal changes, corneal clouding, aortic regurgitation	Keratosulphate
V Scheie	Skeletal changes mild, stiff joints, claw hands, corneal clouding is marked, aortic regurgitation, intellect little affected	Chondroitin sulphate B
VI Maroteaux-Lamy	Dwarfism with severe skeletal changes, hepatomegaly, corneal clouding, intellect normal	Chondroitin sulphate B

examination of lymphocytes, neutrophils,[15] or monocytes from the blood or marrow often reveals characteristic meta-chromatic granules, and (b) skin fibroblasts grown in culture show similar metachromatic granules[16]; the only exception appears to be those cases of the Morquio syndrome in which the defects are restricted to the skeletal system. It is of interest that these abnormal fibroblasts can be cultured from people who are presumed to be carriers as well as from those who are clinically affected.[17]

Diminution in amount of ground substance. This occurs as part of the aging process of connective tissue.

COLLAGEN[18] [20]

Collagen constitutes about one third of the body's protein: it forms a scaffold in all tissues and is the chief component of fascia, dermis, cornea, and tendon giving these structures tensile strength. Isotope studies indicate that although much of the collagen is metabolically stable, some of it is rapidly synthesised and degraded; the excretion of hydroxyproline in the urine gives some indication of the amount of collagen that is being degraded. Thus, the excretion is increased in hyperparathyroidism, Paget's disease of bone, secondary carcinoma, and other destructive bone diseases. Collagen comprises almost 90 per cent of the organic matrix of bone, and its particular composition is adapted for the deposition of the bone salts.

The collagen of connective tissue is synthesised by fibroblasts or similar cells such as are found in tendon, cornea, bone, and cartilage. An exception to this is the collagen component of basement membrane which is formed by the adjacent epithelial or endothelial cells, and differs in several respects from other collagens (see p. 64). Indeed, as more research is carried out on the composition of collagen, it is evident that many forms exist, and it is misleading to talk of collagen as a single entity of fixed composition and structure.

Light microscopic appearance of collagen. By light microscopy collagen is seen to consist of fibres, the arrangement of which varies in different tissues. In tendon the fibres are arranged in parallel bundles, whilst in skin the bundles run in different directions but are mostly parallel to the surface. The fibres have several characteristic *staining properties*:[21]

(a) They stain pink with eosin.

(b) Picric-acid solutions combine with many dyes to form a complex that has a particular affinity for collagen. In *Van Gieson's stain* a mixture of picric acid and acid fuchsin is used, and the fibres are stained red with picrofuchsin.

(c) Aniline blue combined with phosphotungstic or phosphomolybdic acid stains collagen blue. This forms the basis of *Mallory's staining technique. Masson's trichrome stain* is similar, and collagen is stained blue if aniline blue is used or green with light green.

(d) The fibres are not blackened by silver impregnation methods, but are stained a brown colour.

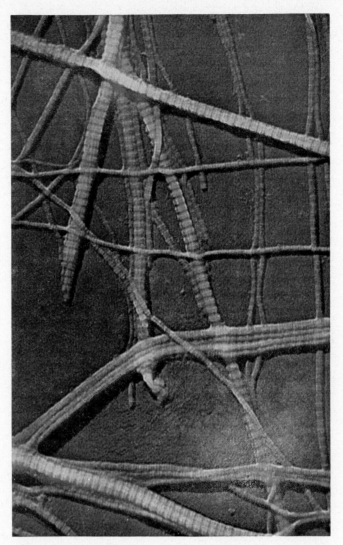

Figure 5.1
Teased preparation of collagen from the *tendo achilles*. The specimen has been shadowed to accentuate the characteristic 64 nm banding. This process involves the throwing of a vaporised heavy metal such as palladium or gold on to the specimen at a small angle. Now that ultra-thin sections can be cut, this technique is not often used. × 34 000. *(Photograph supplied by Dr. C. I. Levene)*

Electron microscopic appearance of collagen. The electron microscope reveals that collagen *fibres* are made up of *fibrils*, which show a cross-banding with a periodicity of about 64 nm (Fig. 5.1). It is thought that these fibrils are made up of tropocollagen molecules each of which is about 280 nm long and 1·4 nm wide. It was at first thought that the molecules were joined together end-to-end with a quarter length overlap with their lateral neighbours. It is now known that there is a gap of about 41 nm between the head of one molecule and the tail of the next as shown in Fig. 5.2. In osteoid tissue, these gaps serve as a nidus for the deposition of bone salts. The thickness of the collagen fibrils varies from

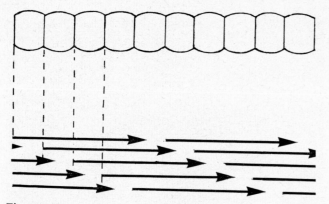

Figure 5.2
Diagram to illustrate how the lateral arrangement of tropocollagen molecules, depicted as arrows, results in the formation of a banded collagen fibril.

tissue to tissue. In cartilage they measure 15–25 nm while in tendon they reach 130 nm in thickness. It is evident that different lateral arrangements of the tropocollagen could form fibrils with different periodicity, and such have in fact been found to exist.

Solubility of collagen. Adult fully matured collagen is very insoluble, and only denaturation by strong acids or heat can render it soluble. The final product is then gelatin. In young collagen a fraction can be extracted by cold neutral buffers. This probably contains tropocollagen, and on warming the solution typical banded fibrils are reformed. An additional fraction can be extracted by dilute acid solutions and this component persists as maturation proceeds. Ultimately the collagen becomes insoluble due to the increasing number of cross-linkages which are formed (p. 63).

Chemical composition collagen. Collagen has a characteristic X-ray diffraction pattern, and from this its structure has been surmised. The basic unit of collagen is called *tropocollagen,* a molecule 280 nm long and 1·4 nm wide, with a molecular weight of about 340 000. Tropocollagen consists of three polypeptide chains: two are identical and called α_1 chains, while the third is different and called an α_2 chain. A third type of chain has been found in cartilage, and others probably exist. The nomenclature of the polypeptide polymers is confusing: a single polypeptide chain is called an α chain, dimers are called β chains, while tropocollagen with three polypeptides is the γ chain. Each of the polypeptide chains is coiled, and the three molecules are wound around a common axis like a three-stranded rope. It is thus a "coiled coil".

Each polypeptide chain consists of about 1 000 amino-acid residues, and has a molecular weight of about 95 000. It is coiled to form a type of helix in which, unlike the usual protein α-helix, there are no hydrogen bonds between adjacent amino acids on the same chain. Each helix is stabilised by hydrogen bonds with adjacent polypeptide chains. Throughout most of the chain every third amino acid is glycine, and a common sequence is glycine-proline-hydroxyproline.

Collagen indeed is characterised by its high content of glycine (33 per cent) and proline and hydroxyproline (which together constitute about 22 per cent). Hydroxyproline is an amino acid which is not found to any extent in other proteins, and an estimation of the amount of it in hydrolysates of tissue may therefore be used to measure the amount of collagen present. It is also noteworthy that collagen contains hydroxylysine, and it is to this amino acid that carbohydrate is attached (either galactose or glucosylgalactose).

Biosynthesis. The primary polypeptide chains are formed in the rough endoplasmic reticulum under the influence of specific mRNA. The three polypeptide chains are probably formed simultaneously, and immediately unite to form a triple helix. The molecule first formed is called *protocollagen*, and it differs from tropocollagen in that it contains no hydroxyproline, hydroxylysine, or glycosylated hydroxylysine. The next step in the formation of collagen is the hydroxylation of proline and lysine (Fig. 5.3).

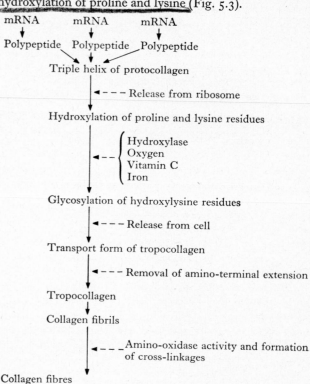

Figure 5.3
Diagram to illustrate the biosynthesis of collagen.

Requirements for hydroxylation. (1) *Specific enzymes*: protocollagen—proline hydroxylase has been isolated, and the presence of a separate lysine hydroxylase seems certain. (2) *α-ketoglutarate*. (3) *Ascorbic acid*. Although this can be replaced by other reducing substances *in vitro*, ascorbic acid is believed to be required *in vivo*. (4) *Iron*. Fibroblasts in culture fail to synthesise collagen in the presence of a metal chelating agent, such as α, α^1-dipyridyl. The cells form protocollagen, and this is released as such from the ribosomes.

(5) *Oxygen.* Likewise fibroblasts in anaerobic culture synthesise protocollagen but not collagen.

Thus the hydroxyproline and hydroxylysine in collagen are formed in the polypeptide chains by hydroxylation of the parent amino acid, and this explains the observation that, in tissue culture experiements, radioactive-tagged proline and not hydroxyproline is the precursor of hydroxyproline in the collagen molecule. Hydroxyproline and hydroxylysine are therefore not directly encoded by specific mRNA, and this raises another problem. What factors determine which proline or lysine is hydroxylated? No definite answer can be given, but it is not surprising that the degree of hydroxylation varies somewhat from one collagen to another even within the same individual.

Glycosylation of hyroxylysine. Glycosylation occurs at some of the hydroxylysine residues, and to some of these sites glucose in further added to the galactose. It has been postulated that in diabetes mellitus excessive glycosylation could lead to the deposition of an abnormal collagen in the basement membrane.

Formation of tropocollagen. The manner by which the three polypeptide chains are formed simultaneously and united is not known. There is some evidence that the first-formed polypeptide chains have an extension at the NH_2-terminal end and that this contains cystine. Hence disulphide bonds could be formed and initiate the formation of the triple helix. This sulphur-containing component probably persists until the tropocollagen molecules finally polymerise into mature collagen. These findings help to explain why sulphur-containing amino acids are necessary for normal wound healing (see p. 113).

Extrusion of collagen from the cell. Tropocollagen is released from the ribosomes into the cisternae of the endoplasmic reticulum. It may then pass into the vacuoles of the Golgi apparatus and finally be extruded from the cell in a manner seen in typical exocrine secretion, e.g. the pancreas. This is not proven, however, and the tropocollagen may pass more directly from the ribosomes to the exterior. Whatever the route, there is some mechanism which controls the type of material which is extruded. Failure in hydroxylation or glycosylation does not immediately inhibit protein synthesis, but the defective product is not extruded and therefore extracellular collagen deposition ceases. This occurs in scurvy.

Extracellular incorporation of tropocollagen into collagen fibrils. Newly synthesised collagen consists of a molecule larger than tropocollagen because of the presence of cystine-containing extensions at the NH_2-terminal ends of the polypeptide chains. This is called *procollagen*, or *transport form*. When the extensions are removed, aggregation occurs. Fibres are formed by the lateral alignment of the molecules with a quarter overlap as shown in Fig. 5.2. This quarter stagger arrangement presents problems if one tries to construct a three-dimensional model with match-sticks. Perhaps four or five polymer chains are arranged so that in cross-section they form a square or pentagon. In this way

G.P.—3*

there is limitation of the points of contact between the chains. Whatever the precise arrangement, the carbohydrate content of the collagen and the mucopolysaccharide composition of the ground substance seem to play a part in the determination of the size of the fibre produced.

Cross-linkage of fibrils to form fibres. The fibrils which are formed when tropocollagen aggregates have little strength. It is by the formation of firm cross-linkages that the tensile strength develops. The first step in the cross-linkage is the production of aldehyde groups on several lysyl or hydroxylysyl residues in the tropocollagen molecules:

$$R—CH_2—NH_3^+ \rightarrow R\text{-CHO} + NH_4^+.$$

The amine oxidase catalyses this reaction, and aldehyde groups of adjacent molecules form cross-links. The process is slow, and it can be readily understood that the tensile strength of collagen in a wound steadily increases over a period of several months (p. 109).

The enzyme amine oxidase is inhibited by the nitriles that produce lathyrism. The enzyme contains copper; this may explain why chronic copper deficiency in animals produces a condition which is indistinguishable from lathyrism. Penicillamine and homocysteine react with aldehyde groups so that they are unavailable for cross-linking (see p. 64).

The first formed collagen fibrils are coated with much ground substance, and it is in this that silver is deposited with suitable silver staining. Bundles of these fibrils form the *reticulin fibres* familiar to the light microscopist. As maturation proceeds the fibres increase in size and there is a diminution in the amount of surrounding ground substance. With light microscopy they are then recognised as *collagen fibres*. With silver stains the metal is deposited mainly in the region of the bands of the constituent fibrils, and the fibres therefore appear brown rather than black.

The maturation of the fibrils is usually accompanied by an increase in size due presumably to the addition of new tropocollagen units. It is only in some sites that full maturation is reached—for example, in tendon, fascia, and sclera. In organs like lymph nodes, lung, and spleen the development tends to halt at the reticulin stage.

Reticulin

Fibres called "reticulin" by histologists are thin (about $1\ \mu$m) and branching. They form a network in many organs, e.g. liver, lung, spleen, and lymph node, and stain an intense black with silver, but faintly with picrofuchsin (in Van Gieson's stain) and eosin.[21, 22] As described above, reticulin is composed of bundles of collagen fibrils which have a characteristic property of external silvering. In granulation tissue the first formed fibres are reticulin, but whether these fibres are precisely the same as those normally found in the organs mentioned above is undecided.

It must be understood that the name "collagen" is used in three different connexions.

To the chemist it is a protein which may exist in solution or in insoluble form.

To the histologist using the light microscope "collagen" exists as broad fibres with special staining properties.

To the electron microscopist it is a fibril of characteristic banded appearance; this corresponds both to the reticulin and "collagen" of the histologist.

Microfibrils[23, 24]

Other fine, branching fibres called microfibrils have been described by electron microscopists. They do not show the banded appearance of collagen, but nevertheless are thought by some investigations to be the precursors of collagen fibrils. Microfibrils tend to be concentrated around elastic fibres and are present also within them. Microfibrils are closely associated with the basement membrane.

Basement Membrane[25]

Under light microscopy the basement membrane is seen as an eosinophilic, hyaline, acellular sheath which is closely applied to epithelium and blood-vessel endothelium. It is PAS-positive, and was at one time regarded as being composed of a condensation of ground substance with reticulin fibres. Electron microscopy has revealed that in reality it has two components: one is a thin band 50–200 nm in width which has a central dense zone, the *lamina densa*, covered on each side by a *lamina rara*. This structure is now regarded as the basement membrane proper, and it can be seen adjacent to epithelial cells, the endothelium of blood vessels, around pericytes, and surrounding smooth muscle cells. It is probably manufactured by these cells, and it is therefore not surprising that antigenic components of one basement membrane are different from those of another elsewhere in the body.[26]

The basement membrane proper contains glycoproteins and collagen. The latter exhibits no fibrillar or banded structure, and differs in other ways from ordinary connective tissue collagen: it contains more carbohydrate, hydroxyproline, and hydroxylysine, and also contains 4–10 cysteine molecules per 1 000 amino-acid residues, so that disulphide bonds can form both between collagen molecules and with glycoproteins.

The second component of the light microscopist's "basement membrane" is an external condensation of microfibrils, reticulin, and ground substance. It is of connective-tissue origin. See Fig. 2.1, p. 12.

Thickening of the basement membrane is a common pathological finding, and has been much studied in diseased glomeruli. It may be due to an increase in the amount of basement membrane material or to the addition of plasma protein components or antigen-antibody precipitates.

ABNORMALITIES OF COLLAGEN

The information regarding the appearance and composition of collagen under pathological conditions is contradictory, confusing, and inadequate. Increase in the amount of collagen, or *fibrosis*, is a common finding in chronic inflammation (see p. 128), and is also a feature of the curious diseases called the fibromatoses (see p. 321). One of these is apparently caused by the administration of methysergide for migraine. It leads to retroperitoneal fibrosis and sometimes mitral regurgitation.[27] In those organs where collagen fibril development is incomplete, the fibrils may mature to form histological collagen. This may explain fibrosis in organs like the spleen and lung.

In old age the cross linkages between the fibrils are thought to be increased, and the amount of intervening mucopolysaccharide decreased. Hence the amount of extractable soluble collagen decreases with age. Unfortunately there is no reliable method of estimating the degree of cross-linkage in collagen.

There are a number of conditions in which the collagen fibres appear normal on microscopy, but are nevertheless abnormal functionally since the affected tissues are weak and can be stretched with undue ease. The defect appears to lie in the intermolecular bonds which are responsible for giving collagen its strength. This group includes three diseases which are inherited (Marfan's syndrome, homocystinuria, and the Ehlers-Danlos syndrome), and an experimentally induced condition (osteolathyrism).

Marfan's syndrome.[28] Affected individuals have long thin limbs, spider fingers (arachnodactyly), redundant ligaments and joint capsules (resulting in double-jointedness and dislocations), hernias, and subluxation of the lens of the eye. In addition, there is weakness of the aorta which leads to aneurysmal dilatation, aortic regurgitation, and the development of dissecting aneurysm. In the aorta there is degeneration of the elastic fibres and a picture resembling Erdheim's cystic medionecrosis. However, the other lesions indicate that there is a major defect in the collagen. The disease is inherited as a Mendelian dominant trait with high penetrance.

Homocystinuria.[29] This resembles Marfan's syndrome, but, unlike it, is inherited as a recessive trait, and there is homocystine in the urine. The skeletal changes are similar, and ectopia lentis occurs. However, the vascular lesions are characterised by thrombosis rather than dilatation; dissecting aneurysm does not occur, but there is increased platelet adhesiveness. Mental retardation is frequent.

Homocysteine probably acts by reacting with aldehydes generated by the amine oxidase reaction so that they are unavailable for cross-linkage. The drug penicillamine has a similar effect, and its use has been advocated in the treatment of scleroderma. Unfortunately the drug cannot be tolerated in the dose necessary, and in any case the effect is difficult to evaluate in a disese as chronic as scleroderma.

Ehlers-Danlos syndrome.[30] In this remarkable condition there is loose-jointedness and great hyperextensibility of the skin (see also p. 619).

Experimental osteolathyrism[31–33] Young rats or chicks fed

---

* Human lathyrism has been described following the ingestion of the chick pea *Lathyrus sativus*, and is characterised by spastic paralysis. The toxin responsible is not known. This neurolathyrism bears no obvious relationship to the osteolathyrism of animals described above.

on sweet-pea (*Lathyrus odoratus*) meal or a lathyrogenic agent like β-aminoproprionitrile develop bony deformities, weakness of tendons and ligaments, and rupture of the aorta. Although the collagen appears normal on electron microscopy, much more of the newly formed collagen is soluble in cold saline. This appears to be due to a defect in the cross-linking of collagen. The urinary output of peptides containing hydroxyproline is increased, due presumably to the fact that uncross-linked tropocollagen is more rapidly degraded than is mature collagen. The synthesis of desmosine and isodesmosine is inhibited, and since these two amino acids are important in the cross-linkages in elastic fibres, it is probable that there is also a defect in the elastic tissue. As noted previously, chronic copper deficiency produces a disease resembling lathyrism; in both conditions there is a tendency towards dissecting aneurysm and rupture of the aorta.[34, 35] The lesions of lathyrism bear some resemblance to those of Marfan's syndrome and medionecrosis of the aorta in man, and this is the major reason for the current interest in the subject.

Hyalinisation

A change which occurs in abnormal deposits of collagen with the passage of time is *hyalinisation*. The individual histological collagen fibres appear to fuse together to form a glassy eosinophilic material. The intervening fibrocytes disappear, and the tissue is converted into an acellular, structureless, inert mass. Such an appearance may also be encountered in muscle fibres, and it must be understood that the term is merely descriptive of a particular microscopic appearance. Hyaline literally means glassy.

Probably several processes are included, but in the hyalinisation of collagen the material appears very uniform. It is seen in a wide array of conditions; in old scar tissue, keloids, and "fibroid" tumours of the uterus (leiomyomata).

The glomeruli of chronic nephritis are converted into hyalinised eosinophilic balls. These usually have two components: the remains of the glomerulus is represented by a mass of basement-membrane-like substance (which is PAS-positive), and the second component is hyalinised collagen produced by the parietal cells of Bowman's capsule. In H. and E. sections the two components cannot be distinguished (Fig. 5.4).

Deposits of hyaline material may also replace epithelial cells. A good example is the hyalinisation of the islets of Langerhans that is sometimes seen in diabetes mellitus (Fig. 5.5). Apparently the substance is laid down around the sinusoids, and eventually replaces the glandular structure. This type of hyaline is probably amyloid. Indeed, amyloid may be considered as a type of hyaline material, but because of its special properties it is considered separately (Chapter 44).

Vascular hyaline. The appearance of homogeneous hyaline material in the subendothelial layer of arterioles is a common event, and in the spleen of adults may be regarded as normal. In the afferent arterioles of the renal glomeruli it is associated

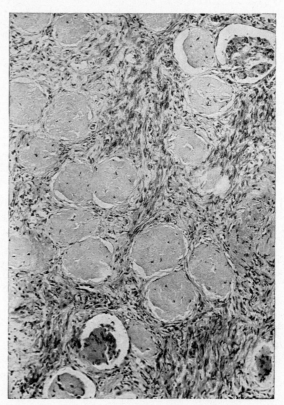

Figure 5.4
Hyalinised glomerular tufts. Most of the glomeruli in this section have been converted into dense, solid balls of hyaline material, almost completely devoid of cellular structure. The patient suffered from chronic pyelonephritis with secondary hypertension. ×65.

with benign systemic hypertension and diabetes mellitus. The nature of this hyaline has been much debated. In the kidney it consists of granular material on electron microscopy; by some it is thought to be material, perhaps fibrin, derived from the blood.[36–39] It has been claimed that fibrin, as it ages, becomes transformed into an acellular substance which has the staining properties of collagen.[40] Other possibilities are that vascular hyaline is derived from smooth muscle,[41, 42] collagen, or that it consists of basement-membrane-like substance.[43]

Necrosis of Collagen

When connective tissue is damaged, its associated fibrocytes undergo necrosis and its fibres appear to degenerate. They break up, and are removed in the course of an inflammatory reaction. This necrosis of collagen differs from hyalinisation in several important respects.

(*a*) Hyaline material appears to be extremely stable; for example, the corpora albicantes seen in an old ovary have presumably been present for many years. Necrotic collagen, on the other hand, is either removed or else organised.

(*b*) Hyaline collagen retains the staining characteristics of

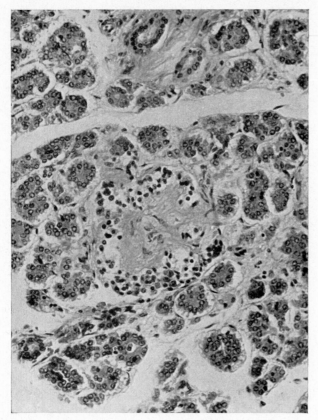

Figure 5.5
Hyalinisation of the islets of Langerhans. This is the pancreas of a
diabetic subject. The central area is an islet largely replaced by
hyaline material; the remains of epithelial cells are visible in the
periphery. ×220.

normal collagen. Necrotic collagen, on the other hand,
becomes Van Gieson negative and PAS positive. It tends to
stain brightly with eosin—in fact, it takes on some of the
tinctorial properties of fibrin. The term *fibrinoid necrosis* is
therefore sometimes applied.

The nature of the change is a matter of much confusion
due mainly to the fact that "fibrinoid necrosis" is a morphological descriptive term of a variety of changes that occur
in various tissues under very dissimilar circumstances; e.g.
in the "collagen diseases", and in tissue damaged by infective agents and ionising radiation. In blood vessels it occurs
in malignant hypertension, the Shwartzman phenomenon,
the Arthus phenomenon, and in polyarteritis.

In rheumatic fever[44] and rheumatoid arthritis the fibrinoid
material has been observed to be continuous with normal
collagen, both on light and electron microscopy.[45] Similar
degeneration of collagen with loss of cross-striations occurs
in the Arthus phenomenon, but in addition antigen-antibody
complexes are present.[46] If antigen is injected into the cornea
of a sensitised rabbit, a visible antigen-antibody precipitate
forms as a ring around the site of injection. This area shows

fibrinoid necrosis on light microscopy. On electron microscopy the precipitate is seen to be coating the collagen fibrils
and filling in the ground-substance matrix. In the Shwartzman phenomenon histochemical studies indicate that the
fibrinoid material contains fibrin, while in the collagen
diseases there is, in addition, immunoglobulin.[47, 48] Another
possibility is that fibrinoid is derived from the smooth-
muscle coat of blood vessels.[41] It must be concluded that
although the term fibrinoid necrosis is useful in a descriptive
sense, it implies no single morphological change or aetiological agent. There may be degeneration of collagen, necrosis
of muscle, deposition of fibrin, precipitation of antigen-
antibody complexes, or any combination of these changes.

Fibrinoid necrosis is encountered in the "collagen diseases", but is certainly not pathognomonic of them. It is
seen when connective tissue is damaged in other ways, for
example, it is a prominent feature of x-ray damage to the
skin (Fig. 5.6). It is also found in the small arterioles in
malignant hypertension, where the damage to the wall is
probably caused by a sudden rise of blood pressure. The
necrotic walls frequently rupture, thereby giving rise to the
haemorrhages in the retina and skin and the haematuria seen
in malignant hypertension.

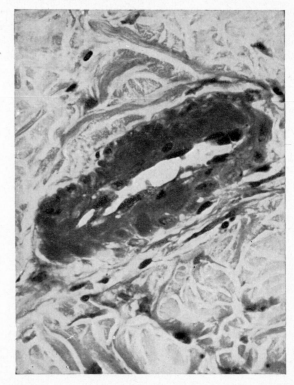

Figure 5.6
Fibrinoid necrosis of arteriole. This section comes from the skin
of a guinea-pig 34 days after irradiation with x-rays. Note the
blurred, deeply staining muscle wall; it has lost its normal structure. It is intensely PAS-positive. ×460. *(From Mellett, P. G.,
Walter, J. B. and Houghton, L. E. (1960), Brit. J. exp. Path.,* **41,** 160)

The term *necrobiosis* is commonly used to describe the fibrinoid necrosis of collagen which occurs in the lesions of certain diseases, for instance in the subcutaneous nodules of rheumatoid arthritis (Fig. 16.7) and the dermal lesions of granuloma annulare. Except for their situation these two lesions cannot be distinguished from each other on microscopy. A somewhat similar appearance is seen in the skin in necrobiosis lipoidica diabeticorum. It is unfortunate that necrobiosis is used in this context, because the term has also been used to describe the physiological death of cells (see p. 296).

ELASTIC FIBRES

The elastic fibres of the aorta and its large branches, the ligamentum nuchae, lung, etc., appear very different from collagen on light microscopy: they stain *deep red with eosin, dark brown with orcein,* and *black with the resorcinol fuchsin stain of Weigert.* Early electron-microscopic studies of elastic fibres showed them to be amorphous and quite unlike collagen. More recent investigations have shown that elastic tissue consists of two components: one is the microfibril and the other is a homogeneous material of variable electron density. The microfibrils are obvious during the formation of elastic, but with aging are more difficult to detect. Elastic tissue is very resistant to digestion by acids and alkalis, but is readily attacked by the enzyme elastase produced by some organisms.

Chemically it thought to consist of a protein, *elastin*, with polysaccharide. Although some authorities regard elastic fibres as being derived from collagen, most maintain that this is unlikely in view of the great difference in amino-acid composition between elastin and collagen. Elastin contains two amino acids, desmosine and isodesmosine, which are thought to be important in forming the cross-linkages which give to elastic tissue the resilience which is its characteristic physical property.[49] With age there is an increase in the content of desmosine and isodesmosine, and this is accompanied by a loss of resilience.[50] Calcification of elastic fibres is another feature of the aging process; it also occurs in metastatic calcification (see p. 570).

Elastic fibres are formed by the activity of smooth muscle cells in some situations, e.g. in the aortic wall and in atheromatous plaques. In other tissues, cells which resemble fibroblasts appear to be involved. No specific "elastoblasts" have been identified. There is little doubt that new elastic fibres can be formed in adult life. Thus degeneration of elastic tissue is sometimes accompanied by new elastic fibre formation, so as to give an appearance of fraying or reduplication.

Elastosis

Although it is sometimes stated that elastic tissue is not reformed in scar tissue in the dermis, this is probably not true. After a long time fibres do appear, and these have the staining properties of elastic. Moreover, there are certain conditions of the skin in which an excess of elastic is formed (actinic elastosis and pseudoxanthoma elasticum[51]). A similar excess of elastic is described in the dermis of skin treated with chemical carcinogens, and indeed has been held to be a step in the development of neoplasia.[52] It is thus evident that elastic fibres can be formed, but the situation is complicated by one uncertainty. Electronmicroscopic examination of some "elastic fibres" has shown that they consist of typical banded collagen fibrils! We are as yet unable to decide whether collagen can change its properties so that it resembles elastic, or whether indeed true "elastin elastic" is itself derived from collagen.

It is apparent from the above account that connective tissue is by no means the inert substance that it is often considered to be. Our knowledge of its basic structure in health and disease is still very inadequate. Changes in it are assuming an ever-increasing importance in the modern concepts of many disease processes ranging from inflammation to neoplasia. There are also a considerable number of obscure chronic inflammatory conditions which are included under the general heading of "collagen disease". These are considered in Chapter 16.

GENERAL READING
WAGNER, B. M. and SMITH, D. E. (1967). (Eds) *The Connective Tissue*, 408 pp. Baltimore: Williams and Wilkins.

REFERENCES
1. SPIRO, R. G. (1963). *New England Journal of Medicine*, **269**, 566 and 616.
2. MEYER, K. (1959). In *Wound Healing and Tissue Repair*, p. 25. Edited by W. B. Patterson. Chicago: University of Chicago Press.
3. MEYER, K. *et al.* (1956). *Biochimica et biophysica acta*, **21**, 506.
4. JEANLOZ, R. W. (1960). *Arthritis and Rheumatism*, **3**, 233.
5. DUNPHY, J. E. (1963). *New England Journal of Medicine*, **268**, 1367.
6. WINDRUM, G. M. (1958). *Laboratory Investigation*, **7**, 9.
7. GROSS, J. I., MATHEWS, M. B. and DORFMAN, A. (1960). *Journal of Biological Chemistry*, **235**, 2889.
8. RAPAPORT, M. (1967). In *The Connective Tissue*, p. 247, *loc. cit.*
9. CATCHPOLE, H. R. (1957). In *The Healing of Wounds*, p. 29. Edited by M. B. Williamson. New York: McGraw-Hill.
10. STEINETZ, B. G., BEACH, V. L. and KROC, R. L. (1959). In *Recent Progress in the Endocrinology of Reproduction*, p. 389. Edited by C. W. Lloyd. New York: Academic Press.

11. Leading Article. (1971). *British Medical Journal*, ii, 294.
12. TRENT, J. K. *et al.* (1970). *American Heart Journal*, **79,** 539.
13. READ, R. C., THAL, A. P. and WENDT, V. E. (1965). *Circulation*, 897.
14. McKUSICK, V. A. (1966). In *Heritable Disorders of Connective Tissue*, 3rd edn, p. 325. St Louis: Mosby.
15. REILLY, W. A. (1941). *American Journal of Diseases of Children*, **62,** 489.
16. MATALON, R. and DORFMAN, A. (1969). *Lancet*, ii, 838.
17. DANES, B. S. and BEARN, A. G. (1967). *Lancet*, i, 241.
18. GRANT, M. E. and PROCKOP, D. J. (1972). *New England Journal of Medicine*, **286,** 194, 242, and 291. This is a review of the biosynthesis of collagen and contains many references.
19. RAMACHANDRAN, G. N. (1967). (Ed.) *Treatise on Collagen*, vol. 1, p. 556. London and New York: Academic Press.
20. GOULD, B. S. (1968). (Ed.) *Treatise on Collagen*, vol. 2, Part A, p. 434 and Part B, p. 488. London and New York: Academic Press.
21. LILLIE, R. D. (1952). *Laboratory Investigation*, **1,** 30.
22. LILLIE, R. D. (1951). *American Journal of Clinical Pathology*, **21,** 484.
23. HAUST, M. D. (1965). *American Journal of Pathology*, **47,** 1113.
24. HAUST, M. D. and MORE, R. H. (1967). In *The Connective Tissue*, p. 352, *loc. cit.*
25. Various Authors (1970). In *Chemistry and Molecular Biology of the Intercellular Matrix*, vol. 1, Chapter III, p. 471. Edited by E. A. Balazs. London and New York: Academic Press.
26. PIERCE, G. B., MIDGLEY, A. R. and RAM, J. S. (1963). *Journal of Experimental Medicine*, **117,** 339.
27. MUNROE, D. S., ALLEN, P. and COX, A. R. (1969). *Canadian Medical Association Journal*, **101,** 536.
28. McKUSICK, V. A. (1966). p. 38, *loc. cit.*
29. McKUSICK, V. A. (1966). p. 150, *loc. cit.*
30. McKUSICK, V. A. (1966). p. 179, *loc. cit.*
31. LEVENE, C. (1967). In *The Connective Tissue*, p. 132, *loc. cit.*
32. BICKLEY, H. (1964). *Journal of the American Geriatric Association*, **12,** 717.
33. BENUSUSAN, H. R. (1966). *Science*, **153,** 322.
34. MILLER, E. J. *et al.* (1965). *Journal of Biological Chemistry*, **240,** 3623.
35. SAVAGE, J. E. *et al.* (1962). *Federation Proceedings. Federation of American Societies for Experimental Biology*, **21,** 311.
36. McKINNEY, B. (1962). *Experimental and Molecular Pathology*, **1,** 275.
37. McKINNEY, B. (1962). *Journal of Pathology and Bacteriology*, **83,** 449.
38. LENDRUM, A. C. (1963). *Canadian Medical Association Journal*, **88,** 442.
39. BIAVA, C. G. *et al.* (1964). *American Journal of Pathology*, **44,** 349.
40. LENDRUM, A. C. *et al.* (1962). *Journal of Clinical Pathology*, **15,** 401.
41. MUIRHEAD, E. E., BOOTH, E. and MONTGOMERY, P. O'B. (1957). *Archives of Pathology*, **63,** 213.
42. SPIRO, D., LATTES, R. and WIENER, J. (1965). *American Journal of Pathology*, **46,** 15a.
43. McGEE, W. G. and ASHWORTH, C. T. (1963). *American Journal of Pathology*, **43,** 273.
44. GLYNN, L. E. and LOEWI, G. (1952). *Journal of Pathology and Bacteriology*, **64,** 329.
45. LANNIGAN, R. and ZAKI, S. (1965). *Nature*, **206,** 106.
46. RICH, A. R., VOISIN, G. A. and BANG, F. B. (1953). *Bulletin of the Johns Hopkins Hospital*, **92,** 222.
47. MOVAT, H. Z. and MORE, R. H. (1957). *American Journal of Clinical Pathology*, **28,** 331.
48. GITLIN, D., CRAIG, J. M. and JANEWAY, C. A. (1957). *American Journal of Pathology*, **33,** 55.
49. PARTRIDGE, S. M., ELSDEN, D. F. and THOMAS, J. (1963). *Nature*, **197,** 1297 and **200,** 651.
50. MILLER, E. J., MARTIN, G. R. and PIEZ, K. A. (1964). *Biochemical and Biophysical Research Communications*, **17,** 248.
51. McKUSICK, V. A. (1966). p. 286, *loc. cit.*
52. GILLMAN, T. *et al.* (1955). *British Journal of Cancer*, **9,** 272.

Chapter 6. The Inflammatory Reaction

INTRODUCTION

One of the characteristics of living tissue is its ability to react to injury. Indeed, the survival of the individual depends upon the ability of his normal cells to respond to damage. The response in the higher animals is complex, involving not only the local cells adjacent to the area of injury, but also the body as a whole. Reaction to injury may therefore be considered under two headings.

Firstly, there is a general body response involving nervous and hormonal adjustments, and resulting in considerable metabolic alterations. At the same time the lymphoreticular system responds by proliferating to provide more phagocytes and antibody-forming cells.

description by Celsus in the first century A.D.: to these has been added a fifth— loss of function.* John Hunter was one of the first to recognise that acute inflammation was not a disease in its own right, but rather a defence mechanism against a variety of injuries.[2]

Definition. Although the features of acute inflammation have been known for a long time, there is no entirely satisfactory definition of the phenomenon. It is commonly defined as "the local response of living tissue to injury", but this wrongly implies that all the succeeding events, like repair and regeneration, are included. Indeed, it also includes the cellular responses to injury, such as those described in Chapter 4, as well as neoplasia. Such a wide definition is therefore misleading and quite unhelpful.

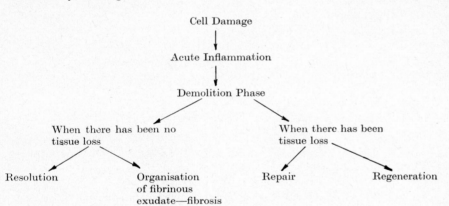

Figure 6.1
Diagram to show the sequence of events which may follow local cell damage.

Secondly, there is a local response. Initially the adjacent living tissues undergo changes which enable phagocytic cells and circulating plasma to enter the area of damage. This phase is known as acute inflammation, and continues so long as tissue damage continues. When the causative agent is withdrawn or removed, the debris of the inflammatory reaction is removed by scavenger cells. The tissue may then return to normal, but when tissue loss has been sustained, there is a final stage of healing by repair, regeneration, or both. The outline of this local reaction to injury is shown in Fig. 6.1. In this chapter we shall deal with the early phase, the acute inflammatory reaction.

ACUTE INFLAMMATION

The cardinal signs of acute inflammation—*calor, rubor, dolor*, and *tumor*—have been known since the original

Some definitions add the rider that the changes are beneficial and protect the tissues from further injury. This is unwarranted since not all the phenomena of acute inflammation, for instance those following the development of hypersensitivity, are necessarily of benefit. In fact, in some infections, e.g. tuberculosis, the cells of the exudate actually spread the organism through the tissues. Acute inflammation must be regarded as a mechanism which has been evolved to protect the individual from a wide range of hazards. On the whole it is a beneficial reaction, but one should not be surprised if under certain circumstances the reaction itself becomes a hazard. The formation of inflammatory oedema

* The origin of this fifth sign is obscure, and to attribute it to Galen is to perpetuate a misconception which has been handed down without verification by many authors, including ourselves in previous editions.[1] To describe it as *functio laesa* is to give it an air of respectability which it ill deserves!

is probably of great importance in the limitation of bacterial infection. In the larynx, however, it may cause rapid death. Opie used the following definition: "Inflammation is the process by means of which cells and serum accumulate about an injurious substance and tend to remove or destroy it." While it is true that in animals which have a circulatory system the predominant features are vascular with the formation of an exudate, part fluid and part cellular, there is no doubt that a primitive type of inflammatory reaction can occur in avascular tissues. In fact, Metchnikoff did much of his work on the starfish, which has no circulatory system.

Nevertheless, it can be argued that this type of response in a lowly creature is not true inflammation comparable with that occurring in the vascular tissues of higher animals. The presence of a vascular system is really a prerequisite for an acceptable inflammatory response. A useful definition is the following:

x *Inflammation is the reaction of the vascular and supporting elements of a tissue to injury, and results in the formation of a protein-rich exudate, provided the injury has not been so severe as to destroy the area.*

In avascular tissue, like the normal cornea,* no true inflammation can occur, although injury may result in changes which include the appearance of phagocytes. This response is comparable with that seen in the lower animals. An attempt to include this type of reaction under the heading of inflammation is unlikely to produce any result other than confusion.

The term *subacute inflammation* is used by some authorities: it appears to mean a mild acute inflammation, but since no exact definition is possible, there seems no good reason for retaining the term.

Causes of Acute Inflammation

Since the inflammatory reaction is a response to injury, its causes are those of cell damage. These may be briefly enumerated:

Mechanical trauma, such as cutting and crushing.

Chemical injury. There are numerous chemicals which injure cells. Many, like corrosive acids, alkalis, and phenol, are general protoplasmic poisons. Others are more selective in their action: thus mercuric chloride causes renal tubular necrosis. Some chemicals are known to act by producing a biochemical lesion, e.g. fluoroacetate. Certain body fluids, like bile and urine, cause damage when they escape into the tissues.

Radiation injury. Heat, ultraviolet light, and all forms of ionising radiations, both electromagnetic and particulate, fall into this category.

Injury due to cold and heat.

Injury due to deprivation of blood supply. Inflammation is a prominent feature around early infarcts.

Injury due to deficiency. Withdrawal of a hormone causes damage to its target cells. The physiological monthly necrosis

* The cornea may become vascularised and is then liable to true inflammation.

of the endometrium following the withdrawal of progesterone is associated with an acute inflammation of the mucous membrane.

Injury due to living organisms. This includes infection with viruses, bacteria, and the larger parasites.

Injury due to antigen-antibody reactions. This includes the diseases mediated by immunological mechanisms as well as those classified as immediate and delayed-type hypersensitivity.

CHANGES IN ACUTE INFLAMMATION

Inflammation is a continuous process, the evolution of which is best studied in the living animal. The transparent web and tongue of the "pithed" frog were originally studied, but in the higher animals the hamster cheek-pouch, the guinea-pig cochlea, the rat mesoappendix, and the rabbit ear-chamber have been used. Cohnheim (1882) gave an admirable description to which surprisingly little has since been added. For descriptive purposes the acute inflammatory reaction may be subdivided as follows:

1. The Vascular Response.
   (i) Change in calibre of vessels.
   (ii) Changes in the vessel wall and flow of blood—stasis.
2. Swelling and Exudation.
   (i) The fluid exudate.
   (ii) The cellular exudate—phagocytosis.
3. Changes in other tissue components.

THE VASCULAR RESPONSE

Changes in the blood vessels are the most obvious manifestations of acute inflammation. They can be considered under two headings:

1. Changes in the vessel calibre.
2. Changes in the vessel wall and the flow of blood.

Changes in the Calibre of the Blood Vessels

Initial constriction. The earliest response to trauma is constriction in the small blood vessels. It can be demonstrated in the skin of man: light stroking produces a white line. This vasoconstriction is apparently due to direct mechanical stimulation of the capillaries. It may also be seen when irritant chemicals are directly applied to a vascular bed. In bacterial inflammation it is questionable whether this initial constriction occurs.

Persistent vasodilatation. Vasodilatation rapidly follows the initial constriction and persists for the duration of the inflammatory process. The first result of arteriolar dilatation is that blood flows by the most direct route to the veins through the *central*, or *thoroughfare*, *channels*. Subsequent opening of the precapillary sphincters allows blood to pass into the capillary bed, and vessels which were temporarily shut down now become functional again. The inflamed part therefore appears to contain an increased number of vessels. In addition their calibre is increased.

The fact that the response of the blood vessels is so constant in acute inflammation suggests that the reaction is mediated by some common mechanism. Lewis (1924) noted that firm stroking of human skin results in a *triple response*, and his analysis of these events led to the hypothesis that histamine liberated from damaged cells was an important factor in the vascular response that follows injury[3] (see p. 79). The features of this triple response to firm stroking of the skin are the red line, the flare, and the weal.

The red line. After a short latent period a red line develops, at first bright red, but later tending to become cyanosed. It is sharply demarcated and is due to capillary dilatation.

The flare. After a further period of 15–30 seconds a flare or flush appears surrounding the red line. It is blotchy and has a crenated outline, and is due to arteriolar dilatation. It has been claimed that if the nerve supply to the skin is sectioned,

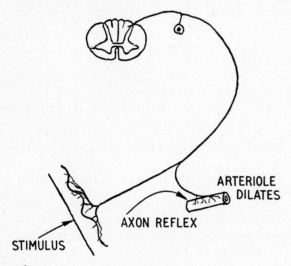

Figure 6.2
The axon reflex. Following stimulation of the skin the impulse passes up the sensory nerve fibre to the point of its division. An impulse then travels to the arteriole and causes it to dilate.

the flare can still be elicited, but if some ten days later the test is performed again, the flare does not appear.[4] This suggests that the flare is caused by a reflex not involving the central nervous system, but mediated *via a local axon reflex*. This is illustrated in Fig. 6.2.

The weal. On the site of the red line a weal may subsequently develop due to an exudation of fluid through the vascular wall. As the oedema increases, the weal becomes paler due to pressure on the capillaries.

It is apparent that simple mechanical injury to the skin can result in vascular changes which are typical of those seen in other types of acute inflammation. The affected part contains more blood and therefore appears red ("rubor").

The arteriolar dilatation increases the blood supply to the area. If the temperature of the part, e.g. skin, is normally below that of the blood due to its contact with the external environment, the increased blood flow that occurs during acute inflammation will be associated with a rise in temperature of the part compared with the adjacent areas. The "calor", or heat, of acute inflammation is seen, therefore, in parts near the body surface—skin, face, ears, fingers, etc. It is not a feature of internal inflammation (Cohnheim).

Although we believe that the vasodilatation is largely mediated chemically (see p. 79), the nervous system plays some part.

Influence of nerve supply on the vasodilatation of acute inflammation. Although inflammation can occur in completely denervated tissues, there is no doubt that nervous influences do modify the response in the intact animal. The axon reflex is one example of this, but the autonomic nervous system can also play a part.

If the vasodilator nerve to a rabbit's ear is sectioned, its vessels become constricted and unresponsive. Injection of a test dose of bacteria produces a slow inflammatory reaction, and there is much more tissue destruction than when a normal ear is infected.[5]

This effect may be correlated with the action of adrenaline. If this drug is injected together with organisms, the inflammatory response is inhibited and a spreading infection ensues. It should, however, be noted that under normal conditions the autonomic nervous system seems to play little part in the inflammatory response. When once inflammation is established, the blood vessels fail to react to sympathetic stimulation or a vasoactive drug like adrenaline.

Changes in the Vessel Wall and the Flow of Blood

Before the changes in the stream of blood in the vessels can be described, the normal flow must be understood.

The normal flow. During normal flow the blood cells tend to occupy the central, or axial, part of the stream (Fig. 6.3). This is best seen in the venules. The clear outer or plasmatic stream has great functional importance, for its viscosity is much lower than that of whole blood, and therefore the peripheral resistance is lower than it would be if the blood components were intimately mixed.

Changes in inflammation. The first change is an increase in blood velocity due to arteriolar dilatation. This phase is short-lived, and is followed by a slowing of the stream. At the same time the white cells are seen to move into the plasmatic zone and to stick to the vessel wall; platelets also stick to the wall. The endothelial cells are swollen and appear to be covered by a gelatinous layer. This sticking of the white cells is highly characteristic of damage to blood vessels, and whereas in the normal stream the white cells cannot be distinguished, in inflammation they roll along the sticky endothelial lining in a leisurely way, quite oblivious of the red cells streaming by. These three features, *stasis, leucocyte adherence*, and *endothelial swelling*, must each be considered separately.

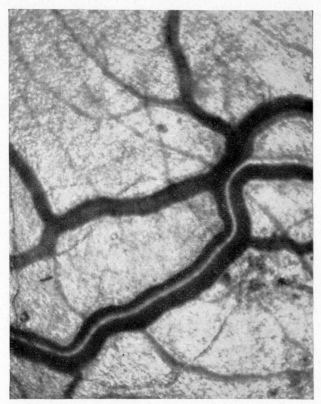

Figure 6.3
Blood flow, from right to left, in small venules seen in a rabbit ear-chamber. Note how the clear plasmatic zones in the two venules join together to produce a well-marked central clear stripe. This was a fortuitous observation which serves to illustrate the streamlining of the circulation as well as the presence of a plasmatic zone. Such a central clear stream is unusual.

Stasis. The dilatation and changes in the endothelial cells may play a small part, but the main factor in the production of stasis is an increase in the vascular permeability. Fluid is lost from the blood, which in consequence becomes more viscid. The lubricating action of the plasmatic zone is impaired or lost, and the blood stream slows down. *Thrombosis* may sometimes supervene, and is then an additional factor in causing further tissue damage.

Adherence of polymorphs. With the occurrence of stasis the red cells tend to come together in the form of rouleaux, a phenomenon noted by Lister. Other factors may also play a part (see sludging, p. 427). These masses of red cells are now the largest components in the blood stream, and the smaller white cells are pushed from the centre of the stream.They impinge more frequently on to the endothelium, which being sticky will tend to retain them. At first the white cells may escape, and either roll gently along the endothelial lining or get swept back into the blood stream. Later, however, the cells become more permanently adherent; they line the endothelium, forming great masses which may even block the lumen. This phenomenon is known as *margination* of the

white cells or *pavementation* of the endothelium. It has been observed that whereas a white cell will stick to endothelium in an area of damage, it will not, if it becomes detached, stick to normal endothelium. Thus the adherence is due to the endothelial change.

Change in the endothelium. Observation of the living tissue shows swelling of the endothelial cells. They appear to be covered by a gelatinous film representing either an exudation from the surface of the injured cells, or an extracellular precipitate such as fibrin. Polymorphs adhere to this damaged area, and also adhere to each other; platelets may also be trapped. An intravenous Indian-ink injection demonstrates this increased adhesiveness very beautifully, for the particles stick not only to the altered endothelium, but also to the polymorphs in the vicinity. However, electron microscopy of such vessels shows carbon particles deep to the endothelial cells (see later). There can be little doubt that there is a change in the blood-vessel lining in acute inflammation, but the nature of the "gelatinous layer" is obscure. A coating, probably of mucoprotein or mucopolysaccharide, has been reported, but most electron-microscopic studies have failed to show any extracellular material covering the endothelial cells. Whether this is due to faulty technique in the method of preparation, or whether the layer does not actually exist, is not definitely decided.

EXUDATION AND SWELLING

The most characteristic feature of acute inflammation in the higher animals is the formation of an exudate. While this usually has a cellular component, it is the exudation of fluid which is the constant feature.

The Fluid Exudate

The formation of the inflammatory exudate is dependent upon several changes. In the first place the arteriolar dilatation not only increases the flow of blood through the part, but also its pressure in the small vessels. The passage of fluid through the blood vessel walls is determined by the resultant of the hydrostatic and osmotic pressures acting upon it (Starling). These are summarised in Fig. 6.4 and described in detail in Chapter 39.

In acute inflammation the pressure in the capillaries even at the venous end may exceed the osmotic pressure of the plasma proteins, and therefore fluid will tend to pass into the tissue spaces. It must not be thought that Fig. 6.4 (*a*) represents the conditions in every capillary; it is known that while one group of vessels may be widely dilated and exuding fluid, another group is shut down. In this way currents of tissue fluid are created, and these may be important in the spread of infection (see p. 97). Furthermore, it must be remembered that the permeability of vessels varies considerably from one tissue to another. Thus the vessels of the brain and thymus are less permeable than those elsewhere. These differences in behaviour of capillaries are finding support from electron microscope studies, which show differences in structure. Fig. 6.4 (*a*) represents a simplification of the conditions which may be expected in an average capillary in a part at heart level.

From the onset, therefore, conditions favour the formation of interstitial fluid of normal low protein content and low specific gravity. However, in inflammation the exudate

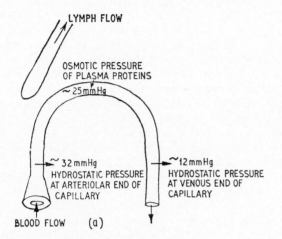

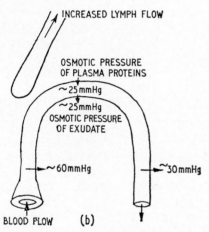

Figure 6.4
Fluid interchanges between blood and tissue spaces:
        (*a*) under normal conditions;
        (*b*) in acute inflammation.

differs from normal interstitial fluid; it has a very high protein content, its fibrinogen leads to clot formation, and it has a high specific gravity (over 1·020). Other important factors must therefore operate.

The crucial factor in the formation of an inflammatory exudate is an increased permeability of the vessel walls to plasma proteins. If trypan blue or pontamine sky blue is injected intravenously into an animal, the dye becomes bound to the plasma albumin and does not readily leave the circulation. When an inflammatory response is elicited, the tagged albumin can be seen to pass into the inflamed area as

the exudate forms. This experimental method is often used to demonstrate an increase in permeability to plasma protein. A similar type of labelling may be done with radioactive iodine.

The conditions in acute inflammation are shown in Fig. 6.4 (*b*). The exudate has virtually the same chemical composition as plasma, with the result that the osmotic effect of the plasma proteins is largely neutralised. In addition, the breakdown of large protein molecules into several smaller ones may further increase the osmotic pressure of the interstitial fluid. Finally, there is yet another factor which may play an important part; one of the first detectable changes in experimental acute inflammation is an alteration in the ground substance, which is rendered more fluid. The effect of this increased fluidity may well be to allow exudate to diffuse more readily, thereby preventing an immediate rise in tissue tension.

To summarise, the mechanisms in the production of the fluid exudate are therefore:

1. Increased vascular permeability to proteins.
2. Increased capillary blood pressure.
3. Breakdown of large-molecule tissue proteins.
4. Increased fluidity of the tissue ground substance.

Since by far the most important of these is the increased vascular permeability, it is not surprising that this has been most extensively studied. In experimentally produced acute inflammation, it has been found that *exudation of fluid occurs in two phases*,[6, 7] an early transient phase which is maximal at 8–10 minutes, and a prolonged delayed phase which requires several hours to develop (Fig. 6.5). The delayed phase may itself have several components. In mild thermal injury to the rat cremaster muscle, the immediate phase is

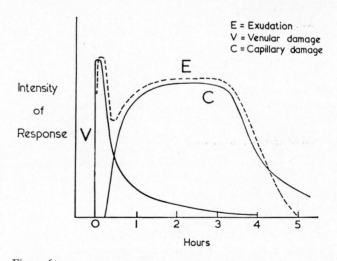

Figure 6.5
Multiphase vascular response to mild thermal injury (54 C for 40 min.) in rat cremaster muscle. *(From Miles, A. A.* (1966), In *Wound Healing*, p. 9, Fig. 4, ed. by C. Illingworth. London: Churchill)

accompanied by venular damage while the delayed response is related to capillary damage.[8] However, in turpentine injury to the rat pleura, both phases are due to venular damage and there is an additional capillary component to the delayed phase.[9] The precise response therefore depends upon the tissue involved, the irritant used, and the species of animal. There is evidence that the two phases are mediated by different agents, and this is described later in the section on chemical mediators.

Vascular permeability in normal tissues.[10] Normally the walls of the capillaries and venules are freely permeable to water and electrolytes but not to proteins and other large molecules. Rapid exchange takes place between intravascular and extravascular water, and in fact about 70 per cent of the water in the blood crosses the vessel wall every minute and is replaced by water from the interstitial space. The mechanism whereby this exchange takes place has been much debated. In most tissues the barriers which must be considered are:

1. The endothelial cell with its attenuated extensions.
2. The basement membrane, which forms a complete sheath.
3. Pericytes, which form a discontinuous outer coat together with connective tissue fibres.

The following possibilities have been suggested:

Direct transport through the cell by simple diffusion. The lipid (and presumably waterproof) nature of the cell membrane has led many authorities to regard this as an unlikely mechanism.

Transport across the endothelial cell by cytopempsis (p. 14). This process probably does take place, but it seems unlikely that it could explain the large volume of fluid which is known to cross the vessel walls. Furthermore, the vesicles formed by micropinocytosis would be expected to contain protein, whereas the fluid which escapes from the blood vessels has a low plasma protein content.

Passage through pores in the endothelial cells. Pores are present in the sinusoids of the liver; in certain other sites, e.g. kidney and intestine, there are fenestrations which are covered by a very thin membrane. In other areas no pores or fenestrations can be seen on electron microscopy.

Passage through spaces between the endothelial cells. The thick cement lines seen in silver-nitrate preparations of endothelium seem to be an artefact, for on electron microscopy the endothelial cells closely adjoin each other and the gap between them is about 15 nm wide. Junctional complexes are present, and in the zonula adherens the central fused membrane is about 4 nm thick. Pappenheimer and his associates have calculated that the properties of the normal vessel wall could be explained by the presence of circular pores with a radius of about 3 nm or slits about 3·7 nm wide.[11] As noted above, no such pores have been seen in the endothelial cells, but it is possible that the junctions between the cells could act as pores or slits. The relative importance of these possible methods of transport is not clear at the present time.

A final consideration concerns the basement membrane, for all substances leaving or entering the vessel must cross it. The membrane appears to have no holes nor does it seem to be a barrier to the passage of water or electrolytes. Cells, large particles, and perhaps the plasma proteins are held back and their passage delayed.

Vascular permeability in inflamed tissue. Examination of the endothelial cells of capillaries in acutely inflamed tissues has revealed several changes—increase in the number and size of the micropinocytotic vesicles, blebs under the luminal cell membrane, and projections or spikes arising from the membrane. The changes are, however, inconstant and seem inadequate to explain the great increase in vascular permeability. On the other hand, it has been shown that when 5-hydroxytryptamine or histamine is applied to rat cremaster muscle important changes occur in the venules. Gaps (0·1–0·4 μm in diameter) appear in the endothelial lining due to the separation of adjacent endothelial cells.[12, 13]

If the animal is first given an intravenous injection of mercuric sulphide suspension, the particles, which are 10–15 nm in diameter, are found to be situated between the endothelial cell and the basement membrane. It appears therefore that in acute inflammation the gap between endothelial cells widens, thereby allowing plasma to reach the basement membrane and escape to the extravascular spaces. The particles of mercuric sulphide being unable to penetrate the intact basement membrane accumulate between it and the endothelial cell (Fig. 6.6).

Similar results are obtained if Indian ink is used and trauma applied to produce an acute inflammation.[14–16] Thus, both the early exudation of acute inflammation and the application of histamine are associated with a separation of the endothelial cells and an escape of plasma. Whether other changes occur, for instance in the basement membrane, and whether the second phase of exudation is associated with other features, are not yet clear.

Function of the fluid exudate. All the constituents of the plasma are poured into the area of inflammation. These include natural antibacterial substances like opsonins and complement as well as specific immunoglobulins. Drugs and antibiotics, if present in the plasma, will also appear in the exudate. The importance of early administration of therapeutic agents is obvious when it is remembered that they are merely carried to the inflamed area in the exudate, and are in no way concentrated. The fluid of the exudate (*inflammatory oedema*) has the effect of diluting any irritant substance irrespective of its origin. Its high fibrinogen content often results in the formation of a fibrin clot. This fibrin has three main functions:

(1) It forms a union between severed tissues, as in a cut.
(2) It may form a barrier against bacterial invasion (p. 98).
(3) It aids phagocytosis (p. 77).

The exudate accounts in part for the remaining cardinal signs of inflammation. It causes swelling ("tumor"), and the

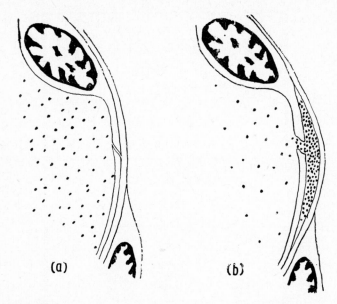

Figure 6.6
Diagrammatic representation of the changes in a venule following the intravenous injection of a suspension of mercuric sulphide (particle size 10–15 nm).

(a) Shows the wall of normal venule with the particles distributed in the plasma.

(b) After the local application of histamine. The appearances suggest that the plasma has leaked through the gap between the endothelial cells, and that the basement membrane has held back the particles but allowed the fluid exudate to pass through.

increased tissue pressure may be an important factor in the production of pain ("dolor") which itself limits activity. In fact, pain is often present before there is much swelling, and the effect of tissue tension on nerve endings cannot be the whole answer. The acid pH of the exudate, an accumulation of K^+ ions, and the presence of chemical mediators like 5-hydroxytryptamine and bradykinin have all been blamed.[17]

Changes in the lymphatics. The small lymphatics of a tissue form a blind-ended system of vessels, which closely resemble the vascular capillaries except that a basement membrane is incomplete or absent and their walls are permeable to proteins. One of their main functions is to allow any plasma protein which has escaped from the blood vessels to drain away and ultimately reach the blood stream again. In acute inflammation the lymph vessels are held widely open and the flow of fluid, containing excess protein, is greatly increased.

The Cellular Exudate

Not only does the vascular wall allow proteins to pass through, but soon the white cells also penetrate it. It has already been described how the white cells come to adhere passively to the sticky endothelium. From there they pass actively by amoeboid motion through the vessel wall. This process is called *emigration* of the white cells into the sur-

rounding tissues. Some authorities* describe this process as diapedesis of the white cells. However, we have followed the common English practice of confining the term diapedesis to the egress of the red cells.

As previously stated, the electron microscope has failed to identify any abnormality of the endothelial surface to account for this. The white cells adhere to the endothelium and push out pseudopodia. One of these enters the gap between two endothelial cells and forces it open. Having penetrated the endothelium, it may travel laterally before bursting through the basement membrane and finally the perivascular sheath.[18]

The first cells involved are the neutrophil polymorphs, and these take 2–9 minutes to penetrate the vessel wall. Later the monocytes predominate, and in the tissues these large cells become phagocytic and are called macrophages; lymphocytes have not yet been observed to migrate in acute inflammation. Some red cells may also escape from the vessels usually following a white cell. They merely spurt through

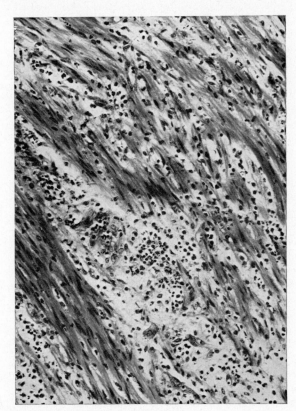

Figure 6.7
Acute inflammation in the muscular coat of the appendix. The muscle fibres are separated by the inflammatory exudate and there is a diffuse infiltration by polymorphs. × 150.

* See Adami, J. G. (1910). "The Principles of Pathology", vol. 1, p. 423, 2nd ed. Philadelphia: Lea and Febiger. Boyd, W. (1961). "A Textbook of Pathology", p. 37, 7th ed. London: Kimpton.

the defect created by the white cells, being ejected as the result of the hydrostatic pressure of the blood. This passive movement is called *diapedesis*, and is to be distinguished from the active emigration of the white cells. In primates organisms may adhere to red cells by the process of immune adherence (p. 148).

The emigration does not stop when the phagocytes have penetrated the vessel wall. The cells then move towards the damaged or infected area, and form a salient histological feature of many acute inflammatory responses (Fig. 6.7).

Chemotaxis.[19, 20] The directional movement of an organism in response to a chemical gradient is called chemotaxis and has been known for some time. The best known example is the attraction of the spermatozoids of the male fern by malic acid, which is present in the female germ cells. The accumulation of polymorphs in acutely inflamed tissues naturally raises the possibility that they are attracted there by some chemical influence. The Boyden chamber has facilated this study.[21] It consists of two tissue-culture chambers placed one on top of the other and separated by a membrane of 3 μm pore size. A suspension of polymorphs is placed in the upper chamber while the test substance is placed in the lower. The number of cells which migrate to the lower surface of the filter is a measure of the chemotactic effect (Fig. 6.8).

Both neutrophil polymorphs and monocytes have been shown to be attracted *in vitro* to a number of agents: these include starch and certain bacteria. Antigen-antibody complexes and dead tissue are chemotactic, but only if complement is activated. Three separate components are involved. One is a soluble activated product of the trimolecular complex termed C$\overline{567}$. The other two are small cleavage products of C3 and C5 which are designated C3a and C5a (see p. 162). Their role *in vivo* is not clear. Leukotaxine and nucleic-acid derivatives like adenosine and adenylic acid have been claimed to be chemotactic *in vivo*, but appear not to be so *in vitro*. The present evidence suggests that polymorphs are attracted to sites of inflammation by chemotactic agents, but the relative importance of the various factors is not known; it probably varies according to the cause of the inflammation.

With monocytes chemotaxis has also been demonstrated, and they appear to react to many of the substances which attract polymorphs. The change in the cells of the exudate from polymorphs in the early stages to monocytes later on has not been adequately explained. One explanation is that the polymorphs, which have only a short life-span, soon die and disappear. The long-lived monocytes remain, an effect that could be accentuated by the presence of migration inhibitory factor (p. 185). The relative number of monocytes would steadily increase. Another possibility is that the monocytes undergo division before assuming macrophage activity (p. 128).

A number of observations now suggest that some chemotactic agents are selective in their action. Thus, when sensi-

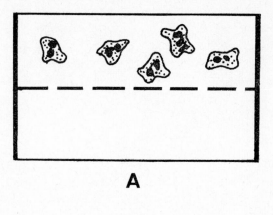

A

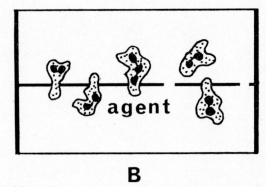

agent

B

Figure 6.8
The Boyden chamber consists of two tissue-culture chambers separated by a membrane of 3μm pore size. If the agent placed in the lower chamber is chemotactic, polymorphs present in the upper chamber migrate through the pores (B). See text.

tised lymphocytes react with antigen, factors called lymphokines are released (p. 149). Some of these are chemotactic agents, and it appears that separate agents affect polymorphs, monocytes, and eosinophils.[22] The reaction of antigen with IgE antibody has also been claimed to release a chemotactic agent for eosinophils, cells which are certainly a feature of human atopic diseases. The varied and changing population of inflammatory cells found in inflammatory disease would be more easily understood if selective chemotaxis were the mechanism. Hopefully future research will clarify this situation. One final point deserves consideration: so far no substance has been found to be chemotactic to lymphocytes. How they traverse the vessel wall and why, are questions which remain unanswered.

The most obvious function of the white cells in inflammation is phagocytosis. Both polymorphonuclears and macrophages may be seen to ingest foreign particles, bacteria, and cell debris.

Phagocytosis. *Opsonins.*[23] The ability of polymorphonuclears to ingest organisms can be tested *in vitro*. It is found that whereas commensals are easily ingested, the presence of serum is necessary before virulent organisms may be phagocytosed. The factor in serum which is necessary is a protein called an *opsonin*. One variety appears to be non-specific and has been called a "natural antibody". It requires the presence of complement, and may be of importance in the recognition and subsequent phagocytosis of foreign antigenic material.[24]

It has been found that some pathogens, usually those with capsules, e.g. pneumococci, are ingested only if specific antibodies are provided. These "immune opsonins" do not require complement, and they are a very important type of antibacterial antibody. It is believed that opsonins coat the surface of the organism, rendering it more readily acceptable to the phagocytes. The more virulent the organism, the more noxious are its surface antigens, and one can easily understand why only "tailor-made", or specific, antibodies are effective in promoting phagocytosis. Phagocytosis is therefore a pominent feature of inflammation occurring in an immune animal. Activation of complement is an important process in the mediation of phagocytosis. The activated trimolecular complex C567, when bound to cells, causes the immune adherence phenomenon and aids phagocytosis.

Opsonisation is also necessary for phagocytosis by cells of the reticulo-endothelial system, as is shown by experiments in which the liver is perfused with fluid containing organisms.[23]

The energy for phagocytosis both by polymorphs and macrophages is derived from anaerobic glycolysis. Phagocytosis of a particle is accompanied by the production of lactate[25] (see p. 96). In polymorphs there is also a dramatic increase in the activity of the hexose monophosphate shunt (Fig. 2.17). This results in the production of NADPH, which is involved in many metabolic reactions including the production of glutathione and hydroxen peroxide. Enzymatic defects in this pathway are associated with an increased susceptibility to infection with certain organisms (see p. 161).

Surface phagocytosis. Although opsonins facilitate the phagocytosis of pathogenic organisms, it has been found that, if a suitable framework is provided *in vitro*, e.g. a fibrin network, the polymorphonuclears may, by trapping an organism in a corner, be able to ingest it without its prior opsonisation. This phenomenon is known as *surface phagocytosis*,[26] and is of importance in the immunity to infection which animals exhibit during the early (and vital) few days before antibodies are produced. When organisms gain entry to an open area like the subarachnoid space, the outcome is more serious than when they infect a compact organ like the skin or lung.

Fate of ingested particles. Ingested material is enclosed in vacuoles, the membranes of which fuse with those of adjacent granules (lysosomes). In this way digestion vacuoles are formed, and the neutrophil becomes degranulated. It is not difficult to envisage how lysosomal enzymes could escape from the cell as lysosomal membranes fuse with those of phagosomes.[50] The cells also release pyrogen, and this is probably a factor in the pathogenesis of the fever which accompanies acute inflammation.[27]

Polymorphs have a short life span, 3–4 days at the most, and when they die, any particles which remain undigested are liberated into the intercellular spaces. Macrophages at this stage form a prominent feature of the exudate, and ingest particles, cell debris, etc. In contrast to the polymorphs they are long-lived, and those that have ingested insoluble particles remain in the tissues for long periods, possibly many years. This is well demonstrated in tattoos.

The fate of ingested organisms and the relationship between resistance to infection and the inflammatory response are considered in Chapter 8.

CHANGES IN OTHER TISSUE COMPONENTS IN ACUTE INFLAMMATION

One of the first changes in inflammation is loss of the specific granules of the tissue mast cells. Since these contain histamine and heparin, they may be a source of chemical mediators. Another early change is an increase in the fluidity of the ground substance.

LOCAL SEQUELAE OF ACUTE INFLAMMATION

The changes which occur following the formation of an acute inflammatory exudate depend upon two major factors:

1. The amount of tissue damage sustained.
2. Whether or not the causative agent remains.

Some agents, e.g. pyogenic bacteria and turpentine, regularly produce considerable destruction of the fixed tissues of an organ. Autolysis of these elements, together with the digestion produced by the ferments of polymorphs ("pus cells"), result in the production of a cavity containing *pus* (suppurative inflammation).

In all cases of acute inflammation, unless tissue death occurs, the initial polymorph exudate is later replaced by a mononuclear one, and this appearance heralds the onset of the demolition phase.

Demolition phase. Macrophages engulf fibrin, red cells, pus cells, foreign material, bacteria, etc. They therefore contain a variety of intracellular structures including fat, haemosiderin, cholesterol, and foreign material. Sometimes the macrophages fuse together to produce giant cells.

Origin of macrophages. The macrophages which accumulate in areas subjected to injury in lower forms of life appear to be derived from histiocytes, which are the resting tissue representatives of the reticulo-endothelial system. In mammals tissue histiocytes may also perform a similar function, but the current evidence suggests that the majority of macrophages present in the stage of demolition are the progeny of monocytes that emigrated from the blood stream. Labelling experiments indicate that monocytes can divide and assume the morphology of histiocytes, macrophages, and lymphocytes.[28] Reports that lymphocytes can change into macrophages may therefore be misleading. The cellular events in small experimental wounds in human skin have been studied by placing glass cover-slips over the wound and examining the cells adhering to the glass.[29] All stages in the transformation of small lymphocytes to macrophages have been described, but it seems unlikely that the cells described as small lymphocytes are the same as those present in the blood and thoracic-duct lymph. Lymphocytes do not readily adhere to glass, and it may well be that the small lymphocytes observed in these experiments are derived from monocytes. It must be concluded that the precise origin of macrophages, histiocytes, and lymphocytes is incompletely understood at the present time.

Resolution

In acutely inflamed tissue in which cellular damage has been relatively slight, the cellular and tissue changes are reversible, and necrosis does not occur. The demolition phase results in removal of the exudate, and the organ returns to normal. To this process the term *resolution* is applied, and one of the best examples is found in lobar pneumonia (see p. 225). *Resolution thus means the complete return to normal following acute inflammation.* Sometimes removal of the exudate appears to be delayed, and then the fibrin becomes invaded by granulation tissue. This sometimes complicates bronchopneumonia, and fibrosis is the result. It often occurs in the fibrinous exudate of inflamed serous cavities; in this manner fibrous adhesions are formed. The process whereby exudate becomes organised in the absence of tissue necrosis is sometimes called "incomplete resolution", but the term is not to be recommended.

It should be noted that while the demolition phase is proceeding, there is a reversed flow of exudate back into the capillaries. Most of the exudate, however, is carried by the lymphatics to the regional lymph nodes. The sinus lining cells remove cellular debris.

Suppuration

When the noxious agent produces much necrosis, resolution is impossible and the process proceeds to *suppuration*. This is typical of staphylococcal lesions, e.g. boils, but can also occur when the agent is a chemical substance, e.g. turpentine.

The first reaction is circumscribed necrosis accompanied by a profuse polymorph infiltration. The agent kills many of these leucocytes—which are called "pus cells" by histologists. The necrotic material undergoes softening by virtue of the proteolytic enzymes released by the dead leucocytes as well as through the autolysis mediated by the tissue's own cathepsins. The resulting fluid material is called *pus* and is contained within a cavity to form an *abscess*. This is lined by a wall, or *pyogenic membrane*, which at first consists of acutely inflamed tissue heavily infiltrated with polymorphs. The copious fibrinous exudate is soon organised into granulation tissue.

The pus itself is made up of (*a*) dead and dying leucocytes, (*b*) other components of the inflammatory exudate—oedema fluid and fibrin, (*c*) organisms, many of which are living and can therefore be cultured. If the pus is chemically induced it is sterile, and (*d*) tissue debris, e.g. nucleic acids and lipids.

The pus tends to track in the line of least resistance until a free surface is reached. Then the abscess bursts and discharges its contents spontaneously—in clinical practice this is usually anticipated by surgical drainage. An abscess when drained heals by repair, but sometimes chronic inflammation ensues due to persisting infection. In this event a chronic abscess results; its wall is composed of fibrous tissue heavily infiltrated by a pleomorphic collection of cells, including polymorphs, macrophages, lymphocytes, and plasma cells. A large quantity of pus is produced, and is discharged through a *sinus* to the exterior or into some hollow viscus.

If, as occasionally happens, the abscess is not drained and remains sequestrated in the tissues, its walls become organised into dense fibrous tissue and the pus undergoes thickening, or inspissation, as the watery part is gradually absorbed. In due course it becomes of porridge-like consistency, and may eventually become *calcified*.

When an acute suppurative inflammation involves an epithelial surface, the covering is destroyed and an *ulcer* is formed. The floor is composed of necrotic tissue and acute inflammatory exudate; this layer of dead tissue forms the *slough*, and is at first adherent because the dead material has not been liquefied. Eventually, however, the slough becomes detached and the ulcer heals by the processes of repair and regeneration, as described in Chapter 9.

Chronic Inflammation

The other sequel of acute inflammation is progression to a state of chronic inflammation, in which the inflammatory and healing processes proceed side by side. This is described

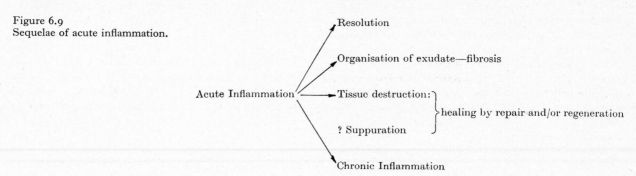

Figure 6.9
Sequelae of acute inflammation.

in Chapter 11. It is worth noting that much chronic inflammation is the result of suppuration which has not been adequately drained. The slough (or sequestrum in osteomyelitis) provides a nidus in which the causative organisms can continue to flourish. Until adequate drainage is provided, there can be no hope of terminating the infection.

Sterile chemical abscesses do not undergo this progressive course. The process is necessarily self-limiting, and apart from the effect of local tissue destruction, there are no permanent sequelae.

THE CHEMICAL MEDIATORS OF ACUTE INFLAMMATION[30-32]

Of all the changes in acute inflammation those affecting the vessels are the most striking. In addition to vasodilatation, the endothelium of the small vessels undergoes changes which not only make it sticky, but also render it more permeable both to blood cells and plasma proteins. These alterations are not solely dependent upon the stretching of the vessel walls consequent on dilatation, for they are not seen in the hyperaemia that accompanies increased tissue activity. Neither are they directly related to the injury itself, as suggested by Cohnheim, for they may extend beyond the area involved (see triple response, p. 7). The most likely explanation for the vasodilatation and the other vascular changes is that they are caused by some chemical mediator. Since the vascular phenomena of acute inflammation are very similar irrespective of the cause, the most likely source of any mediators is the damaged tissue itself.

Sir Thomas Lewis, under the influence of Sir Henry Dale, suggested that *histamine* was an important chemical mediator of the inflammatory response. The first to demonstrate that other factors were also involved was Menkin. The *leukotaxine* which he isolated was later shown by Spector to consist of a mixture of polypeptides. A very potent pure polypeptide, *bradykinin*, was discovered by Rocha e Silva, but whether it is an important factor in inflammation is undecided. It can be generated from plasma by the action of a variety of *kinin-forming enzymes*. One such enzyme is *kallikrein*, which occurs in the blood in an inactive form. Meanwhile it has been found that two other proteolytic enzymes can be formed in the blood. These too may produce vasoactive protein-digestion products. The enzymes are *plasmin* and the *globulin permeability factor*.

Substances which have been claimed to act as chemical mediators may be divided into the following groups:

I. Amines   (a) histamine.
                 (b) 5-hydroxytryptamine (5-HT).
II. The kinins.
III. Kinin-forming
     enzymes   (a) kallikrein.
                 (b) the globulin permeability factor.
                 (c) plasmin.

IV. Biologically active products of the complement system.
V. Biologically active components of polymorphs.
VI. Prostaglandins.
VII. Nucleic acids and breakdown products.
VIII. Others.

The Amines

Histamine. The classical experiments of Lewis on the triple response showed that injury to the skin produced a type of inflammation which had many features in common with the effect of an injection of histamine. Lewis showed that injured skin released some substance ("H" substance) which behaved like histamine.

When histamine is injected into the skin, a bright flare develops and gradually fades. The following ingenious experiment was performed to show that both histamine and "H" substance behave similarly. The circulation to one arm was obstructed, histamine injected, and eleven minutes later the tourniquet was released. The other arm was treated similarly except that the injection was given one minute before releasing the circulation. In both arms the flare developed and faded at the same rate. This experiment indicated that histamine could be retained in the tissues while the circulation was obstructed.

The experiment was repeated except that firm stroking was substituted for the histamine injection. On releasing the tourniquets both arms again developed a flare which faded simultaneously. Lewis concluded from this experiment that injury released a histamine-like substance which produced the flare.

For a time it was accepted that histamine was the most important mediator of the vascular response in acute inflammation. Most workers have been able to identify it in inflammatory exudates, in extracts of inflamed tissues, and in the perfusate of inflamed parts. Further investigation has, however, not confirmed this belief.

(1) Tissues tend to become refractory to continued injections of histamine: the vasodilatation in infection is long-lasting.

(2) Antihistamines only inhibit the very early vascular response to tissue injury. However, antihistamines do not completely abolish the action of known histamine releasers like compound 48/80, and it seems likely that locally-formed histamine may act even when antihistamines are given. Antihistamines are more effective in counteracting inflammation in hypersensitive states. Additional work on turpentine inflammation in the pleural cavity of rats has shown that antihistamines reduce the volume of exudate during the first 30 minutes, but not thereafter. The prior administration of histamine-depleting drugs has the same effect.

Thus, there is good evidence that histamine is liberated in acute inflammation, and that it can mimic some of the vascular events. It seems likely that it is important during the early phase, in initiating the axon reflex, and in certain hypersensitivity reponses (see p. 178).

The actual *mode of formation of histamine* is not known for certain. Although the further breakdown of protein and polypeptides could lead to its production, there is no evidence that this actually occurs. The speed with which histamine appears in acute inflammation suggests that it is liberated either from some more immediate precursor or else from a bound form. It is known that mast cells contain a large quantity of histamine, and it has been suggested that it is held in a loose combination with the basic heparin which these cells also contain.

5-Hydroxytryptamine (5-HT, or serotonin).[33] A smooth muscle contracting substance is found in the early inflammatory exudate of experimentally produced turpentine pleurisy in the rat. It appears that in this species 5-HT rather than histamine is liberated during the early phase of acute inflammation; on theoretical grounds 5-HT could be liberated from mast cells or platelets. It causes either vasodilatation or vasoconstriction, depending both upon the species and its concentration.

Adrenaline and noradrenaline. These substances and their precursors dopamine and DOPA reduce the increased vascular permeability of acute inflammation. They are degraded by the enzyme monoamine oxidase, and an increase in the activity of this enzyme in acute inflammation may release the vessels from the inhibiting effect of this group of amines. This mechanism is probably not of great importance in the pathogenesis of acute inflammation.

The Kinins[34]

The name kinin has been applied to a variety of physiologically-active polypeptides which cause contraction of smooth muscle. One of the first was substance P. *Bradykinin*, so named because of the slow contraction which it induces in the muscle of the guinea-pig ileum, appears to be the active agent in producing the effects of poisoning due to certain snakebites.[35] It may also be concerned in the regulation of blood flow in the salivary glands. This same kinin is formed when human saliva acts upon blood proteins, thereby revealing an unexpected relationship between human saliva and snake venom. Similar substances have been identified from other sources—kallidin, plasma kinin, pain-producing substance, and urinary kinin. It is probable that some, if not all, of these substances are identical. Bradykinin, a nonapeptide, has been synthesised, and is ten times more active as a vasodilator than is histamine (on a molar basis). It is almost certainly the same as pain-producing substance, and is formed in the plasma by the action of plasma kallikrein (see below). Kallidin is a decapeptide, lysyl-bradykinin, and is formed when pancreatic kallikrein acts on plasma. The hormones of the posterior pituitary, oxytocin and vasopressin, both come within this group of physiologically-active polypeptides. Wasp venom contains another kinin.

The part played by these kinins in inflammation is not yet defined. They are capable of causing vasodilatation, increasing venular permeability, and causing pain. It has been suggested that they are responsible for the important prolonged second phase of increased vascular permeability in inflammation, but this seems unlikely, for, as with histamine, tissues become refractory to the action of kinins.

Leukotaxine (or Leucotaxine). In 1936 Menkin[36] described a substance, leukotaxine, which he had isolated from an inflammatory exudate. He found that it was a pure crystalline polypeptide of low molecular weight, and that its main actions were to increase vascular permeability and to attract white cells. The purity of this substance has been questioned, for it now seems evident that it is a mixture of polypeptides and not a single pure substance.

The Kinin-Forming Enzymes

*Kallikrein.** Kallikrein[37, 38] is an enzyme which can form a powerful vasoactive plasma kinin (bradykinin) from an α_2-globulin in the blood. The enzyme exists as a precursor (kallikreinogen, or prekallikrein) which can be activated by an agent called prekallikrein-activator, which itself exists as a precursor (see Fig. 6.10). Kallikrein is one example of a group

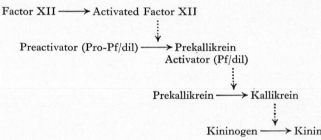

Figure 6.10
Series of proposed interdependent reactions involved in the *in-vivo* generation of kinin. See also Fig. 6.11.

of enzymes which forms kinins from plasma; they occur in blood, urine, pancreas, and snake venom. A number of kallikrein inhibitors are known. One is an α_2-macroglobulin,

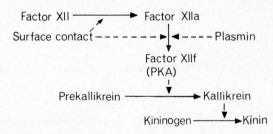

Figure 6.11.
The current hypothesis for the *in-vivo* activation of the kinin system. PKA = Prekallikrein activator

*Kallikrein is so called because it is found in high concentration in pancreas. *Kallikreas* is Greek for pancreas.

another is the Cl-esterase inhibitor, while a third is α_1-antitrypsin.*

The globulin permeability factor. That normal plasma contains a system of permeability factors was first demonstrated by Miles.[39] It was found that normal serum contained a globulin pro-permeability factor which could be activated simply by diluting the serum with saline. Hence it is called Pf/dil. In fact, it is the contact with glass, by activating Clotting Factor XII, which is important. Pf/dil has a powerful action in increasing vascular permeability, and a similar, if not identical, substance has been found in the inflammatory exudate of experimental turpentine pleurisy in rats.

For a while it seemed likely that pro-Pf/dil was identical to the precursor of prekallikrein activator, and that Pf/dil was the same as the prekallikrein activator. The sequential activation of Hageman factor (Clotting Factor XII) prekallikrein activator, and kallikrein appeared to be the mechanism whereby kinin was formed in acute inflammation (Fig. 6.10).

The role of Pf/dil has now been questioned. Prekallikrein activator is believed to be Factor XIIf, which is a fragment of Factor XIIa. It is formed on surface contact and also by the action of plasmin (Fig. 6.11). Pf/dil has never been isolated in a chemically pure form, and it is possible that it represents a mixture of several kinin-forming substances, including Factor XII, plasmin, and kallikrein.

Plasmin.[37] Plasminogen is a normal component of the plasma proteins. It can be converted into plasmin ("activated") by an activator which exists normally as a precursor ("proactivator"). This is described in Chapter 51.

Plasmin itself is a proteolytic enzyme, and digests fibrin as well as other plasma proteins. Plasmin can increase vascular permeability in many ways. It can act directly on kininogen to liberate kinin; this action is slow compared with that of kallikrein. Secondly, it can activate prekallikrein to kallikrein. Finally, it can act on the third component of complement to produce C3a and on Factor XIIa to produce Factor XIIf.

Other proteolytic enzymes have also been described. One is present in skin but its role in acute inflammation is unknown.[37]

BiologicallyActive Cleavage Products of Complement

Activation of the complement system leads to the formation of two anaphylatoxins, C3a and C5a, which cause the release of histamine from mast cells. They also exert a chemotactic influence, as does C567 (p. 76). These components are important in the pathogenesis of aggregate anaphylaxis and in the inflammation present in some lesions of immune-complex disease (p. 182). The alternate pathway of complement activation explains how vasoactive complement components can be formed following tissue damage

---

* The physiological role of these inhibitors is unclear. Patients deficient in Cl-esterase inhibitor are subject to attacks of angio-oedema. Subjects deficient in α_1-antitrypsin are liable to develop hepatic fibrosis in infancy or pulmonary emphysema in adult life.

which is not immunologically mediated. Necrotic tissue e.g. heart muscle,[40] can release enzymes capable of activating C3, and so also can the lysosomal enzymes released from polymorphs. What part they play in inflammation in the non-immune animal and that due to trauma is not known.

Biologically Active Components of Polymorphs

Neutrophils release a variety of agents in acute inflammation. Some are lysosomal enzymes and are credited with the damage which occurs in the Shwartzman reaction and in the vasculitis of immune-complex disease. The activation of kallikrein and the effect on the complement system has already been mentioned. Another permeability factor released by polymorphs during phagocytosis is a group of basic proteins with molecular weights ranging from 6 000 to 12 000. These may act by causing disruption of mast cells and the release of histamine. Lysosomal cathepsins can release kinin from kininogen, but the action is even slower than that of plasmin. Release of SRS-A (p. 178) has also been noted. It is evident than the role of the polymorphs in acute inflammation is very complex. Certainly, under some circumstances, infection introduced into animals rendered leucopenic can be spreading and lethal while a similar infection in a normal animal would lead merely to a local acute inflammation.

The Prostaglandins.[41]

The name prostaglandin was given to a substance found in human seminal fluid by von Euler. The prostaglandins are now known to form a group of at least thirteen chemically related long-chain fatty acid derivatives of prostanoic acid, the 20-carbon parent substance. They are credited with many diverse functions—from acting as chemical transmitters in the nervous system to playing an important role in conception and parturition. They have been isolated in the tissues of human skin in allergic contact dermatitis[42] as well as from inflammatory lesions produced in animals. They may therefore be significant mediators of inflammation.[43] The source of these prostaglandins is not known for certain, but human platelets contain prostaglandin-forming enzymes, and it may be of significance that indomethacin and aspirin both inhibit the formation of prostaglandins from the substrate arachidonic acid.[44] Prostaglandins together with the polymorph lysosomal components are the possible mediators of the delayed second phase of acute inflammation.

Nucleic Acid and Breakdown Products

Many nucleic acid derivatives have been found in inflammatory exudates and perfused tissues. The nucleoside inosine and the nucleotide inosinic acid are both histamine-releasing substances, and they increase vascular permeability. On the other hand, others like adenosine are also active, but are not histamine-releasers.[45] Although present in inflammation, these substances have not actually been shown to be responsible for any phenomena that occur.

Other Possible Mediators of the Inflammatory Response

Menkin in addition to describing leukotaxine (1936) has claimed to have isolated many other active compounds from inflammatory exudate. These may be listed as follows: Leucocytosis-promoting factors and leucopenia factors in both alkaline and acid exudates, necrosin, pyrexin, exudin, and growth promoting and retarding factors. These claims have been neither substantiated nor completely refuted by other investigators. In general, the substances which Menkin claims to have found have not been either well described or identified chemically, and the validity of the biological test systems which show their presence has been questioned. His "exudin" is probably the same as Pf/dil. Another feature emphasised by Menkin is the change of pH of inflammatory exudate which he claims alters the type of cell involved in the exudate. This has not met with general acceptance. *Lactic acid* present in inflamed tissue may, however, play a part in the vasodilatation and change in permeability.

It is possible that some *bacterial toxins* are capable of directly initiating or modifying the inflammatory response. The gas-gangrene organisms, in particular *Cl. oedematiens*, produce toxins which appear to act directly upon blood vessels and increase their permeability. The kinases produced by some organisms, and wasp and snake venom are other examples of exogenous factors.

Extracts of various tissues[46] and a *slow-reacting substance*[47] have also been investigated in the search for chemical mediators in inflammation.

Summary

Although numerous pharmacologically-active agents have been identified in inflammatory exudates, proof that any one of them is actually responsible for any of the phenomena of inflammation is lacking. The reasons for this may be considered under two headings.

Difficulty in identifying the agent. Often the only available methods for identification and estimation are biological. In complex biological mixtures results obtained by these methods may be misleading: several substances may cause the same response in the test system. For instance, both histamine and 5-HT can be estimated by their ability to cause contraction of the smooth muscle of the gut. Recognition of their separate identities may be attempted by testing the additional effect of antihistamine or anti-5-HT

agents. Herein lies a danger, for the action of these agents is not always specific.

Many agents have probably been given different names by separate workers. This is well illustrated by the multitude of names applied to the "kinins".

Failure in correlation between the agent and the effect which it is claimed to produce. Ideally the concentration of the agent should parallel the observed effect under standard conditions. Blocking drugs should not only antagonise the agent, but also inhibit the actions which it is alleged to mediate, in inflammations of a variety of different aetiologies.

There are two major phases in the exudation of acute inflammation.[48] Histamine (and in some species 5-HT) is important in the early phase. The more significant and prolonged secondary phase probably involves a variety of mediators, and it is in this latter group that the greatest confusion exists regarding both the relative importance and the individual identities of the many factors which have been isolated. None of the mediators so far investigated has been proven to play a dominant role in the second phase of acute inflammation. Indeed, it is possible that the increased vascular permeability in the second phase, which involves capillaries as well as venules (whose permeability is essentially affected by chemical mediators), may be the result of the delayed effect of the local injury itself on the vessel wall rather than be due to a mediator.[49]

Although much stress has been placed upon the uniformity of the inflammatory reaction regardless of its cause, it must not be forgotten that there is, in fact, also very considerable individual diversity, both in the amount of exudate and in the type of cell involved. This was stressed by Kettle who recognised that the individuality of an inflammatory reaction was a reflection of the individuality of the agent causing it. It would be hard to deny the importance of many bacterial products; the leucocidins, haemolysins, kinases, permeability factors, etc., must all influence the final outcome. Products of tissue breakdown are not the only agents present in the inflammation of infection. So far, much research has been done on the vasodilatation and increased vascular permeability of acute inflammation caused by trauma or chemical agents. The complex cellular changes and the intricacies of infection have been largely neglected. Until we have much more reliable information, the role of the individual chemical mediators in acute inflammation will remain ambiguous.

GENERAL READING

COHNHEIM, J. (1889). In *Lectures on General Pathology*, p. 248. London: New Sydenham Society. (This is a translation of the 2nd edn of Cohnheim's book published in 1882.)

CURRAN, R. C. (1967). In *Modern Trends in Pathology*, **2,** p. 40. Edited by T. Crawford. London: Butterworths.

FLOREY, H. W. (1970). In *General Pathology*, 4th edn, p. 22 *et seq.* Edited by H. W. Florey. London: Lloyd-Luke.

MILES, A. A. (1958–59). In *Lectures on the Scientific Basis of Medicine*, vol. 8, p. 198. London: Athlone Press.

MOVAT, H. Z. (1971). (Ed) *Inflammation, Immunity and Hypersensitivity*. New York: Harper and Row.

ROBB-SMITH, A. H. T. (1957). *Lancet*, i, 699.

ZWEIFACH, B. W., GRANT, L. and McCLUSKEY, R. T. (1965). (Eds) *The Inflammatory Process*, p. 931. New York and London: Academic Press.

REFERENCES

1. RATHER, L. J. (1971). *Bulletin of the New York Academy of Medicine*, **47**, 303.
2. PALMER, J. F. (1835). In *The Works of John Hunter, F.R.S.*, vol. 1, p. 393. London: Longmans.
3. LEWIS, T. (1927). *The Blood Vessels of the Human Skin and their Responses.* London: Shaw and Sons Ltd.
4. LEWIS, T. and GRANT, R. T. (1924). *Heart*, **11**, 209.
5. ADAMI, J. G. (1909). *Inflammation.* London: Macmillan.
6. SEVITT, S. (1958). *Journal of Pathology and Bacteriology*, **75**, 27.
7. MILES, A. A. (1966). In *Wound Healing*, p. 3. Edited by C. Illingworth. London: Churchill.
8. WELLS, F. R. and MILES, A. A. (1963). *Nature*, **200**, 1015.
9. HURLEY, J. V. and SPECTOR, W. G. (1965). *Journal of Pathology and Bacteriology*, **89**, 245.
10. DAVSON, H. (1970). *A Textbook of General Physiology*, 4th edn, p. 526. London: Churchill.
11. PAPPENHEIMER, J. R. (1953). *Physiological Reviews*, **33**, 387.
12. MAJNO, G. and PALADE, G. E. (1961). *Journal of Biophysical and Biochemical Cytology*, **11**, 571.
13. MAJNO, G., PALADE, G. E. and SCHOEFL, G. I. (1961). *Journal of Biophysical and Biochemical Cytology*, **11**, 607.
14. MARCHESI, V. T. (1962). *Proceedings of the Royal Society*, B, **156**, 550.
15. PAPPAS, G. D. and TENNYSON, V. M. (1962). *Journal of Cell Biology*, **15**, 227.
16. MOVAT, H. Z. and FERNANDO, N. V. P. (1963). *Laboratory Investigation*, **12**, 895.
17. KEELE, C. A. and ARMSTRONG, D. (1964). *Substances Producing Pain and Itch*, p. 268. London: Arnold.
18. FLOREY, H. W. and GRANT, L. H. (1961). *Journal of Pathology and Bacteriology*, **82**, 13.
19. HARRIS, H. (1954). *Physiological Reviews*, **34**, 529.
20. HARRIS, H. (1960). *Bacteriological Review*, **24**, 3.
21. BOYDEN, S. (1962). *Journal of Experimental Medicine*, **115**, 453.
22. WARD, P. A., REMOLD, H. G. and DAVID, J. R. (1969). *Science*, **163**, 1079.
23. HOWARD, J. H. (1963). In *Modern Trends in Immunology*, vol. 1, p. 86. Edited by R. Cruickshank. London: Butterworths.
24. BOYDEN, S. V. (1966). *Advances in Immunology*, **5**, 1.
25. KARNOVSKY, M. L. (1962). *Physiological Reviews*, **42**, 143.
26. WOOD, W. B. (1960). *Bacteriological Reviews*, **24**, 41.
27. BERLIN, R. D. and WOOD, B.W. (1964). *Journal of Experimental Medicine*, **119**, 715.
28. SPECTOR, W. G. (1966). In *Wound Healing*, p. 17, *loc. cit.*
29. REBUCK, J. W. and CROWLEY, J. H. (1955). *Annals of the New York Academy of Sciences*, **59**, 757.
30. Various Authors. (1964). Acute inflammatory response, *Annals of the New York Academy of Sciences*, **116**, 747–1083.
31. MELMON, K. L. and CLINE, M. J. (1967). In *Symposium on Vaso-Active Polypeptides : Bradykinin and Related Kinins, Proceedings of the Third International Pharmacological Congress.* Edited by M. Rocha e Silva. Oxford: Pergamon Press.
32. HERSH, E. M. and BODEY, G. P. (1970). *Annual Review of Medicine*, **21**, 105.
33. CAMPBELL, A. C. P. (1959). In *Modern Trends in Pathology*, p. 231. Edited by D. H. Collins. London: Butterworths.
34. KELLERMEYER, R. W. and GRAHAM, R. C. (1968). *New England Journal of Medicine*, **279**, 754, 802 and 859.
35. ROCHA E SILVA, M., BERALDO, W. T. and ROSENFELD, G. (1949). *American Journal of Physiology*, **156**, 261.
36. MENKIN, V. (1956). *Biochemical Mechanisms in Inflammation*, 2nd edn. Springfield: Thomas.
37. LEWIS, G. P. (1960). *Physiological Reviews*, **40**, 647.
38. ELLIOTT, D. F. (1963). *Annals of the New York Academy of Sciences*, **104**, 35.
39. MILES, A. A. and WILHELM, D. L. (1955). *British Journal of Experimental Pathology*, **36**, 71.
40. HILL, J. H. and WARD, P. A. (1971). *Journal of Experimental Medicine*, **133**, 885.
41. Leading Article (1971). *British Medical Journal*, iii, **61**.
42. GREAVES, M. W., SØNDERGAARD, J. and McDONALD-GIBSON, W. (1971). *British Medical Journal*, ii, 258.
43. MARX, J. L. (1972). *Science*, **177**, 780.
44. VANE, J. R. (1971). *Nature, New Biology*, **231**, 232 and see also 235 and 237.
45. SPECTOR, W. G. and WILLOUGHBY, D. A. (1957). *Journal of Pathology and Bacteriology*, **73**, 133.
46. WILLOUGHBY, D. A. and SPECTOR, W. G. (1964). *Journal of Pathology and Bacteriology*, **88**, 557.
47. SPECTOR, W. G. and WILLOUGHBY, D. A. (1962). *Journal of Pathology and Bacteriology*, **84**, 391.
48. BURKE, J. F. and MILES, A. A. (1958). *Journal of Pathology and Bacteriology*, **76**, 1.
49. HURLEY, J. V. (1972). *Acute Inflammation*, 144 pp. Edinburgh and London: Churchill Livingstone.
50. WEISSMANN, G. *et al.* (1971). Journal of Experimental Medicine, **134**, 149s.

Chapter 7. The Body's Defences Against Infection

Micro-organisms can cause disease in two ways. Either they gain access to the tissues of the host, multiply and cause infection, or they manufacture powerful toxins which are subsequently introduced into the body and produce an intoxication.

Diseases caused by ingestion of preformed toxin need not be considered here in detail. Botulism and staphylococcal enterotoxic food poisoning provide typical examples; neither can be considered as bacterial infections any more than can ergotism be regarded as a fungous infection.

By far the most important method whereby micro-organisms cause disease is by their invasion of and *multiplication in the living tissues of the host*. This is the definition of *infection*, and organisms capable of producing it are termed *pathogens*. With the exception of some rare congenital conditions, all infection is derived from the external environment. The organisms may be injected directly into the host, but more usually they are first deposited on the surface of the body which is thereby contaminated. Infection may or may not follow.

Transmission of Organisms to the Body

The following modes of transmission are important:

Direct skin contact. Wound infection caused by soil or by the contact of a staphylococcal carrier is a most important example; so also are the venereal diseases, e.g. syphilis and gonorrhoea. Contaminated air is important in causing wound infections in hospitals.

Inhalation of droplets and dust.[1] It is generally assumed that influenza, whooping-cough, the common virus diseases of childhood, meningococcal infections, diphtheria, and streptococcal sore throat are spread by droplet infection. Experimental findings have not entirely supported this belief.

Droplets are produced when air passing rapidly over a mucous membrane causes atomisation of the secretion which covers it. A few of these droplets are large (Flugge droplets), and due to the effect of gravity have a limited range. The vast majority are smaller than 100μm in diameter, and dry up almost instantaneously to form droplet nuclei which stay suspended in the air for many hours.

Droplet formation occurs during talking, coughing, and particularly sneezing; the main source is from the *saliva in the front of the mouth*. Only during snorting is the nose an important source of droplets. The viruses of mumps, measles, smallpox, and chickenpox are found in the saliva, and these diseases may well be spread in this way. However, bacteria residing in the nose (*Staph. pyogenes*), nasopharynx (*Strept. pyogenes*), or lung (tubercle bacilli) do not commonly reach the front of the mouth, and it is very unlikely that droplets are an important vehicle of their spread. Some may be expectorated as sputum, but the most important means of dissemination is by the fingers and handkerchief. Using fluorescein or test organisms as markers, it has been found that normal human beings frequently dispense nasal secretions and saliva to their hands, face, and clothing, and to every object that is touched. After desiccation the organisms are readily disseminated in the form of dust particles, and it is these which are important in the transmission of many infections.

Ingestion of contaminated food. Food may be contaminated by a human carrier, e.g. typhoid, or by flies. These insects carry many pathogenic organisms on their hairy legs. Diseases transmitted by food include typhoid fever, bacillary dysentery, and amoebiasis. Poliomyelitis and infective hepatitis are acquired by ingestion. Milk and eggs may contain bacteria because the animal itself is diseased, e.g. bovine tuberculosis, brucellosis, and *Salmonella* infections of fowls.

Inoculation. The agent may be an insect whose bite transmits pathogenic organisms, e.g. arboviruses, *Y. (Past.) pestis*, and rickettsiae, or it may be a needle contaminated with the virus of serum hepatitis.

Transplacental spread. This occurs in secondary syphilis, toxoplasmosis, *Listeria monocytogenes* infection, and also some virus diseases (see p. 279). Disease produced by the infection of a germ-cell before fertilisation is not recorded in human pathology.

Contamination

This is the transfer of organisms on to any object. It may be a surgical instrument, clothing, food, or a body surface.

The contamination of the body, both externally on the skin and internally in the intestinal, respiratory, and other tracts in inevitable, and many of these surfaces are habitually colonised by organisms of low-grade pathogenicity, e.g. *Staph. albus* in the skin and *Strept. viridans* in the mouth and throat. Such organisms are called *commensals*, or "resident flora", and as will be shown later, play an important role in the decontamination of these surfaces against pathogenic organisms. Contamination with virulent organisms is certainly a common event, but infection is rare. Whether contamination with a particular pathogen is followed by infection is dependent upon:

1. *The mechanical integrity* of the body surface.
2. Its powers of removing organisms, i.e. its *powers of decontamination*.

These protective mechanisms vary greatly from one tissue to another, and each will therefore be considered separately.

THE SKIN

The skin is frequently contaminated, and its value as a protective coat ranks second only to its water-retaining properties. Its exposed position renders it liable to both major and minor physical trauma. Its protective function is carried out mainly by the epidermis, and indeed the inability of the subepithelial tissues to resist infection was one of the limiting factors in pre-Listerian surgery. Its defences are:

Mechanical Strength

The many layers of epithelial cells, the tough outer layer of keratin, and the distinct basement membrane all play a part. If this mechanical barrier is impaired, infection is almost inevitable. Excessive sweating may macerate the keratin layer; for this reason skin infections are very common in the tropics, and boils are frequently seen in moist areas like the axillae.

Intact skin appears to be completely impervious to invasion by organisms, and it is only after injury that infection can be established. Even in vaccination minor trauma by pressure is necessary for a successful infection. Following trauma the skin becomes the portal of entry for staphylococci, streptococci, and the clostridia. In the tropics insect bites penetrate the skin barrier, and serve to introduce the causative agents of plague, typhus, yellow fever, malaria, dengue, etc.

Decontamination[2]

The powers of decontamination of the skin may be demonstrated by deliberately contaminating the hands with haemolytic streptococci, and estimating their rate of disappearance by subsequently taking swabs at regular intervals. It is found that the organism can no longer be recovered after 2–3 hours.[3] The actual time taken for the skin to rid itself of organisms depends upon the organism concerned, and in some cases is as short as 10 minutes.[4, 5] The mechanisms involved may be considered under three headings—mechanical, biological, and chemical:

Mechanical. *Desquamation* of the surface squames removes some superficial organisms.

Desiccation is probably of some importance in destroying organisms on the surface of the skin.

Biological. Organisms normally present on the skin constitute the *resident flora*. These include *Staph. albus*, diphtheroids, sarcinae, and aerobic sporing bacilli. In addition about 25 per cent of people harbour *Staph. pyogenes*

particularly on the hands, face, and perineum. It is impossible to remove the resident organisms from the skin; they survive in the gland ducts, and though the surface may be disinfected, the organisms are soon replaced. It is probable that the flora plays an important part in the decontaminating mechanism both by producing antibiotic substances and by competing with other organisms for essential foodstuffs.

Chemical. *Acidity of sweat.*[2] The sweat is normally acid and is unsuitable for the growth of most pathogens The bactericidal activity is probably due to its lactic acid content. If sweating is induced, the pH is said to fall, and may at times be as low as 3. There are certain gaps in this acid coat: these are the alkaline areas where infection is quite common, e.g. axillae, groins, and interdigital clefts of the toes.

Unsaturated fatty acids. These are present in the sebaceous secretion and are bactericidal; it is interesting that some of the diphtheroids grow only in the presence of these fatty acids, so well are they adapted to their environment.[6]

There is no doubt that the mechanical strength together with the decontaminating mechanisms are of great importance in maintaining the integrity of the skin. When one remembers how often it must be contaminated with all types of organisms, and, apart from staphylococci, how rarely it is invaded, one appreciates its efficiency as a protective coat.

THE ALIMENTARY TRACT

The Mouth and Throat

As with the skin the defence mechanism is two-fold:

Mechanical strength. The toughness and integrity of the mucous membrane is important; this mechanical barrier is weakest at two points:

The gingival margin has only a thin epithelium, and is therefore easily traumatised. This is particularly so in the interdental region, where it is believed that a covering epithelium is present only in young healthy adults.[7]

The tonsillar crypts. Here the epithelium is very thin; it has been shown that carmine powder dusted on to the tonsils appears in the underlying cells and connective tissue within 20 minutes.[8, 9] Probably the dye is transported there by phagocytes which are normally resident on the surface. Organisms may similarly reach the subepithelial tissue, and it is therefore these two sites, the tonsils and the gum margins, that are the places where infection occurs when the general body defences are impaired, e.g. in acute leukaemia and agranulocytosis. Nevertheless, it is remarkable how the tissues of the mouth, including the bone, can resist infection even after the contamination that follows dental extraction. Some form of "tissue immunity" must be postulated, but its nature is unknown.

Decontamination

Mechanical. The continual backward flow of saliva traps organisms, which are then swallowed. Carbon particles placed on the mucosa are removed from the mouth in 15–30 minutes.[2]

Biological. As in the skin the resident flora is important. These organisms are α-haemolytic streptococci (*Strept. viridans*), *Neisseria pharyngis*, diphtheroids, lactobacilli* (which have been incriminated as a factor in dental caries), pneumococci, *Borrelia vincenti*, actinomyces organisms, *Candida albicans*, and various *Bacteroidaceae*. Many strains of α-haemolytic streptococci produce hydrogen peroxide,[2] and this has been thought to play some part in the decontaminating mechanism.†

Chemical. The saliva inhibits many pathogens: this may be due to its *mucin*, *lysozyme*, and *antibody* content.

Lysozyme[10, 11] is an acetylaminopolysaccharidase and acts on the muramic acid of the bacterial cell wall. The name *muramidase* has therefore been proposed for this agent which was first described by Fleming. By attacking the cell wall, lysozyme is able to lyse some bacteria, mostly the non-pathogens. With many organisms, however, the cell membrane must be damaged by the activation of complement or by the action of peroxides or other agents before destruction is complete. Lysozyme is present in many of the body's secretions and also in polymorphs.

Antibody.[12] The presence of IgA antibody in many secretions (tears, colostrum, and the secretions of the respiratory, gastrointestinal, and lower urinary tracts) is important in protecting these systems from microbial infection. The antibody is produced locally and is passed into the secretion as a dimer linked to a distinct secretory peptide.

In spite or these mechanisms, potent pathogens can adapt themselves to the mouth and throat, e.g. meningococci, diphtheria bacilli, *H. influenzae*, and *Strept. pyogenes*. These may lead to infection, but if the person has considerable immunity, they may remain as "transients" for a period of time. Such carriers are of great importance in the spread of streptococcal infections, diphtheria, and meningococcal meningitis.

SALIVARY GLANDS

The regular flow of saliva is important, for when secretion is suppressed as in conditions of shock, dehydration, and fever, or as a consequence of infective processes or neoplasia, the lips, tongue, teeth, and remainder of the mouth become coated with a mixture of food particles and dead epithelial cells. If this is not actively removed, it becomes the site of bacterial colonisation. This may result in an ascending

* Lactobacilli are non-sporing, Gram-positive bacilli, usually micro-aerophilic, and conspicuously acid resistant. They are an important element in the commensal flora of the mouth, gastrointestinal tract, and vagina.

† In this connexion the rare Japanese hereditary disorder of *acatalasia* is of interest. The enzyme catalase which normally breaks down H_2O_2 is absent from the blood, and peroxide formed in the mouth produces sufficient damage to cause ulcerating gangrenous lesions in the mouth.

infection of the salivary glands terminating in suppurative sialadenitis.

THE STOMACH

The stomach stands guard over the intestines, and in man is the first part of the alimentary tract not lined by stratified squamous epithelium. It deals not only with food, but also with the secretions of the mouth and swallowed sputum. Its defence mechanisms are:

Mechanical Strength

The continuity of the epithelium is probably not important. Acute erosions are common, and neither these nor the more serious chronic ulcers appear to provide points of entry for organisms.

Decontamination

Mechanical. Vomiting removes chemical and bacterial irritants, but is of little value in combating infection.

Biological. Under normal conditions the gastric juice is sterile.

Chemical. Without doubt the bactericidal activity of gastric juice is due to its hydrochloric acid content and not its enzymes. Proteolytic enzymes do not often kill organisms, and gastric juice loses its bactericidal activity when neutralised.

Fig. 7.1 shows the levels of hydrochloric acid usually attained in the stomach following the ingestion of a meal. It is apparent that organisms such as *Strept. pyogenes*, diphtheria bacilli, and pneumococci are most unlikely to pass through the acid barrier of the stomach into the intestine (the same applies to rhinoviruses). Staphylococci and *Salmonella* organisms will probably pass if ingested with food or large quantities of fluid; likewise enteroviruses can withstand reasonable acidity. Milk with its potent antacid properties is a particularly favourable vehicle for organisms, e.g. *Brucella abortus*, though in fact any food is liable to have a protective action. Coliform organisms in general are able to withstand the acidity of the stomach, as can also the cysts of *Entamoeba histolytica*. The tubercle bacillus can resist acid due to its waxy content, and therefore intestinal tuberculosis may occur when bacilli are swallowed. Gastric aspiration is carried out extensively as a diagnostic procedure in childhood tuberculosis.

The gastric contents are colonised with various organisms, and become very offensive, whenever they are dammed back as the result of pyloric stenosis. This is particularly well marked when the cause is pyloric cancer, where there is often achlorhydria.

THE INTESTINE

The intestine undoubtedly relies upon the stomach's protective action. The minor intestinal upsets of infancy may in part be related to the low gastric acidity in this age-group.[13, 14] Europeans living in tropical climates, especially

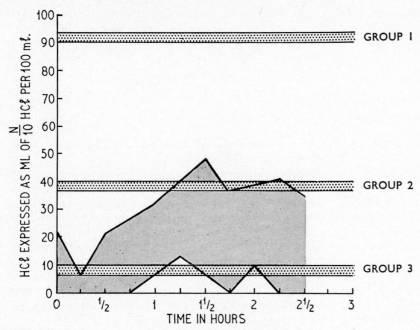

Figure 7.1
The gastric bactericidal barrier. The shaded area represents the limits of free HCl in 80 per cent of normal people following a meal. The horizontal bands are drawn at the average free acid strengths which in 20 minutes are lethal to the three bacterial groups: Group 1. *Esch. coli* and *Kl. pneumoniae*; Group 2. *S. typhi, Shigella* species, and *Staph. pyogenes*; Group 3. *Strept. pyogenes, Strept. viridans*, pneumococci, *N. catarrhalis*, and *C. diphtheriae*. Spore-bearing organisms are resistant to acid and cannot be shown on the chart. *(From Knott, F. A.* (1923), *Guy's Hosp. Rep.,* **73,** 429*).*

before becoming acclimatised, usually develop hypochlorhydria, and this may be a factor in the troublesome diarrhoea that so often afflicts them.[15] The intestine has, however, its own defence mechanism.

Mechanical Barrier

As in the stomach this is probably not important. It is interesting that some organisms, e.g. *S. typhi* and the tubercle bacillus, can penetrate the mucosa without causing obvious damage. Probably phagocytes are normally present on the surface of the gut ready to ingest passing organisms. These are carried into the tissues so that infection follows. This mechanism whereby bacteria and probably also intact protein molecules gain access to the tissues may well be of great importance in the immunological development of the individual.

Decontamination

Mechanical. The development of diarrhoea is common in intestinal infection, and helps to expel the organism. If this symptom is suppressed with drugs, the disease tends to be more severe. Although in minor infections this effect may be unimportant, in typhoid fever it can be serious.

Biological. The small intestine generally contains few organisms, whilst the colon is heavily contaminated with coliforms, faecal and anaerobic streptococci, and clostridia. Spirochaetes (*Borrelia*) have been described.[16] Organisms of the genus *Bacteroides* form an important component of the intestinal flora, but are often forgotten because of the difficulties in their culture. The *Lactobacillus bifidus* occurs in breast-fed infants, and the acidity which it produces is probably beneficial. Although the importance of the flora

is well known, the exact mechanisms involved are not established. Some enteric bacilli release highly specific proteins called *colicines* which can kill other organisms in a variety of ways.[17] When the flora is upset by the broad-spectrum antibiotics, superinfection with *Staph. pyogenes* may be a fatal complication (see p. 218).

Another indication of the importance of the bacterial flora is the experiment in which it was found possible to produce cholera regularly in adult guinea-pigs by preparing them with oral streptomycin. The animals are normally resistant to *Vibrio cholerae*.

Chemical. IgA antibodies secreted locally by plasma cells are important in providing the mucous membranes with local immunity (p. 144). It should also be noted that the lymphoid tissue of the intestine is thought to act as the central organ responsible for the development of the peripheral lymphoid tissues destined to produce all classes of immunoglobulins (p. 149). The bile salts in the intestinal secretion destroy the infectivity of enveloped viruses (p. 272). Hence only enteroviruses, adenoviruses, reoviruses, and the agents of hepatitis reach the intestine.

The appendix is one of the weakest links in the alimentary tract, but the reason for this is not known. Possibly damage by hard concretions and the ease with which its lumen can be obstructed play a part, but it is incredible how little we know about the cause of such a common disease as acute appendicitis.

THE CONJUNCTIVAL SAC

Although the exposed moist surface is subject to frequent contamination, infection is comparatively rare. The conjunctival sac relies partly upon the mechanical washing effect of the tears and partly upon their composition. The tears contain the highest concentration of *lysozyme* of any body fluid examined (see p. 86).

THE EAR[18]

The external auditory canal contains ear wax which is the combined product of sebaceous and ceruminous glands. Most Negroes and Europeans have wet, sticky, honey-coloured ear wax which contains IgA antibody and lysozyme*.[19]

THE RESPIRATORY TRACT

The respiratory tract acts as a whole, the upper part functioning as an air-conditioner for the lungs.[21] The vibrissae filter off large particles, but the main filter is the nasal mucosa itself, covering as it does the complicated ramification of the turbinates. Not only is the inspired air warmed and humidified, but the mucus-covered surface traps organisms and particles just as flies are trapped on fly-paper. The anterior nares are distinct from the remainder of the respiratory tract, because their epithelium and bacterial flora resemble that of the skin. Their great importance lies in their frequent colonisation by *Staph. pyogenes*.

THE NOSE AND NASOPHARYNX

Mechanical barrier. The epithelium of the respiratory tract does not provide an adequate barrier against local infection. This is well demonstrated by the ease with which rhinoviruses and adenoviruses cause acute upper respiratory tract infection. Meningococci are apparently able to penetrate the mucosa of the nasopharynx without much difficulty (see p. 228).

Decontamination. Irritants are expelled by the act of sneezing. If organisms are deliberately implanted in the nose, they disappear within 15 minutes. One of the main mechanisms involved is the continuous flow of mucus backwards to the nasopharynx. The nasal secretion is both bactericidal and virucidal: antibodies have been demonstrated in it against influenza and poliomyelitis viruses (see p. 87). Lysozyme is also present. Nevertheless, pathogens like meningococci and diphtheria bacilli can colonise the nose, and carriers of these constitute an important reservoir of human infection. The fact that the olfactory mucosa is non-ciliated and has beneath it much lymphoid tissue has been held to explain why some organisms gain entry through this area. Experimentally dye, proteins, and viruses can be shown to penetrate the olfactory mucosa and enter the underlying lymphoid tissue.[22, 23]

---

* It is of interest that among the Mongoloid races over 80 per cent of people have grey, brittle, dry wax which contains IgG. Wet ear wax is determined by the presence of a dominant *W* gene.[20] Closely linked is axillary odour. Hence in a race like the Japanese, in whom the *W* gene is uncommon, the few who possess it have wet ear wax and an axillary odour.

The nasopharynx has a resident bacterial flora similar to that of the throat (especially *Strept. viridans* and *Neisseria pharyngis*), and this has a biological decontaminating function.

THE TRACHEA AND LOWER RESPIRATORY TRACT

Mechanical barrier. Below the larynx the respiratory tract should normally be sterile. The mucosa itself forms a poor mechanical barrier as in the nose, and is frequently infected by the influenza virus.

Decontamination. The cough reflex initiated by stimulating the larynx or upper trachea expels irritants, but may also disseminate organisms within the lung. Although the diameter of the air passages decreases steadily with each division from the trachea downwards, the total cross-sectional area increases.[24] Thus it has been estimated that the total cross-sectional area of all the respiratory bronchioles is over 100 times that of the trachea. It follows that the velocity of the inspired air steadily decreases as it passes down the air passages, and this allows particles to fall out of the stream and adhere to the mucus-covered walls.

The film of fluid which covers the mucosa is derived partly by transudation and partly from the secretions of surface goblet cells and the underlying mucous glands. By its chemical composition it protects the epithelial cells from dangerous gases, e.g. SO_2, and its proper consistency allows the cilia to move it on as a continuous sheet.[25] The sheet of mucus ever moving upwards, at a rate of about 2 cm per minute, by ciliary activity is an important decontaminating mechanism, and any obstruction to it impairs the defences of the respiratory tract.

This frequently leads to infection, and is well seen in the bronchopneumonia which follows the obstruction caused by a foreign body or carcinoma. Ciliary action may also be impaired in bronchitis and bronchiectasis, when the normal epithelium is replaced by goblet or squamous cells. Another very important cause of breakdown of the respiratory decontaminating mechanism is the epithelial destruction caused by virus infection, e.g. influenza and measles. A similar effect is seen in whooping-cough and following the inhalation of poison gases, e.g. chlorine, phosgene, and nitrogen peroxide. Chemicals (e.g. sulphur dioxide and tobacco smoke), drugs (e.g. atropine), cold air, and alcohol taken by mouth impair ciliary action and delay clearance from the lung. So also does the inhalation of a high concentration of oxygen; this effect, observed in the experimental animal, may be of clinical significance when giving patients with chronic chest disease oxygen therapy.[26] Alterations in the consistency of mucus, as for example in chronic bronchitis or chronic venous congestion, when there is excessive transudation, may also impair mucociliary action.

In the respiratory bronchioles and alveoli mucociliary streams play little part in the defence of the lung, and it is here that the macrophages, or septal cells, are important.[27]

Bacteria are phagocytosed by these cells and killed in their cytoplasm. The energy for phagocytosis is provided by aerobic metabolism[28] (cf. p. 96), and the hypoxia engendered by collapse or oedema could be a factor in predisposing such an area of lung to infection (Fig. 7.2).

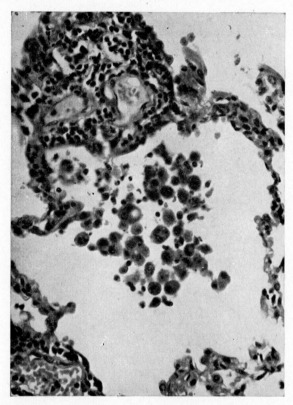

Figure 7.2
Macrophages in alveoli of lung. These large round cells ingest foreign particles inhaled into the lung. They phagocytose organisms, blood pigments, dust, etc. They are known as "heart-failure cells", "dust cells" etc., according to the condition that evokes their outpouring. × 280.

THE URINARY TRACT

Antibacterial and antiviral substances have been found in urine, but in fact the continuous flushing action of urine together with its acidity are probably of much greater importance in maintaining the sterility of the urinary tract. Obstruction always favours infection, as is seen in urethral stricture, prostatic enlargement, pregnancy, stones, and bladder diverticula. The infection is probably blood-borne *via* the kidney more often than "ascending" from the lower urinary tract (see p. 132). The rival view is that organisms enter the bladder *via* the urethra. The greater frequency of urinary infection in the female has been attributed to the shortness of the female urethra. An alternative explanation is that the male is protected by the bactericidal activity of the prostatic secretions rather than the length of the urethra.[29, 30]

Bacteria which remain on the bladder wall are believed to be killed by humoral factors or engulfed by the bladder epithelium.[31] The same probably applies to the upper urinary passages.

THE FEMALE GENITAL TRACT

The vagina is protected by an acid barrier (pH 4·3–5·5)[32] produced by the resident Döderlein's lactobacilli, which ferment glycogen from the desquamated squamous cells to produce lactic acid. As oestrogens are responsible for the glycogen content of these cells, this acid barrier is absent in childhood and old age. Acute vulvovaginitis is therefore seen only in these two age groups.

It will be appreciated that each of the surfaces of the body is provided with a mechanism for either removing micro-organisms or resisting their penetration.

Only after they have penetrated the surface epithelial barrier, either by their own efforts or as the result of trauma, can the organisms exert their influence upon the underlying tissue. If pathogenic, their continued multiplication invariably gives rise to infection.

REFERENCES

1. Hare, R. (1964). *Proceedings of the Royal Society of Medicine*, **57**, 221.
2. Wilson, G. S. and Miles, A. A. (1964). In Topley and Wilson's *Principles of Bacteriology and Immunology*, 5th edn, p. 1251. London: Arnold.
3. Colebrook, L. (1941). *Bulletin of War Medicine*, **2**, 73.
4. Arnold, L. *et al.* (1930). *American Journal of Hygiene*, **11**, 345.
5. Arnold, L. and Bart, A. (1934). *American Journal of Hygiene*, **19**, 217.
6. Pollock, M. R., Wainwright, S. D. and Manson, E. E. D. (1949). *Journal of Pathology and Bacteriology*, **61**, 274.
7. Cohen, B. (1959). *British Dental Journal*, **107**, 31 and *Dental Practitioner*, **9**, 167.
8. Goodale, J. L. (1898). *Archiv für Laryngologie und Rhinologie*, **7**, 90.
9. Hendelsohn, M. (1898). *Archiv für Laryngologie und Rhinologie*, **8**, 476.
10. Chipman, D. M. and Sharon, N. (1969). *Science*, **165**, 454.
11. Glynn, A. A. (1968). *Scientific Basis of Medicine. Annual Reviews*, 31.
12. Tomasi, T. B. and DeCoteau, E. (1970). *Advances in Internal Medicine*, **16**, 401.
13. Blacklock, J. W. S., Guthrie, K. J. and Macpherson, I. (1937). *Journal of Pathology and Bacteriology*, **44**, 321.
14. Miller, R. A. (1942). *Archives of Diseases of Childhood*, **17**, 198.
15. Kligler, I. J. (1936). *Transactions of the Royal Society of Tropical Medicine and Hygiene*, **29**, 531.
16. Lee, F. D. *et al.* (1971). *Gut*, **12**, 126.

17. DAVIS, B. D., DULBECCO, R., EISEN, H. N., GINSBERG, H. S. and WOOD, W. B. (1967). *Microbiology*, p. 767. New York: Harper and Row-Hoeber.
18. Editorial (1971). *New England Journal of Medicine*, **284,** 1099.
19. PETRAKIS, N. L. *et al.* (1971). *Nature*, **229,** 119.
20. MALSUNAGA, E. (1962). *Annals of Human Genetics*, **25,** 273.
21. NEGUS, V. (1958). In *The Comparative Anatomy and Physiology of the Nose and Paranasal Sinuses*, p. 157. Edinburgh: Livingstone.
22. YOFFEY, J. M., SULLIVAN, E. R. and DRINKER, C. K. (1938). *Journal of Experimental Medicine*, **68,** 941.
23. YOFFEY, J. M. and SULLIVAN, E. R. (1939). *Journal of Experimental Medicine*, **69,** 133.
24. STAUB, N. C. (1963). *Anesthesiology*, **24,** 831.
25. Interdepartmental colloquium (1964). *Annals of the Royal College of Surgeons of England*, **34,** 400.
26. Editorial (1968). *New England Journal of Medicine*, **279,** 379.
27. GREEN, G. M. and KASS, E. H. (1964). *Journal of Experimental Medicine*, **119,** 167.
28. HOWARD, J. G. (1963). In *Modern Trends in Immunology*, I, p. 89. Edited by R. Cruickshank. London: Butterworths.
29. STAMEY, T. A. *et al.* (1968). *Nature*, **218,** 444.
30. Leading Article (1968). *Lancet*, i, 1183.
31. Leading Article (1972). *British Medical Journal*, iv, 252.
32. ROGOSA, M. and SHARPE, M. E. (1960). *Journal of General Microbiology*, **23,** 197.

Chapter 8.   The Body's Response to Infection

When organisms gain access to the tissues of the body their fate depends upon the resultant of two factors: the immunity of the host and the virulence of the organism, both of which are in reality different facets of the same thing, as is explained in Chapter 13.

The possible end-results are:

1. Rapid destruction of the organisms, e.g. non-pathogens.

2. The organisms grow for a time, but are soon destroyed, e.g. minor or subclinical infection.

3. The organisms enter into a symbiotic state with the host, e.g. herpes-simplex virus.

4. There is local proliferation of organisms producing tissue damage, but little spread of infection, e.g. a boil due to staphylococcal infection.

5. Organisms may proliferate locally and produce severe damage to distant tissues by means of a soluble exotoxin. The local lesion may be insignificant, as in tetanus, or severe, as in diphtheria.

6. A local lesion is produced, but rapid spread of organisms follows, e.g. cellulitis due to *Strept. pyogenes*.

7. No local lesion forms, but the organism rapidly spreads, e.g. European typhus due to *R. prowazeki*.

8. No local lesion forms initially, but the organism spreads rapidly and later a lesion develops at the portal of entry, e.g. syphilis, typhoid fever, and scrub typhus due to *R. rickettsi*.

9. The organism induces cellular proliferation, e.g. Rous's sarcoma virus. Proliferation may occur and is later followed by necrosis, e.g. smallpox virus.

This list is by no means complete. Thus, the slow viruses produce a type of infection which appears to be unique, but is not well understood. Cholera is peculiar in that the organisms multiply in the gut, produce a toxin which damages the epithelium, but yet never penetrate beyond the basement membrane. It is obvious in this example how difficult it is to separate true infection from intoxication.

Some of these possibilities will be examined in more detail.

If organisms are non-pathogenic they are unable to multiply in the tissues; they are phagocytosed by polymorphs and macrophages and destroyed in the cytoplasm of these cells. It is often difficult to understand why some organisms cannot grow in certain tissues. For example, the gonococcus in unable to grow in animal tissues, and yet is capable of causing human infection. It can grow outside the body on relatively simple media, and yet does not grow in tissues other than those of the human subject. The organisms can multiply in human polymorphonuclear leucocytes, but not in those of other animals. This aspect of host-organism relationship is further considered in connexion with innate immunity (see p. 164).

If an organism is capable of causing disease, it is called *pathogenic* and has the ability to grow in the tissues, and thereby cause infection. The type and severity of this infection depend on the virulence of the organism. The term *virulent* is sometimes applied to strains of an organism which have a special ability to produce severe disease. Certain strains of *C. diphtheriae* are more virulent than others due to their greater ability to produce toxin. This implies that, while all strains of *C. diphtheriae* are pathogenic, some produce a more severe disease than others. Similar variations occur with other exotoxin-producing organisms, e.g. *Cl. welchii*, but the term virulence is also used in connexion with an invasive organism like *Staph. pyogenes*. The ability of virulent strains of such an organism to produce severe disease is often not related to toxin production, but rather to some subtle alteration in the organism itself, probably in its antigenic structure. Virulence in invasive organisms can be considered under two headings:

1. *The ability of the organism to spread.*
2. *The ability of the organism to produce tissue damage.*

The ability to spread, in respect of many organisms, is inversely proportional to their tendency to produce initial local damage and a subsequent inflammatory reaction. Thus pathogenic organisms whose presence seems to excite little immediate inflammatory reaction (like *Mycobacterium leprae*, *Yersinia* (*Pasteurella*) *pestis*, and many rickettsiae and viruses), are able to spread widely without leaving any trace of their site of entry. Some organisms, although behaving essentially in the same manner, do produce diseases in which a lesion later develops at the site of entry. Syphilis is an excellent example of this; the local lesion (chancre) occurs long after the organisms have spread throughout the body, and this is presumably due to a hypersensitivity reaction. Hence, another way in which organisms may produce damage is by interacting with sensitising antibodies.[1] This is best documented with certain virus infections. Measles and respiratory syncytial virus may be more destructive in partially immunised individuals than in the non-immune (p. 279). The subject is further discussed in the section on immune complexes and disease (p. 182).

The existence of L-forms (Appendix 2) raises many possibilities. They are generally considered to be non-pathogenic, but following an overt infection they might remain in the tissues in a dormant form and provide sufficient antigen to sustain an immunological response. Rheumatic carditis and chronic post-streptococcal glomerulonephritis are obvious candidates for such a pathogenesis. L-forms might also revert to type; this could explain recurrent infections, e.g. chronic pyelonephritis and infective endocarditis.

With those organisms which do cause considerable local tissue damage, other mechanisms may enable them to spread. By producing toxins, leucocidins, fibrinolysin, hyaluronidase, etc., they may effectively counteract the body's attempt at localisation. In this way a severe local response will be followed by spread: this type of infection is seen typically with *Strept. pyogenes* and *Cl. welchii*.

Some organisms produce local damage, but have little tendency to spread. The result is a local inflammatory response which may either pass unnoticed (subclinical infection) or else be severe, e.g. a carbuncle due to *Staph. pyogenes*.

Finally, by not causing damage the organism may enter into a symbiotic state with the host. There are many instances of this in the lower animals. The chloroplasts of some protozoa are, for example, symbiotic algae. Many arthropods harbour rickettsiae in their cells, and indeed are infected from the ovum at the time of their conception. Sometimes the relationship is unstable; rats may carry the organism *Bartonella bacilliformis* in their red cells without harm, but if a splenectomy is performed, the animals die of acute haemolytic anaemia. Similarly, man may harbour the virus of herpes simplex without ill effects until the development of some other infection, e.g. pneumonia, malaria, or Weil's disease, causes the characteristic lesion of herpes febrilis to appear. Adenoviruses may also lie latent in the tissues. A factor of great theoretical interest is that the host may exhibit *specific tolerance* to some organisms with which it shares common antigens (see p. 168).

Organisms which resist the decontaminating mechanisms of the body surfaces and are introduced into the tissues, may thus produce a variety of response patterns. The possibilities given on p. 91 are examples of what can happen. Intermediate states also exist; one type of organism may under varying circumstances produce different responses. Thus *Strept. pyogenes* may enter the body through an insignificant lesion, and rapidly kill the patient with septicaemia (pattern 7). Alternately the organism may produce a relatively minor infection such as a sore throat.

The Manner in Which Organisms Produce Damage[2]

Organisms which are capable of causing damage may do this in several ways.

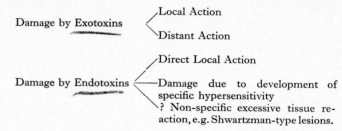

Some organisms form powerful soluble *exotoxins* which produce local tissue damage. Diphtheria and gas-gangrene are diseases in which this occurs. The toxin also acts on distant tissues which it reaches *via* the blood stream. The cardiac and neurological lesions in diphtheria are produced in this way. Sometimes the toxin acts only at a distance (*Cl. tetani*). It should be noted that the lesions produced by circulating toxin are themselves sterile. The distribution of lesions depends on the sensitivity of tissues to the action of the toxin and also on their accessibility. Thus, in the guinea-pig circulating diphtheria toxin can pass the "blood-nerve" barrier and escape into peripheral nerves, but it does not reach the spinal cord.[3]

Exotoxins were the first toxic bacterial products to be identified. They are freely diffusible, and therefore found in the medium of a bacterial culture. They can be purified, identified, and estimated with relative ease. Their mode of action is known in many cases. On a quantitative basis they are very potent—botulinum toxin is the most poisonous substance known. Organisms whose main offensive weapon is an exotoxin are called *toxic organisms*. Examples of these are the causative organisms of diphtheria, tetanus, gas-gangrene, scarlet fever, *Sh. shigae* dysentery, and botulism; the last is not an infection, but an intoxication.

With most other organisms, however, no such powerful toxins have been demonstrated. Cultures may be toxic to animals, but the responsible substances seem to be derived from the bodies of the organisms. These have been called *endotoxins*, but it is probable that in reality they are the complex constituents of the bacterial body. Many substances have been isolated—lipids, carbohydrates, and proteins. The properties or exotoxins and endotoxins are summarised in Table 13.1, p. 165.

Further investigations of the endotoxic group of organisms have shown that some substances do indeed diffuse out of the living cell bodies. The coagulase of *Staph. pyogenes* is one such substance. Some authorities call these substances exotoxins, but this is probably an error of judgement; it is even debatable whether substances like coagulase, hyaluronidase, etc. are "toxins" at all. Therefore whatever the theoretical arguments, in practice the term exotoxins should be restricted to those substances which diffuse easily out of the organism, are highly toxic, causing some or many of the lesions of the disease, and are powerfully antigenic.

Organisms which do not produce exotoxins as defined above are called *invasive*. This term serves a useful purpose, because (with certain exceptions noted below) it emphasises that lesions can be produced only in the actual presence of the organism. Generalised disease can occur only as a consequence of the systemic spread of the organisms. The clostridia of gas-gangrene, typically toxic organisms, can also spread widely in the local tissues, but except as a terminal event they never invade the blood stream and lead to generalised colonisation of the viscera. It should also be noted that *Strept. pyogenes*, an invasive organism, can produce sterile lesions at a distance because of the development of hypersensitivity to its products. In this way acute glomerulonephritis and rheumatic fever are explained. In spite of these difficulties these two terms will be retained, because the division of organisms into "toxic" and "invasive" categories serves many useful purposes, especially in relationship to immunity.

Mechanisms of Damage by Invasive Organisms

The manner in which the invasive organisms produce damage is not clearly understood. Some seem to have a direct action on the tissues, and produce necrosis and acute inflammation. The pyogenic organisms fall into this group. In infection with many other organisms the situation is much more complicated. Typhoid fever illustrates this particularly well.

Typhoid fever. Although the evolution of the human disease is not completely known, experimental work on mice infected with *S. typhimurium* (mouse typhoid) has done much to elucidate the mode of spread of the organism.[4] During the first twenty-four hours following the ingestion of *S. typhimurium* the organisms can be recovered only from the contents of the gut. During the second twenty-four hours they are present in the mesenteric lymph nodes, and by the third day they have reached the blood, liver, and spleen. In the human disease the tempo is slower than this, but by analogy the sequence of events is probably as follows:[5]

After being ingested, the organisms reach the contents of the small intestine; here they are taken up by phagocytes, enter the mucosa, and are carried to the local lymphoid tissue (Peyer's patches). No local damage is done, and no inflammation occurs. The organisms pass on through the lymphatics, through the mesenteric nodes, and finally reach the blood stream *via* the thoracic duct. In this way there develops a transient *bacteraemia* (see p. 99). The blood stream is rapidly cleared by the phagocytic reticulo-endothelial cells of liver, spleen, bone marrow, etc. It is at this stage that the pathogenic properties of the organisms become further manifest: they are able to live and multiply in the RE cells. By about the tenth day the parasitised cells undergo necrosis, and the blood stream is flooded with large numbers of bacilli. This is the end of the incubation period, and the patient becomes seriously ill with *septicaemia* (see p. 100). This phase lasts about one week, and is characterised clinically by a progressive rise in temperature (step-ladder pattern), a relatively slow pulse, and severe constitutional symptoms.

Bronchitis is common and constipation the rule; diarrhoea is not present at this stage. The pathological diagnosis depends on obtaining a positive blood culture.

The next phase of the disease is marked by the onset of diarrhoea due to ulceration of the small intestine and the appearance of organisms in the faeces. The bacilli reach the gut *via* the bile which is heavily contaminated as a result of passage of the bacteria from the RE cells of the liver. The ulceration occurs over the inflamed Peyer's patches, and is associated with mesenteric adenitis (Fig. 8.1). In both the

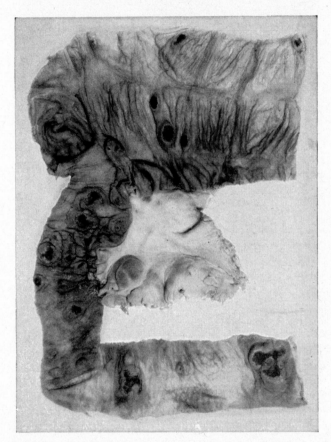

Figure 8.1
Typhoid ulceration of the bowel. There are many ulcers in the terminal ileum and ascending colon. They have retained the shape and size of the inflamed Peyer's patches and lymphoid follicles from which they arose. There is no tendency towards lateral spread. An enlarged lymph node is present in the mesentery. *(A 50.3, Reproduced by permission of the President and Council of the R.C.S. Eng.)*

ulcers and the lymph nodes there is an accumulation of macrophages; polymorphs are almost completely absent (Fig. 8.2). The most likely explanation of these events is that the local lymphoid tissue of the gut has become sensitised to the organism, and that subsequent contact with it produces damage. The local production of sensitising antibodies must be postulated, because the blood level of detectable agglu-

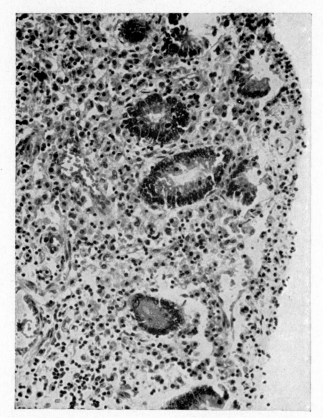

Figure 8.2

Typhoid ulceration of small bowel. There is considerable destruction of the mucous membrane, and an inflammatory infiltrate is present around the remaining glands. Most of the cells are macrophages, but in addition some darkly staining lymphocytes are present. Polymorphs are absent. × 200.

tinins does not rise till later in the course of the disease. During the second week diagnosis depends upon finding the organism in the faeces (and sometimes the urine). By the third week the titre of agglutinins in the serum rises (Widal reaction), and the patient gradually recovers (Fig. 8.3).

Although the nature of the *hypersensitivity* which develops in typhoid fever is not known, a type of bacterial allergy seems probable; a non-specific hypersusceptibility of the Shwartzman type is also possible. There is little doubt that the damage produced during infection is sometimes caused by the body's response to the organism.[6] Such a mechanism should always be suspected in an infective disease that has an incubation period exceeding 7–10 days.

Other invasive organisms. Many *viruses*, e.g. smallpox, behave in a way similar to the typhoid bacillus: they produce no lesion on entry, but after dissemination and multiplication in the body cause extensive tissue damage.

In *syphilis* the organisms rapidly spread from the portal of entry, so that within a few hours they are widely disseminated throughout the body. Two to three weeks later an ulcerating inflammatory reaction occurs at the portal of entry. This

again must be due to some alteration in tissue response to the organism. It certainly is not a primary inflammatory reaction representing an attempt by the body to localise the infection.

Some *rickettsial infections* are also characterised by a lesion at the portal of entry following their widespread dissemination.

The cause of death in septicaemia is poorly understood. The condition has been most studied in *anthrax*.[7] *B. anthracis* produces no exotoxins *in vitro*, and if animals infected with it are untreated, they develop a fatal septicaemia in which there are vast numbers of organisms in the blood. The early administration of antibiotics will save them, but there is a critical time after which treatment is of no avail; although the bacteria may be destroyed, the animal still dies. This may be correlated with the observation that the blood of guinea-pigs dying of anthrax contains a labile toxin which can kill other animals. Thus *B. anthracis*, although a typically "invasive" organism, appears to cause the formation of a toxin *in vivo*. Antibody to this toxin confers good immunity. This state of affairs is very reminiscent of the immunity to toxic organisms.

In *staphylococcal and streptococcal septicaemia* it is reasonable to attribute death to severe toxaemia consequent on the release of endotoxins (see pp. 218 and 220). The cause of death in *pneumococcal septicaemia* is less easily explicable, because this organism does not appear to produce toxic substances.

A final possibility is that some invasive organisms (especially the Gram-negative ones) produce damage by means of a Shwartzman-like reaction.

The local Shwartzman phenomenon.[8–10] The reaction is most easily demonstrated in rabbits. A quantity of bacterial "endotoxin" (lipoprotein extract of certain bacteria) is injected into the skin, and twenty-four hours later an intravenous dose is give. The site of the skin injection then shows necrosis. The following features should be noted.

1. An effective endotoxin can be extracted from many Gram-negative organisms, especially those of the coli-typhoid group.

2. The interval between the first and second dose must be between 12 and 36 hours.

3. The reaction is non-specific, i.e. the two injections can be endotoxins from different organisms. The mechanism involved in this reaction is not understood, and there is little evidence that it is implicated in the lesions of bacterial infection. A similar phenomenon (Sanarelli) is considered in Chapter 32.

Variations of the Acute Inflammatory Reaction due to Infection

Although acute inflammation has been described as a common reaction to cell damage, it is only to be expected that the nature of the irritant causing the damage will influence the final picture. There will be differences depending

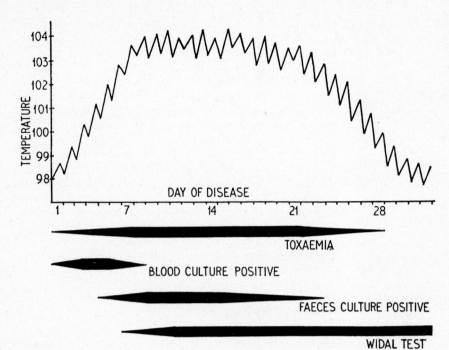

Figure 8.3
Chart correlating the clinical course of a typical case of typhoid fever with the principal methods of bacteriological diagnosis. *(After Harries, E. H. R. and Mitman, M.* (1947), Clinical Practice in Infectious Disease, *3rd edition, p.* 464. *Edinburgh : E. and S. Livingstone Ltd.)*

upon the amount of irritant, and whether it is particulate, like a bacterium, or in solution, like an exotoxin. In respect of bacterial irritants there is the added factor of further growth of the organism. Finally, the presence of immunity or hypersensitivity will alter the tissue response.

In addition to considerations of the causative organism, the inflammatory response also varies according to the tissue involved. Loose tissues tend to show a greater accumulation of inflammatory oedema, and serous sacs may fill with fluid. This is called "serous inflammation". In a compact tissue like bone the amount of swelling is limited, but the inflammatory exudate causes a rise in tissue tension which obstructs the blood supply. Necrosis is therefore a common complication. Certain types of inflammation have been categorised, depending upon the predominance of some particular feature. The terms are useful for descriptive purposes, but are of no fundamental importance.

Suppurative inflammation (Fig. 8.4.) Accumulation of neutrophil polymorphonuclear leucocytes is a feature of inflammation caused by traumatic injury. When tissue necrosis occurs, the disintegrating phagocytes liberate proteolytic enzymes which cause liquefaction. This fluid is pus, and the inflammation is called *suppurative* (see p. 78). Suppuration generally indicates that infection is becoming localised, and therefore in the days before chemotherapy it was regarded as a favourable sign. Hence the origin of the term "laudable pus". Nevertheless, diffuse suppurative lesions do occasionally occur and these are called *phlegmonous.*

Serous inflammation. As stated above, this is encounterd in inflammations involving loose tissues. The fluid component exceeds the cellular one, and a large accumulation of inflammatory oedema results. Infections with *Cl. oedematiens* are also of this type, probably because of the marked ability of the toxin to increase vascular permeability. A characteristic feature of the exudate in gas-gangrene is the absence of polymorphs. The fact that some highly virulent organisms are negatively chemotactic to polymorphs may explain this.

Fibrinous inflammation. Marked fibrin formation is a feature of inflammation in serous sacs and in the lungs. It is well marked in most forms of pericarditis, pleurisy, and peritonitis. It is also frequent in pneumococcal and staphylococcal infections. Often there is considerable serous exudate and the inflammation is then called serofibrinous.

Haemorrhagic inflammation. A haemorrhagic exudate indicates that the irritant has caused severe vascular damage. It is seen in the lung in phosgene poisoning and acute influenzal pneumonia, and is typical of anthrax.

Catarrhal inflammation is seen when a mucous membrane is involved in an acute inflammatory reaction. There is some destruction of the epithelial cells and a profuse mucous secretion from the underlying glands. The common cold provides an excellent example: the running nose exudes a mixture of mucus and inflammatory exudate from the mucosa.

Membranous inflammation. A membrane covering an inflamed area of mucosa is seen in membranous bronchitis and membranous colitis. A complete "cast" of the organ may be expelled; it consists of mucus and fibrinous exudate.

Pseudomembranous inflammation. This differs from the above in that the membrane contains necrotic epithelium as well as fibrin and inflammatory cells. It is seen in diphtheria and *Sh. shigae* dysentery.

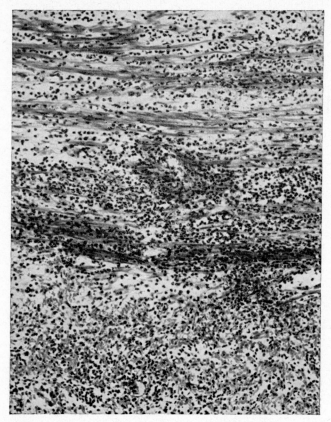

Figure 8.4
Suppurative appendicitis. The structure of the appendix is almost completely destroyed apart from a few muscle fibres. There is a massive infiltration with polymorphs, most of which are disintegrating (pus cells). This is an example of phlegmonous inflammation. ×120.

Gangrene. Gangrene occurs in inflammation whenever the dead tissue is invaded by putrefactive organisms (see p. 55).

Certain inflammations do not show the usual neutrophil polymorph response.

Inflammation characterised by mononuclear response. Typhoid and many virus infections show an inflammatory reaction with virtually no polymorphs. Typhoid bacilli are actively chemotactic to white cells *in vitro*, which makes this even more remarkable. A possible answer is provided by the fact that the typhoid ulcers are not produced during the primary invasion of the organism, but are secondary to a later septicaemic phase with a reinfection from bile-borne organisms. If a delayed type of hypersensitivity is involved, the mononuclear response is to be expected, since this is the characteristic cell-type of that condition.

Inflammation characterised by eosinophils.[11] These cells are found instead of the usual neutrophilis in inflammation produced by helminthic parasites, e.g. ascariasis and schistosomiasis, and also in some allergic conditions (asthma, allergic rhinitis, and hay-fever). The reasons for

this are as yet not understood, but there is evidence that eosinophil production is dependent on the T lymphocytes.[12] Thus, rats to whom larvae of *Trichinia spiralis* are given do not develop an eosinophilia if they have been neonatally thymectomised or treated with antilymphocytic serum, both of which procedures eliminate T lymphocytes selectively (see Chapter 12). On the other hand, such animals can develop a normal neutrophilia if suitably challenged.[12]

The eosinophils are motile, and *in vitro* are attracted by the same agents as are neutrophils. Their granules have been stated to contain both histamine and an antihistamine substance. Other suggested functions of the eosinophil are the processing of antigen as part of the immune response and the ingestion of antigen–antibody complexes.[13] Eosinophils are conspicuous in the retest phenomenon (p. 187) and in a number of skin diseases, e.g. dermatitis herpetiformis.

Inflammation with no cellular exudate. This occurs typically in gas-gangrene.

The Destruction of Organisms in the Acute Inflammatory Exudate

While a wholly teleological view of the inflammatory reaction is unjustifiable, it is generally accepted that the reaction is an adaptive reponse having survival value for the species. It creates around the invading organisms a microenvironment unfavourable for their multiplication and survival.[14] Inhibition of the inflammatory reaction generally decreases resistance to infection. The manner in which organisms are killed in the inflammatory exudate must now be considered.

Part Played by Phagocytes

The polymorphonuclear leucocytes.[15, 16, 17] Although it must be accepted that many pathogenic organisms can multiply in the phagocytes or even be spread by them, their ultimate destruction generally takes place within these cells.

The phagocytosed organisms are at first enclosed in a vacuole, the membrane of which soon fuses with that of a lysosome. In this way the polymorphs become degranulated, and hydrolytic enzymes are poured into the phagosomes.

The factors reponsible for killing ingested organisms are poorly understood and indeed may differ from one organism to another. *Cationic proteins*[18] and *hydrolytic lysosomal enzymes* may be important. In the latter group, *lysozyme* is perhaps important for it is found in high concentration in polymorphs (see also p. 86). *Lactic acid* is produced as a consequence of the glycolysis that accompanies phagocytosis. Lactic acid is bactericidal and its action can be reversed by certain keto compounds and carboxylic acids; this may account for the fact that the leucocytes in experimentally produced diabetes mellitus can still engulf pneumococci, but are less able to destroy them.[19] Various bactericidal compounds of haem, such as *verdohaemoglobin* are produced in the acid medium of the active polymorph. The importance of this is unknown. *Phagocytin*[20] is described as a bactericidal component of lysosomes which is liberated by a fall in pH. Both its composition and importance are unknown.

Most important of all is *hydrogen peroxide*, for the production of which activity of the hexose monophosphate shunt is necessary. Defects in the production of hydrogen peroxide or of its utilisation, e.g. due to myeloperoxidase deficiency,[21] are found in chronic granulomatous disease (p. 161). In this condition *Staph. pyogenes* can be phagocytosed but not killed. Organisms which produce peroxide, such as *Strept. viridans* are killed normally.

The mononuclears. Less is known about the mechanism whereby these cells destroy bacteria. It has been reported that they contain lactic acid and lysozyme.[20] General conditions appear to affect the RE system's ability to destroy engulfed bacteria. Experimentally, haemorrhagic shock and fasting impair the RE system's phagocytic activity. On the other hand, the administration of the endotoxin of coliform organisms and BCG vaccination produce a non-specific rise in resistance to infection. This is mediated by a greater phagocytic activity of the RE system. An anamnestic rise in specific antibody may play some part (see p. 141). Splenectomy in children is sometimes followed by overwhelming infection.[22]

In the immune animal the macrophages appear better able to phagocytose and destroy bacteria.

Part Played by the Extracellular Fluids[14]

Substances like lactic acid found in the phagocytes are liberated into the surrounding fluid, and the pH may fall as low as 5·3. Reduction of the polymorph response, for example by nitrogen mustard administration which causes leucopenia, prevents this acid reaction. Glucose administration, on the other hand, increases it.

The unfavourable conditions in the area of inflammation may kill host cells as well as bacteria. The body may indeed defend itself by a type of "scorched-earth" policy. Necrotic tissue has been shown to contain bactericidal substances. Basic peptides active against the tubercle bacillus have been isolated from caseous debris in tuberculous tissue.

Changes occur in the ground substance, which result in the liberation of, amongst other things, glucuronic acid. This substance is capable of detoxifying certain toxins, and it inhibits the growth of some viruses. Humoral agents, e.g. complement, are also present in the extracellular fluids (see p. 161).

Part Played by Acquired Immunity

It is probable that immunity affords protection by speeding up the inflammatory reaction and with it the normal mechanism of destruction. This may be illustrated by the effect of diphtheria antitoxin. Virulent diphtheria bacilli inhibit the acid reaction in inflammation, but this inhibitory effect can be counteracted by administering antitoxin. Whatever the mechanism there can be little doubt that the immune response plays an important role in the limitation

of the spread of infection. This is most obvious when bacterial allergy is involved, and is considered in Chapter 13.

MECHANISMS WHEREBY ORGANISMS OVERCOME THE BODY DEFENCES

Organisms overcome the body's defences in three ways:
Neutralising action of antigens. There is evidence that organisms release their surface antigens and thereby neutralise antibody. Indeed, the detection of free antigen, by immunoelectrophoresis, in the cerebrospinal fluid has been used as a reliable diagnostic procedure in meningitis, and is comparable in accuracy with Gram's stain and culture.[23] In meningococcal infections the presence of free meningococcal antigen in the blood is associated with a very high mortality.[24] Likewise the SSS (capsular polysaccharide) is liberated in large quantities in pneumococcal infections, and is found in the lungs of fatal cases. It is capable of neutralising antibodies. In the toxic organisms, it is their exotoxins which neutralise the antibodies.

By hindering phagocytosis. Unpleasant surface antigens prevent phagocytosis unless specific opsonin is present. Leucocidins produced by staphylococci and streptococci destroy the white cells. Some organisms secrete substances which *in vitro* repel polymorphonuclears. In general the more pathogenic organisms exhibit this negative chemotaxis.

By spreading and countering efforts at localisation. The factors involved in the spread or localisation of infection are dealt with later (see p. 100). First the methods of spread will be considered.

SPREAD OF INFECTION

Local Spread

The natural cohesion of tissues tends to prevent the spread of organisms. The tissue fluids are, however, in constant motion under normal conditions. Particles, including organisms, will be carried in any stream of fluid which may be present. These streams are created in three ways:

1. *The functional state of the capillaries.*[25] While the vessels in one area are dilated and exuding fluid, those in an adjacent part are at a lower pressure and absorbing fluid. This gives rise to a flow from one area to another.

2. *Pulsations of the vessels* due to the heart's action are important.[26, 27] If a rabbit's ear is perfused with fluid at a constant pressure, it becomes oedematous; injected dyes remain localised. Perfusion with a pulsating pressure simulating the heart's action does not result in oedema formation, and injected dyes diffuse into the tissues.

3. *Movement of muscles* both voluntary and involuntary causes considerable movement of tissue fluid. The time-honoured treatment of inflammatory lesions by rest is based upon this fact.

It should be noted that the motility of the organism appears to play no part in its spread. No correlation can be found between the two features. Of the clostridial group *Cl. tetani* is the most motile, but tetanus is a localised non-spreading lesion. *Cl. welchii* is non-motile, yet produces a rapidly spreading gas-gangrene. Similarly *B. anthracis* is non-motile, but is a very invasive organism.

Local spread may also occur in an entirely different way. Organisms ingested by phagocytes may be transported by these cells. This is an important means of spread in tuberculosis, and almost certainly occurs in many other infections, e.g. gonorrhoea.

The local defence mechanism.[9] The acute inflammatory reaction must be regarded as a defence mechanism although, as we have seen, it is called forth only in the case of certain infections. Much stress has in the past been laid on the fibrin barrier. Certainly fibrin is laid down in localised acute inflammations, particularly in staphylococcal infections. It also forms the adhesions which appear to wall off infection in the serous sacs, e.g. around an appendix abscess. Experimentally in rabbits, when dicoumarol is given to prevent fibrin formation, staphylococcal infections are said to spread and terminate in septicaemia. Similarly urea injected locally prevents fibrin formation, and staphylococcal infections tend to spread just like streptococcal ones.

Staphylococci produce coagulase, and it is tempting to postulate that this is a factor in the production of a fibrin barrier in infections with these organisms. However, it seems unlikely that it is important, because fibrin is also a prominent feature of infections with organisms which do not produce a coagulase, e.g. pneumococci. *Strept. pyogenes* produces streptokinase which activates the plasma fibrinolytic system. It might be thought that this would remove the fibrin barrier and potentiate spread. However, *Staph. pyogenes* produces staphylokinase, which has a similar action, and yet its infections tend to be localised. Moreover, other spreading organisms do not produce a fibrinolytic effect.

The balance of evidence favours the concepts of Menkin. Fibrin formation is evidence of a severe local reaction, and this is associated with localisation of infection. Organisms which spread produce little local reaction, and therefore no "barrier" appears. Fibrin is therefore evidence of an attempt at localisation rather than the main cause of it. It must be admitted that the position is by no means clear. It is certain that if an acute inflammatory reaction remains localised, the exudate plays a part in this localisation. Fibrin itself aids the destruction of bacteria by surface phagocytosis. Hence experimental interference with the formation of fibrin may well upset the balance between organism and host under particular conditions. A localised lesion may thus be converted into a spreading one. On the other hand, fibrin may coat organisms and protect them from phagocytosis.

The present situation may therefore be summed up by saying that a fibrin barrier is good evidence of localisation of an infection, that it plays some part in this localisation, but is only one of the many factors involved in the inflammatory response, the sum total of which effect the destruction of the invading organisms (see also p. 218).

Spread by Natural Spaces

If local spread implicates a natural passage, infection may spread by this route. The following examples may be listed:

Peritoneum. Infection may spread rapidly throughout the peritoneal space from a localised lesion, e.g. acute appendicitis. There is rapid absorption of toxic substances from the large surface involved.

The omentum has properties which tend to limit the spread of infection. It wraps itself around inflamed parts and walls off foci of infection. This may be correlated with the response to irritation. If a chemical irritant is injected into the peritoneal cavity of an animal, the omental and peritoneal vessels all show an inflammatory response and leak protein. The reaction in the omentum persists for longer than that of the other peritoneal vessels, and the fibrin glue which coats it may thus cause it to adhere more readily.[28]

Pleura and pericardium. These sacs are usually infected from an adjacent lung lesion. Adhesions, at first fibrinous but later fibrous, are the usual aftermath.

Meningeal space. The subarachnoid space may be infected from adjacent structures, e.g. a nasal sinus, the middle ear, or brain. Septic thrombophlebitis may complicate facial infections and lead to cavernous sinus thrombosis, while meningitis is often the result of systemic blood spread as part of a septicaemia, e.g. tuberculous, meningococcal, and pneumococcal meningitis. Under these circumstances organisms are probably filtered off in the choroid plexuses, whence they spread directly into the cerebro-spinal fluid.

Although the flow of cerebro-spinal fluid is from the choroid plexus to the venous sinuses, irregular movements due to alterations in blood pressure, respiration, and posture lead to extensive mixing of the fluid. Substances artificially introduced into the spinal theca rapidly reach the ventricles. It is therefore often impossible to locate the area where infection has been introduced into the subarachnoid space.

Joint spaces. Joints may be infected from an osteomyelitis if the metaphysis of the bone is intracapsular. This is, in fact, an unusual anatomical arrangement, and most examples of suppurative arthritis are secondary to blood-borne infection or direct contamination from penetrating wounds.

Bronchi. These are a common route for the spread of invading organisms, e.g. in bronchopneumonia and tuberculosis.

Ureters. Infections of the kidney, e.g. tuberculosis, may spread down the ureters to the bladder.

Gut. This is the route for infection with parasites such as *Ascaris lumbricoides* and *E. histolytica*. Swallowed organisms from pulmonary infections may infect the intestines: a good example of this is the enteritis which occasionally complicates pulmonary tuberculosis.

Tissue planes, synovial sheaths, etc. The psoas abscess is an example of infection spreading in a potential space.

Spread by Lymphatics

The lymphatics form a capillary network almost as extensive as the vascular capillaries. None is present in the spleen, brain, or bone.

In acute inflammation the vessels are held open by the increase in tissue tension.[29] The permeability of their linings is increased, and the flow of lymph increased. Invading organisms frequently gain access to the lymphatics, and are carried to the nearest lymph node. Phagocytes which have ingested organisms, but which are unable to destroy them, also travel to the local nodes, e.g. in tuberculosis. The lymph nodes are thus the *second line of defence* against the spread of infection. Toxins may also be absorbed by the lymphatics. Lymphangitis is therefore a common event in spreading lesions, and when the vessels are near the surface, as in the forearm, they may appear as bright red streaks.

The structure of the lymph node is well adapted to its function as a filter. The afferent vessels pour lymph into the cortical sinus, whence it percolates through a spongework of reticulin fibres, around which there are numerous reticulum cells and RE cells. Finally it is collected in the medullary sinuses, and passes out through the main efferent vessel. The RE cells of the node are therefore in intimate contact with the lymph fluid. When stimulated they are actively phagocytic, and capable of removing particulate matter as well as soluble toxins from the lymph.

Experimentally the efficiency of the lymph node as a filter can be tested by cannulating the efferent and afferent lymph vessels, and then perfusing the node with fluid containing organisms.[30] Experiments of this type show:

1. The efficiency of the filter decreases as the rate of flow is increased.

2. Fatigue develops if the perfusion is continued too long.

It has been shown that exercise increases the lymph flow from a limb. This is another reason why rest is indicated in treating inflamed tissues.

Organisms may become arrested in the lymph nodes and yet not be destroyed. In this way lymphadenitis arises; the filtration will have protected the individual, but at the expense of the node. If organisms pass through the lymphatic barrier, they then enter the blood stream.

Spread by the Blood Stream

The blood stream forms the *third and last defence* against the spread of infection. It has two main defence mechanisms:

1. The circulating blood itself contains a wide array of antibacterial substances. Apart from the circulating phagocytes which probably play little part, there are natural antibacterial substances, like complement, properdin, and opsonins, as well as specific acquired antibodies.

2. The reticulo-endothelial system, especially the sinus-lining cells of the liver, bone marrow, and spleen, forms the main defence against generalised infection. Organisms injected into the blood stream experimentally are rapidly removed. In natural infections with highly invasive organisms, like the typhoid bacillus, early invasion of the blood stream occurs, and the circulating organisms are rapidly taken up by the RE system. These cells ingest foreign materials in the blood stream whether in particulate or soluble form. This is the first step in the afferent limb of the general immune response (see p. 153). The presence of organisms in the blood stream is not an uncommon event; it may occur under several conditions.

1. *Direct invasion of blood vessels*. A few organisms may invade blood vessels in the course of any local infection, e.g. a boil. The infection is often quite trivial, but adjacent blood vessels may be ruptured by trauma, thereby allowing organisms to enter. Gingival infection or apical tooth abscesses are common lesions in which this is thought to occur, e.g. following dental extraction or even chewing hard food. When small numbers of organisms enter the blood stream in this way, they are rapidly phagocytosed by the cells of the RE system and are destroyed. This transient presence of organisms in the blood stream is called *bacteraemia*, and causes few symptoms. Rigors may occur, as in the bacteraemia which follows catheterisation. Its real importance, however, is that under certain conditions it may have serious consequences. Experimentally it has been shown that when an animal has a bacteraemia, histamine injected locally at any site will precipitate a local infection with the organism concerned. Trauma has a similar effect. Staphylococcal osteomyelitis occurs in this way. The patient, usually a child, has a transient bacteraemia usually associated with a septic skin lesion. Trauma to the limbs leads to a mild injury at the metaphysis of a long bone, and this causes localisation of the staphylococci.

In bacteraemia the kidney may filter off the organisms, and a renal infection occasionally results. In this way a carbuncle of the kidney may complicate a staphylococcal bacteraemia. The role of a coliform bacteraemia in the causation of urinary infection is discussed in Chapter 11. *Strept. viridans* bacteraemia is of great importance in the pathogenesis of subacute infective endocarditis. Bacteraemia, especially with Gram-negative bacilli, has been incriminated as a cause of shock, e.g. following operations on the intestine or following the infusion of contaminated fluids (p. 425).

2. *Septic thrombophlebitis*. When thrombophlebitis occurs in the neighbourhood of a pyogenic infection, the thrombus may be invaded by organisms. Softening occurs, and the detachment of pieces of infected thrombus leads to pyaemia. *Pyaemia* is the presence in the circulation of infected thrombus which is carried to various organs where it produces metastatic abscesses or septic infarcts. Which occurs depends on the vascular arrangements of the organ in which the emboli become lodged. Pyaemia is produced after the detachment of infected thrombus either from septic thrombophlebitis or from the heart valves in acute infective endocarditis. If the lesions occur in the systemic circulation, pyaemic lung abscesses occur, e.g. following carbuncles, osteomyelitis, and puerperal sepsis.

Suppuration in the gastro-intestinal tract (acute appendicitis and infected piles) occasionally leads to portal pyaemia with multiple abscesses in the liver. Most pyaemia is staphylococcal, but *Strept. pyogenes*, pneumococci, and the Gram-negative intestinal bacilli may also be responsible.

3. *Spread from lymphatic system.* Organisms which are not held up in the tissues at the portal of entry or in the lymph nodes, reach the venous circulation *via* the main lymphatic ducts. Bacteraemia produced in this way is a common event with many invasive organisms, e.g. *S. typhi*. The number of organisms reaching the blood is small, the condition is symptomless, and the organisms are removed from the blood by the RE cells.

If the phagocytic cells of the RE system are unable to destroy the organisms, they may proliferate in the cells. Following the death of these cells the circulation is flooded with organisms, and the patient becomes gravely ill. This is *septicaemia*. It differs from bacteraemia in the following ways:

1. It is associated with severe clinical symptoms.

2. There are more organisms in the blood.

3. It indicates that the host's resistance to the organism is very inadequate. Bacteraemia is the presence of organisms in the blood of a patient whose defence mechanisms are good. Septicaemia occurs where the defence mechanism has failed; it is therefore a much more serious condition. Septicaemia may be produced by all the pyogenic organisms (see Chapter 17), *S. typhi*, *B. anthracis*, *Y. pestis*, etc. It may sometimes lead to acute infective endocarditis, which in turn causes pyaemia.

Infection via nerves. Some viruses, e.g. rabies virus, are believed to travel up the nerves to reach the central nervous system. Whether they pass up the axoplasm or in the periaxonal spaces is uncertain.[31] Tetanus toxin, injected or formed intramuscularly, almost certainly travels up in the tissue spaces around the axons, driven no doubt by the very high pressures (over 750 mm. water) generated in muscle by its contraction.[32]

Factors Determining the Localisation or Spread of Infection

It is convenient at this point to summarise the factors which determine whether or not a particular organism is likely to spread from its site of primary infection.

Factors Involving the Organisms

Virulence. It should be appreciated that within each species of organism there are many strains with varying degrees of virulence. This may manifest itself both by greater infectivity during epidemics and the ability to produce a very severe spreading infection. Thus some strains of *Cl. welchii* produce a particularly spreading type of lesion, and this is related to toxin production. With *C. diphtheriae* the three strains, gravis, intermedius, and mitis, each produce the same diphtheria exotoxin, but in different amounts.

Dose. Experimentally it can be shown in calves that the lesions produced by injecting tubercle bacilli vary according to the dose. Small doses produce minor local lesions, while large doses result in spreading infections.[33] A similar state of affairs probably exists with respect to many infections. In some cases it seems that there must be a minimum concentration of organisms in the tissues before an infection can be established. This concentration probably varies widely according to the organism. In some instances it has been claimed that a single organism can cause infection (*S. typhimurium* in mice), but this is probably unusual.

Portal of entry. This is a most important factor. Some organisms will cause infection only if administered by a particular route. *V. cholerae* is non-pathogenic if injected subcutaneously, but causes cholera if swallowed. Experimentally the dose of tubercle bacilli necessary to cause infection of the intestine is about 100 times that needed to infect the lungs.[33]

Synergism. The combined effect of two infecting agents may be greater than either one alone. A good example of this is seen in sheep. These animals often harbour *Cl. oedematiens* in their livers, but this is inactive and produces no disease. When, however, the animal becomes infected with the liver fluke *Fasciola hepatica*, local conditions are created which favour growth of the clostridia. The animal develops a fulminating infection of the liver known as "black liver disease".[34]

The presence of two organisms, the one assisting the other, is somewhat unusual in infection. The best-known example is Vincent's infection (*Fusobacterium fusiforme* and *Borrelia vincenti*), which is a common cause of gingivitis. Synergistic gangrene described on p. 221 provides another example. *Haemophilus influenzae* provides an illustration of one organism deriving benefit from the products of another. *H. influenzae* needs for its growth a factor which is produced by staphylococci. This may be demonstrated on a culture plate where the haemophilus organisms grow as satellites around the staphylococcal colonies. Infection of the lung by these two bacteria may occur after a virus infection, e.g. epidemic influenza, and it is possible that the haemophilus organisms are aided by the staphylococci.

Products of the organisms. Spreading factor[9, 35] In 1929 Duran-Reynals showed that vaccinia virus injected subcutaneously produced a widespread infection when mixed with a watery extract of testis. The action of this testicular extract was a local one. It caused liquefaction of vitreous humour, and when injected subcutaneously with dyes led to their more rapid local diffusion. It was shown that some organisms, e.g. clostridia and streptococci, produced the same factor, and that this was related to their pathogenicity. Subsequently the spreading factor was found in some snake venoms and extracts of malignant tumours.

It is generally agreed that the action of these extracts containing spreading factors is due to the enzyme *hyaluronidase*, because there is good correlation between the spreading action and enzyme content. There are, however, exceptions, indicating that other factors may also be involved.

Hyaluronidase is an enzyme which depolymerises hyaluronic acid. Hyaluronic acid forms highly viscous solutions, and is a component of the ground or intercellular substance. The enzyme converts it into a watery fluid, thereby facilitating the diffusion of injected substances.

Its relationship to the spread of infection is debatable.[29] There is some broad correlation between hyaluronidase production and ability to spread. Thus the enzyme is produced by *Cl. welchii*, but not by *Cl. tetani*. However, the amount of hyaluronidase produced by different strains of organisms, e.g. *Cl. welchii*, does not bear any relationship to the observed virulence of the strains. Furthermore, administrations of antihyaluronidase do not hinder the spread of *Cl. welchii* in experimental infections. It should not be forgotten that theoretically hyaluronidase can also be a factor in the limitation of infection. If organisms and toxins are spread too widely, their concentrations at any one point may be too low to cause damage (see p. 100). Until further proof is provided, it must be concluded that hyaluronidase production is not an important factor in the promotion of the spread of natural infection. *Streptokinase* and *staphylokinase* may play a part in the spread of infection, and so, of course, may staphylococcal *coagulase*. These have already been considered in relation to the fibrin barrier.

Factors Involving the Host

GENERAL.[36, 37] *The general state of health* of the host is important. Starvation and haemorrhagic shock have been shown experimentally to render animals more liable to infection. It is frequently observed that patients with chronic debilitating diseases like chronic nephritis and especially diabetes mellitus are less well able to resist infection. The factors involved are complex, but probably involve both humoral factors, e.g. a low complement level, and the phagocytes (see also p. 160).

The immune state. This involves both non-specific factors like complement, and the specific antibodies of acquired immunity. Primary infections tend to spread much more than subsequent ones due to the absence of active immunity. The immunologically deficient states are described on p. 171.

Low white-cell count. Infections tend to spread whenever the neutrophil (polymorphonuclear) leucocyte count is low, e.g. in agranulocytosis or acute leukaemia.

LOCAL. The local blood supply is most important. *Ischaemia* from whatever cause, e.g. injection of adrenaline, nerve lesions, and peripheral vascular disease, adversely affects the inflammatory response designed to destroy the organism. Similarly *foreign bodies* and *chemicals* causing necrosis are harmful. Thus silica potentiates the tubercle bacillus. The action of ionic calcium may also be mentioned in connexion with anaerobic wound infections.

It is evident from this account of the various patterns of infection that the relationship between the host and his infecting organism is extremely complex. This is well illustrated in the case of man and the *Brucella* organism; the infection can vary from an acute illness to a chronic disease or even to a symptomless carrier state in which a symbiotic relationship has been established. Only with the frankly exotoxin-producing organisms is the pathogenesis of the disease which they cause at all clearly understood.

It is not surprising therefore that it is in this group of infections that our understanding of immunity is also most complete.

GENERAL BODY RESPONSES TO INFECTION

The last consideration concerns the general response of the body to infection. There is usually pyrexia, a raised ESR, and an alteration in the white-cell count depending on the organism responsible for the condition. There are various metabolic effects also, e.g. dehydration, protein breakdown with increased nitrogenous excretion in the urine, and a tendency to ketosis. All these features are discussed in later chapters. An attempt should always be made to keep the local and general responses in proper perspective.

REFERENCES

1. WEBB, H. E. (1968). *British Medical Journal*, iv, 684.
2. WILSON, G. S. and MILES, A. A. (1964). In Topley and Wilson's *Principles of Bacteriology*, 5th edn, p. 1228. London: Arnold.
3. WAKSMAN, B. H. (1961). *Journal of Neuropathology and Experimental Neurology*, **20**, 35.
4. ØRSKOV, J. and MOLTKE, O. Z. (1928). *Zeitschrift für Immunitätsforschung und experimentelle Therapie*, **59**, 357. See Wright, G. P. (1958). *An Introduction to Pathology*, 3rd edn, p. 60. London: Longmans.
5. WILSON, G. S. and MILES, A. A. (1964). *Loc. cit.*, p. 1836.
6. COOMBS, R. R. A. (1968). *British Medical Journal*, i, 597.
7. SMITH, H. (1960). In *The Biochemical Response to Injury*: a C.I.O.M.S. Symposium, p. 341. Edited by H. B. Stoner and C. J. Threlfall. Oxford: Blackwell.
8. SHWARTZMAN, G. (1937). *Phenomenon of Local Tissue Reactivity*. Oxford University Press.
9. HADFIELD, G. and GARROD, L. P. (1947). (Eds) *Recent Advances in Pathology*, 5th edn, p. 1. London: Churchill.
10. Annotation (1954). *Lancet*, i, 506.
11. ARCHER, R. K. (1963). *The Eosinophil Leucocytes*. Oxford: Blackwell.
12. Leading Article (1971). *Lancet*, ii, 1187.

13. HIRSCH, J. G. (1965). In *The Inflammatory Process*, p. 266. Edited by B. W. Zweifach, L. Grant and R. T. McCluskey. New York and London: Academic Press.
14. DUBOS, R. J. (1955). *Lancet*, ii, 1.
15. ROBB-SMITH, A. H. T. (1957). *Lancet*, i, 699.
16. SUTER, E. and RAMSEIER, H. (1964). *Advances in Immunology*, **4**, 117.
17. QUIE, P. G. (1969). *New England Journal of Medicine*, **280**, 502.
18. ZEYA, H. I. and SPITZNAGEL, J. K. (1968). *Journal of Experimental Medicine*, **127**, 927.
19. RICHARDSON, R. (1940). *Journal of Clinical Investigation*, **19**, 239.
20. HOWARD, J. G. (1963). In *Modern Trends in Immunology*, 1, p. 86. Edited by R. Cruickshank. London: Butterworths.
21. SCHULTZ, J. *et al.* (1965). *Archives of Biochemistry and Biophysics*, **111**, 73.
22. ERAKLIS, A. J. *et al.* (1967). *New England Journal of Medicine*, **276**, 1225.
23. GREENWOOD, B. M., WHITTLE, H. C. and DOMINIC-RAJKOVIC, O. (1971). *Lancet*, ii, 519.
24. EDWARDS, E. A. (1971). *Journal of Immunology*, **106**, 314.
25. McMASTER, P. D. (1941). *Journal of Experimental Medicine*, **73**, 85.
26. McMASTER, P. D. and PARSONS, R. J. (1938). *Journal of Experimental Medicine*, **68**, 377.
27. PARSONS, R. J. and McMASTER, P. D. (1938). *Journal of Experimental Medicine*, **68**, 353.
28. MAJNO, G. (1964). In *Cellular Injury*, a Ciba Foundation Symposium, p. 87. Edited by A. V. S. de Reuck and J. Knight. London: Churchill.
29. WRIGHT, G. P. (1953). In *Recent Advances in Pathology*, 6th edn, p. 1. Edited by G. Hadfield. London: Churchill.
30. DRINKER, C. K., FIELD, M. E. and WARD, H. K. (1934). *Journal of Experimental Medicine*, **59**, 393.
31. DOWNIE, A. W. (1963). In *Mechanisms of Virus Infection*, p. 136. Edited by W. Smith. London and New York: Academic Press.
32. WRIGHT, G. P. (1953). *Proceedings of the Royal Society of Medicine*, **46**, 319.
33. COBBETT, L. (1917). *The Causes of Tuberculosis*, Cambridge Public Health Series. Cambridge University Press.
34. JAMIESON, S. (1949). *Journal of Pathology and Bacteriology*, **61**, 389.
35. DURAN-REYNALS, F. (1942). *Bacteriological Reviews*, **6**, 197.
36. Annotation (1954). *Lancet*, ii, 908.
37. SMITH, W. (1949). *Proceedings of the Royal Society of Medicine*, **42**, 11.

Chapter 9. Wound Healing

The word *healing*, used in a pathological context, refers to the body's replacement of destroyed tissue by living tissue. It is therefore useful, at the outset, to enumerate the causes of tissue loss or destruction:

1. Traumatic excision, whether accidental or surgical.

2. Physical, chemical, and microbial agents. These all give rise to inflammation, and in sufficient dose lead to necrosis.

3. Ischaemia, which leads to infarction.

4. The body's response to external agents can itself engender necrosis. For example, the inflammatory exudate can interfere with the blood supply of the part, as is seen in acute osteomyelitis. Hypersensitivity reactions to foreign proteins, e.g. the Arthus phenomenon, or to products of organisms, e.g. the caseation of tuberculosis, are other instances of tissue destruction brought about by the body's own vigorous responses.

The healing process has two aspects:

(*a*) *Contraction*, a mechanical reduction in the size of the defect occurring in the first few weeks (see below).

(*b*) *Replacement of lost tissue*, which is brought about by migration of cells as well as division of adjacent cells to provide extra tissue to fill the gap. This can be accomplished in two ways:

Regeneration, the replacement of lost tissue by tissue similar in type. There is a proliferation of surrounding undamaged specialised cells.

Repair, the replacement of lost tissue by granulation tissue which matures to form scar tissue. This is inevitable when the surrounding specialised cells do not possess the capacity to proliferate, e.g. muscle and neurones.

The term *reconstitution* may be used when there is coordinated regeneration of several types of lost tissue resulting in the reformation of whole organs or limbs. Many examples are to be found in amphibians and crustaceans. If, for instance, the limb of a newt is amputated, a new limb-bud appears. Its growth results in the production of a new limb from the stump of the old. The process is well developed in lower forms of life, and crustaceans are capable of reforming limbs, claws, and eyes. These are complicated processes resembling embryonic development or asexual reproduction, and have no exact counterpart in the higher vertebrate animals. The reformation of pancreas and liver following partial resection is the nearest approach to reconstitution seen in man.

It should be noted that the word repair is used in a rather arbitrary way by some surgeons and pathologists. Surgeons refer to the union of fractures or the closure of defects by various inert materials as examples of "repair", but the latter is not even true healing, though it has an ameliorative effect. Some pathologists equate repair with healing and recovery, and describe "repair by resolution", "repair by granulation tissue", and "repair by regeneration". Though it is unwise to be dogmatic, there is no doubt that this variation in nomenclature is confusing; in this book the terms resolution (p. 78), regeneration, and repair are used strictly in accordance with the definitions given above.

It will readily be understood that wound healing is a complicated process involving many changes, e.g. movement of cells, division of cells, rearrangement of tissues, and biochemical changes. Depending upon the manner in which wounds are investigated, various aspects may be accentuated and various stages described.

Before describing the co-ordinated process which occurs during simple wound healing, it is convenient first to describe wound contraction, granulation-tissue formation, and changes in tensile strength.

WOUND CONTRACTION[1, 2]

This is conveniently studied by excising a small, circular, full-thickness disc of skin from the back or flank of a rat. Figs. 9.1 and 9.2 show the results of such an experiment.

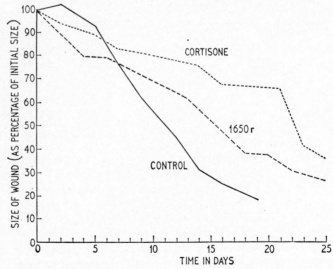

Figure 9.1

Wound contraction in the rat. Daily administration of cortisone acetate causes considerable delay in the process. Irradiation with 1 650 r immediately after inflicting the wounds has a similar delaying effect.

Figure 9.2
Wound contraction in the rat and the effect of x-irradiation. The edges of the skin wounds have been tattooed with carbon so as to render them easily visible. Note how the delivery of 1 650 r to the wound on the right has delayed the contraction process. *(From Blair, G. H., Slome, D. and Walter, J. B. (1961), Review of Experimental Investigations on Wound Healing, British Surgical Practice: Surgical Progress, Ed. by Ross, J. P. London: Butterworths)*

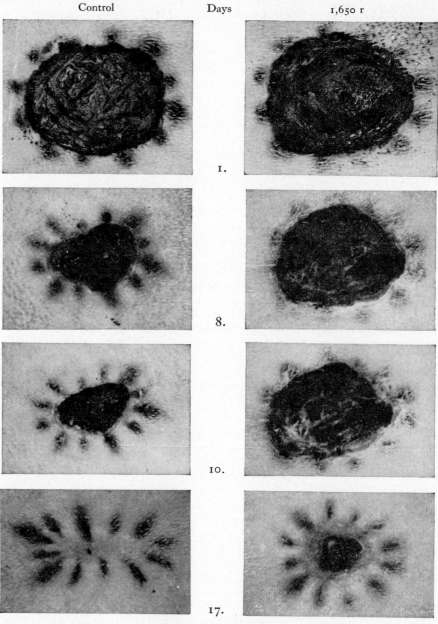

Control   Days   1,650 r

1.

8.

10.

17.

New tissue formation is not included since the measurements are made from the original wound edges. It can be seen that there is an initial *lag period* of 2 to 3 days followed by a period of rapid contraction, which is largely complete by the fourteenth day. The wound is reduced by approximately 80 per cent of its original size.

The magnitude of contraction varies with the species of animal and with the shape, site, and size of the wound. In the rabbit contraction reduces large wounds to a thin linear scar, while in rats the scar occupies 20–30 per cent of the original wound. The importance of contraction is demonstrated in Fig. 9.3.

Contraction results in much faster healing, since only one-quarter to one-third of the amount of destroyed tissue has to be replaced. If contraction is prevented, healing is slow and a large ugly scar is formed. Not only is this cosmetically undesirable, but the large amount of fibrous tissue formed may lead to later complications following cicatrisation.

Cause of contraction. In spite of a great deal of research work neither the mechanism of contraction nor its cause is known for certainty.

Removal of fluid by drying has been suggested as a cause of the diminution in size of wound contents, but this has not been substantiated.

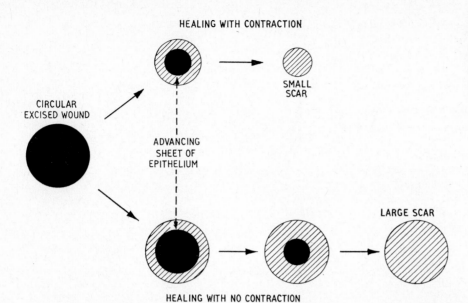

HEALING WITH CONTRACTION

CIRCULAR EXCISED WOUND

SMALL SCAR

ADVANCING SHEET OF EPITHELIUM

LARGE SCAR

HEALING WITH NO CONTRACTION

Figure 9.3
Diagram to show how contraction accelerates the healing of a wound and produces a small scar. It should be noted that in reality a circular wound invariably shows considerable distortion in shape by the time healing is complete.

Contraction of collagen is the time-honoured explanation, but although collagen contracts to one-third of its original length when boiled, there is no evidence that it is capable of contracting *in vivo*.

Wound contraction is actually proceeding at a stage when little collagen is present in the granulation tissue. It is largely completed by the twentieth day, but collagen formation continues after this. Furthermore, in wounded scorbutic animals, although granulation tissue is formed, collagen production is inhibited. Wound contraction, however, proceeds normally, and there seems little doubt that it is not produced by direct contraction of collagen fibres of the granulation tissue.

Contraction of granulation tissue. The fact that contraction occurs at a time when granulation tissue is actively being formed has led many workers to regard the granulations as forming an *organ of contraction*.[3, 4] The observation that contraction occurs normally in the scorbutic animal supports this concept.[5, 6]

The actual location of the contraction mechanism is not known. It seems likely that the process is caused by a general remodelling of tissues rather than a shortening of cells or fibres comparable with contraction of muscle. The granulation tissue in the wound is probably concerned with contraction,[4] and experiments have been carried out which indicate that the contracting mechanism is located in the margins of the wound, the so-called "picture-frame area".[7] Interference with this area delays contraction, whereas careful excision of the granulation tissue of the wound centre has no such effect. Although remodelling of the existing tissues of the wound edge has been suggested as the primary cause, it seems more likely that it is the granulation tissue which is concerned.

Experimental methods of inhibiting wound contraction. *X-irradiation.* Ionising radiation applied to the wounded area at the time of wounding causes a delay in contraction (see Figs. 9.1 and 9.2).

Corticosteroid administration has the same effect[3] (see Fig. 9.1).

Contraction does not proceed normally in *burns*.

Immediate skin grafting of the raw area of a wound prevents its subsequent contraction. It also halts the process if performed in an existing wound during the phase of rapid contraction.[3] The graft must contain dermis.

GRANULATION-TISSUE FORMATION

The ingrowth of granulation tissue into a haematoma can be studied experimentally using the rabbit ear-chamber technique,[8] or by observing the changes in the interstices of an implanted plastic sponge,[9, 10] e.g. Etheron or Ivalon. Three phases may be observed:

1. **Phase of traumatic inflammation.** The damaged cells set in motion the phenomenon of acute inflammation. An exudate of fibrin and polymorphs develops. Haemorrhage also occurs, and the blood clot contributes to the fibrin formation. The ground substance undergoes depolymerisation, and there is loss of granules in the mast cells. These changes have been fully described in Chapter 6.

2. **Phase of demolition.** The dead tissue cells liberate their autolytic enzymes, and other enzymes (proteolytic) come from disintegrating polymorphs. There is an associated macrophage infiltration. These cells ingest particulate matter, either digesting or removing it. They may fuse to form foreign-body giant cells. This demolition phase and the cells involved are described in greater detail in Chapters 6 and 30.

3. **Ingrowth of granulation tissue.** Granulation tissue is formed by the proliferation and migration of the surrounding connective tissue elements; it is composed at first of

capillary loops and fibroblasts together with a variable number of inflammatory cells. It is thus initially highly vascular, but with the passage of time it develops into avascular scar tissue. Two stages in its formation may be recognised: firstly a stage of *vascularisation*, and subsequently a stage of *devascularisation*.

Stage of Vascularisation. The ingrowth of capillary loops and fibroblasts, so that the insoluble fibrin clot is replaced by living vascular granulation tissue, is known as *organisation*, and is conveniently studied in the rabbit ear-chamber.

Fig. 9.4 shows such a chamber in position. It consists of two main parts—a base and a cover-slip—both made of transparent material, usually Perspex for the base and mica

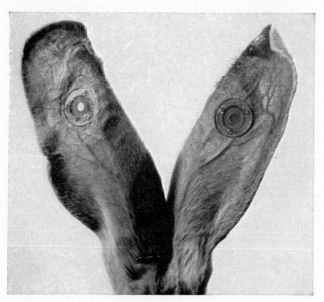

Figure 9.4
Two rabbit ear-chambers in position. The one in the left ear shows the clear central area in which observations are made. In the chamber on the right, the area of the central table is still filled with blood clot. *(From Blair, G. H., van den Brenk, H. A. S., Walter, J. B. and Slome, D. (1961), "Wound Healing", pp. 46–53, in A Symposium organised by Smith and Nephew Research Ltd. Oxford: Pergamon Press)*

for the cover-slip. Between these parts in the central window there is a gap of between 50 μm and 100 μm (Fig. 9.5) which is first filled with blood clot and inflammatory exudate. This fibrin clot is invaded by macrophages, which advance towards the centre table, and they are followed by capillary loops and fibroblasts (Figs. 9.6, 9.7, and 9.8).

Solid buds of endothelial cells grow out from existing blood vessels, undergo canalisation, and by anastomosis with their neighbours form a series of vascular arcades. At first the newly-formed vessels all appear similar, and under the electron microscope show gaps between the endothelial cells, a poorly-formed basement membrane, and long pseudopodia of the endothelial cells which reach out into the

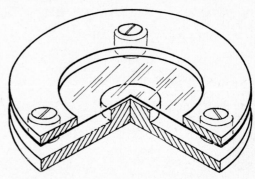

Figure 9.5
Diagrammatic representation of one type of rabbit ear-chamber; a wedge has been cut out to show its construction. The chamber is composed of a Perspex base plate which has a raised central table and three peripherally arranged pillars. The cover-slip consists of a disc of mica supported at the edge by a ring of Perspex. The cover-slip is placed upon the three pillars, and held there in position by screws which are inserted into threaded holes in the pillars. The height of the pillars is such that the gap between the top of the table and the mica is 50–100 μm. *(Drawing by Mr. S. P. Steward)*

connective tissue spaces.[11] These newly-formed vessels leak protein,[12] and it is easy to imagine that the tissue fluid forms a very suitable medium for fibroblastic growth. Very soon differentiation occurs. Some vessels acquire a muscular coat and become arterioles, whilst others enlarge to form thin-walled venules. The remainder either disappear, or persist as part of the capillary bed. The source of the smooth muscle fibres of the arterioles is undecided, since mitosis in the existing muscle fibres is denied by many observers. Cell migration or differentiation of existing primitive mesenchymal cells are two possible though unproven suggestions. Direct arteriovenous shunts are also formed. The fibroblasts which accompany the capillary loops are at first large and plump, but gradually collagenous fibres form around them, and the cells become mature elongated fibrocytes. During this process of fibrogenesis, the pH becomes alkaline. The mode of formation of collagen is discussed in Chapter 5. The first formed fibres are described as reticulin, but these mature to form adult fibrous tissue.

Collagen is usually formed in the body by the activity of fibroblasts (or closely allied cells like osteoblasts). The cells secrete a soluble collagen which polymerises to form fibrils (see p. 62). The soluble collagen might also condense on to pre-existing fibres and thereby reinforce them.[13] Fibroblasts are also thought to be responsible for the production of the mucopolysaccharide ground substance, because during the early phases of organisation the large fibroblasts contain granules which have similar staining reactions to those of ground substance.

Although most authorities regard the fibroblasts of repair as being derived from local cells of a similar nature, there are some who believe that they can be derived from the circulating cells of the blood—either monocytes or large lym-

Figure 9.6
Granulation-tissue formation in the rabbit ear-chamber. Photographs taken at the following times after the insertion of the chamber: (*a*) 9 days, (*b*) 12 days, (*c*) 17 days, (*d*) 21 days, (*e*) 24 days, (*f*) 44 days. At 9 days vessels are seen to be invading the dark blood clot in the centre, and by the 24th day organisation is complete. The large, tortuous vessels are venules; arterioles are more difficult to see at this magnification. The arrow in (*f*) indicates an arteriole which divides almost immediately. Note how by the 44th day changes have occurred in the course of many blood vessels, although the original pattern of certain venules can still be recognised on the left-hand side of the picture. A lymphatic vessel is now visible at the top of the chamber. ×8·5.

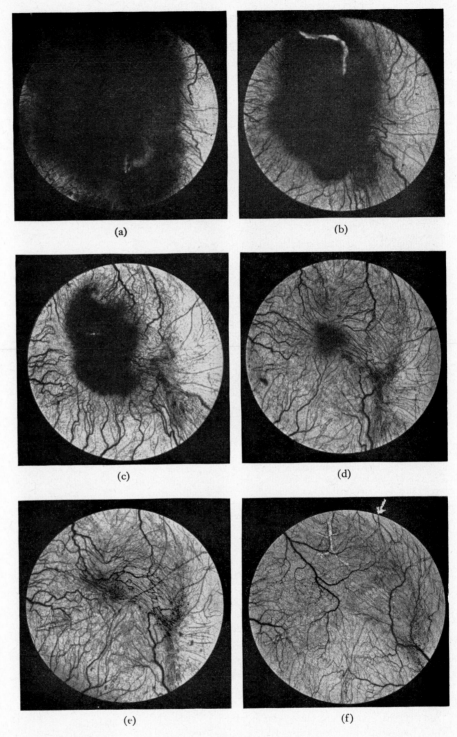

(a)　(b)

(c)　(d)

(e)　(f)

phocytes.[14, 15] Part of the evidence for this is the claim that cultures of blood leucocytes may give rise to fibroblasts and collagen. Probably the cells responsible are endothelial cells or fibroblasts inadvertently introduced during the collection of the blood. However, the matter is not finally settled.

Further changes in granulation tissue. As fibroplasia proceeds, nerve fibres and lymphatics form. The latter develop from existing lymphatics in much the same way as do the blood vessels, only later. With the ingrowth of nerve fibres the arterioles exhibit rhythmic contraction or locomotion.

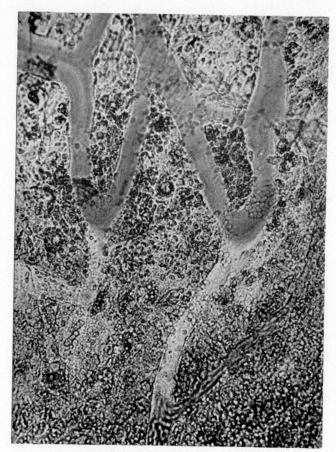

Figure 9.7
The growing edge of granulation tissue in a rabbit ear-chamber. The rapidly moving stream of blood in the capillary loops at the top produces a streaked effect, and individual red cells cannot be distinguished; in the right-hand vessel white cells are adherent to the endothelium, and appear as transparent globules. There is no flow in the capillary buds in the lower half of the picture, and these contain plasma with few cells. Rouleaux formation is seen in one of them.

Mast cells make their appearance, and are a prominent feature of vascular granulation tissue.

As fibroplasia proceeds, some vessels undergo atrophy whilst others show endarteritis obliterans, in which the lumen becomes obliterated due to intimal proliferation. This is the stage of *devascularisation*, and results in the formation of pale, avascular scar tissue. Mast cells disappear, and hyalinisation, calcification, and even ossification may sometimes occur. Coincident with the devascularisation there is often contracture of the scar tissue, with much local tissue distortion. This process is known as cicatrisation, and it must be clearly distinguished from contraction. *Cicatrisation* (or *contracture* as it is sometimes called) is a diminution in size of a *scar*, and is a late event; contraction is a diminution in size of a *wound*, and is an early event.

Although it is generally believed that collagen once formed remains for life, experimental evidence in animals

suggests that it can be removed.[16] The mechanism is not known, but that it does occur in man is suggested by the way in which scars gradually become less obvious and softer. The observation that even healed wounds may break down in scurvy further supports this view, although it is in fact debatable whether mature collagen is removed in this condition. The collagen of bone can certainly be removed in osteoporosis.

Conditions under which granulation tissue is formed (organisation). Organisation is one of the fundamental processes in pathology, and can be defined as the replacement of necrotic tissue, inflammatory exudate, thrombus, or blood clot by granulation tissue. It occurs under four conditions:

In inflammation. It is the fibrinous exudate that is organised if it is not demolished and removed expeditiously. Fibrinous exudates in serous cavities may persist and later be converted into fibrous adhesions. Granulation tissue is an important feature of all chronic inflammatory lesions and in their healing.

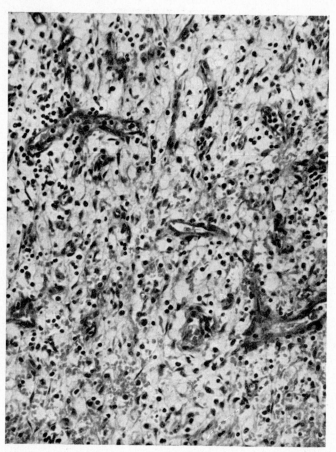

Figure 9.8
Section of young granulation tissue composed mostly of thin-walled capillaries. Several arterioles are also present but at this stage have only a thin muscular coat. Fibroblasts appear as elongated cells, and the small round cells are lymphocytes and plasma cells. × 200.

In wound healing. Both in open wounds and in fractures the initial haematoma between the severed ends is organised as described above. Haematomata in soft tissues (bruises) and even in serous cavities are usually completely absorbed following their demolition by macrophages, and organisation does not generally occur.

In a thrombus.

In an infarct.

Granulation tissue forms an integral part of malignant tumours where it constitutes the stroma. It is particularly prominent in scirrhous carcinoma. The manner of granulation-tissue formation under these circumstances is not altogether clear. The neoplastic cells may excite the formation of an inflammatory exudate which undergoes organisation. Alternatively, the neoplastic cells may in some way directly stimulate a proliferation of the adjacent connective tissue. The latter seems the most likely explanation, and may be likened to the formation of granulation tissue in wound healing (see Fig. 9.11).

Factors Affecting Granulation-Tissue Formation and Maturation

Scurvy. Wounds in scorbutic guinea-pigs do not heal normally owing to the failure of collagen formation. Vascular granulation tissue is formed, but the fibroblasts lack orientation and show a deficiency of phosphatase. Embedded in the ground substance there are abnormal globules and thick fibres of silver-staining material. Hydroxylation of protocollagen does not take place, and since this protein cannot be extruded from the cell, collagen formation does not occur (p. 62). The ground substance itself accumulates in excessive amounts and lacks metachromasia; this is associated with its diminished sulphation, and experimentally a reduced uptake of ^{35}S-labelled sulphate can be demonstrated.

Cortisone administration. Under conditions of excess glucocorticosteroid administration little granulation tissue is formed, fibroblasts remain small, and little collagen is formed. While this effect has been well demonstrated in the experimental animal, glucocorticosteroids in the dosage generally administered do not appear to influence wound healing in man.

Protein starvation. This is considered later (p. 113).

Tensile Strength[17]

Another method of examining a wound, first introduced by Paget in 1853, is estimating its tensile strength. The strength of a healing wound is of great practical importance to the surgeon because it is the main safeguard against wound dehiscence. Experimentally it may be estimated by measuring the force necessary to disrupt the wound. Another technique is to implant two pieces of cellulose sponge held together by a suture. When the animal is killed the sponge is excised and the stitch removed. Part of the specimen is used for chemical estimation of the amount of hydroxyproline, while the other part is distracted on a tensiometer to measure

the strength of the tissue holding the two pieces of sponge together.[18]

During the first few days the strength of a skin wound is only that of the clot cementing the cut surfaces together. There then follows a period of increasing tensile strength which corresponds to the increase in amount of collagen present. If the observations are continued over a long period it is found that whereas the collagen content reaches a maximum at about 80 days, the tensile strength continues to increase for many months thereafter. This is probably due to the reorientation of its fibres and the increase in cross-linkage.

Many factors influence the rate of gain of tensile strength; these are both local and general, but in the main are related to granulation-tissue and collagen formation. Certain additional factors should be noted:

Direction of wound. Skin wounds made in a direction parallel to the lines of Langer heal faster than those made at right angles to them. The tension lines of Langer, first described by Dupuytren in 1832, are due to the orientation of the collagen bundles in the dermis.[19] The skin is less tensile in the direction of the lines than at right angles to them. In general they correspond in direction to the crease lines, although these are in fact related to the movements of the underlying muscles and joints. As skin incisions made across Langer's lines tend to gape, their healing is delayed. When planning a surgical incision the direction of pull of the underlying muscles must also be considered, and as this is related to the crease lines of flexion, the latter constitute the best guide to the placing of the incision. *Wounds parallel to or in the creases are most satisfactory and the scars least visible.* Thus it has been shown experimentally that transverse abdominal incisions produce a stronger scar than do longitudinal ones.[20, 21]

Abdominal support. Abdominal binders reduce the rate of gain of strength of abdominal wounds.[20, 21]

Effect of previous wounding. Pre-existing wounds at a distance do not influence the healing of a further skin wound: there is therefore no evidence of a circulating "wound hormone".[3] Resutured wound do, however, heal faster than those sutured primarily, because the reparative process has already commenced.[22] Severe trauma delays wound healing, presumably because of the adrenocortical response to the stress.

HEALING OF SKIN WOUNDS[23-25]

The histological changes which occur in healing skin wounds have recently been reinvestigated by various workers, and their findings are incorporated in the account that follows.

Healing of a Clean Incised Wound with Edges in Apposition[26]

This process is described as *healing by primary intention*, and is the desired result in all surgical incisions.

The following changes occur:

Initial haemorrhage results in the formation of a fibrin-rich haematoma.

An acute inflammatory reaction occurs, and the fibrinous exudate helps to cement the cut margins of the wound together.

Epithelial Changes. Within 24 hours of injury epithelial cells from the adjacent epidermis migrate into the wound and insinuate themselves between the inert dermis and the

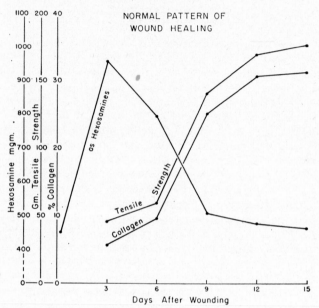

NORMAL PATTERN OF WOUND HEALING

Figure 9.9
The normal pattern of healing in the rat. *(From Dunphy, J. E. and Udupa K. N. (1955), New Engl. J. Med., 253, 847)*

clot (Fig. 9.10(b)). With well-approximated wounds by 24 hours a continuous layer of epidermal cells covers the surface. Overlying the area there is a crust or scab of dried clot. During the next 24–48 hours the epidermal cells invade the space where connective tissue will eventually develop; in this way a spur is formed (Fig. 9.10(c)). The migrating cells of the epidermis do not divide. Mitotic activity occurs in the basal cells a short distance from the edge of the wound, and in the mouse this activity is maximal at 36 hours. Epidermal cells also migrate along suture tracks, and where the suture or the incision encounters a sweat gland or other skin appendage, epithelial cells are contributed from this source (Fig. 9.10(c)). The stimulus for this epithelial growth and migration is not known. Experimentally it has been noted that cells in tissue culture continue to divide until they establish contact with similar cells, at which point mitosis stops. This has been called *contact inhibition* by Abercrombie, but the mechanism is obscure.

A demolition phase follows the acute inflammatory reaction in the area of the wound.

Organisation. By about the third day the wound area is invaded by fibroblasts and capillary buds growing in from the cut surfaces. This ingrowth occurs mainly from the subcutaneous tissues, with little or no contribution from the dense reticular dermis, which appears inert. There may be some contribution from the papillary dermis.

Soon after the granulation tissue appears, collagen formation commences: at first as reticulin fibres but later maturing to collagen fibres. The amount of collagen in a wound can be assessed histologically, but a more objective method is to estimate the amount of hydroxyproline in hydrosylates of the wound contents. By this technique it has been demonstrated that the collagen content closely parallels

Figure 9.10
Diagrammatic representation of the healing of an incised wound held together by a suture, the track of which alone is shown. The wound rapidly fills with clot (A) and shortly afterwards the epithelium migrates into the wound and down the suture tracks (B). Epithelial spurs are formed, and granulation-tissue (gran) formation proceeds (C). In D the suture has been removed, and scar tissue remains to mark the site of the incision and the suture tracks. The epithelial ingrowths have degenerated.

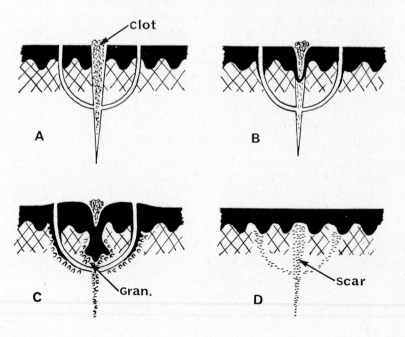

the tensile strength of a wound during the first month. Attempts to demonstrate the amount of ground substance by chemical means have been less successful. The hexosamine content of a healing wound measures not only the hexosamine present in mucopolysaccharides but also that of the plasma glycoproteins in the inflammatory exudate. The total hexosamine level therefore measures the initial inflammatory reaction, rising to a peak at about three days and returning to normal by the ninth day (Fig. 9.9).

The granulation tissue appears to prevent excessive epithelial migration into the wound, and the epithelial cells which form the spurs and the lining of suture tracks degenerate and are replaced by granulation tissue. Only the surface epithelial cells persist, and these divide and differentiate so that a multilayered covering of epidermis is reformed. It first covers a vascular granulation tissue, but as devascularisation proceeds the scar shrinks in size and changes in colour from red to white.

Epithelial cells are thus the first cells to be stimulated, and their presence excites a connective tissue response which in its turn inhibits the epithelial growth. The early role that epithelium plays in the process of wound healing has been stressed by Gillman, and explains the formation of the epidermoid cyst from epithelial remnants (see p. 112), and also the ugly punctate scars which appear if sutures are left in position for any length of time. Punctured wounds due to injections do not form such scars, because the wound is not held open and therefore no epithelial "invasion" occurs. The use of adhesive tapes instead of sutures for closing wounds avoids these marks and produces a better cosmetic result.[27, 28]

Healing of Wounds with Separated Edges
(*Healing by Secondary Intention*)

Although stress is sometimes laid on the difference between healing by primary intention and secondary intention, the pathological changes in both are very similar. When there is extensive tissue loss, either by direct trauma, inflammatory necrosis, or simply failure to approximate the wound edges, a large defect is present which must be made good. The main

bulk of tissue which performs this service is granulation tissue, and this type of healing is therefore sometimes known as *healing by granulation*. The term is, however, misleading, since it wrongly implies that granulations are not formed in the simple incised wound. The differences between healing by primary and secondary intention are quantitative not qualitative.

In healing by secondary intention the wound edges are widely separated, so that healing has to progress from the base upwards as well as from the edges inwards. From the clincal point of view healing of a well-approximated incised wound (primary intention) is fast and leaves a small, neat scar. Healing by secondary intention is slow and results in a large, distorted scar. The difference lies in the type of wound and not in the type of healing.

The following account of the healing of a large uninfected wound is illustrated in Fig. 9.11.

1. There is an initial inflammatory phase affecting the surrounding tissues. The wound is filled with coagulum, as described in simple incisions. This coagulum dries on its surface, and forms a scab in some wounds.

2. An important feature is *wound contraction*, which has already been fully described (see p. 103). Fig. 9.3 (p. 105) shows the changes in size of full-thickness skin loss.

3. As with incised wounds, the epidermis adjacent to the wound shows hyperplasia, and epithelial cells migrate into the wound. They form a thin tongue which grows between pre-existing viable connective tissue and the surface clot with necrotic material. The epithelial cells secrete a collagenase which probably aids their penetration between living and dead connective tissue.

4. Demolition follows acute inflammation, and the clot in the centre of the wound is invaded and replaced by granulation tissue. This grows from the subcutaneous tissues at the wound edge, and is important in causing wound contraction. Granulation tissue is also formed from the base of the wound, the amount from this source depending upon the nature and vascularity of the bed.

When the wound is viewed with a magnifying glass, the

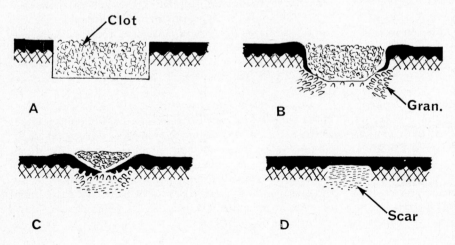

A   B   C   D

Figure 9.11
Diagram to illustrate the healing of an excised wound. The wound is rapidly filled with clot (A). Epithelium soon migrates in from the margins to undermine the clot, which dries to form a crust. Granulation tissue (gran) grows into the wounded area, and is most profuse around the circumference where it is derived from the subcutaneous fat (B). Epithelial ingrowth continued and spurs are produced (C); these, however, do not persist, and the end-result (D) is a scar covered by epidermis which lacks rete ridges. During the healing process contraction has taken place so that the final scar is considerably smaller than the original wound.

surface (under the scab) is deep red and granular, the capillary loops forming elevated mounds. It is very fragile, and the slightest trauma causes bleeding. It was this granularity which was responsible for the name "granulation tissue". The covering of the wound by granulation tissue serves an important protective role. If organisms are introduced into the recent wound, infection is likely to result, but not, however, if the wound is first allowed to granulate. Thus granulation tissue forms a temporary protective layer until the surface is covered by epithelium.

5. The migrating epidermis covers the granulation tissue, and in this way a mushroom-shaped scab is formed with a central attachment, which finally becomes nipped off (Fig. 9.11(c)).

6. The regenerated epidermis becomes thicker, and sends short processes into the underlying tissue. These are transient structures and do not persist as rete ridges, for neither these nor the skin appendages are reformed in man. The epidermal incursions appear to stimulate the formation of granulation tissue, so that the scar gains thickness and is eventually level with the surface of the skin. The scar is at first pink, but the subsequent devascularisation leaves it white.

It can be seen that with full-thickness skin loss, part of the clot occupying the wound is organised but much of it is cast off. With partial-thickness skin loss, as may occur following burns or at the donor site of a Thiersch graft, the area of the wound is covered by epithelium both from the wound edges and from the cut remains of hair follicles and sweat glands. Epithelialisation is therefore very fast, and the granulation tissue which is formed is produced beneath the new epithelium. For reasons which are not known contraction does not occur.

Complications of Wound Healing

Infection. A wound may provide the portal of entry for many organisms. Infection may delay healing, or if severe stop it completely. Scab formation does not occur, and often the base is composed of a slough, underlying which there is granulation tissue. Tissue destruction due to infection is of common occurrence, and a simple incision then heals by secondary intention. Fibrous tissue is formed in excessive amounts, and an ugly scar remains.

Wound dehiscence.[29] Dehiscence, the bursting open of a wound, is particularly important after laparotomy, since the mortality of a burst abdomen is approximately 30 per cent. It occurs in from 0·5 to 5·0 per cent of abdominal operations, and is most common with upper abdominal incisions. Inappropriate suture material and poor surgical technique are important factors, as are also those general conditions which favour poor wound healing, e.g. hypoproteinaemia, lack of vitamin C, and poor general nutrition such as may accompany malignant disease. Local factors such as infection play a part; to this must be added excessive tension due to postoperative ileus, peritonitis, or the effects of

vomiting and coughing. Increased mechanical stress has been found to be a factor in over 90 per cent of cases of burst abdomen.

Implantation (or epidermoid) cysts. Epithelial cells which flow into the healing wound may sometimes persist, and they may later proliferate to form an epidermoid cyst. It should not be confused with a dermoid cyst (see p. 361).

Keloid formation. Occasionally the excessive formation of collagenous tissue results in the appearance of a raised area of scar tissue called a keloid. The cause of this is unknown. Repeated trauma and irritation caused by foreign bodies, hair, keratin, etc., may play a part. They are more common in the young, especially girls, in Negroes, and in tuberculous subjects. They occur most commonly in the region of the neck. They are especially frequent after burns.

Pigmentary changes. Coloured particles introduced into the wound may persist and lead to tattooing. Healed chronic ulcers sometimes have a russet colour due to staining with haemosiderin.

Painful scars. Pain, either local or referred, may be experienced if a neuroma is included in the scar tissue.

Weak scars. If scar tissue is subjected to continuous strain, stretching may result. An incisional hernia develops in this way.

Cicatrisation. This late reduction in the size of a scar is believed to differ from the early contraction of wounds. It is a frequent complication of extensive burning of the skin, and may produce great deformity. Cicatrisation is especially important in hollow viscera such as the urethra, oesophagus, and intestine. It leads to progressive stenosis with stricture formation. The heart valves may exhibit regurgitation as well as stenosis, and in a cirrhotic liver cicatrisation strangles the venous radicles and leads to portal hypertension.

Neoplasia. Trauma may under rare circumstances act as a promoting agent, and squamous-cell carcinoma occasionally develops in scars.

Factors Influencing Repair

Although it would be desirable to analyse the factors which influence repair according to whether they affect granulation-tissue formation, collagen production, contraction, etc., it must be admitted that in many instances we have insufficient information to adopt this policy. In practice the factors which cause delay in wound healing may be divided into two groups: those which act locally, and those whose influence is general.

Local factors. *Poor blood supply.* Wounds with a poor blood supply heal slowly; thus injuries heal much more slowly in the pretibial region than in parts with a good blood supply, e.g. the face. The poor circulation in the skin of the leg in patients with varicose ulcers predisposes to slow healing. Ischaemia secondary to pressure is an important factor in the causation and poor healing of bedsores. Any condition of chronic inflammation is liable to be accompanied by endarteritis obliterans and a poor blood supply to the part;

a good example of this is previous x-irradiation. Finally, the slow wound healing of old age may in part be related to coincidental atheroma.

Adhesions to bony surfaces may, by anchoring the wound edges, prevent contraction and also adequate apposition. This was noted by John Hunter[30] and is well seen in wounds over the tibia, and also in chronic stasis ulcers.

Conditions predisposing to continued tissue breakdown and inflammation. All types of infection come under this heading. Inflammation caused by foreign bodies and irritants like disinfectants is also important. The continued trauma incurred in dressing wounds may cause much damage to the delicate regenerating epithelium.

Movement. Movement may delay wound healing in two ways.

(*a*) By subjecting the wound to persistent trauma and causing acute inflammation.

(*b*) Exercise may act in a systemic way, possibly through the adrenals. It has been shown that animals that are kept on the move show few mitoses in their epidermis.

Neoplasia.

Exposure to ionising radiation. Previous x-irradiation may affect the vascularity of the part, but apart from this x-rays inhibit wound contraction if given at the same time as the injury. The formation of granulation tissue is also delayed.

Ultraviolet light. The exposure of wounds to ultraviolet light is well known clinically to increase the rate of healing, and this has been confirmed experimentally.

General factors affecting wound healing. *Age.* Wound healing is fast in the young, but is normal in old age unless there is some associated debilitating disease or ischaemia.

Nutrition. (*a*) *Protein deficiency.* In starvation or protein depletion there is an impairment of granulation-tissue and collagen formation, resulting in a great delay in wound healing. This may be corrected by the administration of protein containing methionine or cystine. These sulphur-containing amino acids are not present in the mature collagen molecule, but cystine is a vital component of the transport form of collagen or procollagen (p. 63).

(*b*) *Vitamin-C lack.* The observations of Lind on the effect of scurvy in sailors, and the finding that citrus fruit cured the condition is one of the classical descriptions in medicine. In spite of much research there are few who could not re-echo the words of Dr. Grainger, who, writing to Lind concerning scurvy, noted that it was "a subject of which I had read much but knew little".[31]

Experimentally in guinea-pigs (scurvy does not occur in other rodents because they can synthesise vitamin C) wound contraction and epithelial regeneration proceed normally. Granulation tissue is produced, but is abnormal[32] (see p. 109). Dead tissue, catgut sutures, etc., are poorly removed. Capillaries are unduly fragile and haemorrhages occur.

As noted by Lind, healed wounds, even fractures, break down again in scurvy. Young collagen fibres revert to a reticulin-like stage. It is, however, doubtful whether mature established collagen behaves in this manner.

While florid scurvy is uncommon, minor degrees of vitamin-C lack are not infrequent. If guinea-pigs kept on a normal maintenance dose of the vitamin are subjected to burning, they develop a scorbutic state. Wounds then show the characteristic features of scorbutic healing.

(*c*) *The role of zinc.*[33] The addition of zinc to the diet of rats has been shown to promote the healing of thermal burns and excised wounds. The mechanism is not known, but the fact that zinc is an important component of several enzymes may be related. The oral administration of zinc sulphate has been tried in man, and a beneficial effect on wound healing claimed.

Hormones. (*a*) *Glucocorticosteroids.* The effects of cortisone administration on granulation-tissue formation and wound contraction have been previously noted (see pp. 109 and 105).

(*b*) *Deoxycorticosterone acetate* (DOCA) and anabolic steroids like testosterone are claimed to increase the speed of wound healing.

In general the effects of hormone administration in animals are difficult to assess. Their action may be marked, or it may be reversed by a secondary effect upon other endocrines, especially the pituitary.

Temperature. It is general experience that wounds heal much more slowly in cold weather, and experiments on cold-blooded animals (alligators) have shown that the rate of wound healing is proportional to the temperature of the environment at which they are kept. A rise of $10°C$ results in a two-fold increase in the speed of wound healing. In squirrels hibernating at $5°C$ epithelialisation of granulation tissue is completely in abeyance.[34]

Repair in the central nervous system. Repair in the central nervous system follows the same general pattern as that seen in other parts of the body. There are, however, several slight modifications due to its specialised structure. Owing to the abundance of free lipid in damaged brain tissue the macrophages in the demolition phase ingest large quantities of it. They become swollen and their cytoplasm is foamy. They are called compound granular corpuscles, because they contain lipid and haemosiderin. They are probably derived both from microglia (the histiocytes of the brain) and the blood monocytes. In the central nervous system the astrocyte is the counterpart of the fibroblast present in other connective tissues, and therefore glial tissue is found instead of fibrous tissue. Injuries involving the pia may, however, stimulate the production of a granulation tissue containing fibroblasts and collagen as well as neuroglia.

The mechanism of wound healing. When one considers that in a healing wound there is cell and tissue production proceeding at a rate which exceeds that seen in most malignant tumours, it is humiliating to admit how little we know of the mechanisms involved. We understand neither the signal which starts the process, nor the mechanisms which maintain and control it.

Older workers claimed that local wound hormones, or *trephones*, were responsible for healing, but none has been isolated from animal tissue. In the plant world growth factors have, however, been found.*[35] A view more popular at present is that there is a removal of an inhibiting substance normally present. These inhibiting factors are called *chalones*[39, 40] (from the Greek *chalinoein* meaning to bridle or restrain), and they have been isolated from various tissues,

* Somewhat surprisingly, extracts of certain plants, e.g. red kidney beans, have a powerful action in stimulating mitosis of human white blood cells in tissue culture. The extract also causes red-cell agglutination, and is called phytohaemagglutinin.[36-38]

e.g. epidermis, liver, kidney, and circulating granulocytes. The epidermal chalone may be a glycoprotein.[41] Not only could the removal of a chalone be responsible for cell division,[42] but it might also be a factor in neoplasia.[43]

Physical factors may play some part; for instance epithelial cells tend to maintain contact with each other and spread over surfaces. The migration of squamous epithelium in wound healing can thus be understood. However, the subsequent division of the cells and the formation of a multi-layered epidermis cannot be so explained. Although some general factors, such as food supply, hormones, etc., affect wound healing, local factors far outweigh them in potency and probably in importance. In the control of cell division and maturation it is therefore local factors which are most likely to be of major importance.

GENERAL READING

BLAIR, G. H., SLOME, D. and WALTER, J. B. (1961). Review of experimental investigations on wound healing. In *British Surgical Practice*. *Surgical Progress*, pp. 462–505. Edited by E. R. Carling and J. P. Ross. London: Butterworths.

DOUGLAS, D. M. (1963). *Wound Healing and Management: A Monograph for Surgeons*. Edinburgh: Livingstone.

EDWARDS, L. C. and DUNPHY, J. E. (1958). Wound healing. *New England Journal of Medicine*, **259**, 224–233 and 275–285.

LEVENSON, S. M., STEIN, J. M. and GROSSBLATT, N. (1966). (Eds) *Wound Healing, Proceedings of a Workshop*. Washington: National Academy of Sciences–National Research Council.

PEACOCK, E. E. and VAN WINKLE, W. (1970). *Surgery and Biology of Wound Repair*, 630 p. Philadelphia, London and Toronto: Saunders.

RUSSELL, P. S. and BILLINGHAM, R. E. (1962). Some aspects of the repair process in mammals. *Progress in Surgery*, **2**, 1–72.

SLOME, D. (1961). (Ed) *Wound Healing*. Oxford: Pergamon.

REFERENCES

1. VAN DEN BRENK, H. A. S. (1956). *British Journal of Surgery*, **43**, 525.
2. ABERCROMBIE, M. (1966). In *Wound Healing, Proceedings of a Workshop*, p. 193, *loc. cit.*
3. BILLINGHAM, R. E. and RUSSELL, P. S. (1956). *Annals of Surgery*, **144**, 961.
4. ABERCROMBIE, M., JAMES, D. W. and NEWCOMBER, J. F. (1960). *Journal of Anatomy*, **94**, 170.
5. ABERCROMBIE, M., FLINT, M. H. and JAMES, D. W. (1956). *Journal of Embryology and Experimental Morphology*, **4**, 167.
6. GRILLO, H. C. and GROSS, J. (1959). *Proceedings of the Society for Experimental Biology and Medicine*, **101**, 268.
7. WATTS, G. T., GRILLO, H. C. and GROSS, J. (1958). *Annals of Surgery*, **148**, 153.
8. CLIFF, W. J. (1963). *Philosophical Transactions of the Royal Society, Series B*, **246**, 305.
9. BOUCEK, R. J. and NOBLE, N. L. (1955). *Archives of Pathology*, **59**, 553.
10. EDWARDS, L. C., PERNOKAS, L. N. and DUNPHY, J. E. (1957). *Surgery, Gynecology and Obstetrics*, **105**, 303.
11. SCHOEFL, G. I. (1963). *Virchows Archiv für pathologische anatomie und Physiologie und für klinische Medizin*, **337**, 97.
12. ABELL, R. G. (1946). *American Journal of Physiology*, **147**, 237.
13. HADFIELD, G. (1963). *British Journal of Surgery*, **50**, 751.
14. ALLGÖWER, M. (1966). In *Wound Healing, Proceedings of a Workshop*, p. 160, *loc. cit.*
15. GILLMAN, T. and WRIGHT, L. J. (1966). *Nature*, **209**, 1086.
16. WILLIAMS, G. (1957). *Journal of Pathology and Bacteriology*, **73**, 557.
17. DOUGLAS, D. M. (1966). In *Wound Healing*, p. 233. Edited by C. Illingworth. London: Churchill.
18. VILJANTO, J. (1964). *Acta chirurgica scandinavica*, supplement, 333.
19. KAZANJIAN, V. H. and CONVERSE, J. M. (1959). In *The Surgical Treatment of Facial Injuries*, 2nd edn, p. 28. London: Baillière, Tindall and Cox.
20. NISHIHARA, G. and PRUDDEN, J. F. (1958). *Surgery, Gynecology and Obstetrics*, **106**, 305.
21. WIANCKO, K. B., KLING, S. and MACKENZIE, W. C. (1961). *Canadian Medical Association Journal*, **84**, 254.
22. DOUGLAS, D. M. (1961). In *Wound Healing*, p. 62. Edited by D. Slome, *loc. cit.*
23. GILLMAN, T. and PENN, J. (1956). *Medical Proceedings*, supplement, **2**, 121.
24. ORDMAN, L. J. and GILLMAN, T. (1966). *Archives of Surgery*, **93**, 857, 883 and 911.
25. GILLMAN, T. (1968). *Glaxo Volume*, **31**, 5.
26. LINDSAY, W. K. and BIRCH, J. R. (1964). *Canadian Journal of Surgery*, **7**, 297.
27. ROTHNIE, N. G. and TAYLOR, G. W. (1963). *British Medical Journal*, ii, 1027.
28. MURRAY, P. J. B. (1963). *British Medical Journal*, ii, 1030.
29. Leading Article (1972). *British Medical Journal*, iii, 4.
30. PALMER, J. F. (1835). (Ed) *The Works of John Hunter, F.R.S.*, vol. 2, p. 496. London: Longmans.
31. HUNT, A. H. (1940). *British Journal of Surgery*, **28**, 436.

32. STEIN, O. and WOLMAN, M. (1958). *British Journal of Experimental Pathology*, **39,** 418.
33. HALLBÖÖK, T. and LANNER, E. (1972). *Lancet*, ii, 780.
34. BILLINGHAM, R. E. and SILVERS, W. K. (1960). *Annals of Surgery*, **152,** 975.
35. STONIER, T. (1966). In *Wound Healing, Proceedings of a Workshop*, p. 212, *loc. cit.*
36. NOWELL, P. C. (1960). *Cancer Research*, **20,** 462.
37. COOPER, E. H., BARKHAN, P. and HALE, A. J. (1963). *British Journal of Haematology*, **9,** 101.
38. ELVES, M. W. *et al.* (1964). *Lancet*, i, 306.
39. BULLOUGH, W. S. and LAURENCE, E. B. (1960). *Proceedings of the Royal Society*, B, **151,** 517.
40. BULLOUGH, W. S., HEWETT, C. L. and LAURENCE, E. B. (1964). *Experimental Cell Research*, **36,** 192.
41. BULLOUGH, W. S. (1968). In *The Biological Basis of Medicine*, vol. 1, p. 311. Edited by E. E. Bittar and N. Bittar. London and New York: Academic Press.
42. BULLOUGH, W. S. (1966). In *Wound Healing*, p. 43. Edited by C. Illingworth. London: Churchill.
43. Leading Article (1968). *Lancet*, ii, 1126.

Chapter 10. Healing in Specialised Tissues

The healing which follows tissue loss involves two main processes.

1. The wound undergoes contraction; this has been considered in Chapter 9.

2. The defect which remains is filled in by new cells during the processes of repair or regeneration.

Either process may predominate: for instance, repair is a salient feature of healing in excised skin wounds, muscle, and in the central nervous system. In general, tissues composed of cells which are incapable of division (i.e. permanent cells, like neurones and muscle fibres) heal by repair. Regeneration is predominant when the cells comprising the tissue are capable of division (labile and stable cells), and is well illustrated by the healing of a damaged liver. The healing of a wound is therefore a complex process depending upon the types of cells which have been lost; these categories of labile, stable, and permanent cells are further considered on p. 296.

HEALING IN CONNECTIVE TISSUE

BONE

The stages in healing of a fracture are illustrated diagrammatically in Fig. 10.2. It must be remembered that the entire area will not all be at the same stage of healing at the same time; thus, while the centre may be at an early stage, the changes adjacent to the bone ends will be much more advanced. However, for descriptive purposes it is convenient to divide the healing process into separate stages. These can be appreciated only if the normal structure and formation of bone is first understood.

Structure of Bone[1-5]

Bone is composed of calcified osteoid tissue, which consists of collagen fibres embedded in a mucoprotein matrix (osseomucin). It is the special composition of this ground substance which imparts to bone its characteristic properties, and it is here that the bone salts are deposited. Depending upon the arrangement of the collagen fibres, two histological types may be recognised.

Woven, immature, fibrillary, or non-lamellar bone. This shows irregularity in the arrangement of the collagen bundles and in the distribution of the osteocytes. The osseomucin is usually basophilic, and is less abundant than in mature bone. It also contains less calcium. Woven bone is formed under three conditions:

(*a*) When bone forms in a sheet of differentiating mesenchyme. This occurs during embryonic development of the bones of the vault of the skull, the mandible, and the clavicle. These are therefore sometimes called *membrane bones*.

(*b*) When bone forms in the midst of differentiating granulation tissue. This is seen in fracture healing.

(*c*) In osteogenic tumours and other bone disorders.

Figure 10.1
Diagrammatic representation of a transverse section through part of the shaft of a long bone to show the arrangement of lamellar bone.

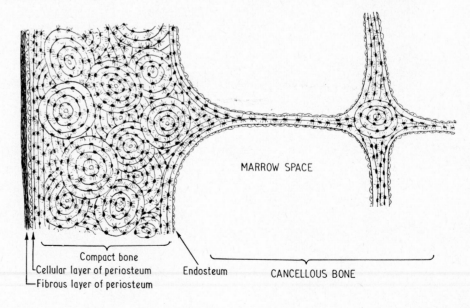

MARROW SPACE

Compact bone
Cellular layer of periosteum
Fibrous layer of periosteum
Endosteum
CANCELLOUS BONE

Lamellar or adult bone. In this type of bone the collagen bundles are arranged in parallel sheets either in the form of concentric Haversian systems or flat plates (see Fig. 10.1).

In the outer dense *cortex* of a long bone Haversian systems predominate, while flat plates are seen under the periosteum and endosteum. This type of bone is called *compact*.

The central portion is hollowed out to form the medullary cavity, which contains marrow. Only a few spicules of bone remain. These are constructed of flat bundles of collagen, although in the wider trabeculae Haversian systems may be found. The central "open" trabeculated part of the bone is called *cancellous*, but it should be noted that, like "compact", this is a term related to the naked-eye appearance of a bone.

Lamellar bone is formed under three conditions:

(*a*) Whenever there has been a previous model of cartilage. Most of the skeleton is formed in this manner, and the process continues at the epiphyseal ends of long bones until adult stature is reached. The process is known as endochondral ossification. It must be understood that the cartilage is not converted into bone, but is *replaced* by bone. The cartilage cells swell up and die, and the intervening matrix then calcifies. This *calcified cartilage* is eroded by osteoclasts, and at the same time osteoblasts lay down lamellar bone.

The cartilage which forms during the healing of fractures is similarly replaced by bone.

(*b*) Lamellar bone is also formed whenever there has been a previous model of woven bone, whether formed during embryonic development or in fracture healing. In the normal adult the entire skeleton is composed of lamellar bone regardless of its developmental origin.

(*c*) When once lamellar bone has been formed, its progressive growth and remodelling result in further adult-bone formation.

Bone, whether woven or lamellar, is made by specialised cells called osteoblasts; microscopically these resemble fibroblasts and they manufacture collagen fibres as well as the osseomucin. They contain alkaline phosphatase, which may play a part in subsequent calcification of the osteoid. It should be noted that osteoid normally calcifies as soon as it is made. When the cells become trapped in the bone they become smaller and inactive, and are called osteocytes. These are enclosed in spaces, or *lacunae*, which intercommunicate by means of fine canaliculi. The latter are formed round the fine cytoplasmic processes of the osteocytes, but when the matrix calcifies the processes are withdrawn leaving an intercommunicating system of channels through which the osteocytes gain nourishment. These lacunae and canaliculi are seen in ground sections of bone and lie between the concentric lamellae of Haversian bone.

Bone is removed by large multinucleate *osteoclasts*, which by resorbing bone are often to be seen lying in small indentations called *Howship's lacunae*. Whether the osteoclast is formed by fusion of macrophages or whether it is a specialised cell related to the osteoblast is undecided, but current opinion favours the first suggestion (p. 398).

In summary, the following classifications of bone are recognised.

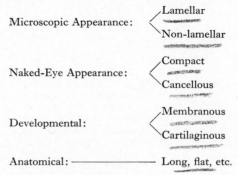

Microscopic Appearance: Lamellar / Non-lamellar

Naked-Eye Appearance: Compact / Cancellous

Developmental: Membranous / Cartilaginous

Anatomical: ——————— Long, flat, etc.

Stages in Fracture Healing (Bone Regeneration)[2, 6, 7]

Stage 1: Haematoma formation. Immediately following the injury there is a variable amount of bleeding from torn vessels; if the periosteum is torn this blood may extend into the surrounding muscles. If it is subsequently organised and ossified, myositis ossificans results.

Stage 2: Traumatic inflammation. The tissue damage excites an inflammatory response, the exudate adding more fibrin to the clot already present. The inflammatory changes differ in no way from those seen in other inflamed tissues. There is an increased blood flow and a polymorphonuclear leucocytic infiltration. This hyperaemia has been held responsible for the decreased density of the adjacent bone ends often noted radiologically. This "decalcification" is presumably due to osteoclastic activity, but the cause of this is not clear. The connective tissue changes accompanying the inflammatory reaction result in a loosening of the attachment of the periosteum to the bone. The haematoma therefore attains a fusiform shape.

Stage 3: Demolition. Macrophages invade the clot and remove the fibrin, red cells, inflammatory exudate, and debris. Any fragments of bone which have become detached from their blood supply undergo necrosis, and are attacked by macrophages and osteoclasts.

Stage 4: Formation of granulation tissue. Following this phase of demolition there is an ingrowth of capillary loops and mesenchymal cells derived from the periosteum and the endosteum of the cancellous bone. The importance of the periosteum in fracture union has been much discussed in the past. The cells of its deeper layer certainly have osteogenic potentiality, and together with its blood vessels contribute to the granulation tissue. Under some circumstances this assumes great importance.

In fractures of the neck of the femur the head is dependent upon the periosteum for its blood supply. If this is damaged, there is ischaemic necrosis of the head. Thus the integrity of the periosteum is of great practical importance. The periosteum alone is capable of effecting complete regeneration of a rib following subperiosteal resection. Here its outer fibrous layer acts by forming a limiting vascular membrane around

Figure 10.2
Stages in the healing of a fracture.

(*a*) Haematoma formation.

(*b*) Stages 2 and 3. Acute inflammation followed by demolition. Loose fragments of bone are removed, and the bone ends show osteoporosis.

(*c*) Stage 4. Granulation-tissue formation.

(*d*) Stage 5. The bone ends are now united by woven bone, cartilage, or a mixture of the two. This hard material is often called callus and can be divided into three parts—internal, intermediate, and external. The intermediate callus is that part which lies in line with the cortex of the bone. The internal callus occupies the original marrow cavity, while the external callus produces the fusiform swelling visible on the outside of the bone.

(*e*) Stage 6. Lamellar bone is laid down; calcified cartilage and woven bone are progressively removed.

(*f*) Stage 7. Final remodelling.

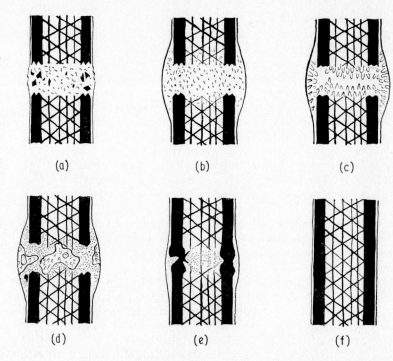

(a) (b) (c)

(d) (e) (f)

the haematoma, while its inner layer provides osteogenic cells for the formation of granulation tissue and bone.

In fractures of the long bones, however, it must not be forgotten that a very extensive area of cancellous bone is exposed. From this the endosteal osteoblasts and the medullary blood vessels grow out to form the granulation tissue. Under these circumstances the periosteum is of much less importance.

During these early phases the pH is low, and this is spoken of as the *acid tide*.

Stage 5: Woven bone and cartilage formation. The mesenchymal "osteoblasts" next differentiate to form either woven bone or cartilage. The term "callus", derived from the Latin and meaning hard, is often used to describe the material uniting the fracture ends regardless of its consistency. When this is granulation tissue, the "callus" is soft, but as bone or cartilage formation occurs, it becomes hard. The word is used loosely by surgeons, radiologists, and pathologists, but exact definition of its various stages is difficult and serves no useful function. If the term is used, it is probably best to apply it to the calcified hard tissue uniting the bone ends.

Formation of woven bone. The osteoblasts form both the collagen fibres and the ground substance osseomucin in which they are embedded. The tissue produced is called *osteoid*, and is formed during maturation of the granulation tissue; as in the repair of ordinary connective tissue progressive devascularisation occurs. The collagen bundles are irregularly disposed with no attempt at lamellar structure. This osteoid undergoes calcification, and is then called woven bone.

After about ten days the pH of the uniting fracture increases. During this *alkaline tide* calcium salts are deposited in the osteoid. Osteoblasts produce an alkaline phosphatase which may play a part in the calcification by leading to a local supersaturation of phosphate following its action on hexose phosphates. However, it must be remembered that in any healing wound the fibroblasts form a similar enzyme, and yet no calcification occurs. The exact function of this enzyme is unknown (see Chapter 47). The resorption of bony spicules may play a part in causing a local supersaturation of calcium salts.

The bone ends thus become united by woven bone. It forms a fusiform mass which may arbitrarily be divided into internal, intermediate, and external callus (see Fig. 10.2 (d)).

Woven-bone formation is found whenever the bone ends are adequately immobilised. It is, therefore, predominant in human fracture healing. In experimentally-produced fractures in animals adequate immobilisation is difficult to attain, and then the granulation tissue matures not to woven bone, but to hyaline cartilage.

Formation of cartilage. The mesenchymal cells ("osteoblasts") behave as chondroblasts and form cartilage, i.e. the cells actively lead to the formation of a specialised ground substance in which the collagen fibres are embedded. These cartilage cells swell and die, and the intervening matrix undergoes calcification. Cartilage formation occurs in fractures in which there is movement, e.g. in experimental animal fractures and human fractures where complete immobilisation is impossible, as in the ribs.

In many fractures cartilage and woven bone are formed; both are merely methods of temporarily uniting bone ends with calcified material. This acts as a scaffold on which the final adult lamellar bone can later be built. The two embryological methods of bone formation, endochondral and intramembranous ossification, are thus faithfully repeated in the bone regeneration of later life.

Stage 6: Formation of lamellar bone. The dead calcified cartilage or woven bone is next invaded by capillaries headed by osteoclasts. As the initial scaffolding ("provisional callus") is removed, osteoblasts lay down osteoid which calcifies to form bone. Its collagen bundles are now arranged in orderly lamellar fashion, for the most part concentrically around the blood vessels, and in this way the Haversian systems are formed. Adjacent to the periosteum and endosteum the lamellae are parallel to the surface as in the normal bone. This phase of formation of definitive lamellar bone merges with the last stage.

Stage 7: Remodelling. The final remodelling process involving the continued osteoclastic removal and osteoblastic laying down of bone results in the formation of a bone which differs remarkably little from the original tissue. The *external callus* is slowly removed, the *intermediate callus* becomes converted into compact bone containing Haversian systems, while the *internal callus* is hollowed out into a marrow cavity in which only a few spicules of cancellous bone remain.

Abnormalities of Fracture Healing

1. **Repair, or fibrous union.** It will be recalled that the mesenchymal cells of the granulation tissue are called osteoblasts, but they are capable of differentiation along several lines. They can form bone, but if immobilisation is not complete, cartilage may develop. When movement is even more free, the cells behave as fibroblasts and the bone ends become united by simple scar tissue. Whether this can ever undergo ossification is debatable. It is claimed by some authorities that fibrous tissue can become replaced by bone, but that it is a very slow process.[7] From a practical point of view fibrous union is an unsatisfactory end-result of fracture healing because in many cases it is permanent.

Occasionally with excessive movement the cells differentiate into synovial cells, and a false joint, or pseudarthrosis, results. This is a well-recognised sequel of fractures of the tibia.

2. **Non-union.** A complete lack of union between the fracture ends results from the interposition of soft parts. Muscle or fascia separating the bone ends may prevent the formation of a uniting haematoma. Under these conditions union of any sort is impossible.

3. **Delayed union.** In the presence of a continuous haematoma any of the causes of delayed healing (see pp. 112) will retard bone regeneration. If the adverse conditions are severe there may be fibrous union rather than delayed union with bone.

In practice the following are the most important:

Movement. Movement of any sort is harmful, because it causes damage to the delicate granulation tissue and thereby excites an inflammatory reaction. In surgical practice every attempt is made to reduce movement to a minimum. In impacted fractures this is usually easy, but where the bone ends are mobile, pins, plates, or other forms of internal splinting may have to be used. The damage caused by overdistraction has been stressed by Watson-Jones as a cause of delayed union or non-union. By contrast, if the bone ends are brought together under high compression, there is rigid immobilisation and healing is accelerated.[40]

Infection. By prolonging the acute inflammatory phase infection is an important cause of delayed union or non-union. Since the tension engendered by the formation of exudate in a bone is particularly liable to lead to extensive ischaemic necrosis, it is especially important to avoid contaminating previously closed fractures during open reduction. Rigorous asepsis must be maintained by employing a no-touch technique.

Poor blood supply. While complete loss of blood supply results in necrosis of bone, poor blood supply leads to slow granulation-tissue formation and therefore delayed union. Certain sites are notorious for this complication, e.g. fractures of neck of femur, shaft of tibia, and the carpal scaphoid. In these situations the avoidance of other causes of delayed healing, e.g. movement, is particularly important. The slow healing of fractures in old age is probably due to ischaemia.

Spontaneous fractures. Sudden unexpected strains may cause fractures in normal bones. The violent convulsive movements of tetanus and strychnine poisoning or elctroconvulsive therapy (ECT) not uncommonly result in the collapse of a vertebral body, causing wedging. Indeed, in patients subjected to ECT without prior anaesthesia it has been estimated that such crush fractures occur in about 20 per cent of cases.[8] Avulsion of the spinous process of the seventh cervical vertebra ("clay-shoveller's disease")[9] and march fracture of the metatarsal[10] are other examples of spontaneous fractures due to muscular stress.

Pathological fracture. This term is applied to fractures occurring in diseased bones subjected to a normal strain. Any lesion which weakens the bones is liable to cause fracture. Generalised conditions, e.g. osteitis fibrosa cystica of von Recklinghausen and osteogenesis imperfecta, are well-known but uncommon examples. Solitary and aneurysmal bone cysts, hydatid cysts, giant-cell tumours, and angiomatous hamartomata are other examples. Secondary tumours must always be borne in mind, and indeed a fracture is often the first symptom of such a tumour. Somewhat surprisingly, most pathological fractures heal well, even when due to metastatic carcinoma.

Cartilage[11, 12]

Regeneration in cartilage is generally poor. In the hyaline cartilage of joint surfaces small defects are made good by regeneration. With larger injuries which damage the underlying vascular bone, a haematoma is formed which becomes vascularised and converted either into fibrous tissue or bone.

Tendon[11, 13]

Regeneration in tendon is good, but the process is slow. It is said that the tendon ends should be accurately united and under some tension, otherwise union is by fibrous scar tissue.

Muscle[14]

It is generally taught that damaged muscle is not replaced, and union is by scar tissue. In large destructive lesions of unstriped muscle a permanent scar remains to mark the site of the original injury, and this is well illustrated in a healed chronic peptic ulcer. Nevertheless, it is not uncommon to find no trace of an ulcer at necropsy despite convincing radiographic evidence that one existed previously. Although unstriped muscle cells appear to have only a limited ability to divide in postuterine life, the arterioles of granulation tissue acquire a muscular coat; the origin of these fibres is debated: perhaps they arise by differentiation of adjacent connective tissue cells.

That smooth muscle cells have definite powers of regeneration has been shown in an experimental crush injury of the taenia of the guinea-pig caecum. Although about 10 000 cells are destroyed, they are so rapidly replaced that by 14 days there is little microscopic evidence of injury. Furthermore, the proliferating cells that fill in the gap show the electron-microscopic features of smooth muscle.[41]

In striated muscle,[11, 15] when part of an individual fibre is damaged, there may be limited regeneration with the production of new myocytes which later fuse to form a syncytial mass. This type of multinucleate giant cell is seen when the muscle damage has been caused by toxins or ischaemia. Cardiac muscle shows no regenerative capacity, and once necrosis has occurred, as in infarction, a permanent scar remains. Under special circumstances cardiac muscle cells may form giant cells similar to those seen in voluntary muscle. It has been suggested that the Aschoff giant cell of rheumatic fever is of this nature.

In a surgical wound of voluntary muscle, the sarcolemmal masses on either side of the incision may unite, so that in time the continuity of the muscle is restored.[16] Similarly, when part of a muscle fibre has been damaged as in Zenker's necrosis, full restoration of structure is possible. However, with extensive damage to muscle the architecture is destroyed, and healing is mainly by scar tissue; this is seen following infarction.

Bone Marrow

Bone marrow provides an excellent example of tissue in which regeneration is complete.

Fat

Although fat cells may appear in fully mature granulation tissue, as sometimes seen in the rabbit ear-chamber, defects in fatty tissue are usually made good by fibrous tissue. The process of repair shows a characteristic feature during the demolition phase: the macrophages ingest large quantities of fat, becoming greatly swollen in the process. These "foam cells" form a prominent feature of traumatic fat necrosis. Fatty acid and cholesterol crystals may also be laid down and excite a giant-cell reaction.

Mesothelial Lining of Peritoneum and other Serous Cavities[17, 18]

Denuded areas are healed by metaplasia of the underlying connective tissue cells, which take on the appearances of flattened mesothelium. It has also been suggested that desquamated mesothelial cells can alight on the raw surface.

Synovial lining cells are also replaced from underlying connective tissue. The adjacent uninjured synovial cells are inert and play no part in the process of healing.[19]

Vascular endothelium.[20] The regeneration of vascular endothelium has been extensively investigated in the hope that it might provide a clue to the pathogenesis of atheroma. Following the mechanical removal of an area of endothelium from the rabbit's aorta, new endothelial cells arise by mitotic division from pre-existing lining cells, and slowly spread over the denuded area covering it in about one year.[21] When a section of baboon aorta is replaced by a knitted fabric prosthesis, a new endothelial lining forms within ten weeks. New endothelial cells are derived from vessels penetrating the fabric as well as from the aorta itself. A similar re-endothelialisation occurs following endarterectomy. The vasa vasorum here contribute to the process.

It has been suggested that endothelial cells can also evolve from deposited circulating mononuclear cells. This view is not supported by the observation that the new endothelial cells can initiate fibrinolysis; it has been found that only endothelial cells in a vessel wall have this property. Flattened monocytes forming a pseudo-endothelium do not have this ability, and they differ also in their electron microscopic appearances.

Nervous Tissue

Adult nerve cells are unable to divide and therefore are incapable of taking part in any regenerative process. In lower animals, e.g. some amphibians, following the loss of the tail, ependymal cells proliferate and later mature into neurones. Thus the spinal cord can be regenerated in these animals; no such phenomenon occurs in man.

When the axon of a nerve cell is severed, changes take place which may result in the reformation of the severed end. The process has been studied most frequently in the peripheral nerves, where the axons are enclosed in the Schwann cells and are myelinated when they exceed 2 μm in diameter.

Peripheral nervous system.[22-24] Following section of the axis cylinder, the nerve cell shows changes described as *chromatolysis*. The cell swells and its Nissl granules disappear. These bodies are zones of endoplasmic reticulum studded plentifully with ribosomes, and their disappearance reflects dysfunction in the protein-synthesising system of the nerve cell. The axis cylinder becomes irregular and varicose, and by 48 hours has become broken up. The surrounding myelin shows splitting of its laminae and later fragmentation. The Schwann cells enlarge, proliferate, and become filled with lipid droplets from the degenerated myelin. These changes were originally described as *Wallerian degeneration*, and affect the nerve fibre distal to the point of section and also, in myelinated fibres, a short area proximally up to the first node of Ranvier. The next stage is described as regeneration, but this entails rather more than a mere replacement of the lost part of an individual cell. From the proximal portion of the cut axon numerous neurofibrils sprout out, and are seen to lie invaginated into the cytoplasm of the Schwann cells. They push their way distally through the Schwann cells at the rate of about 1 mm per day. Many of the fibrils lose their way and degenerate, but some reach an appropriate end-organ and persist to form the definitive replacement axon. It is evident that accurate apposition of the cut ends of the nerve is of great importance in facilitating this process. The final stage involves the reformation of the myelin sheath as the regenerating axon matures and increases in diameter.

The functional end-result of nerve damage depends on various factors: if the axons are damaged but the nerve trunk itself is not severed, an excellent result may be expected. When the nerve is severed, careful suturing and the exclusion of infection are important for good recovery. Functional recovery is more complete when a pure motor or sensory nerve is cut. Recovery from a lesion of a mixed nerve, like the median nerve, is often poor.

Central nervous system.[25, 26] Here oligodendroglia take the place of the Schwann cells in relation to nerve fibres. It is often taught that regeneration of central nerve fibres does not occur: the affected nerve cells show chromatolysis often followed by necrosis, and the destroyed tissue is replaced by proliferating neuroglia to form a dense glial scar. Nevertheless, there is considerable evidence that some regeneration is possible. In the clinical field it is noticeable that in patients with partial spinal-cord lesions, voluntary muscle strength seems to increase steadily for 9 to 12 months.[27] This is generally attributed to improved utilisation of resdual un-damaged pathways, but in addition new fibres may be formed; sometimes these appear to originate from cells in the posterior root ganglia.[28] Certainly in the lower animals regeneration of the long-tract axons in the spinal cord and in the optic nerve is a usual feature, and there is good reason to believe that this can also occur in the higher animals, including man. How important these fibres are from a functional point of view, and whether means could be found to improve regeneration, are subjects which are being studied at the present time. The isolation of a nerve-growth factor in certain tumours, snake venom, and salivary gland has aroused much interest, but the role of this protein, hormone-like substance is at present not known.[29]

HEALING IN EPITHELIAL TISSUES

It is often stated that the greater the degree of specialisation of a tissue, the less well developed are its powers of regeneration. Certainly nerve cells are highly specialised and incapable of division, but degrees of specialisation in cells are as difficult to define as they are amongst human beings. Is a liver cell more or less specialised than a simple unstriped muscle fibre? Liver cells show remarkable powers of proliferation, yet perform functions of which they alone are capable. Similarly, it is impossible to compare the degrees of specialisation of the different types of epithelium, each of which has its own peculiar characteristics. It seems more likely that the power of regeneration is best developed in those organs and tissues which are most liable to injury, and the replacement of which has survival value for the individual.

All covering epithelia show good regenerative power. This is hardly surprising since they are being continuously subjected to trauma, and their integrity depends upon their ability to replace the lost cells.

Skin and Other Squamous Epithelia

These show good regeneration, although specialised structures like the rete ridges, hair follicles, sweat glands, and sebaceous glands are not replaced in man. The details of the epithelial changes in skin wounds, involving both movement and division of cells, have already been described (Chapter 9). Wounds of the oesophagus behave similarly. In both it should be noted that the actively migrating cells do not undergo mitosis; this occurs only when they gain attachment to the underlying connective tissue.

OTHER LINING EPITHELIA[18, 30]

Intestinal Epithelium

Complete regeneration results in perfect replacement of lost epithelium, including in the small intestine the crypts and villi. It is interesting that because there is normally a very high rate of mitotic activity in the epithelium of the small intestine, no further increase occurs at the wound margins. In passing, it should be noted that the remainder of the gut wall, including the muscularis mucosae, heals by scar tissue.

Stomach

Here regeneration is good, and in contrast to stratified squamous epithelium the migrating cells show mitosis. Acute ulceration of the mucosa of the stomach is a common event, but healing occurs rapidly without any scarring because the underlying connective tissue and muscle is not destroyed. In chronic peptic ulcers epithelial regeneration is inhibited, the reason for which is not known. When healing does occur, the newly-formed epithelium may be of intestinal type, showing well-marked villi.

Bladder

In experimental wounds of the bladder mucosa there is active migration and mitosis of cells. As in the intestine and gall-bladder mitosis occurs in the migrating cells. After one month the wound shows characteristic crypt-like downgrowths of epithelium, such as are described in the condition of cystitis glandularis.

Transitional epithelium shows remarkable regenerative capacity after complete removal of the bladder mucosa. In the dog, within 16 weeks the organ is completely relined by epithelium which has grown from the ureters and the urethra.[31] Complete resection of the bladder mucosa has therefore been suggested as a treatment for multiple papillomatous tumours, but whether the new mucosa is any less liable to neoplasia is not known. Another surgical application is the use of vein grafts to replace the ureter, for they are soon lined by transitional epithelium.[32]

Gall-bladder

Regeneration is good, resembling that of bladder.

Respiratory Tract

Loss of epithelium, such as occurs in acute influenzal tracheobronchitis, is quickly followed by the division of basal cells leading to a reformation of ciliated pseudostratified columnar epithelium. Sometimes after repeated damage the new epithelium may change to a simple columnar or squamous type (see metaplasia, p. 306).

GLANDULAR EPITHELIA

Liver[33-36]

The liver has remarkable powers of regeneration. In the rat resection of three-quarters of the organ results in such active division of the remaining cells that within two weeks it is restored to its original size. In dogs, the process is a little slower (6 to 8 weeks). The process could be regarded as a simple type of reconstitution, because it involves the co-ordinated growth of liver cells, bile ducts, blood vessels, etc.

In man regeneration of liver cells is seen following any type of necrosis, provided the patient survives. The end-results of this regeneration vary so widely, depending upon the type of necrosis, that this important subject will be considered in some detail. The clinical manifestations of liver disease are considered in Chapter 43.

Three categories of hepatic necrosis are recognised:

Focal necrosis, in which there are small foci of necrosis scattered throughout the liver. This occurs in many acute infections, e.g. typhoid fever and pneumonia, and may be related to the parasitisation of Kupffer cells during the incubation period. When these are destroyed, the adjacent liver cells undergo necrosis. Healing presumably occurs by regeneration, because old foci of scarring are not found *post*

mortem in such patients when they die of other diseases. Focal necrosis is typical of virus hepatitis.

Zonal necrosis, in which a zone of each lobule throughout the liver undergoes necrosis. Central zonal necrosis is the characteristic effect of many poisons, e.g. carbon tetrachloride, chloroform, muscarine, cinchophen, and hydrazine monoamine-oxidase inhibitors. Midzonal necrosis is characteristic of yellow fever. Peripheral zonal necrosis is seen typically in phosphorus poisoning where there is also severe fatty change, and in eclampsia where there is gross haemorrhage around the portal tracts. Recovery with regeneration is the usual sequel, and during this phase the remaining liver cells undergo division and replace those which have been destroyed. Since the reticulin framework of each lobule is undamaged, the resulting healing leaves a perfectly normal architecture. After repeated attacks of zonal necrosis, however, some distortion of the liver pattern may occur (see cirrhosis).

Centrilobular necrosis also occurs in chronic venous congestion (see cardiac cirrhosis).

Massive necrosis, in which there are extensive areas of necrosis involving the whole liver indiscriminately. It is either idiopathic or the result of severe virus hepatitis or the poisons mentioned above. Death in cholaemia usually ensues within a few days. At necropsy the liver is shrunken, its capsule wrinkled, and the cut surface soft and yellow ("acute yellow atrophy") or dark reddish-brown due to congestion. Sometimes the clinical course is more protracted and there is sufficient time for regeneration to occur. The liver is then small but contains numerous irregular nodules of regenerated parenchyma, many of which also show necrosis. This condition has been called subacute yellow atrophy, but is better named subacute hepatic necrosis. Sometimes the regeneration of liver is adequate to sustain life and further necrosis does not occur. However, large areas of liver have been destroyed and the reticulin framework of the lobules has collapsed. Regeneration from surviving islets of liver cells occurs, but the irregular nodules so produced are not normal lobules. Although this is an excellent example of regeneration, the anatomical and functional end-result is not as satisfactory as that occurring after zonal necrosis.

In addition to the regenerative nodules described above, areas of liver where the lobular structure is preserved also show regeneration. A considerable amount of scar tissue is formed. The bile ducts exhibit hyperplasia, and numerous tubules are present amid the fibrous tissue surrounding the liver nodules. The end-result is a coarsely scarred liver with numerous nodules of parenchyma separated from each other by broad bands of fibrous tissue. The larger nodules show a recognisable lobular pattern. The condition has been given a variety of names—postnecrotic scarring, postnecrotic cirrhosis, and macronodular cirrhosis.

Cirrhosis of the liver. The term cirrhosis was introduced by Laennec who was impressed by the tawny colour of the liver in this condition, but this is due merely to fatty change of the liver cells. The essential feature is diffuse destruction of the parenchyma and its replacement by fibrous tissue which disrupts the normal lobular architecture of the liver. There is usually active regeneration of liver cells occurring at the same time as this fibrous reparative process.

Cirrhosis is best regarded as an *end-stage condition*, as it can be the end-result of liver damage due to many causes—poisons, alcohol, inadequate diet, infection, genetic error, etc. Classifications are very unsatisfactory since in most cases the cause is unknown. A descriptive classification is the most useful:

Macronodular cirrhosis. This has been described above.

Micronodular cirrhosis (portal or Laennec's cirrhosis). The liver shows numerous regenerative nodules which are small and fairly uniform in size, and are separated by strands of fibrous tissue (Figs. 10.3 and 10.4). The condition may be idiopathic but is often found in alcoholics. It is often

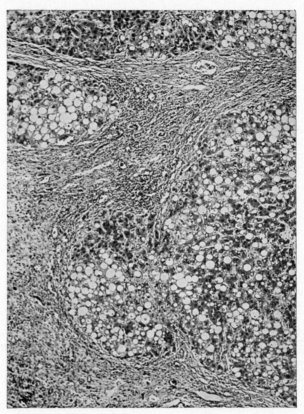

Figure 10.4
Portal cirrhosis. A thick strand of cellular fibrous tissue intersects two nodules, the cells of which show severe fatty change. × 50.

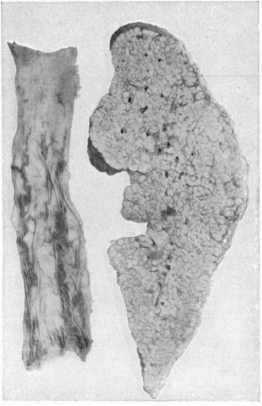

Figure 10.3
Cirrhosis of the liver. The patient was a man of 68 years who died of haematemesis due to a ruptured oesophageal varix, a complication of hepatic cirrhosis. The specimen shows a section through the liver. The edges are irregular and knobbly, and the hepatic substance consists of pale nodules of regenerating parenchyma, interspersed among which there are strands of dense fibrous tissue. The picture is one of micronodular, or portal, cirrhosis. The lower end of the oesophagus has been included. It is opened to reveal a length of dilated, tortuous submucous veins. *(EA 27.1, Reproduced by permission of the President and Council of the R.C.S. Eng.)*

preceded by fatty change which, by leading to necrosis, appears to be responsible for the progressive fibrosis which disrupts the liver lobules.

It must be emphasised that there is no sharp line of division between these two types of cirrhosis. Indeed, some authorities have proposed an intermediate group (*posthepatitic cirrhosis*),[37] but this introduces an unnecessary complication, and is particularly unfortunate since there is no evidence that the condition follows hepatitis. At the present time it is wisest to describe cirrhosis in morphological terms, and accept that any type may follow any cause. Cirrhosis of the liver is a salient feature of haemochromatosis, Wilson's disease, and galactosaemia.

CARDIAC CIRRHOSIS. In prolonged cardiac failure, especially in young people, there may be a fibrous replacement of the destroyed central zones of the lobules. A fine "reversed" type of cirrhosis, i.e. starting from the centres of the lobules instead of the portal tracts, may follow.

BILIARY CIRRHOSIS. In persistent obstructive jaundice due either to intrahepatic or extrahepatic factors, e.g. obstruction to the common bile duct, there is an inspissation of bile in many lobules, and this produces an inflammatory reaction, necrosis of neighbouring cells, and progressive fibrosis. The deeply jaundiced liver is finely granular.

It is evident that although the liver and bile-duct epithelial cells possess remarkable powers of regeneration, destructive liver disease is not always attended by a satisfactory end-result. Some of the factors governing the regeneration of liver are:

Age. Experimentally-induced regeneration is better in young animals.

Blood supply. Interference with the blood supply impairs regeneration; this may be a factor in the production of cardiac cirrhosis.

Maintenance of lobular architecture. The marked difference between the regeneration following zonal necrosis compared with that of massive necrosis has already been mentioned.

Cirrhotic livers have limited powers of regeneration. This may, however, be merely a question of poor blood supply.

Bile-duct obstruction appears to impair healing.

Stimulus for liver regeneration.[35] Small wounds of the liver produced surgically, e.g. when performing a biopsy, heal by granulation tissue and scarring. It is evident that the stimulus for liver regeneration is a metabolic one, but its precise nature remains unknown.

The stimulus for liver regeneration acts on the organ as a whole and comes into play when a mass of liver is *resected*, undergoes *necrosis*, or is induced to *atrophy* as by tying off a branch of the portal vein. It has been postulated that an excessive accumulation of some substance in the blood is the stimulus, but none has been identified. No known hormone plays a significant part. Alternatively, it might be that the liver normally produces some inhibiting substance, the depletion of which allows regeneration to occur. In spite of much experimental work with much conflicting evidence, the metabolic stimulus for liver regeneration is obscure.

Thyroid

Experimentally the thyroid has good powers of regeneration. This may be impaired by the administration of thyroxine, presumably because of pituitary inhibition.[38]

Kidney

The renal tubular epithelium has considerable powers of regeneration; thus in acute tubular necrosis, in spite of extensive damage, complete return to normal may occur. This type of lesion is therefore most eligible for treatment with haemodialysis since recovery is possible. When damage to the kidney results in the destruction of a complete nephron, regeneration does not occur. Glomeruli once destroyed cannot be replaced.

Following unilateral nephrectomy the remaining kidney increases in size. No new nephrons are formed, even in the newborn, and the enlargement is due to an increase in size and number of the cells in the glomeruli and proximal convoluted tubules. The enlargement is greater in young animals than in the old and in well-nourished ones than in the starved. The stimulus for compensatory enlargement is unknown, but is assumed to be humoral.[39]

HYPERPLASIA AND REGENERATION COMPARED

In both conditions there is a division of cells which is kept strictly under control, in contrast with the type of cell division seen in neoplasia. In regeneration there is replacement of lost cells, whilst in hyperplasia there is increased division of cells, resulting in a larger amount of tissue than normal. The stimulus for cell division is probably the same in both conditions and varies from organ to organ; thus it is probably hormonal in the endocrine glands and metabolic in the liver. In most instances we are ignorant of the exact cause. While the distinction between hyperplasia and regeneration is quite clear, the terms are frequently confused. The designation of hepatic cirrhosis as an example of a "hyperplastic regenerative" condition is a reflection of this confusion.

In point of fact the liver cells clearly show regeneration, since the bulk of the liver is not greater than normal in the majority of cases. The bile ducts do show hyperplasia, but nevertheless, the use of the term "hyperplastic regeneration" can only serve to cause confusion and render each word meaningless.

It must be admitted that regeneration and hyperplasia may exist side by side. In a healing skin wound the lost epithelium is regenerated, but the edges of the wound show marked hyperplasia of the squamous cells (see Fig. 9.11). This further stresses the point that the stimulus for both conditions is probably the same. Nevertheless, as long as both pathological terms are used it is desirable that they be used in their correct connotation.

REFERENCES

1. BLOOM, W. and FAWCETT, D. W. (1962). In *A Textbook of Histology*, 8th edn, p. 153. Philadelphia: Saunders.
2. HAM, A. W. (1969). In *Histology*, 6th edn, p. 388. London: Pitman Medical.
3. McLEAN, F. C. and BUDY, A. M. (1959). *Annual Review of Physiology*, **21**, 69.
4. GOLDHABER, P. (1962). *New England Journal of Medicine*, **266**, 870.
5. BAKER, S. L. (1959). In *A Textbook of X-ray Diagnosis*, 3rd edn, vol. 4, p. 55. Edited by S. C. Shanks and P. Kerley. London: Lewis.
6. URIST, M. R. (1959). In *Wound Healing and Tissue Repair*, p. 65. Edited by W. B. Patterson. Chicago: The University of Chicago Press.
7. PRITCHARD, J. J. (1963). In *The Scientific Basis of Medicine Annual Reviews*, p. 286. London: Athlone Press.
8. PALMER, H. A. (1939). *Lancet*, ii, 181.
9. McKELLAR HALL, R. D. (1940). *Journal of Bone and Joint Surgery*, **22**, 63.

10. WATSON-JONES, R. (1952). In *Fractures and Joint Injuries*, 4th edn, vol. 1, p. 345. Edinburgh: Livingstone.
11. WRIGHT, G. P. (1958). In *An Introduction to Pathology*, 3rd edn, pp. 239, 240 and 285. London: Longmans.
12. BENNETT, G. A., BAUER, W. and MADDOCK, S. J. (1932). *American Journal of Pathology*, **8**, 499.
13. BUCK, R. C. (1953). *Journal of Pathology and Bacteriology*, **66**, 1.
14. HAY, E. H. (1971). *New England Journal of Medicine*, **284**, 1033.
15. ADAMS, R. D., DENNY-BROWN, D. and PEARSON, C. M. (1962). In *Diseases of Muscle*, 2nd edn, p. 193. New York: Hoeber.
16. GAY, A. J. and HUNT, T. E. (1954). *Anatomical Record*, **120**, 853.
17. RUSSELL, P. S. and BILLINGHAM, R. E. (1962). *Progress in Surgery*, **2**, 1.
18. JOHNSON, F. R. and McMINN, R. M. H. (1960). *Biological Reviews*, **35**, 364.
19. LEVENE, A. (1957). *Journal of Pathology and Bacteriology*, **73**, 87.
20. Leading Article (1967). *Lancet*, ii, 1239.
21. POOLE, J. C. F., SANDERS, A. G. and FLOREY, H. W. (1958). *Journal of Pathology and Bacteriology*, **75**, 133 and (1959). *Ibid.*, **77**, 637.
22. SEDDON, H. J. (1954). (Ed) *Peripheral Nerve Injuries. Medical Research Council Report.* London: HMSO.
23. GUTH, L. (1956). *Physiological Reviews*, **36**, 441.
24. NATHANIEL, E. J. H. and PEASE, D. C. (1963). *Journal of Ultrastructure Research*, **9**, 511.
25. WINDLE, W. F. (1955). (Ed) *Regeneration in the Central Nervous System.* Springfield: Thomas.
26. McMASTERS, R. E. (1962). *Journal of Comparative Neurology*, **119**, 113.
27. RUSSELL, W. R. (1964). *British Medical Journal*, ii, 403.
28. HUGHES, J. T. and BROWNELL, B. (1963). *Journal of Neurology, Neurosurgery and Psychiatry*, **26**, 528.
29. Leading Article (1972). *Lancet*, i, 1375.
30. McMINN, R. M. H. (1960). *Annals of the Royal College of Surgeons of England*, **26**, 245.
31. SANDERS, A. R., SCHEIN, C. J. and ORKIN, L. A. (1958). *Journal of Urology*, **79**, 63.
32. BOHNE, A. W., OSBORN, R. W. and HETTLE, P. J. (1955). *Surgery, Gynecology and Obstetrics*, **100**, 259.
33. HARKNESS, R. D. (1961). In *The Scientific Basis of Medicine Annual Reviews*, p. 263. London: Athlone Press.
34. HARRISON, C. V. (1960). In *Recent Advances in Pathology*, 7th edn, p. 181. Edited by C. V. Harrison. London: Churchill.
35. WEINBREN, K. (1966). In *Wound Healing*, p. 69. Edited by C. Illingworth. London: Churchill.
36. BUCHER, N. L. R. (1967). *New England Journal of Medicine*, **277**, 686 and 738.
37. GALL, E. A. (1960). *American Journal of Pathology*, **36**, 241.
38. GRAY, S. H. (1929). *American Journal of Pathology*, **5**, 415.
39. MALT, R. A. (1969). *New England Journal of Medicine*, **280**, 1446.
40. MÜLLER, M. E. (1969). In *Recent Advances in Orthopaedics*, p. 79, Edited by A. G. Apley. London: Churchill.
41. McGEACHIE, J. K. (1971). *Experientia*, **27**, 436.

Chapter 11. Chronic Inflammation

The tissue response to injury has been divided into three phases. The initial vascular and exudative phenomena of acute inflammation are followed by a second phase of demolition. This is accomplished by macrophage activity. The third and final phase is one of healing, by which lost tissue is replaced by the processes of repair and regeneration.

It is evident that complete healing can occur only when the acute inflammatory and demolition phases are themselves completed. Since these are the consequences of the initial damage, it follows that healing results only when the cause of the inflammation is removed. If the body is unable to remove the irritant, a disease process develops in which there is present a mixture of the phenomena of acute inflammation, demolition, repair, and regeneration. To such a lesion the term "chronic inflammation" is applied. *Chronic inflammation may therefore be defined as a prolonged process in which destruction and inflammation are proceeding at the same time as attempts at healing.*

Causes of Chronic Inflammation

Since all agents which cause cell damage initiate an acute inflammatory response, they may, if they persist, also lead to chronic inflammation. In this way insoluble particles such as silica, asbestos, and other foreign bodies very readily cause chronic inflammation. Organisms like the tubercle bacillus and actinomyces, against which the body has only a limited resistance, are another important cause. Moreover, if local or general conditions impair the body's defences, an organism which usually produces a self-limiting acute inflammation may persist to cause a chronic one. Any of the causes of delayed healing (p. 112) may so turn the scales against the host that there develops the "frustrated healing" which chronic inflammation has so aptly been called. Finally, a state of hypersensitivity, if persistent, may lead to exuberant chronic inflammatory reactions. This is seen in many chronic infective diseases, of which tuberculosis is the prototype, and is also important in non-infective conditions such as allergic contact dermatitis and hypersensitivity angiitis. The collagen diseases afford excellent examples of chronic inflammation associated with progressive destruction of collagen. It is possible that they too are related to hypersensitivity or autoimmunity (see Chapter 16).

Classification of the Types of Chronic Inflammation

Clinical. Although chronic inflammation may follow obvious acute inflammation (e.g. osteomyelitis), some irritants (e.g. the tubercle bacillus) usually cause only a mild or fleeting acute reaction, but nevertheless persist and lead to the development of a chronic disease.

The initial acute phase is often inconspicuous, and clinically it may be completely missed. It can therefore be induced that two types of chronic inflammation occur: (*a*) following acute inflammation, and (*b*) starting *de novo*.

Specific and non-specific. It is customary to subdivide chronic inflammation in another way: certain irritants cause a tissue reaction which is histologically characteristic. By examining such a lesion, one can infer its origin without either seeing or isolating the causative agent. Such a lesion is said to be *specific*. Tuberculosis, leprosy, and syphilis are included under this heading. In fact, many lesions encountered in these diseases are not histologically characteristic, and therefore, strictly speaking, the term "specific" should not be used. Thus, while the histological appearances of a gumma are fairly typical, the lesions of secondary syphilis are by no means diagnostic. The reaction is "non-specific".

With increasing knowledge it has been realised that tissue reactions which were once regarded as diagnostic of a particular disease are by no means as specific as was once thought. Thus, a "typical tuberculous" lesion may be found in leprosy, sarcoidosis, or even in reactions to a foreign body like talc.

The use of the terms "specific" and "non-specific" are, however, retained, even though it is not really justified in terms of the original conception. Since this convention is so time-honoured, it is unlikely to be altered, but it should be remembered that the distinction between specific and non-specific is quite artificial.

Histological. The histological features of a chronic inflammatory lesion may be used in descriptive classification. Where polymorphs abound and abscess formation is present, the lesion may justly be called a *chronic suppurative inflammation*. Likewise, when epithelioid cells are grouped together in follicles resembling those found in tuberculosis, the term *tuberculoid* is frequently applied. Three variants occur:

Non-caseating tuberculoid reaction, as seen in sarcoidosis (Fig. 21.4), lupus vulgaris, and tuberculoid leprosy.

Caseating tuberculoid reaction, as commonly seen in tuberculosis (Fig. 20.2).

Suppurative tuberculoid reaction, in which small abscesses filled with polymorphs are formed and are surrounded by a mantle of epithelioid cells. This occurs in lymphogranuloma venereum, tularaemia, coccidioidomycosis, and cat-scratch disease (Fig. 21.3).

Some chronic inflammations are characterised by the formation of tumour-like masses composed of granulation tissue which is heavily infiltrated with inflammatory cells. These are sometimes called the *granulomata*. The causative agent is generally an organism, the most frequent examples being those of tuberculosis, syphilis (the gumma), yaws, leprosy, and actinomycosis. By convention these diseases (and other similar protozoan and fungous infections) are often called the "specific infective granulomata". It must be stressed that, in fact, not all lesions in these diseases are "granulomatous", and that tumour-like masses can occur in "non-specific" chronic inflammation. Thus, an apical tooth infection may form a granuloma; there is also the proud flesh in a granulating infected wound. Agents like talc and silica can lead to the production of tumour-like masses: the former is called a talc granuloma, but the nodules of silicosis are not currently named granulomata. Finally there is Wegener's granulomatosis and other variants of poly-arteritis nodosa (see Chapter 16).

Granulomatous inflammation.[1] This is a term frequently used but rarely defined with precision. To some, including Virchow, it implies the presence of granulation tissue, and in this context the term *granuloma* refers literally to a tumour-like mass of granulation tissue, as in the pyogenic granuloma. Most contemporary workers define a granuloma, however, as a chronic inflammatory reaction containing *a predominance of cells of the macrophage series*,[2] and it is probable that this will remain the most widely accepted concept of a granuloma. There are, however, some workers who have restricted the term to lesions characterised by epithelioid cells and giant cells arranged in follicular groups,[3, 4] in which case the terms "granulomatous" and "tuberculoid" would be synonymous. Nevertheless, actinomycosis and sporotrichosis are often included in the group of granulomatous inflammation, even though their lesions are typically suppurative. It is evident that granulomatous inflammation is a term without a precise meaning, and it is wise not to use it without qualification.

It is obvious that many of the terms used in the classification of chronic inflammation are both ambiguous and imprecise.

General Features of Chronic Inflammation

Although there are wide differences between various types of chronic inflammation, depending partly upon the tissues involved and partly upon the causative agent, there are, nevertheless, certain basic similarities. These are best considered under the heading of the three component reactions which together constitute chronic inflammation.

Acute inflammation. Evidence of acute inflammation is frequently seen in chronic inflammation. Exudation is particularly well marked in chronic suppurative disease.

G.P.—5*

Pus, rich in polymorphonuclear leucocytes, is very evident in chronic suppurative conditions such as chronic brain abscess, osteomyelitis, empyema, pyosalpinx, and pyonephrosis, to mention only a few examples. It is also typical of actinomycosis. Fibrin may be seen microscopically, and on occasions forms large masses easily visible to the naked eye. This is prominent in chronic empyema thoracis due to pneumococcal or staphylococcal infection.

Eosinophils are sometimes present in large numbers in the exudate in chronic inflammation. Whether this is a manifestation of hypersensitivity is not known.

Fluid exudation is a feature of draining chronic suppurative lesions, and the continued protein loss may lead to hypoproteinaemia. Accumulations of a protein-rich fluid are frequent in chronic inflammation of the serous sacs, e.g. tuberculous peritonitis, and in some forms of serositis, including that due to tuberculosis, abundant fibrin formation is evident (see Fig. 11.1). The spider-web clot seen in the cerebrospinal fluid of tuberculous meningitis will also be recalled. Usually, however, overt acute inflammation is not an outstanding feature of tuberculosis.

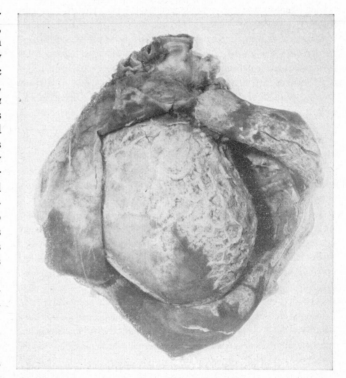

Figure 11.1
Tuberculous pericarditis. The patient was a man aged 22 years, who had had pulmonary tuberculosis for 5 years. The specimen shows the opened pericardial sac, in which the heart is seen to be covered by a thick fibrinous exudate. Over the apex there is a layer of blood clot due to recent haemorrhage. The parietal pericardium is greatly thickened, and is also covered by fibrinous exudate and blood clot. *(EC 12.1, Reproduced by permission of the President and Council of the R.C.S. Eng.)*

Demolition. This is accomplished by macrophages. These cells are derived from emigrating monocytes of bone-marrow origin, and they constitute the bulk of "granulomatous" lesions. By transfusing monocytes labelled *in vitro* with tritiated thymidine to animals bearing granulomata of various types and ages,[5, 6] it has been found that some lesions, notably those due to the local injection of *B. pertussis* vaccine or heat-killed tubercle bacilli in mineral oil, show a high turnover of monocytes. Probably these high-turnover lesions are associated with toxic destruction of monocytes. By contrast a carrageenan (polysaccharide derived from seaweed) granuloma is a low-turnover lesion, and the monocytes remain for many weeks. Monocytes from the blood appear to undergo mitosis soon after leaving the circulation, and then enter a resting phase for several days before further division. The long-lived monocytes neither die nor divide for long periods of time, and are replaced by a local macrophage population (derived from histiocytes) irrespective of the bone marrow. Thus low-turnover granulomata are not affected by bone-marrow x-irradiation, but local x-irradiation reduces DNA synthesis almost completely. The reverse occurs in high-turnover lesions, which need constant replenishment of cells from the marrow.

Chronic inflammatory lesions with a heavy macrophage infiltration are traditionally called "proliferative"; as can be induced from this recent experimental work, the macrophages arise both from an exudation of blood monocytes and their subsequent local proliferation. Nevertheless, an "exudative" lesion is traditionally defined as one showing an exudate of plasma with fibrin and polymorphs (see also pp. 184 and 246). A mononuclear response is a feature of many "specific" chronic inflammations. Well-marked accumulations of macrophages are seen in lepromatous leprosy. A mononuclear response is also found in the lesions of delayed hypersensitivity.

Under certain circumstances the cells become large and polygonal with pale oval nuclei and abundant cloudy eosinophilic cytoplasm whose borders blend imperceptibly with those of their neighbours. These cells are called *epithelioid cells*[7] from a resemblance in appearance to epithelial cells.[1] It has been found experimentally that macrophages become epithelioid cells when they have not undertaken phagocytosis, or have completely digested phagocytosed material, or have successfully extruded material by reverse pinocytosis.[7] Epithelioid cells have lost the power of phagocytosis but can take up material avidly by pinocytosis. The material so taken up can later be extruded either piecemeal or as a whole phagosome together with lysosomal enzymes. Epithelioid cells are typical of the tuberculoid granuloma.

It would appear that they develop when the influx of macrophages exceeds the number required to ingest a non-digestible substance, or when the substance is digestible and not very toxic to the macrophages, but is constantly available so that new macrophages are involved in the process and do not die before they can develop epithelioid features. It may be that epithelioid cells form a barrier between macrophages containing organisms and the host, and that they ingest subparticulate material which is digested, detoxified, or excreted. Their life-span is short, being one to four weeks. The cell either dies or else undergoes mitosis to form small round cells which mature to young macrophages. These may become epithelioid if the circumstances are right.[7]

When macrophages encounter insoluble material, they frequently coalesce to form *giant cells*. It has been found that non-proliferating macrophages may fuse in this way,[8] but despite the darkly-staining, rather inactive appearance of the nuclei of the chronic inflammatory giant cell, DNA synthesis does occur, but only when the cells are 2–4 weeks old.[5, 6] This is associated with a burst of mitotic activity, the nuclei all often entering the mitotic cycle synchronously. Thus it appears that, in an experimental situation, giant cells can renew themselves. Nevertheless, in human tissue one does not see mitotic figures in typical giant cells.

Giant cells are frequently seen around exogenous foreign bodies, e.g. catgut, silk, talc, plastic sponges like Ivalon, etc., and they are also present around such endogenous debris as sequestra, cholesterol crystals, and uric-acid crystals (in gout). They are formed in response to the tubercle bacillus and many other organisms causing chronic inflammation.

TABLE 11.1 Giant cells formed by fusion of macrophages

(1) Reaction to exogenous insoluble material, e.g. talc, silica, and ligatures *(foreign-body giant cells)*.
(2) Reaction to insoluble material formed in the body, e.g. sodium biurate crystals, cholesterol, keratin, and fat.
(3) Touton giant cells.
(4) Reactions to certain organisms, e.g. tuberculosis *(Langhans giant cell)*, fungous infections, and syphilis.

Various types of giant cells are described. In some the nuclei are disposed around the periphery of the cell in the form of a horseshoe or a ring, and these are called *Langhans giant cells*; they are particularly frequent in tuberculous lesions. Another type is the *Touton giant cell* found in xanthomata. Its peripheral cytoplasm has a foamy appearance, and the nuclei surround a central area of clear eosinophilic cytoplasm. In the *foreign-body giant cell* the nuclei are scattered haphazardly throughout the cell, and some are present centrally. In many lesions giant cells of both Langhans and foreign-body type are present. The two types should not be regarded as distinct.

Features of healing. *Repair.* The granulation tissue of repair contains a variety of cells, chief amongst which are:

1. Endothelial cells forming blood and lymphatic vessels.
2. Fibroblasts forming collagen (astrocytes forming a glial scar in the central nervous system).
3. Small round cells—lymphocytes and plasma cells.

These features are all seen in chronic inflammation. In chronic suppuration the pus-filled cavity is lined by acutely inflamed granulation tissue. This is the pyogenic membrane. The vascularity of the granulations predisposes to haemorrhage from the delicate thin-walled capillaries. Repeated haemorrhage is a frequent accompaniment of chronic peptic ulcer, and one of the commonest causes of haemoptysis is the chronic infection invariable in bronchiectasis. It is probable that haemoptysis in cancer of the lung is more frequently due to the associated bronchiectasis than from the tumour itself.

Fibroblasts are prominent in most chronic inflammations. They lay down collagen, which is the product of the repair process that is an integral part of chronic inflammation. Repair is seen in fibroid tuberculosis, chronic peptic ulcer, chronic cholecystitis, in the walls of chronic abcesses, etc. If fibrin is characteristic of acute inflammation, fibrosis can be considered the salient feature of chronic inflammation. The *cicatrisation* that results leads to many of the important complications of chronic inflammation. Thus chronic rheumatic valvulitis leads to valvular stenosis and regurgitation, chronic gastric ulcers may proceed to pyloric stenosis or hour-glass stomach, while fibrous ankylosis with severe limitation of movement is a frequent end-result of rheumatoid arthritis.

A very common feature of chronic inflammation is *endarteritis obliterans*, in which the lumen of the small arteries is gradually occluded as the result of a progressive proliferation of the tunica intima. It is seen in the bed of chronic peptic ulcers, following radiation damage, around gummata, etc.

A feature of chronic inflammation which is worthy of special note is the accumulation of lymphocytes and plasma cells. These are the "cells of chronic inflammation" or "small round cells" (Fig. 11.2). Their significance is poorly understood. Present in the granulation tissue of a healing wound, they are much more numerous in chronic inflammatory granulation tissue. Frequently they assume a perivascular distribution, e.g. in syphilitic aortitis, and are presumably derived from the blood rather than from local lymphoid tissue or stem cells.

A possible function of the lymphocyte is that it forms a mobile reserve for other cells. Some authorities regard it as the precursor of plasma cells, macrophages, and fibroblasts. Lymphocytes have been credited with a growth-promoting function, for they stimulate the growth of fibroblasts in tissue culture, and it has been claimed that their DNA is reutilised by the growing cells. Nevertheless, the evidence is not conclusive, and the role of this enigmatic cell remains undecided.[32]

There is little doubt that plasma cells are concerned with the production of immunoglobulins. Heavy plasma-cell infiltrations are common in chronic inflammatory lesions of juxtacutaneous mucous membranes. In ageing plasma cells there are sometimes intracytoplasmic accumulations of

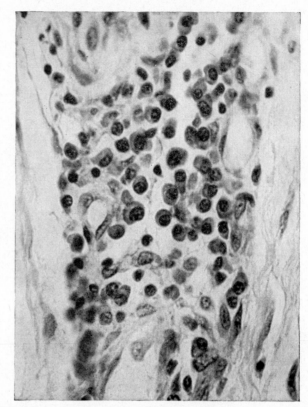

Figure 11.2
Plasma cells. This is the section of a chronic inflammatory response in which plasma cells are predominating. The round and pear-shaped contour of the cells is well marked. Their nuclei are eccentric, and have a conspicuous cart-wheel disposition of clumped chromatin. The cytoplasm is comparatively darkly-staining due to its high content of RNA. The clear area adjacent to the nucleus is the Golgi apparatus. × 400.

strongly eosinophilic material called *Russell bodies*. Despite their prominent appearance they are of no great importance.

Regeneration. When the tissue destroyed in chronic inflammation is of a type capable of division, regeneration rather than repair takes place. This is particularly obvious in surface epithelia. Indeed, regeneration may become so exuberant that the line of demarcation between it, hyperplasia, and neoplasia may be difficult to define. For this reason malignancy has frequently been ascribed to "chronic irritation". A well-known example of this is the regeneration of the epithelium which occurs in ulcerative colitis, and which may progress to polypoid overgrowth and malignancy.

In the gall-bladder chronic inflammation may cause the epithelium to "invade" the wall, giving rise in extreme cases to cholecystitis glandularis proliferans which may easily be mistaken for cancer[9]* (Fig. 11.3). The "tumourlets" seen in

* The normal gall-bladder often shows epithelial-lined diverticula (Rokitansky-Aschoff sinuses) beneath the muscular coat. The possibility that some examples of cholecystitis glandularis proliferans are, in fact, congenital abnormalities (ectopias) cannot be excluded.[10]

Figure 11.3
Chronic cholecystitis with epithelial hyperplasia
(cholecystitis glandularis proliferans). The gall-
bladder wall is thickened, and there is a wide zone
of chronic inflammatory tissue deep to the attenuated
muscle layer. There are many glandular spaces in
this inflammatory zone, and one is connected with
the overlying epithelium by a narrow duct which
penetrates the muscle coat. It is called a Rokitansky-
Aschoff sinus. ×25.

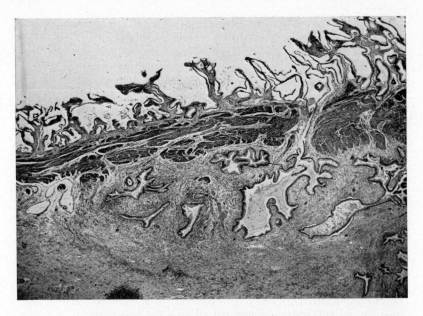

the lung in bronchiectasis are also regenerative and hyperplastic rather than neoplastic[11, 12] (Fig. 11.4). A classical
example of the difficulty in distinguishing the regeneration
and hyperplasia of chronic inflammation from true neoplasia
is the diffuse papillary epithelial overgrowth of the mucosa
of the rat forestomach produced by infestation with the
nematode *Gongylonema neoplasticum*. This was originally
thought by Fibiger to be a true tumour, but it now regarded
as non-neoplastic.[13]

The epithelial overgrowth at the edge of a chronic gastric
ulcer is another pitfall for the unwary. The greatly divergent
views expressed in the past on the frequency of malignant
change in chronic gastric ulcer are largely due to the difficulties in interpreting the microscopic appearances.

General Effects of Chronic Inflammation

The general effects of chronic inflammation depend upon
the nature and extent of the responsible agent. In a localised
foreign-body reaction or a chronic varicose ulcer there is no
noteworthy general response at all. On the other hand, in
chronic infective diseases like tuberculosis or actinomycosis
there may be widespread changes in the reticulo-endothelial
system and in the blood stream. Remarkably little is known
about the exact mechanisms involved.

Changes in the reticulo-endothelial system (see also
Chapter 30). Most chronic inflammatory conditions lead to
hyperplasia of the RE system. The "proliferative" nature of
the local response has already been described. The lymph
nodes draining a chronic septic lesion show hyperplasia
affecting the sinus-lining cells and sometimes the germinal
centres and medullary cords.

If organisms gain access to the blood stream, they are
taken up by the other members of the RE system, namely
the sinus-lining cells of spleen, liver, marrow, etc. General-

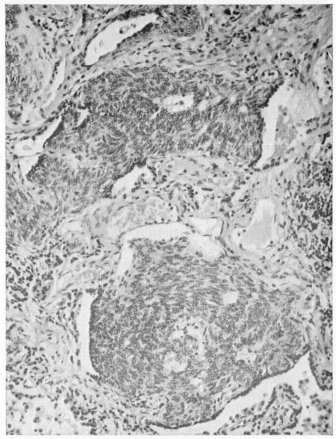

Figure 11.4
"Tumourlet" of lung. This is a section of a fibrosed portion of
lung from a case of bronchiectasis. The groups of epithelial cells
appear to be invading the tissues, but follow-up results indicate
that these lesions are not neoplastic. ×120.

ised parasitisation of the system is seen in kala-azar, miliary tuberculosis, and histoplasmosis. These hyperplastic changes are undoubtedly related to the phagocytic functions of the cells; in addition they also play some part in the immune response. Hyperplasia indeed occurs without obvious widespread dissemination of the organisms, and this may be due to the formation of antigen-antibody complexes in the bloodstream which are subsequently removed by the RE system.

The immune response. Antibody production is a feature of most chronic inflammatory diseases, and the demonstration of specific immunoglobulins is a useful diagnostic procedure. Antibody production may be so marked that the γ-globulin blood level is raised. Kala-azar affords a good example of this.

The antibodies may, on the other hand, be of the lymphocyte or cell-bound type, and be associated with delayed hypersensitivity. Tests like the Mantoux, lepromin, and Frei are based upon this. One wonders whether this delayed hypersensitivity may not be even of broader significance than merely of great use as a diagnostic tool. If the hypersensitive state itself results in tissue damage, then it might be a major factor in the pathogenesis of chronic inflammation. Would tuberculosis be a chronic disease were it not for the development of this type of hypersensitivity? No answer is yet possible, but the relationship between hypersensitivity and the manifestations of infection is further discussed on p. 183.

The immune response may be reflected in definite morphological changes. Hyperplasia of the splenic cells may be sufficient to render the spleen clinically palpable. Splenomegaly is seen in chronic malaria, subacute infective endocarditis, Felty's syndrome, etc.

Finally, the long-continued stress on the antibody producing mechanism may be associated with *amyloid disease* (Chapter 44).

Changes in the blood. The white cells frequently show changes which are related to the causative agent and to the extent of the infection: these are considered in Chapter 50. Anaemia is frequent and usually of the normochromic, normocytic type, but it may become hypochromic and microcytic as a result of repeated haemorrhage, e.g. in peptic ulcer.

The reduction in plasma albumin, the rise in γ-globulin, and other changes that occur in the plasma proteins are described elsewhere (see Chapter 45). A rise in the ESR occurs in many chronic inflammatory diseases, and is commonly used as an aid both to diagnosis and prognosis, e.g. in tuberculosis and rheumatoid arthritis.

Other changes. Although "toxaemia" is put forward as the explanation of many of the general symptoms, it cannot be regarded as anything more than a cloak for our ignorance. The following signs and symptoms are frequent and attributed to this state: tiredness, malaise, headache, anorexia, loss of weight, anaemia, loss of libido, and pyrexia.

Toxaemia is often assumed to be due to the liberation of endotoxins, but although such substances have been identified in some organisms, e.g. staphylococci and *Esch. coli*, there are others, such as *Tr. pallidum*, in which no such endotoxins are known. Possibly toxic substances are formed when tissue is damaged either as a result of direct bacterial action or hypersensitivity. However, there is no direct evidence as to the nature of the endotoxins or products of tissue damage which are responsible for the "toxaemia" of infection.

Examples of Chronic Inflammation

Examples of chronic inflammation can be considered in the following groups:

(*a*) Those due to "non-specific", pyogenic, bacterial agents (*Staph. pyogenes* and *Esch. coli*).

(*b*) Those due to inanimate foreign bodies, e.g. catgut.

(*c*) Those due to "specific" organisms, e.g. tubercle bacillus and *Tr. pallidum*. This third group is so important that it is dealt with separately in Chapters 20 and 21.

(*d*) Those associated with hypersensitivity or autoimmunity. These are discussed in Chapter 16. The collagen diseases can be conveniently included in this group, though their aetiology is obscure.

The first group includes a wide collection of conditions that are very commonly encountered in clinical practice. For the purposes of this discussion a few important examples have been selected.

Osteomyelitis. Acute osteomyelitis occurs most often in children at the metaphysis of one of the long bones of the lower limbs. This is the area which is most easily traumatised, and should this occur during the course of a *Staph. pyogenes* bacteraemia, the organisms may become lodged and produce a metastatic lesion. A typical acute inflammatory reaction occurs, and owing to the rigidity of the bone the increased tension produced by the exudation causes compression of the blood vessels and subsequent ischaemia. Necrosis of bone therefore follows; pus is then formed, and it tracks under the periosteum, thereby further imperilling the blood supply to the cortex. In this way extensive necrosis may occur, sometimes involving the whole shaft. This dead bone acts as a foreign body; it cannot be easily removed, and it not only provides a focus for organismal growth but also prevents adequate drainage of pus. Conditions are ideal for the development of chronic infection.

Pus ruptures through the periosteum into the muscular and subcutaneous compartments. Usually it is discharged on to the skin surface through sinuses. The vascular periosteum attempts to reform the shaft of the bone; in this way the sequestrated shaft becomes encased in a thick bony *involucrum* (Fig. 11.5). The shaft is bathed in pus which escapes through holes, or *cloacae*, in the involucrum, and is then discharged to the surface. Osteoclasts slowly erode the sequestrum, detaching it at each end from living bone and slowly destroying it. This must be completed before healing can be accomplished. In practice this is seldom pos-

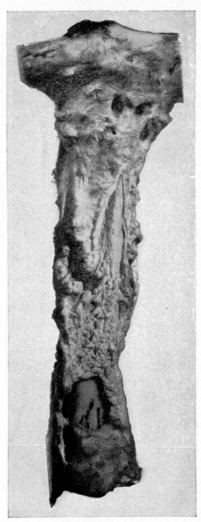

Figure 11.5
Osteomyelitis of tibia. The limb was amputated 6 months after the presence of necrosis was established. In this specimen the extensive central sequestrum is largely concealed by an exuberant involucrum formed from the detached periosteum. There is a cloaca at the base of the shaft (it has been enlarged artificially), and through it the pitted sequestrum is plainly recognisable. (HS 44.1, *Reproduced by permission of the President and Council of the R.C.S. Eng.)*

sible without surgical intervention. If nothing is done, the condition may lead to death as the result of pyaemia, "toxaemia", or amyloid disease.

This chronic infection is fortunately uncommon nowadays since the advent of antibiotic therapy, which is used in combination with early surgical drainage in the acute stage. Once chronicity develops, the outlook for the limb is still very poor.

From a pathological point of view the disease illustrates many points. It shows how an acute infection can become chronic due to the inadequate drainage of pus as well as to the presence of a foreign body, in this case the sequestrum. Moreover, all the features of chronic inflammation are present. Acute inflammation is evidenced by the polymorphonuclear and fluid exudate, demolition by macrophage and osteoclastic activity, regeneration by bone formation, and repair by surrounding scarring.

Chronic pyelonephritis.[14] Chronic pyelonephritis is now recognised as a common cause of chronic renal failure and an important aetiological factor in systemic hypertension.

The organisms usually implicated are the Gram-negative intestinal bacilli, but the exact mode of infection is debated. Certainly urinary obstruction plays an important part. It has been shown in the rabbit that if one ureter is tied, an intravenous injection of *Esch. coli* results in acute pyelonephritis in that kidney.[14]

On the other hand, there is no doubt that organisms can be introduced into the bladder during catheterisation, and that this manipulation is a potent cause of acute cystitis. Some urologists maintain that urine may reflux up the ureters, thereby supporting the theory of "ascending" infection as a cause of acute pyelonephritis.

Chronic pyelonephritis may commence either as an overt acute disease or may appear insidiously. During the acute phase the cortex contains multiple minute abscesses, and the congested medulla shows streaking due to pus cells in the tubules. Why this condition becomes chronic is not altogether clear. Urinary obstruction is liable to perpetuate the infection, and in some cases evidence of this in the form of hydroureter or hydronephrosis may be found. Often, however, there is no obvious obstructive element.

The importance of scars in predisposing to recurrent attacks of pyelonephritis has been stressed by a number of workers. Thus, it has been shown that rabbits whose kidneys have been scarred by electrical burning are very liable to subsequent infection.[15] In another experiment it was found that the intravenous injection of Gram-negative intestinal bacilli produced acute pyelonephritis only in those rabbits whose kidneys already bore the scars of a previous staphylococcal infection.[16] It has been suggested that in man also the presence of old scars predisposes to acute pyelonephritis, and that many such scars are due to congenital abnormalities of the parenchyma.[17] Be this as it may, it seems very probable that one attack of acute pyelonephritis predisposes the patient to repeated ones because of the damage it produces.

In the chronic stage the kidney shows focal scarring and infiltration which chronic inflammatory cells (Fig. 11.6). In the affected areas many glomeruli are hyalinised, and others show typical periglomerular fibrosis. The surviving tubules are often dilated and contain eosinophilic material, producing a picture which resembles normal thyroid tissue. The vessels may show the changes of either benign or malignant hypertension.

Hypertension often occurs, and since this may occasionally be due to unilateral renal disease, and therefore amenable to surgical treatment, it has attained considerable prominence.

The exact incidence is, however, disputed as is its pathogenesis; probably from 15 to 20 per cent of all cases of malignant hypertension are due to pyelonephritis.[14]

Chronic inflammation in the alimentary tract. *The Stomach.* The factors which determine whether the frequently occurring acute gastric ulcers will heal or persist as chronic

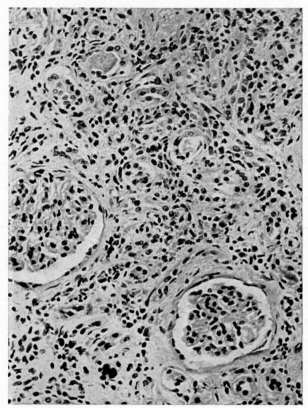

Figure 11.6
Chronic pyelonephritis. Most of the parenchyma of the kidney has been replaced by fibrous tissue heavily infiltrated with small round cells. A few atrophied tubules can still be recognised, and two glomeruli are included in the section. One shows early periglomerular fibrosis. × 220.

ulcers are not known. In chronic ulceration the destructive process penetrates the muscle and destroys it. The ulcer base is then composed of scar tissue, superficial to which there is a layer of vascular granulation tissue heavily infiltrated with pus cells, macrophages, plasma cells, and lymphocytes. Overlying this there is a slough.

Since muscle is incapable of regeneration, it is replaced by scar tissue which remains as a permanent memorial to the chronic inflammatory process even after complete healing has taken place. The epithelium attempts to grow over the ulcer bed; its invaginations at the ulcer edge may simulate neoplastic invasion, and in occasional cases cancer does develop at this site.[18] The incidence is probably low (less than 4 per cent) in gastric ulcers, and never in duodenal ulcers. If heal-

ing does occur, the regenerated epithelium may be of intestinal type with villi, Paneth cells, etc.

The colon.[19] Chronic inflammatory lesions of the colon may follow specific infections by the *Shigella* species or *Entamoeba histolytica*, but in Britain the commonest colonic lesion is *idiopathic ulcerative colitis*. This disease can commence as a fulminating acute condition which either leads to rapid death or else follows a more chronic course. Sometimes the onset is insidious and the disease is chronic from the beginning.

The inflammatory changes are most marked in the mucosa. The earliest lesion is the formation of small abscesses which result from blockage of the openings of the crypts of Lieberkühn. Ulceration follows, and may lead to perforation in the uncommon acute type of disease. The colon becomes rigid and shortened due mainly to hypertrophy of the muscle coat, the cause of which is not known; fibrosis is not marked,

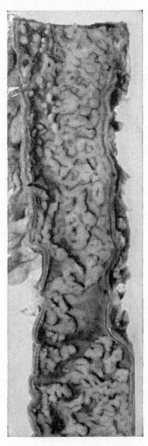

Figure 11.7
Chronic ulcerative colitis with pseudopolyposis. The appearance of these multiple foci of polypoid overgrowth of epithelium is to be distinguished from true polyposis coli. In pseudopolyposis the bowel itself is chronically inflamed, and in this specimen the wall is considerably contracted. Furthermore, the intervening mucosa is roughened and inflamed. In polyposis coli there is no evidence of inflammation. (EA 70.1, *Reproduced by permission of the President and Council of the R.C.S. Eng.*)

and does not affect the muscle. An increase in fat occurs in the subserosal layer. Fat accumulation of this type is a feature of many chronic inflammatory conditions, e.g. chronic pyelonephritis, but the reason for this is not known.

As the disease progresses the outstanding feature is generalised hyperaemia and oedema of the mucosa together with infiltration by lymphocytes. Polymorphs are relatively scanty and are confined to the areas of ulceration which are usually arranged longitudinally over the taeniae coli. The ulceration tends to surround and undermine areas of swollen mucosa which then constitute *pseudopolypi*. This is an example of catarrhal inflammation, for in addition to the pus there is an abundant secretion of mucus. Pus, blood, and mucus are therefore all present in the stools.

In only the very chronic stages of the disease does epithelial overgrowth occur and lead to polypoid excrescences. Although the hyperplastic condition superficially resembles true polyposis coli, the intervening mucosa is normal in polyposis coli, whereas it is inflamed in ulcerative colitis (Fig. 11.7). Ulcerative colitis is sometimes complicated by cancer (see p. 381).

TISSUE RESPONSE TO INSOLUBLE INANIMATE FOREIGN MATERIALS

The tissue response to these substances is very complex, and with the increasing use of metals and plastics in reconstructive surgery is a matter of considerable importance. It is probably true to state that all foreign materials are capable of producing an inflammatory response under certain circumstances. Nothing is truly "inert". The factors which determine the severity of the inflammatory response are not completely understood, but the following are important.[20]

The chemical nature of the material. The chemical stability and solubility are of great importance: thus stainless steel is more inert than ordinary steel.

Physical state of the substance. Smooth, highly-polished surfaces provoke much less reaction than do rough irregular surfaces. It is important to bear this in mind when inserting metallic prostheses or pins. Finely-divided or colloidal substances, e.g. silica, are particularly irritating.

Nylon has been used in joint reconstructions, but the scratching and powdering which occur during use lead to an intense foreign-body reaction.[21]

Electro-chemical potentials set up by the close proximity of dissimilar metals cause tissue damage.[22] This is particularly important in orthopaedic surgery.[20] Plate and screws must be of exactly the same composition.* Otherwise there is sufficient reaction to cause loosening of the screws. Even the metal scraped off the screwdriver may be sufficient to produce this effect.

The relatively insoluble foreign materials cannot be removed by the inflammatory reaction which they excite, and

* It should not be forgotten that there are many different types of "stainless steel".

it follows that the lesions induced are typically chronic in character. Giant cells abound. Most of these are of the foreign-body type, but sometimes Langhans giant cells are also prominent. As already indicated, it is unwise to distinguish categorically between them (Fig. 11.8).

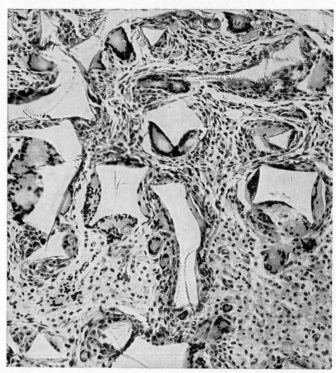

Figure 11.8
Foreign-body reaction. This is a section of an Etheron sponge which had been implanted for 40 days subcutaneously in a rat. The clear areas were occupied by fragments of sponge which have been dislodged during processing. They were surrounded by exuberant giant cells. Many of these have peripherally-disposed nuclei and are of the Langhans type. Only a few have the nuclear arrangement of foreign-body giant cells. × 150.

A few important examples of reaction to foreign materials will be cited.

Carbon. Tattooing consists of introducing carbon into the dermis; it excites little inflammatory reaction, and is soon taken up by macrophages in which it remains in the tissues indefinitely. Inhaled carbon is transported by macrophages to the lymphoid tissues in the lung, where it remains throughout life. Usually there is some dilatation of the respiratory bronchioles ("focal dust emphysema"), which should be distinguished from destructive centrilobular emphysema. Coalminer's pneumoconiosis due to carbon alone produces little disability by itself; it is the associated chronic bronchitis or silicosis which is crippling.

Metals.[20, 22] Vitallium and stainless steel cause little reaction when used in the form of polished plates, Smith-Petersen pins, and arthroplasty cups. Tantalum, titanium, and zirconium are also used because of their inertness. Other metallic objects, e.g. bullets, excite more reaction, and eventually become encapsulated in fibrous tissue. Steel or iron fragments lodged in the eye after penetrating injuries can cause a severe reaction resulting in blindness.

Plastic sponges (e.g. Ivalon, Etheron, and Polyfoam). In surgical practice these materials have been inserted as a means of inducing fibrosis as well as for mammoplasty. There is an initial acute inflammatory reaction with polymorphs, but this is rapidly followed by a macrophage response. Giant cells are formed in abundance, and the interstices of the sponge are invaded by granulation tissue. This matures until eventually dense contracted scar tissue results. For this reason the materials are not uniformly successful for breast reconstruction. Furthermore, there is experimental evidence that in animals they may induce the formation of sarcoma.[23]

Silicones and silastics.[24] Silicones are oily liquids of the basic formula:

$$CH_3\!-\!\underset{\underset{CH_3}{|}}{\overset{\overset{CH_3}{|}}{Si}}\!-\!O\!-\!\underset{\underset{CH_3}{|}}{\overset{\overset{CH_3}{|}}{Si}}\ etc.$$

They are heat stable, chemically non-reactive, and non-toxic, and excite little or no inflammatory or immunological response. Oxygen is ten times more soluble in them than in water, and fish and even small mammals can survive when immersed in them. They have been used in man for many purposes. Injected into arthritic joints, they relieve pain and increase the range of movement. Subcutaneous injections have been used to recontour the face and breasts, but drifting of the fluid is a disadvantage.

Rubbers of varying degrees of hardness and known as *silastics* are formed from silicone by the addition of ferric or aluminium chloride followed by oxidation. They too are inert and can withstand bending without fatigue almost indefinitely. They have been used to form a variety of prostheses—the lens of the eye, the ear drum, breasts, joints, etc.

Suture materials.[25] Catgut excites a brisk acute pyogenic inflammatory reaction which is soon followed by the appearance of macrophages and giant cells. The strength of plain catgut is reduced to half within two days, while for chromic gut the time is ten days.

The tissue reaction to linen, nylon, etc., does not succeed in removing the material, which is therefore retained for a long time.

Silica.[26] Colloidal silica solutions are very toxic to cells, and produce extensive necrosis if injected into the tissues. When silica is inhaled in the form of particles 1–5 μm in diameter, it is taken up by macrophages in the alveoli and carried to the lymphoid tissue of the lung and hilar nodes. Here it excites a foreign-body reaction with macrophages, giant cells, etc., which is later followed by dense fibrosis. The

fibrotic nodules separated by emphysematous lung produce the typical picture of silicosis. The disease is seen in miners, stone-workers, and sand-blasters, and produces great disability due to the extensive lung destruction. The condition predisposes to tuberculosis.

Silica introduced into small cuts, e.g. of the fingers, produces a non-caseating tuberculoid granulomatous reaction resembling sarcoidosis. It is usually stated that the severe chronic inflammatory response to silica is due to the fact that it slowly goes into solution, and that the soluble product is toxic to cells. Experiments in which silica has been placed in diffusion chambers and introduced into the peritoneal cavity have not supported this. Although fluid and proteins can pass in and out of such chambers, no fibrosis occurs around them. Fibrosis occurs only if cells are allowed to enter the chamber and make physical contact with the silica particles.[27]

It has been suggested that the effects of silicosis are due to an autoimmune mechanism, the silica reacting with tissue protein to form an antigen against which antibodies form. It is said that the silicotic nodule contains an unusually high content of globulin.[26]

Asbestos.[28] Another important disease produced by the inhalation of a dust (pneumoconiosis) is asbestosis. The long fibres of asbestos (a complex silicate) are inhaled by workers in the processing plants. They are too large to be removed by

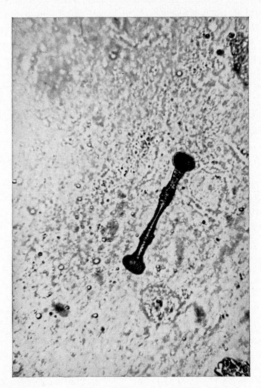

Figure 11.9
Asbestos body in sputum. *(Photograph supplied by Prof. I. M. P. Dawson)*

Figure 11.10.
Starch granuloma. This granuloma was found in the appendix. A central area of necrosis is bounded by a layer of radially disposed macrophages and giant cells. The starch granules, represented as clear oval spaces, are seen within the necrosis and the giant cells. x 150. *(From Neely, J. and Davies, J. D. (1971), British Medical Journal, 3, 625.)*

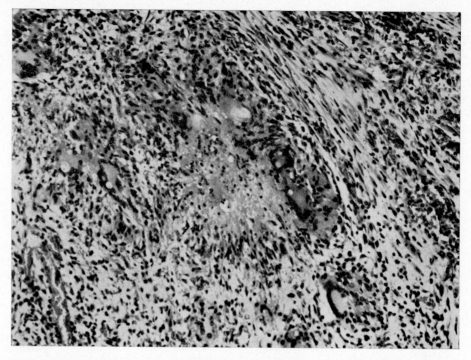

macrophages, and therefore remain in the alveoli where they stimulate a typical foreign-body reaction, which is later followed by diffuse fibrosis of the lung. The fibres themselves become coated with a material containing haemosiderin, giving an appearance which is characteristic. These *asbestos bodies* are dumb-bell shaped, segmented, brown structures, and their presence in the sputum is a useful diagnostic finding (Fig. 11.9), but it does not necessarily indicate active asbestosis.

Unlike silicosis, asbestosis is an important precancerous condition, but it does not predispose so greatly to tuberculosis.

Talc. Talc (magnesium silicate) causes a typical foreign-body reaction which culminates in fibrosis. Its use as a glove-powder is liable to lead to postoperative adhesions following abdominal surgery.[29] Starch powder, although safer, may have a similar effect[30] (Fig. 11.10).

Beryllium.[31] This excites an acute inflammatory response which progresses to chronic inflammation with fibrosis and sometimes a non-caseating tuberculoid reaction. It is seen in the lungs of workers whose occupation entails inhalation of beryllium compounds.

Zirconium. Though metallic zirconium is inert, salts of this metal in deodorant sticks have been reported (mostly from the USA) to produce non-caseating tuberculoid lesions in the skin (see p. 267).

REFERENCES

1. REID, J. D. (1970). *New Zealand Medical Journal,* **71,** 375.
2. TURK, J. L. (1971). *Proceedings of the Royal Society of Medicine,* **64,** 942.
3. EPSTEIN, W. L., SKAHEN, J. R. and KRASNOBROD, H. (1963). *American Journal of Pathology,* **43,** 391.
4. EPSTEIN, W. L. (1967). *Progress in Allergy,* **11,** 36.
5. RYAN, G. B. and SPECTOR, W. G. (1970). *Proceedings of the Royal Society,* B, **175,** 269.
6. SPECTOR, W. G. (1971). *Proceedings of the Royal Society of Medicine,* **64,** 941.
7. PAPADIMITRIOU, J. M. and SPECTOR, W. G. (1971). *Journal of Pathology,* **105,** 187.
8. CARTER, R. L. and ROBERTS, J. D. B. (1971). *Journal of Pathology,* **105,** 285.
9. KING, E. S. J. and MacCALLUM, P. (1931). *British Journal of Surgery,* **19,** 310.
10. YOUNG, T. E. (1959). *American Journal of Clinical Pathology,* **31,** 423.
11. WHITWELL, F. (1955). *Journal of Pathology and Bacteriology,* **70,** 529.
12. CUNNINGHAM, G. J., NASSAU, E. and WALTER, J. B. (1958). *Thorax,* **13,** 64.
13. HADFIELD, G. and GARROD, L. P. (1947). In *Recent Advances in Pathology,* 5th edn, p. 72. London: Churchill.
14. HEPTINSTALL, R. H. (1960). In *Recent Advances in Pathology,* 7th edn, p. 122. Edited by C. V. Harrison. London: Churchill.
15. ROCHA, H. *et al.* (1958). *Yale Journal of Biology and Medicine,* **30,** 341.
16. DE NAVASQUEZ, S. (1956). *Journal of Pathology and Bacteriology,* **71,** 27.
17. MARSHALL, A. G. (1956). *Journal of Pathology and Bacteriology,* **71,** 95 and (1968). *Ibid.,* **95,** 225.
18. NEWCOMB, W. D. (1936). *Proceedings of the Royal Society of Medicine,* **30,** 113.

19. MORSON, B. C. (1966). In *Systemic Pathology*, p. 558. Edited by G. P. Wright and W. St C. Symmers. London: Longmans.
20. WATSON-JONES, R. (1952). In *Fractures and Joint Injuries*, 4th edn, vol. 1, p. 205. Edinburgh: Livingstone.
21. SCALES, J. T. (1953). *Journal of Bone and Joint Surgery*, **35B**, 49.
22. Various Authors (1957). *Lancet*, i, 1174.
23. WALTER, J. B. and CHIARAMONTE, L. G. (1965). *British Journal of Surgery*, **52**, 49.
24. HELAL, B. (1969). In *Recent Advances in Orthopaedics*, p. 91. Edited by A. G. Apley. London: Churchill.
25. LAWRIE, P., ANGUS, G. E. and REESE, A. J. M. (1959). *British Journal of Surgery*, **46**, 638 and (1960). *Ibid.*, **47**, 551.
26. GOUGH, J. (1959). In *Modern Trends in Pathology*, p. 273. Edited by D. H. Collins. London: Butterworths.
27. CURRAN, R. C. and AGER, J. A. M. (1962). *Journal of Pathology and Bacteriology*, **83**, 1.
28. HEARD, B. E. and WILLIAMS, R. (1961). *Thorax*, **16**, 264.
29. SAXÉN, L. and MYLLÄRNIEMI, H. (1968). *New England Journal of Medicine*, **279**, 200.
30. NEELY, J. and DAVIES, J. D. (1971). *British Medical Journal*, **3**, 625.
31. FREIMAN, D. G. and HARDY, H. L. (1970). *Human Pathology*, **1**, 25.
32. Leading Article (1973). *Lancet*, **1**, 409.

Chapter 12.   The Immune Response

One of the characteristic features of the adult vertebrate is its ability to distinguish between its own constituents ("self") and those of external or foreign origin ("non-self"). The reaction to foreign substances ("immune response") may be regarded as self-preservative, evolved as a protection against infection. The reaction involves the elimination of the foreign material,[1] and is an important homeostatic mechanism.*

In the first description of antibody formation by von Behring and Kitasato in 1890, it was shown that animals injected with tetanus or diphtheria toxin produced substances which were capable of neutralising the toxins. The antibodies gave protection against these diseases, and the subject of immunology naturally grew around the central theme of immunity to bacterial infection.

Soon, however, with the description of the tuberculin reaction by Koch and anaphylaxis by Richet, it was realised that the body's reaction to foreign protein was also responsible for the phenomena of hypersensitivity.

More recently it has been recognised that under certain conditions the body is capable of reacting against its own constituents, thereby revealing diseases whose pathogenesis can be explained on an "auto-immune reaction". Great interest is now centred on this aspect, which affords a new pathogenesis to many well-established diseases, and also shows how the body can react against whole living tissues as well as simple protein antigens. The grafting of tissues from one animal to another is a further exploitation of the science of immunology.

Inevitably the highly specific and sensitive methods which have been developed in immunology have been applied to other fields, e.g. in the analysis of protein structure, blood group antigens, etc.

The immune response is therefore a reaction to foreign material which results in the formation of antibodies. These may be either immunoglobulins or cell-bound. It is now believed that two separate systems are involved. The lymphoid tissue associated developmentally with the thymus is responsible for the production of cell-bound antibodies, while the immunoglobulins are synthesised in cells which are dependent developmentally on lymphoid tissue associated with the gut: in birds this is the bursa of Fabricius.

ANTIGENS

Definition of an Antigen

An *antigen* is usually defined as a substance which when introduced parenterally into the tissues stimulates the *production* of an antibody, and when mixed with that antibody *reacts specifically* with it in some detectable way. An *antibody* is a substance produced as a result of the stimulus provided by the introduction of an antigen with which it reacts in a specific way.

These definitions are merely circular, defining the one in terms of the other, and indeed are open to criticism since some antibodies are cellular and are difficult to detect *in vitro*. An antigen may be defined as a substance which when introduced into the body of a susceptible animal leads to an immune response which results in a specific change such that when the antigen is introduced on a subsequent occasion there is a response differing from that seen when the substance was first introduced.† The difference observed may be local or general depending on the route of administration, and the reaction leads to the more rapid elimination from the body, except perhaps in certain cells, and in such a form as to provide for immunological memory.

These definitions of an antigen include two classes of compounds: (a) *haptens*,[2] which show little or no antigenic properties until first combined with protein; this may occur spontaneously *in vivo* when the substance is introduced into the body, or be performed *in vitro* by chemical manipulations, and (b) *true antigens*, which are nearly always proteins. In fact there is no hard and fast line of division between these two classes.

Characteristics of Antigens[3]

True antigens are substances of high molecular weight and are nearly always of protein nature. Not all proteins are antigenic: gelatin, which lacks the amino acids tyrosine and tryptophane, is an example of a protein which is non-anti-

---

* It is of interest to note that there is no immune response in non-vertebrates, and presumably their defences against infection must rely on other mechanisms. The Californian and Atlantic hagfish are primitive vertebrates which occupy a similar position. The sea lamprey can form cellular antibodies but few immunoglobulins. Higher vertebrates produce both types of antibody.

† It is of historical interest that von Pirquet coined the term *allergy* to describe this altered response. It included those changes which led both to immunity and to hypersensitivity. However, by common usage the original meaning has been changed, and allergy is now equated with hypersensitivity (p. 175).

genic, at least so far as the production of immunoglobulin antibodies is concerned.

It is thought that to be antigenic the molecule must have rigidity, and that aromatic-acid residues, like tyrosine, are important in giving the molecule this property. Haemoglobin is an example of a poor antigen, while those found in skin are highly antigenic. It must be appreciated that antigenicity, like pathogenicity with micro-organisms, is not an absolute quality. A substance can be considered antigenic only in relation to a specific host. The skin antigens of an individual are not antigenic to himself, but are highly antigenic to all other individuals (except his identical twin).

The antigenic specificity of each protein is due to specific areas of the molecule called *determinant sites*, or *epitopes*.[4] One protein molecule can have several epitopes, and these may differ from each other not only in specificity but also in antigenic potency. It is therefore an oversimplification to think of a protein like serum albumin as exhibiting a single specificity (see p. 146). The precise nature of the epitopic sites is poorly understood, but the shape of the molecule due to its secondary and tertiary structure is believed to be involved (see footnote, p. 14).

Denaturation of protein involves changes in its secondary structure and changes in antigenicity. New epitopes may be uncovered and old ones lost. A similar phenomenon may occur *in vivo*; antibodies may appear against fragments of an injected antigen due to the exposure of new determinants which were not on the surface of the original molecule.[5]

It has been found that even slight changes in the chemical composition of a protein are capable of altering its antigenic properties. One of the ways in which this may be done is by its conjugation with a second substance known as a *hapten*.[2] This is a non-protein substance which has little or no antigenic properties itself, but which combines with a protein to form a new antigen. The latter is capable of stimulating the production of specific immunoglobulins, the specificity of which depends upon the hapten fraction rather than the carrier protein. This action of haptens may best be understood by a simple illustration (see Table 12.1). Introduction

TABLE 12.1

Antigen	Antibody	Test		
F injected into animal	Anti-F	F	+Anti-F	= precipitate
H injected into animal	Anti-H	H	+Anti-H	= precipitate
		F	+Anti-H	= nil
F^c injected into animal	Anti-F^c	F^c	+Anti-F^c	= precipitate
H^c injected into animal	Anti-H^c	H^c	+Anti-H^c	= precipitate
		H^c	+Anti-F^c	= precipitate
		F^c	+Anti-H^c	= precipitate

of protein "F" into an animal leads to the production of antibody anti-F, which will act as a precipitin when mixed with its antigen "F". Similarly anti-H will act with protein "H", but not with "F". New antigens which are produced by a combination of hapten-C with proteins "F" and "H"

will react specifically with their respective antibodies, anti-F^c and anti-H^c. However, it is found that anti-F^c will also react with antigen-H^c, and similarly anti-H^c will react with antigen-F^c. Therefore the antigenic specificities of "F" and "H" have been suppressed by the hapten "C". This suppression is not necessarily complete, for the antibodies specific for the carrier protein may also appear (p. 184). This applies particularly to the cell-bound type.

Haptens on their own have the property of combining with their specific immunoglobulin, although usually no precipitate is formed. However, the treated antibody is no longer capable of forming a precipitate when added to the antigen–hapten complex. Therefore, while haptens must be combined with protein to elicit their specific antibody response, they do not require the protein to react with the antibody so produced. The more complex haptens, e.g. pneumococcal polysaccharide, do react with their specific antibodies to produce a precipitate.

Carbohydrates and lipids are feebly antigenic alone, but when combined with protein can produce powerful antigens.

The importance of haptens may be illustrated by three examples.

(1) Pneumococci contain an important polysaccharide in their capsules which determines their pathogenicity and antigenicity (see p. 223). Similarly β-haemolytic streptococci contain polysaccharide haptens (see Lancefield grouping, p. 220).

(2) Simple chemicals may combine with body proteins, thereby producing an antigenic complex. This is the basis of allergic contact dermatitis and many types of drug hypersensitivity.

(3) Several important tissue antigens are either haptens or haptens combined with protein. Thus, the blood-group substances (ABO system) are glycoproteins, while transplantation, Forssman, and Wassermann antigens are lipid in nature.

Heterophile antigens.[6] This name is applied to antigens which are identical (or very closely related), and which are found in the tissues of different and unrelated species of animals. Antibodies to them thus appear to be non-specific. The best known is *Forssman antigen*, a lipo-polysaccharide-protein complex, which is widely distributed in nature, being found in certain bacteria, e.g. *Sh. shigae*, and the tissues and red cells of many animals. Guinea-pig kidney is a convenient laboratory source. Other important examples are the antigen shared between (a) *Proteus* organisms and certain rickettsiae (see Weil-Felix reaction, p. 170), and (b) the agent of infectious mononucleosis and sheep red cells (Paul-Bunnell test, Chapter 50).

Alloantigens. Substances which are present in one individual and are antigenic to some (but not all) individuals of the *same species* are termed alloantigens. Good examples are the blood-group and transplantation antigens, and those associated with the genetically determined variants of the immunoglobulins and other plasma proteins. Alloantigens were previously called isoantigens, but this terminology has now been changed to bring it into line with the terms used in transplantation immunology. Likewise alloantibodies replace isoantibodies.

TYPES OF ANTIBODY

The immunoglobulins were for long regarded as the most important products of the immune response, but it is now well established that other types of antibody are produced. One type is confined to the cells, and therefore regarded as *cell-bound*, or *cellular, antibody*. The cells involved in this type of immunity are the lymphocytes. These play an important part in *homograft rejection,* in *delayed-type hypersensitivity*, and in *immunity to microbial infection.*

Interferon may be regarded as yet another mechanism involved in immunity to infection.

The following important types of antibodies may therefore be recognised.

PLASMA ANTIBODIES (Immunoglobulins)

Detectable in vitro

Agglutinins
Precipitins
Amboceptors, e.g. lysins
Opsonins
Blocking antibodies
Neutralising antibodies, e.g. antitoxins and antienzymes

Detectable in vivo

Antibodies causing immunity (see Chapter 13)
Antibodies causing hypersensitivity (see Chapter 14)

CELLULAR ANTIBODIES

Cell-bound antibody (see p. 148 and p. 185)
Interferon (see p. 280)

Figure 12.1
Diagram to show the differences between the primary and the secondary response to an antigenic stimulus.

Factors Influencing Antibody Production

A large number of factors affect the response of an animal to the introduction of an antigen. The following account includes the important generalisations, but as with all generalisations many exceptions will be found.

Previous contact with antigen. When an antigen is introduced into an animal for the first time, there is an interval varying from about four days to four weeks before any immunoglobulin can be detected in the serum. Then follows a rise in antibody titre which reaches a maximum at a time which may vary from 6 days to 3 months. Even then the level reached is comparatively low (*primary response*).

When the same antigen is injected on a second occasion, there is an immediate drop in circulating antibody level due to its neutralisation by the injected antigen. However, after 2–3 days a rapid exponential rise in titre is noted, which reaches a peak after 7–14 days and again falls off, rapidly at first and later more slowly. The final level of antibody is usually above the previous one. The features of the *secondary response* are that a smaller dose of antigen is needed to produce it, the lag period is shorter, and there is a greater production of antibody which is mostly of the IgG type. Thus the prior introduction of antigen has led to a state in which, although the antibody titre is low, the animal is in a particularly favourable position should it ever in the future need to make the same antibody again. This state, usually known as *potential immunity*, is of great importance when considering active artificial immunisation. Potential immunity is dependent upon *immunological memory*, and this appears to reside in small lymphocytes. Thus if small lymphocytes from the thoracic duct of an immunised animal are injected into a syngeneic host, the latter will respond to a first injection of antigen by a typical secondary response. Figure 12.1 contrasts the two responses.

Repeated injections of antigen lead to variable responses depending upon the type of substance used, the frequency of injection, etc. Usually the antibody response is less marked with each injection, and under some circumstances

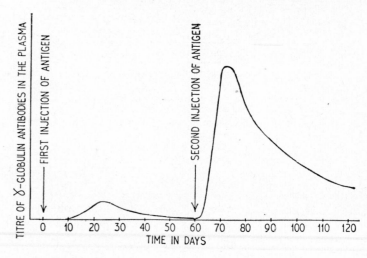

the antibody level may even fall. This may be due to a type of tolerance or immunological paralysis (see below). The unreactive state is not permanent.[7]

Anamnestic reaction. During the stage of potential immunity the production of specific antibodies may also occur in response to the stimulus of an unrelated antigen. The introduction of an antigen may therefore give rise not only to its own specific antibodies but also to others which are specific to the many antigens which the individual has met previously. This "recall" phenomenon is known as the *anamnestic* reaction*; it may also be seen in infection, but fortunately, from a diagnostic point of view, the general rise in titre thereby induced is small.

It is important to remember this phenomenon when interpreting the results of the Widal, Weil-Felix, or other agglutination tests. Any infection is liable to cause an increased production of agglutinins; this affects the anti-H agglutinins especially, and in the Widal test is most marked in those who have been inoculated previously with TAB (p. 170).

The anamnestic reaction has been used to investigate the epidemiology of past influenza epidemics. A person who has suffered from influenza due to one strain of virus will produce antibodies to that strain many years later when infected with an influenza virus of different strain.

Type of antigen. Antigens vary considerably in their ability to elicit antibody production. As a general rule particulate antigen produces a better response than does soluble material. For this reason an antigen precipitated with alum is used for diphtheria immunisation. Another method of improving antibody response is to mix the antigen with Freund's adjuvant† (dead mycobacteria in a liquid oil-in-water emulsion). These methods probably act by delaying the absorption of antigen from the site of injection and from the regional lymph nodes which the adjuvant reaches in one hour,[8] but it has also been suggested that the local inflammatory reaction may play some part in the heightened response. In addition, the inflammatory response may be a factor in stimulating the production of cell-bound antibodies. *Bordetella pertussis* also acts as a potent adjuvant, and is included with diphtheria and tetanus toxoid in triple vaccine. The administration of several antigens together does not always enhance the immune response—sometimes there is inhibition, and the explanation for this competition is unknown.

Quantity of antigen given. Within wide limits the antibody response is not closely related to the quantity of antigen injected. When very large doses are given there may

* Some authorities use this term in a different sense and apply it to the secondary response (see p. 140).

† In the complete "Freund's adjuvant", the acid-fast bacilli are included and a delayed-type hypersensitivity is also induced. The adjuvant is too irritating for human use. The "incomplete" antigen does not contain bacilli, and its use merely augments the immunoglobulin response. Arachis oil is commonly used in Freund's adjuvant.

be a complete failure of antibody production; moreover, the animal may for many months be incapable of reacting to further smaller doses of the same antigen. This phenomenon, known as *immunological paralysis*,[7, 9] is a type of immunological tolerance (p. 156) and has been most studied in mice injected with pneumococcal polysaccharides, substances which are not metabolised and remain in the body for a long period. Immunological paralysis is produced by soluble antigens much more easily than with particulate material. Very small doses of antigen may also induce a state of tolerance.

Route of administration. With some antigens, e.g. bacteria, an intravenous injection gives rise to immunoglobulin production, while subcutaneous or intraperitoneal administration causes, in addition, an immune response associated with delayed-type hypersensitivity. Chemicals applied to the skin are particularly liable to induce delayed-type hypersensitivity.

Duration of antigenic stimulation. The first-formed immunoglobulins are of the IgM type (see Rhesus sensitisation, p. 629). The more usual IgG antibodies appear later, and their presence inhibits IgM production. The IgM antibodies are produced when there is antigen excess as occurs during the early phase of an immune response. If IgG is administered, IgM production is inhibited. The production of IgM antibodies appears to be a primitive response, for this type of antibody is the only one produced in some primitive vertebrates, e.g. sharks. It is the first type of antibody produced by the human fetus whilst *in utero*.

The antibody titre already present.[10, 11] The presence of circulating immunoglobulin may depress or completely abolish the response to injected antigen as expressed by immunoglobulin or cell-bound antibody formation (see also tumour enhancement, p. 379). The explanation for this is not definitely known, but the rapid binding of the antigen by antibody and its subsequent elimination probably play an important part. The implications of this should be remembered when artificial immunisation is being attempted. Thus, the response to diphtheria toxoid is poor in infants who have a high titre of passively transferred maternal antibody (see also tetanus prophylaxis, p. 234). The phenomenon can be used to advantage to prevent sensitisation of Rh-negative mothers who have recently given birth to Rh-positive children. If anti-Rh globulin is administered within 48 hours after delivery, sensitisation is inhibited.[12, 13]

Age of animal. During early fetal life animals will accept foreign protein without antibody production. Furthermore, they may be rendered incapable of reacting to the same antigen on a subsequent occasion. This is *immunological tolerance* and is described in detail later (p. 195). As fetal development proceeds, the ability to produce immunoglobulin appears. At this stage small doses of antigen excite an immune response, while *large* or *very small* doses produce tolerance. The human fetus has the ability to produce antibodies from about the age of 3 months. Nevertheless, it produces little antibody, and the immunoglobulins present in the blood at birth consist almost entirely of IgG of maternal origin. As this is catabolised, endogenous antibody is produced. Adult levels of IgM are attained by one year, IgG by the age of 5 or 6 years, and IgA by 10 years. Infection of the fetus, e.g. with syphilis, leads to IgM antibody production and not tolerance. Indeed, the presence of a high IgM at birth may be used as an indication of intra-uterine infection, since this type of antibody, being unable to cross the placental barrier, cannot be of maternal origin.[14]

Mice are relatively immature at birth, and can be rendered tolerant with small doses of antigen.

Nutrition. Starvation has little or no effect on antibody production. An exception to this is the immunological deficiency exhibited by pyridoxine-deficient rats; the explanation for this is not known.

Anergy. A loss of the ability to express a cell-mediated immune response is called anergy. Thus a person previously sensitive to tuberculin, trichophytin, and mumps antigen becomes negative. Anergy is not uncommon in terminal states due to many causes, e.g. infections and malignancy. In cancer it is associated with a bad prognosis.[15] It is also a well-known feature of sarcoidosis, lepromatous leprosy, and measles. The pathogenesis is not known, and indeed may not be the same in all instances. Destruction of normal lymphoid tissue may be postulated as the mechanism in extensive malignant disease, Hodgkin's disease, and widespread sarcoidosis. However, this cannot be the explanation in early sarcoidosis or measles.

Immunologically deficient diseases. See p. 171.

Artificial Methods Designed to Reduce the Immune Response

Immunological unresponsiveness can be induced in one of two ways. The induction of *tolerance* is described on p. 156. *Immunosuppression* refers to the diminution of the immune response in an otherwise normal animal. The following have been used:

Glucocorticosteroid administration. The continuous administration of a glucocorticosteroid, usually prednisone, impairs the antibody response to a primary antigenic stimulation. The secondary response is not appreciably affected unless large doses are given.

Antilymphocytic serum.[16, 17] The production of anti-lymphocytic serum by the injection of lymphocytes of one species into an animal of another species was described by Metchnikoff in 1899. Administration of the serum blocks the formation of cell-bound antibodies to a much greater extent than that of the immunoglobulins. It prolongs the life of allografts, and has been used in man for suppressing the graft reaction and in treating autoimmune disease. The active factor is a γ-globulin, but serum for human use is difficult to standardise and its adminstration has many unwanted effects, e.g. local pain, anaphylactic shock, thrombocytopenia, and renal damage; this last is due

to a contaminating anti-basement membrane component. Although antilymphocytic serum may produce lymphopenia, this is not invariable, and the degree of suppression of graft rejection does not parallel this effect. It has been suggested that the serum coats the lymphocytes or in some way renders them less active, thus impeding the afferent limb of the immune response. The serum appears to block immunological memory, for if an animal previously sensitised to bovine serum albumin is treated with the serum and subsequently challenged with the antigen, it reacts with a typical primary response. This effect might prove to be of immense value in the treatment of some diseases, but the danger on the other side of the coin is quite considerable: the immunological memory for past infection would also be blocked, and the organisms would promote a primary response.

Total body exposure to ionising radiation.[18] Following exposure to x-rays, animals show a poor response to primary antigenic stimulation. The antibody response to a secondary stimulation is much less inhibited, indicating that it is the development of potential immunity which is affected by the action of ionising radiation. This again stresses the fact that two distinct steps are involved in the immune response. The primary stimulus produces a "conditioning" effect which results in the state of potential immunity. Subsequent stimulation triggers off a different mechanism which leads to the rapid production of antibodies. There is evidence that ionising radiation reduces macrophage activity and that it is this effect which is responsible for inhibiting the primary response (p. 153).

If ionising radiation is given after the injection of antigen, the peak of antibody production may actually be increased.[19] Alkylating agents, such as nitrogen mustard, produce effects similar to those of ionising radiation.

Administration of antimetabolites.[20] The administration of 6-mercaptopurine, or its more potent and less toxic derivative *azathioprine* (*Imuran*), inhibits the primary response; indeed, a state of tolerance may be induced. These agents are most effective if given about two days *after* the administration of antigen, in contrast to ionising radiation which must be given beforehand for a maximal inhibiting effect. Large doses of 6-mercaptopurine also inhibit the secondary response. Actinomycin D has an effect similar to that of 6-mercaptopurine.

Depletion of the body's lymphocytes.[21] This experimental procedure also inhibts the development of a primary response. It may be performed by establishing a thoracic-duct fistula or by the extracorporeal irradiation of blood.

Nature and Properties of Immunoglobulins[22, 23]

Antibody activity in the plasma is due to a group of globulins which, on electrophoretic separation, form a broad band in the γ fraction together with some activity in the α and β regions. They are highly specific and react with their corresponding antigens in various ways, although this action may not always be demonstrable *in vitro*. The *in-vitro* reactions between antigens and antibodies are considered later in this chapter, but it may be noted at this stage that in general the antibodies tend to neutralise their antigens and lead to their elimination.

The antibody produced in an animal after the injection of an antigen is not a single distinct protein, for one antigenic compound may have several epitopes, and therefore antibodies of different specificities are produced. Furthermore, even the antibody possessing a single specificity is heterogeneous and consists of a group of proteins differing somewhat in molecular composition and size, and in electrophoretic mobility.

Nomenclature and Chemical Structure[22, 23]

The estimation of the molecular size led to the recognition of two major groups. The antibodies with a molecular weight of about 150 000 form the 7S group, while the macroglobulins of molecular weight 10^6 form the 19S component. Electrophoresis further subdivided the antibodies into $\gamma1$, $\gamma2$, $\beta1$, $\beta2$, etc., and this led to a complex terminology—thus the macroglobulins were variously called the $\beta2M$, $\gamma1M$, or 19S fraction. It is now agreed that all antibodies be termed *immunoglobulins*, or γ-globulins, with the designation Ig or γ regardless of their electrophoretic mobility. The Ig notation is used in this book.

The work of Porter has shown that each immunoglobulin molecule is composed of four polypeptide chains, one pair half the length of the other—these are called the *light chains* and consist of 217 amino acids, and their molecular weight is 25 000. The longer pair are called *heavy chains* and their molecular weight is 50 000. It follows that the molecular weight of a typical immunoglobulin is 150 000 plus the molecular weight of the attached carbohydrate.

As Fig. 12.2 indicates, the light chains are united to the heavy chains by a single disulphide bond at the carboxy-terminal end of the chain* (here the terminal amino acid has a free carboxyl group, whereas at the amino-terminal end of the chain there is a free amino group). The heavy chains are united together by from 1–5 disulphide bonds (in the diagram two have been depicted). If the molecule is digested with papain, three fragments are produced. Two are identical and have one antibody-combining site each; they are called the *Fab fragments*, and, as can be seen in Fig. 12.2, they consist of the light chains and the amino-terminal portions of the heavy chains. The third fragment is crystallisable (which indicates the homogeneity of the amino-acid sequences in that part of the molecule), and is therefore called the *Fc fragment*. While it has no antibody activity and consists only of part of the heavy chains, it contains many of the antigenic determinants of the molecule as a whole, and is also responsible for the properties of skin fixation, comple-

---

* The carboxy-terminal part of a polypeptide is the first portion to be released from the ribosome, while the amino-terminal portion is released last.

ment fixation, and placental transfer. If the molecule is digested with pepsin, there is a splitting of the heavy chains on the carboxy-terminal side of the disulphide bonds; the remainder of the heavy chains fall apart, and a residue composed of two Fab fragments combined together is left. This acts as a bivalent antibody.

It is evident that the antibody-binding properties of the molecule reside in the Fab fragments at the amino-terminal

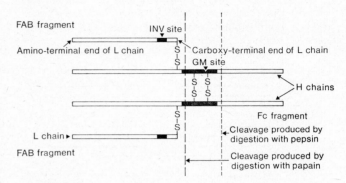

Figure 12.2
Diagrammatic representation of the structure of IgG immunoglobulin. The molecule is composed of two light polypeptide chains and two heavy chains joined together by bisulphide bonds. Digestion with the enzyme papain splits the molecule into three fragments, as indicated by the dotted lines. The two Fab fragments have one antibody-combining site each, whilst the Fc fragment has none. The sites for the antigenic determinants governed by the *Inv* and *Gm* genes are shown.

end. The amino-terminal halves of the light chains and the associated halves of the heavy chains (called the Fd fragments) are described as *variable*, because the amino acids that constitute them vary greatly both in specificity and sequence in each molecule. It is thus that so many different antibodies can be derived from any class of immunoglobulin. The carboxy-terminal halves of the light chains and the Fd fragments are much more constant, and are spoken of as *invariable*. The Fc parts of the heavy chains are the most invariable, hence their tendency to crystallise.

Electron microscopy indicates that immunoglobulins are Y shaped, with the two arms of the Y joining at a hinge area. Movement at this point can result in a change of shape from a narrow Y to a T.

The immunoglobulins are themselves antigenic when injected into other species, and immunoelectrophoretic studies have revealed that the light and heavy chains are not homogeneous. Human antibodies can be divided into classes depending upon specific antigenic determinants on the light and heavy chains. There are five types of heavy chains, which are named: γ, α, μ, δ, and ε. Each antibody molecule has a pair of identical heavy chains and therefore five *classes* are recognised: IgG, IgA, IgM, IgD, and IgE respectively. Each class has been further subdivided into two types: K, for Korngold, and L, for Lipari, after the two workers who first recognised them. The difference lies in the light chains which are termed ϰ (kappa) and λ (lambda). Each molecule, whether IgG, IgA, IgM, IgD, or IgE, has either two ϰ or two λ chains, *but never one of each*. In a normal individual within each class of immunoglobulin, e.g. IgG, IgA, etc., about 70 per cent of the molecules have ϰ light chains and the remainder have the λ. The five classes of immunoglobulins are depicted in Fig. 12.3

Variants of the heavy chains have now been detected. Thus there are four subtypes of the γ chains, called $\gamma_1, \gamma_2, \gamma_3$, and γ_4. Four subclasses of IgG are therefore recognised

Type K   Type L

IgG

IgA

IgM

IgD

IgE

Figure 12.3
Structure of the immunoglobulins. The classes resemble each other in that the molecules are composed of two identical light polypeptide chains and two identical heavy chains. The difference lies in their heavy chains. In any one class there are two types. In the K type there are two ϰ light chains while in the L type there are two λ light chains.

Likewise there are two subclasses of IgA and of IgM to add to the remarkable heterogeneity of the immunoglobulins.

Inherited variation. Inherited antigenic differences have been found in both the light and heavy chains. The first

Figure 12.4
Diagrammatic representation of IgM and IgA. IgM is shown as a pentamer. IgA is a dimer with its two subunits united by a secretory component represented by a triangle. Disulphide bonds are depicted as solid circles.

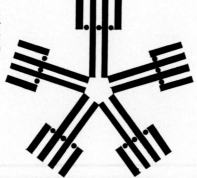
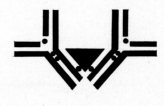

two to be identified were the Gm antigens on the heavy chains, and the InV on the light ϰ chains. These alloantigens are comparable with the alloantigens of the red cells, but naturally occurring alloantibodies are uncommon. They are occasionally produced when immunoglobulin from one individual is transfused into another of different genotype. Alloantibodies also occur in rheumatoid arthritis, and are termed collectively the *rheumatoid factor* (p. 210). A third independent group of genetic markers, called the Am factors, has been described in the IgA molecule. Antibodies occur after transfusion with blood of a different Am type.

Properties of the Immunoglobulin Groups[24]

Ig G Immunoglobulin. This is the slowest component on electrophoresis, forms about 20 per cent of the total plasma proteins (0·6–1·5 g per 100 ml), and contains about 3 per cent of carbohydrate. It is the only immunoglobulin capable of crossing the placenta and is found in all extracellular fluids. It has the longest half life of all the immunoglobulins: about five days.

IgA Immunoglobulin.[25] is present in the plasma (0·2–0·4 g per 100 ml), but its highest concentration is found in secretions (mucus, colostrum, etc.) and it is an important factor in preventing infection of mucous membranes. It contains about 7·5 per cent carbohydrate. Dimers and trimers and higher multimers of the 7S monomers are found in the blood, so that 9S and 11S components are present. Some IgA is made locally in the intestinal wall and secreted as a dimer bound to a third polypeptide called the secretory, or transport, piece, which may serve to stabilise the IgA against proteolysis or to facilitate secretion of this immunoglobulin (Fig. 12.4). The secreted IgA is an 11S component with a molecular weight of 385 000. It does not fix complement by the classical pathway, and it has been suggested that its function is to react with antigens absorbed from the gut and neutralise them without the damaging activation of complement.[26-28]

IgD Immunoglobulin. This has been identified on immunoelectrophoresis of plasma but its function is unknown.

IgE Immunoglobulin is a 7S fraction with a molecular weight of 200 000, which is responsible for human anaphylaxis (p. 178) as well as for hypersensitivity states such as hay-fever and asthma.[29] This immunoglobulin, previously called reagin, has the property of firm fixation to skin, thereby rendering it hypersensitive. It will also fix to leucocytes, and these cells then release histamine when acted upon by antigen. In this way IgE may augment the acute inflammatory reaction. IgE will not fix complement even when aggregated.

IgM Immunoglobulin. This is a 19S globulin containing about 10 per cent carbohydrate, and has a molecular weight of 900 000. It can be dissociated into five 7S subunits, each of which has a similar structure to that of IgG except that the heavy μ chains are present instead of γ (Fig. 12.4). It is largely restricted to the intravascular compartment, and appears in the plasma at the age of 2 to 3 months. Although it might be expected that IgM would have ten combining sites, the antibody is in fact sometimes pentavalent. The explanation for this is not known.

Specificity of Antibodies

The differences between the various chains of the immunoglobulins lie in their amino-acid sequence. Furthermore, the actual specificity of an antibody also lies in its exact chemical composition. Patients with multiple myeloma provide a ready source of homogeneous immunoglobulin whose amino-acid sequence can be analysed. It has been found that there are areas of constant sequence and areas that are variable on both light and heavy chains (p. 143). It is the differences in these variable areas that determine specificity. However, it is not yet possible to identify antibody specifically by chemical analysis; the only method of identification and estimation is by a reaction involving union with the appropriate antigen, either *in vitro* or *in vivo*.

Antigen-Antibody Union

The forces which unite antigen to antibody are not known for certain, but it is generally agreed that non-covalent bonds are involved. The union can certainly be broken; thus potent toxin can be recovered from toxin-antitoxin combinations.

The ability of an antibody to form stable complexes with antigen is termed its *avidity*. Antibodies of high avidity are usually formed in the later stages of an immune response or during a secondary response.

Following the primary union of antibody with antigen secondary phenomena occur; these are of great practical importance and are described below:

Types of Antibodies[30]

Agglutinins. When a particulate antigen is added to its antibody, the particles may adhere together to produce large visible clumps. This clumping is called agglutination, and the antibody is called an agglutinin. The particles may consist of whole organisms, in which case it is a *surface antigen* that is involved. Alternatively, tanned red cells or collodion or polystyrene particles may be coated artificially with antigen, and then used for detecting agglutinating antibodies. This type of haemagglutination technique is very sensitive, being about ten times as effective in detecting antibody as the most sensitive gel-diffusion technique[31] (see p. 146). Coated particles are in common use to detect antibodies in rheumatoid arthritis, infectious mononucleosis, thyroid disease, and systemic lupus erythematosus. Commercial tests are also available for the detection of C-reactive protein and fibrinogen (as a test for hypofibrinogenaemia) in blood, and chorionic gonadotrophin in urine (as a test for pregnancy).

Agglutination is dependent on the pH of the medium, its electrolyte content, and also on the temperature at which it takes place. It may take an appreciable time. It fails to occur if there is great excess of antigen, and also in some cases in the presence of excess antibody (see below). In performing agglutination tests these factors must be taken into account. Estimation of the strength, or titre, of these antibodies is frequently of value, and is performed as follows:

A series of tubes is prepared, the first containing neat serum (left-hand tube, Fig. 12.5), while each subsequent tube contains serum diluted with saline in proportions 1 in 2, 1 in 4, 1 in 8, etc. (doubling dilutions). To each is added an equal volume of a suspension of particles, after which the tubes are incubated at 37°C for a suitable period. The dilution of the serum in the last tube which shows definite agglutination is described as the titre of the antibody. Sometimes the left-hand tubes containing the highest concentrations of antibody fail to show agglutination. This is termed the "prozone" phenomenon.

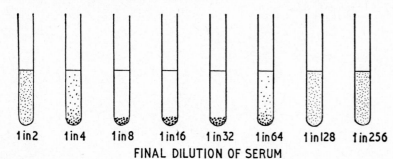

1 in 2   1 in 4   1 in 8   1 in 16   1 in 32   1 in 64   1 in 128   1 in 256

FINAL DILUTION OF SERUM

Figure 12.5
Agglutination test. The titre of the antibody is 1 in 64. The failure of the first tube (1 in 2 dilution) to show agglutination is known as the prozone phenomenon and is not uncommonly seen in *Brucella* agglutination tests and in the standard serological tests for syphilis, such as the VDRL.

Precipitins. Precipitation is the formation of an insoluble product when two soluble substances are mixed together. In this type of reaction the antigen must therefore be in solution. To demonstrate antibacterial precipitins a soluble extract of the organism is first prepared, and then added to the antibody. This may be done by simple mixing, but precipitation does not occur in the presence of excess

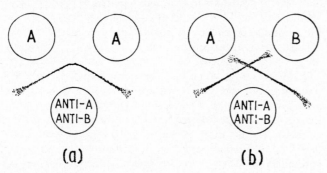

Figure 12.6
Ouchterlony plates showing precipitin reactions. In (a) the precipitin lines join together, as they are both due to the same A-anti-A reaction. In (b) the lines cross, as they are formed by different antigen-antibody reactions.

antibody. A better technique is to layer the one fluid carefully on the other, in which case a precipitate forms at or near the interface. Using this method Lancefield was able to sub-divide the β-haemolytic streptococci into many groups.

Probably the most sensitive method, however, it to perform the reaction in an agar gel (Oudin). If an antigen is placed in a cup cut in an agar plate in which there is incorporated the corresponding antibody, there develops a zone of precipitation which steadily advances with a sharp leading edge. Precipitation occurs where antigen and antibody are in optimal proportions. Another method is to allow antigen and antibody to diffuse towards each other from separate cups (see Fig. 12.6). This technique, developed by Ouchterlony, can be used to identify unknown antigens or antibodies. Thus, if a mixture of antibodies is allowed to diffuse towards different antigens each in a separate cup, lines of precipitation will be formed (see Fig. 12.6). If the lines fuse it may be assumed that they are caused by the same antigen-antibody precipitation, while if they intersect they are due to different reactions.

As with agglutination, electrolyte concentration and pH are important. Precipitation may not occur in the absence of electrolytes, and reactions are usually performed with physiological concentrations of saline.

The investigation of the composition of the precipitate has shown that the ratio of antigen to antibody varies according to the manner in which the precipitate is formed. A plausible hypothesis of the mode of formation of the precipitate is the lattice theory. There is considerable evidence to show that many antibodies are bivalent, while antigens are multivalent. By valency is meant the number of combining units, or arms, attached to each molecule. Thus, when a precipitate is formed with antigen and antibody in optimal proportions, the compound formed has the structure as shown in Fig. 12.7 (A). Less compact precipitates are formed if either antigen or antibody is in excess (Fig. 12.7 (B) and (C)), while soluble products can be explained when either component is present in great excess (Fig. 12.7 (D) and (E)). It should be remembered that one antigen may contain several epitopes, and its introduction into an animal can lead to the formation of separate antibodies each with different specificities. The cooperative action of these may be involved in an antigen-antibody reaction (Fig. 12.8).

Precipitin reactions are used in streptococcal grouping (Lancefield), the medico-legal identification of human blood or semen, and in the diagnosis of syphilis (e.g. the VDRL and

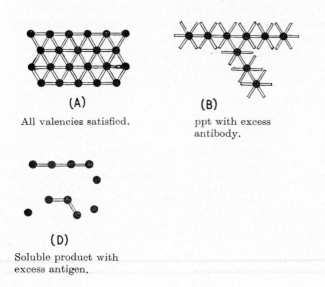

(A) All valencies satisfied.
(B) ppt with excess antibody.
(C) ppt with excess antigen.
(D) Soluble product with excess antigen.

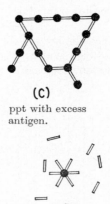

(E) Soluble product with excess antibody.

Figure 12.7
Diagrammatic representation of the composition of various antigen-antibody combinations (see text). Antibody, assumed to be bivalent, is depicted as hollow rods. The solid circles are antigen molecules and have six combining units. *(After Pauling, L. (1940), J. Amer. chem. Soc., **62**, 2643)*

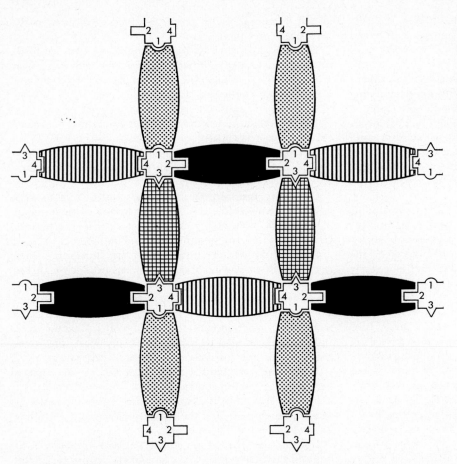

Figure 12.8
Schematic illustration of the diversity of antibodies formed against a pure antigen and their cooperative effects in the precipitin reaction with the antigen. The antigenic determinants (epitopes) are arbitrarily labelled 1, 2, 3, and 4. The diagram is based on Fig. 13.14 in Davis, B. D., Dulbecco, R., Eisen, H. N., Ginsberg, H. S. and Wood, W. B. (1967), "Microbiology", p. 386. New York: Harper and Row-Hoeber.

Kahn tests). In the Kahn test the precipitate is so soft and flocculent that it is usually called a "flocculation test".

Amboceptor. This type of antibody, when combined with its corresponding antigen, can sequentially activate a group of proteins which collectively are called *complement* (see p. 161). The activation of complement may produce some visible effect, for instance the lysis of a bacterium or red cell, or it may be invisible. In such instances the reaction can be detected by using a second "haemolytic system", as in the complement fixation test.

The Wassermann reaction is a good example of this. The test is explained diagrammatically in Table 12.2, in which it will be seen that serum, which has been heated to 56°C for half an hour, is mixed with a standard quantity of complement and antigen. The antigen is in fact a cholesterolised extract of heart muscle. The object of heating the serum is to inactivate the unknown quantity of complement which is normally present, so that a known, measured amount can be added for the reaction. The serum-antigen-complement mixture is allowed to incubate for a standard length of

TABLE 12.2

Wassermann reaction	
First reaction	*Second or detector reaction (haemolytic system)*
Patient's serum with ? antibody heated to 56°C for 30 minutes (to inactivate any complement which is present)	Red cells (sheep)
	Haemolysin (serum of rabbit immunised against sheep red cells). This is inactivated commercially to remove its complement.
Antigen (standard quantity)	
	? complement unused
Complement (carefully measured amount)	

time, e.g. 2 hours at 37°C. If the relevant antibody is present in the patient's serum, the antigen will combine with it, and at the same time "fix", or combine with, the added complement.

The detector system is then added. It is also of an antigen-amboceptor type, and utilises red cells with a corresponding haemolysin. If complement is not used up in the first reaction, it is available for the second system. Therefore, haemolysis of the red cells denotes the absence of syphilitic antibody, and the Wassermann reaction is said to be negative. On the other hand, the absence of haemolysis indicates a positive reaction. The question of false positive reactions is considered on p. 253.

Amboceptors are either IgM or IgG immunoglobulins (IgM is the stronger amboceptor of the two), and the commonly encountered examples are bacteriolysins and haemolysins. Complement fixation tests are employed in the diagnosis of syphilis, gonorrhoea, hydatid disease, and nearly all the virus infections. They are also of diagnostic use in Hashimoto's disease.

Antibodies causing the immune adherence phenomenon.[32] Antigens (e.g. trypanosomes, spirochaetes, bacteria, viruses, or proteins) when combined with antibody are found to adhere to human red cells, thereby causing them to agglutinate. This is due to the activation of complement and the formation of a C3 cleavage component (p. 162). Only primate red cells behave in this manner. In non-primates antigen-antibody-complement complexes adhere to platelets. This adherence can be used *in vitro* as a sensitive means of testing for antibodies, and may also play some part in immunity to infection (see p. 168).

Opsonins.[33] Opsonins are substances which render organisms more readily susceptible to phagocytosis. Polymorphs are in general able to phagocytose virulent organisms only if the latter are first coated with a specific opsonin. This type of opsonin and also the non-specific type are considered in the sections of acute inflammation (see p. 76) and immunity (see p. 163). Opsonisation also aids the clearance of organisms from the blood by the reticulo-endothelial system.

Blocking (or incomplete) antibodies. These combine with their corresponding antigens without visible effect, and prevent the action of some other antibody added subsequently. The best-known antibody of this type is found in cases of Rhesus incompatibility (see Chapter 52); its action may be illustrated as follows:

D cells+Anti-D = agglutination (D-Anti-D combination)
D cells+Anti-D blocking antibody = no agglutination (D-blocking-anti-D combination)
D-blocking-anti-D+Anti-D = no union, no agglutination

The agglutinating action of anti-D is thus blocked by the prior union of blocking anti-D with the red cells. The presence of such an incomplete antibody on the surface of red cells can be detected by the Coombs test (p. 629). In this an anti-human globulin serum is added to the coated red cells and causes their agglutination.

Blocking antibodies are often erroneously assumed to be univalent. A bivalent antibody can combine with its antigen under conditions which are unfavourable for agglutination. Under other conditions agglutination may occur. Thus blocking anti-D antibody causes red-cell agglutination if the test is carried out in a strong albumin solution or if the red cells are first trypsinised.

Precipitin reactions may be blocked by incomplete antibodies. The prozone phenomenon (p. 145) can be due to their action.

Cytotoxic antibodies. Antibodies destructive to cells grown in tissue culture can be demonstrated in the serum of patients with Hashimoto's disease. Bacteriolysins and haemolysins are other examples of this type of antibody.

Antibodies which neutralise the antigen. *Antienzymes and antitoxins.* Many organisms produce toxins or enzymes which are antigenic. The exotoxins, lecithinases, coagulases, haemolysins, leucocidins, hyaluronidases, etc., are examples of these; corresponding antibodies are formed in bacterial infection, and are considered in Chapter 13.

Virus neutralising antibodies probably coat the virus particles and prevent their attachment to cells (see p. 280).

Antibacterial antibodies may have effects not already described, e.g. bactericidal antibodies kill organisms, and these are closely related to the bacteriolysins. Syphilitic antibody causes immobilisation of the organism, a fact utilised in the *Tr. pallidum* immobilisation test.

It cannot be stressed too strongly that the globulin antibodies have been named according to the nature of the test used to detect them. At one time it was thought that each type was distinct, but it is now known that in many cases a single antibody can perform several functions depending upon the conditions under which it is examined. For instance, a substance may be capable of neutralising toxin, e.g. diphtheria toxin, in an *in-vivo* experiment. It is therefore rightly called an antitoxin. However, *in vitro* it can produce a precipitate with its antigen, and may therefore be labelled a precipitin. Some agglutinins, e.g. to red cells, produce agglutination only in the absence of complement. When this is present there is lysis and the complement is fixed.

Nevertheless, such a unitarian theory is too simple, for it is known that a single antigen can lead to the formation of a heterogeneous group of immunoglobulins, each with the same specificity but differing in chemical composition (IgG, IgA, etc.). This is reflected in their avidity and their ability to sensitise, cross the placenta, and engage in the many *in-vitro* activities by which antibodies are detected. Furthermore, antibodies with different specificities may be produced (p. 143).

Cell-bound Antibodies[34, 95]

Cell-mediated immunity and hypersensitivity are related to antibodies residing in lymphocytes. The manner by which such sensitised or immune lymphocytes produce their effect is poorly understood, but it appears that when the cells come into contact with the appropriate antigen, they release a number of effector proteins which can be recognized by their specific actions and are called *lymphokines*. Many such actions have been described, and it is not certain how many agents are involved. One agent may produce several effects, and conversely several agents may produce the same effect. The present situation is very similar to that encountered with the immunoglobulins in the early days of immunology. The following factors may be listed; they are released when specifically sensitised lymphocytes are incubated with the specific antigen, and can be measured by *in-vitro* methods as well as by their effects *in-vivo*.[91]

1. **Migration inhibition factor.** This substance has a molecular weight of 25–55 000. It acts on macrophages and prevents their migration (see Fig. 14.2, p. 186). The agent also seems to activate the macrophages, increase phagocytic activity, and make the cells better able to kill organisms. It may be postulated that this factor causes macrophages to accumulate at a site of infection and overcome it.

2. **Transfer factor.** This has a molecular weight of less than 10 000 and has the property of acting upon uncommitted lymphocytes and rendering them sensitised (see p. 185). The agent may well recruit more immune cells, which are then available to react with further antigen.

3. **Lymphotoxin.** This protein of molecular weight 80 000–150 000 causes a cytopathic effect on cells such as fibroblasts grown in culture as monolayers. *Growth inhibiting factor* is closely related if not identical. There is some evidence that the cytotoxic effect is aided by complement bound to the target cells.[35]

4. **Skin reactive factor.** On injection into the skin, this produces a picture similar to that of a delayed-type hypersensitivity reaction.

5. **Chemotactic factors.** At least two have been described. One affects monocytes while the other attracts polymorphs. Yet another may affect eosinophils.

6. **Mitogenic factor.** This causes lymphocyes to transfer into blast cells and divide. Enhanced incorporation of ^{3}H thymidine can be used to measure this.

7. **Interferon.** See p. 280.

The subject of cell-mediated immune responses is considered in greater detail in the sections on delayed-type hypersensitivity and cell-mediated immunity.

THE ANTIBODY-FORMING TISSUES

Before describing the cellular features of the immune response it is essential to understand the structure and development of the lymphoid tissues of the body.

The Lymphoid Tissues[36–39]

The thymus. The first lymphoid tissue to develop in mammals is the thymus. It contains an epithelial element in the form of reticular cells and Hassall's corpuscles. In addition there are many thymocytes which morphologically resemble lymphocytes. It is taught that germinal centres are not normally present, but this has been disputed.

The bursa of Fabricius. In birds the next lymphoid organ to develop is the *bursa of Fabricius*. This is situated near the cloaca, and, like the thymus, has an epithelial as well as a lymphoid element. It is suspected that mammals have an equivalent tissue, perhaps more widely distributed, and forming the lymphoid tissue of the appendix and colon, and the Peyer's patches of the small intestine.

Lymph nodes. Lymph comes into the lymph node through the peripheral sinus, traverses the cortex, enters the sinusoids of the medulla, and finally leaves through the efferent duct. The sinuses are lined by plump, *littoral*, or *sinus-lining cells*, which have eosinophilic cytoplasm and are phagocytic. Reticulum cells are present and appear to be concerned with the formation of reticulin, which constitutes the connective tissue framework of the node. In the outer part, or *cortex*, of the node there are densely packed lymphocytes which are focally aggregated into *follicles*. In the centre of each follicle there is often a well-defined *germinal centre of Flemming*.[40] This contains large cells which are generally called lymphoblasts. They show a high turn-over rate and therefore mitoses are abundant.

In addition, the centres contain large macrophages which usually contain nuclear debris in their clear, abundant cytoplasm. On microscopy the macrophages produce clear spaces which have been likened to the stars in a starry sky. The purpose of this macrophage activity is probably related to the recycling of DNA. The germinal centres are sites of rapid production of cells which have a short life. Components of DNA such as thymidine are used again, and it follows that measurements of cell proliferation using tritiated thymidine as a marker show a deceptively low uptake because of the existing pool of unlabelled thymidine.

The *medulla* of the node shows prominent sinuses and medullary cords of cells between them. These cells are mainly small lymphocytes together with a variable number of plasma cells and granulocytes.

Between the cortex with its germinal centres and the medulla there is a third zone which is packed with lymphocytes but less densely so than the cortex. There are no follicles in this *paracortical zone*.

T lymphocytes (see p. 150) from the blood normally enter the lymph node by moving through the cytoplasm of the endothelial cells of the post-capillary sinusoids in the paracortical zone and subsequently leave the node in the efferent lymph.[41] The lymphocytes therefore re-enter the blood stream through the thoracic duct. It follows that if this duct is exteriorised and drained, the body is steadily depleted of T lymphocytes.

Blood lymphocytes. The lymphocytes in the blood range from the large to the small variety. The latter have a dense spherical nucleus and little cytoplasm. Lymphocytes are motile cells, and in culture can sometimes be seen to send processes into other cells and even enter their cytoplasm, a process called *emperiopolesis*.[42] Although lymphocytes appear to form a relatively homogeneous group on morphological grounds, it is now appreciated that the population is heterogeneous. Two distinct types have been identified[94]:

T lymphocytes. These cells are thymus dependent and are long lived—in man they live for many months and certainly over one year. The cells continuously recirculate through the paracortical zone of the lymph nodes as described above. T lymphocytes cannot be identified morphologically in man but in the mouse they carry a specific antigen termed theta (θ).[43] The majority of lymphocytes found in the blood are T cells.

B Lymphocytes. B lymphocytes are so named because they are dependent on the bursa, or bursal-equivalent tissue. This type of cell can be found in the blood, but their numbers are small as they tend to remain sessile in the lymphoid tissues. They occupy the primary germinal follicles and are short-lived cells, their life-span being measured in days.

Separation of B and T cells in man.[92] In man is has been found that when blood lymphocytes are mixed with sheep red cells, the red cells adhere to and form *rosettes* around about 30 per cent of the lymphocytes. Since many thymocytes behave in the same way, and rosette formation is not inhibited by anti-Ig serum, it is now presumed that the rosette-forming lymphocytes of the blood are T cells. If blood lymphocytes are mixed with fluorescent labelled anti–IgG or anti–IgM, between 10 and 30 per cent of the cells show membrane fluorescence. These cells with surface immunoglobulin are presumed to be B cells. They do not form rosettes as described above, but may do so in the presence of anti–sheep red-cell antibodies and complement. If these suppositions are true, it is now possible to distinguish B from T cells in the peripheral circulation and investigate their changes in disease. Thus it is now suggested that the cells in chronic lymphatic leukaemia are B cells.[93]

Spleen. In the spleen the blood passes through the central (malpighian) arterioles to enter the sinusoids which are, as in the lymph nodes, lined by phagocytic cells. In the red pulp there are reticulum cells, lymphocytes, and plasma cells as well as occasional granulocytes and megakaryocytes. The lymphoid cuffs are situated around the malpighian arterioles, and the T lymphocytes are derived from the blood as part of the re-circulation of cells as in the paracortical zones of the lymph nodes.[44] Germinal centres may be prominent.

Development of the peripheral lymphoid tissues. The thymus, and in birds the bursa, are well developed and large before the peripheral lymphoid tissue matures. The thymus is the central organ responsible for the formation of the paracortical zone of the lymph nodes and for the sheath of lymphocytes around the central arterioles in the spleen. These are the *thymus-dependent areas*. The bursa is necessary for the formation of the germinal centres in the

spleen and in the cortex of nodes, and also for cells which develop into plasma cells in the splenic red pulp and the medullary cords of the nodes. It is believed that the earliest immunological cell is to be found in the bone marrow (*reticular anlage*). This *stem cell* may differentiate to a haemocytoblast or develop into a lymphoid cell (Fig. 12.9).

It is not known whether the marrow cells migrate to the peripheral tissues and there develop under the influence of a

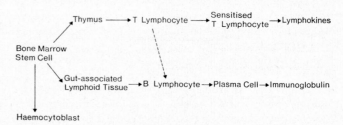

Figure 12.9
Diagram showing the postulated development of the peripheral lymphoid tissue of the lymph nodes.

thymic or bursal hormone, or whether the cells migrate first to the thymus or bursa, develop for a while, and then are released to populate the peripheral lymphoid tissue. There is good evidence that in the mouse, marrow cells migrate to the thymus and develop into lymphoid tissue.[45] It seems likely that in this species there is a continuous replacement of stem cells in the thymus from the marrow.

The Thymus in Relation to the Immune Response[44, 46–48]

If antigen is given intravenously, the thymus does not take part in the immune response unless it is first inflamed: thus there appears to be a blood-thymus barrier which under normal conditions keeps the organ isolated. The thymus undergoes atrophy in the adult animal, and its removal is not associated with any immediate significant depression of the immune response. However, reduced immunological responsiveness is seen after about one year and also following total body irradiation.[47] Recovery from irradiation is impaired as compared with normal animals.

Thymectomy performed shortly after birth can produce dramatic effects in some species. Mice, for example, appear normal for 3–4 weeks, and then a wasting syndome usually develops which closely resembles runt disease (p. 196). This is probably a result of microbial infection, for it does not occur in germ-free animals.* Significantly there is a deficiency of small lymphocytes in the splenic white pulp, the paracortical zones of lymph nodes, and in the circulating blood. The animals exhibit impaired ability to develop delayed-type hypersensitivity, and are tolerant of allografts and sometimes even of xenografts. The production of immuno-

* A germ-free animal is one that has been specially reared under sterile conditions. Caesarian section is generally employed in the initiation of such a colony.

globulins to some antigens is normal, but to others, e.g. sheep red cells, it is impaired.

The implantation of syngeneic thymus tissue will restore the immunological competence of the thymectomised animal, and the graft becomes repopulated by lymphoid cells derived from the *bone marrow of the host*.[49] Even if the thymic implant is enclosed in a Millipore chamber which will not allow the egress of cells, it is reported that it will restore to some extent the immunological competence of the recipient.[50] Presumably the graft cells secrete some substance which allows the animal's lymphoid tissue to develop; the nature of this factor is controversial. A substance called *thymosin*[51, 52] has been isolated by some workers, but as yet the hormonal nature of this is not widely accepted. Its action is weak in relation to its concentration, a property not at all like that of the high potency of a hormone.[53]

Alternative to this humoral theory there is the possibility that the thymus produces lymphocytes which migrate to populate the lymphoid tissues. Experiments using ^{3}H-labelled thymidine indicate that there is very active cell proliferation in the thymus, but that many of the cells die and relatively few leave the organ.[44] A massive overproduction of cells which have a very short life-span is also a feature of lymphoid tissue in the bone marrow and germinal centres.[39] It may be postulated that this apparently wasteful lymphopoiesis serves a purpose in that it provides a constant supply of undifferentiated, uncommitted cells—either marrow stem cells, T cells, or B cells. It is possible that somatic mutation could provide many cell types, as proposed by the selective theory of antibody production (see p. 155). It is also conceivable that abnormal cells could arise and lead to an autoimmune process. Indeed, the thymus has been regarded as an organ commonly involved in autoimmunity.[54]

The Bursa of Fabricius in Relation to the Immune Response

Removal of the bursa, especially if combined with non-lethal total body irradiation, results in an immunologically deficient state characterised by a failure to produce immunoglobulins when suitably challenged by an antigen.[55] It is possible that in mammals the intestinal lymphoid tissue corresponds to the bursa, for its removal in rabbits produces a similar failure in immunoglobulin production. This may be regarded as the *gut-associated central lymphoid tissue*. It is presumed to be responsible for the development of that part of the peripheral lymphoid tissue which is responsible for the production of immunoglobulins, namely germinal centres, B lymphocytes, and plasma cells. The lymphoid aggregates should not be confused with the more diffuse lymphoid tissue and plasma cells which are responsible for the production of IgA.

Lymphocyte Transformation

One of the most remarkable observations of recent times is that the small lymphocytes of the blood and the lymph can

be stimulated *in vitro* to become large cells with basophilic, pyroninophilic cytoplasm containing many free ribosomes and nuclei with nucleoli. These cells have been called *immunoblasts*, pyroninophilic cells, and blast cells. They exhibit DNA synthesis and mitotic activity, a feature which has led to them being intensively used in studies of human chromosomes.

Agents which lead to lymphocyte transformation are:

Phytohaemagglutinin. This is contained in an extract of broad bean, but the active agent has not been identified. Phytohaemagglutinin was used originally to produce agglutination of red cells in experiments designed to facilitate the isolation of white cells from the blood.

Pokeweed mitogen[56]

Streptolysin S

Antilymphocytic serum

Antigen-antibody complexes

Other allogeneic lymphocytes. If small lymphocytes from another individual are mixed with test lymphocytes, both groups of cells undergo blast transformation.

Antigen, if added to the lymphocytes from a sensitised individual. This occurs regardless of whether the sensitisation is of the immediate or delayed type.[57] Although many agents can cause transformation, it does not follow that the process is the same in each instance. Phytohaemagglutinin causes a high percentage of lymphocytes to transform rapidly. Other agents affect fewer cells, and the transformation is slower.

The precise role of the blast transformation phenomenon in the intact animal is not known, but various suggestions have been made:

1. The proliferating cells form the germinal centres. The latter may in fact be clones, producing only one type of antibody.

2. The cells can develop endoplasmic reticulum, manufacture immunoglobulin, and differentiate into plasma cells.

3. They can revert to a type of lymphocyte. Such a cell could have various functions. It could act as a memory cell, so that when next stimulated by antigen it could transform and produce antibody. It could also contain cell-bound antibody and act as an effector cell in cell-mediated responses.

Functional Steps in the Immune Response

The following steps may be postulated as occurring after the introduction of an antigen:

The recognition system. A mechanism must exist for recognising an antigen as foreign. Furthermore, the system must have a *memory* so that the same antigen can be recognised again.

The processing system. Once having been recognised as an antigen, its determinants must be processed in such a way that specific antibody can be produced.

The production system. The final outcome of the immune response is the manufacture of antibody. This often involves synthesis of a range of specific proteins as well as the formation of immune cells. The production system must be *regulated* in some way, so that the immune response can be turned off when the antigenic stimulus is withdrawn.

Anatomical Site of Antibody Production[58], [59]

Antibodies are not produced in any one organ or site. With intravenously administered antigens they are produced in the spleen, liver, and lymph nodes, while locally introduced antigen stimulates antibody production at the local site and in the regional lymph nodes.

Since all antibodies are either cellular or else proteins produced by cells, a complete understanding of the immune response entails an understanding of the cellular events involved. It is generally agreed that the lymphoreticular tissues are of prime importance and that two morphological cell types are concerned. There are the large mononuclear, potentially phagocytic cells grouped together as the RE system, and the lymphocytes. Detailed knowledge about the origin, morphology, and function of these cells is unfortunately lacking, and much confusion has been caused in the past by making wholly unwarranted assumptions. Cells which look alike, e.g. small lymphocytes, do not necessarily have the same origin or function.

The Recognition System

A cell which is capable of recognising antigen and of initiating an immune response, although not necessarily producing antibody itself, is termed an *immunologically competent cell*.[60] There is considerable evidence that such a cell is morphologically a small lymphocyte. The evidence may be summarised as follows: 1. Procedures which deplete the population of small lymphocytes also inhibit the development of a primary response to antigenic stimulation. The following may be mentioned: total body irradiation, administration of drugs (p. 142), thoracic-duct drainage (p. 142), bursectomy, and thymectomy in the neonate (p. 150). 2. Animals rendered tolerant to an antigen (p. 156) can have their immunological responsiveness restored by the injection of lymphocytes from a non-tolerant adult syngeneic animal.

Precisely how the appropriate cells recognise the antigen is not known. One possibility is that the cells have specific immunoglobulin on their surface, and that the stimulus is an antigen-antibody complex. There is evidence that both the T and B lymphocytes have immunoglobulin on their surfaces, but this in itself does not prove that the mechanism outlined above is operative.[61-63], [71]

The process of recognising antigen is sometimes known as the *afferent limb* of the immune response. Actual production of immunoglobulins and effector cells constitutes the *efferent limb*.

Cells Involved in Immunoglobulin Synthesis

There is abundant evidence that immunoglobulins are present in plasma cells. If sections from various organs of an immunised animal are treated with labelled antigen, it is found that the antigen becomes firmly localised to the cytoplasm of the plasma cells. The labelling may be done with fluorescent dye, radioactive iodine or, for electron microscopy, with ferritin.[64], [65] Using this technique, some antibody may also be demonstrated in the germinal centres and in cells which appear to be lymphocytes.

The well-developed endoplasmic reticulum with its ribosomes and the high concentration of cytoplasmic RNA all suggest that the plasma cell is actively engaged in protein synthesis. The evidence all points to its being the major source of immunoglobulin.

The plaque technique.[66] A technique developed by Jerne has shed some light on the morphology of antibody-producing cells. Lymphoid cells from an animal immunised with foreign red cells are poured on to an agar plate containing the same type of red cells. Incubation allows the cells to manufacture antibodies, and when complement is added a clear halo, or plaque of haemolysis, is seen to surround single cells. These have been examined by light and electron microscopy, and found to vary in morphology. Some resemble lymphocytes and others plasma cells. This indicates that immunoglobulins are produced by small lymphocytes which differentiate to form plasma cells.[67] The early stage may be the pyroninophilic cell which develops into a plasmoblast and then a plasma cell. The pyroninophilic cell has a nucleolus and a more vesicular nucleus than a plasma cell, but the same RNA-containing blue cytoplasm. The plasma cell may be regarded as the end-stage of a cell whose function is directed to immunoglobulin production. It has a short life-span—probably two to three days—and is found in conditions in which antibody production is occurring and in sites which are actively engaged in making antibodies, such as splenic pulp, medullary cords of lymph nodes, and chronic inflammatory granulation tissue. Indeed, the plasma cell is the characteristic cell of chronic inflammation.

Morphological Aspects of Immunoglobulin Production

When an antigen such as pneumococcal polysaccharide, which is known to stimulate immunoglobulin production and not delayed-type hypersensitivity, is injected into the skin, some is carried to the regional lymph nodes and is taken up by the sinus-lining cells. There is a dramatic fall in the number of lymphocytes leaving the node, but shortly afterwards the cell count in the efferent lymph rises and reaches a maximum at about 2 days. Many of the cells are large pyroninophilic cells.[68] The lymph also contains specific antibodies. The medullary cords contain pyroninophilic cells, and these appear to mature to adult plasma cells which contain specific immunoglobulin antibody. The germinal centres enlarge and new ones form, but this is a late event in the primary response (Fig. 12.11).

The secondary response has certain distinctive features. Germinal centre formation is a marked feature and occurs early. Antigen can be demonstrated in them, and later on so also can antibody. Antibody formation also occurs in distant sites, e.g. the spleen, and it is possible that the cells responsible for this are derived from the large pyroninophilic cells that migrated from the node during the primary response. A sensitised animal drained of small lymphocytes by thoracic-duct drainage will still give a secondary response to injected antigen. The cells which form antibody in the secondary

centres migrate into the medulla and differentiate into antibody-producing cells.

Number of cell types involved in immunoglobulin production.[39, 69] There is considerable evidence that immunoglobulin formation does not occur as the result of the activity of one cell type acting alone.[69]

It will be recalled that neonatal thymectomy impairs the humoral antibody response to certain antigens, and there is

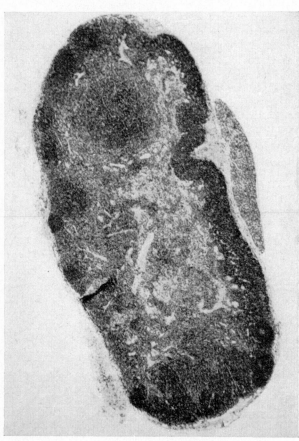

Figure 12.10
Normal auricular lymph node of a guinea-pig showing a small cortex with poorly developed follicles and no germinal centres. ×40. *(From Oort, J. and Turk, J. L. (1965), Brit. J. exp. Path., 46, 147)*

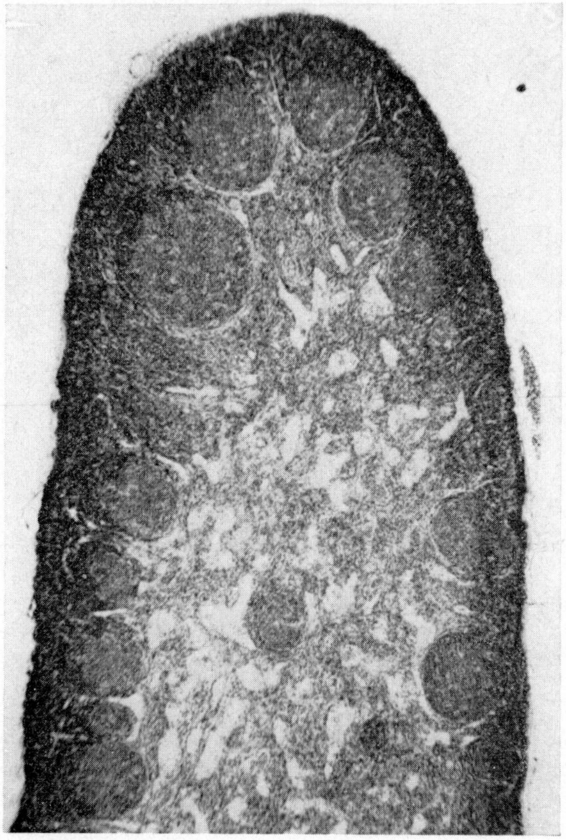

Figure 12.11
Auricular lymph node 5 days after the intradermal injection of 10 μg of pneumococcal polysaccharide into the ear. Note the extensive germinal centre formation and proliferation of cells in the medulla. ×40. *(From Turk, J. L. (1967), "Delayed Hypersensitivity". Amsterdam: North-Holland Publishing Co.)*

response are therefore derived from *sessile cells*: these are the B lymphocytes and cells derived from them.

It is evident that immunoglobulin production is related to the formation of germinal centres, and the greatest amount of antibody is formed in the cells of the medulla which finally appear as plasma cells. These are the bursal, or bursal-equivalent, dependent areas. Whether lymphocytes transform directly into plasma cells perhaps through an intermediate pyroninophilic cell stage, as suggested by Gowans, is not settled. Nor is it clear whether cells from the germinal

considerable evidence that in the production of immuno-globulins by B cells, the T lymphocytes act as helpers.[70] Perhaps they do this by acting as antigen reactive cells and recognising the antigen.[71] Certainly the mobile, recirculating T cells are well adapted to serve this function in contrast to the sessile B cells. Macrophages are also involved in the immune response. Macrophages from a normal mouse, when primed by incubating them with a *Shigella* antigen, will cause specific antibody to be formed when injected into a second, sublethally irradiated (550 r) animal. The antibody

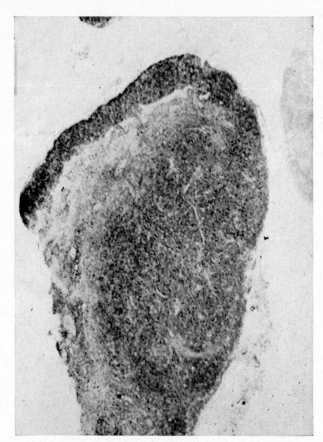

Figure 12.12
Auricular lymph node 2 days after sensitisation with oxazolone.
The cortex is thin and there is an extensive paracortical area. ×40.
(From Oort, J. and Turk, J. L. (1965), Brit. J. exp. Path., **46,** 147*)*

Cell-bound antibody production. This has been studied in experimentally induced allergic contact dermatitis. Oxazolone (p. 184) applied to the skin readily causes allergic contact dermatitis due to the formation of sensitising cell-bound antibodies. The changes in the lymph nodes are instructive[74] (Figs. 12.12 and 12.13). In the paracortical, or thymus-dependent areas, large pyroninophilic cells appear. DNA-synthesis can be demonstrated in them by the usual technique of ³H-thymidine labelling, and they probably arise from small lymphocytes. The number of these pyroninophilic cells reaches a maximum by about the fourth day. Subsequently they disappear, and are replaced by small lymphocyes which are derived from them. At the same time hypersensitivity develops. Excision of the area of skin within 16 hours of application of the sensitising agent, or excision of the regional lymph nodes before three days prevents sensitisation of the animal.[75] An intact lymphatic drainage is therefore necessary for the development of cell-bound sensitising antibodies. With skin allografts the same conditions apply, but a lymphatic connexion is not necessary for sensitisation to occur when grafts are connected by vascular anastomosis, e.g. kidney and heart.

is formed by host lymphoid tissue. Injection of antigen alone, or irradiated primed macrophages, causes no antibody response in such an animal.[72] Furthermore, primed macrophages injected into a *heavily* irradiated mouse (900 r) fail to lead to antibody production since the host's lymphoid tissue is damaged. If the cells are injected together with lymphocytes, an immune response follows. It is thought that macrophages play a vital role by ingesting antigen and manufacturing a specific RNA which evokes antibody formation in lymph-node cells.[73]

If following a primary response to an antigen in an animal, the small lymphocytes are drained from the thoracic duct, it is found that these cells will transfer immunological memory if injected into another animal: administration of antigen will produce a secondary response. Furthermore, the small lymphocytes from the thoracic duct, if incubated with antigen *in vitro*, will themselves evoke a secondary response when injected in another animal. This type of evidence suggests that, *so far as the secondary response is concerned,* an intermediate cell like a macrophage is not required for antibody production.

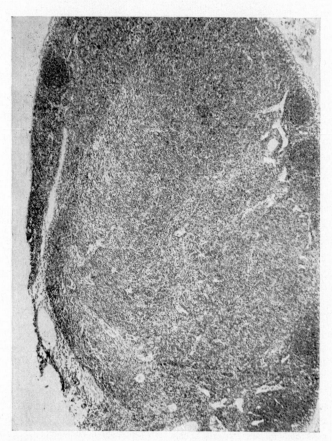

Figure 12.13
Auricular node 4 days after sensitisation with oxazolone. The bulk of the node is occupied by cells derived from the paracortical zone. × 40.
(From Oort, J. and Turk, J. L. (1965), Brit. J. exp. Path., **46,** 147*)*

THEORIES OF IMMUNOGLOBULIN ANTIBODY PRODUCTION

Immunoglobulins are proteins, and it is reasonable to believe that their formation in the rough endoplasmic reticulum of plasma cells is largely determined by genetic information residing in the nucleus. The problem which has taxed immunologists is the mechanism whereby the body can be induced to produce new specific protein following external stimulation by an antigen. Two main theories have emerged.

The Instructive Theory

This classical but improbable theory postulated that an antigen acts as a mould, or template, and that its presence leads to a slight alteration in the chemical composition of immunoglobulin, thereby rendering it highly specific and able to react with that particular antigen. Even a slight difference in the spatial arrangement of the molecule of an antigen leads to the production of a different specific antibody. The template theory assumes that the antigen is present throughout the period of potential immunity, which in many cases lasts for years and possibly the whole life of the animal. Some antigens, e.g. pneumococcal polysaccharides, are known to persist for long periods in an unchanged state, but with others the situation is less clear.

An estimation of the rate of elimination from the blood of injected ^{131}I-labelled antigen (bovine γ-globulin) shows that it is metabolised fastest in the immune animal with circulating antibodies present prior to the injection. In the non-immune, antigen can be detected for seven days and irradiation prolongs the period considerably (see Fig. 12.14 and legend).

It is evident that the development of the immune response leads to the disappearance of circulating antigen. Antigen-antibody complexes in the blood are rapidly taken up and catabolised by the reticulo-endothelial system[76, 77] Nevertheless, there is evidence that small quantites of antigen, or antigen fragments containing the determinant groups, are retained in cells for a long period in the immune animal.[78] It is possible to envisage that, by becoming attached to RNA, they might modify protein synthesis, i.e. lead to antibody production.[79]

An alternative explanation, one not requiring the continued presence of the antigen, is that there occurs a permanent modification of some self-duplicating mechanism in the cell. The nature of this change has, however, never been described in exact terms.

The Selective Theory

An alternative hypothesis is that formulated by Jerne[80] and elaborated by Burnet.[81, 82] It differs from the classical approach in postulating that antigen does not itself determine

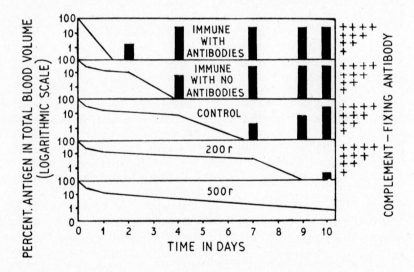

Figure 12.14

Showing the blood levels of antigen (^{131}I-labelled bovine γ-globulin) and antibody in the rabbit following one intravenous injection of antigen. The initial rapid fall in antigen level is due to equilibration between the blood and the tissues. In the group of animals already possessing antibodies due to previous immunisation, the antigen is rapidly eliminated, and antibody appears by the 2nd day. In immunised animals with no circulating antibodies (potential immunity) antigen is eliminated by the 4th day, and antibody production is correspondingly delayed. The control animals show the development of an immune response on the 4th day as evidenced by the rapid elimination of antigen during the next 2–3 days. By the 7th day antibodies appear in the circulation. 200 r delays the immune response till the 7th day, and after 500 r the response is completely suppressed. The slow, steady elimination of antigen in the heavily irradiated group is due to its gradual metabolism, and corresponds to the fall seen in the other groups prior to the development of an immune response. Other experiments show that it also corresponds to the elimination of injected ^{131}I-labelled homologous γ-globulin (this is not antigenic). These results show that the first indication of immune response is the disappearance of antigen from the circulation, and that this precedes the liberation of γ-globulin antibodies. *(From Talmage, D. W., Dixon, F. J., Bukantz, S. C., and Dammin, G. J. (1951), J. Immunol., **67**, 243)* the pattern or the specificity of the antibody, but is only responsible for the amount produced. The chief supposition of this approach is that during the early stages of embryonic development there occur many somatic mutations in the immunologically competent cells (p. 152). This results in the formation of a whole range of cells which between them is capable of mounting an immune response specific for any antigen which the body may subsequently meet. It is postulated that the effect of contact with antigen in the adult is to stimulate the growth of the immunologically competent cells which are capable of making the appropriate response. In this way a body of cells, or clone, develops, and as its size increases so does antibody production appear. A feature of the immune response which is not readily explicable by the selective theory is the interference of the response to one antigen when another unrelated antigen is administered. This suggests that both antigens act on the same cell type, and therefore compete (p. 141).

It is obvious that if somatic mutation occurs so frequently that cells are produced which can form antibodies against all possible antigens, then inevitably some mutations will produce cells capable of forming antibodies against the host's own tissues. It must therefore be postulated that there exists some mechanism during embryonic life for the destruction of these harmful, or *forbidden, clones*: contact with antigen has to destroy the clone rather than stimulate it. This is one explanation of the phenomenon of immunological tolerance.

Specific Immunological Tolerance[83, 84]

The administration of an antigen to an embryo results not in the formation of antibodies but in the acceptance of the foreign substance as "self". The phenomenon was first noticed when embryos were grafted with allogeneic cells, i.e. from an animal of the same species but of a different genetic constitution. So long as the grafted cells survived in the host the animals were tolerant of further grafts from the same donor, but not from those of any other donor. The tolerance was therefore specific and not due to a generalised depression of the immune response. This subject is considered further in Chapter 15.

Specific immunological tolerance to non-living antigens can also be induced, but it persists only for so long as the antigen remains.[7] Repeated injections are therefore usually required.

The theory of Burnet explains how early contact with antigen could destroy the appropriate clone, but in order to explain why tolerance is lost when the antigen is dissipated, it must be assumed that the capacity to relearn "self" from "non-self" is also present during adult life. It could be that new immunologically competent cells are being formed throughout life, and that at an early stage in their development they learn to recognise as "self" those antigens which are present at that time.[83] Thus, during embryonic life when antibody-forming cells are few and many immunologically competent cells are being formed, tolerance is easy to estab-

lish with relatively small doses of antigen. In the adult, on the other hand, there are many antibody-forming cells and few developing immunologically competent cells; therefore tolerance is difficult to establish.

Induction of tolerance. There are various ways in which tolerance may be induced.

(1) Administration of antigen to a fetus or immature animal.

(2) Administration of massive doses of antigen to a mature animal.

(3) Administration of very small, often repeated, doses of antigen to young animals.[83]

(4) Administration of antigen following extensive damage to the lymphoreticular system by ionising radiations or cytotoxic drugs. Antibody formation is temporarily in abeyance, and regeneration of the immunologically competent cells occurs in the presence of antigen.

(5) Administration of antigen to an immunologically defective animal such as one subjected to a neonatal thymectomy.

(6) Administration of certain antigens, e.g. picryl chloride, by mouth.[85, 86]

Tolerance to an antigen can be broken by administering a related antigen or the original one combined with Freund's adjuvent. Guinea-pigs can be rendered so tolerant to bovine serum albumin that they cannot make immunoglobulin or exhibit delayed hypersensitivity. If bovine serum albumin is given with Freund's adjuvant, the animals are then capable of responding to a further injection of antigen by immunoglobulin production, and yet many remain tolerant in respect of delayed hypersensitivity.[87] This dissociation of tolerance has been called *immune deviation*,[88] and again indicates that the two aspects of the immune response, cellular and humoral, are independent of each other.

Maintenance of tolerance. To maintain the state of tolerance the antigen must usually persist in the body, and this can be ensured either by injecting living cells as antigen or by the repeated injection of non-living antigens.

Explanation of tolerance. Two major theories have been put forward.

Production of tolerant cells. Under some circumstances antigen can act on immunologically competent cells to render them unresponsive. It has been suggested that if antigen acts directly on the cells they are rendered tolerant. If antigen is taken up by macrophages first, the immunologically competent cells are stimulated to initiate an immune response. This concept explains how *very large doses* of antigen can produce paralysis, for antigen can act directly on the cells. Likewise *very small doses* of antigen may fail to initiate antibody production and yet can act on the immunologically competent cells to render them tolerant.[83] Another possibility is that antigen-antibody complexes stimulate the immunologically competent cells to divide and lead to further antibody production. Tolerance is easier to produce if specific antibodies are absent and if the animal's capability of producing them is impaired, e.g. in fetal life and following x-irradiation and administration of cytotoxic drugs.

Elimination of potentially reactive cells. It is possible that there is no such thing as a tolerant cell, but rather that the appropriate cell has been eliminated as suggested by Burnet's theory.

An essential clue towards deciding between these two theories would be a knowledge of whether a single cell could produce one or many antibodies. By the use of specific fluorescent antibodies to immunoglobulin, it has been shown that a particular cell always produces one class of antibody, i.e. one type of heavy chain and one type of light chain. As to whether a single cell can produce antibodies specific to more than one antigen is not clear. When an animal is immunised with several antigens, most plasma cells produce an antibody against only one of the antigens.[89] However, some early experiments have shown that some cells produce antibodies against two antigens but not more.[90] Nevertheless, these observations tend to support the theory that tolerance is due to the elimination of the appropriate clone. Although it is usually assumed that the essential recognition unit of immunological competence is a cell, it is quite possible that it is in fact a subcellular component or a chemical mechanism.

It must be concluded that we are very ignorant about the manner in which antigens bring about a lifelong change in immunoglobulin synthesis. Probably the processing of anti-gen by macrophages or some other helper cell is important in producing a primary response, but the stimulation for a secondary response is a direct action of the antigen on sensitised cells, possibly with the formation of an antigen-antibody complex. Tolerance is a state in which a particular antibody mechanism is in abeyance, but whether this is due to chemical repression or to physical elimination of the appropriate mechanism is undecided.

Comparative studies on the immune response in vertebrates have indicated that cell-bound antibodies appear phylogenetically before the immunoglobulins. It has therefore been proposed that these two types of antibody are formed independently of each other. The results of thymectomy and bursectomy support this concept as does the occurrence of certain rare immunologically deficient states in man described in the next chapter. Nevertheless, it is perhaps premature to be too dogmatic, for the line of division between the two systems is by no means as distinct as is sometimes supposed.

In due course it may be expected that the immune response will be understood in proper perspective, for on the one hand it is almost certainly a mechanism evolved to maintain tissue homeostasis so that aberrant cells are eliminated, whilst on the other it has been adapted to aid the body's defences against the intrusion of foreign chemicals and the invasion by micro-organisms.

GENERAL READING

HUMPHREY, J. H. and WHITE, R. G. (1970). *Immunology for Students of Medicine*, 3rd edn, 757 pp. Oxford: Blackwell.

REFERENCES

1. BELLANTI, J. A. and GREEN, R. E. (1971). *Lancet*, ii, 526.
2. LANDSTEINER, K. (1945). *The Specificity of Serological Reactions*. Cambridge: Harvard University Press.
3. DAVIES, D. A. L. (1963). In *Modern Trends in Immunology*, I, p. 1. Edited by R. Cruickshank. London: Butterworths.
4. JERNE, N. K. (1960). *Annual Review of Microbiology*, **14**, 341.
5. LAPRESLE, C. L., KAMINSKI, M. and TANNER, C. E. (1959). *Journal of Immunology*, **82**, 94.
6. JENKIN, C. R. (1963). *Advances in Immunology*, **3**, 351.
7. SMITH, R. T. (1961). *Advances in Immunology*, **1**, 67.
8. FREUND, J. and LIPTON, M. M. (1955). *Journal of Immunology*, **75**, 454.
9. FELTON, L. D. (1949). *Journal of Immunology*, **61**, 107.
10. FINKELSTEIN, M. S. and UHR, J. W. (1964). *Science*, **146**, 67.
11. BRODY, N. I., WALKER, J. G. and SISKIND, G. W. (1967). *Journal of Experimental Medicine*, **126**, 81.
12. FREDA, V. J., GORMAN, J. G. and POLLACK, W. (1967). *New England Journal of Medicine*, **277**, 1022.
13. Leading Article (1968). *British Medical Journal*, i, 659.
14. Annotation (1966). *Lancet*, ii, 1403.
15. EILBER, F. R. and MORTON, D. L. (1970). *Cancer*, **25**, 362.
16. WOLSTENHOLME, G. E. W. and O'CONNOR, M. (1967). (Eds) *Antilymphocytic Serum*, Ciba Foundation Study Group no. 29. London: Churchill.
17. Leading Article (1968). *British Medical Journal*, ii, 507.
18. TALIAFERRO, W. H., TALIAFERRO, L. G. and JAROSLOW, B. N. (1964). *Radiation and Immune Mechanisms*. New York: Academic Press.
19. DIXON, F. J. and McCONAHEY, P. J. (1963). *Journal of Experimental Medicine*, **117**, 833.
20. SCHWARTZ, R. S. (1966). *Federation Proceedings. Federation of American Societies for Experimental Biology*, **25**, 165.
21. McGREGOR, D. D. and GOWANS, J. L. (1963). *Journal of Experimental Medicine*, **117**, 303.
22. Various Authors (1967). *Cold Spring Harbor Symposium on Quantitative Biology*, vol. 32, *Antibodies*. New York: Cold Spring Harbor Laboratory of Quantitative Biology.
23. MARTIN, N. H. (1969). *Journal of Clinical Pathology*, **22**, 117.
24. COHEN, S. and MILSTEIN, C. (1967). *Advances in Immunology*, **7**, 1.
25. TOMASI, T. B. (1972). *New England Journal of Medicine*, **287**, 500.

26. BUCKLEY, R. H. and DEES, S. C. (1969). *New England Journal of Medicine*, **281**, 465.
27. TOMASI, T. B. (1970). *Annual Review of Medicine*, **21**, 281.
28. Editorial (1971). *New England Journal of Medicine*, **284**, 552.
29. Editorial (1969). *New England Journal of Medicine*, **281**, 502.
30. ACKROYD, J. F. (1964). (Ed) *Immunological Methods*, A C.I.O. M.S. Symposium. Oxford: Blackwell. Various authors describe most of the techniques used in detecting antibodies.
31. KABAT, E. A. and MAYER, M. M. (1961). *Experimental Immunochemistry*, 2nd edn, Springfield, Ill.: Thomas.
32. NELSON, D. S. (1963). *Advances in Immunology*, **3**, 131.
33. HOWARD, J. G. (1963). In *Modern Trends in Immunology*, p. 86, *loc. cit.*
34. ROITT, I. M. *et al.* (1969). *Lancet*, ii, 367.
35. PERLMANN, P. *et al.* (1969). *Science*, **163**, 937.
36. YOFFEY, J. M. (1967). (Ed) *The Lymphocyte in Immunology and Haemopoiesis*, 376 pp. London: Arnold.
37. ELVES, M. W. (1972). *The Lymphocytes*, 2nd edn, 604 pp. London: Lloyd-Luke.
38. SMITH, R. T. and MIESCHER, P. A. (1966). *Phylogeny of Immunity*, 276 pp. University of Florida Press.
39. CRADDOCK, C. G., LONGMIRE, R. and McMILLAN, R. (1971). *New England Journal of Medicine*, **285**, 324 and 378.
40. COTTIER, H. *et al.* (1967). (Eds) *Germinal Centers in Immune Responses*, 449 pp. New York: Springer Verlag.
41. GOWANS, J. L. and KNIGHT, E. J. (1964). *Proceedings of the Royal Society*, B, **159**, 257.
42. PULVERTAFT, R. J. V. (1959). *Proceedings of the Royal Society of Medicine*, **52**, 315.
43. RAFF, M. C. (1970). *Immunology*, **19**, 637.
44. MILLER, R. F. A. P. (1967). *Lancet*, ii, 1299.
45. FORD, C. E. (1966). In *The Thymus*, p. 131, see ref. 48.
46. PARROTT, D. M. V. (1968). *Proceedings of the Royal Society of Medicine*, **61**, 863.
47. MILLER, J. F. A. P. and OSOBA, D. (1967). *Physiological Reviews*, **47**, 347.
48. WOLSTENHOLME, G. E. W. and PORTER, R. (1966). (Eds) *The Thymus: Experimental and Clinical Studies*, Ciba Foundation Symposium. London: Churchill.
49. MICKLEM, H. S. *et al.* (1966). *Proceedings of the Royal Society*, B, **165**, 78.
50. OSOBA, D. and Miller, J. F. A. P. (1963). *Nature*, **199**, 653.
51. GOLDSTEIN, A. L. *et al.* (1970). *Journal of Immunology*, **104**, 359.
52. GOLDSTEIN, A. L. *et al.* (1971). *Journal of Immunology*, **106**, 773.
53. REESE, A. J. M. and ISRAEL, M. S. (1969). *British Journal of Experimental Pathology*, **50**, 461.
54. Leading Article (1967). *Lancet*, i, 713.
55. COOPER, M. D. *et al.* (1966). *Journal of Experimental Medicine*, **123**, 75.
56. BÖRJESON, J. *et al.* (1966). *Journal of Experimental Medicine*, **124**, 859.
57. LOEWI, G., TEMPLE, A. and VISCHER, T. L. (1968). *Immunology*, **14**, 257.
58. STAVITSKY, A. B. (1961). *Advances in Immunology*, **1**, 211.
59. WHITE, R. G. (1961). In *The Scientific Basis of Medicine Annual Reviews*, pp. 31–46.
60. WOLSTENHOLME, G. E. W. and KNIGHT, J. (1963). (Eds) *The Immunologically Competent Cell*, Ciba Foundation Study Group no. 16. London: Churchill.
61. BANKHURST, A. D., WARNER, N. L., and SPRENT, J. (1971). *Journal of Experimental Medicine*, **134**, 1005.
62. UNANUE, E. R. *et al.* (1971). *Journal of Experimental Medicine*, **133**, 1188.
63. PAPAMICHAIL, M., BROWN, J. C. and HOLBOROW, E. J. (1971). *Lancet*, ii, 850.
64. SINGER, S. J. (1959). *Nature*, **183**, 1523.
65. DE PETRIS, S., KARLSBAD, G. and PERNIS, B. (1963). *Journal of Experimental Medicine*, **117**, 849.
66. JERNE, N. K. and NORDIN, A. A. (1963). *Science*, **140**, 405.
67. GUDAT, F. G. *et al.* (1971). *Journal of Experimental Medicine*, **134**, 1155.
68. Leading Article (1967). *Lancet*, ii, 974.
09. Leading Article (1968). *Lancet*, i, 185.
70. MILLER, J. F. A. P. *et al.* (1971). *Journal of Experimental Medicine*, **134**, 1266.
71. LESLEY, J. F., KETTMAN, J. R. and DUTTON, R. W. (1971). *Journal of Experimental Medicine*, **134**, 618.
72. FELDMAN, M. and GALLILY, R. (1967). In *Cold Spring Harbor Symposium on Quantitative Biology*, p. 415, *loc. cit.*
73. FISHMAN, M. and ADLER, F. L. (1967). In *Cold Spring Harbor Symposium on Quantitative Biology*, p. 343, *loc. cit.*
74. TURK, J. L. (1967). *Delayed Hypersensitivity*. Amsterdam: North Holland Publishing Co.
75. TURK, J. L. and STONE, S. H. (1963). In *Cell-bound Antibodies*, p. 51. Edited by B. Amos and H. Koprowski. Wistar Inst. Press.
76. BENACERRAF, B., SEBESTYEN, M. and COOPER, N. S. (1959). *Journal of Immunology*, **82**, 131.
77. WEIGLE, W. O. (1961). *Advances in Immunology*, **1**, 283.
78. RICHTER, M. and HAUROWITZ, F. (1960). *Journal of Immunology*, **84**, 420.
79. CAMPBELL, D. H. and GARVEY, J. S. (1963). *Advances in Immunology*, **3**, 261.
80. JERNE, N. K. (1955). *Proceedings of the National Academy of Sciences of the United States of America*, **41**, 849.
81. BURNET, F. M. (1959). *The Clonal Selection Theory of Acquired Immunity*. London: Cambridge University Press.
82. BURNET, F. M. (1967). In *Cold Spring Harbor Symposium on Quantitative Biology*, p. 1, *loc. cit.*
83. MEDAWAR, P. B. (1960). In *Cellular Aspects of Immunity*, Ciba Foundation Symposium, p. 134. Edited by G. E. W. Wolstenholme and M. O'Connor. London: Churchill.
84. HAŠEK, M., LENGEROVÁ, A. and HRABA, T. (1961). *Advances in Immunology*, **1**, 1.
85. CHASE, M. W. (1959). In *Cellular and Humoral Aspects of the Hypersensitive States*, p. 251. Edited by H. S. Lawrence. New York: Hoeber-Harper.
86. CHASE, M. W. and BATTISTO, J. R. (1959). In *Mechanisms of Hypersensitivity*, p. 507. Edited by J. H. Shaffer, G. A. LoGrippo and M. W. Chase. London: Churchill.

87. Turk, J. L. and Humphrey, J. H. (1961). *Immunology*, **4**, 310.
88. Asherson, G. L. and Stone, S. H. (1965). *Immunology*, **9**, 205.
89. Mäkelä, O. (1967). In *Cold Spring Harbor Symposium on Quantitative Biology*, p. 423, *loc. cit.*
90. Mäkelä, O. and Nossal, G. J. V. (1961). *Journal of Immunology*, **87**, 457.
91. Bloom, B. R. and Glade, P. R. (1971). Editors. *In Vitro Methods of Cell-Mediated Immunity*, 578 pp. New York and London, Academic Press.
92. Papamichail, M. *et al.* (1972). *Lancet*, **2**, 64.
93. Wybran, J., Chantler, S. and Fudenberg, H. H. (1973). *Lancet*, **i**, 127.
94. Leading Article. (1973). *Lancet*, **1**, 409.
95. David, J. R. (1973). *New England Journal of Medicine*, **288**, 143.

Chapter 13. Immunity to Infection

The ability to resist infection (immunity) is a property common to all living creatures. It is due in part to the immune response which follows a previous exposure to micro-organisms or their products. This type of immunity is specific, and has been known for a long time. It was well recognised that second attacks of many acute infections were very uncommon, and this observation led to the deliberate infection of the skin with smallpox virus (variolation) as a means of preventing this disease. Although used widely with success its dangers were considerable; the practice fell into disrepute and was made illegal by an Act of Parliament in 1840. Jenner's introduction of "vaccination" in 1796 using the less virulent cow-pox virus proved to be much more satisfactory.

Before describing the various types of immunity, it must be appreciated that the resistance of an animal and the virulence of an organism are merely alternative ways of describing the relationship between host and parasite. The Lancefield Group-B streptococcus is virulent to cows, but not to man. This may be considered from the host's point of view—man is immune, while cows are susceptible. Furthermore, some organisms produce disease only if introduced into a particular tissue. As an example of this, cholera vibrios are harmless when injected subcutaneously, but highly virulent if ingested. Not only is the portal of entry important, but so also is the number of organisms. A dose of tubercle bacilli capable of causing infection in the lung may be insufficient to produce intestinal disease. Some organisms are normally either "avirulent" or produce minor infections, but when the body's defences are weakened can lead to severe disease. This event is called *opportunistic infection*, and good examples are the deep-seated mycoses occurring in patients with one of the immunologically deficient diseases. Immunity, pathogenicity, and virulence are relative terms, which are meaningless unless not only the host and organism are specified, but also the conditions under which the two interact are defined.

Immunity may be divided into two main classes depending on whether or not it is related to previous contact with the organism or its antigens. These types are summarised below.

Immunity not Dependent upon Previous Contact

    Cellular factors

    Humoral factors

    Genetic factors   Species / Racial / Individual

Immunity Dependent upon Previous Contact

    Humoral Factors

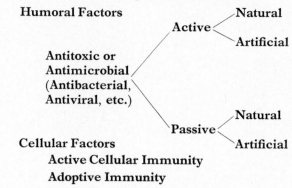

    Active: Natural, Artificial

    Antitoxic or Antimicrobial (Antibacterial, Antiviral, etc.)

    Passive: Natural, Artificial

    Cellular Factors

      Active Cellular Immunity

      Adoptive Immunity

Immunity not Dependent upon Previous Contact with the Organism

All individuals possess an inherent ability to destroy invading micro-organisms which is not dependent on the presence of antibodies. Both cellular and humoral mechanisms are involved, and in the past there has been much discussion as to which is the most important. These arguments are now largely of historical interest, for it is believed that both phagocytes and humoral bactericidal substances are involved, and indeed often work hand in hand.

In addition other factors are involved. An organism may be capable of causing severe infection in one species, and yet incapable of causing disease in others. We are quite ignorant of the reasons for this difference, because neither known humoral nor cellular factors are involved. The tissues of an immune animal appear to be unsuitable for bacterial growth, even though by our present methods of investigation they do not differ from those of a susceptible animal. This type of immunity is probably dependent on subtle biochemical differences, which are generally assumed to be governed by genetic factors. To this type of immunity the terms "innate" or "inborn" are applied.

CELLULAR FACTORS

Foreign particles and organisms are ingested by phagocytes both in the blood and tissues. Polymorphonuclear leucocytes and the cells of the reticulo-endothelial system (monocytes and histiocytes) are involved.

Abnormalities of the Polymorphonuclear Leucocytes:[1, 69, 71]

A variety of patients have been described in whom intrinsic defects in polymorph function appear to be responsible for increased susceptibility to infection. The polymorphs either fail to accumulate, fail to phagocytose the bacteria, or having done so fail to kill them. Infection which normally excites an inflammatory response and is rapidly overcome, therefore persists, becomes chronic, and excites an excessive immune response. Phagocytosis by polymorphs is dependent upon glycolysis for a source of energy.[2] Bactericidal activity, on the other hand, is dependent on oxidative reactions with glucose being oxidised *via* the hexose monophosphate shunt (p. 23). The formation of NADPH is necessary for the generation of hydrogen peroxide, and this is a vital factor in the intracellular destruction of some bacteria, an action potentiated by the enzyme myeloperoxidase.

Failure in Chemotaxis. Two children with recurrent infections have been found in whom there is a failure of polymorphs to accumulate at a site of infection and an associated defect in chemotaxis ("the lazy polymorph syndrome").[3]

Failure in Phagocytosis. Impaired phagocytosis may be due to absence or defective activation of complement components.

Failure in Bactericidal Activity.

Chronic Granulomatous Disease. In this group of conditions polymorphs are capable of phagocytosing bacteria but do not kill them. The most common type is seen in boys who develop repeated infections, often staphylococcal, of the skin, lymph nodes, lungs, and other internal organs. The disease is inherited as an X-linked recessive trait,[4] and the female carriers have been shown to possess two populations of polymorphs in keeping with the Lyon hypothesis. The defect appears to be in the hexose monophosphate shunt, and it can be detected by the failure of the polymorphs to reduce nitroblue tetrazolium dye to blue formazan pigment during the phagocytosis of latex particles.

While the original cases of chronic granulomatous disease were all boys, others have since been described in girls. In these the trait is an autosomal recessive one.[5] The enzyme defect in chronic granulomatous disease has been reported as a deficiency in NADH oxidase,[6] glucose-6-phosphate dehydrogenase,[7] glutathione peroxidase, and myeloperoxidase.

Another condition (*Job's syndrome*[8, 9]) is similar and has been described in girls with red hair. They suffer from recurrent staphylococcal skin infections,* but no defect has yet been demonstrated in their polymorphs.[10] Recurrent skin infections are also seen in the rare *Chediak-Higashi syndrome*,[11] an autosomal recessive trait in which the polymorphs contain large abnormal granules (lysosomes). Its other features are albinism and a fatal termination due to infection or malignant lymphoma.

* "So went Satan forth from the presence of the Lord, and smote Job with sore boils from the sole of his foot unto his crown." Job, xi, 7.

The existence of these rare syndromes indicates the complexity of the mechanisms on which immunity to infection depends. Indeed, it seems likely that the ability to overcome infections varies from one organism to another. It is to be expected that many more cases will be recognised in which individuals are unable to combat particular organisms or groups of organisms.

Congenital Splenic Hypoplasia.[12] One role of the spleen is to phagocytose agents which are not opsonised. Individuals with splenic hypoplasia are therefore particularly susceptible to infection with organisms against which they lack antibodies.

Conditions under which phagocytosis is increased. A non-specific increase in immunity occurs after BCG vaccination. It also follows injections of certain colloids and the endotoxin from Gram-negative bacilli. This appears to be due to an enhanced phagocytic activity of the reticulo-endothelial system which follows an initial period of depression ("RE blockade").[13]

HUMORAL FACTORS

It has been known for a long time that blood and serum possess bactericidal power. For this reason blood is always well diluted with broth when it is cultured bacteriologically. The substances involved are not well understood. In fact, only three have been identified with any degree of certainty: complement, properdin, and the natural opsonin.

Complement[13, 14]

Complement was originally conceived by Bordet as a plasma component which aided or complemented the union of antigen to antibody. It is now known to consist of at least nine components which can be sequentially activated in a cascade manner similar to that described in the clotting of blood. The components of complement are designated C1, C2, etc. The activation of complement involves the formation of enzymes which cleave the next component by limited proteolysis. Cleavage products are suffixed by a lower-case letter, e.g. C3a and C5a are small cleavage products of C3 and C5. Fluid-phase components in an activated state are symbolised by a bar over the component numbers, e.g. $C\overline{42}$. The component of complement which is most abundant is C3, also commonly called $\beta_1 C$, and an antibody to it is commonly used to detect complement deposits (see Coombs's test, p. 629).

The most intensively studied complement reaction is that of immune haemolysis initiated by the interaction of a site on the membrane of an erythrocyte E with a specific antibody A. The antigenic determinant may either be a natural constituent of the red cell membrane or an antigen or hapten artificially attached to it. In either event interaction with specific antibody results in the formation of a complex EA (Fig. 13.1). This so aligns the heavy chains of the antibody molecule that the first component of complement (C1) is

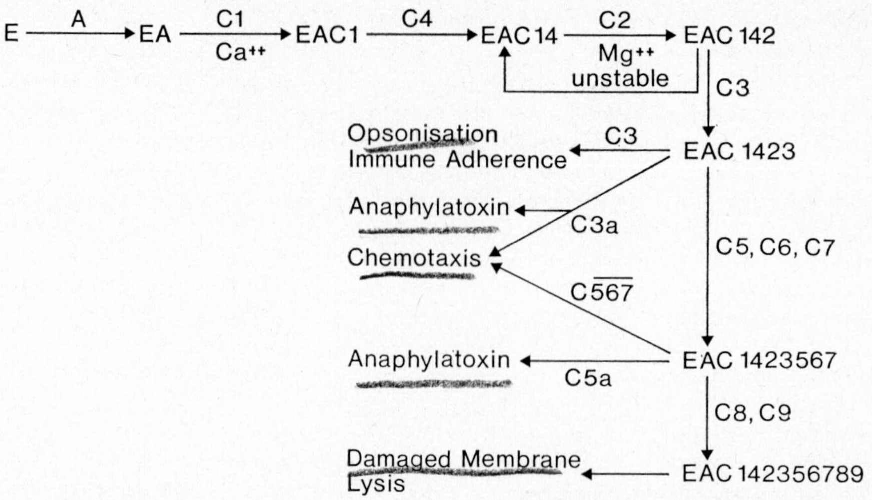

Figure 13.1
Diagram to illustrate the stages in the activation of complement, the components of which are designated C1, C2, etc. E represents a receptor site on a red cell, while A is a specific antibody. The complete reaction results in lysis of the red cell, but intermediate products are formed which result in opsonisation, immune adherence, chemotaxis, and the formation of anaphylatoxin.

$$E \xrightarrow{A} EA \xrightarrow[Ca^{++}]{C1} EAC1 \xrightarrow{C4} EAC14 \xrightarrow[\substack{Mg^{++}\\ unstable}]{C2} EAC142$$

$$EAC142 \xrightarrow{C3} EAC1423$$

Opsonisation / Immune Adherence $\xleftarrow{C3}$ EAC1423

Anaphylatoxin $\xleftarrow{C3a}$

Chemotaxis $\xleftarrow{C\overline{567}}$

EAC1423 $\xrightarrow{C5, C6, C7}$ EAC1423567

Anaphylatoxin $\xleftarrow{C5a}$ EAC1423567

EAC1423567 $\xrightarrow{C8, C9}$ EAC142356789

Damaged Membrane / Lysis $\xleftarrow{}$ EAC142356789

bound to the cell membrane. Actually C1 has three components C1q, C1r, and C1s, but these are held together in the presence of Ca^{++} ions. The bound C1 is an enzyme which acts as an *esterase* and a *protease*. EAC14 is formed by the addition of C4. C2 is the next component to be bound. C2 is probably the natural substrate for the enzyme C1, and is split to produce an active component which is added to the growing complex—now EAC142. This complex is unstable, and may revert to EAC14 with loss of C2. However, under favourable conditions an active component of the complex, $C\overline{42}$, also called C3 convertase, acts on C3 which is activated and split into C3a and C3b. The large fraction C3b is bound to form the complex EAC1423. C1 probably plays no part in this or any subsequent reaction. The next three components exist as a trimolecular complex and are added to form the thermostable EAC1423567. The last stage consists of the addition of the remaining components of complement to form EAC142356789. The details of these two remaining steps have yet to be clarified. The end result is that the receptor site on the cell is so altered that lysis is inevitable. Electron microscopy has revealed the appearance of holes in the cell membrane, 10 nm in diameter, and through these the cell constituents leak out.

Certain features of the complement mediated lysis should be noted:

1. It appears that the activation of one receptor site is sufficient to cause lysis. One hit is enough.

2. One molecule of IgM antibody is necessary to initiate the complement mediated damage at one site on the red cell. Two molecules of IgG1, IgG2, or IgG3 are needed. Thus with IgM antibody, however much diluted, a particular number of red cells is lysed. With IgG the chances of two molecules becoming attached to one receptor site are much less likely as dilution proceeds. IgM antibodies are therefore much more efficient than IgG in sensitising cells. IgG4, IgA, IgE, and IgD do not activate complement in this way.

3. All the components of complement are needed for haemolysis (and bacteriolysis).

During the process of complement activation various soluble components are formed which have important actions. These components are formed not only when the complement is activated at cell receptor sites as in immune haemolysis but also when the reaction takes place in solution. This can be initiated not only by antigen-antibody complexes but also by other mechanisms, for instance by the enzyme plasmin and probably other proteolytic enzymes. Furthermore, the process need not proceed to completion. The components of complement which are released during activation are responsible for:

Opsonisation. Bound C3b is a powerful opsonin and therefore aids *phagocytosis.*

Immune adherence. C3b is also responsible for this phenomenon (p. 148). This is closely related to the opsonic effect, for bacteria adherent to cells are probably more easily phagocytosed.

Chemotaxis. C$\overline{567}$ is chemotactic for polymorphs. This is an important mediator in the Arthus phenomenon (p. 180), aggregate anaphylaxis (p. 178), some types of vasculitis, and probably in acute inflammation in general (p. 81). C3a and C5a are also important chemotactic agents.

Anaphylatoxin production. Anaphylatoxin is an agent which will act on mast cells and lead to the liberation of histamine. At least two types are known; one is a small cleavage product of C3 labelled C3a and the other is C5a derived from C5. Anaphylatoxin can be formed not only by the interaction of antigen with antibody, but also by incubating serum with agar, kaolin, barium sulphate, and inulin, and when the serum proteases are activated (see aggregate anaphylaxis, p. 178; and anaphylactoid reactions, p. 179).

Complement is therefore an important component of plasma, for after its activation it can directly effect the lysis of bacteria; indirectly it can mediate an acute inflammatory reaction by increasing vascular permeability, attracting white cells, and promoting phagocytosis. It might therefore be deduced that complement is a vital factor in the immune mechanism. Nevertheless, a deficiency of various factors has been noted in apparently normal animals. Thus hereditary deficiency of C2 in man, C5 in mice, C4 in guinea-pigs, and C6 in rabbits is not associated with undue liability to infection. Further examples have now been discovered in which the converse is true. In one family, a girl with a dysfunction of C5 activity was found to be unduly susceptible to *Staph. pyogenes* and Gram-negative bacilli.[15] Another case is recorded of a young man with a lifelong susceptibility to infection in whom there was a lack of C3, due apparently to spontaneous activation of the alternate pathway and consumption of C3.[16] It is evident that with such a complex system as complement, subtle errors at critical points can have serious effects, while relatively gross errors at other points can be by-passed or corrected.

Conglutination.[17] This is mentioned here because of its relationship to complement. Red cell-complement-antibody complexes are agglutinated by a protein, *conglutinin*, present normally in the sera of cattle. It is not an antibody and appears to be specific against C3.

A similar substance, termed *immune conglutinin*, appears in the blood in man following many infections and immunisation procedures. It is an antibody directed against epitopic sites on C3 and C4 which are normally hidden, but which become exposed when complement is activated by antigen-antibody complexes. It is therefore a type of autoantibody.

The alternate pathway of complement activation.[14] The observation that bacterial endotoxin and cobra venom can activate the terminal sequence of complement without the consumption of C1, C2, or C4 has led to the discovery of the alternate pathway which is depicted in Fig. 13.2. It will be seen that there is a C3 activator, analogous to $C\overline{42}$, which exists as an inert C3 proactivator. This proactivator

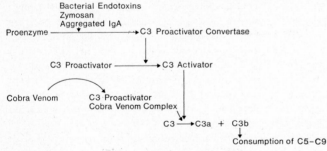

Figure 13.2
Diagram to illustrate alternate pathway for the activation of complement.

can combine with a factor in cobra venom to form a complex which can activate C3. Normally, however, the proactivator is acted upon by a serum activator called C3 proactivator convertase. The latter in turn exists as a proenzyme which is itself activated by bacterial endotoxins, plant polysaccharides like zymosan, and aggregated antibodies including IgA, IgE,[18] and IgG4, immunoglobulins which previously were thought not to activate complement. The precise role

of the alternate pathway has yet to be determined, but abnormalities in it are known to affect immunity to infection (see above), and its activation can explain how defects in the classical pathway may be circumvented. Thus C4-deficient guinea-pigs can exhibit the Arthus phenomenon. The alternate pathway is closely related to the properdin system; indeed the two may be identical. Thus the C3 proactivator has been identified as properdin factor B. The alternate pathway is activated in paroxysmal nocturnal haemoglobinuria.[72]

Natural opsonin. Normal serum contains a protein which can coat relatively avirulent organisms, rendering them more easily phagocytosed by polymorphs. It is said to be heat-labile, and to require the presence of complement. A deficient natural opsonin for pneumococcal phagocytosis is found in patients with sickle-cell anaemia, and these patients are unduly susceptible to infection.[19] The nature of the missing factor is not known. It has been found with *S. typhimurium* infection in animals that serum from a naturally resistant species (the rat) contains an opsonin which will protect a susceptible species (the mouse) from a dose of bacteria that would normally be lethal.[20] How frequently innate immunity is mediated by humoral factors is not decided.

Properdin[21, 22]

Properdin was described by Pillemer in 1954 as a plasma protein which reacts with zymosan, a polysaccharide derived from yeast, in the presence of additional plasma components and magnesium ions, to inactivate the terminal components of complement from C3 to C9. The additional components, Factor A, Factor B, and a euglobulin bear considerable similarity to C4, C2, and C1 respectively.[23] In fact, there has been much controversy regarding the identity of these additional components, for if indeed they are the same as the complement factors, properdin itself might be merely a pool of low-titre antibodies and not exist as a separate entity.[24] For a while it was believed that the properdin system did not exist, but present evidence has led to its reinstatement. Properdin has been isolated in a pure state, and the properdin system may be identical with the alternate pathway for the activation of complement. As such it probably plays a vital part in host immunity, but its precise role in disease has yet to be delineated. Its activation is known to be important in the pathogenesis of paroxysmal nocturnal haemoglobinuria.

Other factors. Bactericidal substances have been extracted from tissue and serum, but in no case has identification been successful. The basic peptides extracted from tuberculous tissue may be cited as an example.

Conditions under which humoral factors are impaired. As many of the humoral antibacterial substances are proteins, it is not surprising that starvation and protein deficiency adversely affect the body's ability to resist infection. Certain metabolic disorders may also upset the basal immune state. Chronic renal disease, diabetes mellitus[25], and alcoholism[26] are good examples, but the exact nature of the upset is not known. In alcoholics with cirrhosis there is defective chemotaxis associated with low C3 levels and also perhaps the presence of an inhibitor.[73]

GENETIC FACTORS—INNATE IMMUNITY

Species. Species immunity is the most absolute immunity known. The human species has almost complete immunity to many animal diseases; distemper and foot-and-mouth disease do not normally affect man, while certain typically human diseases like poliomyelitis, syphilis, and leprosy do not easily affect animals. Humans are immune to Lancefield Group-B streptococci; these organisms are, however, capable of producing mastitis in cattle. On the other hand, Group-A streptococci cause serious human infection, thus illustrating the high degree of specificity of innate immunity. In other words, virulence is sometimes dependent upon quite small changes in antigenic structure. Nevertheless, some organisms do produce disease in several species, a fact utilised by Koch in the formulation of his famous postulates (see Appendix II).

Racial. The selective breeding of disease-resistant plants is well known in agriculture, where it is of great practical importance. Selective breeding in animals is more difficult; the work of Lurie,[27] who succeeded in breeding rabbits of varying degrees of susceptibility to tuberculosis, is a noteworthy achievement in this field. Another instance often cited is that of Algerian sheep, which are said to be immune to anthrax.

In man the position is more difficult to assess. There is considerable evidence to show that individuals with the sickle-cell trait are resistant to malaria.[28] The trait is due to a genetic error, which lends some weight to the thesis that innate immunity is dependent upon inherited characteristics. Other examples are on less firm ground. The European races are said to be more susceptible to yellow fever than are the native races of West Africa. The Irish and the Welsh are generally held to be more susceptible to tuberculosis than are the English. However, the possibility of immunity acquired in early childhood, as well as the question of widely differing social and economic levels in different peoples, make it difficult to prove that these are true examples of innate immunity. Nevertheless, the work with plants and animals would lead us to suppose by analogy that racial differences do exist in man.

Individual. The existence of individual immunity is difficult to prove either in man or animals. The study of tuberculosis in twins has shed some light on this problem.[29] In the case of uniovular twins it is found that when one twin has tuberculosis, the chances of the other twin also having it are over 85 per cent. When, however, one of binovular twins has tuberculosis, the chances of the other twin also having it are only 25 per cent. This percentage corresponds to that which is usually encountered in siblings who are not twins.

Other examples of an individual's genetic make-up affect-ing his response to an infection may be cited.[30] Susceptibility to *H. influenzae* epiglottitis and meningitis has been shown to be related to a major histocompatibility gene in man. In animals it is well known that the immune response to a particular antigen is linked to hereditary factors. A cross-reaction between the bacterial antigen and a tissue antigen, such as a blood-group substance, is sometimes the cause of this.

These examples of innate immunity—species, racial, and individual—are dependent upon genetic make-up. In some instances the ability to mount an immune response is invoked, but usually we are quite ignorant of the mechanism.

Immunity Dependent upon Previous Contact with the Organism or its Antigens—Acquired Immunity

This type of immunity is always associated with the presence of antibodies which may be of either humoral or cellular nature. When the host produces its own antibodies, the immunity is called "active". This may occur naturally or artificially. When the antibodies are donated to the host from another source, e.g. the serum of a convalescent patient or an immunised horse, the immunity is described as "passive". The antibodies are both immunoglobulins and cell bound.

Active Immunity

Natural active immunity follows an overt attack of the disease. Not infrequently people who deny ever having suffered from the infection are found to be immune, and their blood contains specific antibodies. In these cases it is likely that the infection has occurred, but in so mild a form as to escape notice. Subclinical attacks of this type are common in many diseases, e.g. tuberculosis and poliomyelitis, and probably play an important part in preventing epidemics. When an infection is introduced into a virgin population, a widespread, severe outbreak may ensue. This was seen when measles was first introduced into the Fiji Islands (1875),[31] and is also well known with myxomatosis in rabbits: first described in Montevideo by Sanarelli in 1898, devastating outbreaks have since occurred in Australia (by government initiative) and Europe (by private enterprise).[32] Natural selection of individuals having innate immunity is another factor which may operate.

Artificial active immunity follows the injection of toxoids or vaccines. These are considered in detail further on.

Passive Immunity by Transference of Immunoglobulins

Immunoglobulins may be passively transferred either naturally or artificially.

Natural passive immunity:[33-35] although at birth the body is poorly equipped for making its own antibodies, it nevertheless has γ-globulins in considerable quantity, and these confer immunity. They are of maternal origin, and gain access to the child in one of two ways depending upon the species:[34]

In utero, either *via* the placental or the vitelline circulation.

By *absorption through the gut* of antibodies contained in the colostrum and milk.

In man and other primates humoral antibodies are transferred across the placenta, but in guinea-pigs and rabbits absorption is from the uterine lumen through the vitelline circulation. In horses, pigs, and cattle the transfer occurs after birth from the colostrum and milk. Dogs, rats, and mice occupy an intermediate position; some transfer occurs before birth, but most antibodies are received afterwards.

Transmission across fetal membranes is a highly selective affair. IgG globulins tend to be easily transferable, while the IgA, IgM, and IgE fractions are held back. Some antibodies (e.g. diphtheria antitoxin) are found in higher concentration in the offspring than in the mother.[33] There is no adequate explanation for this. Transmission of *antigen* across the placenta is also a possibility, and might lead to the development of potential immunity.[70]

Relationship of immunoglobulins to immunity.[33] Although some antibodies give good protection to the newborn child, e.g. to diphtheria, others do not. Thus, staphylococcal infection is common, although the staphylococcal antihaemolysin titre of the baby is higher than that of its mother. Whooping-cough is another disease for which no protection is afforded.

Artificial passive immunity is deliberately induced by injecting immunoglobulins for prophylactic or therapeutic purposes. The protection afforded is short-lived, because the antibodies are metabolised. It has been shown that in neonatal life the antibodies are destroyed at a slower rate than in the adult. Infants therefore retain their passive immunity for several months, while the effect of a serum injection in adults is measured in days rather than weeks. A plausible but unproven explanation of this is that the infant has acquired tolerance to the "foreign" maternal proteins, and therefore does not react against them.

Passive Immunity by Transference of Cells[36, 37]

If lymph-node cells from an immunised animal are transferred to another animal which is either syngeneic, tolerant, or non-reactive, e.g. due to x-irradiation, the grafted cells lead to the production of immunoglobulins in the new host. This is called *adoptive immunity*. Whether passive cellular immunity, e.g. to tuberculosis, can be transferred by lymphocytes (or in man, transfer factor—see p. 185) is not known.

Before considering the mechanism of acquired immunity, it is important to remember that bacteria produce their harmful effects in two main ways: (1) by elaborating powerful exotoxins; (2) by invading tissues. Although both methods are used by a few bacteria, it is convenient to divide pathogenic organisms into two groups. Those which produce their main effect by means of a soluble exotoxin are called the *toxic organisms*, while those which produce their main effect by means of endotoxins are termed *invasive*. As these two types of organism produce their effects in different ways, it is not surprising that the immunity which the body develops is

TABLE 13.1 Showing the main differences between exotoxins and endotoxins

Property of toxin	Exotoxin	Endotoxin
Liberation	Large amounts liberated in broth culture: easily diffuses out of bacterium	Small amounts liberated with living organisms: liberated when organisms are destroyed.
Composition	Protein (relatively simple)	Complex mixtures containing protein, lipid, and carbohydrate.
Lethal dose	Small. Action specific	Larger. Action not specific.
Action of heat	Heat-labile in general*	Heat-stable in general.
Number of strains producing one toxin	Often all strains*	Often only one.
Ability to stimulate the production of demonstrable antibodies	Strong tendency	Some factors are antigenic (e.g. the surface antigens). Others are poor antigens.
Corresponding antibody	Antitoxin	Many types; some are antibacterial, others (e.g. antihaemolysins) are not.
Value of antibody in infection	Good protection	Variable—some antibodies protective, others are not.
Union with antibody	Simple direct relationship, often precipitation	Complex relationship. Agglutination, complement fixation, etc.

* Botulinum toxin is an exception to these generalisations.

different in the two instances (see Table 13.2). The main differences between exotoxins and endotoxins are shown in Table 13.1.

There are therefore two main subdivisions of this acquired type of immunity:

(1) Antitoxic, against the toxic organisms.
(2) Antibacterial, against the invasive organisms.

because more antibodies are rapidly formed as a result of the stimulus of the infection.

Examples of Antitoxic Immunity

Diphtheria. The exotoxin produced by the diphtheria bacillus is mainly responsible for the organism's ability to survive and multiply at the site of infection. A reasonable

TABLE 13.2   Types of immunity

Type	Due to	Mode of action
Antitoxic	Immunoglobulins (antitoxins)	Neutralises toxin and speeds its elimination. No direct effect on organism.
Antibacterial (and Antiviral)	*Humoral antibodies* Antibacterial Antiviral	Aids phagocytes and activates complement. Prevents attachment.
	Local Tissue Immunity due to IgA	Prevents infection.
	Cellular antibody Immune lymphocytes	Lymphokines: Cytotoxic action or lymphotoxin. Chemotaxis. Macrophage immobilisation. Interferon.

ANTITOXIC IMMUNITY[38]

Toxic organisms produce their effects by means of powerful, diffusible exotoxins which are highly antigenic. The antibodies (antitoxins) are capable of neutralising the toxin, and act in the body by intercepting the toxin before it reaches susceptible tissues. They are commonly of IgG type.

Diphtheria bacilli alighting on a mucous membrane produce their effect, and indeed the disease, by elaborating an exotoxin, which acts upon the local tissues as well as being absorbed by the blood stream and causing damage at distant sites. If the host has a high antitoxin level in the circulation, and therefore in the tissues and mucus, the toxin is rapidly neutralised, thereby leaving the organism without its main offensive weapon. It then becomes in effect avirulent, and is removed by the normal decontaminating mechanism of the part. A virulent organism attacking a host with a high antitoxin level is in the same position as an avirulent organism attacking a normal host.

Virulent organisms may sometimes persist in the nose or throat in spite of a high level of circulating antitoxin. This constitutes the *carrier state*, and although the individual does not suffer any ill-effects from this colonisation, he is nevertheless a source of danger to non-immune contacts. Evidently some type of antibacterial immunity is also involved in diphtheria.

It will be seen that the level of antitoxin in the circulating blood is a good measure of the degree of immunity, and this information is of great value in the assessment of immunity to toxic organisms. The degree of immunity as assessed in terms of an antibody titre is in fact an underestimate,

level of circulating antibody will therefore confer immunity. This forms the basis of the *Schick test*.[39]

A small quantity of toxin* is injected intradermally into the forearm, and the reaction observed after 48 hours. If the individual's blood contains no antitoxin, the introduced toxin causes tissue damage which is manifested by an acute inflammatory reaction (Schick-positive). If, however, the blood contains a fair level of antitoxin, then the introduced toxin is immediately neutralised, and no reaction occurs (Schick-negative).

This type of biological test is found to be most useful in diphtheria; the actual measurement of the antitoxin titre in the blood would be more efficient, though obviously very tedious to perform. The Schick test is usually negative after an attack of diphtheria. Subclinical attacks frequently occur, as evidenced by the fact that many adults are Schick-negative without ever having suffered from a clinical infection. The significance of Schick testing is shown in Table 13.3.

Table 13.3

Schick	Throat swab for Diphtheria bacilli	Condition
+	−	Susceptible
+	+	Diphtheria
−	−	Immune
−	+	Carrier

* The amount used is generally that which is just neutralised by 1/1 000 unit of antitoxin. In the skin of the other forearm a control of heated exotoxin is injected.

Diphtheria can occur in a Schick-negative child, but the infection is not accompanied by generalised toxaemia. This again indicates that there is an antibacterial component to the immunity of diphtheria. However, it cannot be measured, and for practical purposes the antitoxin titre as gauged by the Schick test is of value. It has three uses: (*a*) to assess the general state of immunity to diphtheria in a large community; (*b*) to assess the necessity for active immunisation; (*c*) as a retrospective diagnostic aid in cases suspected of being diphtheria.

Active immunity of the artificial type is produced by the introduction into the body of *toxoid*. If APT (Alum Precipitated Toxoid) is used two doses are given, while with TAF (Toxoid Antitoxin Flocules) three injections are necessary. In practice the toxoid is often given in conjunction with tetanus toxoid, pertussis vaccine, and Salk vaccine.

Antitoxin administration is an essential part of the treatment of diphtheria. It is derived from horses which have been immunised against toxoid (and toxin). By producing a high blood level of antitoxin the toxin liberated at the site of infection is neutralised, and is therefore unable to reach distant organs, e.g. heart, adrenals, and nerves. Toxin which has already reached these tissues is firmly bound to them, and cannot be dislodged by the antibody. Treatment at an early stage of the disease is therefore essential if the full benefits of antitoxin therapy are to be obtained. The organisms themselves are not directly affected, but are destroyed by the acute inflammatory exudate. A carrier state may persist after the attack, and it is therefore advisable to insist on negative throat-swab cultures before discharging the patient.

Scarlet fever. The skin manifestations of this disease are caused by the erythrogenic exotoxin of *Strept. pyogenes*. Immunity may be detected by the *Dick test*,[40] which acts on exactly the same principle as the Schick test. A small quantity of erythrogenic toxin is injected intracutaneously. A positive reaction denotes susceptibility to the effects of the toxin.

The ability of antitoxin to neutralise erythrogenic toxin is used in the *Schultz-Charlton reaction*.[40] In this test some antitoxin* is injected into the skin of a patient who has a scarlatiniform eruption. If the patient has scarlet fever, the toxin is neutralised, and blanching occurs in the region where the antitoxin was injected. Although this reaction has great theoretical diagnostic value, it is not found to be very useful in practice, being positive only in those cases which are fairly obvious clinically.

Many of the different Griffith types of *Strept. pyogenes* produce the erythrogenic exotoxin, which consists of three antigenic types only (see p. 220, but in fact a single attack of scarlet fever is the rule). Therefore a scarlet fever patient infected with any one of these types of streptococcus produces an antitoxin against one of the erythrogenic exotoxins, and is thereafter immune to it. There is, however, no im-

*From animals immunised with erythrogenic toxin

munity to streptococcal infection in general, because this depends on separate antibacterial antibodies against each Griffith type, of which there are about 50. As in diphtheria the antitoxin merely neutralises the toxin, and does not kill the organisms. On the other hand, while the neutralisation of the diphtheria toxin automatically allows the organism to be destroyed by the acute inflammatory exudate, the same does not apply after the neutralisation of the erythrogenic exotoxin of streptococci. The invasiveness of this organism depends on surface antigens, which have to be neutralised by specific antibacterial antibodies (see p. 168).

Tetanus. The tetanus bacillus has limited powers of invasion, and produces a severe disease by liberating a powerful exotoxin. This neurotoxin affects the anterior horn cells; once inside the cells it cannot be neutralised by its antitoxin. As with diphtheria early treatment of the disease is essential. Both horse and human antitetanic sera (ATS) are available, and can be given in large doses to intercept any further toxin which may be liberated. The horse protein is liable to produce hypersensitivity reactions, and its routine use is frowned on by many authorities.

Formaldehyde converts the toxin into toxoid (TT), which is extensively used as an active immunising agent. The prophylaxis and treatment of tetanus are fully considered in Chapter 18.

Gas-gangrene. The clostridia causing this infection produce powerful exotoxins, the α-toxin of *Cl. welchii* being the most important. It is a powerful necrotoxin, and prepares ideal conditions for the invasion of the organisms. Antitoxin prevents this local necrotising action, thereby checking further spread of the bacilli. The antitoxins have no direct effect on the organism.

Botulism. The various strains of *Cl. botulinum* produce toxins which are antigenically distinct. Unless the particular strain involved is known, a polyvalent antiserum must be given. The toxins of this organism are an exception to the general rule that the exotoxins produced by different strains of an organism are identical. In addition, botulinum toxin is very heat stable, unlike most exotoxins (staphylococcal enterotoxin is also thermostable).

Summary of Antitoxic Immunity

(1) Immunity is conferred by circulating immunoglobulins, which are called antitoxins.

(2) The circulating antibody titre is a good measure of the degree of immunity.

(3) Reaction between toxin and antitoxin is a relatively simple, quantitative affair, about which much is known.

(4) Active immunisation with toxoid is reliable.

(5) Passive immunisation is effective in the treatment of the disease, if given early enough.

ANTIBACTERIAL IMMUNITY[38]

Antibacterial immunity is much more complex than antitoxic immunity. The reason for this is the antigenic complexity of organisms, for although they are said to contain "endotoxins", these are in effect the contents of the bacterial cell and many of them are not related to the pathogenic action of the organism. The globulin antibodies which are formed against the invasive organisms are therefore described as antibacterial rather than anti-endotoxic. They are IgM and IgG immunoglobulins.

Antigenic Structure of Invasive Organisms

Bacteria are living unicellular organisms, and as such are composed of a complex mixture of proteins, carbohydrates, and lipids. Many of these substances are antigenic, and one may well regard bacteria as made up of a mosaic of antigens. The virulent or invasive properties are often dependent upon a single substance, which is usually on the cell surface. The polysaccharide hapten capsule of the pneumococcus is a good example of this. Sometimes more than one surface antigen is present, the external one covering those beneath it to a greater or lesser extent. This phenomenon is well shown by the typhoid bacillus. Organisms containing the O surface antigen are virulent, and are agglutinated by anti-O serum. Some virulent strains have an additional Vi antigen coat. They are agglutinated by anti-Vi but not by anti-O. Although it is convenient to consider the Vi antigen as an additional coat which covers the O antigen, it is quite possible that one surface antigenic site can, by its presence, inhibit other antigenic determinants from reacting with their respective antibodies.[20]

It has been reported that bacteria can acquire additional antigens from their surrounding media.[20] Electron microscopy of virus particles escaping from a cell has shown how this can occur with viruses (see Fig. 22.4). If infective agents acquire antigens from their hosts, this might be a factor in promoting their virulence. Thus a future host, by exhibiting tolerance to these antigens, might show a reduced or delayed antibody response to the whole organism. As against this, it must be remembered that with some infections much of the tissue destruction might be caused by the immune response. Thus tolerance would cause immunity.[20, 41] This is well shown in mice with lymphocytic choriomeningitis. Infection *in utero* produces a chronic carrier state (see p. 279), while animals first infected as adults succumb to a severe disease.[42]

It will be seen that there may be considerable variation in the structure of a single bacterial species. Not only does this affect the virulence, but also the colonial appearance of the organisms on a solid medium. For instance, pneumococci whose virulence has been enhanced by animal passage frequently produce *smooth* colonies on plate culture. Continued growth on the artificial media, however, often results in loss of virulence due to a loss of the surface antigen. These colonies appear *rough*. Such attenuated strains may be produced in other ways, e.g. passage through mice in the case of viruses. This change which affects an organism's virulence, colonial appearance, antigenic structure, etc., is known collectively as *microbial variation*.

This multiplicity of antigens leads to the formation of a large number of different antibodies when an animal is infected with the whole organism. As only a few of the bacterial antigens are responsible for invasiveness or virulence, it is only the corresponding antibodies that are of protective value. Many other antibodies may also be present, but in all probability they play no part in immunity. On the other hand, their presence may be of great diagnostic help, e.g. the Widal reaction of typhoid fever.

Organisms in the body are dealt with by two methods: they are destroyed either by phagocytosis or by humoral mechanisms. Both have already been described with regard to innate immunity, and it seems likely that antibacterial antibodies protect merely by aiding or activating these existing mechanisms.

Phagocytosis by polymorphs and macrophages is aided by the action of specific opsonin. Moreover, organisms adherent to red cells (see p. 148) are more easily phagocytosed *in vitro*, an effect which may also occur in the blood stream or in a local area of inflammation.[43] The reticulo-endothelial system clears the blood stream of organisms more quickly in the immune animal.

Examples of Antibacterial Immunity

Pneumococcal infections.[44] Pneumococci produce no powerful toxin, and their virulence depends upon the polysaccharide capsular hapten called the *Specific Soluble Substance* (SSS), which by repelling phagocytes enables the organism to invade the tissues. Pneumococci without capsules are "rough" and avirulent.

Immunity to pneumococcal infection is due to a type-specific antibody, which may be produced both by infection and the administration of the capsular substance. The antibody acts as an *opsonin* both *in vitro* and *in vivo*. It can also act as a precipitin and agglutinin, but is incapable of killing the organism even in the presence of complement. A specific reaction on the capsule can be demonstrated. This is generally described as the "capsular swelling reaction", but in fact there is little or no actual swelling, the appearance being due to an increased opacity of the capsular substance, when it is acted upon by the type-specific antibody. Organisms so treated are still viable, and it seems certain that polymorphs must be present for their destruction.

Immune serum was once used in treating pneumococcal infection, but it has been rendered obsolete by the introduction of sulphonamides and the antibiotics.

Streptococcal infections.[44] The virulence of *Streptococcus pyogenes* is dependent upon its type-specific M protein content, which too is present on the surface of the organism, and like the SSS hinders phagocytosis. Antibodies to it confer good immunity in experimental animals. The organisms produce many toxic and enzymatic products, e.g. haemolysin, hyaluronidase, streptokinase, and sometimes the erythrogenic exotoxin. Antibodies to these are produced, but confer no immunity against streptococcal infection.

Although theoretically useful, the large number of different types of streptococcal antigens makes artificial immunisation by vaccines or sera an impracticable proposition. In any case the organism responds well to chemotherapeutic agents, although early treatment with these agents reduces the immune response.

Staphylococcal infection.[44] Staphylococci are readily phagocytosed by polymorphs, but these may then be killed by the organism, presumably by its leucocidins. The α-toxin, coagulase, and leucocidins are all antigenic; however, their antibodies provide little or no protection. Unfortunately we are ignorant about the antigenic components which are responsible for the virulence of staphylococci, and it is therefore impossible to make effective vaccines. Many preparations have been used, but their value is doubtful.

Typhoid.[44] Typhoid bacilli may be killed by phagocytosis or by humoral mechanisms. Antibodies confer immunity by their opsonic and complement-sensitising effects. The important antigens are not yet clearly defined.[33, 45, 46] Phenolised preparations preserving the O and H antigens are effective. But an acetone killed and dried (AKD) vaccine was superior in a trial conducted in Guyana, and has been adopted by the U.S. Armed Forces. An alcoholised vaccine, high in O and Vi antigens, was introduced for a period during the 1939–45 war, and was of little value.[47] H antibodies do not confer immunity, but nevertheless find great use in the laboratory for the identification of *Salmonella* organisms. Presumably the important antigens in a vaccine are the O and others as yet undetermined.

Whooping-cough. The situation is the same as with typhoid, in that the antigen responsible for virulence has not been identified. Vaccines prepared from freshly isolated smooth strains have, however, proved of great value in prophylaxis.

Tuberculosis. The mechanism of immunity to tuberculosis is not understood; precipitins, agglutinins, and complement-fixing antibodies have been identified, but these do not confer immunity. The Mantoux test is used to detect hypersensitivity to tubercle-bacillus protein, and it is generally assumed that where hypersensitivity exists, so also does immunity. Active immunisation with a living attenuated human strain of bacillus (BCG) is widely used, apparently with good effect, although the degree of protection afforded cannot be directly measured. It is probable that acquired immunity to tuberculosis is due to cellular antibodies. The subject is discussed in Chapter 20.

Virus infections. The immunity to virus infection is considered in detail in Chapter 22. IgA antibodies in the secretions covering mucous membranes prevent initial infection, while IgG neutralising antibodies in the plasma limit dissemination should infection occur. Cell-mediated immunity is also important, since patients with a defect in the thymus-dependent immune response are particularly liable to virus infections. Interferon appears to be a major factor in the recovery from established infection.

Action of the Humoral Antibacterial Antibodies in the Body

Although the action of some antibodies appears to be beneficial, e.g. the opsonins, in others, like the agglutinins and precipitins, the effect is much less clear. Thus, it is possible that agglutinins by causing the organisms to remain localised to one site may so raise their local concentration that in fact infection is favoured. On the other hand, it is possible that agglutination may prevent spread, and help to localise infection and facilitate phagocytosis.

It has already been stressed (p. 148) that antibodies have been named according to the nature of the tests employed to detect them. Furthermore, a single antibody may be detected as a precipitin, agglutinin, or lysin. To attempt to explain antibacterial immunity on the basis of *in-vitro* antibody reactions is not rewarding. It seems certain that the only way in which they can kill bacteria is by aiding one of the normal body defences; thus some antibodies assist complement, while others collaborate with phagocytes in the actual destruction of the organisms. In general, it may be said that the antibacterial antibodies produce their beneficial effect by localising infection.

It has been shown that if an animal is rendered leucopenic, although there may be a high titre of antibacterial antibodies present, injected pneumococci tend to remain localised for only a limited time, and then spread and kill the animal. Therefore, without the intervention of the phagocytes antibacterial immunity is impotent. With other organisms phagocytosis may not be so vital, because humoral bactericidal mechanisms are also effective.

The antigenic structure of most organisms is highly complex, and there are many slight variations which affect their virulence; for instance, antibacterial antibodies to one particular strain of organisms may not protect against other strains. Serum therapy is on this account extremely difficult and rarely efficacious.

In-vitro tests, e.g. agglutination, are dependent on the presence of certain specific antigens present in the organism. It does not follow, however, that these antigens are the ones that confer the property of virulence on the organism. It is very apparent that the titre of antibodies in a patient's serum, as demonstrated *in vitro*, often bears no relationship to the degree of immunity possessed against that particular organism. It often happens that the antigens responsible for an organism's virulence are not the ones investigated in the common *in-vitro* tests. Antibacterial antibodies probably afford as complete a protection against invasive organisms as do antitoxins against toxic organisms. It is unfortunate that the common serological tests investigate the antibody response to antigens that do not concern the organism's virulence. This does not, however, detract from their great value in diagnosis.

Immunity due to IgA antibody in secretions. IgA immunoglobulin is the principal antibody found in the secretions of the nose, salivary glands, and the alimentary tract. Its presence appears to be responsible for the local immunity which follows ingestion of live poliomyelitis vaccine.[48] Antibodies to other viruses have also been detected in the IgA fraction, and it remains to be discovered whether the same mechanism applies to bacterial infection.

Value of Estimating Antibodies in Diagnosis

The Wassermann complement fixation test and Kahn flocculation test are well-known methods of detecting the syphilitic antibody. In typhoid fever agglutinins can be detected against both flagellar H antigens and the somatic O and Vi antigens (Widal test). The titre rises towards the end of the second week of the disease, and particular significance should be attached to a rising titre of anti-O agglutinins. An anamnestic rise following other infections is less liable to affect these than the anti-H agglutinins. In patients previously vaccinated with TAB the Widal test is of much less value in diagnosing typhoid fever, because high titres of antibody may present even before the onset of the infection, and the subsequent anamnestic rise confuses the picture even more.

In the Weil-Felix test advantage is taken of the fact that certain *Proteus* organisms share a common antigen with the rickettsiae; antibodies which agglutinate *Proteus* OX19 are found in European louse-born typhus, while in scrub typhus the antibodies react with *Proteus* OXK.

Cell-mediated Immunity in Bacterial Disease[49]

Although in the past great stress has been laid on the part played by humoral antibacterial antibodies, it is evident that cell-mediated responses are also important. Sensitised lymphocytes in contact with antigen release a number of agents: interferon, lymphotoxin, and factors which augment the inflammatory response and immobilise macrophages. These cells play an important role in immunity.

The increased phagocytic power of macrophages in Mantoux-positive individuals indicates that a change in them may play a part in the antibacterial immunity to the tubercle bacillus.[50] Curiously enough, although the delayed-type hypersensitivity which develops during an infection with the tubercle bacillus is specific, the increased phagocytic activity of the macrophages which accompanies it is much less specific. The cellular immunity is effective against many micro-organisms, and is not specific for the tubercle bacillus that induced it.[51] Indeed, this is the basis for giving BCG in an attempt to control malignant disease. Anergy, indicating a lack of cell-mediated responses, can lead to an increased susceptibility to infection: measles has a reputation for reactivating a tuberculous infection.

It is evident that the interrelationship between delayed-type hypersensitivity, cell-bound antibodies, and immunity is poorly understood. Individuals who display defective cell-mediated immunity show particular susceptibility to certain infections, e.g. to viruses, fungi, and some bacteria (p. 172).

Artificial Antibacterial and Antiviral Immunity

The artificial production of immunity to the invasive organisms is much more difficult than to those of the toxic group. The reasons for this are twofold.

(1) The antigens responsible for the virulence of the organisms are in many cases unknown. Preparations of vaccine may therefore be deficient in vital antigens, and the antibodies which they provoke are then not protective.

(2) Immunity is in part cell mediated, and this is difficult to stimulate other than by infection with living organisms.

The injection of toxins or toxoids is quite unsatisfactory, and it is found that the whole organism, i.e. a *vaccine*,* must be used. Attention has to be paid to the relevant surface antigen of the organism which is used in the preparation of the vaccine. Furthermore, if the strain of organism selected does not happen to be the one which is prevalent at the time, vaccination is unlikely to produce satisfactory immunity, e.g. influenza.

In many diseases dead vaccines are not effective, and a vaccine containing live attenuated organisms is much more efficient.

The artificial induction of local immunity has so far been utilised only in poliomyelitis.

Summary of Antibacterial Immunity

1. Many strains of bacteria exist, and they may differ widely in their antigenic structure and virulence.

2. It is difficult to prepare effective vaccines, because it is not always possible to include all the possible antigenic variants in the preparation.

3. Antibacterial immunity is only partly dependent upon the production of immunoglobulin antibacterial antibodies.

4. It is difficult to measure the immunity because of the wide bacterial variation.

5. Many *in-vitro* actions of humoral antibodies can be demonstrated, but their activity *in vivo* is not necessarily related to their *in-vitro* properties.

6. The effect of the antibodies is to aid localisation of the infection.

7. Local immunity due to local IgA plays a part in some infections.

8. Antibacterial immunity is also related to cellular antibodies.

Artificial Immunisation[46, 52]

Specific immunity to infections may be increased artificially by giving antisera (passive) or by the administration of vaccines or toxoids (active).

A toxoid is a preparation of an exotoxin which has been so treated (usually with formaldehyde) that its toxicity is abolished without impairing its essential antigenic deter-

* The term is derived from the Latin *vacca*, a cow, and was coined by Pasteur in honour of Jenner's observation that an infection with cow-pox protected against smallpox.

minants. Satisfactory preparations of diphtheria and tetanus toxoid are in current use (see pp. 167 and 234).

Vaccines are suspensions of whole organisms either alive or dead. They may be administered orally, but the common route is by parenteral injection. BCG, smallpox, yellow fever, and poliomyelitis (Sabin) are examples of live vaccines; TAB, pertussis, and Salk poliomyelitis are dead.

Although there is general agreement that active immunisation of the population is desirable, there is no unanimity on the schedule to be adopted. With living vaccines one dose is generally sufficient, since the organism multiplies during the course of the subclinical infection which follows and this provides a sufficient antigenic stimulus (but see p. 284). A cellular type of immunity also ensues. With dead vaccines and toxoids a two or three-dose procedure is adopted for primary immunisation. In order to avoid multiple injections, there has been a trend to combine several antigens into one preparation e.g. combined diphtheria, tetanus, poliomyelitis, and pertussis. The pertussis organisms have been found to exercise an adjuvant effect and improve the response to the toxoids.

Maintenance of immunity. Regular booster doses are usually recommended, but there is a tendency to regard these as unnecessary, and indeed, if repeated too frequently, as harmful. Following a satisfactory primary course, immunity to diphtheria and tetanus persists for many years, and booster doses can be given in the event of an exposure to infection.

It is apparent that the immunisation procedures that are adopted are based upon factors determined by administrative convenience, finance, and the patient's comfort as well as on the results obtained from previous experience. The best plan for the individual practitioner is to adopt the procedure which is generally accepted in his own area, and to modify it as the results of well-planned field trials become available.[33]

COMPLICATIONS OF ARTIFICIAL IMMUNISATION[52]

Although serious complications are very uncommon, their occurrence has been a serious handicap to the public's acceptance of widespread immunisation. In some instances particular preparations, e.g. horse ATS, have fallen into disfavour because of their complications. The hazards of artificial immunisation will be summarised here, since many aspects are described in greater detail elsewhere in this book.

Reactions Following the Use of Any Agent:

Infection. With carefully controlled methods of preparation and adequate aseptic technique this is an infrequent complication.

Local acute inflammation due to the irritant properties of the preparation. In severe cases there is also a general reaction with pyrexia, malaise, etc. Such reactions are usually seen after the use of dead vaccines, e.g. TAB, and to a lesser extent alum-containing toxoids.

Provocation poliomyelitis, especially with alum-containing toxoids.

Reactions Following the Use of Specific Agents: Animal Sera.

Hypersensitivity reactions: local reactions, serum sickness, anaphylaxis, and death.

Neurological complications.[53] Encephalitis, myelitis, polyneuritis (of Landry or Guillain-Barré type), neuritis affecting a group of nerves, e.g. "radiculitis" of the brachial plexus, and lesions of individual nerves have all been described. The pathogenesis is obscure; a hypersensitivity reaction may be involved as neurological complications may also occur with serum sickness.

Human Serum

Infection: virus hepatitis is the most important.

Passive transfer of immediate-type hypersensitivity is a minor hazard.

Hypersensitivity reactions to minor genetically-determined protein variants is a possibility.

Live Vaccine.

Excessive local spread of the agent, e.g. BCG and vaccinia.

Widespread dissemination of the organism to produce severe disease, e.g. vaccinia.

Neurological complications, e.g. postvaccinal encephalitis.

Toxoids and Dead Vaccines.

Hypersensitivity. Local reactions due to immediate and delayed-type hypersensitivity. Anaphylaxis is rare. Encephalitis following antirabies injections is probably a reaction to foreign nervous tissue.

Neurological complications resemble those seen following the use of serum. Thus, pertussis vaccine is occasionally followed by encephalitis or blindness.

IMMUNOLOGICALLY DEFICIENT DISEASES[54–56]

In 1952 Bruton[57] described the case of a young boy whose sequence of repeated pneumococcal infections was shown to be related to a very low plasma γ-globulin level. Since that time numerous instances of immunological deficiency disease have been described,[58] and attempts to understand the mechanism in each case have served to test our understanding of the mechanisms involved in the defences of the body against infection.

On the hypothesis that the thymus is necessary for the proper development of cell-mediated immune reactions, while the gut-associated lymphoid tissue is essential for the immunoglobulin responses, attempts have been made to separate the syndromes into groups according to which system is presumed to be at fault. In some cases this has been eminently successful, but there are others in which the defect is such that our knowledge of the immune response is inadequate to explain them. A feature which can cause confusion is a patient with a specific immunological deficiency developing other immunological defects as a secondary event, as the disease and its complications progress.

The term *agammaglobulinaemia* is generally used to describe cases in which the γ-globulin level is very low (under 100 mg per cent). *Hypogammaglobulinaemia* would be more accurate, but is usually reserved for cases in which the level of γ-globulins, although low, is over 100 mg per cent. Although no hard and fast rules can be made, this group of diseases is characterised by repeated pyogenic bacterial infections and also virus hepatitis. When there is a defect in the formation of cellular antibodies, infections with *Myco. tuberculosis*, viruses, and fungi (especially *Candida*) often dominate the picture.

Stem-cell Deficiency

Reticular dysgenesis. This is described in infants who possess no white cells or lymphoid tissue. Presumably the primitive marrow reticular cells failed to develop.

Pure Thymic Deficiency Syndromes[59]

In *thymic alymphoplasia* of Nezelof,[60] sometimes called thymic dysplasia, the thymus is absent or rudimentary and there is a complete absence of all the cell-mediated responses of delayed hypersensitivity. Germinal centres, plasma cells, and the production of γ-globulins are, however, normal. In *thymic aplasia*, described by Di George, there is in addition absence of the parathyroid glands.

Pure Immunoglobulin Deficiency Syndromes

Bruton's congenital sex-linked agammaglobulinaemia. This is restricted to males, and usually appears at about the age of six months when maternally derived immunoglobulins are exhausted. There is a striking absence of plasma cells everywhere and atrophy of the lymphoid tissue of the tonsils, appendix, and Peyer's patches. The thymus is normal and cell-mediated responses are normal. There is, however, a virtual absence of the three main classes of immunoglobulins, and this is associated with a liability to repeated, serious infections which invariably lead to death. Fulminating hepatitis may occur. Curiously enough, if these patients are given human γ-globulin they sometimes manufacture antibodies to it.[61] Polyarteritis and rheumatoid arthritis are more frequent in these patients, indicating perhaps that this is not simply a disease in which there is a failure of immunoglobulin synthesis.

Acquired agammaglobulinaemia and hypogammaglobulinaemia of late onset. A variety of syndromes have been described in which a low immunoglobulin level is first detected in childhood or adult life. The disease is sometimes called acquired, but probably inherited factors are involved in many cases. Plasma cells are not formed in response to antigenic stimulation, but germinal centres are seen and may even be hyperplastic.

Dysgammaglobulinaemia. This term is used to describe the condition in which there is a low level or absence of one or more, but not all, of the γ-globulin classes. So far as the three main classes of immunoglobulins are concerned, there are six possible combinations. Thus in the most common type affecting male infants, IgG and IgA are low or absent while IgM is elevated.[62] Isolated IgA deficiency is not uncommon and usually presents no characteristic syndome. Some cases suffer from sinusitis and pulmonary infections with intestinal malabsorption and a sprue-like syndrome, and also show a tendency to develop rheumatoid arthritis or other autoimmune disease.[55] Several other types of dysgammaglobulinaemia are known, and some exhibit a malabsorption syndrome—steatorrhoea with nodular hyperplasia of the intestinal lymphoid tissue[63] or lymphadenopathy and hepatomegaly. Liability to infection is common.

This group of immunoglobulin deficiency syndromes may be regarded as disorders of the gut-associated lymphoid tissue. In some cases all classes of antibody are reduced, while in others the defect spares some subclasses of antibody. In many instances the defect appears to be inherited, but some are probably acquired; virus infection, e.g. rubella, has been implicated. An interesting but unexplained feature of this group is that the patients or their families exhibit a high incidence of rheumatoid arthritis, systemic lupus erythematosus, Crohn's disease, lymphoma, and thymoma.

Deficiency Syndromes of Mixed Type

In this group, in addition to thymic hypoplasia and defective cell-bound antibody production, there is also depression of some or all of the immunoglobulins.

Swiss-type lymphopenic agammaglobulinaemia. This form of deficiency shows a total lack of both cell-mediated and humoral immunity, and is the most severe immunological defect known. The disease is noticed during the first few weeks of life. There is a failure to thrive, infection particularly by viruses, *Candida albicans*, and *Pneumocystis carinii* (see p. 265), and diarrhoea. The infants seldom survive more than two years. The thymus and all the lymphoid tissue are hypoplastic, and both cell-mediated and humoral immune responses are absent. Allografts are not rejected. Administration of fresh blood to these patients often leads to a fatal *graft-versus-host* reaction beginning in 7–10 days with a high fever, morbilliform rash, hepatosplenomegaly, and diarrhoea. Pancytopenia develops and death occurs within 15 days. In some patients who have not been transfused, a skin rash similar to that of the GVH rash has been seen, and it is suggested that it is due to a GVH reaction by maternal lymphocytes.[56, 64]

Swiss-type lymphopenic agammaglobulinaemia is inherited as an autosomal recessive character. Other types are now recognised, and one is sex linked.

Ataxia telangiectasia. This is inherited as an autosomal recessive character and is characterised by progressive cerebellar ataxia, oculocutaneous telangiectasia, and recurrent sinus and pulmonary infections by viruses and bacteria.

The onset is in early childhood and death usually occurs by adolescence. The thymus is absent or hypoplastic, and delayed-type reactions are markedly depressed. In addition there is a low level of plasma IgA and often IgE. Unexpectedly, plasma cells are present in the alimentary tract, but they contain IgM rather than the normal IgA immunoglobulins.[65] A considerable number of patients develop a malignant lymphoma or other tumour.

Wiskott-Aldrich syndrome.[66] This is characterised by atopic *eczema*, bleeding due to *thrombocytopenia*, and an increased susceptibility to *infection*. It is inherited as a sex-linked recessive character, and death usually occurs in infancy. The major defect appears to be in the afferent limb of the immune response such that the individual fails to react to polysaccharide or lipopolysaccharide antigens. This leads to a low IgM level. As the disease progresses, there is a failure in T-lymphocyte development. Infection with a wide range of viruses, fungi, and bacteria occurs, and patients rarely survive over 10 years of age.[55]

Treatment of immunological-deficiency diseases. Patients who lack particular immunoglobulins can be treated by the administration of suitable antibody concentrates. When cell-mediated function is defective, marrow and thymic grafts have been used. The administration of transfer factor has also been tried both in some primary immunological deficiency states and in acquired ones such as lepromatous leprosy.[74] Results are being assessed, and such treatment is at present the task of specialised centres.[67]

Acquired Immunological Deficiency[68]

Antibody levels are low in a number of naturally occurring diseases.

Secondary to infection. During measles, German measles, and following measles vaccination there is depression of cell-mediated hypersensitivity. There is a similar anergy in lepromatous leprosy (p. 184).

Hodgkin's disease. The major defect is suppression of the reactions dependent upon cell-bound antibodies. There is an increased liability to infection with tubercle bacilli, viruses, and fungi, a liability sometimes aggravated by the treatment.

Sarcoidosis. The defect is as in Hodgkin's disease.

Multiple myeloma and *Waldenström's macroglobulinaemia.* Both exhibit impairment of normal immunoglobulin production.

Lymphosarcoma and chronic lymphatic leukaemia. There is depression of both immunoglobulin and cell-bound antibody production.

Intestinal lymphangiectasia. The dilated, abnormal lymphatic vessels leak fat, plasma proteins, and lymphocytes into the intestine. Cell-mediated responses are particularly affected. Since the long-chain fatty acids are absorbed into the lymphatics and increase the lymph flow, their administration worsens the disease. A low-fat diet, or one containing medium-chain triglycerides which are absorbed into the portal vein system, has a beneficial effect.

Iatrogenic immunological deficiency. In the treatment of patients with grafts or "autoimmune" diseases, deliberate suppression of the immune response is often attempted by the administration of corticosteroids, cytotoxic drugs, anti-lymphocytic serum, and ionising radiation. The results of this are often disappointing in relation to the aims of the treatment and devastating in terms of the infections that result.

REFERENCES

1. BAEHNER, R. L. (1969). *New England Journal of Medicine*, **280**, 1355.
2. KARNOVSKY, M. L. (1962). *Physiological Review*, **42**, 143.
3. MILLER, M. E., OSKI, F. A. and HARRIS, M. B. (1971). *Lancet*, i, 665.
4. LANDING, B. H. and SHIRKEY, H. S. (1957). *Pediatrics (Springfield)*, **20**, 431.
5. HOLMES, B. *et al.* (1970). *New England Journal of Medicine*, **283**, 217.
6. BAEHNER, R. L. and KARNOVSKY, M. L. (1968). *Science*, **162**, 1277.
7. BELLANTI, J. A., CANTZ, B. E. and SCHEGEL, R. L. (1970). *Pediatrics Research*, **4**, 405.
8. DAVIS, S. D., SCHALLER, J. and WEDGWOOD, R. J. (1966). *Lancet*, i, 1013.
9. WHITE, L. R. *et al.* (1969). *Lancet*, i, 630.
10. Editorial (1968). *New England Journal of Medicine*, **279**, 1053.
11. STEGMAIER, O. C. and SCHNEIDER, L. A. (1965). *Archives of Dermatology and Syphilology*, **91**, 1.
12. MILLER, M. E. (1970). *Medical Clinics of North America*, **54**, 713.
13. MÜLLER-EBERHARD, H. J. (1968). *Advances in Immunology*, **8**, 1.
14. RUDDY, S., GIGLI, I. and AUSTEN, K. F. (1972). *New England Journal of Medicine*, **287**, 489, 545, 592 and 642.
15. MILLER, M. E. and NILSSON, U. R. (1970). *New England Journal of Medicine*, **282**, 354.
16. ALPER, C. A. *et al.* (1970). *New England Journal of Medicine*, **282**, 349.
17. LACHMANN, P. J. and COOMBS, R. R. A. (1965). In *Complement*, A Ciba Foundation Symposium, p. 242. Edited by G. E. W. Wolstenholme and J. Knight. London: Churchill.
18. ISHIZAKA, T., SIAN, C. M. and ISHIZAKA, K. (1972). *Journal of Immunology*, **108**, 848.
19. Editorial (1968). *New England Journal of Medicine*, **279**, 489.
20. JENKIN, C. R. (1963). *Advances in Immunology*, **3**, 351.
21. PENSKY, J. *et al.* (1968). *Journal of Immunology*, **100**, 142.
22. LEPOW, I. H. and ROSEN, F. S. (1972). *New England Journal of Medicine*, **286**, 942.
23. GOODKOFSKY, I. and LEPOW, I. H. (1971). *Journal of Immunology*, **107**, 1200

24. Austen, K. F. and Cohn, Z. A. (1963). *New England Journal of Medicine*, **268**, 933, 994 and 1056.
25. Mowat, A. G. and Baum, J. (1971). *New England Journal of Medicine*, **284**, 621.
26. Brayton, R. G. *et al.* (1970). *New England Journal of Medicine*, **282**, 123.
27. Lurie, M. B. (1950). *American Journal of Medicine*, **9**, 591.
28. Roberts, J. A. F. (1967). In *An Introduction of Medical Genetics*, 4th edn, p. 67. London: Oxford University Press.
29. Kallmann, F. J. and Reisner, D. (1943). *American Review of Tuberculosis and Pulmonary Diseases*, **47**, 549.
30. Leading Article (1971). *Lancet*, ii, 914.
31. Burnet, F. M. (1962). *Natural History of Infectious Disease*, 3rd edn, p. 205. Cambridge University Press.
32. Fenner, F. (1959). *British Medical Bulletin*, **15**, 240.
33. Cruickshank, R. (1963). In *Modern Trends in Immunology*, I, p. 107. Edited by R. Cruickshank. London: Butterworths.
34. Brambell, R. W. R. (1961). *Proceedings of the Royal Society of Medicine*, **54**, 992.
35. Bangham, D. R. (1961). *Proceedings of the Royal Society of Medicine*, **54**, 993.
36. Harris, T. N. and Harris, S. (1960). In *Cellular Aspects of Immunity*, Ciba Foundation Symposium, p. 172. Edited by G. E. W. Wolstenholme and M. O'Connor. London: Churchill.
37. Cochrane, C. G. and Dixon, F. J. (1962). *Advances in Immunology*, **2**, 205.
38. Wilson, G. S. and Miles, A. A. (1964). In *Topley and Wilson's Principles of Bacteriology*, 5th edn, p. 1261. London: Arnold.
39. Cruickshank, R. (1965). In *Medical Microbiology*, 11th edn, p. 183. Edited by R. Cruickshank. Edinburgh: Livingstone.
40. Gillies, R. R. (1965). In *Medical Microbiology*, p. 152, *loc. cit.*
41. Rowley, D. and Jenkin, C. R. (1962). *Nature*, **193**, 151.
42. Wagner, R. R. and Snyder, R. M. (1962). *Nature*, **196**, 393.
43. Nelson, D. S. (1963). *Advances in Immunology*, **3**, 131.
44. Gladstone, G. P. (1970). In *General Pathology*, 4th edn, p. 860. Edited by H. Florey. London: Lloyd-Luke.
45. Cvjetanovic, B. and Outschoorn, A. S. (1963). *British Medical Journal*, i, 609.
46. Various Authors (1969). *British Medical Bulletin*, **25**, 119–212.
47. Leading Article (1967). *Lancet*, ii, 1075.
48. Ogra, P. L. *et al.* (1968). *New England Journal of Medicine*, **279**, 893.
49. Rowley, D. (1962). *Advances in Immunology*, **2**, 241.
50. Howard, J. G. (1961). *Scottish Medical Journal*, **6**, 60.
51. Dannenberg, A. M. (1968). *Bacteriological Reviews*, **32**, 85.
52. Wilson, G. S. (1967). *The Hazards of Immunisation*, 324 pp. London: Athlone Press.
53. Miller, H. G. and Stanton, J. B. (1954). *Quarterly Journal of Medicine*, **23**, 1.
54. Sell, S. (1968). *Archives of Pathology*, **86**, 95.
55. Bergsma, D. and Good, R. A. (1968). (Eds) *Immunological Deficiency Diseases in Man*, Birth Defects, Original Articles Series, vol. IV, no. 1. New York: National Foundation—March of Dimes.
56. Gatti, R. A. and Good, R. A. (1970). *Medical Clinics of North America*, **54**, 281.
57. Bruton, O. C. (1952). *Pediatrics*, **9**, 722.
58. Good, R. A. (1966). In *The Thymus*, A Ciba Foundation Symposium, pp. 470–1. Edited by G. E. W. Wolstenholme and R. Porter. London: Churchill.
59. di George, A. M. *et al.* (1967). *Lancet*, i, 1387.
60. Nezelof, C. *et al.* (1964). *Archives Françaises de Pédiatrie (Paris)*, **21**, 897.
61. Editorial (1968). *New England Journal of Medicine*, **278**, 1174.
62. Stiehm, E. R. and Fudenberg, H. H. (1966). *American Journal of Medicine*, **40**, 805.
63. Hermans, P. E. *et al.* (1966). *American Journal of Medicine*, **40**, 78.
64. Kadowaki, J.-I. *et al.* (1965). *Lancet*, ii, 1152.
65. Eidelman, S. and Davis, S. D. (1968). *Lancet*, i, 884.
66. Leading Article (1968). *British Medical Journal*, ii, 66.
67. Leading Article (1969). *Lancet*, i, 243.
68. Hobbs, J. R. (1968). *Proccedings of the Royal Society of Medicine*, **61**, 883.
69. Windhorst, D. B. (1970). *Advances in Internal Medicine*, **16**, 329.
70. Gill, T. J. (1973). *Lancet*, i, 133.
71. Brewer, D. B. (1972). *British Medical Journal*, ii, 396.
72. Götze, O. and Müller-Eberhard, H. J. (1972). *New England Journal of Medicine*, **286**, 180.
73. DeMeo, A. N. and Andersen, B. R. (1972). *New England Journal of Medicine*, **286**, 735.
74. Bloom, B. R. (1973). *New England Journal of Medicine*, **288**, 908.

Chapter 14. Hypersensitivity

Hypersensitivity is a state in which an animal exhibits an excessive reactivity to the introduction of an antigen or hapten. The mechanisms involved are poorly understood, and there are few subjects in pathology over which so much confusion exists; even the terminology is confusing. Strictly speaking, *hypersensitivity* means excessive reaction, e.g. anaphylaxis, while *allergy* implies an altered reaction as exemplified by the Mantoux test. It is debatable whether such a distinction can be justified, and for practical purposes the two words are best regarded as synonymous. The excessive or altered reaction to bacteria as seen in the Koch phenomenon is conventionally called *bacterial allergy*. However, diseases like asthma and hay-fever are also called "allergic", although in fact they differ markedly from the bacterial allergies. It is obvious that the two terms mean different things to different people, and therefore no useful purpose is served by trying to distinguish between them, even if this were desirable on theoretical grounds.

Two distinct types of hypersensitivity can be recognised. In one the reaction to administration of antigen is immediate (within minutes), while in the other it is delayed for 24 to 48 hours. The distinction between these two types is of fundamental importance. The *immediate-type* hypersensitivities are related to the formation of sensitising immunoglobulins. In *delayed-type* hypersensitivity, the reaction is cell mediated.

It is now realised that immunoglobulins can cause hypersensitivity in various ways and that in only one of these is the reaction immediate in the sense that this term is usually used. Indeed, injury due to immunoglobulins can be caused in three distinct ways, and these have been classified thus:

Type I, immediate hypersensitivity. This is commonly mediated by IgE and is typified by acute anaphylaxis in man.

Type II, or cytotoxic reaction. Antibodies, IgG or IgM, are directed against cellular or tissue antigens, e.g. as in haemolytic anaemia.

Type III, due to antigen-antibody complexes. IgG is mainly involved.

In the *delayed-type* hypersensitivities no such sensitising antibodies can be demonstrated, and the hypersensitivity is cell-mediated. This type of hypersensitivity is classified as *Type IV*.

TYPE I IMMEDIATE HYPERSENSITIVITY

Many examples of this type of hypersensitivity occur in man; the offending antigen is usually a dust, food, or drug.

The features of immediate-type hypersensitivity have been the subject of intensive experimental study in animals. Anaphylaxis, which represents the most severe manifestation, will be described in some detail, because it illustrates the main features of this group.

ANAPHYLAXIS[1, 2, 3]

The term "anaphylaxis" was first used to describe the severe reaction classically described by Richet and Portier in 1902. Since that time a localised, usually cutaneous, manifestation of hypersensitivity has been labelled *cutaneous anaphylaxis*, and it is therefore advisable to describe the generalised form as *generalised*, or *systemic, anaphylaxis*.

Systemic Anaphylaxis

Richet and Portier were attempting to immunise dogs against the toxins of the sea-anemone, and noted that animals which had survived a sublethal injection of toxin were unduly sensitive to a second injection—so sensitive indeed that quite small doses produced a severe reaction, often resulting in death. At first the phenomenon was explained on the basis of the toxic nature of the extract, but subsequent work showed that other antigenic proteins could produce the same effect, even though they were not in themselves toxic. Richet called the reaction anaphylaxis because it seemed to represent the antithesis of immunity (Gr. *ana*—against, *phylaxis*—protection).

Anaphylaxis may be elicited by giving a single large, *shocking* dose of antigen at a suitable interval after one or more *sensitising* doses.

Active sensitisation. The first dose of antigen must reach the tissues in an unaltered state. It may be injected, but as the dose need only be small, a sufficient amount may be absorbed by inhalation or ingestion, provided the antigen is not denatured during absorption. Haptens may induce anaphylactic sensitisation if injected into the skin, because they may combine with body proteins to produce complete antigens; in some instances, e.g. neoarsphenamine, intravenous injection leads to sensitisation. Presumably the drug combines with a body protein, thereby becoming antigenic.

Although some animals, e.g. guinea-pig, are easily sensitised by one small injection, others like the rabbit respond less readily, and may require several sensitising doses combined with an adjuvant.

Development of hypersensitivity. Anaphylactic shock can be demonstrated only if the shocking dose is given some time after the sensitising dose. The period is usually 8 to 10 days. The existence of this latent interval strongly suggests that an immune mechanism is involved. Once established, the state of hypersensitivity remains unaltered for a long time.

Production of shock. Following the injection of the second or "shocking dose" of antigen, the animal develops a state which closely resembles acute histamine poisoning. The following features of the shocking dose should be noted:

Specificity. The same antigen must be used, a fact which indicates that the sensitisation is specific.

Dosage and rate of administration. The shocking dose must be administered quickly so that the damaging antigen-antibody reaction can produce systemic effects. In experimental work the intravenous route is used. The dose of antigen to be given varies with the type of anaphylaxis. It is often large when compared with the sensitising dose (in aggregate anaphylaxis), but enormous doses must not be given because antigen-antibody union is less damaging when there is great antigen excess, and shock may not occur.[4]

Action of haptens. Haptens will induce shock provided they are capable of causing precipitation when mixed with their corresponding antibodies. Haptens which do not precipitate in this manner will not produce shock; instead they induce a refractory state to the subsequent injection of whole antigen. This state lasts only a few hours.

The shock.[3] The manifestations of anaphylactic shock resemble those of histamine poisoning. They vary considerably in different species, but in any one species the reaction is fairly constant.

Guinea-pig. A few seconds after the injection of the shocking dose, the animal begins to twitch its nose. It rapidly develops respiratory distress, having great difficulty in expiration. Cyanosis appears, and death from asphyxia usually occurs within 5–10 minutes. The symptoms are due to severe bronchospasm, and over-distension of the lungs can be demonstrated at necropsy.

Rabbit. The onset of shock is slower than in the guinea-pig. The animal becomes unsteady, rests on the ground, and frequently urinates and defaecates. Cyanosis develops, consciousness is lost, and in well-sensitised animals death follows. There is generalised arteriolar constriction which affects the pulmonary vessels in particular. Measurements of pulmonary blood pressure reveal hypertension, and death is usually ascribed to acute cor pulmonale.

Dog. The dog shows a fall in systemic blood pressure. It is believed that the hepatic veins undergo constriction, leading to acute venous congestion of the liver and organs drained by the portal system. Vomiting of blood and diarrhoea occur before death.

Rat. The animal exhibits prostration, rapid and laboured breathing, cyanosis, hypotension, hypothermia, and marked haemoconcentration.

Man. The symptoms of anaphylaxis in man closely resemble those of the guinea-pig, being characterised by acute respiratory distress of an asthmatic type. Generalised oedema develops, causing obvious swelling of the eyelids and dependent parts. Oedema of the larynx may add to the respiratory distress caused by bronchospasm. Itching and diffuse erythema of the skin may occur. Anaphylaxis is rare in man and usually follows the injection of horse serum, e.g. ATS, either intravenously or intramuscularly. It may also follow bee stings and the administration of drugs, e.g. penicillin and neoarsphenamine. In one case, which must surely be unique, it followed sexual intercourse, and was due to antibody directed against mucoprotein in seminal fluid.[5] Occasionally the shock resembles that seen in the dog, rabbit, or rat.

It has been suggested that sudden death in infancy ("cot death") is due to hypersensitivity to milk.[6] The sensitised child is presumed to inhale regurgitated milk during sleep and to die of acute anaphylaxis. But this hypothesis has received little direct support, and the cause of cot death still awaits solution.[6] Infection may be important in some cases.[6]

Although the manifestations of anaphylaxis vary in different species, the disturbance is fundamentally the same in all of them. The two main effects are:

(1) *Spasm of smooth muscle*—either blood vessel or bronchial.

(2) *Damage to small blood vessels and an increase in their permeability.* Generalised oedema, although not obvious in animals, may nevertheless be demonstrated.

Systemic anaphylaxis is a generalised reaction affecting all parts of the body, though not with equal intensity. Some organs appear to be particularly sensitive, and the disturbances produced in them not only dominate the clinical picture but may also cause death. This is well illustrated by anaphylaxis in the dog. The liver is the organ most affected; obstruction to the hepatic venous outflow causes circulatory failure followed by death. In hepatectomised dogs anaphylaxis can still be demonstrated, but with much greater difficulty.

Cutaneous Anaphylaxis

If a small quantity of antigen is injected into the skin of a sensitised animal, an immediate local reaction occurs which is characterised by erythema and increased vascular permeability. A weal forms in man but not in animals, and intravenous trypan blue is given to detect the increase in vascular permeability (p. 73).

This type of reaction may be used clinically to detect sensitisation before giving a large therapeutic dose of foreign serum, thereby avoiding acute anaphylactic shock and possibly death.

Unfortunately, the results of such skin tests are not a reliable indication of a possible sensitisation to anaphylaxis. The antibodies which cause skin sensitisation are not necessarily the same as those responsible for anaphylaxis. It is suggested that the safest procedure when administering foreign sera is to give a small test dose subcutaneously and watch for any mild general reaction. Adrenaline and a syringe should, of course, be at hand (see p. 234).

Pathogenesis of Anaphylaxis[1, 2]

There is abundant evidence that anaphylaxis is initiated by the interaction of antigen with antibody; this leads to the release of pharmacologically active compounds which are directly responsible for the characteristic features of the syndrome. There has been much speculation in the past concerning the type of antibody involved, the site of the interaction, and the nature of the chemicals released. *It is now evident that at least two groups of antibodies are concerned and that there are at least two distinct mechanisms whereby the shock is produced.* Much of the experimental work performed in the past was on actively sensitised animals in which both mechanisms were involved, either separately or in combination. The anaphylactic shock produced under one set of circumstances was not identical with that produced under different experimental conditions; thus many apparently conflicting findings were published. Sometimes complement was shown to be involved in anaphylaxis and sometimes not. Likewise, antihistamine drugs may or may not protect. The use of passively sensitised animals has clarified the situation, because relatively pure antibody can be administered in known quantity and its role in sensitisation to anaphylaxis can be assessed.

Cytotropic anaphylaxis. Anaphylaxis is described as *cytotropic* when it is the result of antigen reacting with immunoglobulin (IgE in man) fixed to cells—usually mast cells. When the antibody is manufactured by the test animal itself, or in passive anaphylaxis by an animal of the same species, the antibody is termed *homocytotropic*. When the antibody is derived from a different species it is called *heterocytotropic*. Cytotropic anaphylaxis is the classical type of reaction as exemplified by anaphylaxis in the actively sensitised guinea-pig.

Aggregate anaphylaxis. This type of anaphylaxis occurs in the actively sensitised rabbit, and is due to the formation of antibody-antigen aggregates in the circulation. Fixation of antibody to cells plays no part in the pathogenesis of aggregate anaphylaxis, but activation of complement is vital and polymorphs are essential.

Both types of anaphylaxis must be examined in more detail.

Cytotropic Anaphylaxis

This type of anaphylaxis is dependent upon immunoglobulin in the circulating blood becoming attached to certain target cells and thereby sensitising them.

Evidence that circulating antibodies are involved. (1) The blood of a sensitised animal contains antibodies which precipitate with the corresponding antigen or hapten.

(2) That these antibodies are related to the sensitisation is indicated by the evidence derived from passive sensitisation.

Passive sensitisation. Serum from one sensitised animal will, if injected intravenously, sensitise another animal to anaphylaxis. The passive sensitisation is made manifest only after a time-interval of several hours. It appears therefore that the mere presence of circulating antibody is not sufficient, and that some other conditions have to be fulfilled before sensitisation can occur. The present evidence suggests that antibody has first to be fixed to cells. The Schultz-Dale phenomenon and passive skin sensitisation provide more conclusive evidence.

Schultz-Dale phenomenon. If a piece of the uterine muscle is removed from a sensitised guinea-pig, it is found to contract vigorously when placed in contact with the antigen. The muscle is first thoroughly washed in Tyrode solution to remove blood and serum, and then suspended in a bath containing Tyrode solution at 37°C. The addition of antigen to the bath results in contraction, which can be recorded by means of a suitable system of levers. The Schultz-Dale reaction can also be carried out on uterine muscle sensitised *in vitro* by immersing it in sensitising antibody, and also by using the uterus removed from a passively sensitised animal. Isolated intestinal muscle behaves in the same way as myometrium. As under the conditions of these tests no blood or plasma is present, it seems certain that the antibody is firmly fixed to the cells.

Passive cutaneous anaphylaxis.[7, 8] A small amount of serum from a sensitised animal* is injected into the skin of a guinea-pig, and this is followed a few hours later by an intravenous injection of antigen mixed with Evans blue. Within a few minutes an exudative reaction is detectable by the leakage of the dye into the skin site.

Reversed passive cutaneous anaphylaxis. If *antigen* is injected into the skin of an animal it will sensitise the skin provided it is itself an immunoglobulin which will fix on to the tissues, e.g. rabbit serum injected into guinea-pig skin. When a specific antibody is injected intravenously some hours later, a local reaction is seen at the site of the injected skin. This is termed reversed passive cutaneous anaphylaxis. *Reversed systemic anaphylaxis* may similarly be produced by injecting antigen intravenously followed some time later by a specific antibody.

Guinea-pigs sensitised to anaphylactic shock can be desensitised by repeated small injections of antigen. In this way a very high titre of circulating antibody is produced. Administration of antigen to such an animal does not produce anaphylaxis, because the circulating antibody is sufficient to neutralise all the injected antigen, none being left over to react with fixed antibody.

Target cells involved in cytotropic anaphylaxis. Although it seems certain that anaphylaxis is produced by an antigen-antibody interaction in close association with cells, precisely which cells are involved is by no means certain. Mast cells are important in the guinea-pig, rat, dog, and

* This test will not detect the reagins responsible for human anaphylaxis.

mouse; these show degranulation and are presumed to release histamine. In the rat 5-hydroxytryptamine is released, while in the dog sufficient heparin enters the circulation to cause prolongation of the clotting time. In man the polymorphs are thought to be involved, and in the rabbit both polymorphs and platelets. Whether fixation occurs in other cells, e.g. the liver macrophages, argentaffin cells, or the parenchymal cells of skin and muscle, is not known. It is evident that very considerable species differences exist, and that if human disease is to be elucidated, man himself must be investigated.

Mediators of cytotropic anaphylaxis.[9] *Histamine*. Histamine can be detected in the blood in acute systemic anaphylaxis, and is released if antigen is applied to sensitised tissue *in vitro*. Antihistamine drugs inhibit the production of acute anaphylactic shock, and likewise if a sensitised animal is depleted of histamine by the administration of a histamine-releasing agent like compound 48/80, it is protected temporarily.

5-Hydroxytryptamine (serotonin). This is present in the platelets of all species and in the mast cells of rats and mice. Its release may be important in anaphylaxis of these rodents. *Slow-reacting substance of anaphylaxis (SRS-A)*. If the lungs of a sensitised guinea-pig are perfused with a fluid containing antigen, histamine can be demonstrated in the fluid issuing at the beginning of the experiment. Alternatively, antigen can be added to lung chopped into small pieces. Later, another substance appears, which, when applied to isolated uterine muscle, causes a slow sustained contraction, unlike the more rapid "kick" produced by histamine.[10, 11] This substance is a lipid of unknown composition,[12] and might be responsible for the bronchospasm seen in man. Histamine is not so important in this connexion; histamine-releasing compounds given to humans cause pruritus, oedema of the face, and hypotension, but not bronchospasm.[13]

Kinins. There is evidence that kinin-forming enzymes are activated in anaphylactic shock.

If one compares the mediators of cytotropic anaphylaxis with those of acute inflammation, one is struck by the similarity of the factors involved. Indeed, the main reactions are very similar in both phenomena, for both are characterised by an increased vascular permeability. However, in our present state of knowledge it would be unwise to pursue the analogy too far.

Species variation. In addition to the species variation as regards the target cells and the nature of the mediator released, there is very considerable difference in the type of response and sensitivity of different species to these agents. Thus man and the guinea-pig are highly sensitive to histamine, while the mouse and rat are very insensitive. The reverse is true of serotonin. It is hardly surprising that the manifestations of anaphylaxis vary so greatly from one species to another (p. 176).

Protracted anaphylaxis. Although the manifestations of anaphylactic shock in the guinea-pig are very similar to those of histamine poisoning, antihistamine drugs do not completely counteract the shock. Indeed, when death in the acute phase is prevented, the animal sometimes dies of protracted shock some hours later. The cause of this syndrome of *protracted anaphylaxis* is not known, but it has been suggested that a continuing production of kinin is responsible. The animals show hypotension and hypothermia. At necropsy there is congestion of and haemorrhage into the abdominal viscera but no overinflation of the lungs. A similar prolonged anaphylaxis has been demonstrated when antigen is given to a sensitised animal by the intraperitoneal or subcutaneous route so that its absorption is delayed.

Aggregate Anaphylaxis[2]

The recognition of this type of anaphylaxis was based on various observations which were contrary to what would be expected in the classical anaphylaxis of the guinea-pig. In the rabbit the sensitivity to anaphylactic shock is proportional to the level of plasma antibody; a high level does not confer immunity. Passive transfer in this species is best accomplished by injecting a large dose of antibody, and the sensitisation is immediate, indicating that cell fixation is not a prerequisite. Furthermore, complement is required, and sensitisation to shock can be abolished by depleting the animal of complement, e.g. by injecting zymosan.

Aggregate anaphylaxis is a type III reaction, and the damaging antigen-antibody complexes are produced in the circulating blood. Precipitates are formed, and the complement system is activated. Anaphytatoxins are produced, and they lead to the release of histamine from mast cells. C567 component causes polymorphs to join the aggregates, and these can be seen in the circulation. They plug the capillaries in many organs, but more important than the mechanical interference with the circulation is the liberation of their damaging lysosomal contents.

Antibodies Concerned in Anaphylaxis[2]

All animals so far examined produce at least two types of antibody, and it seems likely that further investigation will reveal an even greater heterogeneity. Nevertheless, the antibodies may be divided into two groups: the *cytotropic antibodies*, which are responsible for cytotropic anaphylaxis, and a second group responsible for *aggregate anaphylaxis*.

Cytotropic anaphylaxis antibodies. In the guinea-pig and the mouse the important antibody is a 7S, γ_1 or fast γ-globulin. It is thermostable and will sensitise animals of the same species to cytotropic anaphylaxis. This type of antibody is therefore called a *homocytotropic antibody*, and a similar type of immunoglobulin is produced in other species. In man the important antibody concerned in anaphylaxis is thermolabile, and is a IgE immunoglobulin. It is generally called a *reagin*, and is non-precipitating. It has the unusual property of *firm, long-lasting fixation to skin*, and on this property the

Prauznitz-Küstner reaction is based (p. 180). It cannot be detected in serum by the commonly used *in-vitro* tests, but can be recognised and measured by highly sensitive methods such as the radio-immuno-inhibition technique and by the use of living cells (p. 180).

Aggregate anaphylaxis antibody. This is a γ_2 or slow γ-globulin which acts as a precipitin and can *fix complement*. It can passively sensitise an animal of the same species to aggregate anaphylaxis. A confusing facet of this subject is that this antibody, when injected into an animal of a *different species*, will sometimes sensitise it to cytotropic anaphylaxis. The latter type of anaphylaxis is therefore called *hetero-cytotropic anaphylaxis.*

Conclusion

The precise manifestation of anaphylaxis exhibited by an actively sensitised individual depends upon the relative proportions of the various sensitising antibodies which are produced. It is probable that all commonly used laboratory animals can manufacture antibodies for both cytotropic and aggregate anaphylaxis, but that preference is often shown for one of them. Thus, γ_1-globulin predominates in the guinea-pig, γ_2-globulin in the rabbit, and IgE-reaginic antibody in man.

Anaphylactoid shock.[14] A condition very like anaphylactic shock can be produced by the intravenous injection of the following substances:

1. Antigen-antibody mixtures—especially those with moderate antigen excess.[15–17] This in fact is a type of aggregate anaphylaxis.

2. Serum which has been incubated with kaolin, starch, and other polysaccharides—this procedure leads to the formation of kinins and anaphylatoxin[3] by the activation of complement *via* the alternate pathway.

3. Forssman antibody. Some writers refer to this as an example of "cytotoxic anaphylaxis". It is a type II reaction.

4. Trypsin. This leads to the formation of kinin.

5. Peptone.

6. Salts of heavy metals.

DUST AND FOOD HYPERSENSITIVITY AND ATOPY[25]

This group of hypersensitivity reactions occurs after the ingestion of certain foods and the inhalation of antigens like pollen and dust. The symptoms differ according to the route of absorption, and there is considerable variation from one person to the next. The offending chemical may be a complete antigen or a hapten: the latter presumably combines with tissue or plasma proteins to produce a complete antigen.

Types. *Inhalation* of antigens like pollen, horse dander, and dust, usually produces symptoms referable to the respiratory tract, e.g. allergic rhinitis, hay-fever, and asthma of the extrinsic type.

Ingested substances produce either gastro-intestinal symp-toms or skin eruptions. Shellfish, mushrooms, strawberries, and milk are among the numerous foods to which some people are sensitive.

Nature of the lesions. The lesions are exudative, and frequently contain eosinophils. The appearance of these cells in the secretions in hay-fever and asthma is of diagnostic value. Blood eosinophilia may also be conspicuous, but its significance is unknown. It will be recalled that eosinophils are also present in many parasitic diseases, in which allergic manifestations are often prominent. Eosinophils are not, however, a feature of atopic dermatitis.

Characteristics. *Genetic influence.*[26] Patients with this type of hypersensitivity frequently give a family history of similar complaints. The pattern of reaction differs in members of the same family; one may have hay-fever, another asthma, and another atopic dermatitis. What is inherited is the capacity to react to antigens in this peculiar way. The antigens involved may vary, because they are presumably determined by environmental factors. Nevertheless, families are on record in which there has been a constantly recurring response, e.g. hypersensitivity to a particular food.

Hypersensitivity in which there is a strong hereditary element and expressed in hay-fever, asthma, and atopic dermatitis, is called *atopy*. The basis for this may be an overproduction of sensitising IgE, perhaps accompanied by a deficiency of IgA, IgG, or IgM.[27] Thus atopy is often a feature of immunological deficiency states, e.g. the Wiskott-Aldrich syndrome, IgA deficiency, and Bruton's agammaglobulinaemia.

Sensitisation. Previous contact with either antigen or hapten is necessary, but as only small quantities are needed, the event may be forgotten. Nurses who spill streptomycin on their fingers may react with skin eruptions to subsequent injections of the drug; they would, however, deny any previous streptomycin treatment.

Detection. A scratch test or intradermal injection with the antigen produces an immediate-type reaction with a weal appearing in a minute or two. This occurs whether the hypersensitivity is of respiratory, alimentary, or cutaneous type. Haptens may not produce a positive test until they are first conjugated with protein. Some, e.g. aspirin, produce a reaction if applied to the buccal mucous membrane or the tongue.

Skin testing is of limited value in atopic patients. Such individuals tend to make sensitising IgE against many antigens, and it is often impossible to decide which of the positive results is of significance in relation to the current illness.

The sensitivity shown by some individuals is extreme.[28] Thus the active antigens in the grass pollens are polypeptide or protein carbohydrate substances of low molecular weight, and doses of the order of $10^{-7}\gamma$ to $10^{-8}\gamma$ are sufficient to elicit and intradermal reaction in a sensitive person; 10 000 times this dose given intravenously can be fatal.

Passive transfer. Although for a long time antibodies could not be detected in the serum by the ordinary *in-vitro* techniques, serum will passively sensitise a normal person. This was first demonstrated by Prausnitz and Küstner.

Prausnitz-Küstner (P-K) reaction. Küstner was hypersensitive to cooked fish. Some of his serum was injected into Prausnitz's skin, and after 24 hours this area responded to the local injection of an extract of cooked fish by the immediate formation of a weal. The ingestion of fish was also capable of eliciting an urticarial reaction in the local area. This passive hypersensitivity remained for weeks, but was dissipated after eliciting the P-K reaction. The P-K test is still performed, but is inconvenient and exposes the test subject to the danger of virus hepatitis. Monkeys may be used, but they are now more scarce than humans!

Reagins.[29] The antibodies detected by the P-K reaction are called reagins. They have a strong affinity for human and monkey skin but not that of other species. A reliable *in-vitro* method of detecting reagins would be of great value in the investigation and treatment of patients with hypersensitivity, and many techniques, none of them very satisfactory, have been devised. Thus in ragweed-sensitive people it is found that the addition of antigen to the patient's white cells leads to the release of histamine.[3, 30] Chopped human lung can be sensitised passively *in vitro* so that, on addition of antigen, histamine and SRS-A are released. This release can be inhibited by β-adrenergic drugs such as adrenaline, and the action has been ascribed to an increase in the cell's content of cyclic AMP. α-Adrenergic stimulation has the reverse effect.[31] A rather similar observation is that the basophils of penicillin-sensitive patients show degranulation when mixed with the drug.[32] Monkey ileum can be sensitised with human reagin and can be used in a Schultz-Dale reaction.

Another method is the exposure of the patient's serum to red cells to which antigen has been attached. Reagin coats the cells but, being an incomplete antibody, causes no agglutination. Addition of anti-human IgE globulin causes agglutination. In this way the IgE levels in the blood may be measured, and the results in one group of patients (exposed to castorbean extract) with asthma correlated well with the clinical state and with the level of reagin as measured by passive cutaneous anaphylaxis using the baboon.[33] IgE protein obtained from a patient with myeloma will specifically inhibit the P-K reaction, presumably by competing with reagin.[34] Indeed, there seems little doubt that human reaginic antibody is a IgE immunoglobulin, and that the level of this antibody is raised in asthma, hay-fever, and atopic eczema.[35]

Desensitisation in man. Very small doses of antigen administered at 30-minute intervals may be given without the occurrence of anaphylactic shock. Fixed antibody is steadily neutralised, but the desensitisation is of temporary duration and the method is not recommended for it may be followed by accelerated serum sickness (see also p. 234).

Antigen administered in weekly doses of increasing size confers some degree of desensitisation. This method is used in hay-fever and asthma, but the results are not uniformly satisfactory. The mechanism involves the production of excess antibody, some of which is of the blocking type. This type of antibody, when injected into a P-K prepared site, will desensitise the skin so that the antigen no longer provokes the response, i.e. it "blocks" the reaction. This it does by competition for antigen. The degree of hypersensitivity which an individual exhibits may thus be related to the relative proportions of heat-labile sensitising reagin and heat-stable blocking antibody.[36]

As previously pointed out, the hypersensitivity under consideration is of the immediate type. Histamine and a slow-reacting substance are probably released. Antihistamines counteract the vascular effects, but, as would be expected, not the bronchial muscle spasm (see p. 178). Cortisone, however, has the reverse effect, and finds an important place in the treatment of asthma.

Infection

Immediate-type hypersensitivity to microbial products may develop during the course of an infection. Thus, during convalescence from lobar pneumonia, an injection of the capsular polysaccharide (SSS) of the causative organism into the skin produces an immediate-type reaction (weal). The Casoni test is a similar reaction, and is used in the diagnosis of hydatid disease. Whether this type of sensitisation plays any part in the pathogenesis of lobar pneumonia is not known (see p. 224).

HYPERSENSITIVITY MEDIATED BY ANTIBODY-ANTIGEN COMPLEXES

The Arthus phenomenon: This can be demonstrated both in man and animals. Repeated weekly subcutaneous injections of antigen even into different areas lead to progressively more severe local reactions. Oedema and erythema appear within one hour, and over the next few hours haemorrhage and necrosis develop. Microscopically, there is an acute inflammatory reaction with a massive accumulation of polymorphs both within the vessels and their walls. Necrosis of the vessel wall leads to haemorrhage, and completes the picture of an acute vasculitis.

Pathogenesis. The interaction of antigen with antibody in the vessel walls leads to the formation of complexes which activate complement and leads to the accumulation of polymorphs. Antigen, antibody, and complement can be detected in the vessel walls by immunofluorescent techniques and electron microscopy. The polymorphs release their lysosomal enzymes, and the damage produced leads to an increase in vascular permeability and the tissue necrosis. There is no evidence that histamine is a mediator, nor do antihistamine drugs inhibit the reaction. The Arthus reaction cannot be elicited in an animal depleted of polymorphs, nor in one depleted of complement by the prior administration of zymosan or the venom of the cobra *Naja naja*.

The antibody concerned in the Arthus reaction is a precipitating IgG immunoglobulin. Passive transfer (passive

Arthus reaction) can be demonstrated by the intravenous injection of antibody, e.g. 10 mg in the rabbit. This large dose contrasts with the much smaller quantities required to transfer sensitivity to anaphylaxis of either the cytotropic or the aggregate type. No latent period is required, and there is no cell fixation.

This explanation is supported by the phenomenon of the *reversed passive Arthus reaction*. This is demonstrated when a local injection of antibody (obtained from a sensitised animal) is introduced into the skin of a normal animal, which is then given a large intravenous dose of corresponding antigen. Thus, an Arthus-type reaction can be produced whenever antigen and appropriate complement-fixing antibody meet in the vessel wall.

SERUM SICKNESS[1]

Serum sickness differs from most other forms of hypersensitivity response in that only one dose of antigen is necessary to produce it. It usually appears between the 7th and 14th day after the administration of a foreign protein, e.g. therapeutic serum of horse origin. The reaction may be accelerated, appearing after 3 or 4 days, in patients who have had serum previously; occasionally it may occur immediately. The main features are fever and a skin eruption which is sometimes first apparent at the site of injection. A generalised urticarial or morbilliform eruption is frequently seen. The skin lesions often cause intense irritation. Other features are generalised lymphadenopathy, joint pains, oedema of the eyelids and dependent parts, albuminuria, and early leucopenia followed by leucocytosis. Increased vascular permeability accounts for many of the signs of the disease. Polymorphonuclear leucocytes leave the circulation, and can be found in the oedema fluid.

Experimental production. A single large injection of foreign protein in a rabbit produces a disease with lesions similar to those described in the few fatal cases of human serum sickness. By using ^{131}I-labelled antigen the following sequence of events may be observed (Fig. 14.1):

1. There is an immediate drop in the blood level of antigen due to equilibration with extravascular, extracellular fluids.

2. During the first 10 days the blood level of antigen is high, but shows a slow progressive fall because of its metabolism.

3. From the 10th to 13th day antigen is rapidly metabolised, and by the 13th day none is present in the circulation. This rapid disappearance of antigen is called *immune catabolism*. During this period even the antigen which is still present in the blood is bound to antibody, and fluorescent techniques have demonstrated that soluble antigen-antibody complex is also found in the affected inflamed arteries.

4. From the 13th to 14th day the disease abates, all antigen is eliminated, and precipitating antibodies appear in the blood.

On the basis of these observations the following mechanism is postulated: the disease is caused by persistence of circulating antigen which reacts with newly-formed antibody. As only one exposure to antigen is given, the delay of 7 to 14 days is easily explicable in that this is the usual time-interval for antibody production after a primary injection. The damaging antigen-antibody reaction occurs in certain tissues, but when once the antigen is combined with antibody, it is rapidly metabolised. The disease is therefore self-limiting. Finally excess antibody is produced, and appears in the circulation.

Antigen-antibody complexes are formed in the circulation and are deposited in the vessel walls. As in the Arthus reaction, complement is fixed, polymorphs accumulate and

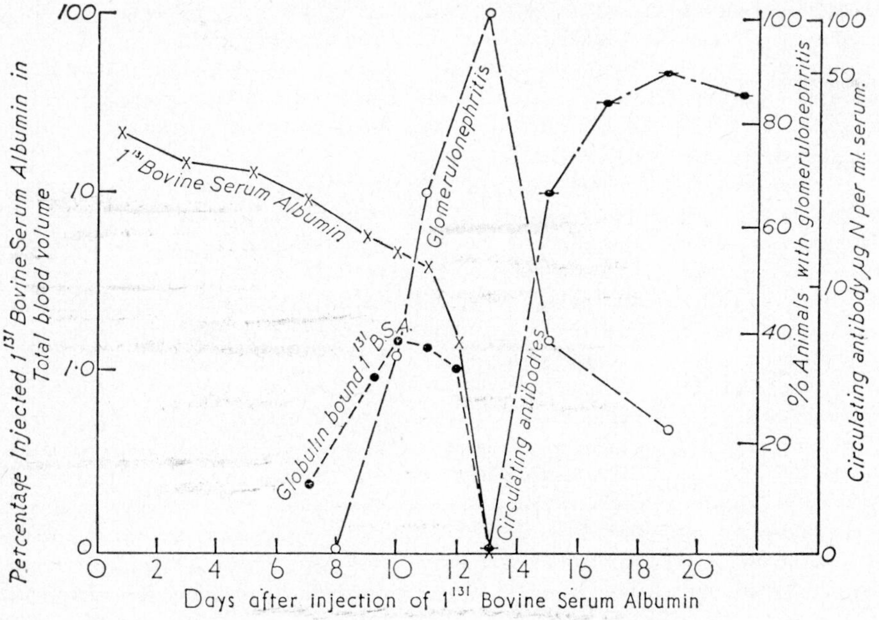

Figure 14.1
Time relations between fall of circulating antigen, formation of antigen-antibody complexes, lesions of serum sickness, and rise of circulating antibody in rabbits injected with large doses of ^{131}I-labelled bovine serum albumin. *(From Gladstone G. P. (1961) in Florey, H. W.* General Pathology, 3rd edn., *after Dixon, F. J. et al. (1959) in Lawrence, H. S.* Cellular and Humoral Aspects of the Hypersensitive States, p. 354. *New York: Harper and Row)*

release their enzymes, and tissue damage results. An acute vasculitis is the characteristic lesion and is seen in many organs, for instance the skin and heart. The development of these lesions can be prevented by the prior depletion of complement or polymorphs. Another characteristic lesion of experimental serum sickness is glomerulonephritis; immune complexes are deposited in the glomerular basement membrane as granular deposits. There is a proliferation of glomerular cells but, unlike the other vascular lesions, polymorphs do not accumulate. Increased vascular permeability accounts for the proteinuria.

The deposition of antigen-antibody complexes in the vessel wall is probably due to a local increase in vascular permeability mediated by histamine. Antihistamine drugs therefore inhibit the development of the lesions of acute serum sickness. In the rabbit it is believed that the histamine is derived from platelets which adhere to the complexes by the process of immune adherence (p. 148). An alternative explanation is that leucocytes sensitised by specific IgE release soluble factors when acted upon by antigen. The factors cause the clumping of platelets and the release of histamine and serotonin.[18] Whatever the mechanism, a local increase in vascular permeability appears to be the important event which localises the lesions of serum sickness.

The pathogenesis of the Arthus reaction and acute serum sickness both involve the formation of immune complexes which initiate complement activation and result in vascular damage. They are conveniently grouped together under the term *immune-complex disease*, and it is instructive to consider some other examples at this point.

Chronic immune-complex disease. If daily injections of antigen are given to animals in doses such that antigen-antibody complexes with antigen excess are formed in the blood, a chronic glomerulonephritis develops. Histologically there is thickening of the basement membrane (membranous change), and fluorescent studies reveal a coarsely granular deposit containing antigen, antibody, and complement. This "lumpy-bumpy" deposit can be located electromicroscopically on the epithelial side of the basement membrane. The pathogenesis is similar to that of acute serum sickness, but the dominant lesion is renal—a localisation which is not explained. It appears that the kidneys are readily damaged by circulating immune complexes; this mechanism may be the explanation of the renal component of many diseases, particularly those associated with a chronic infection (often viral) and in individuals with a defective immune response, e.g. the *glomerulonephritis* of lupus erythematosus, post-streptococcal nephritis, NZB and NZB/NZW mice, Aleutian mink disease, and lymphocytic choriomeningitis[19] of mice.

Other organs may be affected. After the use of killed measles vaccine a natural infection with measles can cause an excessive *lung lesion* due to immune complexes:[20] a similar response can be seen with respiratory-syncytial-virus infection.[21] *Immune-complex arthritis*[22] may occur with virus hepatitis, especially in association with Australia antigen.

Polyarthritis, urticaria, and angio-oedema are the main features of this syndrome, which has also been noted with other virus diseases, e.g. rubella, mumps, vaccinia, and variola.

Some Clinical Examples of Hypersensitivity mediated by Immunoglobulins

In clinical practice it sometimes happens that hypersensitivity reactions are mediated by several mechanisms, commonly a combination of type I and type III responses. Two subjects will be described: drug hypersensitivity and allergic lung disease.

Drug Hypersensitivity[23, 62]

Hypersensitivity to drugs is a common clinical event and is due to the drug, or one of its degradation products, acting as a hapten and stimulating the formation of sensitising antibodies. Virtually any drug can produce a reaction, but common offenders are penicillin,[63] sulphonamides, aspirin, para-aminosalicylic acid (PAS), barbiturates, and quinine. Relatively few people given a drug manifest hypersensitivity, and the tendency to do so is probably inherited. Thus atopic individuals are particularly at risk especially in respect of IgE-mediated effects.

Types of drug reaction. The reaction may be *immediate*: if the drug is given by injection it can occur within a few minutes. Urticaria is common and in more severe cases laryngeal oedema, asthma, hypotension, and death complete the features of acute anaphylaxis. Immediate reactions are due to the formation of sensitising IgE antibodies.

Later drug reactions begin several days after the administration of the drug and have the features of immune-complex disease. Urticarial, morbilliform, petechial, and other types of skin eruptions are common, and the addition of arthralgia, renal damage, and fever produce a disease resembling serum sickness. Sometimes the eruption is fairly specific, e.g. that produced by ampicillin especially in patients with infectious mononucleosis.[24] In other cases individual features may occur alone, e.g. renal damage, drug fever, or acute vasculitis of the skin. Antibodies concerned in these reactions are either IgG or IgM.

Late drug effects are thrombocytopenia (p. 619), haemolytic anaemia (p. 594), erythema multiforme (which if severe and affecting the mucous membranes is called the Stevens-Johnson syndrome), cholestatic jaundice, and a syndrome resembling systemic lupus erythematosus. The pathogenesis of many of these effects is obscure. In some instances, e.g. haemolytic anaemia, cytotoxic antibodies are present (type II reaction); they may be directed against the drug as in penicillin-induced haemolytic anaemia, or against the red-cell surface antigens, an effect induced by α-methyldopa (p. 594).

Detection of drug sensitisation. With most drugs it is not possible to detect sensitisation other than by giving a test dose. The sensitivity to penicillin has been the most studied. Benzylpenicillin is broken down to several products. The major component forms a benzylpenicilloyl haptenic group which appears to be unimportant, because not only does it induce the formation of IgE antibodies but also IgG blocking ones. A minor breakdown product is benzyl penamaldic acid mixed disulphide group which acts as a hapten for the formation of sensitising IgE only. It is possible to perform skin tests using these components, but the test itself can lead to sensitisation. This may be avoided by using a reagent composed of the haptenic group attached to a small synthetic polypeptide. Nevertheless, skin tests detect only IgE sensitising antibody, and do not eliminate the possibility of the presence of IgG or IgM, which can lead to immune-complex effects. Skin testing is therefore not a routine clinical procedure. *In-vitro* tests are described below.

Allergic Lung Disease[64–66]

Lung tissue is constantly confronted with airborne, antigens, and it is not surprising that allergic disease is common. Several patterns of reaction can be found:

The extrinsic type of bronchial asthma. This is a component of atopy and is a type I reaction mediated by IgE. It has been described above.

External allergic alveolitis. This disease is due to the inhalation of fine particles of organic material and the subsequent development of precipitin, IgG, sensitising antibodies. The later exposure to the same dust results in an immune-complex reaction in the alveoli (type III reaction). Clinically there is a sudden onset of fever, headache, dyspnoea, and cough coming on 4–6 hours after exposure. The lung compliance is decreased and the pulmonary defect is restrictive in contrast to the airways obstruction of bronchial asthma. The best known example of external allergic alveolitis is *farmer's lung*; the antigen is derived from fungal spores in mouldy hay. Many other examples are known and are related to occupation, habit, or hobby. The antigen can be fungal (baggassosis and malt-worker's lung) or of insect or animal origin (bird fancier's lung, pituitary-snuff taker's lung, etc.).

Asthma with pulmonary infiltrates and eosinophilia. This is a mixed group and is mediated by a combination of types I and III hypersensitivity. The term Loeffler's syndrome has been applied but this is not a defined entity. Some cases are due to parasites. *Broncho-pulmonary aspergillosis* is due to colonisation of cavities or bronchi by *Aspergillus fumigatus* and the development of sensitising IgE and IgG. Skin tests reveal an immediate reaction followed later by an Arthus type response.

There are other types of lung disease in which an allergic basis has been postulated with varying degrees of conviction. Thus there is Goodpasture's syndrome (type II reaction) and the various forms of pulmonary vasculitis (see p. 213).

DELAYED-TYPE HYPERSENSITIVITY[37–39]

As the main features and pathogenesis of anaphylactic and immune-complex hypersensitivity became clarified, it

became evident that there also existed a separate, completely distinct type of hypersensitivity. Its recognition stemmed from the early observations of Robert Koch on the effects of tuberculous infection in guinea-pigs. Since similar reactions were noted in other infections the term *bacterial allergy* was applied. However, the term is not appropriate because immediate-type hypersensitivity may also be induced by bacteria. **Delayed-type** is a more acceptable term, and it can occur not only as the result of infection but also as a response to antigens of non-bacterial origin. **Cell-mediated hypersensitivity** is another term which is commonly used to describe these reactions, since it is currently believed that they are mediated by the activity of cellular antibodies. The term is useful in that certain immune-complex reactions which are related to humoral antibodies may take many hours to develop, and therefore difficult to distinguish if the classification is based strictly on the time taken for the reaction to appear. In this book the terms delayed-type, cell-mediated, and type IV reactions are used synonymously. The subject is most easily understood by first considering Koch's observations.

The Koch Phenomenon

If tubercle bacilli are injected into a normal guinea-pig, there is an incubation period of 10 to 14 days followed by the appearance of a nodule at the site of injection. Ulceration follows and persists till the death of the animal. The bacilli spread to the local lymph nodes, finally reach the blood stream, and produce generalised miliary tuberculosis and death. The injection of tubercle bacilli into an animal infected 4 to 6 weeks previously evokes a different type of response. A nodule appears in 1 to 2 days, ulcerates, and then heals. There is little tendency to spread to the local lymph nodes. This second type of response was described by Koch, and it should be noted that the reaction of a tuberculous animal to tubercle bacilli differs from that of a normal one in three important respects:

1. The incubation period is greatly shortened—this may be described as hypersensitivity.

2. The lesion heals quickly.

3. There is no spread. These are the features of immunity.

The heightened tissue response of the tuberculous animal can be demonstrated not only to the living tubercle bacillus, but also to dead organisms and extracts of organism. Koch originally used "old tuberculin", but more recently a Purified Protein Derivative (PPD) has been introduced.

The injection of a small quantity of PPD into a normal animal results in a negligible inflammatory response. In the tuberculous animal, however, there develops a raised erythematous lesion **appearing within 24 hours and reaching a peak by 72 hours.** This is the *Mantoux test*, and a positive result indicates the existence of hypersensitivity to tuberculoprotein. The delay in the appearance of the reaction is noteworthy, and contrasts with the rapid appearance of anaphylactic reactions. The injection of a larger quantity of PPD into a tuberculous animal may result in a flare-up of the tuberculosis lesion. Attempts to "immunise" patients may therefore do more harm than good.

Tuberculin shock. Injection of a relatively large dose of PPD into a highly sensitised animal will produce a systemic reaction characterised by prostration, hypothermia, and death within 30 hours. Inhalation of an aerosol can have the same effect.

Although tuberculoprotein is capable of eliciting the Mantoux reaction in a sensitised subject, it does not induce this delayed type of hypersensitivity. It is antigenic, but its use as a sensitising agent results in the development of immediate-type hypersensitivity.

Under natural conditions bacterial allergy occurs only as a result of infection with the organism. A conversion from Mantoux-negative to positive during the course of an undiagnosed illness is therefore good evidence of its tuberculous aetiology. If the infection is completely eradicated the test may, over a period of years, revert to negative. Nevertheless, the Mantoux test is of great importance clinically because a positive reaction indicates a past or present tuberculous infection.

Delayed-Type Hypersensitivity in Other Infections

Hypersensitivity reactions akin to the Mantoux test are of diagnostic value in other infections, and indicate the existence of sensitisation. The following tests may be cited: Frei (lymphogranuloma venereum), coccidioidin (coccidioidomycosis), histoplasmin (histoplasmosis), and blastomycin (blastomycosis).

The injection of lepromin elicits a tuberculin-like reaction at 24–48 hours (Fernandez reaction), and a more significant papular lesion which develops in about four weeks (Mitsuda). The lepromin test is negative in lepromatous leprosy and positive in the tuberculoid type* as well as in many non-lepers. Hypersensitivity to Candida antigen, mumps antigen, streptokinase, streptodornase, and trichophytin is very common in normal people. A negative response to these, and to tuberculin and coccidioidin in California, indicates an abnormal state (see anergy, p. 142).

It seems certain that this type of hypersensitivity develops in many chronic infections, and indeed plays an important part in the production of the lesions. Even in acute infections delayed-type hypersensitivity may occur. Thus, following lobar pneumonia a delayed-type skin reaction can be demonstrated by injecting the specific pneumococcal protein. Delayed-type hypersensitivity to antigens of infective agents is seen after recovery from many, if not all, virus infections. This aspect is further discussed in other parts of this book (see lobar pneumonia, p. 224, syphilis, p. 253, typhoid, p. 93, and smallpox, p. 279).

* The Mantoux test may also be positive, and the two mycobacteria concerned appear to have antigens in common. BCG vaccination has been advocated in leprosy prophylaxis.

Features of Delayed-Type Hypersensitivity

Active induction. Delayed-type hypersensitivity may be induced in man or animals by the following methods:

Infection. This has been described above.

Injection of antigen with adjuvants. Delayed-type hypersensitivity develops if antigen is injected together with Freund's complete adjuvant (p. 141). The essential component of the tubercle bacillus appears to be a high-molecular-weight mycoside, termed Wax D. The explanation of this observation is not known, but there is some evidence to suggest that the local tissue response to the injection is of some importance. If a simple antigen, e.g. egg albumin, is injected into a tuberculous focus in an animal, both immediate and delayed-type hypersensitivities develop to the egg protein.

Application of simple chemicals to skin. Hydrophobic compounds are most effective since they penetrate the skin more readily than do hydrophilic substances. Detergents aid absorption and, therefore, sensitisation. Sensitisation by skin application, e.g. of picryl chloride, dinitrochlorobenzene, and 2-ethoxymethylene-5-oxazolone (oxazolone),[40] have been used extensively in animal experimental work (p. 154). In man many agents lead to allergic contact dermatitis (p. 186).

Tissue grafting. See Chapter 15.

Time of appearance of reaction. The reaction is not visible before 12 hours and is maximal at 24–72 hours. Injected antigen finds no antibody with which to interact and there is no immediate reaction. The reaction is dependent upon an intact blood supply to the part, and presumably sensitised cells, lymphocytes and macrophages, are brought to the site. The stimulus for this emigration is not known, but one may suppose that the cells accumulate slowly and that this is the explanation of the delay which is typical of all cell-mediated hypersensitivity responses.

Type of tissue response.[37] An early acute inflammatory response with oedema and polymorph infiltration is soon followed by an accumulation of macrophages, lymphocytes, sometimes eosinophils and mast cells, and later epithelioid cells and giant cells. The predominant reaction is mononuclear in contrast to the exudative response of anaphylaxis and the polymorph accumulation of the immune-complex reaction. In severe reactions necrosis is prominent.

Inhibition of reaction. Glucocorticosteroid administration inhibits delayed-type responses, but the effect is non-specific since many inflammatory responses are also affected. The effect is temporary and reactivity returns on withdrawing the drug. Antihistamine drugs produce no inhibition.

Specificity. With few exceptions, the delayed-type hypersensitivity responses are even more specific than the usual serological and immediate-type reactions. When hapten-protein conjugates are used, the sensitisation is directed against both the hapten and the carrier protein.

Tolerance. Delayed-type hypersensitivity cannot be induced in animals rendered tolerant by the procedures listed on p. 142. A curious feature noted in guinea-pigs is that animals given picryl chloride by gastric tube, to avoid contact with skin, are permanently tolerant to this chemical, so that subsequent application to the skin does not produce sensitisation. The mechanism is not understood.

Passive transfer. Although antibodies of precipitating, agglutinating, and complement-fixing types can be found in the serum, they are not causally related to the hypersensitivity. An injection of these immunoglobulins into a normal animal does not passively transfer the state of hypersensitivity. This contrasts markedly with the immediate-type sensitisation which is transferable by serum. It seems certain that immunoglobulins are not concerned, and this is supported by the observation that patients with agamma-globulinaemia can become Mantoux-positive, although they are virtually incapable of forming immunoglobulin antibodies.

Delayed-type hypersensitivity can be transferred to another animal by transferring living cells. Intraperitoneal injections of splenic or lymph-gland cells from a tuberculous animal will confer passive hypersensitivity. There is no appreciable latent period, and the hypersensitivity lasts for as long as the grafted cells survive, e.g. months if syngeneic cells are used. Passive transfer has been reported in guinea-pigs using serum from irradiated sensitised donors.[41] It is postulated that a cell-bound factor can be released into the circulation by the irradiation.

The mechanism whereby transferred lymphocytes render the host hypersensitive is poorly understood. One possibility is that the specific sensitised lymphocytes accumulate selectively at the site of antigen administration, and are therefore responsible for the positive reaction. By labelling lymphocytes with tritiated thymidine in the donor the fate of injected cells can be followed. Results are contradictory—some workers claim that donor cells accumulate specifically at the site of a skin test,[42] while others maintain that the majority of cells are of host origin.[43-45] The latter is almost certainly correct and supported by the following experimental observation: if lymphocytes from an immunised host are injected into an x-irradiated animal, immunoglobulin antibody formation can be detected[46] (see adoptive immunity, p. 165). The transferred cells do not, however, support the transfer of delayed-type hypersensitivity,[47] indicating that host cells are necessary. These results apply to animals; in man host cells are certainly involved, for the injection of small numbers of white cells from the blood of a sensitised person (e.g. 0·1–0·5 ml of a concentrate) will transfer hypersensitivity of bacterial, fungal, viral, and contact dermatitis types. This passively induced, delayed-type hypersensitivity is generalised, appears within 24 hours, and lasts for many months. Furthermore, in contrast to the findings in animals, transfer can be effected by extracts of white cells. The nature of the agent, called the *transfer factor*, is not known. It is unaffected by deoxyribonuclease,[48] and appears to be dialysable, stable on prolonged storage, and has a molecular weight of less than 10 000. A possibility which has not been ruled out is that the transfer factor is RNA with an attached fragment of the original antigen.

Antibody involved. There are two theories:

Serum antibody. It has been suggested that delayed-type hypersensitivity is, like other immune phenomena, mediated by serum antibodies, and that since passive transfer by serum cannot be demonstrated, the antibodies must be in very low concentration and of high avidity.[49] Alternatively the antibodies might be of a special class (*cytophilic antibody*) such that they have a high affinity for lymphocytes and macrophages. Another variant of this theory is that antibody is produced locally by lymphocytes when stimulated by antigen. The antibody reacts locally, and does not appear in detectable amounts in the serum. It seems unlikely that any of these explanations is true.[50]

Cellular antibody. The alternative and currently accepted hypothesis is that the antibody concerned in delayed-type hypersensitivity is entirely *cell-bound*.[51] This theory is attractive in that it explains the failure of serum transfer, and also that it presupposes the existence of a completely separate type of antibody. The unsolved mystery of the transfer factor certainly indicates that the mechanisms involved in delayed-type hypersensitivity are separate from those related to immunoglobulin production. So also do the effects of thymectomy and bursectomy (pp. 150–1).

In spite of the potent effects exhibited by sensitised lymphocytes *in vivo*, the manner by which they produce tissue damage is poorly understood. As described on page 149, when T-lymphocytes come into contact with specific antigen, a number of potent low-molecular-weight factors called lymphokines are liberated.[67] Insofar as cell-mediated hypersensitivity is concerned, lymphotoxin is probably the most important, but the other factors may recruit cells and augment the inflammatory reaction. In practice, the most useful *in-vitro* test has been one that measures the migratory inhibitory factor.[52]

This can be demonstrated by packing the lymphocytes and macrophages from the peritoneal exudate of a sensitised guinea-pig into a capillary tube and incubating it in a suitable chamber containing culture fluid. Normally the cells migrate from the free ends of the tube to form tufts. These tufts do not appear if the cells from a guinea-pig showing delayed-type hypersensitivity are incubated in the presence of antigen (Fig. 14.2). If cells from a normal animal, mixed with about 10 per cent of cells from a sensitised one, are placed in a tube and cultured in the presence of antigen, *none* of the cells migrate. Hence a few sensitised cells can transfer information to other cells *in vitro*, just as they can *in vivo*. It should be noted that lymphocytes from an animal sensitised towards immunoglobulin production and not delayed hypersensitivity do not show this phenomenon.

The effect of antigen on sensitised human cells can be assessed by using white blood cells from the buffy coat. If these are packed into capillary tubes as described above, their

Figure 14.2
Specific inhibition by antigen of the migration of cells from sensitised animals. The cells, mostly macrophages and lymphocytes from a peritoneal exudate, are placed in capillary tubes and incubated in a micro-chamber. Normally the macrophages migrate from the open end and produce a tufted appearance. The cells derived from animals with delayed-type hypersensitivity show no migration in the presence of the specific antigen. *(From David, J. R., Al-Askari, S., Lawrence, H. S. and Thomas, L.* (1964), J. Immunol., **93**, 264)

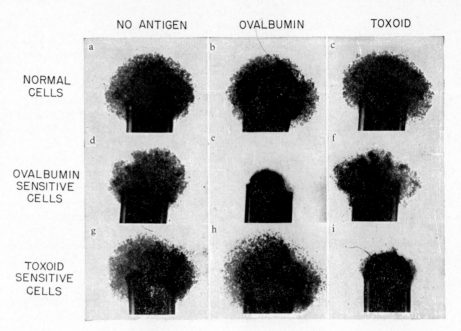

NO ANTIGEN   OVALBUMIN   TOXOID

NORMAL CELLS

OVALBUMIN SENSITIVE CELLS

TOXOID SENSITIVE CELLS

migration is inhibited by antigen to which the patient is sensitive.

Allergic Contact Dermatitis[53]

The occurrence of a localised dermatitis following the repeated exposure of the skin to a chemical is a frequent event. Sensitisation may occur to a wide variety of substances-tulips, primulas, poison ivy, wool, iodine, atropine, para-phenylenediamine (used as a hair dye), and nickel are common examples. The last is usually seen in women; cheap jewellery and the nickel-plated buckles of suspenders and brassières cause dermatitis where they come into contact with the skin.

Heredity is sometimes involved, but the liability to become hypersensitive is not related to atopy. The reaction is essentially local, and consists of intra-epidermal oedema with vesiculation and a dermal inflammatory reaction. The lesions are therefore dermatitic. The offending substance taken by mouth is harmless. Only direct application to the skin is effective.

Sensitisation can be detected by a *patch test*: the suspected agent is kept in contact with the skin for 24 hours, and a positive reaction is indicated by the appearance of swelling and redness about 24 hours later.

Performing a patch test is not without its disadvantages, for the test may itself induce hypersensitivity in persons not previously sensitive. Sometimes following a negative response a *flare reaction* occurs at the site of the test 10–20 days later. This is due to persistence of the antigen at the test site, and the mechanism is therefore analogous to that of serum sickness. The ability to develop hypersensitivity to dinitrochlorobenzene is used clinically to test the cell-mediated immune response.

The patch test can be demonstrated on any part of the body surface, and has the characteristics of delayed-type hypersensitivity. Passive transfer can be obtained only by injecting sensitised cells or transfer factor. The condition therefore closely resembles other cell-mediated reactions, except that the skin is the only tissue where this hypersensitivity is normally manifested.

The offending chemical probably acts as a hapten, and by combining with skin protein produces a potent antigen. A plausible explanation of the delayed-type hypersensitivity which develops is that this new antigen is in fact a living skin cell, and is therefore treated like a foreign graft. Once sensitisation has occurred, further application of the chemical to the skin results in the reformation of the abnormal cells, and therefore a "graft rejection" phenomenon occurs. An alternative but less satisfactory explanation is that lipids of the skin act as adjuvants in much the same way as perhaps the wax of tubercle bacillus.

It is interesting that atopic eczema of children, although generally linked with asthma, appears to be due to a delayed-type hypersensitivity. Indeed, it has been reported that lymphocytes from atopic patients sensitive to grass pollen, when cultured in the presence of specific antigen, show blast transformation and the formation of IgE antibody.[54, 55] The atopic diseases, although classified as examples of immediate hypersensitivity, are clearly complex and poorly understood. Since they are so common they are deserving of careful study.

Experimentally-Produced Autoimmune Disease

There is considerable evidence that autoimmune encephalomyelitis is cell mediated (see Chapter 16).

Homograft Rejection

The hypersensitivity which develops during the rejection of a homograft is of the delayed type. This is considered in Chapter 15.

The Retest Phenomenon[56]

If a positive tuberculin test is performed on a hypersensitive person, and the same site is retested with tuberculin at a later date, an accelerated reaction is observed. It appears at 2 hours and is maximal at 8 hours. The lesion is characterised by exudation of fluid and massive accumulation of eosinophils. Immediate-type hypersensitivity is not involved, but the mechanism concerned in the retest reaction is not known. Perhaps a specific chemotactic lymphokine for eosinophils is liberated[57] (p. 149). This phenomenon deserves further study, for eosinophils develop in response to repeated injections of antigen or antigen-antibody complexes, and many human diseases of an "allergic" nature are also characterised by exudation and eosinophil infiltration. These are curiously unresponsive to antihistamine drugs (e.g. asthma, allergic rhinitis, nasal polyps, etc.).

The Jones-Mote Reaction[58]

If repeated small doses of protein antigen are injected into the skin of guinea-pigs or man, a state of delayed-type hypersensitivity develops. This phase is usually transient and is soon replaced by Arthus-type hypersensitivity as immunoglobulins appear in the blood. It seems unlikely that this Jones-Mote type of delayed hypersensitivity is the same as the classical delayed type; the skin reactions tend to develop rather more quickly and to fade earlier. Histologically they are characterised by the accumulation of basophils, and the term *cutaneous basophil hypersensitivity* has been proposed.[59, 60] Its role in human pathology remains undetermined, but it may be related to the presence of basophils in some inflammatory lesions, e.g. in the lesions of allergic contact dermatitis.[61]

SUMMARY

It is evident that in response to antigenic stimulation the body is capable of reacting in a variety of ways. Antibodies are produced which have the effect of altering the individual's response to the same antigen should this substance be introduced on a subsequent occasion. The best-known antibodies are the immunoglobulins found in the plasma. These may neutralise toxins or aid in destroying micro-organisms and thereby confer immunity on the individual. Alternatively the immunoglobulins may lead to sensitisation of the immediate type. The difference between those antibodies which confer immunity and those which cause hypersensitivity appears to be qualitative rather than quantitative. The liability of an individual to produce sensitising antibodies is, to some extent at least, determined by genetic factors.

The role of the cell-bound type of antibody is more difficult to understand. The sensitised lymphocytes release factors which can kill cells and induce an inflammatory reaction. In particular the macrophages are affected, and they are more phagocytic to bacteria, and by remaining localised may be an important factor in the localisation of infection. Sensitised lymphocytes are responsible for the features of delayed-type hypersensitivity. It is not known whether immunity and delayed-type hypersensitivity are two aspects of one process or whether they are distinct and separable components of the cell-mediated immune response. At first sight the tissue destruction of allergic contact dermatitis or at the site of a positive Mantoux reaction may seem to be of no advantage to the individual. The process may be seen in a different light when it is remembered that cellular antibodies are usually produced against living cells (see p. 201). These cells may be foreign, as with bacteria and grafts, or they may be host cells altered by contact with chemicals or following degenerative or neoplastic changes. Destruction of these cells would be of great survival value to the individual. The value of immediate-type hypersensitivity is more difficult to see, but it is possible that the inflammatory reaction which results is of advantage in that cells and plasma are brought rapidly to the site of bacterial invasion. Nevertheless, of the two types of hypersensitivity the delayed type appears to be more closely related to immunity than does the immediate type.

REFERENCES

1. DAVIS, B. D., DULBECCO, R., EISEN, H. N., GINSBERG, H. S. and WOOD, W. B. (1967). *Microbiology*. New York: Harper and Row-Hoeber.
2. MIESCHER, P. A. and MUELLER-EBERHARD, H. J. (1968 and 1969). *Textbook of Immunopathology*, vols 1 and 2. New York and London: Grune and Stratton.
3. AUSTEN, K. F. and HUMPHREY, J. H. (1963). *Advances in Immunology*, **3**, 1.
4. LIACOPOULOS, P., HALPERN, B. N. and FRICK, O. L. (1963). *Journal of Immunology*, **90**, 165.
5. HALPERN, B. N., KY, T. and ROBERT, B. (1967). *Immunology*, **12**, 247.
6. Leading Article (1970). *Lancet*, ii, 1021.
7. OVARY, Z. (1964). In *Immunological Methods*, A C.I.O.M.S. Symposium, p. 259. Edited by J. F. Ackroyd. Oxford: Blackwell.
8. WEIR, D. M. (1963). In *Modern Trends in Immunology*, I, p. 77. Edited by R. Cruickshank. London: Butterworths.
9. BROCKLEHURST, W. E. (1968). In *Clinical Aspects of Immunology*, 2nd edn, p. 611. Edited by P. G. H. Gell and R. R. A. Coombs. Oxford: Blackwell.
10. BROCKLEHURST, W. E. (1962). *Progress in Allergy*, **6**, 539.
11. BROCKLEHURST, W. E. (1960). *Journal of Physiology*, **151**, 416.
12. BROCKLEHURST, W. E. (1963). *Biochemical Pharmacology*, **12**, 431.

13. LECOMTE, J. (1956). In *Histamine*, Ciba Foundation Symposium, p. 173. Edited by G. E. W. Wolstenholme and M. O'Connor. London: Churchill.
14. WILSON, G. S. and MILES, A. A. (1964). *Topley and Wilson's Principles of Bacteriology and Immunity*, 5th edn, p. 1402. London: Arnold.
15. WEIGLE, W. O. (1961). *Advances in Immunology*, **1**, 283.
16. DIXON, F. J. (1962). In *Mechanism of Cell and Tissue Damage Produced by Immune Reactions*, p. 71. Edited by P. Grabar and P. Miescher. Basle: Benno Schwabe.
17. CAMPBELL, D. H. (1962). p. 67, *ibid.*
18. COCHRANE, C. G. (1971). *Journal of Experimental Medicine*, **134**, 75S.
19. OLDSTONE, M. B. A. and DIXON, F. J. (1971). *Journal of Experimental Medicine*, **134**, 32S.
20. FULGINITI, V. A. *et al.* (1967). *Journal of the American Medical Association*, **202**, 1075.
21. CHANOCK, R. M. *et al.* (1968). *Perspectives in Virology*, **6**, 125.
22. KOFF, R. S. (1971). *New England Journal of Medicine*, **285**, 229.
23. LEVINE, B. B. (1968). *Annals of the New York Academy of Sciences*, **151**, 988.
24. Annotation (1969). *Lancet*, ii, 993.
25. Various Authors (1968). In *Clinical Aspects of Immunology*, pp. 633–59 and 693–755, *loc. cit.*
26. DE GARA, P. F. (1959). In *Mechanisms of Hypersensitivity*, p. 703. Edited by J. H. Shaffer, G. A. LoGrippo and M. W. Chase. London: Churchill.
27. KAUFMAN, H. S. and HOBBS, J. R. (1970). *Lancet*, ii, 1061.
28. RAFFEL, S. (1963). In *Modern Trends in Immunology*, p. 184, *loc. cit.*
29. Leading Article (1968). *Lancet*, ii, 1131.
30. STANWORTH, D. R. (1963). *Advances in Immunology*, **3**, 181.
31. ORANGE, R. P. AUSTIN, W. G. and AUSTEN, K. F. (1971). *Journal of Experimental Medicine*, **134**, 136S.
32. SHELLEY, W. B. (1963). *Journal of the American Medical Association*, **184**, 171.
33. COOMBS, R. R. A. *et al.* (1968). *Lancet*, i, 1115.
34. STANWORTH, D. R. *et al.* (1967). *Lancet*, ii, 330.
35. JOHANSSON, S. G. O. (1967). *Lancet*, ii, 951.
36. CHAN, P. C. Y. (1963). Ph.D. thesis, University of London, quoted in *Advances in Immunology* (1964). **4**, 335.
37. TURK, J. L. (1967). *Delayed Hypersensitivity*. Amsterdam: North Holland.
38. UHR, J. W. (1966). *Physiological Reviews*, **46**, 359.
39. CHASE, H. W. (1965). *Medical Clinics of North America*, **49**, 1613.
40. OORT, J. and TURK, J. L. (1965). *British Journal of Experimental Pathology*, **46**, 147.
41. DUPUY, J.-M., PEREY, D. Y. E. and GOOD, R. A. (1969). *Lancet*, i, 551.
42. NAJARIAN, J. S. and FELDMAN, J. D. (1961). *Journal of Experimental Medicine*, **114**, 779 and (1963), **117**, 775 and (1963), **118**, 341.
43. McCLUSKEY, R. T., BENACERRAF, B. and McCLUSKEY, J. W. (1963). *Journal of Immunology*, **90**, 466.
44. TURK, J. L. and OORT, J. (1963). *Immunology*, **6**, 140.
45. PRENDERGAST, R. A. (1964). *Journal of Experimental Medicine*, **119**, 377.
46. HARRIS, T. N. *et al.* (1954). *Journal of Experimental Medicine*, **100**, 289.
47. CUMMINGS, M. M. *et al.* (1955). *Journal of Immunology*, **74**, 142.
48. LAWRENCE, H. S. (1970). *New England Journal of Medicine*, **283**, 411.
49. KARUSH, F. and EISEN, H. N. (1962). *Science*, **136**, 1032.
50. SILVERSTEIN, A. M. and BOREK, F. (1966). *Journal of Immunology*, **96**, 953.
51. AMOS, B. and KOPROWSKI, H. (1963). (Eds) *Cell Bound Antibodies*. Philadelphia: Wistar Inst. Press.
52. DAVID, J. R. (1966). *Proceedings of the National Academy of Sciences of the United States of America*, **56**, 72.
53. CALNAN, C. D. (1968). In *Clinical Aspects of Immunology*, p. 756, *loc. cit.*
54. BROSTOFF, J., GREAVES, M. F. and ROITT, I. M. (1969). *Lancet*, i, 803.
55. WARD, P. A. (1971). *Journal of Experimental Medicine*, **134**, 109S.
56. ARNASON, B. G. and WAKSMAN, B. H. (1963). *Laboratory Investigation*, **12**, 737.
57. COHEN, S. and WARD, P. A. (1971). *Journal of Experimental Medicine*, **133**, 133.
58. JONES, T. D. and MOTE, J. R. (1934). *New England Journal of Medicine*, **210**, 120.
59. RICHERSON, H. B., DVORAK, H. F. and LESKOWITZ, S. (1969). *Journal of Immunology*, **103**, 1431.
60. RICHERSON, H. B. (1971). *Journal of Experimental Medicine*, **134**, 630.
61. DVORAK, H. F. and MIHM, M. C. (1972). *Journal of Experimental Medicine*, **135**, 235.
62. DASH, C. H. and JONES, H. E. H. (1972). *Mechanisms in Drug Allergy*, 208 pp. Edinburgh and London: Churchill Livingstone.
63. LEVINE, B. B. (1972). *New England Journal of Medicine*, **286**, 42.
64. McCOMBS, R. P. (1972). *New England Journal of Medicine*, **286**, 1186 and 1245.
65. Leading Article (1969). *Lancet*, i, 1195.
66. Leading Article (1970). *British Medical Journal*, i, 708.
67. Leading Article (1973). *Lancet*, **1**, 1490.

Chapter 15. The Graft Reaction

Having described the immunological response to bacteria and simple antigens, no study of immunity would be complete without including the body's response to complex living cells. This includes the allied subjects of graft immunity and autoimmunity.

TRANSPLANTATION OF TISSUES[1, 2]

Although it is usually assumed that the art of grafting is a modern one, it is interesting to note that it has been performed for over two thousand years. Local skin flaps were used by Indian surgeons for the operation of rhinoplasty, and

grafting has done much to extend our knowledge of the body's response to foreign tissues.

Classification of Transplants

The terms transplant and graft are used synonymously. They may be conveniently classified in the following ways[3]:

Species of origin. Grafts may be classified as autologous, homologous, or heterologous.

An autograft is a transplant made from one site to another site in the same individual.

A homograft is a transplant made from one individual to another of the same species. If the two individuals are

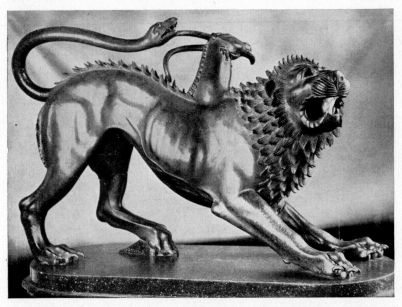

Figure 15.1
The Chimera, a mythical monster who dwelt in Lycia, was the terror of the neighbourhood, until she was killed by Bellerophon mounted on his winged steed, Pegasus.

> A mingled monster of no mortal kind:
> Behind, a dragon's fiery tail was spread,
> A goat's rough body bore a lion's head,
> Her pitchy nostrils flaky flames expire,
> Her gaping throat emits infernal fire.
>   Iliad, VI, 180.

Quoted in Precope, J. (1954), *Medicine, Magic and Mythology*, p. 160. London: Heinemann.
The term *chimera* is now used in medicine to describe an animal which for long periods contains living, viable cells belonging to another individual who is genetically different. The condition may arise naturally, as in the case of binovular twins sharing a common placenta, artificially by the immunological tolerance technique of Medawar, or by the induction of irradiation chimerism. *(Photograph of an Etruscan bronze provided by the director of The Archaeological Museum, Florence)*

the techniques were described by Celsus. During the fifteenth century the use of pedicle flaps was devised in Italy, but the practice fell into disrepute because of the opposition of surgeons and the Church. For nearly 300 years no further advance was made, until in 1794 two Army doctors stationed in India witnessed the operation of rhinoplasty performed by an Indian surgeon, and reintroduced the art into England. With the development of anaesthesia in the nineteenth century and the advent of two world wars in the twentieth century plastic surgery came into its own, and with it extensive transplantation of tissue. In addition to the practical value in surgery of transplantation of tissue, recent work on

syngeneic (isogeneic), i.e. of identical or nearly identical genetic structure, then the terms *isograft* or *syngeneic homograft* are used. In man this applies only to grafts from one identical twin to another. In all other instances, when the two individuals are of different genetic make-up, the terms *allograft* or *allogeneic homograft* are used. In practice the unqualified term homograft is generally taken to refer to the latter type of graft.

A xenograft, or *heterograft*, is a transplant from one animal to another of a different species.

Nature of the tissue transplanted. Tissue may be fetal, normal mature, or neoplastic. It may be transplanted directly from the donor, or there may be some intermediate period of storage or growth *in vitro*.

Viability of the graft. Those grafts whose function is dependent upon the continued survival of their cells are called *vital*. This contrasts with a *static* graft in which the cells die, but the matrix performs an important function, e.g. many bone grafts. Thus, one may have homovital and homostatic grafts if the material is derived from a member of the same species.

Method of grafting. Grafts are called free, when they are completely disconnected from the donor before subsequently being implanted in the host site. They may be grafted by means of pedicle transplants, in which case they remain partially attached to the donor's site for a while. In general such grafts are autologous, although homologous pedicle transplants have been tried, and are called parabiotic transplants.

A third manner of transplantation is by vascular anastomosis: the major blood vessels of the transplant are connected with those of the host at the time of operation. This method is used for transplanting kidney, liver, and heart.

Site of grafting. An *isotopic* graft is one which is placed in an anatomical position similar to that from which it came, e.g. the cornea to cornea. An *orthotopic* graft is one which is surrounded in the host by the same kind of tissue as that previously present in the donor, e.g. skin grafted from the leg to the arm. A *heterotopic* graft is one which is placed in a situation which differs from that of the donor site. An example of this is the transplantation of cornea to a subcutaneous situation.

For practical purposes the most important feature of any graft is its origin. Therefore it is convenient to subdivide grafts into the three main groups—autografts, homografts, and heterografts.

AUTOGRAFTS[1]

Autotransplantation, the transplantation of tissues from one site to another in the same individual, occurs spontaneously in a variety of conditions. It is a familiar feature of malignant tumours when they metastasise, but also occasionally occurs with some normal tissues. It is believed, for instance, that the cells of the haematopoietic tissues are capable of circulating in the blood and settling down in abnormal sites. Rupture of the spleen is occasionally followed by the implantation and growth of splenic tissue in the peritoneal cavity (*splenosis*).

Deliberate autotransplantation is frequently carried out surgically, and such grafts survive provided they once become established; the conditions necessary for this may be classified as follows:

Tissue must be healthy. Transplants do not survive if the tissue is subjected to undue mechanical or chemical trauma.

Freedom from infection. Sepsis effectively prevents vascularisation, and leads to rapid necrosis of the graft.

Adequate nutrition. In tissues which have a reasonably high oxygen requirement, large free transplants undergo central necrosis because vascularisation does not occur sufficiently fast to prevent death of tissue.

Hormonal stimulation. Free transplants of endocrine glands are more likely to be successful if the animal is deficient in that type of tissue. This is sometimes known as *Halsted's law*, but it is neither strictly true nor was it first described by him; it was noted in 1905 by Cristiani. It is not the deficiency of the endocrine secretion itself which stimulates the growth of the graft, but rather the excess of pituitary hormone which is attendant upon the deficiency.

Nervous stimulation. Muscle grafts, even when embryonic, die unless left attached to their nerve supply.

Mechanical stimulation. Bone grafts persist only if subjected to a mechanical stimulation. Heterotopic grafts in soft tissue tend to disappear.

Temperature. Free testicular grafts take only if placed in sites where the temperature is lower than that of the remainder of the body; thus in the rabbit testicular grafts can grow in the ears.

Other factors. Free autografts of pieces of kidney, liver, and pancreas may survive for a while, but always die later. The whole organs can be transplanted successfully if connected by vascular anastomosis.

FATE OF AUTOGRAFTS[1]

The body does not respond by any immunological mechanism, and provided the local conditions are satisfactory, most autografts survive. Avascular tissue, like cartilage and cornea, can live without vascularisation, but with all other grafts survival is dependent upon the acquisition of an adequate blood supply.

Vascularisation. It has long been debated whether the vessels which supply autografts are those of the original transplant, or whether they are new ones derived from the local site. It appears that vascularisation occurs in two phases. During the first three days new host capillaries develop and anastomose with the existing vessels of the graft. In this way rapid vascularisation is accomplished. During the second phase which occurs from the fourth day onwards, the graft is invaded by new host vessels. Some of these grow along the lumina of the original vessels of the graft. It seems fairly certain that the small capillaries of the graft persist, but that larger vessels, although they may develop a circulation during the first phase, do not long persist.

Tissue induction. The term *induction* is used to describe the changes which occur in one tissue as a result of the juxtaposition of other tissues. The best-known example is the ossification which is induced in connective tissue by heterotopic autotransplants of urinary-tract epithelium. It is also found that fascia used to suture bladder injuries may undergo ossification; gall-bladder epithelium has similar "osteogenic" properties.

Creeping substitution. This process, although not the same as induction, has many features in common with it. It is applied to the process whereby a graft is gradually replaced by host tissue. It is, for instance, believed that grafts of bone are steadily replaced by host bone. Similarly, nerves are invaded by axons from the host, and transplanted blood vessels appear to be steadily replaced by host tissue.

FUNCTIONS OF GRAFTS

Autografts usually function in exactly the same way as do normal tissues. However, skin and bone function only if transplanted orthotopically. The endocrine glands present certain special problems. If ovarian, testicular, and possibly thyroid tissue is transplanted into an area which is drained by the portal vein, their secretions are carried to the liver and inactivated. Although the graft may function normally, it fails to produce the expected, generalised hormonal effect. Although the anterior pituitary may survive if transplanted heterotopically, its function is retained only when it is placed under the median eminence of the tuber cinereum; only in this situation does it receive the necessary hormonal stimulation.

HOMOGRAFTS (ALLOGENEIC) [1,4]

Great interest is at present centred around the fate of homotransplants. There are two main reasons for this. In the first place, the potentialities of grafting tissue from one individual to another are of enormous practical importance. Secondly, the study of homograft reaction has revealed fundamental biological properties having far-reaching effects in all branches of medicine.

FATE OF HOMOGRAFTS

Homografts are usually rejected and three patterns may be recognised: 1. *Hyperacute rejection*, 2. *Acute rejection*, and 3. *Chronic rejection*.

Hyperacute rejection. [5] Free grafts are not vascularised, and the graft dies—see white graft reaction, p. 193. With transplants attached by vascular anastomosis, the graft vessels become obstructed by polymorphs and fibrin until the circulation through them ceases—see hyperacute renal rejection. Humoral antibodies are mainly responsible for hyperacute rejection.

Acute rejection. Free homografts become vascularised in much the same way as autografts. The graft, however, remains viable for only a limited period. This varies from about 8 days in mice to 13–14 days in rats and 2–3 weeks in man: rarely this period may extend to 6 weeks in the human subject. The first sign of rejection of a homograft is infiltration with lymphocytes and pyroninophilic cells, so called because their cytoplasm stains with pyronin due to the presence of many free ribosomes. These cells are of host

G.P.—7*

origin, and are almost certainly derived from small lymphocytes by transformation (p. 151). This is followed by stasis in the vessels of the graft, thrombosis both in the graft and the bed, haemorrhage, and oedema. Finally the whole graft becomes necrotic, and there follows an acute inflammatory response with an infiltration of polymorphs, which may include a large number of eosinophils. The graft is cast off if on the surface, while in the deeper parts of the body it is invaded by macrophages and granulation tissue.

The survival time of homografts is related to the size of the graft. Thus in rats small grafts may remain viable for 22 days, while large grafts survive only for 8 days. It is also worthy of note that where two grafts are applied to the same animal from the same donor, even though the grafts are of a different size, they are both rejected at the same time. These features all point to graft rejection involving an immunological mechanism. The cell-mediated response is the most important.

When the transplant is attached by a vascular anastomosis, the changes are similar. These have been studied most extensively by transplanting kidneys in dogs. It is found that the homotransplanted kidney begins to function within an hour or even less. During the next 3 or 4 days although the organ functions, it increases in weight and becomes swollen. The cortex is wider than normal and is somewhat nodular.

By the second to third day the cortex shows cellular infiltration with lymphocytes and pyroninophilic cells; later cells of the plasma-cell series appear. The kidney becomes oedematous, and vascular damage leads to a reduction in blood flow, tubular necrosis, and haemorrhage. In the terminal stages there is an inflammatory response with polymorph infiltration. The glomeruli tend to remain intact until quite late in the process.

The route by which graft antigen reaches the host immune mechanism varies. With skin grafts the presence of intact lymphatics at the host site is important—if these are blocked sensitisation is impeded. [6] With kidney grafts the lymphatics are not important, and activation of the immune response either depends on host cells passing through the kidney [7] or on the release of antigen into the plasma leaving the graft. [8]

Chronic rejection. The graft appears to be accepted, but its vessels gradually become obstructed by intimal thickening. This type of rejection has been most studied in patients with renal and heart transplants.

Factors Which May Determine Long Survival of Homotransplants

Although homotransplants are usually rejected as described above, there are conditions under which the graft may survive for a long period. These are best divided into three groups.

1. Factors which affect the graft itself. Certain tissues are found to behave differently and to be capable of long survival.
2. Grafts in certain situations behave differently.

3. Condition of the recipient may alter the fate of the graft.

SPECIAL PROPERTIES OF CERTAIN TISSUES

Normal tissues. *Cartilage.* Homotransplants of cartilage may remain intact with viable cells for months or even years. It is found also that grafts of dead cartilage may remain intact for very long periods. The reason for this long survival is not known, but is presumed to be related to its peculiar composition. It is suggested that its avascularity may play a part, but this explanation is hardly convincing when it is remembered that epidermis is also avascular and yet rapidly rejected.

Cornea. Homotransplants of cornea remain intact only if grafted isotopically—that is to say, into the eye. Heterotopic transplants are rapidly destroyed. Isotopic grafts of cornea may go cloudy prior to their rejection. Those, however, which do not behave in this way may remain clear and functional for a long time. It is found that when a successful corneal graft is applied to an animal, and some 2–6 weeks later a skin graft is applied from the same donor, not only is the skin graft rejected, but at the same time the cornea becomes opaque and is rejected. It therefore appears that the cornea grafted isotopically is nevertheless vulnerable to the rejection mechanism that can be evoked by skin grafting.

It is, however, found that if the skin graft from the same donor as that from which the cornea is obtained is applied 6 weeks or more after the corneal graft, it has no effect on that graft. It would therefore seem that in the rabbit the corneal graft is in danger only during the first 6 weeks, but thereafter is protected from any immunological mechanism which may subsequently be elicited. The explanations offered are:

(*a*) the graft becomes walled off by fibrous tissue;

(*b*) the graft is steadily replaced by host cells or at least its epithelial and endothelial component;

(*c*) the graft undergoes a change known as *adaptation*, in which it is presumed that the foreign cells are gradually modified to become more acceptable to the mechanisms of the host.

Ovary. There is a vast literature on the results of homo-transplanting ovarian tissue; it appears that occasional grafts may survive permanently, or more probably that occasional grafts may survive for a long time. It seems certain that ovarian grafts remain viable longer than do skin grafts.[9, 10]

Tissues from embryos and immature individuals. It is generally stated that fetal tissues grow better and survive longer than do normal mature tissues, but there is much conflicting evidence. There seems little doubt that in the anterior chamber of the eye fetal tissue does grow better. Such a transplant may increase in size 1 000 times, while a normal adult tissue increases only three times.

Neoplastic tissue. Under some circumstances there is no doubt that homotransplants of tumours can grow quite easily. A good example of this is the Brown-Pearce carcinoma of rabbits.

TRANSPLANTATION TO SPECIAL SITES

Anterior chamber of the eye. It is well known that transplants grow particularly well in the anterior chamber of the eye. Medawar has shown that in the rabbit homografts survive indefinitely in this situation, so long as they are not vascularised. Woodruff,[1] on the other hand, has demonstrated survival and vascularisation of homotransplants of thyroid tissue in the guinea-pig. Fetal tissue may also grow well in the anterior chamber and become vascularised. The actual results of transplanting tissue into the anterior chamber of the eye therefore depend largely upon the species involved and the tissue which is transplanted.

In general it appears that grafts in the anterior chamber excite a slow immune response, that is, slow as compared with grafts placed in other situations. Any immunity already present as the result of previous grafting is made manifest also in the anterior chamber. In addition, it seems likely that the first few weeks in the anterior chamber are critical for the graft. If it survives this period, it is capable of withstanding any immune response. It can even be removed from the anterior chamber and placed in another site, and still grow. This is another good example of a graft showing adaptation.

Brain. Brain, and to a lesser extent testis, kidney, and uterus, are sites where homotransplants seem to survive longer than elsewhere.

FACTORS CONCERNING THE HOST

The antigenic compatibility between graft and host is the single most important factor in determining the fate of a graft. The antigens concerned are the *transplantation antigens*, and are considered on p. 194. Since the antigens are determined by *histocompatibility genes*, it follows that the genetic compatibility between graft and host is important. Thus a graft from one identical twin to another (syngeneic homograft, or isograft) excites no immune response and is treated as an autograft. It is also found that with highly inbred strains of animals, tissues may be freely interchanged between individuals. An exception to this is that in certain strains of mice, grafts donated from males to females die. This is sometimes known as the *Eichwald and Silmser effect*,[11] and is due to a histocompatibility gene on the Y chromosome.

Constitutional abnormalities of the host. A variety of conditions may cause prolonged survival of homografts.

Immunological deficiency syndromes. The graft rejection mechanism is impaired in the syndromes described on pp. 171 to 173, in which the thymus-dependent system is affected; of the acquired conditions, Hodgkin's disease is the best documented.

Uraemia. It is well known that kidney and skin transplants last longer in uraemic patients.

Pregnancy. Pregnant animals seem more tolerant to homotransplants (see also p. 196).

Experimental procedures. Experimental procedures

including specific immunological tolerance are described later (see pp. 195–6).

HOMOGRAFT IMMUNITY

If following the rejection of a homograft another graft is applied to the same animal from the same donor, this second graft is rejected even more rapidly. This is known as the *second set phenomenon.*

The application of a second skin graft within a short time (about 12 days) of the rejection of the first results in the *white graft reaction*: the graft is not vascularised, but becomes pale, undergoes necrosis, and is cast off. If the second graft is applied after a longer interval, it shows early vascularisation, but suddenly by the fourth to fifth day it becomes cyanosed and the surrounding skin shows marked erythema and oedema. The vessels thrombose and the graft undergoes necrosis. This is termed the *accelerated graft rejection phenomenon*. At the same time the site of the original graft becomes inflamed (*recall flare*) due, it is thought, to persistence of graft antigen.

The same type of rapid rejection has been shown to occur with kidney transplants. If a second kidney from the same donor is grafted into a dog, it begins to secrete urine like the first kidney, but the flow diminishes after 12 hours and stops completely after 24 hours. Histologically there is severe tubular damage with haemorrhage, oedema, and fibrinoid material in the glomeruli. It should be noted that skin grafts will immunise an animal against kidney and *vice versa*.

The leucocytes of the blood are also capable of causing immunisation against skin, and appear to act much more rapidly than do skin grafts. Thus, if white cells are given intraperitoneally, a state of immunity rapidly develops. If white cells are injected intraperitoneally at the same time as skin is grafted, it is found that the skin graft is rejected much more rapidly than a first graft ought to be. This is easily explained by the fact that the injection of leucocytes causes the rapid development of a state of immunity.

It is not difficult to show that the second set rejection phenomenon is dependent upon the development of an immunological reaction. Both humoral and cellular factors have been implicated, and it is instructive to examine the evidence on which the various hypotheses have been based.

Humoral Factors[12]

Following the rejection of a first skin graft there appear in the blood stream a variety of immunoglobulins. Some are capable of agglutinating the red cells of the donor and are therefore called *haemagglutinins*. Haemolysins, leucocytic agglutinins, complement-fixing antibodies, and precipitins, have all been described. Factors have also been found in the plasma which are toxic to donor cells grown in tissue culture.

Attempts to transfer the state of immunity to another animal by the injection of serum have not generally been successful, and confirmatory evidence that immunoglobulins

were not important in causing graft rejection came from diffusion-chamber experiments. These chambers are composed of a Millipore membrane of a porosity chosen to allow the inward diffusion of soluble substances but to prevent the entry of host cells. Homografts enclosed in such a chamber and placed in the peritoneal cavity of an incompatible host were found to survive even in animals previously immunised.[13] These results have been challenged on the grounds that the pores of the chamber do not allow antibodies and complement to penetrate easily. Furthermore, it has been found that some grafts, usually of tumour tissue, can be destroyed within a diffusion chamber.[14]

It is evident that the immunoglobulins play some role in the rejection of certain grafts under certain circumstances. The following factors are concerned[15]:

1. The amount of transplantation antigen on the cell surface. Cells with a large amount combine with a large amount of antibody, activate complement, and are thereby lysed. Cells with little antigen are protected against complement lysis.

2. The complement-fixation properties of the antibody involved.

3. Physical factors; thus the injection of antibodies in and around a graft can lead to its rejection.[16, 17] Likewise dissociated cells are more readily killed than are solid grafts. The hyperacute rejection in both skin and kidney is mediated by humoral antibodies, and they may also play some part in chronic rejection.

Immunoglobulins sometimes have a second and quite opposite effect on a graft: the life of the graft is sometimes prolonged in an animal which has been passively immunised. This phenomenon is known as *enhancement*.[18, 19] Two mechanisms at least are involved.[15]

1. The antibody may combine with antigenic sites without harming the graft by activating complement. By covering the sites, the immune response is inhibited by blocking the *afferent* pathway so that complement-fixing and cellular antibodies are not produced.

2. The immunoglobulin may compete with immune lymphocytes for the receptor sites on the graft cells. Since immunoglobulin formation will continue, the state of enhancement can be self-perpetuating.

The phenomenon of graft enhancement has a simile with infection by the tubercle bacillus. The preliminary immunisation of an animal with tuberculoprotein interferes with the development of delayed tuberculin reactivity induced by the administration of BCG.[20]

Cellular Factors[21]

As the relationship between immunity and humoral antibodies is complex, it was not unnatural that cellular factors should be considered. There is much evidence to show that the type of immunity is cell mediated and indeed, the state of immunity to grafts can be passively transferred by the conveyance of lymphoid tissue from an immune animal to a normal one which is syngeneic (*adoptive immunity*). If animals sensitised to a graft are injected intradermally with cells or extracts of cells from the donor strain, an inflammatory reaction akin to the tuberculin reaction ensues. A similar reaction is seen if lymphocytes from the sensitised host are injected into an animal of the donor strain. This is called the *transfer reaction*, and may be regarded as a local graft-versus-host reaction. This occurs only if the animal's own lymphocytes are active, and it can be abolished by prior irradiation.

Passive transfer of homograft immunity can be performed by an intravenous injection of lymphocytes prepared from the regional lymph nodes and spleen of an animal which has rejected a graft. If the transferred cells are suitably labelled, they can be found in the lymph nodes and spleen of the recipient (see Fig. 15.2). They do not, however, appear

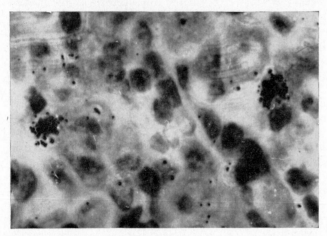

Figure 15.2
Passive transfer of homograft immunity. A guinea-pig sensitised to an allograft was given injections of tritiated thymidine to label its dividing cells. The animal was then killed, and a suspension of regional lymph node and splenic cells prepared. About 20 per cent of the cells were found to be labelled. The suspension was injected into a normal guinea-pig and 24 hours later this animal was killed and autoradiographs prepared. This section of lymph node shows two heavily labelled lymphocytes. ×1 000. (*From a slide of Dr. J. S. Najarian. See Najarian, J. S. (1962), Plastic and Reconstructive Surgery, 30, 359*)

preferentially in a graft when the animal is challenged even though the graft is rapidly rejected. Adoptive immunity of this type cannot be induced in an animal if it has been irradiated previously. Host cells are essential, and it seems that the injected sensitised lymphocytes alter the host's own lymphocytes. Such a transfer of information from sensitised to non-sensitised lymphocyte can also be demonstrated *in vitro* as with the transfer factor of delayed-type hypersensitivity.

There seems little doubt that small lymphocytes are capable of causing the rejection of a graft. Thus, if a tolerant animal with an established graft is injected with syngeneic small lymphocytes from either a normal or a previously

immunised animal, the graft is promptly rejected. If the antibodies which cause the accelerated graft rejection are closely associated with the lymphoid series of cells, it is curious that these cells are not always in evidence histologically. The accelerated reaction is characterised by vascular damage and necrosis. The explanation of this is not at all clear.

Antigens concerned.[4] The antigens in tissue grafts which are responsible for the development of homograft immunity are termed the transplantation antigens. They are associated almost entirely with the cell membrane and are of lipoprotein nature, but they have not yet been isolated with any degree of purity.

The transplantation antigens are determined genetically. In the mouse 15 separate loci have been identified, and are designated H-1, H-2, etc. Of these the H-2 locus is the most important, for the antigens to which the genes give rise are capable of exciting a strong graft reaction. Thus skin exchanged between mice that differ only at the H-2 locus is rejected in about 10 days, whereas with differences at the H-1 locus the range of survival of the grafts is 32–91 days. At least 20 alleles are recognised at the H-2 locus.

In man the transplantation antigens are determined by a number of genes situated at independent loci. However, only one of these is of great importance, and this consists of a complex of linked genes at two regions of the chromosome termed segregants, or sub-loci. As with the Rh system, there is no crossing over between these linked genes, and many alleles are known. The antigens determined by this gene complex are termed the *HL-A antigens*, and over 30 have been identified. In contrast with the mouse H-2 antigens, those of the HL-A system do not occur on the red cells; haemagglutinins are not produced, and it is difficult to investigate them since cellular antibodies must be studied (see below).

Distribution of Antigens.[22] Transplantation antigens appear to be present in all nucleated cells of the body, but the quantity varies from one tissue to the next. Thus some tissues, e.g. skin and spleen, are rich in antigens, while others are poor, e.g. aorta, muscle, and fat. Liver and lung occupy an intermediate position.

Identification of transplantation antigens. As noted previously, the white cells contain transplantation antigens, and these have been used extensively in attempts to identify human T antigens. Multiparous women and patients who have had numerous transfusions of whole blood or who have rejected grafts have anti-leucocytic antibodies in their serum. Two types of test have been employed to detect them:

Leucoagglutination test. The antibodies detected in this test are capable of agglutinating the leucocytes of some individuals. Unfortunately the test has several technical drawbacks, and the cells utilised must be fresh—no reliable method has yet been devised for preserving them. Donors must therefore be bled for each testing session.

Cytotoxicity test.[23] The antibodies detected in this test are capable of activating complement and killing lymphocytes. This is detected by the uptake of supravital stain or by changes seen on phase-contrast microscopy. Lymphocytes can be stored at the temperature of liquid nitrogen, and cells from one donor can be utilised when required and sent to other laboratories for their use.

These two methods are in current use, and by suitable absorption methods specific antisera have been prepared. The supply of these is very limited, and for each purified serum the actual specificity is not known. A sample of "specific" serum can have antibodies against several antigens, but by extensive computer analysis it has been possible to define fairly clearly more than 20 leucoagglutinins.

Conclusions. The pathogenesis of homograft rejection is still poorly understood. As with bacterial immunity both humoral and cellular factors have been implicated, but their relative importance differs according to the particular circumstances. It may well transpire that, as in bacterial immunity, cellular and humoral factors work hand in hand. It has for instance been found in tumour transplantation work that normal macrophages can be so changed by the addition of specific immunoglobulins that they are enabled to phagocytose tumour cells.[24] They thus behave in the same manner as do the macrophages of an immune animal. It is evident that much careful work has yet to be done before the problems of transplantation immunity can be solved.

Experimental Procedures Which Affect Behaviour in Homografts

Procedures affecting primarily the host. *Total body irradiation.* Although total body irradiation impairs the body's capacity to form antibodies to bacterial toxins and red cells, its effects on grafts are more complex. Total body irradiation does indeed prolong the life of a primary homograft. It does not, however, seem to affect the survival time of second set grafts even though the lymphocyte count is much reduced.

Cytotoxic chemicals. Nitrogen mustards and aminopterin are said to be without effect on the life of homografts. But, other drugs, e.g. azathioprine, are being used clinically for their effect on the survival of kidney and other transplants (see pp. 142 and 198).

Lymphocyte depletion by chronic thoracic-duct drainage impairs the rejection of first set homografts in rats.[25]

Antilymphocytic serum, see p. 142.

Reticulo-endothelial blockade. The results obtained by RE blockade are somewhat conflicting, but most workers claim that blockade does prolong graft survival. Most of this work has, however, been done on transplantable tumours, e.g. Brown-Pearce carcinoma in rabbits.

Glucocorticosteroids. While these can prolong the life of homografts in some animals, there is much species variation. Steroids, e.g. prednisone, are used in man in transplant work (pp. 198–9).

Enhancement. This has been described on p. 193.

Procedures affecting the transplant. Procedures designed to alter the antigenicity of the transplant with a view to prolonging its life have been largely unsuccessful.

Specific Immunological Tolerance of Homotransplants[26]

The acceptance of foreign tissue by immature animals has been known to experimental embryologists for many years. The grafting of parts of one embryo on to another was carried out without realising its more general biological significance. In 1948–49 Burnet and Fenner[27, 28] predicted that immature animals would be capable of accepting foreign tissues. They postulated that the tissues of an animal and their breakdown products possessed "self-markers", which were recognisable to its reticulo-endothelial system. In this way animals did not make antibodies against their own tissue components. These workers further postulated that the capacity to learn to recognise these "self-markers" is present only during embryonic and early post-natal life. The presentation of foreign antigens to a developing embryo could therefore be expected to lead to their being recognised as "self" throughout the rest of the life of the individual. Owen,[29] in 1945, described red-cell chimerism in cattle. This condition results when binovular twins share a common placenta. The blood cells from each twin are shared, and each is born with two sets of red cells. It has since been shown that the state may exist throughout life, due to the fact that each twin has accepted and become tolerant to the erythrocyte-forming tissue of its fellow. This type of chimerism has been described in cattle, lambs, and chickens, and several instances are on record of its occurrence in man.[30–32]

However, the fundamental significance of these facts was not fully realised until 1952, when Medawar showed that red-cell chimeras could also exchange skin grafts. It was later shown that they also exchanged kidney grafts. Then Medawar and his colleagues, Billingham and Brent,[33] undertook a series of experiments upon which our understanding of immune tolerance is based. In their early experiments they injected mouse embryos of CBA strain with cells of the testis, kidney, and spleen from mice of strain A. The injection of this mixture of cells was given with a fine needle inserted through the abdominal wall, after an incision had been made into the skin of the pregnant CBA mice. Many of the embryos survived this injection, and were subsequently born as normal mice which were then allowed to grow up. When 8 weeks old they were challenged with skin grafts from strain A mice, and it was found that these grafts behaved like autotransplants, i.e. they survived. This experiment clearly demonstrated the existence of a specific immune tolerance, which developed in response to intra-uterine contact with foreign cells.

Further experiments have shown that the injection of foreign cells into young animals, e.g. the rat, at birth may also induce tolerance. Cortisone treatment does not interfere with the development of tolerance; in fact it permits tolerance to be induced for up to two weeks when given from the time of birth onwards. A direct proof that tolerance is acquired during early life has been provided by an ingenious experiment performed on the tree frog *Hyla regilla*.[34] The buccal part of the pituitary was removed from an embryo, maintained in culture, and later replaced in the same animal when it had attained maturity. There was a typical homograft reaction to the implant, which was not seen when only a part of the buccal pituitary was removed beforehand.

It should be noted that immunological tolerance is not an all-or-nothing affair. There are varying degrees of tolerance, and these are manifested as gradations of prolongation of graft survival. When fully developed, tolerance is attended by the permanent survival of homografts.

Maternally-induced tolerance. It has been suggested that maternal cells enter the fetal circulation, and the fetus should therefore be tolerant to maternal tissue. Although it is known that this may occasionally happen, it does not seem likely that it is a common event. It may, however, explain the occasional case in which grafts from a mother have been accepted by her child.

Induction of Tolerance after the Development of Immunological Maturity

Enhancement.[18, 19] The growth of tumour homografts may be enhanced by the prior injection of killed cells of the prospective donor. This effect is probably due to the formation of haemagglutinins. The effect is much less marked when normal tissue is used as a graft.

The survival of skin grafts in rabbits may be prolonged by a previous intravenous injection of a suspension of dissociated epidermal cells of the donor (Billingham-Sparrow phenomenon).[1, 35] A second graft may survive even longer than the first. The explanation of these findings is not clear, but this is probably related to enhancement.

Induction of tolerance after irradiation. It is known that total body irradiation of lethal dose will inhibit the immune response. Under these circumstances the injection of foreign bone-marrow cells, either homografts or heterografts, results in the repopulation of the bone marrow with foreign cells. The animal may survive in this state for some time, and can accept grafts, e.g. skin grafts, from the same donor as the marrow cells. Frequently, however, these *x-ray chimeras*, as they are called, die of *secondary disease*, a condition which closely resembles runt disease and is due to a GVH reaction (see below).

The administration of cytotoxic drugs, see p. 195.

Pregnancy.[36, 37] It is a remarkable fact that pregnancy, even repeated, rarely causes the mother to react immunologically against her developing fetus. Furthermore, females pretreated with tissue antigens of the breeding male can have normal offspring. Although the pregnant female shows some immunological unreactivity, this non-specific effect is quite inadequate to provide the whole explanation. In some cross-matings the pregnant animals develop specific tolerance to the transplantation antigens of the fetuses. But this is not a general rule. The fetus itself develops transplantation antigens at an early stage of development, but the placenta, although of fetal origin, is antigenically inferior. The placenta is usually credited with some barrier function, but the nature of this is obscure. The popular concept is that the barrier is non-cellular and consists of the fibrinoid layer which covers the trophoblast, thereby preventing the cell-to-cell contact which is necessary for initiating the immune response.[38] Nevertheless, although fetal tissues, e.g. red cells, lymphocytes,[39] and trophoblast, often enter the maternal circulation, it is remarkable how little the mother reacts against them (see also Rhesus sensitisation, Chapter 52).

In summary, therefore, it must be accepted that the remarkable mutual forebearance exhibited between mother and fetus is not due to any one known mechanism. To describe it as multifactorial should not delude one into thinking that the subject is understood, nor deter the investigator from giving this phenomenon the attention it deserves.

The ease with which tolerance can be induced is therefore related to many factors. The antigenic differences between graft and host are very important. Thus, it is relatively easy to produce tolerance in mice when they differ at the H-1 or H-3 locus, but difficult when the difference lies at the H-2 locus. Tolerance is easier to induce in immature animals than in adults unless the immune response has been depressed. Large doses of antigen tend to produce tolerance, although the curious fact that very small quantities can do the same has been noted on p. 156. Finally, the route of administration plays a part, the intravenous route sometimes leading to tolerance when an intraperitoneal injection results in immunity.

Graft-Versus-Host Reaction

It was soon found that the injection of foreign cells into young or embryonic animals was not free from danger. Some died, and the percentage mortality varied considerably according to the exact circumstances of the experiment. In some instances the injected animals developed a disease which was characterised by wasting, atrophy of the lymphoid tissue, and a liability to intercurrent infection. The condition has come to be known as *runt disease*,[40–42] and is due to the graft cells reacting immunologically against the host. It is an example of a graft-versus-host (GVH) reaction, and occurs when the following conditions are fulfilled:

(1) If the host is tolerant of the grafted cells.

(2) If the graft cells are immunologically competent. Indeed, the ability to produce a GVH reaction can be used to assess immunological competence. Thus, adult small lymphocytes from the thoracic duct are effective.

(3) If the host contains antigens which are not present in the grafted cells and to which the grafted cells are not tolerant.

When the antigenic difference between the host and the graft is great, as when there is a difference at the H-2 locus in mice, there is a severe GVH reaction and the animals die. When the difference is slight the grafted animals may survive.

A local method of demonstrating a GVH reaction in guinea-pigs is to inject lymphocytes into the skin of an allogeneic host.[43] After 24–36 hours a reaction develops which resembles a positive Mantoux test. This test has been used as a means of selecting suitable donors for renal transplantation in man. Thus, if lymphocytes from the proposed recipient are injected into the skin of a panel of willing donors, the intensity of the reactions is a measure of the future reaction to the transplanted kidney. Although of great theoretical interest, this test, sometimes called the *normal lymphocyte transfer test*, presents obvious difficulties and dangers. Its value in predicting the fate of a graft in man has not been established, and tissue typing is more commonly used.

The pathogenesis of runt disease is not understood. It can be shown that the injected cells populate the host.[44] If small lymphocytes from the thoracic duct of a rat are injected into lethally irradiated mice, it can be shown that the mouse spleens contain many pyroninophilic cells of rat chromosomal type. By administering tritiated thymidine 12 hours before examination it is evident that most of these cells are synthesising DNA. Furthermore, 12 hours later the labelled cells are all small lymphocytes. This and other experiments[45] indicate that the small lymphocytes can change into pyroninophilic cells, divide, and produce small lymphocytes again. Nevertheless, the splenic enlargement which is a characteristic feature of runt disease is not only due to this effect, for there is considerable evidence that many of the proliferating cells are of host origin.[46] How the cells, whether of host or donor origin, produce the lesions of runt disease is not known.

GVH reactions in man. A GVH reaction is seen in man when allogeneic marrow is given after the heroic treatment of leukaemia with total body irradiation or with cytotoxic drugs. It can also follow the administration of fresh whole blood to cases of immunological deficiency (see p. 172). The reaction occurs even when the recipient and donor are siblings and compatible insofar as the HL-A antigens are concerned.[47] Salient features of the syndrome are wasting, anorexia, diarrhoea with malabsorption, exfoliative dermatitis, liver damage with jaundice, and an increased susceptibility to fungous and virus infections.

HETEROGRAFTS[1]

Heterotransplants are destroyed even more rapidly than are homotransplants. They are indeed treated like "second-set" homografts. There is no vascularisation, and the graft undergoes necrosis which stimulates an acute inflammatory reaction. The rejection certainly involves an immunological

mechanism, but there is no reason to assume that this is the only mechanism involved. The ultimate consequences of bringing together tissues of very dissimilar genetic constitution are not known and cannot be foreseen.[48]

Heterotransplants of living skin usually die within a few days, while cartilage may last for up to three weeks. Heterostatic grafts of cartilage may remain in the body much longer and, as with arteries, dead material is usually more satisfactory than is a fresh living graft.

Special sites. Tumour heterotransplants may grow in the anterior chamber of the eye, brain, testis, hamster cheek-pouch, and in the yolk-sac. Heterotransplants of embryonic

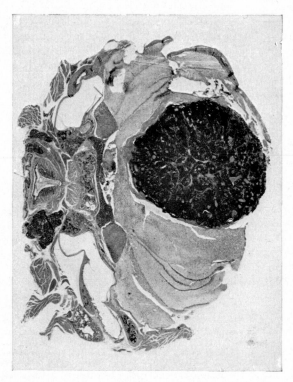

Figure 15.3
Coronal section through the head of a mouse which 66 days previously had been given an intracerebral inoculation of human oat-cell carcinoma of the lung. The heterotransplanted tumour showed active growth, and produced the large circular tumour mass which is here seen in section. ×9. (*From Chesterman, F. C. (1955), "Intracranial heterotransplantation of human tumours", Brit. J. Cancer, **9**, 51*)

tissue may also survive in these sites, but normal adult tissue does not usually do so.

Second set phenomena. Second grafts are probably destroyed even more quickly than are the first, but this is difficult to assess in view of the rapidity with which even first grafts are eliminated.

Antibodies concerned. Many antibodies have been identified in animals which have rejected heterotransplants. These include haemolysins and cytotoxic factors. They may be species-specific and sometimes even organ-specific. Immunoglobulins can in fact be present even in normal animals, and are perhaps induced by previous contact with heterophile antigens. Thus, many human sera contain lymphocytotoxic and haemagglutinating activity against sheep's cells and pig's cells.[49] It is worth noting that heterotransplants in diffusion chambers are killed in immunised animals. It is therefore probable that heterotransplant immunity is effected by humoral antibodies, but cellular antibodies have not been excluded.

Cortisone has been administered in the study of the heterotransplantability of tumours; human tumours may be grown in animals treated with cortisone. Total body x-irradiation has similarly been used. Animals subjected to total body irradiation of lethal dose may be made into red-cell chimeras as described in connexion with homografts. These heterograft chimeras will accept other grafts from the same donor, so long as the state of chimerism persists.

CLINICAL USE OF GRAFTS IN SPECIAL SITUATIONS[1, 2]

Grafting has now become an established procedure. With some tissues, e.g. heart valves and cornea, immediate rejection is not a problem, while with skin no practical means have been found to prevent it. With renal transplants a fair degree of success has been obtained; tissue matching and immunosuppressive therapy have played an important part in this, and no doubt the methods evolved will be applicable to the grafting of other organs, e.g. liver, lung, and heart, which is at present in an experimental stage. Renal grafts will therefore be considered in some detail.

RENAL TRANSPLANTATION[50-52]

Renal transplantation is now a common procedure, and a one-year survival time can be expected in over 50 per cent of cases if the donor is a living relative (and in 65–75 per cent of cases when the donor is a parent or sibling). With unrelated donors the figure is lower—about one third. With sibling grafts the results are much better when there is compatibility for the HL-A locus. How important compatibility is when the donor is not related is debated.[53] The risk of rejection is greatest during the first year, and few grafts fail after the second year; indeed, sepsis is then the problem. Grafted kidneys appear to exhibit adaptation, for when one is accepted, a subsequent kidney graft or skin graft from the same donor can be rejected and yet the original graft remains unaffected.

Renal Complications of Grafting

Acute tubular necrosis. This is liable to occur regardless of the origin of the kidney. It is due to the hypoxia sustained during the transfer of the organ from the donor to the patient.

Recurrence of the original renal disease. In patients with chronic glomerulonephritis the grafted kidney may develop the same disease. This is seen more frequently with syngeneic grafts, when no immunosuppressive drugs are given, than with allografts. Presumably the additional therapy prevents the development of the disease.

Rejection. *Hyperacute rejection.* This occurs immediately, and the kidney becomes swollen and congested. The vessels in the graft become blocked by fibrin and polymorphs. The reaction is due to major ABO incompatibility or the presence of immunoglobulin antibodies to the graft, e.g. following the rejection of a previous graft. The reaction is complement dependent. Antigen-antibody-complement complexes are deposited and lead to polymorph and platelet deposition in the vessels, as in the Arthus reaction (p. 180).

Acute rejection. This may occur at any time from days to months after the operation. The lesion is brought about by infiltrations of host lymphocytes reacting against the endothelium of the capillaries and venules situated around the tubules in the cortex. The capillary walls are disrupted with extravasations of blood in the interstitial tissue. The kidney shows infiltration by mononuclear cells (p. 191) and severe tubular damage. Fibrinoid necrosis may occur in the arterioles. Clinically there is fever, tenderness of the graft, a raised blood urea, and oliguria.

Chronic rejection. This occurs at any time after one year. One type of chronic rejection is due to platelet thrombi in the capillaries of the glomeruli; these can be rapidly reversed by glucocorticosteroids. A later type of chronic rejection is due to a lesion resembling membranous glomerulonephritis, and is caused by a deposit of IgM on the capillary walls. This is of linear deposition, as in Goodpasture's syndrome. It may be that the IgM forms against components of the basement membrane. Clinically there is proteinuria and progressively decreased renal function.

Non-Renal Complications

Infection is a constant danger in patients on immunosuppressive therapy, and may be due to a wide variety of opportunistic organisms. Various late syndromes have been described in patients with renal grafts—the symptoms include splenomegaly, fever, synovitis, and muscle pains. Pulmonary changes may occur ("transplantation lung"). It is not clear whether these syndromes are caused by an immunological reaction and comparable to Goodpasture's syndrome, or by an undetected infection, such as with *Pneumocystis carinii.*[54]

Immunosuppressive Therapy

The early attempts at immunosuppression utilised total body irradiation, but although some long-term survivors appeared, the risk of marrow aplasia was great, and the balance between survival of the patient and acceptance of the graft was too precarious. The method is therefore no longer used. 6-Mercaptopurine was introduced in 1959, and later replaced by the less toxic azathioprine ("Imuran"). This, together with steroids, is now the mainstay of therapy. Antilymphocytic serum is under study at some centres. In the experimental animal it greatly prolongs the life of homografts and heterografts. Its action seems to be directed against the mobile long-lived lymphocytes which recirculate through the lymph nodes.[55] Anti-thymus serum is reported as being superior in that it also abolishes the second set rejection.[56]

The administration of prednisone and actinomycin C, and the local irradiation of the graft are additional measures which are often instituted if signs of acute rejection occur.

An unfortunate effect of immunosuppressive therapy is an increased susceptibility to infection, e.g. cytomegalovirus and herpes simplex.[57] Nearly half the patients treated for over one year develop recurrent crops of warts.[58]

Another problem which accompanies immunosuppresive therapy is the development of malignant tumours.[59] A number of patients have developed a lymphoma within one year of grafting. There are several reports of malignancy present in the graft which has spread and killed the recipient of a renal transplant.[60] In one case where the kidney contained a secondary carcinoma of the lung, withdrawal of immunosuppressive therapy resulted in rejection of both the kidney and the carcinoma.[61] It seems possible that immunosuppression encourages the growth of tumour cells and that organ replacement with homografts is unlikely to be of value in the treatment of cancer.

Enhancement. This has been used experimentally as a means of preventing graft rejection. The animal may be given tissue antigen, or antibody can be administered passively.[62]

Tests of Tissue Compatibility

The following tests have been employed to assess the antigenic compatibility between graft and host.

ABO blood grouping. Success is unlikely if the donor blood group is not compatible with that of the host.

Normal lymphocyte transfer test (p. 197). One drawback of this test is that the lymphocytes of uraemic patients react poorly.

Mixed leucocyte culture. If donor and recipient lymphocytes are cultured together, both undergo transformation and division (p. 151). This may be measured by the uptake of tritiated thymidine. The test can be made one-way and more specific if the donor cells are treated with mitomycin C prior to mixing, so that only the recipient's reaction to the donor is measured. The test probably detects antigens determined by the HL-A locus, and about 25 per cent of siblings are compatible. Unrelated individuals are rarely compatible.

Detection of preformed serum antibodies in the recipient which are cytotoxic to the lymphocytes of the donor.

Tissue matching. Tissue typing has been described previously, and an attempt is made to match the donor and recipient as closely as possible. In general, it has been found that the best matches are obtained between siblings and that these give the best clinical results.[63] Antigenic matching of graft with host appears to be the most promising development in recent years. The techniques are, however, complex, and the supply of donor material erratic; there is no satisfactory way of preserving tissue. The organisation of a transplantation unit is now beyond the resources of a single hospital, and regional co-operation is essential.[64]

Bone[65]

Bone grafts have in the past been used to provide internal fixation, but advances in metallurgy have largely obviated this function. Grafts are now commonly used to provide a temporary scaffold to fill a cavity, to bridge the gap between an ununited fracture, or to fuse a joint in the operation of arthrodesis. Free grafts are unable to acquire a blood supply sufficiently fast to prevent necrosis of most of the bone cells. With fresh autografts some of the superficial osteocytes and the endosteal and periosteal osteoblasts may survive, but their contribution to the subsequent healing process is probably small. Blood vessels grow into the Haversian canals, and the bony matrix is slowly eroded by osteoclasts and subsequently replaced by living lamellar bone. With solid cortical bone grafts this process may take many months, but with cancellous bone the process is quicker; cancellous bone is therefore preferred. In addition to the slow replacement of the graft by this process of creeping substitution, the presence of the graft excites the formation of granulation tissue around it. This is derived from the vascular medullary cavity and to a lesser extent from the periosteum. The granulation tissue matures to form woven bone, and this is replaced by lamellar bone. Coincidentally, there is a general remodelling process as the area adapts to the local stresses to which it is exposed. It will be seen that a bone graft has an inductive effect on local tissues and can lead to the formation of new bone. This can occur even if the bone graft is embedded heterotopically in an extra-skeletal site.

In clinical practice *fresh autografts* are most satisfactory, and some of the osteogenic cells which take part in the incorporation process may be of graft origin. *Fresh homografts* excite an inflammatory reaction due to rejection and this delays healing. Homografts preserved by various means, e.g. freezing, freeze-drying, and X-irradiation, can be stored in bone banks. In some hands their use has been satisfactory. *Heterografts*, usually calf, are less useful. Preserved bone grafts of any origin serve as a temporary scaffold on which host bone can be formed, but there is no agreement as to the best method of preservation. In clinical work there are so many variables, such as the age of the patient, the site of insertion of the graft, the technique and skill of the surgeon, etc., that evaluation of the results obtained is virtually impossible. There is, however, general agreement that fresh autografts of cancellous bone are better than any other type.

Blood Vessels

Both autografts and homografts have been used in the replacement of blood vessels in man, and it seems likely that in all cases the cells of the graft die. They therefore behave as static grafts. For obvious reasons autografts of large arteries are not practicable in man, and homografts are therefore the only material available. There is considerable evidence to show that freeze-dried material is superior to both frozen and fresh grafts. This is possibly due to its lack of antigenicity.

The tissue of the graft remains in an unaltered state for a long period, but is eventually replaced by the host tissue. It appears therefore that arterial grafts act merely as mechanical dead tissues, and recent workers have favoured their substitution by synthetic plastic material.

The main problems involved in both types of grafts are mechanical, i.e. fitting the graft or prosthesis, and subsequently preventing rupture or thrombosis.

Heart[66, 67]

The recent heart transplants have been attended by more publicity than success. Of over one hundred cases very few long-term survivors are recorded. The graft may fail within the first month, and the microscopic signs of rejection comprise infiltration of the myocardial interstitial tissue by lymphocytes, macrophages, and polymorphs. Late rejection is characterised by intimal thickening and fibrosis of the coronary vessels, and an infiltration by lymphocytes, plasma cells, and macrophages. Somewhat unexpectedly, the heart appears to be more vulnerable than the kidney to rejection, and histocompatibility is the critical factor in the survival of the patient. With our present immunosuppressive agents there seems to be no reliable method of preventing rejection of a heart that is a poor antigenic match.

Heart-valve grafts,[68, 69] mostly aortic, have been in use since 1955,[70] but the best technique is difficult to assess because of the many variables which have been introduced. The aortic valve may be inserted isotopically or be placed in the descending aorta. It may be fresh or freeze-dried and sterilised by β-propiolactone, ethylene oxide, formaldehyde, or γ-rays. The major complications are incompetence, endocarditis (often an infection by an organism not generally encountered), and thrombosis with subsequent embolism. In spite of these hazards many valves have remained functional for several years. It appears that there is little or no homograft reaction, for the valve is virtually avascular and it remains acellular. This being so, it is probable that heterografts will also be satisfactory; indeed pig valves have been used.

Nerves

Much work has been done on the replacement of a resected portion of nerve by either autografts, homografts, or heterografts of nerve tissue.

Autografts. A living autograft shows classical Wallerian degeneration with proliferation of Schwann cells, into which regenerating nerve fibres of the host nerve subsequently penetrate. When large nerve grafts are used, there is some danger of necrosis of the central portion, and for this reason several smaller strands or cables are used to bridge the defect. The good results obtained with experimental autografts are reflected in equally good results obtained in human beings, although many early reports were extremely pessimistic. There is little doubt that, provided the segment of nerve is not too long, fresh autografts can be invaded by regenerating nerve fibres, and the results can be at least as good as those obtained after suture of a severed nerve.

Homografts. A homograft also shows Wallerian degeneration, but the process is much slower than with autografts. The Schwann cells proliferate, but subsequently die as the graft becomes infiltrated with lymphoid cells. The dying graft is invaded by host Schwann cells and axons; with small segments there may be sufficient invasion to bridge the gap. Homografts have been of some use experimentally where small defects have to be bridged, but are valueless where the segment to be replaced is long.

In clinical work homografts have produced extremely disappointing results. It seems probable that attempts at homografting with suppression of the homograft reaction might produce better clinical results, but no reports are as yet available.

Heterografts. These show Wallerian degeneration with some degree of proliferation of Schwann cells in certain species. There is little tendency for the graft to be invaded by host axons, and in general heterografts fail. Their use is therefore not to be recommended in man.

Skin

Autografts take readily, the only limiting factor being the readiness with which the graft acquires a blood supply. Split skin grafts have been extensively used, and readily take on a suitable bed. Free whole-thickness, or Wolfe grafts, if stripped of subcutaneous fat, take well on fresh, clean surfaces, but survive much less readily on granulation tissue. Pedicle grafts are extensively used in plastic surgery.

Isografts in man take as readily as autografts. Allografts are almost invariably rejected except in non-identical twins showing blood chimerism. In about 25 per cent of homografts from mother to child, and less commonly in homografts from child to mother, survival has been reported for periods up to one year. Homografts between other individuals, however, are usually rejected from 1–4 weeks, and rarely survive longer than 10 weeks.

Various attempts have been made to prolong the life of homografts. The most valuable appears to be the use of grafts from multiple donors. This work is based upon the fact that the immune response is to some extent related to the size of the graft. Several small grafts from a number of donors therefore excite less response than does a large graft from a single donor. The use of fetal tissue or skin from infants has been tried, but no convincing evidence has been forthcoming that it is of any value. This also applies to pure epidermal grafts. At the present time the value of human homografts is to provide temporary cover when this is needed, e.g. for patients with extensive burns. Heterografts are invariably rejected, but in recent years the use of embryo calf skin has been advocated for severely burned patients. The graft persists for periods ranging from 12–17 days, and may therefore provide a temporary cover, much the same as a homograft.

The Cornea[71, 72]

The privileged position which isotopic corneal grafts enjoy is an important factor in their clinical use. Under normal conditions host lymphocytes are unable to reach the graft, but should iritis occur, inflammatory cells enter the anterior chamber, and this is followed by oedema of the graft.

The fate of the grafted cells has been the subject of much speculation. It is generally agreed that the surface epithelial cells are soon replaced by those of the host. With full-thickness grafts the endothelial cells remain viable for many months, but it is likely that they too are replaced. Since the integrity of the graft is dependent on the presence of a healthy layer of endothelial cells, it is evident that this component of the graft must be viable. At present only the use of fresh material can ensure this; freeze-dried grafts are of no value.[73] They may, however, be successful as lamellar, or partial-thickness, grafts.

OTHER ORGANS

Other organs which have been transplanted include liver[74–76] and lung.[77] The number of cases is small, and although some long-term survivors are recorded, the procedures are still experimental. Thymus, spleen, and bone-marrow grafts have been employed in some cases of immunological deficiency, e.g. Di George's syndrome, and have been found useful.[78] Another potential value of grafting is to supply enzyme-forming tissue to patients with inborn errors of metabolism. Renal transplantation has been carried out in patients with Fabry's disease and cystinosis. Advanced Wilson's disease has been treated by liver transplantation.

Very few cases have been treated in this manner, and the value has yet to be proven.[80]

It is evident from this brief account that the fate of a homograft is dependent upon a large number of factors. The genetic difference between host and graft is most important. The content of antigen varies from one tissue to another, and the graft may show adaptation. The site of grafting is sometimes important, and also whether the graft establishes lymphatic or vascular connexion with the host. Finally, there is the host response, humoral and cellular, both of which can be modified by therapy. Tolerance may develop to graft antigens. It is hardly surprising that in human transplantation there is enormous variation in the end-result, so that some grafts function for years while others are rejected immediately. The complexity of the homograft reaction is to be regarded as a challenge, for as its intricacies are being unravelled, so is homotransplantation finding a valuable place in clinical medicine.

One final point deserves consideration. Why do the vertebrates possess such an efficient mechanism for the rejection of grafts, bearing in mind that such a function could have had no obvious survival value in the past? Various suggestions have been made, but none is satisfactory. The invasion by organisms which characteristically multiply in the host macrophages may have prompted the development of a cellular immune response. Another suggestion is that the mechanisms of cellular immunity have been evolved in mammals (and other live bearers) to prevent invasion of the mother by fetal cells during gestation. Yet another possibility is that the graft rejection phenomenon is a manifestation of a homeostatic mechanism whereby damaged or abnormal cells, such as those of neoplasia, are destroyed and eliminated. Although there has been no dramatic increase in the incidence of malignancy in patients on immunosuppressive therapy, lymphomata have been reported,[81] and there is one case of a reticulum-cell sarcoma developing at the site of injection of antilymphocytic serum.[79] The long-term effects of powerful immunosuppressive therapy may well provide an answer to this problem.

REFERENCE

1. WOODRUFF, M. F. A. (1960). *The Transplantation of Tissues and Organs.* Springfield, Ill.: Thomas.
2. RAPAPORT, F. T. and DAUSSET, J. (1968). *Human Transplantation*, 278 pp. New York and London: Grune and Stratton.
3. GORER, P. A., LOUTIT, J. F. and MICKLEM, H. S. (1961). *Nature*, **189**, 1024.
4. RUSSELL, P. S. and WINN, H. J. (1970). *New England Journal of Medicine*, **282**, 786, 848 and 896.
5. Editorial (1968). *New England Journal of Medicine*, **279**, 657.
6. BARKER, C. F. and BILLINGHAM, R. E. (1967). *Transplantation*, **5**, 962.
7. STROBER, S. and GOWANS, J. L. (1965). *Journal of Experimental Medicine*, **122**, 347.
8. NAJARIAN, J. S. *et al.* (1966). *Annals of the New York Academy of Sciences*, **129**, 76.
9. AMOS, B. (1964). In *Progress in Medical Genetics*, vol. 3, p. 106. Edited by A. G. Steinberg and A. G. Bearn. New York: Grune and Stratton.
10. HICKEN, P. and KROHN, P. L. (1960). *Proceedings of the Royal Society, B*, **151**, 419.
11. EICHWALD, E. J. and SILMSER, C. R. (1955). *Transplantation Bulletin*, **2**, 148.
12. STETSON, C. A. (1963). *Advances in Immunology*, **3**, 97.
13. PREHN, R. T., ALGIRE, G. H. and WEAVER, J. M. (1955). *Transplantation Bulletin*, **2**, 147.
14. AMOS, D. B. and WAKEFIELD, J. D. (1959). *Journal of the National Cancer Institute*, **22**, 1077.
15. Leading Article (1969). *Lancet*, ii, 1111.

16. Stetson, C. A. and Demopoulos, R. (1958). *Annals of the New York Academy of Sciences*, **73**, 687.
17. Kretschmer, R. R. and Peréz-tamayo, R. (1961). *Journal of Experimental Medicine*, **114**, 509.
18. Kaliss, N. (1962). *Annals of the New York Academy of Sciences*, **101**, 64.
19. Kaliss, N. (1965). *Federation Proceedings. Federation of American Societies for Experimental Biology*, **24**, 1024.
20. Boyden, S. V. (1957). *British Journal of Experimental Pathology*, **38**, 611.
21. Wilson, D. B. and Billingham, R. E. (1967). *Advances in Immunology*, **7**, 189.
22. Berah, M., Hors, J. and Dausset, J. (1968). *Lancet*, ii, 106.
23. Terasaki, P. I., Vredevoe, D. L. and Mickey, M. R. (1967). *Transplantation*, **5**, 1057.
24. Bennett, B., Old, L. J. and Boyse, E. A. (1963). *Nature*, **198**, 10.
25. McGregor, D. D. and Gowans, J. L. (1964). *Lancet*, i, 629.
26. Silverstein, A. M. (1964). *Science*, **144**, 1423.
27. Burnet, F. M. and Fenner, F. (1949). *The Production of Antibodies*, 2nd edn. London and Melbourne: Macmillan.
28. Glynn, L. E. (1963). In *Modern Trends in Immunology*, I, p. 206. Edited by R. Cruickshank. London: Butterworths.
29. Owen, R. D. (1945). *Science*, **102**, 400.
30. Dunsford, I. *et al.* (1953). *British Medical Journal*, ii, 81.
31. Nicholas, J. W., Jenkins, W. J. and Marsh, W. L. (1957). *British Medical, Journal* i, 1458.
32. Booth, P. E. *et al.* (1957). *British Medical Journal*, i, 1456.
33. Billingham, R. E., Brent, L. and Medawar, P. B. (1953). *Nature*, **172**, 603.
34. Triplett, E. L. (1962). *Journal of Immunology*, **89**, 505.
35. Billingham, R. E. and Sparrow, E. M. (1955). *Journal of Embryology and Experimental Morphology*, **3**, 265.
36. Hašek, M. *et al.* (1962). In *Transplantation*, Ciba Foundation Symposium, p. 118, *loc. cit.*
37. Anderson, J. M. (1971). *Lancet*, ii, 1077.
38. Currie, G. A. and Bagshawe, K. D. (1967). *Lancet*, i, 708.
39. Walknowska, J., Conte, F. A. and Grumbach, M. M. (1969). *Lancet*, i, 1119.
40. Simonsen, M. (1960). In *Cellular Aspects of Immunity*, Ciba Foundation Symposium, p. 122. Edited by G. E. W. Wolstenholme and M. O'Connor. London: Churchill.
41. Simonsen, M. (1962). *Progress in Allergy*, **6**, 349.
42. Nisbet, N. W. and Heslop, B. F. (1962). *British Medical Journal*, i, 129 and 206.
43. Brent, L. and Medawar, P. B. (1963). *British Medical Journal*, ii, 269.
44. Gowans, J. L. *et al.* (1962). *Nature*, **196**, 651.
45. Porter, K. A. and Cooper, E. H. (1962). *Journal of Experimental Medicine*, **115**, 997.
46. Nowell, P. C. and Defendi, V. (1964). *Transplantation*, **2**, 375.
47. Graw, R. G. *et al.* (1970). *Lancet*, ii, 1053.
48. Lance, E. M. and Medawar, P. B. (1968). *Lancet*, i, 1174.
49. McKenzie, I. F. C. *et al.* (1968). *Lancet*, ii, 386.
50. Calne, R. Y. (1967). *Renal Transplantation*, 2nd edn. London: Arnold.
51. Merrill, J. P. (1967). *Advances in Immunology*, **7**, 275.
52. Porter, K. A. (1966). In *Pathology of the Kidney*, p. 601. Edited by R. H. Heptinstall. London: Churchill.
53. Leading Article (1971). *Lancet*, i, 639.
54. Slapak, M., Lee, H. M. and Hume, D. M. (1968). *British Medical Journal*, i, 80.
55. Leading Article (1968). *Lancet*, i, 1238.
56. Nagaya, H. and Sieker, H. O. (1966). *Transactions of the Association of American Physicians*, **79**, 205.
57. Montgomerie, J. Z. *et al.* (1969). *Lancet*, ii, 867.
58. Spencer, E. S. and Anderson, H. K. (1970). *British Medical Journal*, iii, 251.
59. Leading Article (1969). *Lancet*, i, 505.
60. Hume, D. M. (1966). In *Advances in Surgery*, vol. 2, p. 419. Chicago: Year Book Medical Publishers.
61. Wilson, R. E. *et al.* (1968). *New England Journal of Medicine*, **278**, 479.
62. Stuart, F. P., Saitoh, T. and Fitch, F. W. (1968). *Science*, **160**, 1463.
63. Stickel, D. L. *et al.* (1967). *Transplantation*, **5**, 1024.
64. Terasaki, P. I., Wilkinson, G. and McClelland, J. (1971). *Journal of the American Medical Association*, **218**, 1674.
65. Burwell, R. G. (1969). In *Recent Advances in Orthopaedics*, p. 115. Edited by A. G. Apley. London: Churchill.
66. Fernbach, D. J., Nora, J. J. and Cooley, D. A. (1969). *Lancet*, i, 425.
67. Nora, J. J. *et al.* (1969). *New England Journal of Medicine*, **280**, 1079.
68. Barratt-Boyes, B. G. (1967). *Modern Concepts in Cardiovascular Disease*, **36**, 1.
69. Ross, D. (1967). *British Journal of Surgery*, **54**, 842.
70. Murray G. (1956). *Angiology*, **7**, 466.
71. Rycroft, B. W. (1955). *Corneal Grafts*. London: Butterworths.
72. DeVoe, A. G. (1961). *Archives of Ophthalmology*, **66**, 652.
73. Bacsich, P. and Wyburn, G. M. (1955). *Transplantation Bulletin*, **2**, 144.
74. Leading Article (1969). *Lancet*, i, 868.
75. Williams, R. *et al.* (1969). *British Medical Journal*, iii, 12.
76. Williams, R. (1970). *British Medical Journal*, i, 585.
77. Leading Article (1970). *British Medical Journal*, iii, 600.
78. Leading Article (1969). *Lancet*, i, 243.
79. Deodhar, S. D. *et al.* (1969). *New England Journal of Medicine*, **280**, 1104.
80. Leading Article (1972). *Lancet*, ii, 1235.
81. Leading Article (1972). *British Medical Journal*, iii, 713.

Although it is evident that under normal conditions the body does not make antibodies against the antigens of its own tissues, the mechanisms which prevent their formation may on occasion break down.

It is assumed that an individual's proteins have "self" markers, which are recognised by the immunologically competent cells. If the theory of Burnet is true, the ability to recognise these "self" markers is learned by the contact of immunologically competent cells with the antigens during embryonic development and is maintained during life by continued contact.

It may be postulated that antibodies against the individual's own tissues (*autoantibodies*) may be manufactured under three circumstances.

Alteration in antigenicity of tissue proteins. This may be due to:

Degenerative lesions, e.g. lens protein in cataracts and skin in burns.

Attachment of hapten, e.g. allergic contact dermatitis.

Specific antibodies should be formed against the affected tissue or the hapten.

Release of an antigen which has always been "isolated" from the immunologically competent cells or which has become "sequestrated" during development, e.g. lens protein. Such a protein will be labelled "non-self", and the antibody produced should be specific for it.

Loss of tolerance. Tolerance of self proteins might be expected to be lost in a variety of ways.

Forbidden clones might be formed as a result of some disease of the lymphoreticular system, e.g. lymphoma. Alternatively the defect might be a failure to eliminate a forbidden clone due to disorder of the regulating mechanism —this might reside in the thymus.[1] Tolerance can also be broken due to the formation of an antigen which closely resembles self protein. This can occur as a result of some degenerative process, the attachment of a hapten, or by infection with an organism which has an antigen in common with its host.

If it is assumed that the continued presence of antigen in reasonable quantity is necessary for the maintenance of tolerance, then the atrophy of any tissue (e.g. adrenal or thyroid) might cause the level of relevant antigen to fall below the critical point, and tolerance would be lost.

Types of antibody. It may be postulated that the autoantibodies will either be immunoglobulins or cell-bound.

The immunoglobulins might be of any class and of one of two types:

1. *Organ-specific* immunoglobulins, whose specificity is directed against a determinant present in one organ, e.g. haemolysins and antithyroid antibodies.

2. *Non-organ specific.* Antibodies directed against DNA, mitochondria, smooth muscle, and immunoglobulin determinants (rheumatoid factor) fall into this group.

ROLE OF AUTOANTIBODIES IN DISEASE PROCESSES

Antibodies may directly attack a tissue and cause damage. The immunoglobulins acquire destructive properties by activating complement; an obvious example is an acute haemolytic anaemia due to a haemolysin. Cell-bound antibodies can also destroy cells; experimental allergic encephalomyelitis is the most clear-cut example. Diseases in which the major lesions are caused by an immune mechanism may with justification be called autoimmune diseases. However, it must be stressed that the autoimmunity merely provides a mechanism in the pathogenesis of a disease. It does not provide the cause, which as noted later may be inherited or acquired.

Autoimmune mechanisms may cause lesions which are minor manifestations of the disease, e.g. the vasculitis of leprosy. Clearly, there is no sharp line of distinction between this group and those described above. Sometimes the autoantibodies appear to play no part in the disease process. The Wassermann antibody in syphilis may provide an example of this.

An important mechanism whereby antibodies produce pathological lesions is by forming damaging immune complexes with antigen. This has been described under immune-complex disease (p. 182).

AETIOLOGY OF IMMUNOLOGICALLY MEDIATED DISEASES

1. **Genetic factors.** Antigen-antibody complexes are damaging when in antigen excess. An inherited defect in antibody production may favour this, and indeed some autoimmune diseases tend to be familial, e.g. lupus erythematosus and rheumatoid arthritis. Furthermore, these diseases are common in patients with immunological deficiency, e.g. agammaglobulinaemia (p. 172).

2. **Acquired factors.** Any of the extrinsic causes of disease can precipitate an autoimmune process. Thus, drugs (e.g. hydralazine) and sunlight can precipitate the onset of

lupus erythematosus. Infection, particularly with viruses, can lead to the formation of autoimmune haemolytic anaemia (e.g. in mycoplasmal pneumonia) or renal damage of immune-complex type, e.g. NZB mice. Tissue damage however caused can presumably so alter the tissue's antigenicity that antibodies are formed. These may aid the elimination of the dead tissue and provide the basis for useful diagnostic tests. Sometimes they may themselves cause further lesions, e.g. the post-cardiotomy syndrome following heart-muscle damage.

When the aetiology of a disease is clearly established, as in smallpox, the immunologically mediated manifestations of the disease, such as the skin eruption, are readily accepted as part of the whole condition. It is when the cause of a disease is not known, e.g. rheumatoid arthritis, that stress is laid on the autoimmune component of the illness. The label "autoimmune disease" should not, however, delude one into thinking that one knows the cause of the disease—one has only described part of its pathogenesis.

It is instructive to describe some diseases in which there is a prominent autoimmune component.

RENAL DISEASE[2]

Nephrotoxic nephritis (Masugi type). The injection of heterologous antibody against glomerular basement membrane produces a glomerulonephritis; rats have generally been used and injected with duck anti-rat serum. The antibody becomes attached to the basement membrane and appears as a linear ribbon on immunofluorescence. A similar effect can be induced in animals if they are given basement-membrane substance with Freund's adjuvant. In the Masugi type of nephrotoxic nephritis the initial glomerulonephritis due to heterologous antibody is soon followed by a second phase— the autogenous phase—as antibody to the foreign immunoglobulin is produced and deposited in the basement membrane.

The linear pattern of immunoglobulin deposition in the glomeruli is seen in some types of human glomerulonephritis. The best known is *Goodpasture's syndrome*. This is an acute disease which generally attacks males of the age-group 25–35 years and is characterised by extensive pulmonary haemorrhage (resembling idiopathic pulmonary haemosiderosis, p. 563) combined with a rapidly progressing glomerulonephritis. Immunoglobulin is deposited in the basement membrane of lung and glomeruli; presumably the damage caused by this explains the lesions, but the aetiology of the disease is unknown; a respiratory virus infection has been suggested. Apart from Goodpasture's syndome, a linear pattern of immunofluorescence is uncommon in human glomerulonephritis.

Serum sickness. Glomerulonephritis due to non-glomerular antigen-antibody complexes occurs in this condition (p. 182). It appears that the complexes first accumulate between the endothelial cells and the basement membrane, then pass through the membrane, and finally lie beneath the epithelial

cells as "lumpy-bumpy" deposits. Glucocorticosteroids tend to hold up the passage of the complexes through the membrane, and the mesangial cells are able to phagocytose and eliminate them. Steroid administration therefore tends to prevent renal damage. Immune-complex glomerulonephritis can be produced most easily in animals which have a poor immune response to the given antigen. This underlines the fact that immune complexes are most damaging when in antigen excess. Administration of steroids can indeed increase the incidence of nephritis by inhibiting the immune response.

Immune-complex glomerulonephritis can be produced in animals in many ways, e.g. after injection of brush-border antigen, or indeed many other antigens such as thyroglobulin, when combined with Freund's adjuvant. It occurs spontaneously in NZB/NZW hybrid mice and in NZB mice infected with murine leukaemia virus. In man it is seen in serum sickness itself, in secondary syphilis, quartan malaria, and in allergic drug reactions. The most important example, however, is post-streptococcal glomerulonephritis.

Post-streptococcal glomerulonephritis. Like acute rheumatic fever, *acute glomerulonephritis* usually occurs after an obvious *Strept. pyogenes* infection. After pharyngitis the mean period is about 10 days, whereas after impetigo it is generally three weeks or longer.[3] The glomeruli exhibit "lumpy-bumpy" immunoglobulin deposits situated between the epithelial cells and the basement membrane. Streptococcal antigen cannot, however, be demonstrated, and the precise pathogenesis of the disease is not known. Some streptococci have antigens in common with kidney,[4] and this may lead to the formation of anti-kidney antibodies. Alternatively, streptococcal antigen may act as a hapten. An impaired immune response by the patient is another possibility. However the damage is produced, there is an infiltration of the glomeruli with polymorphs and a proliferation of mesangial cells. The glomeruli are enlarged, relatively bloodless, and hypercellular (Fig. 16.1). Resolution usually ensues, but sometimes the disease progresses. With severe glomerular damage the parietal epithelial cells of Bowman's capsule proliferate to produce characteristic crescents (Fig. 16.2). This is *rapidly progressive chronic glomerulonephritis,* * and death occurs within two years. More usually the disease progresses slowly over a period of many years until the glomeruli are converted into hyaline functionless masses. Uraemia, hypertension, or heart failure are the clinical accompaniments. Before reaching this stage the glomeruli may take on a lobular appearance (*lobular nephritis*), and the patients often exhibit a nephrotic syndrome.

Acute nephritis most often follows a type-12 streptococcal infection. Rabbits given a culture filtrate of type-12 strepto-

---

* In the past this type of lesion has been called subacute nephritis and linked with a nephrotic syndrome. While the patient may pass through a nephrotic phase, this is not invariable, and the characteristic clinical feature is progressive renal failure terminating in uraemia.

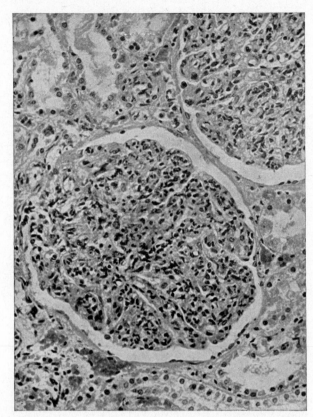

Figure 16.1
Acute glomerulonephritis. The glomerulus is greatly enlarged, and is hypercellular due to an infiltration of polymorphs and a proliferation of mesangial cells. The vascular lumina have been occluded, with the result that few red cells are present in the tuft. ×220.

cocci intravenously develop a nephritis-like condition after an incubation period of ten days.[5, 6] A polypeptide extracted from the filtrate has been found to produce typical glomerulonephritic lesions in rabbits and *Rhesus* monkeys.[7] The interpretation of these findings is, however, complicated, for they may all be examples of non-specific immune-complex damage.

Other types of glomerulonephritis. Other types of nephritis are not post-streptococcal in type and their aetiology is unknown. Glomerulonephritis occurs in *anaphylactoid purpura* (p. 620), and deposits of IgG and complement are found in the glomeruli. The pattern is neither linear nor "lumpy bumpy", for the deposits are seen in the mesangium and are not related to the basement membrane.

Liver disease.[8, 9] Non-organ-specific autoantibodies are found in active chronic hepatitis, primary biliary cirrhosis, and some cases (cryptogenic) of cirrhosis. These have been grouped as "autoimmune liver disease", but the relationship between the antibodies and the pathogenesis of the diseases in unknown. Rheumatoid factor and antinuclear antibodies may be found, but the most frequent are anti-smooth

muscle (in active chronic hepatitis) and anti-mitochondrial antibody (in primary biliary cirrhosis).

Skin diseases.[10] Antibodies to skin components have been reported in burns and a number of skin diseases. The best documented examples are to be found in the bullous

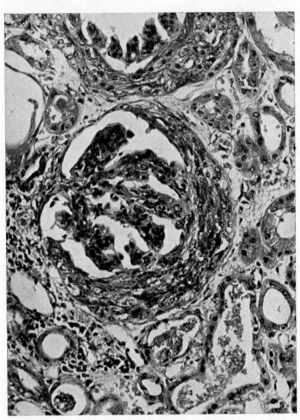

Figure 16.2
Chronic glomerulonephritis of the rapidly progressive type. The cells of the parietal layer of Bowman's capsule have proliferated to produce a crescent, and adhesions are present between this and the glomerulus. The glomerular tuft itself is reduced in size, hypercellular, and shows a forked or lobular shape similar to that seen in lobular nephritis. The proximal convoluted tubules are atrophic, and there is some increase in the amount of interstitial tissue. ×220.

diseases. In bullous pemphigoid antibody is present in the basement membrane of the skin in the lesions (Fig. 16.3), and it can also be detected in the serum. Likewise in pemphigus vulgaris there is antibody directed against the intercellular substance of the epidermal cells. Dermatitis herpetiformis is the latest disease to join this group, for IgA has been detected in the early characteristic papillary lesions of this condition.[11, 12] The antibodies in lupus erythematosus are noted on p. 211.

Haemolytic anaemias. There is no doubt that some haemolytic anaemias are caused by autoantibodies. Some are frank autoagglutinins, while others act *in vitro* as incomplete antibodies. Both types of antibody cause red-cell destruction *in vivo*. The Donath-Landsteiner antibody is a true haemo-

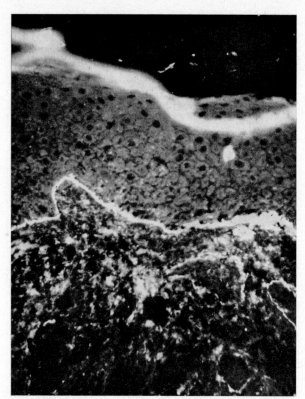

Figure 16.3
Deposition of IgG antibody in the basement membrane of skin in bullous pemphigoid. A frozen section of skin taken adjacent to a recent vesicle was stained with fluorescein-labelled anti-IgG and examined microscopically under untraviolet light. The linear staining of the basement membrane is characteristic of this disease. The ill-defined fluorescence on the surface of the skin is non-specific staining of the stratum corneum.

lysin. Viral, mycoplasmal, and rarely spirochaetal infections may lead to autoimmune haemolytic anaemia.

Autoimmune haemolytic anaemia may be due to an abnormality in the recognition system, as in reticulum-cell sarcoma or chronic lymphatic leukaemia, or there may be some obscure defect in the red cells themselves. Alternatively, a foreign factor may act as a hapten and render the cells antigenic, e.g. penicillin (p. 594).

Agranulocytosis and thrombocytopenia may also be associated with autoantibodies (see Chapters 50 and 51).

Thyroid disease. *Hashimoto's disease.*[13] The finding of antithyroglobulin antibodies in this condition has led to the hypothesis that it is an autoimmune disease. It is argued that the thyroglobulin is normally sequestrated from the body as a whole, and therefore not recognised as "self". Damage to the gland (possibly due to a virus infection like mumps) might cause a release of thyroglobulin, and the body then responds by making antibodies. If these cause further damage to the gland, a vicious circle is established. Histologically the gland shows atrophy of its epithelial elements, together with a dense infiltration of lymphoid cells often

with germinal centres. There are also many plasma cells (Fig. 16.4). These findings are very suggestive of local antibody production.

Antithyroglobulin antibodies are found in about 90 per cent of cases of Hashimoto's disease, and in addition other factors are also present. Antibodies to microsomal fractions occur, but these may be found in some cases of *primary myxoedema, thyrotoxicosis*, and even in normal people. Other antibodies are present which are cytotoxic to thyroid cells grown in tissue culture. An agglutination test using coated latex particles or red cells is used extensively as a diagnostic procedure. On the other hand, the injection of serum from patients cannot reproduce the disease in animals.

The possibility of cellular antibodies has been investigated, and lymphocytes from cases of Hashimoto's disease are said to behave abnormally in tissue cultures of thyroid cells. It is evident that there is some abnormality in the immunological mechanism in Hashimoto's disease, but the nature of this error is obscure. For the present it is safest to regard the serum antibodies as of great diagnostic value, but not necessarily related to the pathogenesis of the disease.

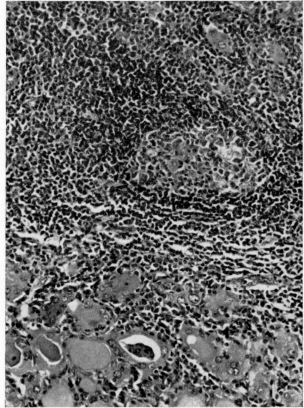

Figure 16.4
Hashimoto's disease. One portion of the thyroid gland is completely replaced by a mass of lymphoid tissue in which there is a prominent germinal centre. The remainder of the acini are atrophied, and in between them there is a profuse small round cell infiltration consisting of lymphocytes and plasma cells. × 160.

Eye diseases. *Sympathetic ophthalmia.*[14] This condition follows perforating injuries of the eye involving the uveal tract. A chronic inflammatory granulomatous lesion commences in the injured eye, and is followed one to two months later by a similar reaction in the other eye. The second eye is usually more severely damaged than the first, and blindness often results. The "sympathetic" inflammation can be prevented by removal of the injured eye within one to two weeks of injury. The condition is rare, and occurs in less than 2 per cent of penetrating injuries.

The lesions are caseating tuberculoid granulomata, but no causative organism has been isolated. There is evidence to suggest that the lesions might be due to the development of hypersensitivity to uveal pigment[15] or the matrix of the pigment granule. This would certainly explain the bilateral nature of the disease, and its favourable response to ACTH and glucocorticosteroids. If uveal pigment is regarded as sequestrated and "non-self", it is easy to see how an injury could result in the formation of antibodies. What is less simple to explain is why the other eye is subsequently involved, because if it is postulated that the pigment is sequestrated from the immunologically competent cells, it is difficult to imagine how the antibodies (which may be of a cellular type) can gain access to the normal uveal pigment.

Phako-anaphylactic endophthalmitis[14, 16] (lens-induced endophthalmitis). This name is applied to an inflammatory reaction in the region of the lens capsule which occasionally occurs following the extracapsular extraction of a cataract, or sometimes after an injury involving the lens. It is thought to be due to the development of antibodies to lens protein, which by becoming sequestrated from the immune mechanism during development, is treated as "non-self". However, an alteration in the antigenicity of the lens protein itself may also be an important factor.

Other conditions. Autoantibodies have been described in numerous conditions, but there is little evidence that they are causally related. The following may be cited: Addison's disease, ulcerative colitis, and pernicious anaemia.

Experimentally-produced autoimmune diseases. Injections of emulsions of normal tissues, usually mixed with Freund's adjuvant, into animals sometimes produce characteristic lesions. If brain is used, a demyelinating *allergic encephalomyelitis* is produced.[17] Nerve tissue produces an *allergic neuritis*.[18, 19] With thyroid a condition somewhat resembling Hashimoto's disease results.[20, 21] Damage can be produced against other tissues, e.g. testis[22] and uveal tissue,[23] by this type of experiment. Passive transfer experiments indicate that the antibodies involved are cell bound and not immunoglobulins.

What relationship these experimental lesions have to any human disease is not known. Certainly the encephalitis following immunisation against rabies (due to its rabbit spinal cord content) may fall into this group, but there is no evidence that other demyelinating conditions, e.g. multiple sclerosis, can also be included. The typically relapsing course of the human disease is not seen in experimental autoimmune encephalitis.

Post-vaccinal encephalitis is also characterised by perivascular demyelination, and although an autoimmune mechanism is postulated, direct evidence is lacking.

Conclusions

It is obvious that under a wide range of conditions the body can produce antibodies to its own normal or slightly altered tissue antigens. The immunoglobulins that appear in the circulation are of interest in diagnosis, and sometimes play an important role in the pathogenesis of the disease.

The association of cell-mediated antibody with disease is much less clear. In the experimentally-produced autoimmune conditions they appear to be of great importance. Unfortunately methods of detecting this type of antibody are not reliable and have only recently been applied to human disease; for the present no categorical statement can be made about the role of cellular autoantibodies in human disease.

THE COLLAGEN DISEASES

In 1933 Klinge first drew attention to the damage to the fine collagen framework of the myocardium that occurs in *acute rheumatic fever*, and suggested that this condition was fundamentally a disease of collagen.[24] In 1942 Klemperer and his colleagues were struck by the many morphological features that were common to diseases as distinct as acute rheumatic fever, *rheumatoid arthritis, systemic lupus erythematosus*, and *polyarteritis nodosa*.[25] They felt that this group could be classified under the heading of the "collagen diseases". Indeed, the feature common to all these diseases is extensive fibrinoid necrosis involving collagen, though this is also invariable in malignant hypertension, which is never classified in the group. A fifth member, *scleroderma*, was later added, but here atrophy and condensation of collagen is much more typical than fibrinoid necrosis, which is present only in certain uncommon lesions of the disease.

The term "collagen disease" has been a convenient repository for a number of conditions of obscure aetiology in which there is a chronic inflammatory reaction and widespread parenchymatous destruction. The presence of autoantibodies in some of these conditions has confused the issue still further, so that the collagen diseases have been regarded as important examples of autoimmune processes. There is little evidence that any of the five diseases mentioned above, in which there is damage to collagen, are caused by autoantibodies, nor does the collagenous lesion appear to be primary. The present consensus of opinion favours an immune-complex type of allergy as the basis of most of these conditions, and it seems that the concept of collagen disease will pass into disuse. It has been retained here because of its past association and its value in linking the five conditions closely together.[26]

Acute Rheumatic Fever

This is typically a disease of childhood, and it is closely related to a *Strept. pyogenes pharyngitis* which usually occurs about three weeks before the onset of the disease. It almost never follows streptococcal impetigo or pyoderma.[3] The present view is that there is an immune-complex reaction between large amounts of streptococcal antigen and small amounts of antibody in the patient's serum. The formation of soluble antigen-antibody complexes, and their localisation on the walls of small blood vessels in the heart and joints predominantly, leads to the activation of complement and tissue damage (see p. 182). The peculiar localisation of these complexes is not understood; in the other streptococcal immune-complex disease, acute glomerulonephritis, the localisation is entirely glomerular.

The tissue reactions of this group of diseases usually start as acute inflammation which persists and enters a chronic stage. Instead of an organismal agent being the cause of the reaction, the precipitating factor is a focus of damaged connective tissue.

The basic lesion of rheumatic fever is the *Aschoff body*,[27] which is typically situated in the interstitial tissue of the

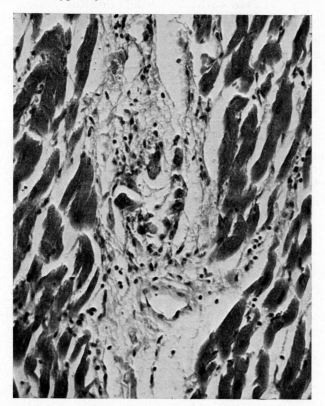

Figure 16.5
Aschoff nodule in myocardium. In the connective tissue between two muscle bundles there is a fusiform lesion arranged near to a small blood vessel. It consists of a minute focus of damaged connective tissue surrounded by typical Aschoff giant cells and a non-specific small round cell infiltration. × 180.

myocardium close to a coronary arteriole (Fig. 16.5). It is fusiform in shape and microscopical in size, and consists of a small area of necrotic connective tissue. Around this there is a pleomorphic cellular infiltration, of which the most characteristic elements are large cells with basophilic cytoplasm and vesicular nuclei having prominent nucleoli. These nuclei are sometimes multiple, in which case the cell is called an "Aschoff giant cell". The origin of these cells has given rise to much debate. They are generally regarded as myocardial histiocytes, though a rival school of thought believes that they are derived from damaged heart muscle.[28] The other cells present are lymphocytes, macrophages, and occasional polymorphs and eosinophils. These foci are also present under the pericardium and the endocardium. Furthermore, there is extensive oedema of the entire heart muscle in the acute stage. Indeed, in those uncommon cases of death from fulminating rheumatic fever, the oedema is the most prominent feature, the cellular infiltration is diffuse, and there are no true Aschoff bodies.

The cause of heart failure in acute rheumatic fever is unknown. The muscle fibres themselves look normal; perhaps there is a more subtle biochemical type of lesion. Mitral regurgitation is the common valvular defect in the acute disease and is due to dilatation of the valve ring.

As recovery occurs, so these foci heal to form scars. This is of great importance in the endocardium and valves. Even in the acute stage the inflammatory oedema leads to endocardial damage, which is most severe around the mitral and aortic valves. The formation of rheumatic vegetations is the result of this. As healing occurs there is progressive scarring and shrinkage of the valve cusps and the chordae tendineae. In due course valvular stenosis or regurgitation ensues. The mitral valve is most commonly attacked in acute rheumatic fever, and then the aortic valve. The right side of the heart is only occasionally affected.

There may be an acute sero-fibrinous pericarditis which is organised to form pericardial adhesions. These are of little functional importance, and should not be confused with constrictive pericarditis which is never due to acute rheumatic fever; it is usually tuberculous or pyogenic in origin.

Essentially similar lesions may occur in the joints, producing a characteristically flitting *arthritis*. Rheumatic *pleurisy* is an occasional feature, and from time to time lesions in the *aorta* and the *medium-sized arteries* have been reported. Cerebral involvement gives rise to *Sydenham's chorea*; vague lesions have been described in the basal ganglia and the cortex.

A more typical lesion is the *rheumatic nodule* (Fig. 16.6). Crops tend to erupt subcutaneously along tendons and over bony pressure points. Histologically they are merely florid Aschoff bodies with little central necrosis. The lesions merge into the surrounding tissue. Rheumatic nodules are typically transient, usually disappearing after a few days. In this respect it is interesting that the lesions of acute rheumatic fever do not appear to leave significant residual foci of dam-

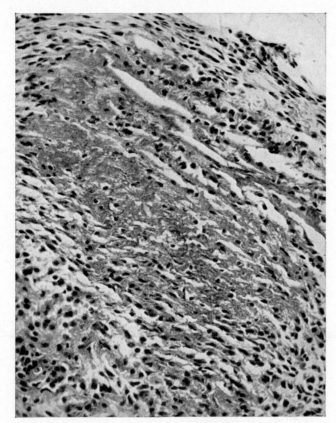

Figure 16.6
Rheumatic nodule. The section shows a small central lattice of degenerating collagen, surrounded by a zone of small round cells. There are no Aschoff giant cells; these are found only in cardiac lesions. ×200 approx. *(From Bywaters, E. G. L. and Scott, F. E. T. (1960), "Rheumatism and the connective tissue diseases", in* Recent Advances in Clinical Pathology, *Series III, edited by S. C. Dyke, p. 301, Fig. 6. London: Churchill)*

age; for instance, the arthritis does not cause chronic crippling. Unfortunately the heart is an exception to this dictum.

The significance of acute rheumatic fever lies in the chronic heart disease that it produces. It is interesting how mild the disease is nowadays, a tendency noticeable with regard to streptococcal lesions generally (see p. 220). Most cases of rheumatic heart disease survive nowadays to middle age, and not infrequently, old age.[29]

Rheumatoid Arthritis

This disease has its maximal incidence during early adult life, and it afflicts women much more frequently than men. The lesions are characteristically polyarticular, and the smaller joints tend to bear the brunt of the disease. Clinically it starts as an acute arthritis, and this is reflected histologically in an acutely inflamed synovial membrane. There is proliferation of the synovial lining cells and a heavy infiltration of lymphocytes, plasma cells, macrophages, and numbers of polymorphs. The synovial fluid contains many pus

cells. As the disease progresses, the synovial membrane becomes crowded with lymphocytes. Sometimes lymphoid follicles develop in their midst.

There is later an ingrowth of granulation tissue from the perichondral margins. This spreads over the articular surfaces in the form of a pannus, and eventually destroys them completely. Progressive deformity and ankylosis follow. Associated with this there is atrophy of the neighbouring bones and muscles, and the overlying skin becomes smooth and shiny.

In the articular lesions there is little evidence of necrosis, but a very characteristic feature of the disease is the appearance over bony prominences of large *rheumatoid nodules*. These are composed of an extensive central area of necrotic connective tissue which is surrounded by a zone of erectly-orientated fibroblasts, which forms a "palisade" around it. In the periphery there is an infiltration of lymphocytes, plasma cells, and macrophages. Rheumatoid nodules persist for years. The large amount of necrotic material is probably the cause of this (Fig. 16.7). Similar nodules may sometimes be found in the internal viscera.

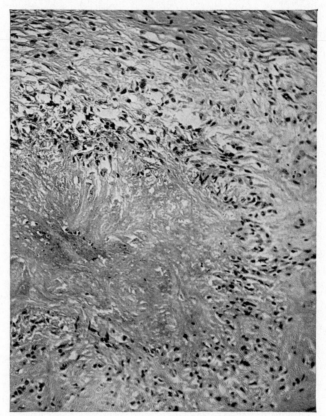

Figure 16.7
Rheumatoid nodule. There is an extensive central area of necrotic connective tissue surrounded by a palisade layer of fibroblasts. In the periphery there is reparative fibrosis and a moderate small round cell infiltration. ×200 approx. *(From Bywaters, E. G. L. and Scott, F. E. T. (1960), "Rheumatism and the connective tissue diseases", in* Recent Advances in Clinical Pathology, *Series III, edited by S. C. Dyke, p. 301, Fig. 6. London: Churchill)*

More knowledge is being accumulated about the visceral lesions of rheumatoid arthritis. The *heart* is not uncommonly involved, the most frequent lesion being pericarditis[30] which may sometimes be constrictive.[31, 32] Myocardial lesions[33] are rarer, and may take the form of diffuse small round-cell infiltrations, fusiform foci reminiscent of Aschoff bodies, and even discrete rheumatoid granulomata. Some authorities believe that there is a relationship between rheumatic fever and rheumatoid arthritis, despite the fact that streptococcal infection does not play a part in rheumatoid arthritis. A rare, progressive arthritis affecting especially the hands is known to follow rheumatic fever. Its crippling effects resemble those of rheumatoid arthritis; this *Jaccoud's arthritis*[34–36] might conceivably be a link between the two conditions.

Necrotising arteritis,[37] rather similar to that of polyarteritis nodosa, occasionally affects the vessels of the heart, bowel, nerves, and muscles, and infarction may complicate rheumatoid arthritis.

The pulmonary lesions of rheumatoid arthritis are important.[38] The commonest is pleurisy, with or without an effusion.[39] A type of diffuse fibrosis (or fibrosing alveolitis) may occur, and also the more typical rheumatoid pneumoconiosis (Caplan's syndrome).[40] This occurs in coalminers who are afflicted with rheumatoid arthritis. In the lungs there are nodular foci composed of a large area of central necrosis, which is surrounded by inflammatory cells and fibrous tissue. It seems that the pneumoconiosis acts as a local precipitating factor for the development of rheumatoid nodules in the lungs. Much more rarely nodules develop in previously normal lungs.

There is often *regional lymphadenitis* in rheumatoid arthritis. Sometimes this is generalised, and there may be moderate enlargement of the liver and spleen also. The histological changes are those of nonspecific reactive hyperplasia. This may occur at any age, but is most prominent in the childhood condition (Still's disease). If it is accompanied by leucopenia and melanotic pigmentation of the skin, it is called Felty's syndrome.[41]

Ocular lesions are sometimes present. The commonest is keratoconjunctivitis sicca,[42] others are uveitis and scleromalacia perforans.[43] In this condition true nodules form in the sclera; they break down and often destroy the use of the eye.

The combination of keratoconjunctivitis sicca, xerostoma, and rheumatoid arthritis forms *Sjögren's syndrome*, or the *sicca complex*. It is common in many of the diseases associated with non-organ specific autoantibodies and in liver disease.[44]

Generalised amyloidosis is an important complication of rheumatoid arthritis.

The nature of rheumatoid arthritis is unknown. It has been placed in the autoimmune group because there may be autoantibodies present, though there is no evidence that these play a causative part in the disease process. About three-quarters of patients with active disease have the *rheumatoid factor* in their sera. This is an IgM antibody which reacts against human IgG containing the corresponding Inv or Gm specificity (see p. 144). In practice the globulin is adsorbed on to red cells or latex particles; these are then agglutinated by the rheumatoid factor. Anti-nuclear antibodies are found in about 20 per cent of cases, but the LE-cell phenomenon is seldom present.

On a number of occasions mycoplasma has been isolated from rheumatoid joints; whether these organisms are of importance aetiologically is debatable, but it would not be surprising if the cause of rheumatoid arthritis were an allergic reaction to foreign infective antigen.

Systemic Lupus Erythematosus (SLE)

For a long time the skin disease *chronic discoid lupus erythematosus* has been known to dermatologists. It consists of plaques of scaling erythema on the skin of the exposed parts, notably the face and hands. These lesions persist for long periods and heal by scarring. Histologically there is atrophy of the epidermis, hydropic degeneration of the basal cells, a tendency to plugging of the hair follicles with horny material, and an infiltration of small round cells (mostly lymphocytes) in the dermis. It is particularly dense around hair follicles and sweat glands. Foci of altered collagen may be present in the dermis, but this is inconstant.

It was known that occasionally this chronic disease could spread rapidly, especially after prolonged exposure to sunlight. Then a "sub-acute" or even an "acute" type of lupus erythematosus could supervene, in which there were severe constitutional disturbances. Death frequently ensued.

More recently the incidence of the acute disseminated or "systemic" type of disease has increased considerably. It almost always arises *de novo*, though there is no doubt that the chronic discoid type of the disease is related to the systemic variety, for there are subtle gradations in severity between these two extremes.[45] The question arises whether this great increase in incidence of systemic lupus erythematosus is a true indication of establishment of a new disease, or whether it was always present but remained unrecognised. The disease is much commoner in women than in men, and the age group 20–40 years is most often affected.

The manifestations of this disease are very protean. There may be widespread *erythematous eruptions* (involving especially the exposed areas) but on the whole it is the visceral manifestations which predominate. Of these the most important are *arthritis, pericarditis, pleurisy, endocarditis*, and *nephritis*. Fever is present during active phases, and there is usually leucopenia. The disease runs an erratic course, and over 40 per cent of cases survive 15 years. Nephritis is the commonest lethal lesion, and glucocorticosteroids also contribute to the mortality figures.[46]

The characteristic histological lesion of the systemic disease is fibrinoid necrosis of the connective tissue under the endothelium of the serous sacs (e.g. pleura and pericardium), beneath the synovial lining cells of joints, and under the endocardium.[47, 48] The disease also attacks the walls of small arterioles. In the kidney a characteristic appearance is produced in the glomeruli because of a thickening of the basement membrane of the capillaries. The process is focal, and the affected vessels have a brightly eosinophilic thickened wall thereby resembling the bacteriologist's wire loop: this is called the *wire-loop lesion* (Fig. 16.8). Many glomeruli show foci of mesangial proliferation, and ultimately undergo necrosis. Another characteristic but distinctly uncommon lesion may be seen in the splenic arterioles situated in the

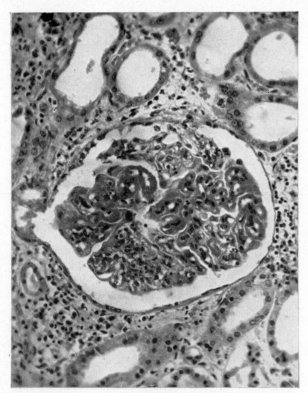

Figure 16.8
Systemic lupus erythematosus. This glomerulus shows the typical "wire-loop" lesion. The thickened capillary wall stains brightly with eosin, because there is fibrinoid necrosis of the underlying collagen. Not all the basement membrane is affected. This accounts for the patchy appearance of the lesion in the glomerulus. ×240. *(From Heptinstall, R. H. (1960), "Diseases of the kidney", in Recent Advances in Pathology, 7th edition, edited by C. V. Harrison, p. 103, Fig. 4.11. London: Churchill)*

centre of the lymphoid follicles: a concentric laying-down of collagen fibres without much necrosis, producing an onion-skin appearance.

In the heart the necrotic connective tissue under the endocardium may erupt through on to the surface and lead to the formation of vegetations. These may be mural or valvular, and unlike rheumatic disease, both sides of the heart are equally affected, the brunt being borne by the mitral and tricuspid valves. This lesion is called *Libman-Sacks endocarditis*,[49] and is a characteristic, though uncommon, mani-

festation of SLE. The myocardium is not primarily affected, though foci of necrotic connective tissue may be found in it.

Around the areas of fibrinoid necrosis there is an inflammatory reaction in which lymphocytes and plasma cells are present. A very important diagnostic feature of the disease is the presence of lilac-staining *haematoxyphil bodies* amid the necrotic debris. They are foci of degraded nuclear material, and are the histological counterpart of the "LE cell'. These bodies are small, round, and homogenous.

A prominent feature of the condition is the presence of many autoantibodies in the serum. Acute haemolytic anaemia is common, and the Coombs test is sometimes positive. Circulating anticoagulants may be present, and there may also be thrombocytopenic purpura due to platelet antibodies. These patients are also prone to develop alloantibodies against transfused red cells, and if they require a transfusion expert selection of blood and cross-matching is essential. The serological tests for syphilis may be falsely positive, and the rheumatoid factor is present in about a third of the cases.

The most important antibodies from a diagnostic point of view are those which are active against nuclear components.[50] These may be detected by immunofluorescence, which is the most sensitive test, being positive usually even when the disease is inactive, or else by the *LE-cell phenomenon*, which was the first specific laboratory test described for the diagnosis of SLE.[51] It is found that when normal leucocytes are incubated with the serum of a patient for about 2 hours at 37°C, some of the neutrophils contain a homogeneous mass of uniformly purplish material (using a Romanowsky stain) in their cytoplasm. The mass consists of altered nuclear material. The neutrophil is called a "LE cell", and it must be distinguished from a "tart cell", which is a monocyte which has phagocytosed a nuclear fragment, the basic structure of which is still recognisable. It is the homogeneous structureless nature of the inclusion that is typical of the LE cell. The exact nature of the phenomenon is ill-understood. The current view is that the patient's serum contains an antibody against a component of nucleo-protein—probably a nucleo-histone. When the leucocytes die, e.g. after prolonged incubation, the antibody reacts with this component. The nucleus is then ingested by a polymorph. Apparently the process of ingestion causes the alteration in the nuclear appearance.

These antinuclear antibodies are very useful in the diagnosis of SLE. The LE-cell phenomenon is not commonly present in the other "collagen diseases", but it is usually found in active chronic hepatitis (see p. 537).

The wide range of antibodies present in SLE react with widely distributed antigen, and are non-organ specific.[52] There is no evidence that the antibodies against intracellular fractions are active against living cells. It is interesting that the relatives of patients with SLE show an increased incidence of autoantibodies and related diseases (see also pp. 172 and 215).

There is good evidence that lupus nephritis is an immune-complex disorder due to the localisation of soluble complexes of nuclear antigen and antinuclear antibody in the glomeruli.[53, 54] The nuclear antigen is DNA, and it may be autologous or foreign, e.g. from a bacterium or virus. Patients with active lupus nephritis almost invariably have a reduced serum level of complement.[53] It seems probable that the protean manifestations of SLE are all attributable to damaging immune complexes in the small blood vessels of the viscera, e.g. heart, joints, and serous cavities. The agent is thought to be a drug or an organism which acts on autologous DNA or contributes its own DNA. The antihypertensive agent hydralazine stimulates antibodies to native DNA when it produces a lupus syndrome.[55] In a number of cases of lupus nephritis filamentous tubular structures have been seen in the glomerular endothelial cells and these have been interpreted as being viral, e.g. myxovirus or paramyxovirus.[56] It now seems more likely that they are modified endoplasmic reticulum.[57] In a recent case haemobartonella-like organisms have been found in the red cells.[58] In other cases high titres of antibodies to various viruses, especially EB virus, have been reported.[59] There has been a swing away from associating SLE with autoimmunity, and the autoantibodies present are believed to be the results of diffuse tissue damage. In all cases of SLE it is most important to eliminate drugs and organisms as the cause of the condition.

Polyarteritis Nodosa

Polyarteritis nodosa of the classical, or Kussmaul-Maier, type is a *necrotising arteritis* affecting the *medium-sized muscular vessels* of the heart, kidneys, bowel, liver, spleen, pancreas, and also the nutrient arteries of the peripheral nerves. The usual victims are middle-aged men, and the clinical manifestations are a febrile, wasting illness to which the effects of regional vascular occlusion are added. Multiple asymmetrical neuritis (*mononeuritis multiplex*) due to ischaemia of peripheral nerve trunks is a common finding.[60] The effects of polyarteritis nodosa are extremely widespread; recovery is exceptional.

Histologically there is an extensive zone of fibrinoid necrosis involving a segment of the artery. The whole thickness of the wall is affected (i.e. it is a panarteritis), and there is a profuse inflammatory response with infiltrations of lymphocytes, plasma cells, macrophages, polymorphs, and often many eosinophils as well. The weakened wall tends to yield to the intra-arterial pressure, and small nodular aneurysms may form (hence the name polyarteritis nodosa) and subsequently rupture. An even commoner complication is thrombosis and infarction. At necropsy there are often large extravasations of blood, e.g. around the kidneys and in the wall of the bowel, as well as extensive areas of infarction of the kidneys, spleen, and other organs. The lesions may heal, especially under the influence of steroid therapy, and then the arterial wall is invaded by granulation tissue. This in no way lessens the danger of infarction; indeed, the worst ischaemic effects may be seen in the healing stage.

The renal lesions of polyarteritis are particularly severe,[61, 62] not only is there often necrosis of the arcuate and interlobular arteries, but there is also much fibrinoid necrosis of individual glomeruli. Hypertension is commonly present, especially as the renal lesions heal.[63]

Variants of polyarteritis nodosa. A type of polyarteritis occurs which affects small vessels and spares those of larger calibre. This *microscopical polyarteritis*[63] is characterised by vascular necrosis and an accompanying acute inflammatory reaction (Fig. 16.9). This is often marked, and the initial

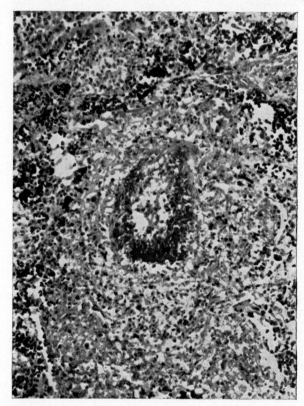

Figure 16.9
Polyarteritis nodosa with pulmonary involvement. This small pulmonary artery shows severe fibrinoid necrosis. It is surrounded by a heavy cellular infiltration. ×198. *(From Harrison, C. V. (1960), "Diseases of arteries", in* Recent Advances in Pathology, *7th edition, edited by C. V. Harrison, p. 172, Fig. 5.8. London: Churchill)*

polymorph exudate is followed by a mononuclear one sometimes with epithelioid-cell and giant-cell formation. Vascular obstruction leads to tissue necrosis, and later there is granulation-tissue formation. The lesions may therefore show extensive necrosis and chronic inflammation and resemble those produced by bacteria and fungi. These granulomatous variants generally are examples of Wegener's granulomatosis or allergic granulomatous vasculitis (Churg and Strauss), as described below. The aetiology of polyarteritis is unknown in most cases, but sometimes hypersensitivity to drugs, e.g.

sulphonamides, phenylbutazone, tetracyclines, and thiazides,[64] appears to be the precipitating factor. A variety of names has been attached to this group of conditions, e.g. necrotising arteritis (or vasculitis, if small veins are also involved) and hypersensitivity angiitis. In the latter, described by Zeek, the lesions all tend to be at the same stage. The distribution of the lesions varies from case to case and a large number of clinical syndromes are recognised. In some, e.g. Wegener's granulomatosis, the lesions are severe and, if untreated, the disease is invariably fatal. In others the arteritis is confined to one area and the disease is benign and self-limiting, e.g. erythema nodosum and Henoch-Schönlein purpura (p. 620). In the syndromes which affect the kidney the characteristic lesion is glomerulonecrosis and capsular crescent formation, very much like that seen in rapidly progressive glomerulonephritis.

Recognised syndromes. A few only of these will be outlined.

Lethal midline granuloma or *malignant granuloma*. This affects males rather more frequently than females, and usually in the 20–50 age group. It often commences with epistaxis, and is characterised by inflammatory granulation-tissue formation in the nose and nasopharynx. This is combined with necrosis and gangrene, so that eventually the palate and nasal structures are destroyed. This terrible disease usually kills by local infection or haemorrhage.

Progressive allergic granulomatosis. This variant often starts with the development of asthmatic attacks. Nodular necrotic lesions are present in the lungs, and these are accompanied by chronic inflammation with epithelioid cells and giant cells (Fig. 16.10). The lesions therefore resemble those of tuberculosis.

Wegener's granulomatosis.[65, 66] This is usually defined as a polyarteritis affecting amongst other organs the *kidney, lungs,* and *upper respiratory tract.* In the last site the lesions resemble those described in lethal midline granuloma. Death is usually due to renal failure.

Although many separate syndromes are described, the validity of regarding them as separate entities must be questioned. On the one hand, it is common to encounter cases in which the features, although clearly those of a vasculitis, do not fit readily into any one of the described syndromes. On the other hand, it is also doubtful whether the custom of including these many syndromes under the heading of polyarteritis is a valid basis for classification. In some instances the disease appears to be a manifestation of hypersensitivity to drugs, food, or infection. The only feature which is common to all members of this group is a morphological one—namely the presence of an arteritis.

Although the precipitating agent is usually not discovered, the morphology of the lesion and its not infrequent association with hypersensitivity make an immune-complex mechanism the most probable. Lesions of experimental serum sickness in animals closely resemble human polyarteritis nodosa. Of great interest is the occasional association

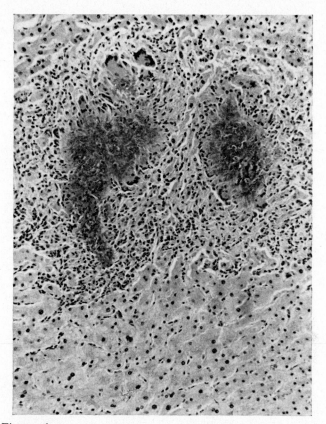

Figure 16.10
Two allergic granulomata in the portal area of the liver. Note the central necrosis and the surrounding zone of macrophages and giant cells. The small cells at the periphery of the lesions are eosinophils, plasma cells, and macrophages. × 135. *(From Abell, M. R. et al. (1970), New England Journal of Medicine, 282. 665).*

of Australia antigen with polyarteritis nodosa.[67] In the incubation period of serum hepatitis the following immune-complex lesions have been described: polyarteritis, glomerulonephritis, urticaria, and arthritis.[68]

Another example of vasculitis due to the deposition of immune complexes is erythema nodosum leprosum;[69] this is seen in lepromatous leprosy when treated with dapsone. There is a cutaneous vasculitis manifest as erythematous indurated areas which may ulcerate. Fever, lymphadenopathy, albuminuria, and arthritis are present, as in serum sickness.

Polyarteritis nodosa is not usually associated with autoantibodies. The diagnosis is histological from a skin or muscle biopsy, or from a deep-seated lesion.

Scleroderma

As with LE, scleroderma was first described as a skin disease. Two types are recognised: circumscribed scleroderma, or morphoea, and systemic scleroderma, or progressive systemic sclerosis.[70, 71]

Morphoea. The disease is usually restricted to the skin.

Well-demarcated plaques are formed which are stiff and firm. These lesions are of little significance unless they are extensive, when they are associated with atrophy of the underlying subcutaneous tissue and skeletal muscles. If the face is affected there may be hemiatrophy. Morphoea rarely, if ever, progresses to the systemic form.

Progressive systemic sclerosis. The skin lesions may start centrally on the trunk and spread peripherally, or they may start on the face and hands. The latter type is usually associated with Raynaud's phenomenon, and calcification may occur particularly in the pulp of the fingers. The affected skin becomes indurated, stiff, and tight so that if the area involved is great, considerable impairment of movement ensues. This is accentuated by atrophy of the subcutaneous tissues, so that the skin is bound to underlying muscles. Muscle weakness due to *myositis* is common and often severe. In contrast to morphoea, the skin lesions are poorly defined. Nevertheless, the changes which occur are very similar in both types of disease.

In the skin lesion of scleroderma the collagen fibres are at first swollen and oedematous, and there is a small round cell infiltration which is most heavy around the blood vessels. Later on the collagen fibres become condensed into compact masses in which the normal spaces between individual bundles are greatly reduced in extent. New collagen is formed, and this results in the thickening of the dermis. In due course the fibroblasts become very scanty and the cellular infiltration disappears. The hair follicles and sebaceous glands atrophy. The elastic tissue may also disappear, but more usually it persists. Hyperelastosis is occasionally reported. There is also a tendency towards increased melanin pigmentation over the affected areas of skin, and Addison's disease may be simulated.

Visceral lesions.[72–74] *Skeletal muscle* is nearly always affected. There is degeneration of muscle fibres with an associated inflammatory response, and ultimately replacement by fibrous tissue occurs. Similar changes are often seen in the smooth muscle of the *gastro-intestinal tract*. The oesophagus is the most common site and dysphagia and regurgitation of food result. *Cardiac muscle* may be affected and heart failure occurs. The *lungs* often suffer, not only as the result of the oesophageal lesion, but also primarily. Diffuse fibrosis leads to contraction of the lung substance, and there may be the formation of cysts lined by bronchiolar epithelium surrounded by dense fibrous tissue (honeycomb lung).

The smaller *arteries* in sclerodermatous lesions show intimal proliferation (endarteritis) with medial hypertrophy and a mild inflammatory reaction around them. In the extremities this may lead to Raynaud's syndrome, which sometimes precedes overt disease.

A similar type of lesion is occasionally found in the interlobular arteries of the *kidney*,[75] and the thickened tunica intima contains large amounts of an acid mucopolysaccharide. Distal to this there may be fibrinoid necrosis of the arteries which can extend to the afferent glomerular arterioles and the glomeruli. The appearance is identical to that of severe malignant hypertension, but in scleroderma the blood pressure is usually normal. This renal lesion is rare, and when present is rapidly fatal.

Of all the "collagen diseases" scleroderma is the most chronic. Inflammatory change is seldom conspicuous, and apart from the renal lesion, the process is a very prolonged one.

The nature of the condition is obscure, but some authorities consider the vascular lesion to be the primary one. On electron microscopy similarities have been noted in the small vessels of cases of SLE, dermatomyositis, and scleroderma.[76] The last shows more advanced changes than those of the first two. In one case of scleroderma that progressed to a fatal polyarteritis nodosa, immunoglobulin and complement were found free within the acutely inflamed small arteries,[77] but there is no evidence that scleroderma itself is an immune-complex disease.

Polymyositis[78] is frequently included among the collagen diseases. Histologically there is a diffuse inflammatory infiltration affecting many skeletal muscles, accompanied by destruction of muscle fibres. There may also be a non-specific acute inflammatory reaction in the dermis, in which case the condition is called *dermatomyositis*. In chronic cases this may proceed to a stiffening of the skin. Though the disease bears a resemblance to scleroderma, and may complicate SLE and polyarteritis from time to time, it is preferable not to include it in the "collagen" group of disorders. It probably has an allergic origin. There is a well-recognised association between dermatomyositis and deep-seated malignant disease.[78, 79]

Conclusions

The "collagen diseases" comprise a group of conditions that have the following features in common:

There is widespread degeneration of collagen, and fibrinoid necrosis is present in all of them. The necrosis is greatest in polyarteritis and SLE, and is least conspicuous in scleroderma. Nevertheless, degeneration of collagen can occur following many types of injury, and it is difficult to accept that these conditions are primarily diseases of collagen. They do, however, involve the connective tissues of many organs in addition to being associated with parenchymal damage, e.g. epidermis in SLE. Collagen, like its derivative gelatin, is feebly antigenic,[80] but it could possibly become more antigenic with ageing or pathological change.[81] Be this as it may, there is no evidence that anticollagen antibodies are formed.

They all respond well to glucocorticosteroids and ACTH. Their action is presumably not only anti-inflammatory but also inhibitory to auto-antibody formation. More recently *immunosuppressive agents* have been used, e.g. cyclophosphamide and azathioprine, and good results have been reported, especially in polyarteritis nodosa and its more lethal variants.[82] Once again the effect is anti-inflammatory as well as immunosuppressive.

There is a marked constitutional effect typified by a greatly raised red-cell sedimentation rate. This is useful prognostically in gauging the progress of the condition. In scleroderma the ESR may be normal, as it is the most torpid of all these conditions. There is a general tendency to hypergammaglobulinaemia, which is most pronounced in rheumatoid arthritis and SLE.

There is an inter-relationship between the disorders. Some cases of rheumatoid arthritis develop features of SLE, and polyarteritis nodosa may complicate SLE or rheumatoid arthritis. Scleroderma occasionally merges into rheumatoid arthritis and SLE. Furthermore there is sometimes an increased familial incidence of this group of diseases. The increased incidence in patients with certain congenital immunological deficiency syndromes has been noted on p. 172. The explanation of this is not known, for while it might be taken to support the thesis that an altered immune response is of prime importance, an increased liability to infection with an unidentified agent is equally possible.

The initial enthusiasm for including the collagen diseases under the heading of autoimmunity has now waned.

Certainly autoantibodies are present in SLE and rheumatoid arthritis, and hypersensitivity is important in some types of polyarteritis. Scleroderma appears to be the exception. An alteration in the immune response is a feature of this group of diseases, but its relationship to their pathogenesis is obscure.

It is of interest to conclude with a brief account of certain animal diseases which closely mimic the human collagen diseases.[83] *Aleutian mink disease* resembles SLE and is due to a virus infection. The *auto-immune haemolytic anaemia* which develops in New Zealand black (NZB) mice is suspected of being a virus infection, perhaps acquired *in utero*, because the disease still develops if the animals are reared under germ-free conditions.[84] The NZB mice occasionally, and the hybrids NZB/NZW frequently, develop an immune-complex nephritis which closely resembles human lupus nephritis. Genetic, viral, and immunological factors are therefore involved. Swine develop a polyarthritis due to an infection with *Erysipelothrix insidiosa*, while *equine viral arteritis* resembles human polyarteritis. An arteritis is also a feature of equine infectious anaemia (a virus disease) and Aleutian mink disease. Now that an autoimmune aetiology for this group of diseases is no longer favoured, there is a search for similar infective agents in man.

GENERAL READING

ASHERSON, G. L. (1967). *British Medical Journal*, iii, 417 and 479.
GLYNN, L. E. and HOLBOROW, E. J. (1965). *Autoimmunity and Disease*, 420 pp. Oxford: Blackwell.
MACKAY, I. R. and BURNET, M. (1963). *Autoimmune Diseases*. Springfield, Illinois: Thomas.

REFERENCES

1. Leading Article (1967). *Lancet*, i, 713.
2. CARPENTER, C. B. (1970). *Annual Review of Medicine*, **21**, 1.
3. WANNAMAKER, L. W. (1970). *New England Journal of Medicine*, **282**, 23 and 78.
4. ZABRISKIE, J. B. (1967). *Advances in Immunology*, **7**, 147.
5. REED, R. W. and MATHESON, B. H. (1954). *Journal of Infectious Diseases*, **95**, 191 and 202.
6. MATHESON, B. H. and REED, R. W. (1959). *Journal of Infectious Diseases*, **104**, 213.
7. REED, R. W. and MATHESON, B. H. (1960). *Journal of Infectious Diseases*, **106**, 245.
8. DONIACH, D. *et al.* (1966). *Clinical and Experimental Immunology*, **1**, 237.
9. HOBBS, J. R. (1970). *British Journal of Hospital Medicine*, **3**, 669.
10. BEUTNER, E. H., CHORZELSKI, T. P. and JORDAN, R.E. (1970). *Autosensitisation in Pemphigus and Bullous Pemphigoid*. Springfield, Illinois: Thomas.
11. DICK, H. M., FRASER, N. G. and MURRAY, D. (1969). *British Journal of Dermatology*, **81**, 692.
12. VAN DER MEER, J. B. (1969). *British Journal of Dermatology*, **81**, 493.
13. Annotation (1962). *British Medical Journal*, i, 1467.
14. HOGAN, M. J. and ZIMMERMAN, L. E. (1962). *Ophthalmic Pathology*, 2nd edn, pp. 367 and 153. Philadelphia: Saunders.
15. FRIEDENWALD, J. S. (1934). *American Journal of Ophthalmology*, **17**, 1008 and (1949). Ibid., **32**, 1699.
16. WOODS, A. C. (1959). *American Journal of Ophthalmology*, **48**, 463.
17. PATERSON, P. Y. (1966). *Advances in Immunology*, **5**, 131.
18. WAKSMAN, B. H. (1963). In *Mechanisms of Demyelination*, p. 170. Edited by A. S. Rose and C. M. Pearson. New York: McGraw-Hill.
19. WAKSMAN, B. H. and ADAMS, R. D. (1956). *Journal of Neuropathology and Experimental Neurology*, **15**, 293.
20. TERPLAN, K. L. *et al.* (1960). *American Journal of Pathology*, **36**, 213.
21. LERNER, E. M., McMASTER, P. R. B. and EXUM, E. D. (1964). *Journal of Experimental Medicine*, **119**, 327.
22. FREUND, J., THOMPSON, G. E. and LIPTON, M. M. (1955). *Journal of Experimental Medicine*, **101**, 591.
23. VANNAS, S., NORDMAN, E. and TEIR, H. (1960). *Acta Ophthalmologica (KBH)*, **38**, 618.
24. KLINGE, F. (1933). *Ergebnisse der allgemeinen Pathologie und pathologischen Anatomie*, **27**, 1.
25. KLEMPERER, P., POLLACK, A. D. and BAEHR, G. (1942). *Journal of the American Medical Association*, **119**, 331.
26. KLEMPERER, P. (1950). *American Journal of Pathology*, **26**, 505.
27. ASCHOFF, L. (1904). *Verhandlungen der Deutschen Pathologischen Gesellschaft*, **8**, 46.
28. MURPHY, G. E. (1960). *Medicine (Baltimore)*, **39**, 289.
29. KERR, J. W. (1963). *Journal of Clinical Pathology*, **16**, 529.

30. WILKINSON, M. (1962). *British Medical Journal*, ii, 1723.
31. SUTTON, R. A. L. (1967). *Proceedings of the Royal Society of Medicine*, **60**, 339.
32. HARROLD, B. P. (1968). *British Medical Journal*, i, 290.
33. LEBOWITZ, W. B. (1963). *Annals of Internal Medicine*, **58**, 102.
34. BYWATERS, E. G. L. (1950). *British Heart Journal*, **12**, 101.
35. TWIGG, H. L. and SMITH, B. F. (1963). *Radiology*, **80**, 417.
36. GRAHAME, R. (1968). *Proceedings of the Royal Society of Medicine*, **61**, 1109.
37. CRUICKSHANK, B. (1954). *Annals of the Rheumatic Diseases*, **13**, 136.
38. SCADDING, J. G. (1969). *Proceedings of the Royal Society of Medicine*, **62**, 227.
39. Leading Article (1972). *Lancet*, i, 480.
40. CAPLAN, A. (1953). *Thorax*, **8**, 29.
41. Leading Article (1971). *British Medical Journal*, iv, 379.
42. THOMPSON, M. and EADIE, S. (1956). *Annals of the Rheumatic Diseases*, **15**, 21.
43. ROSENTHAL, J. W. and WILLIAMS, G. T. (1962). *American Journal of Ophthalmology*, **54**, 862.
44. GOLDING, P. L. *et al.* (1970). *British Medical Journal*, iv, 340.
45. COHEN, H. and CADMAN, E. F. B. (1953). *Lancet*, ii, 305.
46. Leading Article (1971). *Lancet*, i, 1283.
47. GROSS, L. (1940). *American Journal of Pathology*, **16**, 375.
48. KLEMPERER, P., POLLACK, A. D. and BAEHR, G. (1941). *Archives of Pathology*, **32**, 569.
49. LIBMAN, E. and SACKS, B. (1924). *Archives of Internal Medicine*, **33**, 701.
50. Leading Article (1967). *British Medical Journal*, ii, 654.
51. HARGRAVES, M. M., RICHMOND, H. and MORTON, R. (1948). *Proceedings of Staff Meetings of the Mayo Clinic*, **23**, 25.
52. ASHERSON, G. L. (1967). *British Medical Journal*, iii, 479.
53. Leading Article (1971). *Lancet*, ii, 964.
54. CHRISTIAN, C. L. (1969). *New England Journal of Medicine*, **280**, 878.
55. HAHN, B. H. *et al.* (1972). *Annals of Internal Medicine*, **76**, 365.
56. KAWANO, K., MILLER, L. and KIMMELSTIEL, P. (1969). *New England Journal of Medicine*, **281**, 1228.
57. PINCUS, T. *et al.* (1970). *Lancet*, ii, 1058.
58. KALLICK, C. A. *et al.* (1972). *Nature New Biology*, **236**, 145.
59. EVANS, A. S., ROTHFIELD, N. F. and NIEDERMAN, J. C. (1971). *Lancet*, i, 167.
60. BLEEHEN, S. S., LOVELACE, R. E. and COTTON, R. E. (1963). *Quarterly Journal of Medicine*, **32**, 193.
61. DAVSON, J., BALL, J. and PLATT, R. (1948). *Quarterly Journal of Medicine*, **17**, 175.
62. WAINWRIGHT, J. and DAVSON, J. (1950). *Journal of Pathology and Bacteriology*, **62**, 189.
63. ROSE, G. A. and SPENCER, H. (1957). *Quarterly Journal of Medicine*, **26**, 43.
64. BJÖRNBERG, A. and GISSLÉN, H. (1965). *Lancet*, ii, 982.
65. GODMAN, G. C. and CHURG, J. (1954). *Archives of Pathology*, **58**, 533.
66. Leading Article. (1971). *British Medical Journal*, iii, 446.
67. GOCKE, D. J. *et al.* (1970). *Lancet*, ii, 1149.
68. Leading Article (1971). *Lancet*, ii, 805.
69. WEMAMBU, S. N. C. *et al.* (1969). *Lancet*, ii, 933.
70. GOETZ, G. H. (1945). *Clinical Proceedings*, **4**, 337.
71. FARMER, R. G., GIFFORD, R. W. and HINES, E. A. (1960). *Circulation*, **21**, 1088.
72. TUFFANELLI, D. L. and WINKELMANN, R. K. (1962). *American Journal of the Medical Sciences*, **243**, 133.
73. TUFFANELLI, D. L. and WINKELMANN, R. K. (1962). *Annals of Internal Medicine*, **57**, 198.
74. MIDDLETON, W. S. (1962). *Annals of Internal Medicine*, **57**, 183.
75. HEPTINSTALL, R. H. (1960). In *Recent Advances in Pathology*, 7th edn, p. 104. Edited by C. V. Harrison. London: Churchill.
76. NORTON, W. L. (1970). *Laboratory Investigation*, **22**, 301.
77. TOTH, A. and ALPERT, L. I. (1971). *Archives of Pathology*, **92**, 31.
78. WALTON, J. N. and ADAMS, R. D. (1958). *Polymyositis*. Edinburgh: Livingstone.
79. AZZOPARDI, J. G. (1966). In *Recent Advances in Pathology*, 8th edn, p. 101. Edited by C. V. Harrison. London: Churchill.
80. STEFFEN, C., TIMPL, R. and WOLFF, I. (1964). *Journal of Immunology*, **93**, 656.
81. HELLER, P. and YAKULIS, V. J. (1963). *Proceedings of the Society for Experimental Biology and Medicine*, **112**, 1064.
82. Leading Article (1972). *Lancet*, ii, 519.
83. LEADER, R. W., GORHAM, J. R. and WAGNER, B. M. (1967). In *The Connective Tissue*, pp. 95–131. Edited by B. M. Wagner and D. E. Smith. Baltimore: Williams and Wilkins.
84. EAST, J. *et al.* (1967). *Lancet*, i, 755.

The organisms responsible for suppuration account for some of the most important lesions seen clinically.[1] Although most of these bacteria respond to antibiotic therapy, surgical drainage of abscesses caused by them is still often necessary. The most important members of this group are:

The pyogenic cocci, viz. *Staphylococcus pyogenes, Streptococcus pyogenes*, pneumococcus, meningococcus, and gonococcus.

The Gram-negative intestinal bacilli, viz. *Escherichia coli, Proteus* species, *Pseudomonas pyocyanea* (*Ps. aeruginosa*), and organisms of the genus *Bacteroides*.

Of these it is the staphylococcus, streptococcus, and Gram-negative bacilli that produce the most widespread lesions. Not only do they infect wounds, burns, and chronic ulcerative skin lesions secondarily, but they can also spread to any organ of the body. No tissue is exempt from these non-specific bacterial infections.

By contrast, the pneumococcus nearly always affects the lungs. Though an initial septicaemia is characteristic of lobar pneumonia, the organism produces metastatic lesions only exceptionally. Likewise, the meningococcus and gonococcus usually confine themselves to the meninges and genital tract respectively.

The local tissue response to each of these bacteria is similar: acute inflammation with a copious outpouring of neutrophil polymorphs. The process and its possible sequelae have been described in Chapter 6. If the organisms are destroyed early by the inflammatory response, there is resolution; otherwise the condition proceeds to suppuration with abscess formation. If the pus is successfully drained healing follows; otherwise the lesion becomes chronic. Many of the common chronic inflammatory lesions due to non-specific bacterial infections come into this category, e.g. chronic pyelonephritis, chronic diverticulitis, chronic cholecystitis, and chronic osteomyelitis. It should be remembered, as stressed in Chapter 11, that a neutrophil infiltrate is not pathognomonic of a simple acute inflammatory reaction, for it occurs in chronic abscesses and in other chronic infections such as actinomycosis and sporotrichosis. When a pyogenic lesion becomes chronic there is an admixture of other cells, e.g. lymphocytes, plasma cells, macrophages, and eosinophils, as well as a proliferation of connective tissue and specialised cells.

In generalised pyogenic infections there is a severe constitutional reaction with fever and a neutrophil leucocytosis. The ESR is raised, and immunoglobulins are produced which are important in the defence against the organisms (see Chapter 13). The diagnosis is generally made by isolating the organism either from a local lesion or by blood culture. Nevertheless, in some instances serological methods are of value. Thus the gonococcal complement fixation test may be indicative of the aetiology of an obscure arthritis and the anti-staphylococcal haemolysin titre rises in patients with deep-seated staphylococcal abscesses. A rise in anti-DNAse and anti-streptococcal haemolysin O (commonly shortened to ASO) is seen following streptococcal pharyngitis and tonsillitis, and this may help to confirm the diagnosis of acute glomerulonephritis and rheumatic fever. With streptococcal skin infections no such rise in ASO titre is seen[2] (see also p. 204 and 208).

GENERAL BACTERIOLOGY OF PYOGENIC ORGANISMS

It is important to note the salient bacteriological features of these organisms because of the frequency with which they cause infection. By examining the properties of each organism an attempt can be made to understand the type of disease it causes.

STAPHYLOCOCCI[3]

Morphology. They are Gram-positive, spherical organisms about 1 μm in diameter, which are arranged in grape-like clusters. They are non-motile, non-sporing, and non-capsulate.

Cultural characteristics. They grow easily on most media. They are aerobic organisms, but can tolerate an anaerobic atmosphere quite well, i.e. they are facultative anaerobes. They grow best at 37°C. On blood agar, shiny, convex colonies about 3 mm in diameter appear within 24 hours, and these are pigmented. Most have a creamy white or dull yellow colour, but some species are golden, lemon yellow, and even red. Though pigmentation is no longer regarded as important, the organisms are still called *Staphylococcus albus* when non-pathogenic (whatever the actual colour of the colony) and *Staphylococcus aureus* when pathogenic. In this book such pathogenic organisms are called *Staph. pyogenes*. Staphylococci are divided into these two groups according to their production of coagulase in the laboratory. The term non-pathogenic is not strictly true, for *Staph. albus* can produce infection (p. 219).

Coagulase production. Coagulase is an enzyme, a precursor of a substance like thrombin, which coagulates plasma even in the absence of calcium ions. *Staph. albus* does not produce it but *Staph. pyogenes* does. It can be demonstrated by a slide test, in which a suspension of staphylococci in water is mixed with a drop of plasma. The organisms clump together at once if coagulase is present, because fibrin sticks to the surfaces of the cocci and makes them adhere to one another.

Typing of staphylococci. Not all varieties of *Staph. pyogenes* are equally virulent. Some are associated with superficial skin lesions only, while others may lead to disastrous ward epidemics. In such an epidemic of hospital infection it is necessary to type the staphylococcus to see whether all the patients are infected with a single strain or with a number of strains, as explained in Chapter 19. Staphylococci are typed with a bacteriophage (which is a virus that parasitises bacteria) that acts specifically against staphylococci. Some bacteriophages, however, lyse more than one strain of staphylococcus, and some strains of staphylococci are lysed by a number of bacteriophages. However, the number of bacteriophages lysing a particular strain of staphylococci is constant, and the organism is typed according to the *pattern* of lysis. For example, a well-known epidemic strain of staphylococcus is lysed by phages 47, 53, 75, and 77, and is therefore typed 47/53/75/77. One of the most notorious epidemic strains is the phage type 80 staphylococcus. This was first recognised in Australia in 1953,[4] and has since then wreaked havoc in many hospitals throughout the world.

Toxin production. The staphylococcus is an invasive organism, but the factors responsible for its virulence are not clearly defined. Nevertheless, some toxins are known, and these mainly have the properties of endotoxins. The most important of these is the *α-toxin*, which produces local tissue necrosis, and is lethal when injected intravenously. It is also haemolytic to red cells, and destroys white cells, i.e. it is a haemolysin and a leucocidin.

Another staphylococcal toxin acts only on white cells, and is called the *Panton-Valentine leucocidin*. Three other endotoxins are also described, and these have haemolytic and necrotising actions. An erythrogenic factor has also been described on a few occasions (see footnote, p. 221).

In addition three enzymes are produced by staphylococci:
Coagulase.
Staphylokinase, which lyses fibrin by activating the plasmin system.
Hyaluronidase. Both staphylokinase and hyaluronidase are produced only by some strains and seldom in large amounts.

Some strains also produce an exotoxin called *enterotoxin*, which produces symptoms of food-poisoning when ingested. It is the only exotoxin produced by the staphylococcus, and unlike most exotoxins it is thermostable.

Lesions produced by staphylococci.[1, 5] The typical staphylococcal lesion is a *circumscribed abscess*. Coagulase production has been suggested as an important factor in the localisation of the infection by virtue of the copious fibrin formation that it induces (see fibrin barrier, p. 98). On the other hand, some authorities regard coagulase as a factor aiding the spread of infection, because the deposition of fibrin acts as a protective covering for the organism. It is evident that our ideas on the importance of coagulase in staphylococcal infection are still purely speculative. It seems likely that the local damage inflicted by the α-toxin leads to a marked inflammatory reaction, which in its turn successfully localises and overcomes the infection.

Staphylococcal skin lesions are very frequent and include boils, carbuncles, paronychia, impetigo, and its bullous variant in the newborn.

In *impetigo* the organism invades the superficial layers of the skin and produces characteristic superficial, intraepidermal bullae and pustules.

A deeper infection is the common *boil*, or *furuncle*, in which a hair follicle is involved. Suppuration is the usual result, and pus is discharged from a single opening. A well-known regional boil is the stye, or hordeolum, in which an eye-lash is implicated. Boils are particularly common in the axillae and the back of the neck, and they are often multiple in these sites due to the regional concentration of hair follicles and sebaceous glands. Nevertheless, each boil has its own "head", through which pus is discharged.

In a *carbuncle* the infection extends to the underlying fatty subcutaneous tissue. The anatomical arrangement of the superficial fascia is such that it is divided into compartments by dense fibrous septa which extend from the deep fascia up to the dermis above. This is particularly well marked in the back of the neck. It therefore follows that when infection spreads to the subcutaneous tissue, many separate loculated abscesses form, and each bursts on to the surface through its own "head", or sinus. In this way a single carbuncle has multiple heads, one for each loculus.

Staphylococci are the commonest causal organisms in *infected wounds*, usually the result of hospital infection.

*Bullous impetigo of the newborn** is the result of similar cross-infection in maternity wards. Many infants become carriers and may transmit the staphylococci to their mothers during breast feeding. A *breast abscess* may result if the nipple is cracked.

Two other important examples of cross-infection are pneumonia and enterocolitis. *Staphylococcal pneumonia*[6] is due to the inhalation of virulent organisms, and is characterised by the development of lung abscesses which may spread to the pleural cavities and lead to empyema. *Staphylococcal enterocolitis*[7, 8] is an occasional complication of gastrointestinal surgery, especially in patients who have been given antibiotics. There is an acute, patchy inflammation

---

* The alternative name pemphigus neonatorum is best abandoned, since the condition is in no way related to the pemphigus group of diseases.

of the intestinal mucosa, which causes severe diarrhoea. The shock engendered by this in a patient in the early post-operative period is an important cause of the very serious *pseudomembranous enterocolitis*, in which long strips of mucosa undergo necrosis and remain attached to the wall to form a membrane. Most cases die rapidly of the combined effects of diarrhoea and intestinal haemorrhage, and microscopically there is often thrombosis of the mucosal and submucosal vessels.[9]

Staphylococci are the most important causal agents in *acute osteomyelitis*, a disease commonest in growing children (see p. 131). It is believed that a few organisms, probably

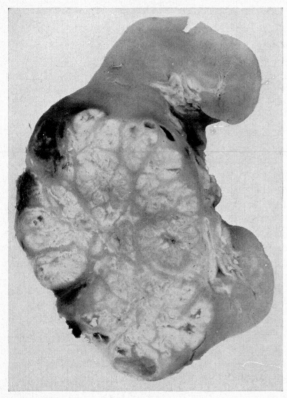

Figure 17.1
Carbuncle of kidney. The kidney is the seat of a large loculated cortical abscess which has extended as far as the hilum. *(U 15.1, Reproduced by permission of the President and Council of the R.C.S. Eng.)*

derived from the skin, during the course of a bacteraemia[10] infect the metaphysis of a long bone that may have been mildly injured during play. Sometimes the lesion becomes circumscribed and chronic leading to a *Brodie's abscess*.

In similar fashion staphylococci may produce a spreading cortical abscess in a kidney. This is called a *renal carbuncle*; it may lead to a large perinephric abscess (Fig. 17.1).

If the blood stream is massively invaded during the course of a staphylococcal infection, a fatal *septicaemia*[10] or pyaemia will ensue. *Pyaemia* is not uncommon, and follows a sup-

purative thrombophlebitis which may complicate any staphylococcal infection.

Staphylococcal food-poisoning is the only condition due entirely to the exotoxin, enterotoxin. It follows the ingestion of food products contaminated by toxin-producing strains. The resulting gastroenteritis is severe, but is seldom fatal. The condition is a true intoxication (see p. 84), and is to be contrasted with enterocolitis, in which there is an invasion of the bowel wall by staphylococci.

Occurrence. The reservoir of pathogenic staphylococci is the anterior nares. About 40 per cent of healthy adults are nasal carriers, and in a hospital population the figure may rise to over 70 per cent. From the nares they are transferred to the skin, particularly of the hands and perineum. Staphylococci are also present in the faeces, but this is probably not an important source of infection except in patients with enterocolitis.

Staphylococcus albus. This organism is coagulase negative and a universal commensal of the skin. It has become important as a cause of opportunistic infection especially following surgery when foreign material is inserted. Thus it causes endocarditis following open-heart surgery, and may colonise the artificial shunts (Spitz-Holter valves) inserted into the brain to relieve congenital hydrocephalus. It causes urinary-tract infection especially in association with stones. Occasionally it produces septicaemia. One variety of coagulase-negative staphylococcus has a lemon-yellow colony and is called *Staph. citreus*.

STREPTOCOCCI[11]

Morphology. These too are Gram-positive, spherical organisms, slightly smaller than staphylococci. They tend to be arranged in chains, but this is conspicuous only when the organisms are cultured in fluid media. These chains vary in length, and some are very short indeed. Sometimes the organisms are disposed simply in pairs. They are non-motile and non-sporing. Some strains possess very thin capsules called microcapsules.

Cultural characteristics. They grow less easily than staphylococci, but are also aerobes and facultative anaerobes. A few strains are obligatory anaerobes.

They can be cultured on blood agar at 37°C, and within 24 hours, transparent colonies 0·5–1 mm in diameter develop. Around these there may be a zone of haemolysis, and according to this the organisms are classified into three main groups:

α-haemolytic streptococci, which produce an ill-defined zone of partial haemolysis, which may be yellow or green in colour. These organisms are often reported as *Strept. viridans*.

β-haemolytic streptococci, which produce a sharply demarcated zone of complete haemolysis. These organisms are sometimes called "*Strept. haemolyticus*", a confusing name.

Non-haemolytic streptococci. These are also called "*an-haemolytic*" or γ-type streptococci.

Although both the first two varieties produce a haemolytic effect on blood agar, it is only the β-haemolytic group that possesses a soluble haemolysin capable of completely lysing horse red cells in suspension. β-haemolytic streptococci are particularly important in producing serious pyogenic infections. Not all, however, are pathogenic to man; some produce disease only in cattle and other animals. It is therefore important to distinguish between the different groups of β-haemolytic streptococci. One point of difference is the greater sensitivity of the human pathogen to *bacitracin*, but of more importance is serological grouping.

Lancefield grouping of streptococci. Lancefield found that β-haemolytic streptococci could be divided into 15 groups according to the presence of a specific carbohydrate hapten (called the C antigen) present in the wall of the organism. The vast majority of human pathogens fall into Lancefield's group A, and a group-A organism is called *Strept. pyogenes*. To perform this test, the carbohydrate is first extracted from cultures of the organism, and the extract is then superimposed on a layer of specific antiserum (from rabbits previously immunised against different groups of streptococci) contained in a length of capillary tube. A precipitate forms at the interface of the antigen and the corresponding antibody within five minutes.

Griffith typing. *Strep. pyogenes*, like its staphylococcal counterpart, may give rise to epidemics of hospital infection and also acute nephritis in army camps, schools, and similar institutions. Typing is carried out, not by bacteriophage lysis, but by serological methods. Griffith discovered that group-A streptococci could be subdivided into over 50 different types depending on the presence of protein antigens, called M and T antigens, on the surface of the organism. The M antigen is particularly important because its presence is related to virulence (see p. 168). Typing is carried out by agglutination and precipitation tests using type-specific rabbit antisera. The T antigen is demonstrated by agglutination and the M antigen by precipitation. There seems to be little variation in the virulence of the different types, except that a few, especially type 12, are related to acute glomerulonephritis.

Toxin production. Like the staphylococcus, *Strept. pyogenes* is an invasive organism that produces powerful endotoxins and a single exotoxin. There are two haemolysins designated *streptolysin O* and *streptolysin S*. Streptolysin O is also cardiotoxic and leucocidic, whereas streptolysin S is a pure haemolysin. As the chemical nature of endotoxins is generally so poorly understood, it is right to include the M protein among them. This is powerfully antigenic. It acts by interfering with phagocytosis, and the antibody formed against it is an opsonin.

The organism produces the following enzymes:

Hyaluronidase.

Streptokinase, which induces fibrinolysis by activating the plasmin system.

Streptodornase, which depolymerises DNA. The name streptodornase is derived from the first letters of the syllables **de**oxyribo**n**ucle**ase**.

The exotoxin referred to is the *erythrogenic toxin* responsible for the punctate erythema characteristic of scarlet fever. There are three antigenic types of erythrogenic toxin. The toxin is produced by some strains only, and those that do so are lysogenic.* Virulent strains of *C. diphtheriae* are also lysogenic, and it seems that the production of exotoxin is related to the presence of prophage in the organism's DNA.

Lesions of Strept. pyogenes.[12] The typical streptococcal lesion is a *spreading cellulitis*. The poor localising tendency has been associated with the hyaluronidase and streptokinase produced by most strains, often in large amounts (but see p. 101). Abscesses occur much later than in staphylococcal infections, and the pus is watery and often bloodstained. It is probable that the streptodornase and streptokinase are responsible for this, because the viscosity of pus is due to DNA and fibrin.

In recent years the virulence of *Strept. pyogenes* has declined so markedly that many of its classical lesions which produced so much damage in the past are now rarely seen. By contrast, staphylococcal lesions are commoner and more severe than ever.

Streptococci are occasional causes of *wound infection* and are also responsible for some cases of *impetigo*. *Erysipelas*, a cellulitis of the dermis, is a classical streptococcal lesion.

Necrotising fasciitis[13–15] is usually caused by *Strept. pyogenes*, but occasional staphylococcal cases have been described. The condition was first described by Meleney as haemolytic streptococcal gangrene. It is an uncommon fulminating infection which follows trauma, sometimes quite trivial. There is a rapidly spreading infection of the subcutaneous fatty layer. Thrombosis of the dermal vessels causes a red discoloration of the skin with bulla formation and necrosis. The skin lesions are ill defined in contradistinction to erysipelas, and if the patient survives there is extensive sloughing. Although the infection is due to an organism which is sensitive to antibiotics, surgical relief is also necessary.

Streptococci are important causes of tonsillitis and pharyngitis (*streptococcal sore throat*), and these may be complicated by *otitis media*. In the 1918 influenza pandemic many people died of a complicating *streptococcal pneumonia*. Streptococcal infection has a great tendency to invade the blood stream with the development of *septicaemia*. *Strepto-*

---

* A bacterium is *lysogenic* when it harbours a bacteriophage which lies latent in its DNA. Such a bacteriophage is said to be *temperate*, and it lies latent in the bacterium as *prophage*. Some external circumstances, e.g. exposure to ultraviolet light, may cause the bacteriophage to become *virulent*, whereupon it promptly lyses the organism. Although prophage causes no obvious damage to the bacterium, it may alter or modify some of its functional characteristics. Lysogeny is an example of a latent virus infection (see p. 277).

coccal puerperal sepsis killed thousands of women before the introduction of the sulphonamides, but today it is very uncommon.

If an infecting streptococcus produces the erythrogenic exotoxin, and if the patient has no circulating antitoxin, the local lesion will be complicated by the effects of this toxin. A punctate erythema appears, and the condition is called *scarlet fever*.*

There is a more indirect relationship between streptococcal infections on the one hand and *rheumatic fever* and *acute glomerulonephritis* on the other. These two conditions may occur about 3 weeks after the initial infection, and it is generally held that they are manifestations of allergy to the streptococcus or its products. Some cases of *erythema nodosum* are similarly related to streptococcal infection.

Occurrence. *Streptococcus pyogenes* is found in the throats of about 10 per cent of people, and in from 2 to 5 per cent it is present also in the anterior nares.

Other β-haemolytic streptococci. Organisms of groups C and G can be isolated from the throat and are a cause of pharyngitis. Group C organisms may cause puerperal sepsis.

Infections Due to α-haemolytic Streptococci

The α-haemolytic streptococcus (*Strept. viridans*) is an invariable commensal of the mouth and throat, and has been incriminated in apical tooth infections. A bacteraemia occurs quite frequently after dental extraction, and this is dangerous in people with congenitally-deformed or rheumatically-damaged heart valves. The organism tends to settle on such areas of abnormal endocardium, and causes *subacute infective endocarditis*.

Infections Due to Non-haemolytic Streptococci

The non-haemolytic streptococcus is always present in the colon, hence its alternative names *Strept. faecalis* and *enterococcus*. If it leaves its normal habitat, this organism can cause suppurative lesions of a type and distribution similar to *Esch. coli*. It is a common cause of *urinary-tract infection*. Occasionally *Strept. faecalis* produces a true β-haemolysis on blood agar, but it does not possess a soluble haemolysin. It belongs to Lancefield's group D.

Anaerobic Streptococcal Infections[17]

Anaerobic streptococci are normal inhabitants of the bowel and vagina. They are occasionally associated with *infected wounds*, and in civilised countries used to be an important cause of *puerperal sepsis*. *Suppurative myositis*[18] is an unusual condition caused by these organisms.

Meleney's postoperative synergistic gangrene[14, 19] usually follows the drainage of a deep abscess, either peritoneal or in the chest. There is a slowly spreading infection of the skin;

* A scarlet-fever-like illness due to staphylococci has also been described. A filtrate of the *Staph. pyogenes* contained an erythrogenic factor, which was antigenically distinct from the streptococcal erythrogenic toxin.[16]

the margin of the area is bright red and as the lesion expands this becomes purple, then black and gangrenous, and finally the necrotic skin is sloughed off leaving a granulating surface (Fig. 17.2). The infection is caused by a microaerophilic

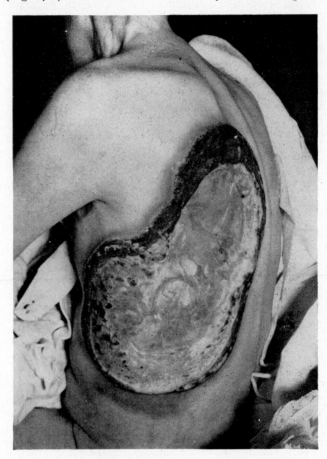

Figure 17.2
Meleney's postoperative synergistic gangrene. This patient developed an empyema as a complication of bronchopneumonia with abscess formation. Attempts to drain this resulted in a spreading gangrene which finally involved a large area of the chest wall.

non-haemolytic streptococcus acting synergistically with *Staph. pyogenes*. *Meleney's chronic undermining, or burrowing, ulcer* is a different condition. It usually follows an operation on the intestinal or genital tract, and is caused by an infection with a haemolytic microaerophilic streptococcus. It involves the subcutaneous tissues and burrows deeply into the pelvis. The condition is very painful.

THE GRAM-NEGATIVE INTESTINAL BACILLI[20]

In the account that follows no attempt has been made to delineate the features of each genus, for this is the task of the bacteriologist. For the present the clinician must be prepared to accept a nomenclature which varies from one centre to another depending on the classification adopted and the effort which the laboratory is prepared to put into the typing of each isolated "coliform organism".

Most of the members of this group belong to the family *Enterobacteriaceae*.[21] The important pus-forming genera are *Escherichia*, *Klebsiella* and *Enterobacter* (sometimes grouped together as *Aerobacter*), *Citrobacter*, *Hafnia*, and *Proteus*. Other important members of the family *Enterobacteriaceae* are *Salmonella*, responsible for typhoid fever and food poisoning, and *Shigella*, responsible for bacillary dysentery; these two groups of organisms are not distinguished by suppuration and are not described further. Another important Gram-negative intestinal genus that causes suppuration is *Pseudomonas*. It does not belong to the *Enterobacteriaceae*, for although it may occur in the intestine of man, this is not its natural habitat. It is found widely distributed in nature. Of the many *Pseudomonas* species only one, *Ps. pyocyanea* (commonly called *Ps. aeruginosa*) is pathogenic to man.

There are a number of *Proteus* species, e.g. *Pr. mirabilis*, *Pr. vulgaris*, *Pr. morganii*, and *Pr. rettgeri*, and they can be distinguished by biochemical reactions.

Morphology.* They are all Gram-negative rods 1–4 μm long, with a tendency to considerable variation in size. With a few exceptions, e.g. *Klebsiella*, they are vigorously motile. *Klebsiella* also differs from the others in having a capsule. None of these organisms forms spores.

Cultural characteristics. These organisms grow well at 37°C, being aerobic and facultatively anaerobic. On blood agar most members of this group produce greyish, shiny colonies 3–5 mm in diameter within 24 hours. Some *Proteus* species are distinctive in spreading over the surface of the agar in a confluent layer and submerging other colonies that may be present. This is called *swarming*. *Ps. pyocyanea* produces a bluish-green pigmentation due to the formation of the pigments fluorescin and pyocyanin. These are best seen on nutrient agar, because the haemoglobin in blood agar obscures them. In addition, colonies of *Ps. pyocyanea* have a characteristic fresh odour resembling fruit.

Biochemical reactions.* The most important ones are the sugar fermentation tests. Nearly all ferment some sugars, e.g. glucose, often with the production of gas (see p. 650). But it is the fermentation of lactose which is most distinctive. *Esch. coli* ferments lactose vigorously with the production of acid and gas, and most of the related coliform group do likewise, but in some instances without gas formation.

The distinctive property of lactose fermentation by some organisms is made use of in MacConkey's selective medium, the composition of which is described in Appendix II. The lactose in this medium is fermented by *Esch. coli* and most coliform organisms, and the lactic acid produced turns the

* *Salmonella* and *Shigella* are not considered here. Both genera are characterised by a failure to ferment lactose (except *Sh. sonnei*). The *Salmonellae* are motile, while the *Shigellae* are non-motile (see p. 650).

neutral-red indicator a pink colour. Therefore these colonies are pink, while those of *Salmonella*, *Shigella*, *Proteus*, and *Pseudomonas* are colourless.

Occurrence. Unlike the pyogenic streptococci and staphylococci, these organisms may be regarded as normal inhabitants of the body, causing disease only when they leave their normal habitat.

Esch. coli is always present in the bowel, and about a third of all human faeces harbour *Proteus* species. *Ps. pyocyanea* is less commonly present, being found in from 3 to 16 per cent of faeces.[22]

Pathogenicity. The pathogenic action of these organisms is believed to be due to an endotoxin, which as yet has been poorly defined. When they escape from the lumen of the bowel and invade the tissues, they lead to suppurative lesions. *Ps. pyocyanea* produces an elastase, which may explain the organism's tendency to invade blood vessels.[23]

Esch. coli and the **coliform organisms** always predominate in infective lesions associated with the bowel, e.g. *appendix abscess*, *acute diverticulitis*, *ischiorectal abscess*, and *generalised peritonitis following perforation of a hollow viscus*. They frequently infect penetrating *wounds* of the abdomen and furthermore are the commonest agents in *urinary-tract infections*, reaching the kidney as part of a normal bacteraemia from the colon, or else being introduced into the bladder following catheterisation. They are also a common cause of *acute cholecystitis*, presumably reaching the gall-bladder from the liver to which they are conveyed by the portal vein. The alternative route of infection *via* the bile duct seems unlikely.

Esch. coli is often cultured from sputum and is a cause of bronchopneumonia. The genus *Klebsiella* is a more notorious cause of lung infection, *Kl. pneumoniae*, or Friedlander's bacillus, causing a particularly dangerous bronchopneumonia characterised by a very slimy exudate. *Klebsiella* is not confined to the lung, but shares the full range of pathogenicity of other coliform organisms.

Proteus organisms and **Ps. pyocyanea** have a similar range of pathogenicity, but they are less frequently commensals of the bowel, and are much more often transmitted by cross-infection. This is particularly true of *Ps. pyocyanea*, which is the commonest cross-infecting organism after *Staph. pyogenes*. Serological and bacteriophage typing has been used in investigating hospital epidemics.[23]

Proteus organisms are very important causes of *urinary-tract infection*, due especially to cross-infection during catheterisation and bladder drainage. They decompose urea readily and produce ammonia. The urine therefore becomes alkaline, a factor favouring the formation of phosphate calculi in the bladder (see Chapter 48). *Proteus* organisms are important agents in *wound infection*, and secondary invaders of chronic ulcerative skin lesions.

Ps. pyocyanea[23] is even more widespread in its infecting tendencies, and is easily recognisable clinically by the bluish-green pus it produces. It frequently *infects the urinary tract*, and it can spread through a urological ward very rapidly. It is of great importance in *wound infection* and *eye infection* (see p. 237), and is frequently the cause of *chronic otitis media* and *otitis externa*. Like the *Klebsiella* and *Proteus* organisms, it is an important cause of *respiratory infections*. It is very invasive, and can produce a fatal *septicaemia*.[24, 25] A characteristic feature of this is an acute necrotising angiitis due to the invasion of vessel walls by the organisms. This leads to the formation of large areas of haemorrhagic infarction in the skin and internal organs, particularly the lungs and kidneys. The skin lesions appear as black nodules and consist of foci of necrosis teeming with bacilli (*ecthyma gangrenosa*).[26]

It should be noted that although *Esch. coli* is an inevitable and harmless inhabitant of the bowel, there are a few well-recognised enteropathogenic strains.[27] These are of no special importance as causes of suppuration, but they may produce epidemics of *gastro-enteritis amongst infants*. Only a few enteropathogenic types are described, e.g. 026, 055, 0111, 0119, and 0128, and they are typed serologically by agglutination tests. The condition is most common in artificially-fed babies, and is probably spread by fomites and contaminated food.

Gram-Negative Anaerobic Intestinal Bacilli

The Gram-negative intestinal organisms of the genus *Bacteroides* are an important group, for they form the bulk of organisms in the intestine as well as being present as part of the normal flora of the vagina. They are non-sporing, strict anaerobes, and are very sensitive to the toxic effect of oxygen. They cause infection of wounds, the peritoneal cavity, and the uterus following labour or abortion (see p. 56).

They may invade the blood stream, and are a cause of Gram-negative shock—as are also the other Gram-negative intestinal bacilli. Infections by *Bacteroides* are probably missed quite frequently because of the extreme oxygen sensitivity of this group of organisms. Not only must culture be performed under anaerobic conditions, but oxygen must also be excluded from the specimen during its transit to the laboratory. The ordinary type of swab is therefore quite inadequate for isolating this organism.

THE PNEUMOCOCCUS[28]

Diplococcus pneumoniae is closely related to the streptococci, and is sometimes called *Strept. pneumoniae*, but it is better to regard it as a separate genus.

Morphology. It is oval or lance-shaped, and is arranged in pairs with the long axes in line with each other. It is the same size as the streptococcus, and like it is Gram-positive, non-motile, and non-sporing. An important feature is the presence of a prominent capsule.

Cultural characteristics. It resembles the α-haemolytic streptococcus very closely, and like it produces a diffuse greenish haemolysis of the surrounding blood agar. Its colonies are somewhat larger than those of *Strept. viridans*, and have raised margins. They resemble in shape the chequers used in a game of draughts.

Unlike the streptococcus, the pneumococcus is soluble in bile, being lysed by bile salts very rapidly. Another point of difference is the great sensitivity of the pneumococcus to *optochin* (ethyl hydrocuprein hydrochloride).

Typing of pneumococci. Type-specificity depends on

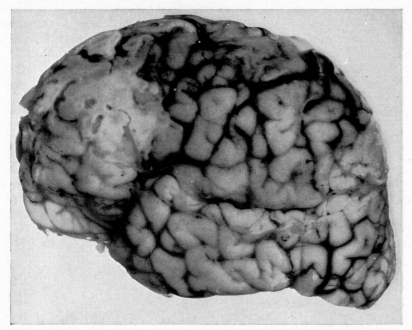

Figure 17.3
Pneumococcal meningitis. The patient was an infant of 8 months who had had recurrent attacks of pneumonia, the last of which was complicated by meningitis. The specimen is the left cerebral hemisphere, and the sulci of the frontal portion are filled with a thick, opaque layer of inflammatory exudate. *(N 6.2, Reproduced by permission of the President and Council of the R.C.S. Eng.)*

the polysaccharide hapten (the specific soluble substance, or SSS) present in the capsule of the organism, and it is this that determines its virulence (see p. 168). When a type-specific rabbit antiserum is mixed with a suspension of pneumococci, their capsules become opaque and give an appearance of swelling if the SSS corresponds to the antibody in the serum. Over 70 different types of pneumococci have been recognised, but pneumococcal typing is seldom carried out nowadays because serum therapy is obsolete in lobar pneumonia. Types 1, 2, and 3 are the most virulent, and are responsible for most cases of lobar pneumonia. The remainder used to be called "Type 4", but nowadays each type is given a number of its own. Types 5, 7, and 14 are also quite virulent, but the others appear to be commensals of the nose and throat, and cause little harm in healthy people.

Pathogenic lesions. The most important pneumococcal lesion is *lobar pneumonia*, which will be described in detail. Other primary pneumococcal conditions are *otitis media* and *suppurative sinusitis*, both of which may lead to *meningitis* (Fig. 17.3). Pneumococci may cause *purulent conjunctivitis*. Another interesting condition is the *primary pneumococcal peritonitis* which is described in young girls. Whether it is really primary, the organism gaining entrance to the peritoneal cavity by way of the fallopian tubes, or whether it is blood-borne from a lesion in the respiratory tract, is undecided.

Lobar Pneumonia[29, 30]

This is a disease especially of healthy young adults. The organism is a pneumococcus of high virulence, usually type 1, 2, or 3, and it is acquired from another victim or a convalescent carrier. "Contact" carriers, i.e. those who have never had clinical infection, may also transmit the organisms. The infection is exogenous, and the contending parties are a virulent organism and a healthy, though unimmunised, host.

The infection is acquired by inhalation, and once the pneumococci reach an area of lung parenchyma, they elicit an acute inflammatory reaction. If immunity is good, the condition may never pass beyond this stage, but otherwise a rapidly-spreading inflammatory oedema soon implicates a whole lobe, and sometimes several lobes (Fig. 17.4).

The rapid spread of the infection to the periphery in a gigantic wave of oedematous exudate suggests that allergy is involved in the process. Perhaps the patient has already had a minor pneumococcal infection sufficient to initiate an immune response. When now attacked a second time, a reaction of hypersensitivity complicates and augments the inflammatory response. Alternatively, the organisms may have passed through the lungs symptomlessly, proliferated in the RE system, and then returned to the blood, thereby causing septicaemia. When they reach the lungs again, an allergic episode follows the recently acquired immune response. This mechanism would be analogous to that described in typhoid fever (p. 93) and syphilis (p. 253).

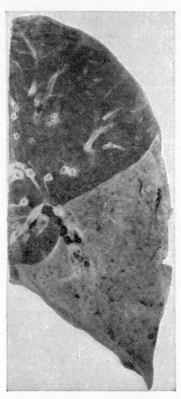

Figure 17.4
Lobar pneumonia. The left lower lobe is completely consolidated while the upper lobe is unaffected. *(R 30.2, Reproduced by permission of the President and Council of the R.C.S. Eng.)*

Whatever the mechanism there is no doubt that during this acute stage there is septicaemia, and sometimes the pneumococci may become localised and produce *meningitis, acute infective endocarditis, peritonitis,* and *suppurative arthritis.* For the first week the organism has the upper hand, and if death occurs, it is due to overwhelming "toxaemia" (though the nature of the toxic principle is unknown) sometimes accompanied by the metastatic lesions already named. After a week the titre of antibodies (opsonins) in the circulation rapidly rises, and with their aid the polymorphs are able to phagocytose the organisms (see Chapter 13). The disease resolves dramatically, and the fever abates precipitously by "crisis".

Corresponding with this general effect, the local lesion in the lungs passes through four stages:

(1) **Inflammatory oedema.** There is engorgement of the alveolar capillaries which show margination of leucocytes. In the alveoli there is an oedematous exudate containing macrophages ("septal cells") and a few polymorphs. The oedema fluid spreads rapidly through the entire lobe *via* minute openings in the alveolar walls (the pores of Kohn) and through the lumina of the alveolar ducts. At this stage it is teeming with pneumococci.

(2) **Red hepatisation.** The capillary engorgement persists,

while the oedema in the alveoli coagulates into fine skeins of fibrin. The alveoli are crowded with polymorphs, and there are also considerable numbers of red cells present (Fig. 17.5). These enter by diapedesis, and their products of haemolysis

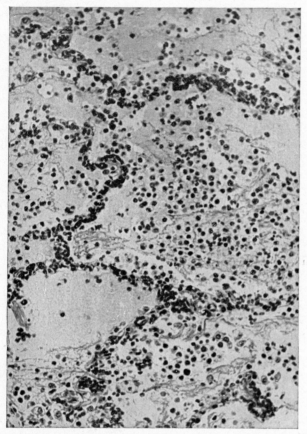

Figure 17.5
Lobar pneumonia. The alveoli are filled with a loose fibrinous exudate in which there are many pus cells. The alveolar capillaries are dilated, and are distended with red cells. This corresponds to the stage of red hepatisation. × 220.

are responsible for the rusty colour of the sputum that is coughed up. It is very tenacious due to the large amount of fibrin present.

The lobe itself is firm (consolidated), airless, and red in colour. In consistency it resembles liver (red hepatisation).

(3) **Grey hepatisation.** This follows on the red stage. The alveolar capillaries are now closed down, partly because the acute inflammatory reaction has to an extent spent itself, and partly because of pressure exerted on the capillaries by the distended, solid alveoli. These are full of dense inspissated fibrin, around which there are numerous degenerating and dead polymorphs (Fig. 17.6). At this stage bacteria and red cells are scanty. The fibrin tends to retract from the alveolar walls, and then the capillary circulation becomes active again.

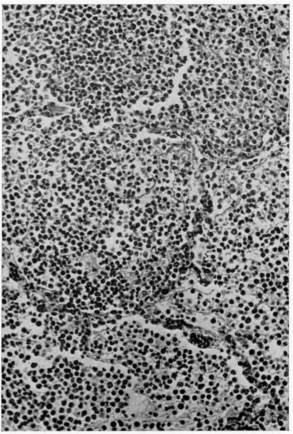

Figure 17.6
Lobar pneumonia. The alveoli are crowded with pus cells, and the fibrinous exudate has been condensed into thick strands. The alveolar capillaries are inconspicuous, and appear to have shut down. This corresponds to the stage of grey hepatisation. × 220.

The lobe is even firmer now than before, and it has a grey colour due to the relative bloodlessness. It is so voluminous that the ribs indent the lateral surfaces.

(4) **Resolution.** This is carried out by macrophages as part of the process of demolition. The inspissated fibrin is removed with great rapidity, and all remaining debris is cleared away. The fluid exudate and macrophages leave the alveoli mainly *via* the lymphatics, and they are intercepted at the hilar lymph nodes which show the features of reactive hyperplasia (see p. 399). Some of the exudate leaves *via* the alveolar capillaries, and so re-enters the blood stream.

During the process there is an acute fibrinous pleurisy over the affected lobe. Because the fibrinous exudate is so extensive it is unusual for it to be completely "demolished" by macrophages during resolution. Remnants of it persist long enough to undergo organisation into permanent pleural adhesions. These are of little functional significance.

Though the stages of lobar pneumonia have been described sequentially, it must be remembered that biological processes rarely proceed as methodically as this. While one part of a lobe shows red hepatisation, an adjacent area will be grey and solid, while elsewhere resolution may be progressing. Nevertheless, in contradistinction to bronchopneumonia, it it usual for all the alveoli in one low-power microscope field to be at one stage. The stages described above are seldom seen nowadays, because the infection is curtailed by chemotherapy.

Local sequelae of lobar pneumonia. (*a*) The commonest sequel is *resolution*, which is usually so complete that only the residual pleural adhesions remain as a testimony to the attack of pneumonia.

(*b*) Rarely the fibrinous exudate in the alveoli does not undergo demolition, but persists and is organised into fibrous tissue, a process called *carnification*. Fibrosis of the lung results.

(*c*) *Suppuration* with the production of a lung abscess is also very uncommon in lobar pneumonia, but it may be encountered in individuals with a poor resistance to infection, e.g. alcoholics and diabetics. There is usually an associated pneumococcal empyema, and the pericardial sac may be involved by direct contact.

Bronchopneumonia[30]

In bronchopneumonia, unlike lobar pneumonia, there are numerous discrete foci of inflammation around terminal bronchioles. As the disease progresses these tend to become confluent, and occasionally the process becomes so extensive that a whole lobe is consolidated. However, the wildfire spread of lobar pneumonia is not present.

There are many varieties of bronchopneumonia. They are best considered as follows:

Endogenous bronchopneumonia due to commensal organisms of the upper respiratory passages. Of these the pneumococci of low-grade virulence are by far the most important. The host is invariably in a poor state of health. The antagonists are therefore a poorly virulent endogenous organism and an enfeebled host (cf. lobar pneumonia). The following conditions in the host predispose to endogenous bronchopneumonia:

Extremes of age. It is commonest in infancy and old age.

General debilitating illness. It is a common terminal event in cancer, cerebral vascular accidents, and uraemia.

Pre-existing respiratory disease, e.g. chronic bronchitis, influenza, measles, whooping-cough, and mycoplasmal pneumonia.

Local obstruction to the upward flow of mucus which is wafted along by ciliary action (see Chapter 7). The dammed-up secretion forms an admirable medium for baterial growth. Examples of such conditions are foreign bodies and tumours of the bronchi.

Pulmonary oedema, e.g. after chest injuries, ether anaesthesia (which also damages the cilia), heart failure, and in any terminal condition ("hypostatic pneumonia").

The untreated disease lasts much longer than does lobar pneumonia. If the primary condition is fatal and the pneumonia is merely a terminal event, there will be little attempt at cure, but even in the childhood bronchopneumonia that follows measles and pertussis, a prolonged course is the rule and is often punctuated by relapses and remissions, depending on whether the organism or the host is gaining the upper hand. The fever gradually subsides in step-like fashion, a process described as "lysis".

The general pathological process is, of course, similar to that of lobar pneumonia, but there is no attempt at the orderly sequence described in that condition. The disease is usually basal and bilateral in distribution.

If an area of bronchopneumonia is examined microscopically, it is found to consist of acutely inflamed bronchioles full of pus. Some of the surrounding alveoli contain oedema fluid in which there are macrophages and polymorphs, while others are filled with a dense fibrinous exudate in which there are innumerable polymorphs. Some are collapsed as the result of the absorption of air distal to the blocked bronchioles ("absorption collapse"), whereas neighbouring alveoli are empty and distended due to compensatory emphysema. As the process proceeds, some of the alveoli show evidence of demolition of exudate by macrophages, but in others there is progressive organisation.

SEQUELAE OF BRONCHOPNEUMONIA

(*a*) *Resolution.* This is less frequent than in lobar pneumonia.

(*b*) *Progressive Fibrosis of the Lung.* This is correspondingly more frequent, and is due to the organisation of fibrinous exudate. In addition there is often a continuance of the inflammatory process, so that the lung is progressively destroyed and converted into fibrous tissue. This is, of course, chronic inflammation, and bronchopneumonia often becomes chronic. In due course the infection spreads, and the muscle and elastic tissue of the adjacent bronchi are destroyed and replaced by granulation tissue. In consequence the lumina widen, and eventually the dilatation becomes so extensive that secretion accumulates, forming the nidus for further infection and inflammatory destruction. This is the pathogenesis of *bronchiectasis*, which is both a sequel of bronchopneumonia and a predisposing cause of further attacks of it.

(*c*) *Suppuration.* This is also not uncommon, particularly when the host's resistance is exceptionally poor.

Table 17.1 contrasts untreated pneumococcal lobar pneumonia and endogenous bronchopneumonia.

Another type of endogenous bronchopneumonia follows the inhalation of material from the mouth. The root of a tooth inhaled during extraction under general anaesthesia is a classical example of this. It lodges in a bronchus, and the *Bacteroides* organisms present in it lead to a putrid type of pneumonia which terminates in abscess formation (see p. 56).

Exogenous Bronchopneumonia. A large variety of virulent organisms, when inhaled, can lead to severe

TABLE 17.1 A comparison of lobar and endogenous bronchopneumonia

	Lobar	*Bronchial*
Host	Healthy young adult	Enfeebled patient at extremes of life or chronically ill; after virus infections or with bronchial obstruction
Organism	Highly virulent exogenous pneumococcus	Poorly virulent endogenous pneumococcus and other organisms
Type of lesion	Rapid spread throughout an entire lobe	Discrete foci, usually basal, around bronchioles. Affects several lobes. Bilateral.
Progress	Wildfire spread with resolution after a week. Fever falls by crisis	Prolonged course with slow convalescence. Fever falls by lysis
Sequelae	Resolution and organised pleural exudate. Fibrosis of lung and suppuration exceptional.	Complete resolution uncommon. Residual fibrosis and bronchiectasis frequent. Suppuration is not uncommon
Mode of death	Toxaemia Metastatic pneumococcal lesions, e.g. meningitis, peritonitis, and acute infective endocarditis	Precipitating condition, e.g. cancer. Progressive lung damage

bronchopneumonia. The host may be a healthy adult, or he may be enfeebled as the result of a previous disease.

Examples of virulent organisms causing exogenous bronchopneumonia are:

Staph. pyogenes, as a result of hospital cross-infection (Fig. 17.7).

Strept. pyogenes, e.g. during the 1918 influenza pandemic.

Kl. pneumoniae; and also *Esch. coli*, *Proteus* organisms, and *Ps. pyocyanea*.

Yersinia (*Pasteurella*) *pestis* ("pneumonic plague").

B. anthracis ("woolsorter's disease").

Myco. tuberculosis (see Chapter 20) and the deep-seated fungous diseases (see Chapter 21). This type of disease is quite distinct, as the lesion produced is always chronic. Furthermore, the cellular response is not pyogenic.

Most of these organisms are very virulent, and suppuration or necrosis is usual. There is generally an accompanying septicaemia, and only the most vigorous treatment will prevent death. Apart from the extremely destructive potentialities of these agents, the pneumonia they produce is basically similar to that of endogenous pneumococci. Streptococcal and *Klebsiella* pneumonia may be so extensive as to simulate lobar pneumonia.

Primary atypical pneumonia. This term was used to include those acute pneumonias which were not pyogenic in type. Nowadays they are named after the causal organism: (a) mycoplasmal pneumonia[31] due to *Mycoplasma pneumoniae*, (b) rickettsial pneumonia due to *Cox. burneti* and the psittacosis agent, (c) virus pneumonia due to numerous agents, e.g. adenoviruses, myxoviruses, respiratory syncytial virus, and certain enteroviruses. These are discussed in

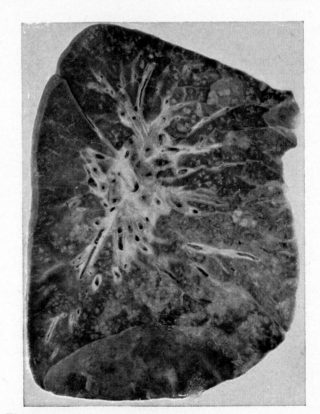

Figure 17.7
Staphylococcal bronchopneumonia. There are discrete foci of consolidation scattered throughout the lung. (R 29.3, *Reproduced by permission of the President and Council of the R.C.S. Eng.*)

Chapter 23. Histologically these pneumonias are characterised by moderately heavy macrophage and lymphocyte infiltrations in the alveolar walls, and to a lesser extent in the alveoli. Polymorphs are scanty, unless there is a secondary bacterial pneumonia. A hyaline membrane lining the alveoli is a common finding.

THE NEISSERIAL ORGANISMS[32]

The genus *Neisseria* includes a large number of Gram-negative cocci. Many of these are commensals of the mouth, nose, and throat, and are named collectively *N. pharyngis*. There are in addition two highly pathogenic members of the group, *N. meningitidis* (meningococcus) and *N. gonorrhoeae* (gonococcus), which merit a brief consideration.

Morphology. These two organisms are kidney shaped and arranged in pairs with their concave surfaces opposed. They are non-motile and non-sporing. The meningococcus has a very fine capsule. Both organisms are encountered most typically within the cytoplasm of polymorphs, and it is impossible to distinguish between them morphologically.

Cultural characteristics. Many *Neisseria* organisms grow quite easily on blood agar at $37°C$ under aerobic conditions, but the two pathogens are much more demanding in their requirements than the others. An atmosphere of 5 per cent CO_2 is essential for the gonococcus and helpful for the meningococcus, which is the more easily cultured of the two. Both grow quite well on blood agar, chocolate agar, and serum agar (see Appendix II). The colonies are small, translucent, circular discs rather like those of the streptococcus. They do not produce haemolysis.

It is evident that there is great similarity between the meningococcus and the gonococcus; one point of difference is that whereas the meningococcus ferments both glucose and maltose, the gonococcus ferments only glucose.

Typing. As with the pneumococcus typing plays very little part in the study of these organisms. The meningococcus can be divided into four types (nowadays designated A, B, C, and D) using special agglutinating antisera.

Pathogenicity. In man both are invasive organisms, and both produce an ill-defined endotoxin. Neither organism is found naturally in any other host, but a typical meningitis follows the injection of the meningococcus into the cerebrospinal fluid of rabbits and monkeys. It has recently been claimed that urethritis can be produced in the chimpanzee by the local inoculation of gonococcal pus.[33]

Meningococcal Infections[34]

From 5 to 10 per cent of healthy individuals carry the meningococcus in the nasopharyngeal area. Epidemics of meningococcal infection are prone to occur when a large number of people are herded together in cramped quarters, e.g. barracks. Under these conditions the carrier rate may rise to over 50 per cent, and then the danger of infection becomes great. This state of affairs also occurs in pneumococcal lobar pneumonia.

It is possible that there is first an insignificant infection in the nasopharynx, but it must be admitted that the factors involved in the invasiveness of the organism are ill-understood. It may be that the meningococcus invades the cranial cavity directly through the cribriform plate,[35] because the olfactory area of the nasal mucosa appears to be specifically vulnerable in that it does not possess cilia.

More usually, however, there is a stage of *septicaemia*, during which the patient develops severe constitutional symptoms and a profuse petechial eruption.[36] Occasionally the septicaemia may be so fulminating that death occurs before there is much evidence of meningeal infection. Under such conditions there is an extensive bleeding tendency with bilateral adrenal haemorrhages (Waterhouse-Friderichsen syndrome).

The septicaemia is rapidly succeeded by meningeal involvement. The reason for this specific localisation is unknown. There is a generalised fibrinous *meningitis* which rapidly becomes purulent. As in other types of meningitis the exudate is most abundant over the base of the brain because of the arrangement of capacious cisternae in this area. The pia mater acts as an efficient barrier against the invasion of the brain by organisms; the cerebral substance is merely congested and oedematous. In untreated cases death occurs either in the acute stage, or else following the organisation of adhesions in the area of the cisterna magna. The severe hydrocephalus that results is soon fatal.

More rarely the meningococcus also becomes localised in other tissues, in which case such complications as *arthritis*, *endocarditis*, and *otitis media* occur. *Primary meningococcal conjunctivitis* is a rare, though well-recognised, condition. *Chronic meningococcal septicaemia* is a rare variant; there is a remittent fever resembling malaria, a maculopapular skin eruption that fades and recurs, and migratory arthralgias.[37]

Gonococcal Infections[38]

The usual manifestation of gonococcal infection is the venereal disease *gonorrhoea*. In the male it commences as an acute suppurative urethritis, which if untreated spreads rapidly to the prostate, seminal vesicles, and epididymes. The destruction of tissue and the subsequent scarring lead to such permanent sequelae as urethral stricture and sterility.

In the female the disease is often less acute, and it affects the urethra, vulvovaginal glands of Bartholin, and cervix primarily. The vagina is characteristically immune because of its acidity (see Chapter 7), except in young girls. The disease may spread to the endometrium and lead to salpingitis and pelvic peritonitis. The subsequent occlusion of the fallopian tubes is an important cause of sterility.

Other venereal presentations of gonorrhoea are *proctitis* in those, commonly male homosexuals, who practise sodomy, and *pharyngitis* and *tonsillitis* in those who practise oral methods of intercourse. Such manifestations are not rare nowadays, and should always be remembered when a throat lesion is accompanied by a marked systemic reaction which does not respond promptly to chemotherapy.[39, 40]

The gonococcus is much more invasive locally but much less so systemically than is the meningococcus. Nevertheless, gonococcal *septicaemia* is becoming more common nowadays. A conspicuous feature of this is a rather scanty maculopapular and pustular skin eruption found especially on the extremities.[45] *Acute infective endocarditis* is a rare complication.

Another important gonococcal lesion is *purulent conjunctivitis*. This occurs classically in the newborn, whose eyes are contaminated during passage through the birth canal. A patient with gonorrhoea may also develop conjunctivitis by contaminating his eyes with his hands. The invasive character of the organism is obvious in gonococcal ophthalmia; the infection starts as a superficial conjunctivitis, but it soon implicates the cornea, the substance of which is rapidly destroyed and converted into scar tissue. Blindness was almost invariable, but the prognosis has completely changed since the introduction of penicillin.

An important later complication of gonorrhoea is *arthritis*.[41] It is typically monarticular, and is said to be commoner in women and in Negroes. It must be distinguished from the joint lesions of *Reiter's syndrome*,[42–44] which comprises a diagnostic triad of non-gonococcal urethritis, conjunctivitis, and arthritis, and may manifest uveitis and a horny thickening of the skin of the palms and soles called keratoderma blenorrhagica. This condition is of unknown aetiology, and may be acquired non-venereally—sometimes there is a history of dysentery beforehand. The arthritis is polyarticular, and men are much more commonly affected than are women.[41] As gonorrhoea and Reiter's syndrome can both occur at the same time, it is wiser not to diagnose gonococcal arthritis until the organisms are isolated from the synovial fluid. It is probable that in both types of arthritis there is an immune-complex type of allergic reaction in addition to the possible presence of an infective agent in the joint.

TREATMENT OF THE PYOGENIC INFECTIONS

It is in the treatment of the pyogenic group of infections that chemotherapy has had its greatest triumph. The sulphonamides have been extremely valuable (especially in meningococcal infections), but they are now largely superseded by the vast range of newly-discovered antibiotics.

Against the pyococcal infections generally penicillin is the drug of choice. Tetracyclines are also very useful. The Gram-negative intestinal bacilli are penicillin resistant, but respond well to the tetracyclines and the streptomycin group, especially kanamycin and gentamicin. *Ps. pyocyanea* is a very resistant organism, but responds to polymyxin and gentamicin.

An advance of great importance has been the development of new penicillins which have extended properties over the generally employed penicillin G. Some of the broad-spectrum penicillins, e.g. ampicillin, are effective against many Gram-negative intestinal bacilli, and one, carbenicillin, can be used in *Ps. pyocyanea* infections.

REFERENCES

1. WILSON, G. S. and MILES, A. A. (1964). In *Topley and Wilson's Principles of Bacteriology and Immunity*, 5th edn, p. 1788. London: Arnold.
2. WANNAMAKER, L. W. (1970). *New England Journal of Medicine*, **282**, 23 and 78.
3. GOULD, J. C. (1965). In *Medical Microbiology*, 11th edn, p. 134. Edited by R. Cruikshank, Edinburgh: Livingstone.
4. ROUNTREE, P. M. and FREEMAN, B. M. (1955). *Medical Journal of Australia*, **2**, 157.
5. ROGERS, D. E. (1956). *Annals of Internal Medicine*, **45**, 748.
6. EDE, S., DAVIS, G. M. and HOLMES, F. H. (1959). *Journal of the American Medical Association*, **170**, 638.
7. ALTEMEIER, W. A., HUMMEL, R. P. and HILL, E. O. (1963). *Annals of Surgery*, **157**, 847.
8. GARDNER, R. J., HENEGAR, G. C. and PRESTON, F. W. (1963). *Archives of Surgery*, **87**, 58.
9. Leading Article (1971). *British Medical Journal*, iii, 132.
10. SKINNER, D. and KEEFER, C. S. (1941). *Archives of Internal Medicine*, **68**, 851.
11. GILLIES, R. R. (1965). In *Medical Microbiology*, p. 149, *loc cit.*
12. WILSON, G. S. and MILES, A. A. (1964). p. 1763, *loc. cit.*
13. MELENEY, F. L. (1924). *Archives of Surgery*, **9**, 317.
14. MELENEY, F. L. (1933). *Surgery, Gynecology and Obstetrics*, **56**, 847.
15. STRASBERG, S. M. and SILVER, M. D. (1968). *American Journal of Surgery*, **115**, 763.
16. DUNNET, W. N. and SCHALLIBAUM, E. M. (1960). *Lancet*, ii, 1227.
17. HARE, R. (1967). In *Recent Advances in Medical Microbiology*, p. 284. Edited by A. P. Waterson. London: Churchill.
18. HAYWARD, N. J. and PILCHER, R. (1945). *Lancet*, ii, 560.
19. MELENEY, F. L., FRIEDMAN, S. T. and HARVEY, H. D. (1945). *Surgery*, **18**, 423.
20. GILLIES, R. R. (1965), pp. 249–261, *loc. cit.*
21. WILSON, G. S. and MILES, A. A. (1964), p. 806, *loc. cit.*
22. WILLIAMS, R. E. O., BLOWERS, R., GARROD, L. P. and SHOOTER, R. A. (1966). In *Hospital Infection*, 2nd edn, p. 43. London: Lloyd-Luke.
23. LOWBURY, E. J. L. (1968). In *Recent Advances in Clinical Pathology*, Series Five, p. 2. Edited by S. C. Dyke. London: Churchill.
24. CURTIN, J. A., PETERSDORF, R. G. and BENNETT, I. L. (1961). *Annals of Internal Medicine*, **54**, 1077.
25. RABIN, E. R. *et al.* (1961). *New England Journal of Medicine*, **265**, 1225.

26. Forkner, C. E. *et al.* (1958). *American Journal of Medicine*, **25**, 877.
27. Hutchinson, R. I. (1957). *Journal of Hygiene*, **55**, 27.
28. Gillies, R. R. (1965). p. 165, *loc. cit.*
29. Wilson, G. S. and Miles, A. A. (1964). p. 2018, *loc. cit.*
30. Reimann, H. A. (1962). *Annals of Internal Medicine*, **56**, 144.
31. Chanock, R. M. *et al.* (1961). *Journal of the American Medical Association*, **175**, 213.
32. Cruikshank, R. (1965). In *Medical Microbiology*, p. 169. *loc. cit.*
33. Lucas, C. T. *et al.* (1971). *Journal of the American Medical Association*, **216**, 1612.
34. Wilson, G. S. and Miles, A. A. (1964). p. 1736, *loc. cit.*
35. Fairbrother, R. W. (1947). *Journal of Clinical Pathology*, **1**, 10.
36. Banks, H. S. (1948). *Lancet*, ii, 635 and 677.
37. Nielsen, L. T. (1970). *Archives of Dermatology and Syphilology*, **102**, 97.
38. Wilson, G. S. and Miles, A. A. (1964). p. 1755, *loc. cit.*
39. Brø-Jorgensen, A. and Jensen, T. (1971). *British Medical Journal*, iv, 660.
40. Metzger, A. L. (1970). *Annals of Internal Medicine*, **73**, 267.
41. Wright, V. (1963). *Annals of the Rheumatic Diseases*, **22**, 77.
42. Weinberger, H. W. *et al.* (1962). *Medicine (Baltimore)*, **41**, 35.
43. Leading Article (1971). *British Medical Journal*, iii, 386.
44. Csonka, G. W. (1972). *British Journal of Hospital Medicine*, **7**, 8.
45. Shapiro, L., Teisch, J. A. and Brownstein, M. H. (1973). *Archives of Dermatology*, **107**, 403.

Chapter 18. Wound Infections: The Clostridia

THE SOURCE OF WOUND INFECTION

The most important organisms responsible for wound infection are (*a*) *Staph. pyogenes*; (*b*) *Strept. pyogenes*; (*c*) Gram-negative intestinal bacilli; and (*d*) clostridia. Certain uncommon wound infections should be noted. *Anaerobic streptococci* and *Bacteroides* are described in Chapter 17. *Fusospirochaetal* infections have been noted following human bites, as has also *actinomycosis*. In tropical countries wounds are occasionally infected with *Corynebacterium diphtheriae*, producing cutaneous diphtheria. Other tropical oddities are *mycetoma* (see p. 258) and *myiasis*, the infestation of a cutaneous wound with fly larvae.

Wounds may be infected primarily at the time of injury or else secondarily at a later date; either infection may be derived from the patient himself or from an outside source. The types of wounds most liable to primary infection are those that follow battle or agricultural accidents, when gross soiling is almost inevitable. Likewise wounds implicating the bowel are contaminated by the patient's faeces. The organisms found in such wounds include clostridia and Gram-negative intestinal bacilli. On the other hand, wounds following industrial accidents may be only lightly contaminated with staphylococci, and clean surgical wounds should, at least theoretically, be free of pathogens.

It is regrettable that wounds that were primarily sterile, or else rendered sterile by appropriate antibiotic therapy, often become infected during convalescence. The source of such infection may be the patient himself, as a result of touching his injuries, but more commonly the infection of a wound is from an extrinsic source following cross-infection. The most prevalent wound infections nowadays are the result of cross-infection in hospital wards, and the organisms usually responsible are *Staph. pyogenes* and *Ps. pyocyanea*. These are considered in Chapter 19. The remainder of this chapter is devoted to anaerobic wound infections due to the clostridial group of organisms.

ANAEROBIC WOUND INFECTIONS

These infections are of great clinical importance, and with few exceptions, e.g. those due to anaerobic streptococci, actinomyces, and bacteroides, all are due to the clostridial group of anaerobic spore-bearers. The clostridial organisms are responsible for two extremely serious conditions, *gas-gangrene* and *tetanus*. Gas-gangrene is produced by the combined action of a number of clostridia, the most important of which are *Cl. welchii*, *Cl. oedematiens*, and *Cl. septicum*, whereas tetanus is caused by a single organism, *Cl. tetani*. The rare, lethal form of food-poisoning, botulism, is produced by another clostridium, *Cl. botulinum*.

BACTERIOLOGY OF THE CLOSTRIDIAL ORGANISMS[1]

Morphology. They are large, Gram-positive bacilli approximately 5 μm long. The most characteristic feature is the spore, which is produced whenever the organism is placed in adverse conditions. It is usually central or subterminal, but in *Cl. tetani* it is situated terminally producing a characteristic drum-stick appearance. These organisms are all motile and non-capsulate with the exception of *Cl. welchii* which is non-motile and capsulate.

Cultural characteristics. They all grow easily but demand absolute anaerobiosis, i.e. they are obligatory anaerobes. They are most conveniently cultured at 37°C on blood agar in the anaerobic atmosphere afforded by a McIntosh and Fildes jar. There appear flat, rather irregular colonies, and these may be surrounded by a zone of haemolysis, depending on the species.

Robertson's meat medium, which consists of cooked meat suspended in infusion broth, is useful in that it allows the growth of both anaerobes and aerobes (see Appendix II). The anaerobes can then be subcultured anaerobically on to blood agar to obtain pure colonies.

Biochemical reactions. These are of considerable importance. Clostridia are divided into two categories, saccharolytic and proteolytic.

Saccharolytic clostridia ferment many sugars, e.g. lactose and glucose. They do not break down proteins, and they merely turn the meat in Robertson's medium a pink colour due to the production of acid. The true pathogens of gas-gangrene, viz. *Cl. welchii*, *Cl. septicum*, and *Cl. oedematiens*, come into this category.

Proteolytic clostridia. These break down protein and produce foul-smelling gases like hydrogen sulphide and ammonia. The meat in Robertson's medium becomes black due to the formation of iron sulphide. Some of these organisms are also able to ferment sugars, but they are less active than the first group. The secondary putrefactive saprophytes of gas-gangrene, e.g. *Cl. sporogenes* and *Cl. histolyticum*, come into this category. *Cl. tetani* does not ferment sugars at all, and is only feebly proteolytic.

Toxin production. The clostridia are typical toxic organisms, the lesions they produce being due entirely to exotoxins. The infection is localised, but the systemic effects are far-reaching.

Of the gas-gangrene group *Cl. welchii* is the most important. Five types are described, and type A is the human pathogen, causing gas-gangrene and food-poisoning. The other four types affect sheep and cattle. The toxin of type A is called *α-toxin*. It is lethal for laboratory animals and is necrotising. It is a lecithinase, and attacks the phospholipid constituents of red cells thereby causing severe haemolytic anaemia. This lecithinase is used in detecting *Cl. welchii*: if egg-yolk, which is rich in lipoprotein, is incorporated into nutrient agar, it is rendered opalescent by *Cl. welchii* by virtue of its lecithinase. This effect is prevented if the agar plate is first treated with an antitoxin to the α-toxin. This is called *Nagler's reaction*.

In addition, some strains of type-A *Cl. welchii* produce variable amounts of haemolysin (θ-toxin), collagenase (ϰ-toxin), hyaluronidase (μ-toxin), and deoxyribonuclease (ν-toxin).

Cl. septicum produces various toxins: one that is lethal and haemolytic, a haemolysin, a deoxyribonuclease, and a hyaluronidase. *Cl. oedematiens* produces a toxin that is haemolytic and has a lecithinase activity and is also necrotising and lethal.

By contrast, *Cl. tetani* produces only two exotoxins. The important one is a neurotoxin called *tetanospasmin*, which is responsible for the convulsions of tetanus. Tetanospasmin has been separated in a pure crystalline form. It is an immensely potent poison, being second only to the exotoxin of *Cl. botulinum* in this respect. The other exotoxin is haemolytic, and is known as *tetanolysin*.

Occurrence. The spores of these organisms are widely dispersed in nature, and are especially plentiful in soil. They are contaminants of the human and animal intestine, and are excreted in the faeces and returned to the soil in the form of manure. *Cl. welchii* is an invariable inhabitant of the human bowel, but tetanus spores occur somewhat more sporadically. These organisms must be expected in all environments, including the air and furniture of wards and even operating theatres.[2] As regards the latter, plenum filtration systems (see p. 238) are important in preventing the entry of spores from the atmosphere.

By virtue of their ability to form spores in adverse circumstances, these organisms are resistant to heat and desiccation. Only well-devised sterilising methods can destroy them.

Apart from the role played by *Cl. welchii* in gas-gangrene, certain specific strains are an important cause of *food-poisoning* when they contaminate meat in heavy culture. The symptoms, which may be quite severe and occasionally fatal, are dysenteric in type. The causal organisms are isolated with ease from the meat and the patient's faeces.[3, 4, 5]

GAS-GANGRENE[6]

Gas-gangrene may follow the contamination of a wound with the spores of the pathogenic clostridia. Considering the very widespread distribution of these spores and the rarity of gas-gangrene in civilian practice, it is evident that the contamination of a healthy incised wound is not followed by infection. The factor essential for spore germination is a reduced oxygen tension. This is present in severely contused or lacerated wounds containing much dead tissue, which has been devitalised as a result of compression or impaired blood supply. Deep punctured wounds are particularly dangerous. Foreign bodies like shrapnel or pieces of clothing exert local pressure, and also favour pyogenic infection. Soil is particularly dangerous, for its ionisable calcium salts and silicic acid lead to tissue necrosis. Finally, any coincidental infection by aerobic organisms serves to augment the anaerobiosis. The local injection of adrenaline has a similar effect by causing vasoconstriction, and this drug should not be injected into the buttocks where the skin is liable to be contaminated with clostridial spores.[7]

It therefore follows that most gas-gangrene is exogenous in origin, and is due to the contamination of large wounds. It is seen typically in battle casualties or in agricultural accidents. An appreciable amount of gas-gangrene is, however, endogenous from the bowel. Examples of this are the clostridial puerperal sepsis that follows criminal abortion, and the gas-gangrene of the high thigh stump after amputation of the lower limb for peripheral vascular disease. The stump is often soiled with faeces, especially in an elderly, incontinent patient.[8]

Spores of clostridia have been known to remain dormant in healed wounds, and to have germinated following surgical intervention. This is particularly important with regard to tetanus, and immunisation is always advisable before surgery is performed on old war and agricultural wounds.

Pathogenesis. Gas-gangrene is not due to infection by a single clostridial organism; it is the consequence of a combined assault by numerous saccharolytic and proteolytic organisms. The true pathogens, *Cl. welchii*, *Cl. septicum*, and *Cl. oedematiens*, germinate, and the powerful exotoxins which they liberate produce local tissue necrosis. At this stage the proteolytic saprophytes, such as *Cl. sporogenes* and *Cl. histolyticum*, flourish on the dead material, and break it down into putrid products.

If the wound is merely superficial, it will discharge foul-smelling fluid in which there are bubbles of gas (anaerobic cellulitis), but if it is extensive enough to implicate the underlying muscles, the anaerobic myositis typical of gas-gangrene develops.[9, 10]

(*a*) There is a rapidly progressive necrosis of muscle fibres due to the necrotising exotoxins of the saccharolytic clostridia.

(*b*) The muscle carbohydrate is fermented by these organisms. Lactic acid and gas (mostly hydrogen and carbon dioxide) are formed. This is the origin of the "gas" in gas-gangrene. At this stage it is odourless.

(*c*) There is rapid spread of infection due to the breaking down of intercellular ground substance and local tissue barriers (e.g. endomysium and perimysium) by the hyaluronidase and collagenase produced by the organisms. A whole muscle bundle may be affected with great rapidity. Indeed, gas-gangrene resembles an invasive infection in the extent of its local spread, but the organisms show no tendency towards blood-stream invasion, except perhaps at the time of death. This accounts for the gas bubbles in the liver (*foamy liver*) and other organs sometimes found at necropsy. Moreover, this appearance is not confined to gas-gangrene; clostridial organisms may also enter the blood stream from the bowel as an agonal phenomenon during the course of any fatal disease.

(*d*) As the infection spreads, so the necrosis increases both by toxic action and the ischaemia following pressure by the gas and exudate on the surrounding blood vessels. The area is tense, oedematous, and crepitant, and the muscle is odourless and brick-red in colour.

(*e*) Following the extensive necrosis there is progressive putrefaction, which is brought about by the proteolytic clostridia. These thrive on and decompose the dead muscle, which becomes greenish-black in colour. Necrosis with superadded putrefaction is called gangrene (see p. 55), and these saprophytes complete the evolution of "gas-gangrene". It is at this stage that the characteristically foul odour appears.

(*f*) During this local process there is severe toxaemia due to circulating exotoxins. It is manifested by profound shock and a rapidly-developing haemolytic anaemia (see p. 232). It is this toxaemia which brings about the death of the patient.

The local pathological effects of gas-gangrene are acute inflammation with much muscle necrosis and spreading oedema.[11, 12] Polymorph infiltration is not conspicuous while the process is advancing, a point of difference between clostridial and streptococcal myositis. In the oedema fluid there are large numbers of organisms. The severe oedema may be related to the permeability factor produced by some clostridia, especially *Cl. oedematiens*. The absence of polymorphs is strange; perhaps the powerful exotoxins exert a negative chemotactic influence.

Treatment of gas-gangrene.[13] It is usual to give a polyvalent anti-serum against the exotoxins of the three main pathogens, as well as penicillin or a tetracycline. For prophylaxis in cases of grossly contaminated wounds penicillin has replaced antiserum therapy. There is no doubt, however, that a proper wound toilet is the most important aspect of prevention and treatment.

TETANUS[14]

The spores of *Cl. tetani* not infrequently contaminate wounds, but as with the gas-gangrene organisms a reduced oxygen tension is essential for their germination. The conditions conducive to tetanus infection are therefore similar to those already described. Quite often the degree of trauma is very mild, because an insignificant punctured wound like the prick of a contaminated thorn can be the site of origin of a fatal tetanus infection.

Exogenous infection has also resulted in *surgical tetanus*,[15, 16] i.e. the introduction of spores into a wound during the course of a surgical operation. For such spores to germinate they must be presented with a nidus where conditions are relatively anaerobic. Contaminated foreign materials embedded in the tissues, e.g. catgut, talc, or cotton-wool, provide the necessary nidus, and are the causes of surgical tetanus, which nowadays is very rare. Catgut, which is made from the intestine of sheep, is almost inevitably contaminated, but fortunately modern processes of sterilisation during its manufacture are so effective that it has ceased to be a hazard in most countries.

The umbilical stump of newborn babies is another potential site of infection, and *tetanus neonatorum* has killed many infants in primitive communities where dung is used as a dressing.

In the USA the condition of *4th of July tetanus* is recognised. Apparently the wads used in the manufacture of fireworks can contain spores, and tetanus may complicate firework injuries. The condition seems to have no British counterpart on November 5th!

Endogenous tetanus infection is rare, but it has been reported after septic abortions.

Pathogenesis

Tetanus is clinically a disease of the central nervous system. The local lesion may be so mild that only very careful search will reveal it, yet the exotoxin produced may be sufficient to cause death.

After peripheral absorption, the toxin reaches the central nervous system probably by passing along the motor trunks; it spreads up the spaces between the nerve fibres.[17, 18] It acts by interfering with the inhibition processes at the motor neurones. This accounts for the generalised increase in tone, and also explains *local tetanus*.[19] This is the early tendency to spasms of those muscles controlled by the same spinal segment as that supplying the area infected.

The incubation period varies from a few days to several weeks, and the shorter it is, the worse the prognosis. Tetanus developing from wounds of the upper extremities, neck, and face is said to be more frequently fatal than that arising after injuries to the lower parts of the body.

The condition usually commences with stiffness and spasm confined to the area of infection (local tetanus). This is soon followed by severe trismus due to masseteric spasm (lock-jaw), dysphagia, spasm of the facial muscles producing the characteristic *risus sardonicus*, and finally generalised tetanic convulsions, in which there may be opisthotonos. The picture resembles strychnine poisoning quite closely, but unlike it there is residual muscle stiffness between periods of convulsion. Death is due to asphyxia following involvement of the respiratory muscles. There are no characteristic *post-mortem* findings.

Prophylaxis of Tetanus[20-23]

Since tetanus may occur following quite trivial wounds, by far the best method of prophylaxis is active immunisation. This is carried out by a course of three injections of tetanus toxoid, a formolised preparation of the exotoxin adsorbed on to aluminium hydroxide or phosphate.[21] The second injection is given about 8 weeks after the first, and the third from 6–12 months after the second.

When a person is severely wounded, tetanus prophylaxis is essential. If there has been a complete course of active immunisation previously, all that needs to be done, apart from proper excision of the wound, is to give another injection of toxoid provided a booster has not been given within the last three years[21, 23] when another dose is unnecessary. In unimmunised people with fresh, clean wounds, excision alone may suffice, but if more than six hours have elapsed before treatment, or if the wound is extensive or likely to have been contaminated, some additional form of prophylaxis is necessary. The usual treatment is the administration of horse antitetanic serum (ATS) in a dose of 1 500 units that can be increased to 10 000 units if the danger of tetanus is judged to be great.

The difficulty about horse antitoxin is that it may lead to severe allergic reactions, notably immediately dangerous anaphylaxis and delayed serum sickness. Whenever horse serum is administered, a small test dose should first be given subcutaneously, and if after half an hour there are no general symptoms such as tachycardia or dyspnoea, the remainder can be given. One ml of 1 in 1 000 adrenaline solution should always be close at hand for *intramuscular* injection in case anaphylactic symptoms, namely dyspnoea, pallor, and collapse, develop.[24]

The duration of passive immunity shows great individual variation, and is in general related to the reaction engendered by previous sensitisation to horse protein, e.g. by a previous injection of ATS. Among non-reactors antibodies can usually still be detected at 10–16 days. But when a systemic reaction occurs, the antitoxin is rapidly removed, none being present 10–12 days later. It therefore follows that people who react to a test dose will obtain little benefit from the antitoxin, even if the full dose is given in such small repeated

doses that a serious reaction is averted. Such people include those previously given horse serum, and also some atopic subjects. These people may develop tetanus despite attempted passive immunisation with ATS. The horse serum combines with preformed anti-horse antibody, and the complex is rapidly eliminated from the body (see Fig. 12.14, p. 155).

In view of the danger of hypersensitivity reactions (occurring in about 12 per cent of patients[22]) and the unpredictability of the immunising action of horse ATS, there has been a move against using it and instead relying on surgical excision and antibiotic cover. But in extensive wounds excision may, despite all care, be incomplete, and antibiotics (chiefly penicillin), apart from their own tendency to produce allergy, have also been known to be ineffective in preventing tetanus. Horse ATS is still recommended for large wounds and those whose treatment has been delayed. A better antiserum is that derived from hyperimmunised human volunteers; it does not cause allergy, and persists in the circulation longer than horse serum. Its value, both prophylactic and therapeutic, has been commended, but unfortunately it is still not universally available. It should be given whenever possible to all patients and particularly to those who are hypersensitive to horse ATS and are severely wounded.[22]

In all patients who have not been actively immunised, the first dose of tetanus toxoid should be given while the wound is being treated, whether or not ATS has been administered. Provided adsorbed toxoid is used, its action is not interfered with by the antitoxin in the circulation. The patient must be instructed to report back for the remainder of the course of injections.

Treatment of Tetanus

The treatment of established tetanus is still unsatisfactory. Large doses of antitoxin (even up to 100 000 units) are recommended, sometimes even intravenously after preliminary subcutaneous and intramuscular test doses, but by the time the disease is clinically manifest much of the exotoxin is firmly bound to the affected cells, and is therefore invulnerable to the action of circulating immunoglobulins. The therapeutic value of antiserum is, however, not accepted by all workers.[25] Penicillin and a tetracycline should also be given. The most important factor is undoubtedly the maintenance of respiratory function; on this especially does recovery depend.[26]

REFERENCES

1. COLLEE, J. G. (1965). In *Medical Microbiology*, 11th edn, pp. 308 and 327. Edited by R. Cruikshank. Edinburgh: Livingstone.
2. LOWBURY, E. J. L. and LILLY, H. A. (1958) *Journal of Hygiene*, **56**, 169.
3. HOBBS, B. C. *et al.* (1953). *Journal of Hygiene*, **51**, 75.
4. Annotation (1963). *Lancet*, ii, 991.
5. Annotation (1963). *British Medical Journal*, ii, 1604.
6. WILSON, G. S. and MILES, A. A. (1964). In *Topley and Wilson's Principles of Bacteriology and Immunity*, 5th edn, p. 2124. London: Arnold.
7. HARVEY, P. W. and PURNELL, G. V. (1968). *British Medical Journal*, i, 744.

8. Leading Article (1969). *British Medical Journal*, ii, 328.
9. MacLennan, J. D. (1943). *Lancet*, ii, 63, 94, and 123.
10. Wilson, T. S. (1960). *Canadian Journal of Surgery*, **4**, 35.
11. Robb-Smith, A. H. T. (1945). *Lancet*, ii, 362.
12. Govan, A. D.T. (1946). *Journal of Pathology and Bacteriology*, **58**, 423.
13. Altemeier, W. A. *et. al.* (1957). *Archives of Surgery*, **74**, 839.
14. Wilson, G. S. and Miles, A. A. (1964). In *Topley and Wilson's Principles of Bacteriology and Immunity*, 5th edn, p. 2095. London: Arnold.
15. Williams, R. E. O., Blowers, R., Garrod, L. P. and Shooter, R. A. (1966). In *Hospital Infection*, 2nd edn, p. 141. London: Lloyd-Luke.
16. Report of the Public Health Laboratory Service (Medical Research Council, London). (1959). *British Medical Journal*, i, 1150.
17. Wright, E. A., Morgan, R. S. and Wright, G. P. (1950). *Journal of Pathology and Bacteriology*, **62**, 569.
18. Ibid. (1951). *British Journal of Experimental Pathology*, **32**, 169.
19. Ibid. (1952). *Lancet*, ii, 316.
20. Williams, R. E. O., Blowers, R., Garrod, L. P. and Shooter, R. A. (1966), p. 286, *loc. cit.*
21. Leading Article (1967). *Lancet*, ii, 662.
22. Leading Article (1967). *British Medical Journal*, iv, 635.
23. Leading Article (1969). *Lancet*, i, 763.
24. Parish, H. J. and Cannon, D. A. (1962). *Antisera, Toxoids, Vaccines and Tuberculins*, 6th edn, p. 31. Edinburgh: Livingstone.
25. Vaishnava, H. *et al.* (1966). *Lancet*, ii, 1371.
26. Leading Article (1963). *British Medical Journal*, i, 558.

Chapter 19.   Hospital Infection ✓

The present pre-eminence of surgery can be attributed to advances in the two ancillary fields of anaesthesia and microbiology. The advisability of analgesia on the grounds of humanity and cleanliness on the grounds of necessity was recognised by surgeons at least as early as the third millennium B.C., yet even in the nineteenth century these were blatantly ignored. A change was precipitated by Ignaz Semmelweiss in Vienna and Oliver Wendell Holmes in Boston. Independently they revived the idea of the contagious nature of wound infection by showing that puerperal sepsis was related to the unclean hands and clothing of the obstetrician rather than to an act of God. The idea was unacceptable to the medical establishment of the day: Holmes was ignored but did at least live to see his ideas vindicated; Semmelweiss, on the other hand, was derided and dismissed from his post, and he subsequently died insane.[1] A century later we fully appreciate the dangers of hospital infection.

Hospital infection is the result of the transmission of pathogenic organisms to a previously uninfected patient from a source in the environment of a hospital. If the organisms are derived from some external source the infection is called *cross-infection*; if they are derived from the patient himself, it is called *auto-infection*. In *maternity wards* epidemics of staphylococcal bullous impetigo of the newborn (and subsequent maternal breast abscess) may be encountered, while amongst the older infants explosive epidemics of gastro-enteritis due to enteropathogenic species of *Esch. coli* and to *Salmonella* and *Shigella* organisms are not uncommon. In a *children's ward* the common virus diseases like chickenpox and measles, when once introduced, will spread like wildfire, and epidemics of infective hepatitis may also occur. In *mental hospitals*, *Shigella* diarrhoea is often a great nuisance. Even in *general medical wards* the menace of cross-infection is always present. A patient with open pulmonary tuberculosis is an obvious source of danger, and should be isolated as soon as possible. It is quite common for patients admitted with cerebral vascular accidents to succumb to staphylococcal pneumonia, and for patients with neurological disorders like multiple sclerosis and cauda equina lesions, who require repeated catheterisation, to develop intractable *Ps. pyocyanea* infections of the urinary tract.

It is, however, in *surgical and maternity wards* that the incidence of cross-infection reaches its peak, because the patients often have large areas of denuded integument as a result of wounds and extensive burns, or following delivery.

These provide an admirable avenue for bacterial invasion. The most common infecting organisms are *Staph. pyogenes* and the Gram-negative intestinal bacilli. *Strept. pyogenes* has had an evil reputation for producing wound infections and puerperal sepsis, but nowadays streptococcal lesions of this type are uncommon. When present, streptococci are usually found in association with staphylococci.

Staphylococcal cross-infection manifests itself as (*a*) wound infection; (*b*) skin infections, e.g. boils and bullous impetigo of the newborn; (*c*) enterocolitis; (*d*) pneumonia; (*e*) breast abscesses in lactating women; (*f*) acute conjunctivitis in the newborn. The Gram-negative bacilli are the usual causes of urinary-tract cross-infection, and they are also responsible for much wound infection. Herpesvirus infection has been described as a complication of burns.[2]

The incidence of hospital wound infection varies from 2 to 20 per cent, and it depends on such variable factors as the patient's age, the size of wound, the duration of operation, the presence of drainage tubes, the normal bacterial flora of the part, and the hospital in which the patient is treated.

SOURCE OF AND TRANSMISSION OF ORGANISMS

Staph. pyogenes.[3] The reservoir is the anterior nares, from where the organisms are conveyed to the skin of the hands. The hands and perineum[4] are areas on which staphylococci tend to multiply with greatest readiness. The organisms are excreted either from overt lesions like boils and pustules, or else they may be discharged from the skin of symptomless carriers. The nose is the ultimate reservoir, but is of less importance in the actual transmission of the organism, except perhaps during heavy breathing and snorting.[5]

The staphylococci are transferred either by direct contact on to a patient, or else to objects that may come into contact with patients (*fomites*). A perineal carrier is very liable to contaminate his bedclothes, sheets, and blankets.[6] Bedclothes and sheets are boiled, and thereby sterilised during laundering, but blankets retain their organisms because they are not boiled routinely owing to the damage such treatment would inflict on the fabric. Such blankets act as additional reservoirs of infection when they are placed on the beds of other patients. A carrier may likewise contaminate a communal bath or bowl.

It is important to realise that not all carriers are equally efficient excretors, nor does it necessarily follow that carriers who suffer from recurrent overt lesions are more dangerous than those who are symptomless. Some of the most virulent staphylococcal cross-infections have been transmitted by carriers who have not even exhibited evidence of local nasal infection. These dispensers of staphylococci are particularly dangerous.[6, 7] The nature of local immunity to staphylococcal infection and the relationship between carriage and excretion are ill-understood at present.

Finally, excretors of staphylococci may contaminate the air around them both directly and indirectly from their sheets and blankets. It is well recognised that movement in bed increases the number of organisms in the surrounding air.[8]

There are two good methods of assessing the bacterial content of the air, the *settling* or *sedimentation plate* and the *slit-sampler*. The former consists of a culture plate of standard diameter, on which the organisms in the air are allowed to settle. This is a time-consuming procedure but is particularly valuable in operating theatres, where the danger is most liable to arise from particles settling on the area of incision. The exposed plate is comparable with the exposed wound. The slit-sampler consists of a narrow slit through which air is sucked on to a rotating culture plate beneath it. This is a very efficient method of collecting most of the organisms in the sampled volume of air, and is speedy as compared with the settling plate.

Air-borne staphylococci are particularly liable to contaminate wounds in the operating theatre, where the area of incision must of necessity be exposed for some time; even in a ward these bacteria can contaminate wounds while being dressed. Furthermore, staphylococci will almost certainly be inspired by other patients and attendants, whose anterior nares may then be colonised. In this respect it is most important to note that a considerable amount of staphylococcal auto-infection from the nose is really the result of cross-infection at a slightly earlier period. Many patients become nasal carriers during the pre-operative period, and subsequently contaminate their wounds. Air-borne organisms may be inspired or swallowed and lead to staphylococcal pneumonia or enterocolitis.

Some types of staphylococci spread much more rapidly than others. The type-80 staphylococcus is notorious for the severity of its lesions as well as for its speed of spread. Most epidemic strains are resistant to the commonly-used antibiotics, but it does not follow that sensitive organisms are necessarily less virulent than resistant ones. With the constant use of antibiotics over the years most of the sensitive strains have been eliminated, so that a predominantly resistant population has been left behind. This is one of the results of the abuse of antibiotics. Once a resistant population has developed, it is perpetuated by infecting new victims. In this way cross-infection plays a major part in maintaining resistant strains.

The two cardinal hazards of hospital practice, the abuse of antibiotics and the presence of cross-infection, tend to reinforce each other and set up a vicious circle.

Strept. pyogenes. The reservoir is the throat, but it is particularly those people who harbour streptococci in their noses who are likely to transmit infection. The important mode of transmission is by close direct contact. Unlike staphylococci, these organisms do not survive long on the skin, nor is the transmission of infection by fomites of much importance. There is good experimental evidence that blankets heavily contaminated with streptococci do not infect people who sleep in them.[9–11] The part played by airborne transmission in streptococcal cross-infection is also not of great moment, except perhaps in extensive burns.

Gram-negative intestinal bacilli. *Esch. coli* is a universal commensal of the bowel, and *Proteus* organisms are present in about a third of all specimens of faeces. It is probable that a considerable amount of wound infection caused by these organisms is the result of true auto-infection, but until the established methods of typing come into general use, the actual amount of cross-infection produced by them will remain unknown. It is also important to note that the anterior urethra is frequently colonised by *Esch. coli*, *Proteus* organisms, and *Strept. faecalis*,[12] and that these organisms can be forced into the bladder during catheterisation.[13, 14] Cystitis may then ensue.

Faecal carriage of *Ps. pyocyanea* is uncommon enough to make it unlikely that auto-infection is the explanation of the majority of infections it causes. The reservoirs are the infected wounds and urinary tracts of individual patients. Most urinary cross-infection is carried by the hands of attendants from urine bottles to bladder drainage apparatus connected to indwelling catheters.[15, 16] The role played by inadequately-sterilised cystoscopes has also been demonstrated.[16, 17]

The Gram-negative intestinal bacilli can be shed quite easily into the air, but they are much less resistant to drying than are the staphylococci and streptococci. Therefore airborne spread is not so important as with these cocci. On the other hand, stagnant water affords a suitable environment for the Gram-negative organisms, especially *Ps. pyocyanea*, which has been known to contaminate the humidifiers of operating theatres and infant's incubators. It can survive in certain disinfectants, notably cetrimide, and has caused suppurative panophthalmitis (with the loss of the eye) when contaminated eye-lotions have been used to irrigate eyes on which surgery had been recently performed. Similar ocular infection has been described in a special-care nursery among neonates, and the source was contaminated resuscitation apparatus.[18]

MODE OF CROSS-INFECTION

In surgical cases cross-infection may occur either in the operating theatre or else later in the ward. Infections acquired during the period of operation usually manifest themselves within the next seven days, whereas later manifestations are more likely to be due to subsequent ward infection. Both ward and operating-theatre infections may be superficial in nature, but if the infection is obviously deep-seated, it is almost certain to have been acquired during the operation.

Cross-Infection in Operating Theatres

The three methods of theatre cross-infection are (*a*) *by direct contact from the surgeon or attendants*, (*b*) *from the air*, and (*c*) *from contaminated instruments*.

The surgeon[19] may have overt infection on his hands or another part of his body, or more likely be a nasal carrier with contaminated hands. The most dangerous areas for transmitting staphylococcal infection are the hands and wrists. Even the most scrupulous "scrubbing up" cannot sterilise the skin, for some organisms are bound to find shelter in its pores. Impermeable gloves are therefore essential for all surgical procedures, and they must be changed at once if they are perforated during the operation. The sweat that accumulates under the glove is bound to contain many organisms. The area of the wrist just above the rim of the glove is also dangerous to the patient. The sleeve of the theatre gown soon becomes sodden with blood, and organisms can penetrate it with ease, and so be introduced into the wound. By contrast the nose is less dangerous as an immediate source of infection, but should be masked in order to obviate the danger of violent expulsion of droplets during sneezing or coughing.[20]

Much interest has been centred around the problem of the *air-borne transmission of infection*,[21] which is particularly important in operating theatres. In poorly ventilated rooms there is a progressive accumulation of pathogenic organisms derived in part from the patient and his clothes and in part from the attendants and spectators[22] who have gathered around to watch the operation. All movements of the specta-tors cause settled organisms to rise in the air, from where they may alight on to the wound.

Efficient ventilation is obviously necessary to remove these organisms, but unless intelligently devised, it may cause more harm than good. In the past there have been epidemics of theatre infection due to suction of air from an adjacent contaminated source by means of a reduced pressure exhaust system of fans. In fact the air that is drawn in comes from near-by wards, and is heavily contaminated with staphylococci.[21, 23] Clostridia are the commonest pathogens found in the outside air. The inlet for fresh air to the air-conditioning plant should be as high as possible.

Inadequately sterilised instruments are of the greatest danger in transmitting infection. The role played by cysto-scopes has already been mentioned.

Prevention of Theatre Cross-Infection

Architecture and design of theatre. In theory it is best either to have the theatres completely separate from the wards, or else in one composite block. In practice the most that

can be hoped for is that a single floor may be reserved entirely for a suite of theatres, adequate in number for the size of the hospital. It is better situated in a cul-de-sac than near a main thoroughfare.

The *accessory compartments*, e.g. the scrub, sterilising, and sink rooms, should be separate from, though connected to the theatre. In this way the splashes produced during "scrubbing up" will not contaminate the theatre, nor will the contamina-ted instruments washed up in the sink room come in contact with the theatre environment. The heat engendered by autoclaving, and the steam subsequently produced, make a separate sterilising room desirable, and furthermore the dirty atmosphere of the theatre may contaminate sterilised instruments. In fact, sterilisation ought to be done in a central sterile supply away from the theatre. The anaesthetic room is useful for transferring a patient on to the operating table prior to his entry into the theatre. It should have close access to the theatre.

The *walls* and fittings of a theatre should be smooth and easy to wash down. There should be no ledges to collect dust. The *floors* should have a smooth finish, and slope gently towards a gully so that they can be swilled down with ease.

The *temperature* most suitable for work varies according to the country; in temperature climates 65–70°F is a good air temperature for a theatre, and the *relative humidity* should be about 55 per cent.

Ventilation is of paramount importance. Not only is it essential for the comfort of the staff, but it also serves to remove anaesthetic gases. The air admitted must be free of pathogenic organisms, so that it does not endanger the area of operation or the sterile equipment.

A positive pressure (plenum) system is essential,[21] and the air should be filtered before admission. Positive pressurisation serves to prevent contaminated air infiltrating into the theatre. It is also necessary to direct the air flow, so that any organisms released in the theatre may be removed as ex-peditiously as possible. There are two methods of distribut-ing the incoming air. In one, turbulent ventilation, the air is rapidly mixed with that already present in the theatre, while in the other, displacement ventilation, the air is introduced gently, and merely displaces that in the theatre by quiet downward movement. In both types of ventilation the air is introduced at ceiling-level. It is customary to extract some of it by exhaust fans situated near the floor. It is said that displacement ventilation is better in a room which is gener-ally contaminated, whereas turbulent ventilation is preferable if the source of contamination is confined to the area of the operating table, for it will produce less contamination of the incision. In practice either is acceptable.

The *filter* itself should have pores of about 5 μm in diameter. At first sight this seems very large in relation to the size of the organisms, but in fact they seldom occur singly as unattached particles in the air.[24] They are usually attached to particles of dust which are considerably larger than 5 μm.[25] Filters made of disposable fabric and oiled mesh are very effective; they must be adequately maintained, otherwise there may be heavy contamination of air entering the theatre, or else the pores may become so blocked that no air can enter at all.

The surgeon and attendants.[26] Nobody with overt staphylococcal infection, whether a boil or a superficial skin lesion anywhere on the body, should be allowed into the theatre. Streptococcal sore throat is another contraindication, but the common cold is less dangerous. It may, of course, be transmitted to the patient and lead to a chest infection. It is impractical to exclude staphylococcal carriers unless they bear epidemic strains.

The ritual of a shower bath before operating is useless, and indeed increases the dispersal of bacteria, particularly staphylococci, in the air for some hours. Even washing with a hexachlorophane soap is not helpful. The removal of underclothes is another ritual; it does not decrease the infectivity of the surgeon because the underlying skin is the source of the organisms. The surgeon should be gowned and masked to prevent direct contact between the incised area and his own skin. Theatre gowns are unfortunately inefficient in preventing the escape of organisms, which penetrate between the pores of the fabric and at the trouser openings at the ankles. New theatre garments with a finer pore mesh and closed ankle openings are being devised.

The method of washing up, no matter how painstaking and prolonged, will remove only those "transient" organisms which are picked up adventitiously; it will reduce but cannot eliminate the "resident" flora. A six-minute scrub with soap and water reduces the bacterial flora by about 50 per cent, while a two-minute handwashing in one of the liquid preparations containing hexachlorophane or iodophors can reduce the population to as little as 1 per cent. Rinsing in a 0·5 per cent solution of chlorhexidine is equally effective. Liquid soap or detergent preparations are more effective than are antiseptic bar soaps. Prolonged washing is not only unnecessary but is indeed harmful to the skin if frequently carried out. Recently it has been recommended that two or three minutes' scrubbing, with careful attention to the nails, before the first operation, and two or three minutes' washing without a brush before the subsequent operations of a list should be an adequate routine for a surgeon.[27] Rings should be removed from the fingers before washing up.

Caps are important as the hair often harbours staphylococci and a mask should be worn to protect the wound from salivary droplets and mucus emitted during talking or sneezing. Cotton masks with impervious material inserted between the two layers are simple and adequate. Some paper masks are also suitable. Finally, intact gloves must be worn; the pretested ones are best. A waterproof fabric is useful for protecting the sleeve area.

The spectators.[26] These should wear masks and caps and be gowned. Shoes should be removed, and theatre boots or shoes worn. Above all there should be as little movement as possible, and this means limiting the number of spectators and assistants. The surgical team should be as small as possible, and the equipment so well placed that extraneous movements are unnecessary.

The patient.[26] His bedclothes and blankets should not be allowed into the theatre. The disinfection of his skin can be carried out for some days in advance with hexachlorophane soap to cut down the staphylococcal flora. This is done particularly in orthopaedic cases but could be applied to other types of surgery. Skin disinfection at operation is discussed on p. 642.

Surgical equipment.[26] The amount of theatre equipment present should be limited, for all objects accumulate organisms. Sterile packs should have a double wrapping and must be kept dry, as organisms move by capillary action through moist porous material. All equipment should be disinfected, or sterilised if it comes into contact with the incision. This is described in Appendix I.

Chemoprophylaxis.[26] The use of a cream containing chlorhexidine and neomycin (or preferably gentamicin) can reduce the staphylococcal population of the nose when inserted locally. Likewise oral antibiotics reduce the flora of the bowel before resection. The widespread use of antibiotics is harmful by encouraging the emergence of resistant organisms, and this practice can lead to serious outbreaks of infection. It has been reported that such an outbreak can be controlled by discontinuing the use of all antibiotics.[28, 38] Prophylactic chemotherapy is justified in particular circumstances, e.g. before dental extraction in patients with valvular heart disease, in open-heart surgery especially if valve prostheses are being inserted, and in diabetics undergoing amputation for peripheral vascular disease.

Cross-Infection in Surgical Wards[29]

The modes of staphylococcal cross-infection in a ward are not very different from those in a theatre, except that many other patients are also present. They are potential sources of infection.

Patients with obvious septic lesions,[30, 31] e.g. extensive skin infections with a copious purulent exudate or chronic osteomyelitis with pus seeping through the plaster, are particularly dangerous. The organisms soon contaminate the bedding, and are shed into the air. The same applies to patients suffering from staphylococcal pneumonia or enterocolitis. Others may merely be carriers, but of these a few may harbour virulent strains, which can lead to a ward epidemic.

The *air* may be sufficiently contaminated to endanger wounds during dressing, especially such complicated lesions as extensive burns. In this respect it is important that sterilised dressings which have been exposed to the air should be discarded if not used at the time of exposure. It is bad practice to keep a large supply of dressings in metal drums, using some as required and keeping the remainder. If small packages are used, there will be less temptation to retain any dressings that are left over.

Another source of mischief is contaminated bedclothes,

especially blankets. Apart from the possible danger of direct contact with patients, contaminated blankets are of even greater importance in shedding staphylococci into the air. An experiment in which woollen and cotton blankets were heavily contaminated with *Staph. citreus* demonstrated the great speed with which the organisms were dispersed throughout the ward. When the blankets were covered by a counterpane, the dispersion was even greater; this was attributed to friction on the surface of the blankets.[32]

It must finally be reiterated that much postoperative infection due to organisms in the patient's nose or on his skin is really the result of initial cross-infection and subsequent auto-infection.

Quite apart from direct implantation into the wound, it is possible that nasal carriers are subjected to a period of bacteraemia during the inexpert insertion of endotracheal tubes. The tissue damage in the wound could be sufficient to localise infection there.

Prevention of Cross-Infection in Surgical Wards

Isolation policy.[33] Under ideal circumstances all patients harbouring staphylococci should be isolated from the remainder of the hospital community, but in practice this is impossible. There is no doubt, however, that patients suffering from extensive discharging staphylococcal lesions should be separated from uninfected patients. Carriers of virulent strains, e.g. the type-80 staphylococcus, should be treated likewise.

On the other hand, there are patients who are particularly susceptible to infection, and they too should be isolated in their own interests. Patients who have undergone extensive skin grafting or organ transplantation, or who are suffering from agranulocytosis or immunological deficiency disease fall into this category.

The type of isolation recommended is again subject to the criterion of practicability. *Complete isolation* in an air-conditioned cubicle in a special hospital is an ideal but is rarely practical, and it may have the additional disadvantage of necessitating a break in the continuity of the medical attendants responsible for the patient's treatment. *Ward side-rooms*, on the other hand, are convenient and practical, but it is important to ensure that the flow of air is in the right direction. If the patient is excreting large numbers of staphylococci, the ventilation must be adjusted so that the air is discharged without contaminating the main ward. Care must also be taken to prevent the nursing staff from contracting infection from the patient. The use of protective clothing is advisable.

Communal segregation of infected patients in "septic wards" is another possibility. It protects the uninfected, but entails the risk of the infected patients acquiring each other's infection. In practice it is very useful in times of emergency. Barrier nursing in open wards, so useful in an intestinal infection like typhoid fever, is of no value in preventing staphylococcal cross-infection. In an epidemic of staphylo-coccal infection the whole ward may have to be evacuated and then disinfected.

Dressing technique. The danger of doctors and attendants who have overt infection, or who carry virulent staphylococci on their skin, has already been discussed. People who have infected lesions should not dress wounds. All dressers should be properly clothed and masked, and a *rigorous no-touch technique* should be employed by the use of sterile forceps. Alternatively gloves should be worn.

It is bad practice to dress wounds in general wards if there is no evidence of overt infection among the patients. It is far better to use separate, well-equipped, properly ventilated *dressing rooms*. The question of ventilation is particularly important if infected wounds are being dressed in the room. In a short time there will be an accumulation of pathogenic organisms in it, and they must be discharged to the outside atmosphere and not into the general ward. Likewise it is foolish to allow ward air to contaminate the dressing room.

Urinary drainage. Catheterisation should be avoided whenever possible because of the danger of cystitis (see p. 237), but when the use of the catheter is necessary the operator should be gloved. Where continuous bladder drainage is necessary, the weight of evidence incriminates open systems for cross-infection. The use of *closed drainage systems*, especially those which do not need to be disconnected periodically during bladder irrigation, has reduced the amount of urinary cross-infection very considerably.[34-36]

Disposal of contaminated articles. Wound dressings should be placed in paper bags and burnt. They should not be left lying around the wards. Used instruments should be sterilised without delay, and dirty bedclothes should be sent to the laundry as soon as possible.

General cleaning and disinfection of the ward. This includes the disinfection of bedding and the cleaning of the ward furniture, walls, and floors. It is a counsel of perfection to advocate disinfected blankets, mattresses, and pillows for each new patient, and the most that can be hoped for is a general cleaning every few months, or when the bedding is obviously soiled. *Bedding* used by patients who are infected severely enough to warrant isolation should be disinfected before further use, and a general disinfection is mandatory in cases of ward epidemics. Bedding used by patients suffering from particularly dangerous diseases like staphylococcal enterocolitis and tuberculosis must be disinfected before it is sent to the laundry. In cases of smallpox the bedding is best burnt.

It has been shown that the disinfection of blankets before use by each patient does not significantly reduce the general bacterial or *Staph. pyogenes* counts on exposed culture plates placed in the ward.[37] The blankets themselves become heavily recontaminated from other bedding and patients after a few days. It would seem that the rate of recontamination is so great that the air does not show any permanent diminution in bacterial content.[33] Cotton blankets are recontaminated as rapidly as are woollen ones,[33] but as they can be cleaned after each patient, they are more desirable from an aesthetic point of view. On the other hand, woollen blankets are more comfortable than are cotton ones.

Screens and *curtains* should be disinfected at monthly intervals. They should be made of cotton, for they can then be boiled during the laundry process. *Communal baths* should be disinfected after use. The *walls, floors*, and *furniture* of wards should be cleaned so frequently that there is no visible dirt on them. This entails the daily washing of floors and dusting of furniture. Walls and ceilings should be cleaned at least once a year.

It is easy to adopt a sanctimonious attitude towards ward hygiene. A state of mind may result in which the staff are more concerned about preventing infection than about treating patients under their care. A sense of perspective is always essential. The scope of hygiene depends on the size and position of the hospital, and the nature of the surgery that is performed in it. Hospital infection will be overcome only when aseptic methods are used by every member of the staff as part of an unwritten, instinctive routine in the treatment of each patient that is admitted.

Investigation of an Epidemic of Surgical Cross-Infection

First of all, the infecting organism must be isolated, and it should then be typed.

Secondly, it should be decided by clinical assessment whether the infections occurred during the time of operation or later on in the ward. The time of first appearance of the lesions and their depth are good indications.

If all the organisms are all of one type, it is strong presumptive evidence that the infection has originated from a single source. It is therefore important to swab the anterior nares of the relevant theatre and ward staff, and also to examine any overt or healing infected lesions that may be present on their skin. In ward infections all the patients should be similarly investigated.

If a carrier is found, he should be isolated and treated. Sometimes there may be several carriers, or else the source of infection may not be discovered. All the infected individuals may have to be isolated, and the ward closed and sterilised. When it is re-opened, it should be barred to the previous patients and all articles that may have been in contact with them. Only thus can the effectiveness of the disinfection be assessed.

If the organisms are of different types, it is futile to engage in exhaustive searches for carriers. If the infection occurred in the theatre, it is far better to investigate the ventilation system and to check details of general hygiene as regards the patients' bedclothes and the movements of spectators. In ward infections of this type the various hospital routines should be critically examined.

GENERAL READING

WILLIAMS, R. E. O., BLOWERS, R., GARROD, L. P. and SHOOTER, R. A. (1966). *Hospital Infection*, 2nd edn, 386 pp. London: Lloyd-Luke.

REFERENCES

1. INGLIS, B. (1965). *A History of Medicine*, p. 152 *et seq.* London: Weidenfeld and Nicolson.
2. Leading Article (1970). *British Medical Journal*, ii, 618.
3. BARBER, M. (1960). In *Recent Advances in Clinical Pathology*, Series III, p. 2. Edited by S. C. Dyke. London: Churchill.
4. RIDLEY, M. (1959). *British Medical Journal*, i, 607.
5. SHOOTER, R. A. *et. al.* (1958). *British Medical Journal*, i, 607.
6. HARE, R. and THOMAS, C. G. A. (1956). *British Medical Journal*, ii, 840.
7. HARE, R. and RIDLEY, M. (1958). *British Medical Journal*, i, 69.
8. MILES, A. A. *et al.* (1940). *British Medical Journal*, ii, 855.
9. PERRY, W. D. *et al.* (1957). *American Journal of Hygiene*, **66**, 85.
10. PERRY, W. D., SIEGEL, A. C. and RAMMELKAMP, C. H. (1957). *American Journal of Hygiene*, **66**, 96.
11. RAMMELKAMP, C. H. *et al.* (1958). *Journal of Hygiene*, **56**, 280.
12. SHACKMAN, R. and MESSENT, D. (1954). *British Medical Journal*, ii, 1009.
13. GUZE, L. B. and BEESON, P. B. (1956). *New England Journal of Medicine*, **255**, 474.
14. KASS, E. H. and SCHNEIDERMAN, L. J. (1957). *New England Journal of Medicine*, **256**, 556.
15. DUTTON, A. A. C. and RALSTON, M. (1957). *Lancet*, i, 115.
16. MILLER, A. *et al.* (1958). *Lancet*, ii, 608.
17. GILLESPIE, W. A. *et al.* (1960). *Journal of Clinical Pathology*, **13**, 187.
18. DREWETT, S. E. *et al.* (1972). *Lancet*, i, 946.
19. DEVENISH, E. A. and MILES, A. A. (1939). *Lancet*, i, 1088.
20. SHOOTER, R. A., SMITH, M. A. and HUNTER, C. J. W. (1959). *British Journal of Surgery*, **47**, 246.
21. BOURDILLON, R. B. and COLEBROOK, L. (1946). *Lancet*, i, 561 and 601.
22. DUGUID, J. P. and WALLACE, A. T. (1948). *Lancet*, ii, 845.
23. SHOOTER, R. A. *et al.* (1956). *Surgery, Gynecology and Obstetrics*, **103**, 257.
24. BLOWERS, R. and CREW, B. (1960). *Journal of Hygiene*, **58**, 427.
25. NOBLE, W. C., LIDWELL, O. M. and KINGSTON, D. (1963). *Journal of Hygiene*, **61**, 385.
26. A Report of the Medical Research Council (1968). *Lancet*, i, 705, 763 and 831.
27. Leading Article (1970). *British Medical Journal*, iii, 418.
28. PRICE, D. J. E. and SLEIGH, J. D. (1970). *Lancet*, ii, 1213.

29. Leading Article (1963). *Lancet*, i, 537.
30. GIRDLESTONE, G. R. and BOURDILLON, R. B. (1951). *Lancet*, i, 597.
31. VOGEL, R. A. *et al.* (1959). *New England Journal of Medicine*, **261**, 1301.
32. RUBBO, S. D., STRATFORD, B. C. and DIXSON, S. (1962). *British Medical Journal*, ii, 282.
33. WILLIAMS, R. E. O. *et al.* (1962). *British Medical Journal*, ii, 275.
34. PYRAH, L. N. *et al.* (1955). *Lancet*, ii, 314.
35. MILLER, A. *et al.* (1960). *Lancet*, i, 310.
36. Leading Article (1963). *British Medical Journal*, ii, 332.
37. Newcastle Regional Hospital Board Working Party (1962). *Journal of Hygiene*, **60**, 85.
38. LOWBURY, E. J. L., BABB, J. R. and ROE, E. (1972). *Lancet*, ii, 941.

Chapter 20. Tuberculosis, Syphilis, and Actinomycosis

Whereas the acute pyogenic infections produce an inflammatory reaction which may or may not terminate in resolution, there are many other infections which commonly proceed to chronicity. In these there is usually such great tissue destruction that resolution is impossible and a chronic course invariable. During the progress of these infections acute exacerbations of an exudative type may occur, and these are usually due to allergy. Tuberculosis, syphilis, actinomycosis, and the fungous, protozoan, and helminthic infections all come into this category.

There are no histological features common to all these infections: in tuberculosis, leprosy, histoplasmosis, and leishmaniasis the macrophage is the prominent cell type and the infiltrate may be either diffuse or tuberculoid (p. 126); in actinomycosis and sporotrichosis there is a polymorph infiltration; in syphilis there is an infiltration of lymphocytes and plasma cells. The helminthic diseases are often associated with heavy eosinophil accumulations.

In the acute bacterial infections the causal organisms appear to produce damage by some direct action often by producing powerful toxins. From many of the micro-organisms responsible for chronic infection no definite toxin has been isolated. Their pathogenic action is probably the result of allergy of the cell-mediated type. Skin tests of a type similar to the Mantoux test are used in their diagnosis (see Chapter 14). Erythema nodosum,[1] which sometimes accompanies these conditions, is an allergic vasculitis of the skin and subcutaneous tissues due, at least in leprosy, to a deposition of immune complexes on the vessel walls.[2]

In many acute bacterial infections a long-lasting immunity is produced, and this is due to circulating immunoglobulins. In chronic infections there may also be antibodies in the circulation, but though these can be valuable in diagnosis, e.g. in the serological diagnosis of syphilis, they do not necessarily produce immunity against the disease. In some of these infections, notably tuberculosis, a degree of immunity is acquired after an infection; it is not due to immunoglobulins, but is mediated by lymphocytes.

If these infections are generalised there is pyrexia; severe constitutional disturbances are invariable in miliary tuberculosis, leishmaniasis, and trypanosomiasis. The ESR is considerably raised, and there is usually hypergammaglobulinaemia. The white-cell count often indicates the course of the local infection. In active tuberculosis and protozoan diseases there is often a monocytosis, in actinomycosis a neutrophil leucocytosis, and in the helminthic infections an eosinophilia. Secondary syphilis may be accompanied by an absolute lymphocytosis, a change also noted on occasions in healing tuberculosis (see Chapter 50).

TUBERCULOSIS

There are at least five distinct strains of *Mycobacterium tuberculosis* as well as a sixth group of unclassified mycobacteria.[3] The *human* and *bovine* strains are potential human pathogens, and the *murine* strain ("vole bacillus"), which is endemic in wild voles, has been used as an alternative to BCG in active immunisation against tuberculosis. *Myco. avium* is pathogenic to birds and may occasionally cause human infection.[4] The fifth strain of mycobacteria affects the *cold-blooded vertebrates*, and is of no human importance. The bovine organism is excreted in the milk of infected cows, and was once an important cause of intestinal and tonsillar infection in childhood. Nowadays bovine tuberculosis in man has almost completely disappeared in civilised countries following the eradication of tuberculous herds and the pasteurisation of milk. It therefore follows that nearly all tuberculosis is caused by the human strain. The mode of infection is by the inhalation of organisms present in fresh droplets or the dust of dried sputum expectorated from an open case of pulmonary tuberculosis. There are three possible methods of acquiring infection: inhalation, ingestion, and inoculation. Inhalation is all-important, since ingestion is now rare and inoculation of the skin from *post-mortem* material is little more than a curiosity. Congenital tuberculosis has been described in a few cases as a result of transplacental spread.

Bacteriology.[5] *Myco. tuberculosis* is a slender bacillus about 3 μm long, non-motile and non-sporing. Its most conspicuous feature is its waxy content which makes it impermeable to the usual stains. It slowly takes up heated stains, e.g. carbol fuchsin in the Ziehl-Neelsen method (see Appendix II), and then resists decolorisation even by strong acids and alcohols, i.e. it is acid-fast and alcohol-fast. It is Gram-positive, but Gram-staining is not performed because the methyl violet penetrates only with great difficulty.

It grows very slowly, and then only on very complex artificial media which should contain, amongst other things, egg-yolk and glycerol. The Löwenstein-Jensen medium is one that is commonly used, and it takes several weeks at 37°C in an aerobic atmosphere for any growth to appear. It is necessary to wait six weeks before discarding the culture as negative. Colonies can be recognised much earlier than this if micro-methods are used. Growth is faster in fluid media containing Tween 80 and albumin.

The organism is pathogenic to the guinea-pig, and when injected subcutaneously, it leads to the animal's death within a few months. Necropsy reveals widespread miliary tuberculosis. A greatly enlarged spleen is characteristic; it contains many caseous foci crowded with acid-fast bacilli. Rabbits are highly susceptible only to the bovine strain.

The bovine strain grows less readily than the human strain, and glycerol does not favour its growth as in the human strain.

Myco. tuberculosis is very resistant to drying, and it can survive in dust for several months. It is, however, very sensitive to the effect of ultraviolet radiation, and is rapidly killed in sunlight.

Atypical or anonymous mycobacteria.[6] Occasionally cases of human tuberculosis are encountered in which atypical bacilli are isolated. They differ from *Myco. tuberculosis* in being non-pathogenic to guinea-pigs and resistant to anti-tuberculous drugs, especially isoniazid. In the past such organisms have often been discarded as non-pathogens, but it is now accepted that they can cause disease, generally milder than classical tuberculosis. This is a good example of the futility of attempting to define pathogenicity in terms of one or two properties of an organism without considering its host. The atypical bacilli have been subdivided provisionally into four groups.

Group I, Photochromogens. These organisms produce a yellow pigment if the culture is grown continuously in light. *Myco. kansasii* is the best known.

Group II, Scotochromogens. Pigment is produced regardless of whether the growth is in the light or dark.

Group III, Nonchromogens. The Battey bacillus is in this group; it was named after the Battey Tuberculosis Sanatorium in Georgia where it was first isolated. Organisms in this group are closely related to the avian bacillus. No pigment is produced and, like groups I and II, growth in culture is slow and occurs at 37°C.

Group IV, Fast-growing Organisms. This group differs from the others in that there is rapid growth at 25°C as well as at 37°C. It includes *Myco. phlei* and *Myco. smegmatis.* Organisms in this group are the least pathogenic, but occasionally cause adenitis in children.

Some idea of the frequency of infection with these atypical organisms has been obtained by testing US Naval recruits with tuberculin derived from the various strains.[7] Whereas only 8·6 per cent reacted to tuberculin of *Myco. tuberculosis*, 35 per cent gave a positive reaction to that of the Battey bacillus. There is considerable cross-reaction to tuberculins derived from the various strains and it has been suggested that subclinical infection with an anonymous mycobacterium may give a degree of immunity to tuberculosis.

Mycobacteria causing skin infection. In addition to the cutaneous infections with *Myco. tuberculosis*, such as

lupus vulgaris, two other organisms have been implicated in chronic ulcerations of the skin. Both organisms are characterised by growing best at 31–33°C, a property which was responsible for them being overlooked until 1948.

Myco. ulcerans.[8, 9] This organism causes chronic ulceration most commonly of the limbs. The lesion commences as a subcutaneous nodule in which there is necrotic fat but little inflammatory reaction. The necrosis spreads laterally and deeply, and the undermined skin breaks down into an ulcer with an overhanging edge. After several weeks healing commences, but may take several months or even years for completion. The disease is remarkable for the lack of inflammation considering the extent of the necrosis. It bears little resemblance histologically to tuberculosis. The disease was first recognised in Australia but is known to occur elsewhere. It is common in Uganda, where in retrospect it was probably described as long ago as 1897; it is called Buruli ulcer.

Myco. balnei.[10, 11] This organism causes infection of abrasions, and may be acquired in swimming pools (hence its name) or occasionally from tropical fish tanks.[12] The ulcers are usually solitary, and the elbow or knee is a common site. Microscopically a chronic inflammatory reaction, perhaps

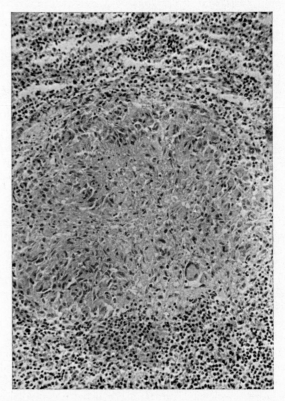

Figure 20.1
A tubercle follicle. There is a small area of caseation in the centre, and it is surrounded by an ill-defined zone of epithelioid cells, in the midst of which a Langhans giant cell is present. There is a diffuse infiltration of small round cells in the periphery. × 120.

with a non-caseating tuberculoid reaction, is seen. The lesions tend to heal spontaneously.

Pathogenesis of the tuberculous lesion.[13] The following sequence of events occurs when tubercle bacilli are introduced into the tissues:

1. A transient acute inflammatory reaction with an infiltration of polymorphs. These cells are rapidly destroyed by the organisms.

2. A progressive infiltration of macrophages derived from the local histiocytes and the monocytes of the blood. The macrophages are responsible for the destruction of the organism.

3. The macrophages phagocytose the bacilli. In a short time their character changes: their cytoplasm becomes pale and eosinophilic and their nuclei elongated and vesicular. Their appearance bears a resemblance to the epithelial cell, and they are called *epithelioid cells* (see p. 128).

4. Some macrophages, instead of becoming epithelioid cells, fuse to form Langhans giant cells (see p. 128).

5. Surrounding this mass of altered macrophages there is a wide zone of small round cells, mostly lymphocytes, and fibroblasts.

6. Within 10–14 days necrosis begins in the centre of this mass, which consists of altered macrophages and cells peculiar to the tissue of the part. This is a firm, coagulative necrosis called *caseation*, and it is characterised by a high content of lipid and a tendency to resist autolysis and demolition. Histologically the necrosis is structureless and eosinophilic, but with silver stains reticulin fibres can sometimes be demonstrated.

Caseation appears to be caused by allergy to products of the bacilli, notably tuberculoprotein. It is not produced directly by toxins, nor can it be explained on an ischaemic basis, because it precedes vascular injury.[13]

There is now produced the *tubercle follicle* (Figs. 20.1 and 20.2), which consists of a central mass of caseation surrounded by epithelioid and giant cells, which in turn are enclosed in a wide zone of small round cells. The appearance is characteristic of tuberculosis, but a rather similar picture is seen in some of the deep-seated mycoses (see Chapter 21). For a diagnosis of tuberculosis organisms must be found in

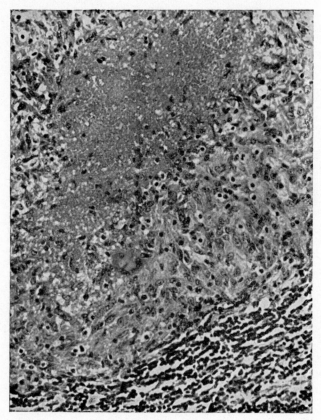

Figure 20.2
A tubercle follicle. The large central area of structureless caseous necrosis is surrounded by a zone of epithelioid cells in which a Langhans giant cell is present. In the periphery there is a small round cell infiltration. × 230.

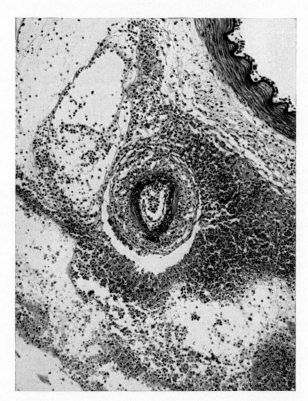

Figure 20.3
Tuberculous meningitis. In this section of the meninges of the base of the brain a small central vessel is seen to be surrounded by small round cells (perivascular cuffing), and in the proximity there is a large area of dense cellular infiltration, much of which is the seat of early caseous necrosis. In the periphery there is an open space meshed with strands of fibrin, in which there are collections of small round cells. This is a typical example of the exudative type of tuberculous reaction seen in a serous cavity. The absence of giant cells is noteworthy. × 100.

the lesion. This is very difficult at this stage, and culture must be employed in parallel with Ziehl-Neelsen staining of smears or sections.

Variations in the reaction to the tubercle bacillus. The common type of lesion described above is called *productive* or *proliferative*, because its main components are cells rather than a fluid exudate.

Another type of lesion is the *exudative* form of tuberculosis. It is characterised by the out-pouring of an inflammatory exudate rich in fibrin. There is a considerable infiltration of lymphocytes, and often polymorphs are present, but epithelioid and giant cells are rather scanty (Fig. 20.3). Exudative lesions are typical of tuberculosis of serous cavities. They are not necessarily more serious than productive ones. It was well recognised in the pre-antibiotic era that the so-called "primary pleural effusion" of young adults was one of the most favourable types of pulmonary tuberculosis, and that recovery usually occurred. Tuberculosis involving epithelial surfaces also assumes an exudative character. This accounts for the "sterile" pyuria that is such an important diagnostic feature of open renal tuberculosis.

In compact organs like the liver and kidney the lesions are almost always productive. In the lungs either type of reaction is possible, but here exudative phenomena are particularly serious, because they are attended by extensive caseation and a rapid spread of infection. Indeed, it is usual to classify pulmonary tuberculosis into the following categories, depending on the reaction of the tissue:

Acute caseous tuberculosis. There is confluent caseation of much of a lobe, producing caseous bronchopneumonia (Fig. 20.4). This is seen when large amounts of caseous debris are insufflated down a large bronchus, and a vigorous response is elicited as the result of intense hypersensitivity. A similar type of reaction may occur if the host's immunity is feeble, or if the organism is particularly virulent. The constitutional effects are very severe ("galloping consumption").

Chronic tuberculosis. Here the immunity of the host is adequate to cause some destruction of the bacilli, and healing by repair (fibrosis) occurs side by side with caseous destruction. Three types of chronic pulmonary tuberculosis are recognised: caseous, fibro-caseous, and fibroid, depending on the relative degrees of caseation and fibrosis. In long-standing fibroid tuberculosis the lung may be converted into a contracted mass of dense fibrous tissue in which there may be little recognisable evidence of active tuberculous infection. Bronchiectasis is a frequent complication of this type of disease.

The most serious type of lesion is *non-reactive tuberculosis*.[14] This consists of extensive foci of caseation teeming with bacilli, but with virtually no cellular reaction around them. This type of disease is seen as a complication of leukaemia, and is also met with from time to time in elderly people. It may be associated with severe aplasia of the bone marrow (see Chapter 50), and the presenting symptoms may be those of an obscure blood dyscrasia. The tuberculin

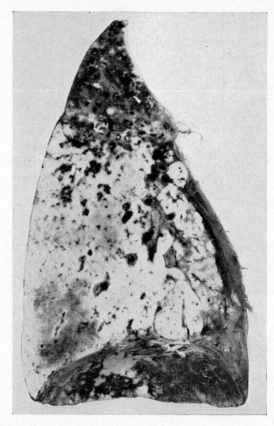

Figure 20.4
Confluent tuberculous bronchopneumonia. The whole of the lower lobe and much of the upper lobe shows caseous consolidation. (R 36.2, *Reproduced by permission of the President and Council of the R.C.S. Eng.*)

reaction is sometimes negative; this may be due to an overwhelming infection impairing the immune response or alternatively there may be an initial immunological deficiency that predisposes to a non-reactive state. In either event the prognosis is very grave.

The fate of the tuberculous lesion. The caseous focus may either cease to progress and heal by fibrosis, or it may soften and spread.

The hallmark of healing is fibrous tissue, and this is produced by the proliferating fibroblasts at the periphery of the lesion. In due course the area of caseation may be replaced by a solid fibrous nodule. Sometimes only a rind of fibrous tissue forms around the periphery, while the central mass of caseation undergoes slow dystrophic calcification. In this calcareous nodule organisms can still survive, and years later, when the resistance of the host breaks down, they may become active again. Sometimes the nodule ossifies.

The hallmark of activity is caseation and softening. If the lesion is spreading, bacilli are carried by macrophages into the surrounding lymphatics and tissue spaces. There they settle and set up satellite follicles, which by fusing with the primary enlarging lesion, produce a conglomerate tubercle follicle. Caseous material does not soften rapidly, due possibly to phosphatides that inhibit autolytic enzymes.[15] Sometimes, however, liquefaction does occur, and this is attended by serious consequences.

There is no really satisfactory explanation for this softening. There is no doubt that it is associated with spread, and that the liquefied debris contains many bacilli, but it is not known whether this multiplication of organisms is the cause or the result of the softening. It has been suggested that the liquefaction is due to secondary infection, but this is untrue. Pyogenic infection may certainly complicate a tuberculous lesion, but liquefaction often occurs in the absence of such infection. Hypersensitivity is probably of considerable importance.

Once liquefaction has occured, the debris contains large numbers of tubercle bacilli, and the whole is called a *cold abscess*. Unlike a pyogenic abscess it contains few cells, and most of these are disintegrating. The term "pus" is therefore inapplicable, as there are no pus cells. The term "cold abscess" is equally inapplicable. In practice it is reserved exclusively for tuberculous lesions, even though other suppurative lesions such as actinomycosis may also be "cold", inasmuch as neither the heat, pain, nor redness of acute pyogenic infection is marked in them. The liquefied debris ("pus") tracks towards a free surface and discharges there. In a lesion of the lung rupture soon occurs into a bronchus, and the disease spreads to other parts of the lung; much infectious material is also coughed up.

In areas such as the bones and joints, lymph nodes, and epididymis, where there are no immediately available passages, large cold abscesses often accumulate, e.g. the collar stud abscess of the neck secondary to infection of a cervical lymph node. In due course these abscesses track through the tissues, the substance of which is destroyed in the path of the advancing tuberculous lesion. In this way sinuses are formed, which are lined by *tuberculous granulation tissue*. This consists of systems of tubercle follicles irregularly disposed in a mass of newly-formed fibrous tissue which is heavily infiltrated with lymphocytes and macrophages. Sometimes the "pus" may track for longe distances, e.g. it may enter the psoas sheath from an infected vertebra, spread down as a psoas abscess, and finally point below the inguinal ligament.

Whenever a tuberculous abscess opens to the exterior, the disease becomes more serious, firstly because of its *open*, infectious character, and secondly because the tubercle bacillus is an aerobic organism and proliferates much more profusely in an atmosphere of air. These features are well illustrated in the open, cavitating type of pulomonary tuberculosis. Much of the value of artificial pneumothorax therapy was due to the fact that it prevented the aeration of the affected lung.

Spread of tuberculosis in the body. The principles differ in no significant way from those of other infections.

Local spread by macrophages has already been described.

Lymphatic spread is a continuation of local spread. The result is a regional tuberculous lymphadenitis which is typical of childhood infections. The primary focus with its attendant lymphangitis and lymphadenitis is called the *primary complex*. Nowadays nearly all primary complexes are pulmonary.

Blood spread occurs as an extension of lymphatic involvement. In an overwhelming infection the organisms escape from the lymph nodes and enter the blood stream to produce *miliary tuberculosis*, which in extreme cases is of the nonreactive type. The lungs, spleen, liver, kidney, and to a lesser extent other organs, are seeded with tubercle bacilli which produce numerous follicles of millet-seed size. Blood spread also occurs when caseous hilar nodules directly implicate an adjacent pulmonary vein. If there is a discharge of large numbers of organisms into the blood stream, miliary tuberculosis occurs, but the lungs are often spared.

Miliary tuberculosis is seen in young children as an extension of a primary complex. However, tuberculosis is now less frequent in children and it is not rare to encounter miliary tuberculosis in adults, especially the elderly and those on glucocorticosteroid therapy.[16] It produces fever, wasting, hepatosplenomegaly, leucopenia, and thrombocytopenia. The absence of classical miliary mottling in the chest radiograph and a negative tuberculin test render diagnosis difficult.[17, 18] Bone-marrow examination, liver biopsy, or a therapeutic trial with specific antituberculous drugs such as PAS and isoniazid, are the most successful diagnostic procedures. *Tuberculous meningitis* is a very frequent accompaniment of miliary tuberculosis, and is due either to direct involvement of the choroid plexus, or else to a small subcortical lesion (*Rich's focus*) rupturing into the subarachnoid space.[19]

In older children and adults it sometimes happens that a tuberculous focus implicates a small pulmonary vein in the vicinity, and then only a few bacilli invade the systemic circulation. These may be destroyed by the RE system, or else become lodged in various sites to give rise to metastatic disease. Such a lesion may progress immediately to produce clinical effects, or else remain quiescent, only to undergo reactivation years later. This type of lesion is called *local metastatic tuberculosis*, and it accounts for most of the disease seen in surgical practice (Fig. 20.5). Organs sometimes involved in this way are the kidneys, adrenals, fallopian tubes, epididymes, and the bones, joints, and tendon sheaths. Curiously enough, the thyroid, pancreas, heart, and voluntary muscles are seldom affected. The spleen is not commonly the seat of extensive caseous tuberculosis, though in miliary tuberculosis it is almost invariably affected.

Spread in serous cavities is seen in the pleurisy that may complicate lung lesions, the localised peritonitis found around tuberculous salpingitis, and in tuberculous meningitis.

Spread along epithelial-lined surfaces is typified by the intrabronchial spread of tuberculosis that occurs when

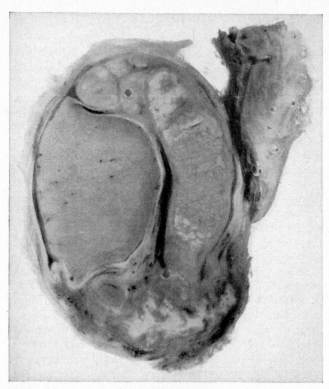

Figure 20.5
Tuberculous epididymitis. The enlarged, cowl-shaped epididymis shows diffuse caseous necrosis. (*M* 5.3, *Reproduced by permission of the President and Council of the R.C.S. Eng.*)

sputum is inhaled into adjacent lung segments. If the sputum is coughed up it can produce tuberculous laryngitis, and when swallowed, the bacilli may infect the ileo-caecal area of the bowel and lead to tuberculous enteritis. Rectal involvement is manifested by ischiorectal abscesses.

Likewise tuberculosis of the kidney can spread down the ureter to implicate the trigone of the bladder, and tuberculous salpingitis can lead to endometrial disease.

Factors determining the response of tissues to tuberculous infection.[3] It is apparent that sometimes there is healing by fibrosis of a small caseous focus, and on other occasions a rapidly spreading fatal disease. The factors that determine the tissue response are:

(*a*) The dose and virulence of the organism. Virulent strains tend to produce rough colonies, and when cultivated on solid media aggregate to grow in long cords. Pathogenicity is not, however, closely correlated with growth characteristics. Pathogenicity to animals is discussed on page 244.

(*b*) The innate and acquired resistance of the body. This is a very important consideration.

Innate immunity is of great importance in tuberculosis and is discussed on page 164. Amongst the most susceptible groups are the Negroes, American Indians, and Australian Aborigines.

Age and sex. During the first five years of life the body's resistance is poor and the mortality rate is high. From 5–15 years resistance is at its peak, but it breaks down during the early adult period of 15–30 years, particularly in women. After the age of 30 years resistance is quite high, but it breaks down again in old age, particularly in men.

General health of the individual is also of great importance. Malnutrition and overcrowding in prison camps and slums predispose to spreading tuberculosis. Psychological stress and chronic debilitating diseases also lower the resistance. Diabetes mellitus is particularly notorious in predisposing to a rapidly spreading type of infection. Thyroxine increases tissue resistance to the tubercle bacillus,[20] while adrenal steroids lower it.[21] Glucocorticosteroids should be used with great caution in tuberculosis.

Occupational factors influence the resistance: for instance, those whose work carries the hazard of silicosis, e.g. tunnellers, miners, and quarrymen, are liable to a spreading type of disease. Asbestosis is a less serious predisposing factor.

The effect of previous infection. A second infection shows a completely different pathogenesis to the primary one. This was demonstrated by Koch in guinea-pigs, and the *Koch phenomenon* is described in detail on page 183. It will be remembered that the secondary response is accelerated, a manifestation of baterial allergy, and that it does not spread to the lymph nodes but remains localised and heals, an indication of acquired immunity. The animal becomes hypersensitive to a protein fraction of the organism called *tuberculoprotein* or *tuberculin*. Koch's *Old Tuberculin* (*OT*) is now superseded by *Purified Protein Derivative* (*PPD*). The administration of tuberculin to a hypersensitive person, whether by the Mantoux intradermal method or the Heaf multiple puncture technique, produces a local area of inflammation within 48 hours. Necrosis may ensue in very hypersensitive people, therefore a very small initial dose should be used. The *tuberculin unit* (*TU*) has been introduced to standardise the relative doses of OT and PPD. One TU is equivalent to 0·1 ml of a 1 in 10 000 solution of OT, or 0·000028 mg of PPD. It is recommended that 3–5 TU should first be given, and if the result is negative the dose should be raised to 100 TU.[5]

It is evident that when a sensitised person is exposed to tuberculoprotein, whether in a skin test or through a second infection, a delayed hypersensitivity reaction occurs, which in extreme cases (when the dose of tuberculoprotein is great or if it is given intravenously) produces fever and a flare-up of other foci. Indeed, the reaction may be so severe that it kills the patient, an event sometimes noted when tuberculin was used therapeutically in the belief that the allergic inflammation helped to destroy the bacilli. Tuberculous allergy develops within a month to six weeks of infection, and is of cell-mediated (lymphocytic) type (see p. 183). It has been found that the hypersensitivity declines with age, especially from the fifth decade onwards.[22] This may be due to decreased contact with the organism.

It is the acquired immunity of the Koch phenomenon which is particularly interesting. It is not as effective as that which follows smallpox or diphtheria, and furthermore is not due to circulating immunoglobulins; though these are present and can be demonstrated serologically, they play no part in immunity. The immunity of tuberculosis is cell mediated: the altered lymphocytes enable the macrophages to destroy the bacilli more effectively than they do in a primary infection. The macrophages of rabbits previously immunised with BCG, when grown in tissue culture, withstand parasitisation by tubercle bacilli, whereas the macrophages from unimmunised animals have no such power.[23] The precise nature of these cellular changes is unknown. In addition, the sensitised lymphocytes liberate lymphokines in the vicinity of the tubercle bacilli; these by inhibiting the random movement of the macrophages probably augment their local phagocytic activity. It is possible that the lymphokines have a directly lethal effect on the organisms as well.

Although allergy and acquired immunity are clearly closely related, they are also distinct; thus it has been found that the degree of immunity that follows BCG vaccination is not related to the degree of tuberculin sensitivity induced.[24] It has also been noted that guinea-pigs can be immunised with methyl-alcohol extracts of tubercle bacilli without the development of allergy,[25] whereas hypersensitivity without immunity can be induced by injecting a mixture of tuberculoprotein and a waxy extract from the bacilli.[26] It would appear that allergy is harmful in that, by causing caseation, it leads to the destruction of fibrous tissue barriers which might limit the spread of infection. On the other hand, it has been argued that the inflammation it induces does bring macrophages into contact with the bacilli—and these are the cells that destroy them. It appears that following BCG immunisation the protective value of an accelerated macrophage response far exceeds any tendency to necrosis and spread of the infection engendered by the allergy.

It should finally be noted that the acquired immunity is only of partial degree, and has no effect in overcoming the primary infection. Despite Koch's phenomenon, the guinea-pig still dies of its first infection. This may indicate that an important mechanism of the immunity is the localisation of the organism at a very early stage of the infection.

Morphology of Tuberculous Infection

It is well recognised that the morbid anatomy of pulmonary tuberculosis in children differs from that of adults. At all ages the lung is the organ principally affected.

(*a*) *Childhood.* In childhood the primary focus (Ghon focus) is a small, wedge-shaped area situated at the periphery of the lung field usually in the mid-zone. This subpleural focus may heal, or else the infection spreads to the hilar nodes, which become greatly enlarged and caseous. A conspicuous primary complex is the result. It either heals and calcifies, or else it spreads, and the child dies of miliary

tuberculosis with meningitis. The lung lesion is usually of little importance in causing death, but the enlarged hilar nodes may compress a bronchus sufficiently to lead to segmental collapse.

In days gone by the alimentary tract was frequently the site of childhood tuberculosis, and this was due, of course, to infection by bovine bacilli. In abdominal disease the primary focus in the bowel is so small that it is rarely identifiable, and the first manifestation of the infection is great enlargement of the mesenteric lymph nodes, giving rise to the clinical picture of *tabes mesenterica*. These may occasionally rupture into the peritoneal cavity, and cause acute tuberculous peritonitis. Usually calcification ensues and recovery follows, but otherwise there is a progressive lymphatic spread to the thoracic duct culminating in miliary tuberculosis.

More rarely the primary focus is tonsillar. This usually passes unnoticed, until progressive enlargement of the

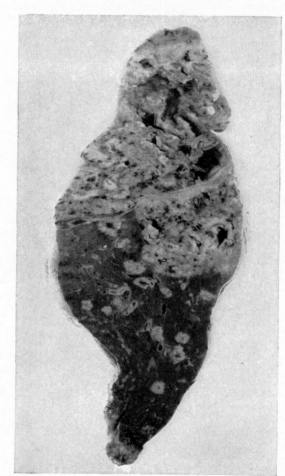

Figure 20.6

Caseous tuberculosis of lung. In this section the entire upper lobe is consolidated with extensive tuberculous bronchopneumonia, and at the apex there is a large, ragged-walled cavity. The adjacent upper part of the lower lobe is also affected. (R 37.1, *Reproduced by permission of the President and Council of the R.C.S. Eng.*)

cervical lymph nodes and their softening and discharge through the skin (*scrofula*) make the disease obvious.

In all childhood lesions the feature in common is the small size of the primary focus, and the tendency to extensive lymph-node involvement (as in the guinea-pig).

(*b*) *Adult life.* In adult life the focus is almost always apical or subapical (*Assmann focus*), particularly involving the right lung. The reason for this apical situation is unknown. The lesion either heals, or else it progresses, softens, and produces a cavity. Depending on the resistance of the patient, there is a tendency either to fibrosis or extensive cavitation. In severe cases great destruction of lung tissue results. A large cavity may be produced, and a vessel in its wall may be eroded, leading to haemoptysis. If caseous debris is inhaled into other bronchi tuberculous bronchopneumonia develops. This may occur on a small scale and result in extension of the disease, but if widespread it causes massive caseation of a great area of lung tissue. This is a fulminating allergic response, and the disease remains localised to the lungs. Lymph-node involvement is inconspicuous, and bloodspread dissemination is unusual. Death is due to the local lung lesion (Fig. 20.6).

A similar pathogenesis occurs in other organs in the adult. Tuberculous enteritis due to swallowing infected sputum is characterised by ulceration of the wall of the ileum (Fig. 20.7). There is a localised peritonitis and an insidious tendency for strictures and fistulae to develop, but local lymph-node involvement is only slight. The contrast between this and the childhood abdominal lesion is obvious.

Renal tuberculosis usually starts as a cortical focus, which spreads to destroy the surrounding renal parenchyma. Other lesions develop in the medulla due to the passage of bacilli down the renal tubules, and eventually cavitation into the pelvis ensues. The destructive lesion of tuberculous pyelonephritis ultimately converts the kidney into a ragged cavity lined by tuberculous granulation tissue, and spread down the ureter may follow (Fig. 20.8). If it is occluded, a large tuberculous pyonephrosis is produced.

Skeletal tuberculosis usually starts in the metaphyseal area of a bone, and it causes great local destruction. Unlike pyogenic osteomyelitis it destroys the epiphyseal cartilage with

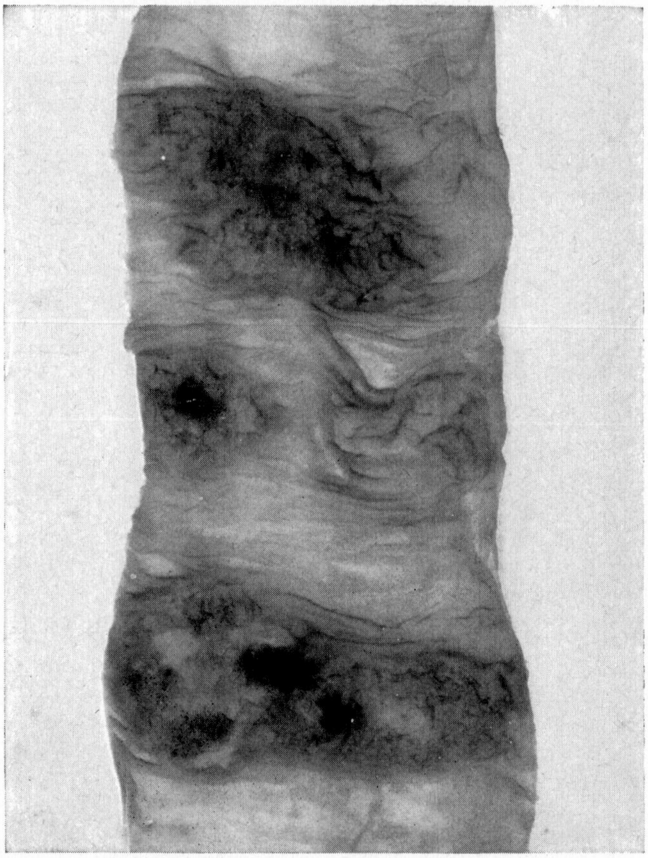

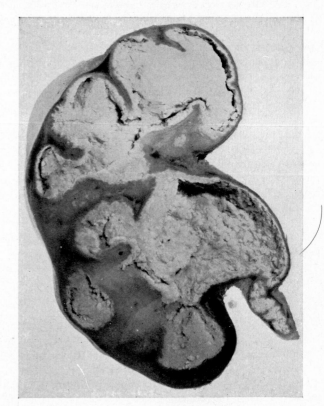

Figure 20.7
Tuberculous ulceration of ileum. In this specimen of ileum there are several extensive tuberculous ulcers. They have arisen from Peyer's patches, but unlike typhoid ulcers they have spread laterally and have encircled the lumen; this is due to lymphatic involvement. (A 51.1, *Reproduced by permission of the President and Council of the R.C.S. Eng.*)

Figure 20.8
Tuberculous pyelonephritis. Most of the kidney has been destroyed, and is replaced by large ragged cavities full of putty-like caseous debris. The pelvis is greatly dilated and filled with similar material. (U 16.1, *Reproduced by permission of the President and Council of the R.C.S. Eng.*)

great ease, and soon the neighbouring joint is affected (Fig. 20.9).

The feature that all these adult lesions have in common is the tendency to extensive local destruction with little lymphatic involvement.

It is traditionally believed that the adult lesion is always secondary to a primary lesion acquired during childhood, and that the difference in course of the two infections can be

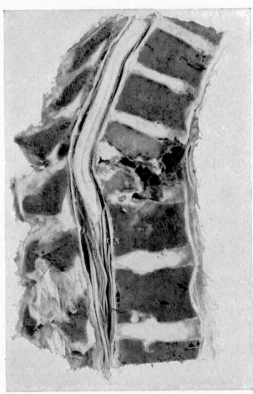

Figure 20.9
Tuberculosis of the spinal column (Pott's disease of the spine). Two adjacent vertebral bodies have been destroyed by progressive caseous necrosis, and the intervening intervertebral disc has disappeared in the debris. Tuberculosis not only destroys bone, but also invades and destroys cartilage. The result has been collapse of the two vertebrae with acute angulation of the spine (gibbus). (S 49a.4, *Reproduced by permission of the President and Council of the R.C.S. Eng.*)

explained on the basis of allergy and immunity acquired during the primary infection. Just as in the Koch phenomenon, where the second dose of organisms remained localised and did not spread to the regional nodes, so it is that the secondary adult lesion remains localised to the lungs and does not spread further afield.

It has, however, become apparent that even when a previously Mantoux-negative young adult develops tuberculosis, the lesion approximates more to the adult type than the "primary" Ghon type with prominent hilar lymphadenopathy. Thus there is usually an apical focus without

much lymph-node enlargement. Furthermore, there are very definite differences between the adult lesion and the Koch phenomenon. There is lymph-node involvement in the adult, though it is of a microscopic extent only; also the lesion shows no particularly tendency to heal. The difference in behaviour between childhood and adult lesions appears to be due to tissue maturation;[13] the older the patient the less is the tendency towards marked lymph-node involvement. The effect of a previous infection, perhaps with a relatively avirulent atypical bacillus, as an additional modifying factor cannot be excluded, but it is unjustifiable to label all adult lesions as secondary. The terms *childhood* and *adult* tuberculosis are much more accurate than primary and secondary tuberculosis.

The source of the organisms causing adult-type tuberculosis has been the centre of much discussion in the past. The pulmonary lesions were regarded as due either to *reactivation* of a quiescent primary lesion or to the development of a new lesion produced by a *reinfection* from some external source. In the past reinfection was probably of great importance, but nowadays it seems that many adult-type lesions are themselves primary infections. In other organs, e.g. kidney and bone, it is almost certain that tuberculosis is due to the reactivation of small lesions which were produced during a bacteraemic phase of a previous primary infection.

Incidence of tuberculosis. Tuberculosis is still widespread despite the great advances that have been made both chemotherapeutically and immunologically. It is the poorer countries that show the highest incidence, and as most of these are in Africa, Latin America, and Asia, tuberculosis has now the predominant distribution of a tropical disease. Its incidence continues to be an accurate reflection of the social standards of a community.

In Britain it would appear that most of the population is infected during some period of life, but that the disease usually remains subclinical. This is induced from the high frequency of positive tuberculin reactions in adults. However, it is now recognised that infection with other mycobacteria, especially the avian bacillus and *Myco. balnei*, can also cause Mantoux conversion, though usually the reaction is weak.[27] A strongly positive reaction to the standard PPD is considered good evidence of past infection with the human bacillus; indeed, it calls for further investigation of overt infection, especially in children, young adults, and the elderly. The interpretation of a weakly positive reaction is difficult, and a differential skin test using tuberculin made from *Myco. avium* and other atypical bacilli might be of help. Other evidence of past infection is the presence of calcified hilar lymph nodes, but in North America these may be due to mycotic infection, often histoplasmosis. Likewise calcified mesenteric nodes in the elderly bear witness to infection from contaminated milk in their childhood.

Clinical tuberculosis is infrequent in Britain. Amongst the indigenous population the reservoir is predominantly in the elderly, particularly old men. It is, however, constantly being reinforced by younger immigrants who bring their infection in with them.[28]

The Registrar-General's Statistical Review for England and Wales for 1969 reveals the current trend in tuberculous mortality very eloquently. During that year 1 325 men and 515 women died of the disease. In the first 35 years of life the mortality rate was low in both sexes. After this age there was a much greater mortality. The peak death rate in both sexes occurred in the age-group 50–70 years, and it was three times greater in men than in women. Nearly all fatal tuberculosis nowadays is pulmonary, but amongst the less common extrapulmonary types of disease the sex incidence is equal. It is probable that some tuberculosis in the elderly is due to the reactivation of foci acquired at an earlier period of life, but the breakdown in immunity in old age as well as poor social conditions make reinfection an important alternative.

The Eradication of Tuberculosis

There are three main principles:

A general improvement in social conditions. The importance of overcrowding and malnutrition in the spread of tuberculosis has already been indicated.

The treatment of patients. There are no "carriers" of tuberculosis comparable with the nasal carriers of staphylococci or the faecal carriers of typhoid bacilli. The source of infection is always an "open" case, and his sputum, sometimes after drying into dust in the atmosphere, is inhaled by another person. It is therefore important to diagnose the disease as early as possible. Mass radiography is very useful especially in screening large populations. Patients must be isolated and treated as expeditiously as possible.

Streptomycin, para-aminosalicylic acid (PAS), and isonicotinic acid hydrazide (isoniazid) have been the main antituberculous drugs, but they are being supplemented or replaced by other agents, e.g. ethambutol (to replace PAS) and rifampicin. If possible the patient should not be allowed back into the community until his sputum is negative for tubercle bacilli on many occasions.

Prophylactic active immunisation. The strain commonly used is the BCG (*Bacille-Calmette-Guérin*), a bovine strain attenuated by prolonged culture on a bile-potato medium.* It is administered intradermally and it produces a mild localised infection. A successful result is indicated by a conversion in the tuberculin reaction. This is, of course, purely an indication of hypersensitivity, but it is assumed that there is also a concomitant acquisition of immunity.

There is now a general consensus of opinion that BCG vaccination is a valuable method of establishing immunity to tuberculosis and that it should be offered to all tuberculin-negative reactors. The reports of the Medical Research Council Clinical Trials Committee indicate that in Britain the incidence of tuberculosis in vaccinated children is a fifth

that in tuberculin-negative controls.[29] Those whose profession brings them in contact with the disease and who are tuberculin negative should be immunised without delay. The value of BCG vaccination in other communities is still being assessed.[29] The question of weak tuberculin reactors is arousing interest; as already noted, many of these may have been infected with avian and other mycobacteria. These infections may conceivably add their quota to the patient's immunity to tuberculosis, but it seems to be quite in order to offer them BCG in addition. Data are needed about the relative efficiency of BCG and other mycobacterial infections as immunisers against tuberculosis. In strongly tuberculin-positive reactors BCG is both unnecessary and potentially harmful.

The complications of BCG are a tuberculous abscess at the site of inoculation, sometimes with associated axillary lymphadenitis severe enough to require chemotherapy, and very rarely a generalised infection with progressive pulmonary lesions.[30] Sarcoidosis is an occasional sequel of BCG vaccination.[31]

SYPHILIS

The causative organism *Treponema pallidum*[32] is a delicate spiral filament, or spirochaete, about 10 μm long. It cannot be stained by the usual techniques, and is demonstrable in the exudate of chancres and secondary lesions by means of dark-ground illumination and fluorescent antibody techniques. In histological sections it is stained by special silver impregnation methods.

The organism has never been cultured artificially even in fertile eggs or tissue-culture systems, nor does animal inoculation play any part in the diagnosis of the disease. In fact, rabbits develop acute orchitis after the intratesticular inoculation of the organisms. This method is used to obtain a supply of spirochaetes for such procedures as the *Treponema pallidum immobilisation* (*TPI*) *test* and the *fluorescent treponemal antibody* (*FTA*) *test.*

During the course of infection the patient develops immunoglobulins of great importance.[33–35] Two groups are recognised:

The Wassermann antibody. This antibody, formerly called reagin, was described by Wassermann as a complement-fixing antibody to an antigen present in extracts of human syphilitic liver. Subsequently an alcoholic extract of normal tissue was found to contain a similar antigen, and nowadays an extract of beef heart, to which cholesterol and lecithin have been added, is used. It is called *cardiolipin*, and the active component has been identified as *diphosphatidylglycerol*. This antigen is used in the *standard tests for syphilis*, namely the *Wassermann complement-fixation test* and the *flocculation tests*, of which the *Kahn* and the *Venereal Disease Research Laboratory* (*VDRL*) *tests* are the most widely used. They are more sensitive than the complement-fixation test but are no more specific.

* Vole bacillus is an effective alternative. Earlier batches occasionally produced severe local lesions, and the vaccine has never been as popular as BCG.[29]

Whether the Wassermann antibody is induced in the patient by an antigen of the treponeme or of damaged host tissue is not clear. The antigen is certainly not specific for *Tr. pallidum*, for not only are the serological tests positive in other treponemal diseases, such as yaws, pinta, and bejel, but false positive reactions may occur in non-treponemal diseases, notably malaria, leprosy, infectious mononucleosis, mycoplasmal pneumonia, trypanosomiasis, systemic lupus erythematosus, and autoimmune haemolytic anaemia, as well as occasionally in pregnant women, and in over 25 per cent of normal subjects after vaccination with vaccinia.[36] In a recent epidemic of Coxsackie B infection there was a remarkably high incidence of positive reactions.[37] The occurrence of these false positive reactions suggests that tissue damage by a variety of agents can stimulate the formation of Wassermann antibodies. This correlates well with the observation in experimental syphilis in rabbits that the standard tests tend to be positive during active phases of the disease but negative during the latent periods, when presumably tissue damage is at a minimum. In human disease the flocculation tests are often positive even when the disease appears inactive.

Treponemal antibody. The second group of antibodies which is formed reacts with treponemal protein. Some antibody activity is directed against protein common to several treponemes (group protein), while others are more specific. The following tests are employed.

Reiter Protein Complement-Fixation (RPCF) Test. The Reiter strain, unlike the pathogenic *Tr. pallidum* strains, can be cultured artificially under strictly anaeorbic conditions, and so the antigen can be obtained quite easily. The RPCF test is more specific than the standard tests for syphilis and therefore gives fewer false positive results.

Treponema Pallidum Immobilisation (TPI) Test. This employs the ability of antibody to immobilise *Tr. pallidum* in the presence of complement. A concentrated suspension of organisms is incubated for 18 hours with guinea-pig complement and serum, and motility is assessed under darkground illumination. Positive sera can be adsorbed with cardiolipin without diminution of the titre, thereby showing that the antibody detected is not the same as the Wassermann antibody. The TPI test becomes positive a little later in the disease than do the standard tests, but it remains positive for a prolonged period, even during latent stages of syphilis. Being more specific, it is useful when there is a suspected false serology. Unfortunately the test is technically difficult to perform and needs a supply of pathogenic organisms.

Fluorescent Treponemal Antibody (FTA) Test. Specific antibody adheres to *Tr. pallidum*, and can be detected by applying fluorescein-labelled anti-human γ-globulin. Two antibodies are involved; one is group specific, reacting with *Tr. pallidum* and other treponemes, while the other is specific for *Tr. pallidum*. Both are formed in syphilis. The group-specific antibody can be absorbed by Reiter treponemes, and the test (FTA-ABS) is as sensitive and specific as the TPI.

These two specific tests are performed only when the standard tests are equivocal, or when the results do not correlate with the clinical features of the case. No test is absolutely reliable, and none can distinguish between syphilis and yaws, which is caused by *Tr. pertenue*.

The disease.[38, 39] The infection is almost always acquired venereally, though on rare occasions the primary lesion may occur on the lips, tongue, or even on a finger. Unlike the tubercle bacillus, *Tr. pallidum* is very rapidly destroyed both in water and by drying. Intimate direct contact is therefore necessary for infection to occur. The spirochaete is one of the most invasive organisms known. Once it penetrates the surface integument, it spreads along the lymphatics to the regional lymph nodes, and finally reaches the blood stream within a matter of hours. There is therefore systemic dissemination long before any local manifestation appears.

Syphilis may also be transmitted by blood transfused from an infected donor.[40] The organisms are destroyed after storage of the blood in a refrigerator for about four days,[41] but, of course, in practice a syphilitic donor should not be accepted.

The disease is divisible into three stages with a latent period between each of them.

Primary syphilis. The typical lesion of primary syphilis is the *chancre*, which usually appears 2–4 weeks after exposure to infection. It is an indurated papule which breaks down to form an ulcer. It is characteristically painless, and is accompanied by a considerable regional lymphadenitis which is also painless.

The histological appearance is non-specific, consisting merely of a dense infiltration of lymphocytes, plasma cells, and a few macrophages in the dermis. There is a tendency towards a perivascular accumulation or "cuffing" of these cells, but this is not peculiar to syphilis. Even without treatment the chancre gradually heals, and it leaves little scarring.

The painlessness of the chancre (and the later lesions of syphilis) is best explained in terms of its cellular, or proliferative, nature. There is little fluid exudate, which contains pain-producing substances in acute inflammation. The digital chancre is painful—it is called a syphilitic whitlow—due to raised tissue tension in a confined space.

The fact that the spirochaetes become disseminated in the blood stream long before there is any local lesion suggests that allergy plays an important part in the process. The chancre is not comparable with a boil, for it is not a local inflammatory reaction tending to limit the infection. A possible explanation is that sensitising antibodies are first formed in the cells at the site of entry and in the regional lymph nodes. During the incubation period the spirochaetes multiply in the RE system, and when liberated react with the sensitised tissue. This would explain the chancre and the lymphadenopathy quite well.

At a later stage the other tissues of the body become sensitised, and then the generalised lesions of secondary syphilis become manifest.

Diagnosis. The laboratory diagnosis depends on demonstrating spirochaetes in the exudate from the chancre by dark-ground illumination.

One to three weeks after the appearance of the chancre both Wassermann and antitreponemal antibodies first appear in the blood. Blood serology should never be neglected in practice.

Secondary syphilis. Within 2–3 months after exposure the disease becomes clinically generalised. When syphilis was first introduced into Europe, this stage was severe enough to warrant the name "the great pox". Nowadays it is much milder, and is characterised by the development of a skin rash. This is widespread, symmetrical, usually not pruritic, and commonly present on the face, palms, and soles. The lesions are generally erythematous papules, but may be of any type except vesicular or bullous. Mucosal lesions in the form of condylomata lata, mucous patches, and snail-track ulcers are less frequent. The muco-cutaneous lesions may be accompanied by constitutional symptoms which include low-grade fever, myalgia, arthralgia, moderate anaemia, iritis, and a generalised painless lymphadenopathy. Histologically the secondary lesions show an infiltration by lymphocytes, plasma cells, and macrophages. They resolve spontaneously and do not form scars. This is the phase of maximal infectivity; spirochaetes ooze out of condylomata and mucous patches.

Diagnosis. The serological tests are always positive in overt secondary syphilis. If a negative result is reported in the face of strong clinical indications of syphilis, *the prozone phenomenon should be suspected* (p. 145) and the test repeated with suitable dilutions, so that the titre of antibody can be measured.

Organisms can be demonstrated with ease in the exudates from mucosal lesions and the condylomata. They can also be shown in histological sections of primary and secondary lesions using silver impregnation methods. But in practice it is unnecessary to demonstrate the spirochaete in secondary syphilis.

Tertiary syphilis. Local destructive lesions of a truly chronic inflammatory nature may begin to appear 2–3 years after exposure, and may continue to erupt sporadically for at least 20 years. The lesions are presumably due to marked hypersensitivity, since spirochaetes are few and the reaction is excessive. Two forms of lesions occur: localised gummata and diffuse inflammatory lesions characterised by parenchymatous destruction.

Localised Gummata. The *gumma* is the classical lesion of tertiary syphilis. It is usually solitary, and consists of a large area of coagulative necrosis very similar in appearance to caseation, except that the tissue destruction is usually not quite so complete. Details of architecture can therefore still be faintly distinguished amid the debris. It is surrounded by an extensive zone of lymphocytes, plasma cells, and macrophages. Proliferating fibroblasts are plentiful, and much reparative fibrous tissue is laid down. Giant cells are much

less numerous than in tuberculosis (Fig. 20.10). The arteries in the vicinity show marked endarteritis obliterans.

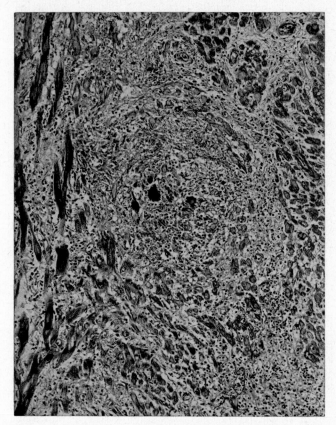

Figure 20.10
Gumma of heart. There is a central area of coagulative necrosis in which several darkly-staining giant cells are prominent. Surrounding it there is a diffuse infiltration of small round cells in vascular fibrous tissue. At the periphery the remains of muscle fibres are still present. The lesion was discovered during the course of a necropsy on a man who died of a ruptured aortic aneurysm. × 115.

Gummata are particularly liable to occur in the liver, testes (Fig. 20.11), subcutaneous tissues, and in bones, notably the tibia, ulna, clavicle, calvaria of skull, and the nasal and palatal bones. The destruction produced by gummata is exemplified by the perforated palate and the saddle-shaped nasal deformity so characteristic of tertiary syphilis. In the liver gummata are often multiple, and as they heal by fibrosis, a scarred, deformed *hepar lobatum* is left.

The mechanism of gummatous necrosis is probably allergy to products of the spirochaete. As in tuberculosis the necrosis probably precedes interference with the blood supply.

Spirochaetes are demonstrated only with great difficulty in the wall of a gumma. Tertiary syphilis is much less infectious than are the two preceding stages of the disease.

Diffuse lesions of tertiary syphilis. The really baneful effects of tertiary syphilis fall on the cardio-vascular and nervous

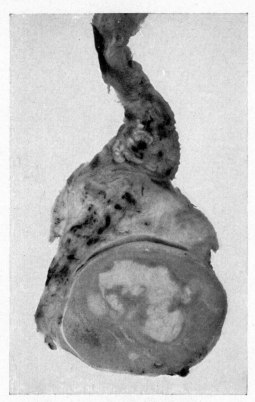

Figure 20.11
Gumma of testis. The testis is enlarged, and its substance is replaced by a diffuse area of gummatous necrosis, the edges of which are irregular. (EM 6.1, *Reproduced by permission of the President and Council of the R.C.S. Eng.*)

systems. In the former it is the ascending part of the thoracic aorta which usually suffers first. An infiltration of lymphocytes and plasma cells accumulates around the vasa vasorum of the tunica adventitia, and soon spreads inwards into the tunica media, where it destroys much of the elastic tissue on which the integrity of the aorta depends. Occasionally there is frank gummatous necrosis in the area of cellular infiltration, but usually the tissue of the aorta appears to disintegrate in front of the advancing cells.

The *syphilitic aortitis* that results weakens the media so much that aneurysmal dilatation eventually ensues. Sometimes the disease extends to the aortic ring, which dilates leading to aortic regurgitation. If the ostia of the coronary arteries are occluded at the same time there is severe myocardial ischaemia as well. It is hardly surprising that cardiovascular complications are responsible for most of the deaths directly attributable to syphilis. The abdominal aorta is rarely attacked in syphilis.

Cerebral syphilis may be *meningo-vascular* or *parenchymatous*. In the former type there is focal meningitis and vascular occlusion due to endarteritis obliterans of the small vessels. Isolated cranial nerve palsies are quite common.

Parenchymatous neurosyphilis includes the two well-

known conditions, *general paralysis of the insane* and *tabes dorsalis*. General paralysis of the insane is a chronic syphilitic meningo-encephalitis, and spirochaetes can be demonstrated in the frontal lobes, which are particularly severely affected. Tabes dorsalis is essentially a degenerative condition of the posterior columns of the spinal cord and the posterior roots of the spinal nerves. There is severe demyelination of the posterior columns which is followed by gliosis.

The osseous system is also frequently affected by a diffuse type of syphilitic inflammation. There may be widespread periostitis involving especially the tibia and the bones of the calvaria of the skull. The irregular thickening that is very apparent clinically is due to the laying down of new bone. This gives rise to the classical *sabre tibia*. Unlike the tibial deformity of rickets or Paget's disease, where there is true bowing due to softening of the bone, the lesion of syphilis is a mere "pseudo-bowing" due entirely to the irregular deposition of new periosteal bone. In the skull a worm-eaten appearance is produced by the concurrent effects of gummatous destruction and new-bone formation (Fig. 20.12).

Diagnosis. The diagnosis of tertiary syphilis is primarily clinical, but it may often be substantiated by serological examination of the blood and cerebro-spinal fluid. In most cases of overt syphilis this examination is strongly positive, and in neuro-syphilis the cerebro-spinal fluid is generally more helpful than the blood. In at least 20 per cent of cases of tabes dorsalis serological examination both of blood and cerebro-spinal fluid is negative. An additional aid is the presence of spirochaetes in histological sections of gummata, but as already mentioned these are very scanty.

Congenital syphilis. An untreated syphilitic mother is very liable to transmit the disease to her fetus during the first two years of infection, particularly after the fourth month of pregnancy, when the Langhans layer of the placenta disappears. Abortion may result, or else a severely affected infant may die soon after birth. There is marked syphilitic inflammation of most of the organs, notably the liver, pancreas, lungs, and bony epiphyses. A characteristic lesion is *pericellular fibrosis of the liver*, in which innumerable groups of liver cells are isolated and surrounded by syphilitic granulation tissue.

More frequently the child survives, and it may then show early stigmata of infection like skin eruptions, snuffles, epiphysitis of the elbows, and marasmus. Sometimes stigmata appear only in later childhood. The notched, peg-shaped Hutchinson's incisor teeth due to syphilitic infection of the tooth germs during fetal life are well-known examples of this type of lesion, as are also interstitial keratitis, tibial periostitis (sabre tibia), and eighth-nerve deafness.

The histological appearances of these various lesions are all very similar, being combinations of the heavy cellular infiltration of secondary syphilis together with the gummatous destruction typical of the tertiary phase. In fact, congenital syphilis may be regarded as a combined secondary

Figure 20.12
Gummatous osteo-periostitis of skull. The calvaria
of the skull shows multiple areas of gummatous
destruction, many of which are overhung by extensive
layers of new bone. The total effect is one of a worm-
eaten skull, which is greatly thickened. (S 50a.2,
*Reproduced by permission of the President and Council
of the R.C.S. Eng.)*

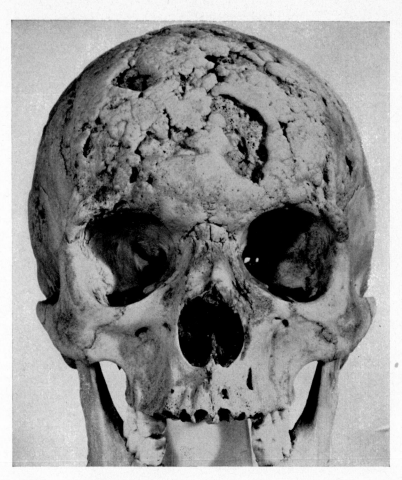

and tertiary syphilis occurring in a child whose primary lesion
was placental.

Diagnosis. This depends on serological examination of the
blood of the child and its parents. In the more florid lesions
spirochaetes abound, and are demonstrated with ease.

Immunity to syphilis. There appears to be a resistance
to further infection while treponemes are present in the
tissues. Two chancres may develop if the second infection
precedes the appearance of the primary lesion, but once this
has appeared, further infection fails to produce another
chancre.[38] There is no doubt that asymptomatic infection
may coexist with the presence of treponemes in the tissues;
these can produce syphilis when transferred to other
animals.[38] There is no spontaneous cure of the disease, and
therapeutic cure occurs only in the early stages.

In some patients with good immunity the infection remains latent for long periods, its existence being indicated
by the specific serological tests. In the tertiary stage there is
good evidence that treponemes are sequestrated in the
tissues,[42] often remaining latent, but always liable to flare up
in new lesions. In a case of tabes it has been possible to
demonstrate treponemes in the anterior chamber of the eye,
the cerebrospinal fluid, and the liver despite completely

negative serology.[43] The immunity is presumably cell
mediated, but macrophages are not as prominent as they are
in tuberculosis. There is little evidence that immunoglobulins are important. The maximum immunity develops
in the later stages—after two years in man—and it is never
absolute.[38]

Incidence of syphilis. After a prolonged period of
decline, the incidence of syphilis has risen in many parts of
the world over the last decade. Due to the great therapeutic
value of penicillin, syphilis accounted for the death of only
229 people in 1969 in England and Wales, the Registrar-
General's Statistical Review revealing that 153 men and 76
women died of the disease. Of these 65 per cent succumbed
to cardiovascular syphilis and the remainder to neuro-
syphilis; none died of congenital syphilis.

ACTINOMYCOSIS[44]

Actinomycosis is characterised by chronic, loculated foci
of suppuration occurring particularly in the region of the
lower jaw. It is seen in cattle, dogs and cats, and human
beings. The causal organisms are *Actinomyces bovis* (in

cattle), *Actinomyces baudeti* (in dogs and cats), and *Actinomyces israeli* (in human beings).[45, 46]

The disease in cattle is called *lumpy jaw*. It is often confused with another chronic suppurative condition of cattle called *woody tongue*. This is caused by a completely different organism, *Actinobacillus lignieresi*, a small Gram-negative bacillus.[45] Actinobacillosis has many points of similarity to actinomycosis, but it does not usually invade bones, and it has a tendency to spread along the lymphatics.

Bacteriology.[47] These organisms are Gram-positive branching filaments which show a tendency to break up into bacillary and twig-like forms. The filaments are much thinner than those of the fungi, and the organism is now classified as a bacterium in the family *Actinomycetaceae*, which also includes the genus *Nocardia* (Table 20.1). In

from the abscess sinuses. These are then crushed between two slides and stained, and also cultured anaerobically on blood agar (see Appendix III). The demonstration of antibodies plays no part in the diagnosis.

Pathogenesis. *Actinomyces israeli* is a normal commensal of the mouth, and it is found especially in the tonsils and carious teeth. Actinomycosis is an endogenous infection,[48] and is not transmitted by contaminated pieces of straw and grass that have been sucked by cattle. It can follow a dental extraction,[49] though considering the widespread distribution of the organism, the disease is surprisingly infrequent. It is not understood what local conditions must be fulfilled before the organism can invade the tissues of the gingiva and set up a progressive inflammatory reaction. It has been known to produce infection in a hand wound caused by

TABLE 20.1 Members of the order Actinomycetales

Order	Family	Genus
Actinomycetales	*Mycobacteriaceae*—no mycelium, acid fast	*Mycobacterium.*
	Actinomycetaceae—branching filaments which break up into bacillary elements	{ *Actinomyces*—not acid-fast { *Nocardia*—somewhat acid-fast
	Streptomycetaceae—mycelium with filaments which do not break up readily. Not acid-fast	*Streptomyces*—spores formed in chains

animal tissues the organisms grow in colonies consisting of a densely felted mass of filaments* matted together in an amorphous matrix. Such a colony appears in the pus of actinomycotic lesions in the form of a small granule which is greyish-yellow in colour. This is called a *sulphur granule*. In artificial culture this colonial tendency is less pronounced, and the individual filaments remain more separate.

A colony formed in the tissues tends to be surrounded by a radially projecting fringe of club-shaped excrescences (*clubs*). These "clubs" are Gram-negative, and are not formed in artificial culture. It is believed that they are produced as the result of deposition on to the colony of lipid material derived from the host's tissues. This radiating fringe around the colony gave rise to the alternative name *ray fungus* which has been loosely applied to *Actinomyces* organisms.

The pathogenic actinomyces organisms are anaerobic or, at the most, micro-aerophilic. They grow best at 37°C on ordinary media like blood agar or glucose agar, though a few days may elapse before colonies appear. Aerobic actinomyces organisms, e.g. *Actinomyces graminis*, may sometimes also be found in actinomycotic lesions, but they are apparently secondary contaminants.

Diagnosis. The diagnosis of actinomycosis depends on finding sulphur granules in the copious pus that exudes

* Often called a *mycelium*, although this term is often restricted to fungal growth.

hitting an assailant in the teeth ("punch actinomycosis").[50]

The actinomycotic lesion starts as an acute suppurative inflammation, which then persists and progresses to intractable chronicity. As the organisms spread by direct continuity, large numbers of abscesses are produced. Some of these fuse together, but there is a tendency for individual foci of suppuration to remain discrete owing to the persistence of fibrous septa. This produces a characteristically loculated appearance, which is seen most typically in actinomycotic lesions of the liver (*honeycomb liver*).

Histologically the abscess cavities are crowded with pus cells which surround actinomycotic colonies (sulphur granules—Fig. 20.13). The narrow septa between the abscesses are composed of fibrous tissue which is heavily infiltrated by polymorphs with some lymphocytes, macrophages, and plasma cells. These fibrous septa are not merely the remains of destroyed parenchyma; they represent attempts at repair, and the entire lesion is surrounded by a dense zone of fibrous tissue.

Spread of infection. About 65 per cent of clinical actinomycosis starts in the cervico-facial area, 20 per cent is primarily ileocaecal, and the remainder commences in the lungs.

The main mode of spread of the disease is by direct contact. Whereas other organisms move in the tissue spaces along preformed planes, the actinomyces extend slowly and inexorably ever onwards. In cervico-facial actinomycosis

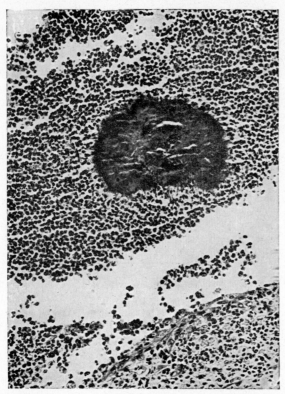

Figure 20.13
Actinomycotic pus. The section shows a dense infiltration of pus cells, in the centre of which there is a colony of actinomyces (sulphur granule). The peripheral clubs are evident as areas of darker staining. ×150.

there is direct spread to the adjacent muscles and bones, so that eventually the spinal column and skull are invaded.[51] There is also progressive cutaneous involvement, and the abscesses discharge through multiple sinuses. In the pus that exudes numerous pin's-head sized, yellowish or greyish sulphur granules are discharged. The appearance of a diffuse, indurated, painless area of suppuration in the area

of the neck, discharging to the exterior through multiple sinuses, is characteristic of actinomycosis.

Similarly ileo-caecal actinomycosis spreads through the anterior abdominal wall with the development of discharging sinuses, and pulmonary actinomycosis erupts through the wall of the chest. When tuberculosis implicates a serous sac, there is usually a widespread involvement; actinomycosis on the other hand, spreads directly from visceral to parietal layers and then invades the body wall and discharges externally. In abdominal actinomycosis fistulae develop between loops of bowel as in Crohn's disease and tuberculosis.

Lymphatic spread does not occur in actinomycosis; perhaps the filaments are too large to be accommodated in the lymphatic channels. Any regional lymphadenitis that may occur is attributable to secondary bacterial infection.

Blood-borne spread, on the other hand, is important, and is typified by the spread of ileo-caecal disease by the portal vein to the liver, where the loculated actinomycotic abscesses of *honeycomb liver* are produced. Likewise pulmonary actinomycosis may disseminate in the systemic circulation and produce lesions in the kidneys, brain, bones, and other parts. Occasionally a honeycomb liver implicates the lung above it by direct spread of infection through the diaphragm.

Treatment.[52, 53] Actinomyces organisms are very sensitive to the commonly-used antibiotics, especially penicillin. The prognosis of cervico-facial disease is very good, but the abdominal and pulmonary infections are sometimes fatal.

Incidence. This is a rare disease in Britain. The Registrar-General's Review for 1969 has recorded six deaths only.

Mycetoma[54, 55]

The term mycetoma is used to denote a localised infection of the subcutaneous tissues, usually of the hands or feet, that follows the introduction of the specific causal organisms from the exterior. The organisms responsible fall into two groups, one bacterial and the other fungal.

Figure 20.14
Mycetoma of hand. The hand has been sectioned to show the wide-spread ramifications of the infection in the deeper tissues, which have been destroyed by masses of black material. (S 52.2, *Reproduced by permission of the President and Council of the R.C.S. Eng.)*

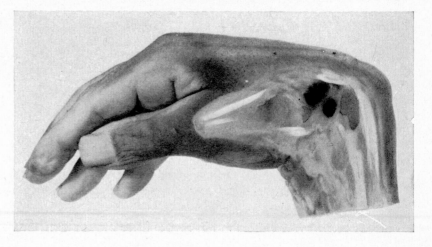

Bacterial mycetoma. Nocardia and streptomyces in the order *Actinomycetales* are involved. Nocardia are aerobic, Gram-positive, and often acid-fast. They grow as branching filaments which tend to break up into bacillary forms. *N. asteroides* and *N. brasiliensis* are the best known. The streptomyces, e.g. *S. madurae*, grow as stable filaments, and are on the borderline of the bacteria and fungi.

Fungal mycetoma (maduromycosis). At least thirteen species of fungi have been identified as causes of mycetoma. These include *Madurella mycetomi*, *Allescheria boydii*, and *Aspergillus nidulans*.

The habitat of all these organisms is the soil, and they may be introduced into the skin and subcutaneous tissues as the result of trivial injury. The condition occurs mainly in tropical countries, and is endemic in India. The foot is most commonly involved (*Madura foot*).

The pathogenesis and spread of the disease is similar to that described in actinomycosis except that blood-spread does not occur. There is widespread destruction of tissue and the appearance of multiple sinuses through which coloured granules are discharged. These are large and often black in colour. If the disease is left unchecked, the patient eventually dies of cachexia.

Suphonamides are useful in *Nocardia* infections[52] but are of no value against fungi. The affected part may have to be amputated (Fig. 20.14).

REFERENCES

1. VESEY, C. M. R. and WILKINSON, D. S. (1959). *British Journal of Dermatology*, **71**, 139.
2. Leading Article (1972). *Lancet*, ii, 580.
3. WILSON, G. S. and MILES, A. A. (1964). In *Topley and Wilson's Principles of Bacteriology and Immunity*, 5th edn, p. 1588. London: Arnold.
4. MARKS, J. and BIRN, K. J. (1963). *British Medical Journal*, ii, 1503.
5. CRUICKSHANK, R. (1965). In *Medical Microbiology*, 11th edn, p. 194. Edited by R. Cruickshank. Edinburgh: Livingstone.
6. DAVIS, B. D., DULBECCO, R., EISEN, H. N., GINSBERG, H. S. and WOOD, W. B. (1967). *Microbiology*. New York: Hoeber and Row.
7. EDWARDS, L. B. (1963). *Annals of the New York Academy of Sciences*, **106**, 32.
8. MacCALLUM, P. *et al.* (1948). *Journal of Pathology and Bacteriology*, **60**, 93.
9. CONNOR, D. H. and LUNN, H. F. (1966). *Archives of Pathology*, **81**, 183.
10. LINELL, F. and NORDÉN, Å. (1954). *Acta Tuberculosea Scandinavica*, Suppl. 33.
11. PHILPOTT, J. A. *et al.* (1963). *Archives of Dermatology and Syphilology*, **88**, 158.
12. Leading Article (1970). *British Medical Journal*, ii, 438.
13. POOLE, J. C. F. and FLOREY, H. W. (1970). In *General Pathology*, 4th edn, p. 1190. Edited by H. W. Florey. London: Lloyd-Luke.
14. OSWALD, N. C. (1963). *British Medical Journal*, ii, 1489.
15. WEISS, C. and HALLIDAY, N. (1944). *Proceedings of the Society for Experimental Biology and Medicine*, **57**, 299.
16. Leading Article (1969). *British Medical Journal*, ii, 265.
17. GOLD, J. *et al.* (1957). *Gastroenterology*, **33**, 113.
18. KORN, R. J. *et al.* (1959). *American Journal of Medicine*, **27**, 60.
19. RICH, A. R. and McCORDOCK, H. A. (1933). *Bulletin of the Johns Hopkins Hospital*, **52**, 5.
20. LURIE, M. B. and NINOS, G. S. (1956). *American Review of Tuberculosis and Pulmonary Diseases*, **73**, 434.
21. MOLOMUT, N. and SPAIN, D. M. (1953). *American Review of Tuberculosis and Pulmonary Diseases*, **67**, 101.
22. JOHNSTON, R. N., RITCHIE, R. T. and MURRAY, I. H. F. (1963). *British Medical Journal*, ii, 720.
23. FONG, J., SCHNEIDER, P. and ELBERG, S. S. (1957). *Journal of Experimental Medicine*, **105**, 25.
24. Leading Article (1969). *Lancet*, i, 192.
25. WEISS, D. W. and WELLS, A. Q. (1960). *American Review of Respiratory Diseases*, **82**, 339.
26. RAFFEL, S. (1948). *Journal of Infectious Diseases*, **82**, 267.
27. GALBRAITH, N. S. *et al.* (1972). *British Medical Journal*, i, 647.
28. SPRINGETT, V. H. (1972). *British Medical Journal*, i, 422.
29. Leading Article (1972). *Lancet*, ii, 168.
30. MARKS, J. *et al.* (1971). *British Medical Journal*, iii, 229.
31. ELLMAN, P. and ANDREWS, L. G. (1959). *British Medical Journal*, i, 1433.
32. SWAIN, R. H. A. (1965). In *Medical Microbiology*, p. 342, *loc. cit.*
33. Annotation (1968). *Lancet*, i, 1187.
34. Leading Article (1967). *British Medical Journal*, ii, 394.
35. SPARLING, P. F. (1971). *New England Journal of Medicine*, **284**, 642.
36. LYNCH, F. W., KIMBALL, A. C. and KERNAN, P. D. (1960). *Journal of Investigative Dermatology*, **34**, 219.
37. Leading Article (1971). *Lancet*, i, 1170.
38. WILSON, G. S. and MILES, A. A. (1964). p. 2170, *loc. cit.*
39. BEERMAN, H. *et al.* (1960). *Archives of Internal Medicine*, **105**, 145 and 324.
40. RAVITCH, M. M., FARMER, T. W. and DAVIS, B. (1949). *Journal of Clinical Investigation*, **28**, 18.
41. MOLLISON, P. L. (1972). In *Blood Transfusion in Clinical Practice*, 5th edn, p. 613. Oxford: Blackwell.
42. Leading Article (1968). *Lancet*, ii, 718.
43. SMITH, J. L. and ISRAEL, C. W. (1967). *Journal of the American Medical Association*, **199**, 980.
44. COPE, V. Z. (1938). *Actinomycosis*. Oxford University Press.
45. WILSON, G. S. and MILES, A. A. (1964). p. 1563, *loc. cit.*
46. PEABODY, J. W. and SEABURY, J. H. (1957). *Journal of Chronic Diseases*, **5**, 374.
47. GILLIES, R. R. (1965). In *Medical Microbiology*, p. 303, *loc. cit.*

48. Utz, J. P. (1962). *Laboratory Investigation*, **11**, 1018.
49. Lesney, T. A. and Traeger, K. A. (1959). *Journal of Oral Surgery*, **17**, No. 1, 51.
50. Winner, H. I. (1960). Quoted in *Lancet*, ii, 907.
51. Intile, J. A. and Richert, J. H. (1962). *Journal of the American Medical Association*, **181**, 724.
52. Peabody, J. W. and Seabury, J. H. (1960). *Journal of the American Medical Association*, **28**, 99.
53. Spilsbury, B. W. and Johnstone, F. R. C. (1962). *Canadian Journal of Surgery*, **5**, 33.
54. Ochoa, A. G. (1962). *Laboratory Investigation*, **11**, 1118.
55. Mackinnon, J. E. (1962). *Laboratory Investigation*, **11**, 1124.

In the previous chapter the inflammatory reactions associated with tuberculosis, syphilis, and actinomycosis were studied, and three responses were described:

The tuberculoid reaction, which consists of an epithelioid cell–giant cell follicle sometimes with central caseation and surrounded by lymphocytes. It is seen in tuberculosis.

The small round cell reaction, which consists of a diffuse lymphocyte–plasma cell infiltration. It is seen in syphilis.

The pyogenic reaction, which consists of a loculated abscess crowded with polymorphs. It is seen in actinomycosis.

It was noted that none of these reactions was strictly specific. Indeed, they can all be produced by different types of foreign bodies introduced into the tissues, though admittedly caseation is peculiar to tuberculosis and a few uncommon fungous diseases. In the conditions about to be described these reactions are often reproduced and sometimes combined, while on other occasions there may be very little tissue reaction at all. The theme of this discussion is the versatile response of the body to noxious agents of various types.

SOME DEEP-SEATED FUNGOUS INFECTIONS

The first three infections considered here are cryptococcosis, histoplasmosis, and coccidioidomycosis. They are all caused by yeast-like fungi* present in the soil, which when inhaled may produce a pulmonary lesion. It usually heals, but occasionally systemic spread to the viscera ensues, and the outcome is often fatal. The parallel between these diseases and tuberculosis is very close; many of the histological features of tuberculosis are encountered in the deep-seated mycoses. Candidiasis is also described because the systemic variety is becoming increasingly common.

CRYPTOCOCCOSIS[1]

The causative organism *Cryptococcus neoformans* (formerly called *Torula histolytica*) is a true yeast, i.e. it reproduces by

---

* A *fungus* is a member of the vegetable kingdom, devoid of roots, stems, and leaves, and incapable of photosynthesis. Some are parasites, others saprophytes. They may be unicellular (e.g. yeasts), or else consist of branching filaments *(hyphae)* aggregated into a mass *(mycelium)*. The walls tend to be rigid. Multiplication is by budding in yeasts, and spore formation (sexual and asexual) in the higher fungi.

---

budding and does not form a mycelium. It is a spherical cell, 4–12 μm in diameter, Gram-positive, and surrounded by a thick gelatinous capsule which stains for mucus using the PAS or mucicarmine methods. This characteristic makes it easily demonstrable in histological sections.

The organism has been found in soil, in the droppings of birds, particularly pigeons, and also on fruit and in milk. It causes sporadic disease in horses, cattle, and pigs, and is characteristically pathogenic to mice. In animals and human beings it is rarely isolated except from overt lesions. The human disease has a world-wide distribution and occurs at all ages. The sporadic cases that occur are probably due to inhalation of organisms from the soil. The condition is not infectious.

The primary lesion is pulmonary,[2] usually a single subpleural mass called a "toruloma". It is very chronic and is usually symptomless; it occasionally undergoes cavitation. Spread to the hilar nodes is very uncommon. Healing by fibrosis without much calcification may occur, but sometimes the disease is disseminated by the blood stream. The central nervous system is then usually invaded, and more rarely lesions may be encountered in the skin,[3] bones[4], and lymph nodes.

The leptomeninges of the base of the brain are usually first affected. There is widening of the infiltrated subarachnoid space, and the colonies of cryptococci may proliferate so rapidly as to rupture through the pia arachnoid into the brain substance. The exudate is gelatinous in consistency, and there may be cystic spaces in the underlying brain, filled with aggregations of the organisms and their mucoid capsules. Clinically the disease resembles tuberculous meningitis, and the effects are due to a raised intracranial pressure. Untreated cases always die.

The tissue reactions to the cryptococcus.[5] Most commonly there is no reaction at all. Masses of organisms resembling a pure culture are found in the subarachnoid spaces, and there is no inflammatory or glial reaction (Fig. 21.1).

Occasionally there is an accumulation of giant cells both of foreign body and Langhans type, containing many phagocytosed organisms.

Sometimes a collection of organisms is surrounded by a diffuse small round cell infiltration composed of lymphocytes and plasma cells. This is common in pulmonary torulomata.

An epithelioid-cell infiltration with Langhans giant cells and a surrounding zone of small round cells is occasionally

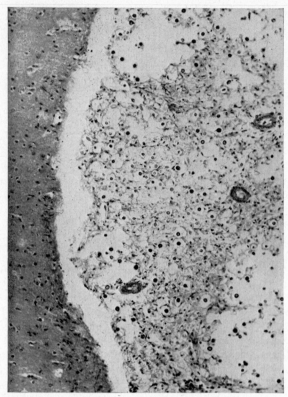

Figure 21.1
Cryptococcosis. In the meninges overlying the brain there is a gelatinous inflammatory exudate in which the conspicuous yeast *Cryptococcus neoformans* abounds. As there are virtually no inflammatory cells in this exudate, the nucleate structures are nearly all cryptococci. × 170.

seen in cryptococcosis. This tuberculoid reaction is diffuse, and lacks the circumscribed follicular pattern typical of tuberculosis. Caseation is uncommon except in conglomerate torulomata. The cryptococci are present in the inflammatory tissue.

In addition to producing primary disease cryptococci are important causes of opportunistic infection in cases of T-lymphocyte deficiency (see p. 172). There may be a generalised infection or else the disease may remain localised to a few lymph nodes.

The diagnosis of cryptococcosis depends on isolating and culturing the organisms from the sputum or cerebro-spinal fluid. Serological methods are not helpful.

HISTOPLASMOSIS[6, 7]

The causative organism *Histoplasma capsulatum* is a dimorphic fungus, i.e. it exists in yeast form when cultured at 37°C and in animal tissues and in mycelial form in saprophytic life. It is a small, oval yeast cell, 1–5 μm in diameter, surrounded by a thin capsule which consists of mucoid

material. Like the cryptococcus it is found in the soil, and it produces disease in various animals, e.g. dogs, rodents, cattle, and horses.

The disease has a world-wide distribution, and is endemic in the Mississippi Valley area of the USA. A special African type of histoplasmosis due to *Histoplasma duboisi* has been described. This organism is distinctly larger than *Histoplasma capsulatum*.

Infection may occur at any age, but children are particularly susceptible. The inhalation of contaminated soil dust appears to be the mode of infection. The disease is not infectious.

The primary lesion is pulmonary. There is a transient infection with hilar-gland involvement, usually followed by rapid healing with residual calcification; only occasionally does a chronic lesion with cavitation persist.[8] Rarely the disease becomes disseminated by the blood stream, and the organisms are carried to various viscera. Systemic histoplasmosis[9] is a fatal disease, and it resembles leishmaniasis, a protozoan disease that is also spread throughout the body by macrophages. The organs most heavily involved are the spleen, liver, lymph nodes, and bone marrow, and therefore severe anaemia and leucopenia are prominent features. Mucosal ulceration of the mouth and gut is a common manifestation. Adrenal destruction may lead to Addison's disease.

The tissue reaction typical of histoplasmosis[5] is intracellular parasitisation within macrophages (Fig. 21.2). In the African variety giant cells may also be formed. In the liver and spleen there are usually large areas of necrosis surrounded by the parasitised macrophages.

A tuberculoid reaction is rather uncommon, but occasionally affected lymph nodes may contain follicles reminiscent of sarcoidosis. Caseation is most uncommon except in solitary lung lesions. Like cryptococcosis, histoplasmosis may occur as an opportunistic infection where there is T-lymphocyte deficiency.

The diagnosis is made by finding the yeast-form of the organism as an intracellular parasite. Smears made from the blood, bone marrow, sputum, and scrapings from mucosal lesions may all show parasitised macrophages. The organism is easily cultured.

Serological methods help to confirm the diagnosis. Within a few weeks complement-fixing antibodies appear in the serum, and their titre is an indication of the activity of infection. At the same time hypersensitivity to the antigens of the organism develops, and this forms the basis of the *histoplasmin* skin test. A positive result indicates past or present infection.

COCCIDIOIDOMYCOSIS[10]

The causative organism *Coccidioides immitis* is a dimorphic fungus. In the tissues the organism appears typically as a large, spherical, non-budding structure about 50 μm in

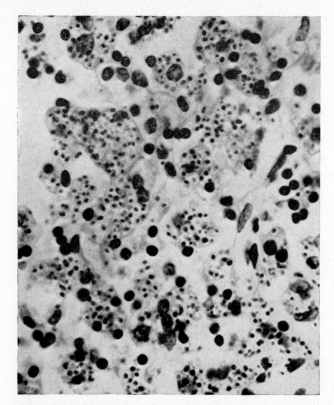

Figure 21.2
Histoplasmosis. This is a section of spleen from a patient who died of generalised histoplasmosis. There is a profuse infiltration of macrophages which are crammed with *Histoplasma capsulatum* organisms. ×400.

diameter. It has a thick wall and is called a sporangium. In it there are many small, spherical endospores from 2 to 5 μm in diameter. When the sporangium ruptures, these spores are released and then develop into new sporangia. This mode of reproduction contrasts sharply with the simple budding encountered in the *Cryptococcus* and *Histoplasma* species.

It too is a soil saprophyte, and it causes disease in rodents, dogs, and cattle. The distribution is fairly widespread, but the great bulk of the disease occurs in the South-West of the USA, especially Arizona and California where it is endemic. It is estimated that over three-quarters of the population of the San Joaquin Valley of California have had the disease as indicated by skin tests. It is also seen in South America and Italy.

As in the other two mycotic diseases infection is due to the inhalation of soil dust. All age-groups are afflicted, and patients are not infectious.

The primary lesion is a pulmonary complex very similar in morphology to tuberculosis. There is considerable mediastinal lymphadenopathy. The condition is generally benign and heals with calcification. It is often subclinical, but sometimes it is attended by a mild febrile illness called "valley fever". About 3 weeks after this there is often a sharp attack of erythema nodosum. This is much less common in cryptococcosis and histoplasmosis. The patient usually recovers completely, but in a few instances there follows the generalised disease of progressive coccidioidomycosis[11] with destructive lesions in the viscera, skin, and bones. This is usually fatal, there often being a terminal meningitis. Generalisation is said to occur most frequently in dark-skinned races. Opportunistic infections may occur, but are less common than with cryptococcosis and histoplasmosis.

The tissue reaction of coccidioidomycosis.[5] Of all the fungous diseases coccidioidomycosis resembles tuberculosis most closely in histological appearance. Complete tuberculoid systems with variable amounts of caseation are present, especially in lung lesions.

Often, however, there is a suppurative element: micro-abscesses filled with pus cells lie centrally, and are surrounded by epithelioid cells and scanty giant cells. Such lesions are encompassed by extensive infiltrations of small round cells, and may fuse to form large conglomerate masses. Organisms may be found in the central abscesses.

Diagnosis. This depends on the isolation and culture of the organism. The disease is notorious for the ease with which laboratory workers may become infected.

Complement-fixing antibodies appear in the serum after a few weeks, and a skin test using an extract of organism (*coccidioidin*) gives a positive result. Patients with the progressive disease may not react, a state of affairs that is reminiscent of fulminating tuberculosis.

CANDIDIASIS[12, 13]

Infection with the *Candida* species is becoming one of the most frequent fungous diseases in man. The organism most frequently involved is the dimorphic funigus *Candida albicans*. The common yeast form is found in superficial lesions, and it is 1·5 to 5·0 μm in diameter and intensely Gram positive. It reproduces by budding, but sometimes the bud elongates to form a mycelium. This form can occur in cultures, and is also seen in invasive candida infections, especially in systemic candidiasis.

The organism is a common commensal in the mouth, alimentary tract, and vagina. The superficial infections of the mucous membranes appear as white patches called *thrush*. In the mouth this is very common in infants, especially premature ones, and it may be accompanied by perianal lesions. Oral candidiasis can occur at any age in the course of a debilitating illness. Vaginal thrush is common during pregnancy and in diabetes mellitus. In both conditions there is excess glycogen in the vaginal cells; this the fungus ferments, and the acidity of the vagina increases. The organism grows well in an acid pH, and is in fact best cultured on an acid medium (Sabouraud's medium, see p. 647). The glycosuria in diabetics also favours the growth of *Candida albicans* in the vagina. *Cutaneous candidiasis* occurs around the mouth (perlèche), in other moist intertriginous areas, and in the nail folds (chronic paronychia).

The importance of candidiasis is that it is a serious opportunistic infection. In any condition of impaired cell-mediated immunity, e.g. lymphomata and after the administration of glucocorticosteroids or cytotoxic durgs, oral lesions can extend down the alimentary or respiratory tracts to produce fatal results. The most serious type is *generalised, systemic candidiasis* in which there is haematogenous spread to many organs; renal lesions are prominent, but almost any organ may be affected and endocarditis is sometimes seen. Generalised candidiasis is sometimes a salient feature of those immunological deficiency syndromes in which there is a T-lymphocyte defect, e.g. Nezelof's syndrome (see p. 172). Less extensive candidal infections are seen in particular circumstances. *Endocarditis* can occur as an isolated event, particularly in addicts who inject themselves intravenously with narcotics. Oral lesions can spread to produce extensive *gastro-intestinal infection* following the prolonged use of oral broad-spectrum antibiotics.

Finally there are some types of primary immunological deficiency disease affecting T lymphocytes in which widespread *chronic mucocutaneous candidiasis* is seen.[14] The type of defect varies from case to case. In some patients there is a lymphocyte defect such that the cells are unresponsive to phytohaemagglutinin. In others, such stimulation produces a normal transformation but the cells are unresponsive to *Candida* antigen. The treatment of this latter group with transfer factor may be successful. In some patients endocrine abnormalities, particularly hypoparathyroidism, may coexist. Chronic mucocutaneous candidiasis is therefore a manifestation of several distinct disease processes. It lasts for many years and does not terminate in generalised spread, nor is there usually a tendency for other infections to occur.

The tissue reaction to *Candida* varies. In minor and superficial infections there is some tissue necrosis accompanied by a pyogenic response; intra-epithelial pustules are seen in the cutaneous lesions. When the infection is overwhelming, as in generalised candidiasis, there is much necrosis and very little inflammatory reaction. Indeed, the lesions show massive accumulations of fungus and few host cells.

Treatment of Deep-Seated Fungous Infections

The local pulmonary lesions usually heal spontaneously, though a toruloma, if diagnosed clinically, should be resected in view of the danger of systemic spread. For generalised infections of these organisms the antibiotic *amphotericin B* offers hope where once there was none.

5-Fluorocytosine is a new, less toxic drug which promises to be useful in treating fungous diseases, especially cryptococcosis and candidiasis.[15] Topical nystatin is used for superficial *Candida* infections, but cannot be administered systemically.

SOME PROTOZOAN INFECTIONS

The most important protozoan diseases of man are malaria, leishmaniasis, trypanosomiasis, and amoebiasis. These are not discussed here because detailed accounts of their pathology are available in standard text-books of tropical medicine. Instead, two rather uncommon diseases are touched on, toxoplasmosis and pneumocystis pneumonia, both of which are encountered in Britain from time to time.

TOXOPLASMOSIS[16]

The causative organism *Toxoplasma gondii* belongs to the subphylum *Sporozoa* and probably to the genus *Isospora*. It is crescentic in shape and about 7 μm long. It is stained by the usual Romanowsky methods used for malarial and leishmanial parasites; the nucleus is red and the cytoplasm blue. When introduced into an animal host, it parasitises many of the nucleated parenchymatous cells. By repeated binary fission it soon proliferates and kills the cell, whereupon the liberated organisms infect other cells both locally and by carriage in the blood and lymph. This stage of parasitaemia is accompanied by focal cell necrosis. The animal either dies, or else becomes immune to the organism. In this case the intracellular parasites encyst themselves in the tissues. Such a cyst may at first be less than 10 μm in diameter, but soon the parasites inside it start dividing, and the cyst may eventually attain a size of 100 μm. Cysts are found especially in the brain, but may also be encountered in the heart muscle, liver, lungs, spleen, and lymph nodes. As immunity increases, so the number of cysts decreases. A breakdown of immunity may be followed by a recrudescence of overt disease.[17]

A sexual phase of development has been described in cats:[18, 19] if they are fed on toxoplasma-infected mice, the organisms parasitise the cells of the bowel mucosa where both schizogony and gametogony occur. Oocysts are produced which are excreted in the cat's faeces. These can then divide into two sporocysts each containing four sporozoites when the cyst is ingested by another animal. It seems probable that man becomes infected through ingesting oocysts from the excreta of domestic animals. What is strange in human infections is the tendency for the products of schizogony to penetrate the bowel wall and be carried in the blood and lymph to different organs. Here they end their existence as cysts. Well over half the populations of many communities have been exposed to infection, usually during later childhood and at adolescence, by the evidence of serological tests.

The vast majority of human infections are subclinical, a state of affairs reminiscent of tuberculosis. Occasionally an adult may suffer from overt toxoplasmosis.[20] Very rarely this may take the form of a fulminating typhus-like disease, and such features as interstitial pneumonia and encephalitis may be superadded. A much more usual event, however, is a mild though prolonged, febrile illness in which lymphadenopathy is a prominent manifestation. The disease is easily mistaken for infectious mononucleosis,[21] but the Paul-Bunnell reaction is negative.

The histological changes seen in an affected lymph node are those of pronounced reactive hyperplasia (see Chapter 30). In addition there are often small collections of epithelioid cells scattered throughout the lymph node.[22] The appearance may resemble sarcoidosis, except that the aggregations are smaller, and there are no giant cells. Very occasionally a toxoplasma cyst may be included in the section. Both clinically and histologically toxoplasmosis may be confused with Hodgkin's disease.

The tragedy of toxoplasmosis lies in its tendency to be transmitted transplacentally to the fetus. The mother is usually healthy though infected, and there is often no transmission in succeeding pregnancies.

The effects on the fetus vary. A very severe infection may precipitate abortion, but this is not common. More often the child survives, and develops a severe generalised disease a few weeks after birth. The lungs, liver, spleen, and lymph nodes are severely affected. Acute peritonitis and pleurisy are common features, and there may also be skin eruptions of various types.

In other cases the disease appears later, when central nervous system and ocular lesions predominate. A severe choroidoretinitis is characteristic, and this may proceed to microphthalmos and blindness. On the other hand, a focal scotoma may be the only residual feature. Toxoplasmosis is a very important cause of posterior uveitis, and recrudescences are common. It is possible that some toxoplasmal uveitis is secondary to disease acquired in adult life.

The cerebral infection produces necrotic nodules in the meninges and brain substance, particularly around the walls of the lateral ventricles. Necrotic material may be shed into the ventricles and lead to obstructive hydrocephalus, which may also be produced as a result of fibrinous meningitis around the base of the brain. Sometimes necrosis is so extensive that microcephaly ensues. In patients who survive calcification in the area of the necrotic tissue is prominent. It is seen radiologically as sharply-outlined, curved ridges situated in the para-ventricular areas of the cerebral hemispheres. Severe cases die in a few months, while others may be left with various residua, including paralysis and idiocy.

Pyrimethamine (Daraprim) and *sulphonamides*, especially sulphadiazine, are of some value in treatment.

The histological features of these severe congenital lesions are not pathognomonic. Focal necrosis may be found in the liver, spleen, and lungs, and this is surrounded by non-specific small round cell infiltrations that include polymorphs. Haemorrhagic extravasations are common, and the fibrinous pleurisy that often occurs may also be haemorrhagic. The brain likewise contains necrotic foci surrounded by small round cells and proliferating glial tissue. Dystrophic calcification is a prominent sequel.

The lymph nodes show no necrosis, but only a reactive change similar to that of the adult lesion.

Diagnosis.[17] *Demonstration of the organism in lesions.* It is uncommon to find the toxoplasms in histological section, and they are furthermore very difficult to identify. Occasionally cysts may be found in areas that are quiescent.

Isolation of the organism. The mouse is very susceptible to infection. It is inoculated with a test suspension, and a rapidly fatal disease usually ensues. Smears of the spleen, lung, liver, and brain should reveal large numbers of organisms within the cells of the organ.

A rising titre of antibodies is the most important diagnostic test. These can be demonstrated by means of complement-fixation tests using a toxoplasmal antigen. The *dye-test* is also very useful. Normally extracellular toxoplasms stain easily with a methylene-blue buffer solution, but in the presence of the specific antibody and free complement, staining is impaired, due apparently to a modification induced in the cytoplasm of the organisms. The organisms for this test are obtained from the peritoneal exudates of infected mice.

A skin test can also be done, and is said to be especially useful in epidemiological surveys.

PNEUMOCYSTIS PNEUMONIA[23]

This is a pulmonary disease characterised by a progressive pneumonic infiltration which was first described in debilitated and premature infants. Treatment is unsatisfactory, but recently pentamidine isothionate has been used with encouraging results.

The lungs are firm, dry, and homogeneous in consistency and grey in colour. On section the alveoli are seen to be filled with a foamy, reticulated, eosinophilic exudate. If examined carefully, this apparently acellular honeycomb exudate is found to contain many punctate bodies. Special staining techniques, e.g. Gomori's methenamine silver method, the PAS method, and the Romanowsky stains, reveal the exudate crowded with parasites. The other prominent feature in some cases is an abundant plasma-cell infiltration of the interalveolar septa.

The parasite is called *Pneumocystis carinii* and is a protozoon, but it has never been successfully cultured.

There is a close relationship between this disease and immunological deficiencies, especially those involving T lymphocytes.[24] Hence pneumocystis pneumonia is not infrequently seen in patients with impaired cell-mediated immunity, and less often in cases of Bruton's congenital agammaglobulinaemia.[24] It is thus an important opportunistic infection, and has been described occurring together with cytomegalic inclusion disease in this context.[25]

SOME CHRONIC INFLAMMATIONS OF DOUBTFUL AETIOLOGY

CAT-SCRATCH DISEASE[26-28]

This is an unusual inflammatory condition of lymph nodes, and there is reason to believe that it is caused by an agent allied to that of lymphogranuloma venereum.

The disease is found almost invariably in people who come into contact with cats, and there is often a history of a cat-scratch. About a week later a sore develops locally, and there may be variable constitutional symptoms. About 3 weeks later there is painful regional lymphadenitis with considerable reddening of the skin over the nodes, and suppuration may occur if these are not excised.

The histological picture approximates closely to that described in coccidioidomycosis, namely a suppurative tuberculoid reaction. It starts with collections of epithelioid cells in the substance of the node, and these soon undergo central necrosis while a polymorph infiltration develops in their midst. After a few weeks these foci increase greatly in size and number. The larger ones collapse due to the extensive central necrosis, and so tend to assume a flattened shape. The surrounding layers of epithelioid cells arrange themselves in a palisade around the collapsed centre. A few Langhans giant cells may appear among them, but they are never numerous (Fig. 21.3). Associated with this destruction of the

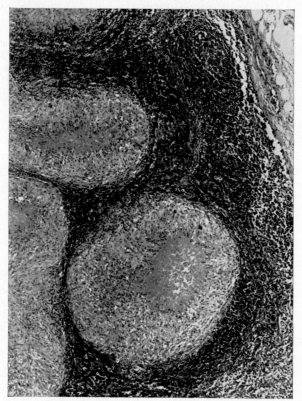

Figure 21.3
Cat-scratch disease. In this lymph node there are follicles typical of cat-scratch disease. In the centre there is a large area of necrosis in which the nuclei of disintegrating polymorphs are barely recognisable, and surrounding this there is an exuberant zone of epithelioid cells. There are few giant cells in this area. The evenly palisaded arrangement of the epithelioid cells perpendicular to the surrounding lymphoid tissue is very characteristic of the condition, and is in marked contrast to the irregular disposition of the cells in tuberculosis. × 50. *(Photograph supplied by Dr. A. D. Thomson)*

node there is severe periadenitis with an infiltration of lymphocytes, plasma cells, and macrophages into the surrounding connective tissue. There is eventual healing by fibrosis, but suppurative foci persist for many months.

This picture is seen also in lymphogranuloma venereum, and in the acute mesenteric adenitis caused by *Yersinia (Pasteurella) pseudotuberculosis* that resembles acute appendicitis clinically.[29] An extract of pus from a lymph node removed from a case of cat-scratch disease produces a positive reaction when injected intradermally into a fresh case. This closely resembles the Frei test of lymphogranuloma venereum.

SARCOIDOSIS[30]

This is a systemic disease of unknown aetiology in which characteristic epithelioid-cell follicles are scattered throughout many organs. It is quite common in Northern European communities.

The unit of sarcoidosis is a discrete follicle composed of plump epithelioid cells, in the midst of which a few Langhans giant cells may be found. Sometimes these giant cells contain star-shaped acidophilic bodies, or *asteroids*, and spherical basophilic masses, or *Schaumann bodies*. These inclusions are in no way pathognomonic of sarcoidosis, being found in the Langhans giant cells of other conditions from time to time. The follicle is surrounded by a narrow rim of lymphocytes. It is very like the tubercle follicle, but differs in that there is never any true central caseation (Fig. 21.4). In very florid cases of sarcoidosis some of the follicles may contain small central areas of necrosis. The extensive small round cell infiltration of tuberculosis is lacking in sarcoidosis. Individual follicles often undergo partial coalescence to form conglomerate masses, a feature seen particularly in pulmonary sarcoidosis. The course of the lesions is towards healing. In them there are many reticulin fibres, and the follicles are gradually replaced by dense fibrous tissue. Ultimately a hyalinised scar remains.

Though the lesions are generalised,[31] the lungs bear the brunt of the disease. Chest radiography reveals miliary (and sometimes conglomerate) mottling of both lung fields with considerable hilar lymphadenopathy. The pulmonary symptoms are often initially very mild in comparison with the extent of the disease. In appearance the sarcoid tissue is pearly-grey in colour, and forms discrete or confluent masses in the lungs, especially in the mid-zones and bases. Other organs frequently involved are the lymph nodes, spleen, and liver, all of which may be clinically palpable. In the bones small cysts may be produced (*osteitis cystica multiplex*). The phalanges are most commonly affected. A considerable range of cutaneous lesions is due to sarcoidosis; a well-known one is *lupus pernio*, in which soft, infiltrated, violaceous plaques with superficial telangiectasia are present, especially on the nose, ears, or fingers ("chilblain lupus"). Furthermore, *erythema nodosum* is a common accompaniment: indeed, in Northern European countries sarcoidosis and tuberculosis are the most frequent precipitating factors of

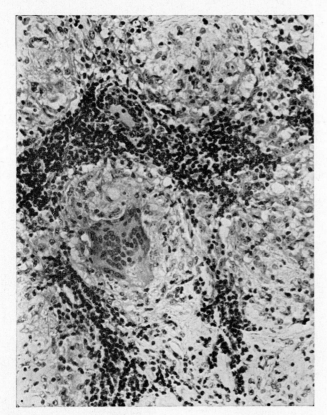

Figure 21.4
Sarcoidosis. In this section of lymph node there are semi-confluent follicles consisting of epithelioid cells. A large giant cell is present in one follicle; it resembles a foreign-body cell rather than a Langhans one. There is no central caseation. ×230.

erythema nodosum. Patients who develop erythema nodosum have a good prognosis, and their lung lesions tend to heal without the severe fibrosis which is a common sequel to sarcoidosis.[32] Other important manifestations of sarcoidosis are uveitis and salivary-gland and lacrimal-gland enlargement (when the three occur together it is called *Heerfordt's syndrome*).[33] The central nervous system is occasionally implicated, and diabetes insipidus due to involvement of the posterior pituitary may occur. Despite the benign course of the lesions, sarcoidosis can be a serious condition attended by an appreciable mortality rate.[34]

An occasional feature is hypercalcaemia. This is due to an increased sensitivity to the action of vitamin D, which is absorbed in normal amounts from the bowel. The nature of this sensitivity is unknown. A more constant biochemical finding is hypergammaglobulinaemia.

A noteworthy feature of many cases of sarcoidosis is a depression of cell-mediated immunity. Thus the tuberculin reaction is frequently negative. This fact has been invoked to establish a relationship between sarcoidosis and tuberculosis, but current thinking is critical of this connexion. It is known that sarcoidosis can sometimes be complicated by

tuberculosis, but this is proabably merely a reflection of poor lymphocytic immunity. Indeed, patients with sarcoidosis treated with corticosteroids are liable to severe opportunistic infection, e.g. cryptococcosis.

An interesting diagnostic adjunct is the *Kveim test*,[35] in which an extract of sarcoid tissue (usually obtained from a patient's spleen) produces a very delayed inflammatory reaction composed of sarcoid lesions when injected intradermally into a patient with sarcoidosis. At one time the test was regarded as virtually pathognomonic when positive (it is occasionally negative in longstanding disease), but it has become evident that a considerable number of other diseases can also give a positive result depending on the source of the material used.[36] The classical Chase-Siltzbach suspension is said to be diagnostic of sarcoidosis when positive,[37, 38] but clearly much more work remains to be done on this fascinating, if obscure, test. The test is read by sectioning a biopsy of the lesion 4–6 weeks after injection.

It has been found that if immunologically deficient mice (thymectomised a few weeks after birth and then subjected to whole body radiation) are injected with extracts of sarcoid material in their footpads, they develop disseminated granulomatous lesions resembling sarcoidosis and the Kveim test becomes positive. Material from one mouse may be transmitted to another immunologically deficient one in this way and the lesions are reproduced.[39, 40] This technique is very valuable for infecting mice with organisms that they would not tolerate in a healthy state, and has been used for the cultivation of *Myco. leprae*. It remains to be seen whether a specific infective agent is responsible.

Many different agents can produce local sarcoid tissue reactions. The lymph glands draining cancerous foci occasionally contain follicles indistinguishable from those of sarcoidosis, and a similar appearance is sometimes encountered in the outlying lymph nodes in Hodgkin's disease. Various organs occasionally contain sarcoid follicles in the course of chronic inflammatory conditions. Sometimes tuberculosis, leprosy, leishmaniasis, histoplasmosis, and berylliosis give rise to focal lesions indistinguishable from sarcoidosis.[41] So also may zirconium compounds used in deodorant preparations,[42] and silica implanted in the skin.

It follows that the diagnosis of idiopathic sarcoidosis is a combined histological and clinical one, in which chest radiography plays an important part. It is particularly important to exclude tuberculosis and berylliosis before making a final diagnosis of sarcoidosis. The lesions of sarcoidosis are reversed by glucocorticosteroids. This forms a useful diagnostic test in distinguishing the hypercalcaemia of sarcoidosis from that of hyperparathyroidism, which is quite unresponsive to these drugs.[43]

CROHN'S DISEASE[44]

This chronic granulomatous disease of unknown aetiology usually affects the terminal ileum, but it may also occur elsewhere in the small bowel and in the colon. It has even been described in the mouth, oesophagus, and stomach, and when it involves the colon, anal fistulae are quite common. These may cause extensive skin involvement.[45]

The affected bowel is swollen, its wall thickened, and its lumen considerably stenosed. A characteristic feature is a cobblestone mucosa between which linear ulcers extend into the bowel wall. These form the basis of fistulae between loops of bowel and to the abdominal skin. The mesentery is thickened and the local lymph nodes are enlarged. A feature of the disease is the tendency to affect several areas of the bowel—with normal intervening *skip areas*. There is often

seen in this disease is not found in Crohn's disease. The lymph nodes may also contain tuberculoid granulomata. The mucosa is often fairly normal apart from the intersecting fissures that may be lined by epithelioid cells or polymorphs.

The nature of the disease is obscure. As in sarcoidosis there is often hypergammaglobulinaemia and a tendency to impaired cell-mediated immunity. A transmissable agent has been demonstrated in immunologically deficient mice as in sarcoidosis,[40, 46] and the Kveim test has often been reported positive with certain batches of reagent.[36] But the condition does not resemble sarcoidosis clinically, for it is nearly always confined to the gastro-intestinal tract. Crohn's

Figure 21.5
Resected specimen of the terminal ileum, ileo-caecal junction, caecum, and a small portion of the ascending colon from a man aged 22 years. The terminal ileum shows great thickening and rigidity of its wall and the lumen is reduced in size. The mucosa has a characteristic cobble-stone appearance and the disease stops sharply at the ileo-caecal valve. Microscopically, the affected bowel showed transmural oedema, fibrosis, and the presence of non-caseating tuberculoid granulomata. *(Photograph supplied by Dr. J. B. Cullen).*

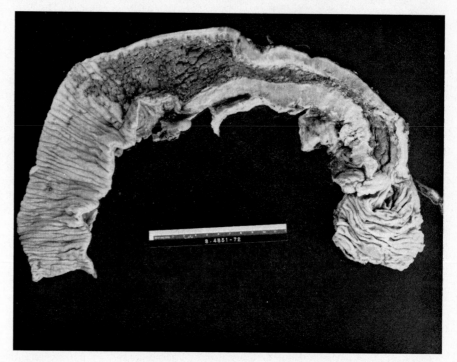

a sharp line of demarcation between diseased and healthy segments (Fig. 21.5).

Histologically there is a chronic inflammatory reaction involving the whole wall, but it is the submucosa that is especially involved. It is widened by oedema and later fibrosis, and there are many plasma cells and lymphocytes infiltrating it. Polymorphs, macrophages, and eosinophils are more scanty. A conspicuous feature in many cases is the development of lymphoid follicles in the submucosa and deeper in the wall. These may assume a tuberculoid character with epithelioid cells and Langhans giant cells, as in sarcoidosis, but the circumscribed arrangement of follicles

disease closely resembles intestinal tuberculosis, and it is important to rule out this infection by repeated faecal cultures. Ileo-caecal disease in the dark-skinned races is more often due to tuberculosis than to Crohn's disease.

When it affects the colon alone it may be difficult to distinguish from ulcerative colitis, but the mucosal lesions of this disease, particularly the crypt abscesses, contrast with the generalised involvement of the wall in Crohn's disease. In addition, there are no fistulae or giant-cell systems in ulcerative colitis. Crohn's disease of the colon is a much less serious carcinogenic hazard than is ulcerative colitis.

REFERENCES

1. Cox, L. B. and Tolhurst, J. C. (1946). *Human Torulosis.* Melbourne University Press.
2. Knudson, R. J., Burch, H. B. and Hatch, H. B. (1963). *Journal of Thoracic and Cardiovascular Surgery,* **45,** 730.
3. Rook, A. and Woods, B. (1962). *British Journal of Dermatology,* **74,** 43.
4. Durie, E. B. and MacDonald, L. (1961). *Journal of Bone and Joint Surgery,* **43B,** 68.

5. SYMMERS, W. StC. (1960). In *Recent Advances in Clinical Pathology*, Series III, p. 304. Edited by S. C. Dyke. London: Churchill.
6. SCHWARZ, J. and BAUM, G. L. (1963). *Archives of Internal Medicine*, **111,** 710.
7. SCHWARZ, J. and BAUM, G. L. (1963). *Archives of Pathology*, **75,** 475.
8. SALIBA, A. and BEATTY, O. A. (1960). *Thorax*, **15,** 204.
9. EARLE, J. H. O., HIGHMAN, J. H. and LOCKEY, E. (1960). *British Medical Journal*, i, 607.
10. FIESE, M. J. (1958). *Coccidioidomycosis*. Springfield, Illinois: Thomas.
11. COLWELL, J. A. and TILLMAN, S. P. (1961). *American Journal of Medicine*, **31,** 676.
12. WINNER, H. I. and HURLEY, R. (1964). *Candida Albicans*, 306 pp. London: Churchill.
13. STIEHM, E. R. *et al.* (1972). *Annals of Internal Medicine*, **77,** 101.
14. HOLT, P. J. L. *et al.* (1972). *British Journal of Clinical Practice*, **26,** 331.
15. Editorial (1972). *New England Journal of Medicine*, **286,** 777.
16. Toxoplasmosis Symposium (1961). *Survey of Ophthalmology*, **6,** 699–972.
17. BEVERLEY, J. K. A. (1960). In *Recent Advances in Clinical Pathology*, Series III, p. 38 *loc. cit.*
18. HUTCHISON, W. M. *et al.* (1970). *British Medical Journal*, i, 142.
19. Leading Article (1970). *British Medical Journal*, i, 126.
20. BURFORD, F. and SUTCLIFF, W. D. (1960). *Archives of Internal Medicine*, **106,** 835.
21. REMINGTON, J. S. *et al.* (1962). *Archives of Internal Medicine*, **110,** 744.
22. STANSFELD, A. G. (1961). *Journal of Clinical Pathology*, **14,** 565.
23. BAAR, H. S. (1955). *Journal of Clinical Pathology*, **8,** 19.
24. ROSEN, F. S. (1972). *British Journal of Clinical Practice*, **26,** 315.
25. SYMMERS, W. StC. (1960). *Journal of Clinical Pathology*, **13,** 1.
26. HARRISON, C. V. (1960). In *Recent Advances in Pathology*, 7th edn, p. 36. Edited by C. V. Harrison. London: Churchill.
27. NAJI, A. F., CARBONELL, F. and BARKER, H. J. (1962). *American Journal of Clinical Pathology*, **38,** 513.
28. SNYDER, J. N. (1962). *Journal of the American Medical Association*, **180,** 780.
29. KNAPP, W. (1958). *New England Journal of Medicine*, **259,** 776.
30. SCADDING, J. G. (1967). *Sarcoidosis*, 542 pp. London: Eyre and Spottiswoode.
31. MAYOCK, R. L. *et al.* (1963). *American Journal of Medicine*, **35,** 67.
32. Annotation (1967). *Lancet*, i, 373.
33. Leading Article (1967). *British Medical Journal*, ii, 459.
34. SONES, M. and ISRAEL, H. L. (1960). *American Journal of Medicine*, **29,** 84.
35. MITCHELL, D. N. (1968). In *Recent Advances in Clinical Pathology*, Series Five, p. 431. Edited by S. C. Dyke. London: Churchill.
36. Leading Article (1971). *Lancet*, ii, 750.
37. SILTZBACH, L. E. *et al.* (1971). *Lancet*, ii, 634.
38. Leading Article (1972). *Lancet*, i, 188.
39. MITCHELL, D. N. and REES, R. J. W. (1969). *Lancet*, ii, 81.
40. MITCHELL, D. N. and REES, R. J. W. (1971). *Proceedings of the Royal Society of Medicine*, **64,** 944.
41. JONES WILLIAMS, W. (1971). *Proceedings of the Royal Society of Medicine*, **64,** 946.
42. EPSTEIN, W. L. and ALLEN, J. R. (1964). *Journal of the American Medical Association*, **190,** 940.
43. ANDERSON, J. *et al.* (1954). *Lancet*, ii, 720.
44. Various Authors (1971). *Proceedings of the Royal Society of Medicine*, **64,** 157.
45. Leading Article (1972). *British Medical Journal*, iii, 658.
46. MITCHELL, D. N. and REES, R. J. W. (1970). *Lancet*, ii, 168.

Chapter 22. Virus Disease

I. THE PRINCIPLES OF VIROLOGY

INTRODUCTION

The properties of viruses are best understood when they are compared with those of other organisms.

Bacteria are generally unicellular, but even the smallest is within the range of the light microscope (which resolves up to about 0·2 μm in diameter). They grow with variable ease on artificial, cell-free media, though in this respect *Myco. leprae* and *Tr. pallidum* are exceptions, and have as yet not been cultured artificially. The baterial cell contains DNA in its nuclear body and RNA in its cytoplasm (see Appendix II).

Rickettsial organisms.[1] The order *Rickettsiales* comprises genera occupying an intermediate position between the smallest bacteria and the viruses. Their main features are a small size (250–500 nm in diameter), visibility under light microscopy using Macchiavello's stain,* a rigid cell wall containing muramic acid, the presence of DNA and RNA in the protoplasm, division by binary fission, sensitivity to antibiotics (notably tetracyclines), and nearly always an inability to grow on cell-free media. They are cultured in animals, the yolk-sac of fertile eggs, and in tissue-culture systems. The most important genera are:

Rickettsiae. These cause the typhus fevers, transmitted by the arthropods lice, fleas, ticks, and mites (*R. prowazeki* causes epidemic louse-borne typhus). This group shares a heterophile antigen with a strain of *Proteus* organism (see Weil-Felix reaction, p. 170).

Coxiella. The causative agent of Q (query) fever is *Coxiella burneti*, a somewhat smaller organism than the *Rickettsiae*, and very resistant to environmental adversity and disinfectants. It is transmitted by the inhalation and ingestion of infected tick and cattle excreta, e.g. in milk. Q fever gives a negative Weil-Felix reaction.[2] There are pulmonary manifestations but no skin eruption.

Bartonella. The important species is *Bartonella bacilliformis*, which parasitises red cells and tissue cells, causing the severe Oroya fever of the Andean area of South America with its haemolytic anaemia, and the benign cutaneous variant verruga peruana. This organism is distinctive in being able to grow on cell-free media, although it shows a marked tendency to multiply within host's cells in nature.

---

* In this method a smear is stained with basic fuchsin, decolorised by citric acid, and counterstained with methylene blue. Rickettsiae are stained red and the cells blue.

Chlamydia (*Bedsonia*). These cause psittacosis, lymphogranuloma venereum, and trachoma. They are the smallest of the organisms mentioned above (250–300 nm in diameter), but share their general properties. Psittacosis, a type of pneumonia, is responsive to tetracyclines, and lymphogranuloma venereum and trachoma to sulphonamides as well as tetracyclines. Basophilic inclusion bodies are found in the cytoplasm of infected cells.

An agent closely related to that of trachoma causes inclusion conjunctivitis (blenorrhoea), which is severe but does not produce a pannus or lead to scarring, as in trachoma. The trachoma-inclusion conjunctivitis agents are together called the *TRIC agents*. Inclusion conjunctivitis agent also causes a venereal urethritis and cervicitis, and eye infections may be contracted in swimming-baths following the contamination of the water with infected discharges.

Mycoplasmas[3] (pleuropneumonia-like organisms, or PPLO). This is a remarkable group of bacteria completely lacking a rigid cell wall and enclosed by a thin cytoplasmic membrane only. The result is extreme fragility and pleomorphism. Their size ranges from about 0·1 μm to over 1 μm, and the smallest granules, which pass through bacterial filters easily, are called elementary corpuscles. The shapes include coccoid forms, clubs, rings, and long fine filaments. They are Gram-negative, but are stained best with Giemsa's stain. They can be grown on cell-free media, the colonies being very small and having a "fried-egg" appearance. Many mycoplasmas also thrive in tissue culture systems. Like bacteria and rickettsiae they contain both RNA and DNA. Their mode of reproduction is unique: the granules become round and then filamentous, after which segmentation takes place and the fragments condense to form new granules.

The important human pathogen is *Mycoplasma pneumoniae*,[4] also known as the *Eaton agent*[5, 6] after the worker who first isolated it in the bronchial mucosal cells of chick embryos following the inoculation of infective material into fertile eggs. At that time it was classified as a virus, and the disease it caused was erroneously called virus pneumonia. Mycoplasmal pneumonia[7] presents clinically as a pyrexial disease in which the radiological signs in the chest are out of all proportion to the pulmonary symptoms. Patients usually have a high titre of cold autohaemagglutinins (directed against the I antigen widely present in adult red cells) and agglutinins against streptococcus MG in their serum. The mycoplasma presumably shares an antigen with this non-haemolytic and non-pathogenic streptococcus. The Coombs test and the serological reactions for syphilis may also be positive. These, like the cold haemagglutins, are auto-immune phenomena following tissue damage by the myco-plasma. The infection responds well to tetracyclines.

Other strains of mycoplasma are found in the mouth and genital tract,[43] and have been implicated in cases of non-specific urethritis. Likewise Reiter's syndrome and the Stevens-Johnson syndrome have on occasion been associated with strains of *M. pneumoniae*, but the aetiological connexion is not proven. Mycoplasmas have been isolated from neo-plastic tissue, but are probably secondary invaders.[8] Some observers believe that there is a relationship between mycoplasmas and rheumatoid arthritis, because they are sometimes found in affected joints.[9]

Viruses.[10] These are smaller than rickettsiae, but some of them are larger than the mycoplasmal organisms; size, there-fore, is not an absolute criterion in defining a virus. Like rickettsiae they are obligatory intracellular parasites. The one feature common to all viruses is a conversion to a non-infec-tive form during the process of multiplication; this non-infective "eclipse phase" is the essential difference between viruses and rickettsiae. Viruses do not possess all the enzyme systems necessary for the synthesis of new viral material; they are therefore dependent on the parasitised cell for survival and multiplication. Indeed, the essential differ-ence between viruses and other organisms is that the syn-thetic processes that attend multiplication take place within the protoplasm of the infected cell in viruses, but in the body of the organism itself in all other infective agents.

PROPERTIES OF TRUE VIRUSES

Size and Shape

Amongst the largest of the true viruses are the pox group responsible for smallpox, vaccinia, and similar diseases in other species of animals. These are about 250 nm in size, and a single virus particle, or elementary body (called a *Paschen body* in vaccinia), is just visible under the light microscope using special staining techniques, e.g. Gutstein's method.*

The remainder cannot be seen by light microscopy, and therefore other methods of measurement are used.

(*a*) Their size can be assessed by their capacity to pass through specially graded filters. This is rather inaccurate.

(*b*) A more precise method is ultracentrifugation using high-speed centrifuges. The larger the particle, the faster it falls.

(*c*) The most accurate method at present available, how-ever, is direct observation under the electron microscope, which is capable of demonstrating objects as small as 0·5 nm

---

* This method is admirable for staining Paschen bodies in skin scrapings. The smear is fixed in methyl alcohol and stained with a mixture of methyl violet and sodium carbonate. The Paschen bodies are stained purple.

in diameter. Electron microscopy has imparted fundamental information about virus size, shape, and chemical con-figuration. Most viruses are less than 200 nm in size: varicella virus is 150–120 nm, mumps virus 120–80 nm, adenovirus 90–70 nm, bacteriophage 100–50 nm, entero-viruses about 30 nm, and one of the smallest, that of foot-and-mouth disease, only 20 nm.

Many viruses are spherical in shape, e.g. enteroviruses, herpesviruses, and adenoviruses. Some are filamentous, e.g tobacco-mosaic virus and myxoviruses. Bacteriophage has a characteristic tadpole shape (Fig. 22.1) and poxviruses are brick-shaped.

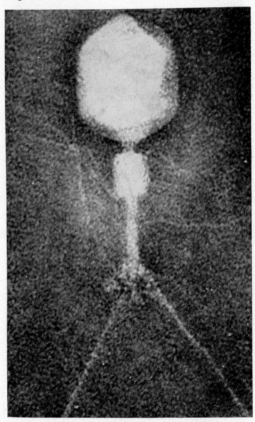

Figure 22.1
The bacteriophage particle viewed under the electron microscope after negative staining. The following structures are visible:

The head, a bipyramidal hexagonal prism. This contains the viral DNA.

A central rigid core.

The tail sheath which surrounds the central core. In this picture the sheath is contracted to the upper part of the core. The sheath has a helical symmetry. It is attached to a hexagonal plate structure at the extreme end of the tail—in this picture it is diffuse and unrecognisable.

Tail fibres (6 altogether) associated with the plate structure.

It is suggested that the plate and fibres may be a means of attach-ment to the host. The components of bacteriophage have been compared to a microsyringe system serving to inject the viral DNA into the host bacterium. × 300 000. *(From Brenner, S., et al. (1959), J. molec. Biol., **1**, 281)*

Chemical Constitution

A single virus particle, alternatively called a *virion* or an *elementary body*, consists basically of a core of a single nucleic acid and a surrounding protein shell called a *capsid*.

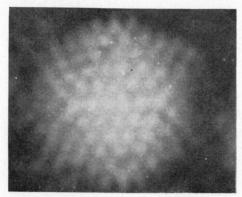

Figure 22.2
A single particle (elementary body) of adenovirus embedded in electron-opaque phosphotungstate. The negatively-stained particle viewed under the electron microscope is seen to be composed of morphological units (capsomeres) of spherical shape packed in a symmetrical arrangement. It has been calculated that the total number of capsomeres around the central core of an adenovirus is 252. ×480 000. *(From Horne, R. W., Brenner, S., Waterson, A. P. and Wildy, P. (1959), J. molec. Biol., 1, 84)*

Plant viruses all contain RNA, whereas nearly all bacteriophages contain DNA. Of animal viruses the adenoviruses, poxviruses, herpesviruses, and papovaviruses contain DNA, whereas the myxoviruses, picornaviruses, arboviruses, reoviruses, rhabdoviruses, and arenoviruses contain RNA. It is

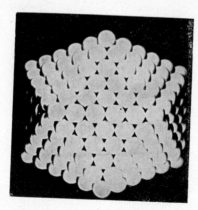

Figure 22.3
A model of the icosahedron formed by the capsomeres of an adenovirus using 252 table-tennis balls. When viewed along an axis through the vertices of the faces, the solid has five-fold rotational symmetry; along an axis through the centre of a face, three-fold symmetry; along an axis through the middle of an edge, two-fold symmetry. The icosahedron shows the highest form of cubic symmetry, described as 532 symmetry. *(From Horne, R. W., Brenner, S., Waterson, A. P. and Wildy P. (1959), J. molec. Biol., 1, 84)*

this nucleic acid that controls the synthesis of new viral material in an infected cell.

The capsid is composed of a specific number of identical subunits called *capsomeres*, which are built up regularly to form a compact mass. Spherical viruses have their capsomeres arranged in the form of a regular solid with twenty equilateral triangular faces. This is called an *icosahedron*, and the symmetry is described as being *cubical*. Rod-shaped filamentous viruses have their core of nucleic acid in the form of a spiral, and this is invested by a capsid composed of wedge-shaped capsomeres. This is called *helical* symmetry. The tadpole-shaped bacteriophage has a *binal* symmetry in its capsid, meaning that it is arranged differently around the head as compared with the tail (see Fig. 22.1).

Some viruses are also ensheathed in one or more outer membranes, or envelopes, composed predominantly of lipid, derived in part from the host cell membrane prior to the release of the virus. Enveloped viruses, e.g. herpesviruses, myxoviruses, and arboviruses, are vulnerable to fat solvents such as ether and bile salts. The larger viruses, especially poxviruses, also contain carbohydrates, coenzymes, and even some enzymes, e.g. lipase, catalase, and phosphatase, but none contains all the enzymes necessary for the metabolism of its own substance. It is for this reason that viruses are obligatory intracellular parasites.

The Life-Cycle and Reproduction

The knowledge about the life-cycle of a virus in a cell is still far from complete, and most of it has been gained from research into individual viruses, notably bacteriophage, vaccinia, and poliovirus.

Attachment.[11] The first step is the attachment of the virus to a specific *cell receptor*, or *receptor site*, on the cell membrane. This appears to be a necessary precursor of penetration and is related to the absorption of complementary areas of the virus coat on to the cell receptors. Influenza virus attaches to the cell membrane by the action of neuraminidase which combines with mucopolysaccharide on the cell surface. Bacteriophage (Fig. 22.1) attaches by its tail fibres to specific receptor sites on the bacterial wall, which are weakened by a hydrolytic enzyme present in the phage tail.

Penetration.[11] With bacteriophage the naked DNA is injected into the interior of the bacterium, while the protein coat, which acts as a microsyringe, remains exterior attached to the bacterial wall. The mode of penetration of animal viruses is probably different, and both pinocytosis and phagocytosis are involved. With vaccinia virus in tissue cultures, the next step is removal of the protein coat and release of the nucleic acid.

Eclipse phase.[12] Once the nucleic acid has been released it becomes unidentifiable for a few hours. This is the all-important *eclipse phase* characteristic of viruses, and the nucleic acid is not infectious during this period.

It appears that the free nucleic acid is engaged in redirecting the cell's metabolism so that more viral nucleic acid and protein are produced. The eclipse phase takes from one to thirty hours. In DNA-containing viruses the DNA directs the formation of mRNA as well as virus specific enzymes which take part in the formation of new virus material. With RNA-containing viruses the single-stranded RNA appears to act as mRNA.[13] In some instances it directs the formation of DNA (p. 385). It is remarkable that a minute quantity of foreign nucleic acid can so dominate the cellular metabolism that, instead of forming normal cell substance, the cell is perverted into forming large amounts of the virus. This mode of reproduction (or replication) contrasts strongly with the binary fission of higher organisms.

Maturation and replication of the virus.[12] Much remains to be known about the formation of the virion. In

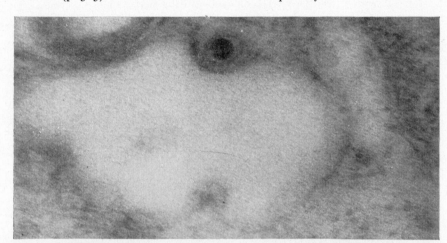
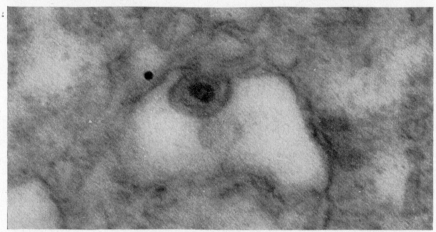
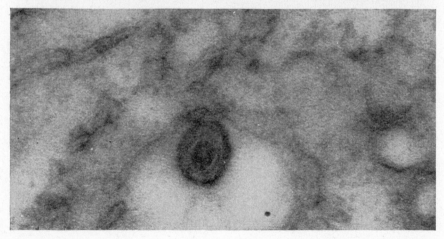

Figure 22.4
Small areas of cytoplasm from HeLa cells infected with herpesvirus. Immature particles can be seen in various stages of budding out through cytoplasmic membranes, from which they acquire in the process an outer covering, and thus the morphology of the free virus. × 120 000. *(From Epstein, M. A. (1962), J. Cell Biol.,* **12**, 589)

some viruses the components are formed in the nucleus, in others in the cytoplasm, and in yet others in both cytoplasm and nucleus. When the components are assembled into mature infective virus, they are soon recognisable as elementary bodies and escape from the cell either in a dramatic burst—as with poliovirus—or in a steady release from the cell surface—as with herpesviruses and myxoviruses—or else very tardily after accumulating in the cell, as with adenoviruses. The myxoviruses and herpesviruses incorporate lipid from the cell membrane into their outer envelopes during the period of release, which takes about an hour (see Fig. 22.4). The virus then enters other cells either by direct contact or after carriage by the body fluids.

Some viruses produce globular intracellular masses which are easily visible under the light microscope. These are called *inclusion bodies*. Some, like the intranuclear inclusions of herpesviruses, are formed as a result of cell degeneration. A few, like the inclusions of adenoviruses and reoviruses, are crystalline aggregates of virions. Most are composed of aggregations of developing virus particles bound together in a gelatinous matrix (Fig. 22.5). Unlike *elementary bodies*, which are single mature virus particles, inclusion bodies are large (up to 20 μm in size). Some are acidophilic and others basophilic; some intracytoplasmic and others intranuclear. At one time they were of great moment in the diagnosis of virus disease; nowadays they are mostly of historical interest. Nevertheless, a few are worth noting:

(*a*) *Negri body*, an acidophilic body found in the cyto-

Figure 22.5
Nuclear inclusion induced by adenovirus 12. The virus crystals in the centre are surrounded by very dense material with irregular contours. Many virus particles are dispersed in the nucleoplasm. × 24 000. *(From Bernhard, W. (1964), In "Cellular Injury", a Ciba Foundation Symposium, p. 215. Edrs de Reuck, A. V. S. and Knight, J. London : Churchill)*

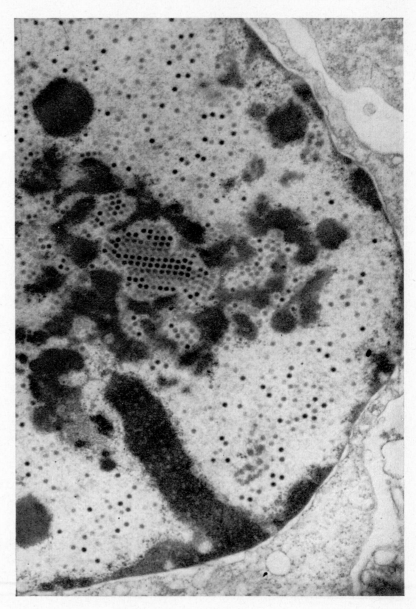

plasm of neurones in cases of rabies. The hippocampus is particularly involved.

(*b*) *Guarnieri body*, an acidophilic body seen in the cytoplasm of epidermal cells in vaccinia and smallpox.

(*c*) The enormous intranuclear body seen in various parenchymatous cells in *cytomegalic inclusion disease* (Fig. 22.6). Smaller ones are found in the cytoplasm.

(*d*) The intranuclear bodies found in the epidermal cells in *zoster* and *herpes simplex*, the respiratory mucosal cells in

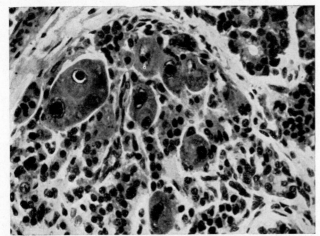

Figure 22.6
Cytomegalic inclusion disease. This is a section of the pancreas of an infant who died of this condition. The acinar cells are enormously swollen, and their enlarged nuclei are distended with darkly-staining inclusion bodies, while the remainder of the nuclear chromatin is pushed out to the nuclear membrane. Surrounding these cells there is an inflammatory exudate. × 330.

adenovirus infections, and the anterior-horn-cell neurones in the later stages of *poliomyelitis*.

The nucleic-acid composition of the virus does not determine whether the inclusion body is intranuclear or intracytoplasmic.

Reaction to Environment

Unlike bacteria, most viruses are easily inactivated even at room temperature, and care must be taken to keep specimens frozen, if possible at −70°C. A few viruses are much more stable than this, however, and the viruses of poliomyelitis and vaccinia can survive at ordinary atmospheric temperatures for some weeks. The agents of hepatitis are very resistant to heat (see p. 289), but the most resistant agent is that of scrapie which withstands boiling for three hours.

Reaction to Chemicals

Viruses are rapidly destroyed by disinfectants used against bacteria; the scrapie agent is an exception, surviving in strong formalin solutions. It is noteworthy that viruses are resistant to a 50 per cent solution of glycerol—vaccinia virus is preserved in it—while non-sporing bacteria are killed quite

rapidly. Antibiotics and sulphonamides are powerless against viruses, but some chemotherapeutic agents are now known (p. 280).

Inactivation of Viruses[14]

The question of virus destruction is, in fact, less simple than would appear at first sight. If activity is defined as the ability of a single virus particle to multiply in and produce lesions in a cell, there is no doubt that inactivation is quite easily achieved. But inactivated virus can undergo reactivation under certain circumstances. A bacteriophage inactivated by ultraviolet light and then introduced into a bacterium can sometimes be reactivated if the bacterium is exposed to visible light. Again, ultraviolet-light inactivated bacteriophage, myxoviruses, and poxviruses can sometimes achieve activation if a large dose is introduced into a cell system. This is called *multiplicity reactivation*. The explanation is that the nucleic acid which carries the genetic information of the virus is damaged by ultraviolet light, so that the *genome* (complete set of hereditary factors) is disrupted. If a large number of ultraviolet-light inactivated viruses are in close contact, a common pool of nucleic acids is produced. As these are likely to show different disturbances of their genomes, it is possible for two nucleic acids to mate and constitute an uninjured genome by complementing each other's deficiencies. Another genetic type of reactivation is *cross-reactivation*, in which an inactivated particle is rendered active by a closely related active virus. The explanation is as described above. It is an example of *recombination* (a phenomenon also described in bacteria and important in the transference of drug resistance).

A non-genetic type of reactivation is seen in the case of heat-inactivated myxoma virus injected into a rabbit with active fibroma virus (both are poxviruses). The animal dies of myxomatosis, and does not develop a fibroma (*Berry-Dedrick phenomenon*).[15] The essential transfer factor is a protein.

Cultivation of Viruses

As viruses multiply only in susceptible living cells, the provision of suitable systems is of great importance. At first the only living systems that could be used were experimental animals and chick embryos. The discovery by Enders and his colleagues in 1949[16] that the virus of poliomyelitis could proliferate in tissue cultures of non-neuronal origin, e.g. human prepuce, made modern virus research possible. Nowadays the vast majority of viruses are cultivated in tissue culture, a method which is cheap, simple, and efficacious.

(*a*) At present *animal inoculation* is reserved for those viruses which do not grow satisfactorily in tissue culture. Most Coxsackie A viruses do not grow in any cell systems, but when injected into suckling mice produce a characteristic fatal myositis. There is still a place for the use of suckling mice in isolating arboviruses. An intracerebral injection of material from a rabid animal into adult mice produces a characteristic encephalitis. Animal isolation is slow, expensive, and useful for only a limited number of viruses.

(*b*) The *chick embryo* has been a very useful medium for virus cultivation. Many myxoviruses can be cultured in the amniotic cells, while the poxviruses and herpes-simplex virus produce characteristic lesions on the chorioallantoic membrane. The fertile egg is used comparatively infrequently in virology nowadays.

(*c*) The method of choice is *tissue culture*. In this technique living cells are grown on the sides of test-tubes (see p. 8). Many viruses are able to multiply in the cells, in which they produce destructive changes (*cytopathic effects*). These are sometimes characteristic of a certain virus, but in any case the virus must be accurately identified by complement fixation and neutralisation tests using specific rabbit antisera. If, for instance, a specific antiserum prevents a cytopathic effect in a cell system (or for that matter, if it prevents a lesion in an egg or a test animal), the virus is typed accordingly. The fluid in the tissue culture system provides the virus material, which is also used as the source of antigen for complement fixation tests. The cell systems commonly employed in this way are derived from monkey kidney, human amnion, and strains of cancer cells, e.g. the "HeLa cell" derived from a carcinoma of the cervix[17] of a woman named *He*len *La*ne. Among the many viruses that can grow

in such systems are the enteroviruses, adenoviruses, herpesviruses, and poxviruses (Figs. 22.7–22.9).

Organ culture can be used to cultivate some viruses that do not flourish in cell systems. Thus some rhinoviruses have been isolated in organ cultures of adult and fetal trachea.[18]

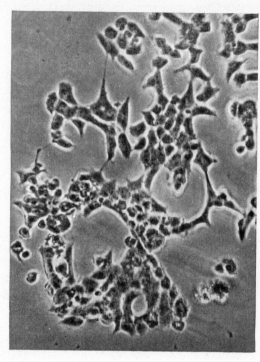

Figure 22.8
HeLa cells infected with adenovirus. The sheet is broken up, and the swollen, refractile cells have fused to form irregular masses. (McCarthy phase contrast × 200)

Some viruses produce damage to the epithelium which can be determined histologically after the culture is fixed. The respiratory syncytial virus and some para-influenza viruses grow in the tracheal cells and cause the cilia to cease moving.[18]

Infectivity

Viruses produce disease even in minute quantities, and their degree of infectivity is so high that epidemics are very common, e.g. smallpox, influenza, and the common virus diseases of childhood.

Virus disease is by no means confined to vertebrates; there are insect infections like silkworm jaundice and sacbrood of bees, plant diseases like tobacco-mosaic disease, and also the very important group of bacterial infections due to bacteriophage. Sometimes a virus disease of an animal may be transmitted to man. A harmful transmission is rabies from a dog, while a beneficial one is cow-pox as in the classical Jennerian vaccination technique.

Of the viruses pathogenic to man many seem to attack one

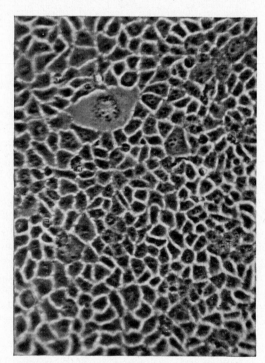

Figure 22.7
Normal HeLa cells. The confluent sheet is composed of plump, polygonal cells derived from a malignant epithelial cell line. A giant form is conspicuous in this field. (McCarthy phase contrast × 200)

organ specifically, but the once fashionable concept of *tropism* is no longer adequate. A "neutrotropic" virus like poliovirus multiples in the cells of the small intestine, while the "dermatotropic" virus of herpes simplex can produce

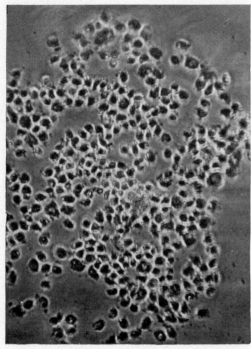

Figure 22.9
HeLa cells infected with poliovirus. The cells have undergone profound disintegration, so that only a few shrunken survivors are still present. The polioviruses have a much more destructive effect on cell cultures than the adenoviruses. (McCarthy phase contrast ×200)

encephalitis. It is helpful to enumerate the main viruses pathogenic to man in terms of the organ principally attacked:

Viruses attacking the skin: vaccinia, herpes-simplex, varicella-zoster, and the viruses of verruca vulgaris and molluscum contagiosum.

Viruses attacking the central nervous system: enteroviruses, varicella-zoster, rabies, lymphocytic choriomeningitis, arboviruses causing encephalitis, mumps, and occasionally herpes simplex, measles, influenza, and vaccinia.

Viruses attacking the liver: hepatitis and yellow fever.

Viruses attacking the respiratory tract: myxoviruses, reoviruses, adenoviruses, and common cold viruses (rhinoviruses).

Viruses attacking the conjunctiva: herpesviruses and adenoviruses.

Viruses attacking the salivary glands and other secreting organs: mumps virus and cytomegalovirus.

Generalised virus diseases often producing characteristic skin eruptions: smallpox, measles, rubella, chickenpox, dengue, and some enterovirus infections.

TISSUE REACTIONS TO VIRUSES

The effects of viruses on the tissues of the body all start at a cellular level; viruses are intracellular parasites, and the damage they produce is directed primarily at the cell. This is followed secondarily by a local inflammatory reaction.

Cellular reaction. A cell infected with a virus may necrose at once, or it may undergo proliferation which may or may not be followed by later necrosis, or it may show no change whatsoever.

This last effect is typical of *latent virus* infection.[19] It is well known, for example, that the epithelium of the lips and face may harbour herpes-simplex virus without showing any lesion. A febrile incident, e.g. a cold, precipitates an attack of herpes febrilis. It clears up, and recurs when the precipitating factor operates again. Similarly, many children are infected with certain types of adenoviruses early in life. These remain in their tonsils and adenoids without producing conspicuous lesions, but if such organs are grown in tissue culture, the emerging cells rapidly disintegrate because the virus released is now active and destructive.

Whether a cell necrosis or proliferates depends on the type of cell involved and on the nature of the infecting virus. Labile cells like those of the epidermis undergo continuous division throughout life, and if infected with virus may exhibit a proliferative tendency, e.g. verruca vulgaris. On the other hand, the foot-and-mouth disease virus causes rapid necrosis of the epidermal cells. Other cells described as permanent, e.g. neurones, cannot divide after birth, and virus infection of these is necessarily always destructive in tendency.

Taking a tissue in which the gamut of changes from immediate necrosis to indefinite proliferation is possible, Wright has considered five virus infections of the skin:[20]

Foot-and-mouth disease causes a rapid swelling and necrosis of epidermal cells.

Vaccinia causes an early proliferation of the cells with necrosis following about 3 days later.

Fowl-pox causes a much more prolonged proliferation with necrosis supervening some weeks later.

Verruca vulgaris produces a marked proliferation which may last many months before involution occurs.

The Shope papilloma of wild cottontail rabbits is manifested by a neoplastic proliferation of cells, and squamous-cell carcinoma may occur.

This is an extremely instructive list, but most of the diseases mentioned are not relevant to man. In fact, human virus disease is generally destructive to cells, and only a few skin conditions, e.g. verruca vulgaris and molluscum contagiosum, are attended by proliferation of any extent or persistence. There is as yet no human neoplasm directly attributable to viruses, a very important difference between human and animal virus disease.

A few other skin infections exhibit early proliferation followed by rapid necrosis, e.g. vaccinia, smallpox, zoster, chickenpox, and herpes–simplex infections, but on the whole virus disease of other tissues is always primarily necrotising. The respiratory viruses destroy the surface epithelium, a tendency well marked in influenza; the viruses of hepatitis and yellow fever produce necrosis of the liver; mumps and cytomegalic inclusion disease lead to destructive lesions of the acinar cells of the salivary glands and sometimes the pancreas, while the central nervous system may sustain permanent neuronal loss as a result of poliomyelitis and virus encephalitis.

Once the infection is overcome there is rapid regeneration due to proliferation of neighbouring cells. The focal necrosis of infective hepatitis heals so rapidly that needle biopsy of the liver performed after a few months may reveal no abnormality whatsoever. Neuronal destruction can be healed only by gliosis, and hence permanent paralysis, or sensory loss in zoster, must sometimes be expected. However, not every neurone infected with poliovirus is doomed. Many recover completely after undergoing the degenerative change of chromatolysis (disappearance of Nissl granules from the cytoplasm).

Inflammatory reaction. Secondary to the cellular damage (and sometimes to allergy) there is an acute inflammatory reaction in the vicinity. This consists of vascular dilatation and an exudate containing moderate numbers of lymphocytes and macrophages. Polymorphs are scanty except in superficial skin lesions like smallpox and herpes simplex, where they are present even before secondary bacterial infection complicates the picture.

Virus disease of the central nervous system, typified by poliomyelitis, is accompanied by an active phagocytosis of neuronal debris by macrophages, some of which are mobilised microglial cells. This is called "neuronophagia". In the vicinity the blood vessels are dilated, and there is a heavy small round cell infiltration. This also accumulates around small blood vessels, especially those under the meninges, and is called "perivascular cuffing"; it is by no means pathognomonic of virus infection, occurring also in cerebral syphilis and tuberculous meningitis. Most of these cells are lymphocytes and macrophages, but sometimes a few polymorphs are also present.

Similarly the focal necrosis of viral hepatitis is accompanied by a moderate small round cell infiltration, not so much in the area of damage as in the portal tracts.

One of the few virus diseases that produces a diagnostic lesion is measles. There is generalised lymphoid hyperplasia, most marked in the tonsils and appendix. In the midst of the active germinal centres there are characteristic giant cells with bunched-up, hyperchromatic nuclei. These are called *Warthin-Finkeldey giant cells*, and are pathognomonic of measles (Fig. 22.10).[21, 22]

Virus infection of epithelial surfaces is usually complicated by secondary bacterial infection, and this is accompanied by a pyogenic reaction.

It is noteworthy that most virus disease is acute; it either

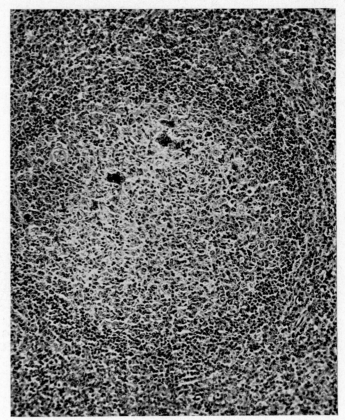

Figure 20.10
Lymphoid hyperplasia in measles. The germinal centre is enlarged, and amid the palely-staining lymphoblasts there are several giant cells with crowded, darkly-staining nuclei. These hyperchromatic Warthin-Finkeldey giant cells are typical of measles. × 150.

kills rapidly or else is followed by recovery. Exceptions are those animal tumours due to viruses and also molluscum contagiosum and verruca vulgaris. The neurological conditions caused by slow viruses would be another exception if these agents are indeed true viruses.

THE GENERAL BODY REACTION TO VIRUS INFECTION

Localisation.[23] Like all foreign organisms viruses first contaminate and infect a surface integument, either by inoculation (e.g. vaccinia), or by ingestion (e.g. poliomyelitis), or by inhalation (e.g. influenza), or by the bite of an arthropod vector (e.g. yellow fever). Some viruses remain localised to their tissues of entry, e.g. that of verruca vulgaris and rhinoviruses, while others become disseminated throughout the blood stream and produce lesions in an organ remote from the sites of primary infection, e.g. poliomyelitis and yellow fever, or else lead to a generalised infection involving many organs, e.g. smallpox and measles.

The systemic type of infection is associated with much more pronounced constitutional symptoms than is the localised one, and a characteristic feature is the presence of high fever during the early viraemic phase followed by a remission, which is then succeeded by another spurt of pyrexia when the virus becomes clinically localised at its organ of destination. Localised diseases like upper respiratory tract and eye infections cause little constitutional upset. Systemic virus infection is associated with leucopenia during the prodromal period. Once the typical lesion appears (e.g. the eruption in smallpox or jaundice in infective hepatitis) the white-cell count returns to normal, and there may be a moderate neutrophil leucocytosis.

Dissemination. The mode of dissemination of a virus in the body has been investigated in mouse-pox.[24] This virus enters the mouse's body through an abrasion on its skin, and multiplies there. Within 8 hours the virus reaches the local lymph nodes, from where after further multiplication it invades the blood stream* and is taken up by the RE cells of the liver and spleen. There it multiples once more, invades the blood stream in large amounts, and settles selectively in the epidermal cells of the skin. This process takes about 6 days; still another 4 days elapse before the skin eruption appears. Before this, however, inclusion bodies can be demonstrated in these cells.

The 6 days prior to final skin localisation constitute the *incubation period*, and the 4 days of severe illness, which may prove fatal in overwhelming infections, are the *prodromal period*. During this time virus material may still be cultured from the blood, but once the eruption appears there is a rapidly rising level of neutralising antibody in the circulation. Human diseases like smallpox and measles probably have a somewhat similar pattern of dissemination, but the route of infection is apparently through the respiratory tract.

Transplacental infection[23] of the fetus is important in rubella infections and in addition may lead to congenital abnormalities (p. 292). Other generalised virus diseases in the mother do not appear to be teratogenic, but it may be that they kill the fetus, and the subsequent abortion is dismissed as "inevitable". Other virus diseases that may be transmitted across the placenta are cytomegalic inclusion disease, Coxsackie myocarditis of the newborn, herpes infection, and vaccinia. In mice the lymphocytic choriomeningitis virus is likewise transmitted transplacentally.

Antibody response. Virus infections are accompanied by a high titre of immunoglobulins during the period of convalescence. The highest antibody response is encountered in those viruses which are widely disseminated in the circulation, and a life-long *immunity* may be expected after poliomyelitis, smallpox, measles, and mumps. Localised infections, like the common cold, herpes simplex, and verruca vulgaris, also induce antibodies, but probably because the

* This stage corresponds to the primary bacteraemia of typhoid fever. The next stage of blood-borne spread corresponds to septicaemia.

virus does not enter the blood stream in large amounts, the degree of immunity is small and recurrence is common. Some viruses, e.g. adenoviruses and rhinoviruses, have many serotypes, and these are responsible for the tendency to recurrent upper respiratory-tract infections.

Allergy is also noteworthy in virus infections. The accelerated reaction following a second vaccination is a good example. The lesion appears within a day or two and resolves after about a week, while a primary vaccination reaction appears only on the fourth or fifth day and reaches its zenith on about the tenth day. It takes about 3 weeks to heal, and is occasionally complicated by systemic lesions. The close resemblance of this to the Koch phenomenon is obvious, except that here the immunity is much greater than in tuberculosis. There is a strong allergic element in the exanthem that occurs in the course of generalised infections like smallpox and measles. In these there is an incubation period of about a fortnight, and it seems likely that the skin is sensitised to viral products before the virus reaches it in full force. The analogy to the later intestinal ulceration of typhoid fever is very close.

There are certain occasions when antiviral antibody appears to augment the damage inflicted by a virus.[25] Thus lymphocytic choriomeningitis virus produces a very severe disease in normal adult mice: many die, but the survivors have a permanent immunity to the virus. On the other hand, neonatal or fetal mice, or adults who have been given X-irradiation or glucocorticosteroids, or have been subjected to neonatal thymectomy, when similarly infected get a symptomless condition and may indeed develop tolerance. Thus delayed hypersensitivity has been invoked as the major cause of the effects of this virus. In postvaccinal encephalomyelitis the immune response also appears to be involved, since the condition occurs late in the course of the vaccination reaction. Another important example is with respiratory syncytial virus infection; the presence of IgG antibody augments the damage caused by the virus to the lower respiratory tract. Specific immunoglobulins may be detrimental in another way: viral antigen acting in excess with antibody can be the cause of some immune-complex reactions (p. 182).

The pathogenic effects of viruses.[26] Viruses produce their harmful effects by virtue of the cell destruction they cause; no factors comparable with bacterial toxins have been demonstrated. The cytotoxic effect of viruses is due in part to complex biochemical disturbances that accompany virus replication. The cause of death in acute virus disease is obvious enough when vital organs are damaged, e.g. the liver in hepatitis, and the central nervous system in polimyelitis and encephalitis. In the pox diseases the mode of death is less easily explained. Clinically there is "shock" reminiscent of the toxaemia of invasive bacterial infections, and it is suggested that this is due to virus invasion and damage of vascular endothelial cells.

It is becoming obvious that viruses may produce damage

by immunological means, as noted above. Furthermore, chronic virus diseases are now recognised as not uncommon, and their effects are wide ranging. Immune-complex reactions, recrudescent infection as in measles and varicella-zoster, and the slow-virus infections are examples, and their existence points to the range of virus disease expanding to include many more examples—perhaps multiple sclerosis and malignant disease.[44]

IMMUNITY TO VIRUS INFECTIONS[27]

The mechanism of immunity to virus infection is complex and has several components.

(a) **Immunoglobulins** play an important part. Viruses have a number of antigens, some associated with the nucleo-protein and others with the capsid and outer envelope. It is against these last two antigens that immunoglobulins act; by neutralising them they prevent the virus attaching itself to a cell receptor. The extracellular complex is phagocytosed and destroyed. Intracellular virus is invulnerable to antibody.[28]

The classes of antibody that act against viruses are IgG and IgA; In the circulation the virus-neutralising antibodies are IgG, whereas the antibodies in the secretions that prevent infection of the mucous membranes belong to class IgA (see p. 144). In this respect it is noteworthy that an attack of poliomyelitis or the administration of the oral vaccine confers a local intestinal immunity as well as a circulating one, whereas the parenteral vaccine has no effect on the local proliferation of the virus, but merely intercepts it when it has become systematised. This is because the live oral virus, whether virulent or attenuated, stimulates IgA as well as IgG, whereas the dead parenteral vaccine stimulates only IgG. A similar state of affairs holds for virus infections of the respiratory tract, except that in this situation IgA is more immediately important than IgG, because the effects of these viruses are more localised than are those of the entero-viruses.[29–31]

(b) **Cell-mediated immunity** plays an even more important role in virus infections than do the immunoglobulins. Thus in states of pure immunoglobulin deficiency (hypo-gammaglobulinaemia) there is usually an effective host response to systemic virus infections, whereas in states of T lymphocyte deficiency chronic, progressive, fatal virus infections, e.g. vaccinia, chickenpox, herpes simplex, and cytomegalic inclusion disease, are extremely common.[27] The part the lymphocyte plays in virus infection is still obscure. It is known that a sensitised lymphocyte secretes interferon[32] as well as lymphokines; in addition, it is possible that the lymphocyte destroys the virus-infected cell directly, thereby killing intracellular virus.

(c) **Interferon.**[33] The interferons are a family of antiviral proteins varying in molecular weight from 20 000 to 160 000 which are produced by cells infected with a virus. This protein is non-toxic and non-antigenic to the host (and only feebly antigenic to other species), and has a remarkable effect in making the cells resistant to further virus infection. It "interferes" with the proliferation of a second virus in the affected cell, and this effect has a very broad spectrum of activity. Inactivated virus is as effective in stimulating interferon production as is living virus. Interferon can be produced in many tissue culture systems, but its action is specific for the animal from which it was derived. There can be little doubt that it is important in checking the course of many virus infections.[34] Whether it plays any part in the acquired cellular immunity of virus disease is uncertain. The administration of glucocorticosteroids inhibits the production and action of interferon,[35] pyrexia, on the other hand, stimulates it.[34] Interferon is thought to act by inhibiting the translation of viral mRNA. This it does not directly, but by inducing the formation of a second cellular protein called translation-inhibitory protein. Translation of host-cell mRNA is not interrupted; this explains why interferon is non-toxic.

Interferon is potentially an important therapeutic agent, and there have recently been a few encouraging reports of its use in human disease.[33] Unfortunately the active interferon for such investigations must come from a primate source, preferably human. It has also been found that many substances other than live virus induce the formation of interferon. Among these are some bacteria, rickettsiae, mycoplasmas, malarial parasites, and *Toxoplasma gondii*. A few chemicals are also active, notably bacterial endotoxin and phytohaemagglutinin. None of these could be used therapeutically because of their toxicity. Two products of fungal fermentation called *helenine*[36] and *statolon*[37] (derived from *Penicillium funiculosum* and *Penicillium stoloniferum* respectively) are powerful interferon inducers, and in both the active principle is a double-stranded RNA molecule, which is a fungal virus. Synthetic double-stranded RNA molecules are also important interferon inducers; the most effective is a complex of polyinosinic acid and polycytidylic acid called *poly I:C*. These agents have given promising results in animal virus infections, but their effect in man is still under trial. It should be noted that interferon is not only actively formed by cells, but can also be released preformed from lymphocytes and possibly RE cells.[32] This method of promoting interferon formation seems better than the administration of extraneous interferon, but it must be given about a day before the infection starts.[38, 39]

Chemotherapy of Virus Diseases[40, 41]

Virus multiplication is so intimately bound up with normal cell metabolism that the possibility of finding effective chemotherapeutic agents seemed remote a few years ago. This gloomy forecast has proved to be ill founded and a number of effective agents have been discovered. Unfortunately many of them are unsuitable for systemic use in man, but there is every indication that new less toxic agents will be found.

Chemotherapeutic agents may act at any stage in the life-

281

cycle of the virus from its initial attachment to the cell to the final stage of assembly of mature virus particles and their subsequent release. Some agents appear to act at different or several stages according to the particular virus infection. The following account must therefore be regarded as provisional.

Interference with virus entry into cells. *Amantadine* (*α-adamantanamine*) inhibits the penetration of influenza virus in tissue culture and in mice. Preliminary trials in man indicate that it can prevent contacts from developing clinical influenza. The main side-effect is somnolence.

Inhibition of replication of viral nucleic acids. Agents may block the formation of viral nucleic acid for viral replication, the formation of mRNA, or in the RNA oncogenic viruses, the production of viral DNA.

5-Iodo-2'deoxyuridine (*IUDR, 5-IDU,* or *Idoxuridine*) has two actions. It inhibits the enzyme thymidic acid synthetase which converts deoxyuridilic acid to thymidilic acid. The latter is necessary for DNA synthesis. In addition, 5-IDU is incorporated into DNA instead of thymidine to produce a non-functional DNA. This is an example of Peters's lethal synthesis (p. 46). The drug inhibits the growth of vaccinia and herpes-simplex viruses *in vitro*. It has been used in herpetic encephalitis but its toxicity is a grave disadvantage. Locally 5-IDU finds its greatest use in the treatment, and prevention of spread, of herpes-simplex infection of the skin, mucous membranes, and cornea (dendritic ulcers).

Cytosine arabinoside (*cytarabine*) is another nucleoside analogue which acts on DNA-core viruses. It has been tried with some success in severe progressive herpes-simplex and varicella-zoster infections and in congenital cytomegalo-virus infections. Like 5-IDU it is too toxic to be a useful systemic agent except in desperate situations.

2-(α-hydroxybenzyl) benzimidazole (*HBB*) is active against picornaviruses and inhibits viral RNA synthesis. It is less active in the intact animal and has not been used clinically.

Inhibition of Synthesis of Viral Proteins. *N-methylis-atin β-thiosemicarbazone* (*methisazone* or *marboran*) inhibits the formation of viral protein necessary for completing the assembly of viral particles. It is active against smallpox, and its administration prevents the development of clinical disease in contacts; when once the disease has developed, methisazone is much less effective. It has also been tried in vaccinia gangrenosa and eczema vaccinatum. Toxic effects include vomiting, skin eruptions, and jaundice.

Rifampicin, a derivative of rifamycin. Both drugs have been used in the treatment of tuberculosis and leprosy, and are relatively non-toxic. Rifampicin is effective against a number of viruses and appears to act at various points; with vaccinia virus it interferes with the final assembly of virus particles. It also inhibits DNA-dependent RNA polymerase. Another derivative, N-demethylrifampicin, inhibits RNA-dependent DNA polymerase in RNA oncogenic viruses, and is therefore being studied as a possible agent in cancer chemotherapy.

Interferon and the *interferon inducing agents* have been described on p. 280.

THE DIAGNOSIS OF VIRUS DISEASE

In only a few virus infections can the agent be demonstrated in the lesions by the presence of typical inclusion bodies, e.g. rabies and cytomegalic inclusion disease, or by characteristic histological features, as for example the measles giant cell. Electron microscopy can be used to identify viral bodies in infected tissue, and although absolute identification is not possible at present, much useful information can be obtained. Thus smallpox can easily and quickly be distinguished from chickenpox; the fluid or scraping of the lesions is examined using the technique of negative staining (see Fig. 23.1, p. 285). Fluorescent antibody techniques are also useful in identifying virus from suitable materials.[42]

An important diagnostic procedure is the isolation of the virus from the patient's secretions using the living cell systems already described. The virus may then be typed by means of complement fixation and neutralisation tests using specific rabbit antisera.

In convalescent patients there is invariably a rise in titre of antibodies against the agent, and these too may be demonstrated by complement fixation, haemagglutination inhibition, and neutralisation tests against the specific viruses. It is important to collect a specimen of the patient's serum during the acute phase so that a rise in antibody titre can be recognised. The greatest rise will be encountered in systemic infections like smallpox, mumps, measles, and poliomyelitis. In clinical practice it may be difficult to isolate the causal virus from the patient or his secretions during the acute phase, because it is often so evanescent that no virus is demonstrable by the time the clinician's attention is drawn to the necessity of searching for it.

It follows that retrospective diagnosis made on serological grounds is the most important clinical method of diagnosing virus disease.

REFERENCES

1. WILSON, G. S. and MILES, A. A. (1964). In *Topley and Wilson's Principles of Bacteriology and Immunity*, 5th edn, p. 1134. London: Arnold.
2. MARMION, B. P. and STOCKER, M. G. P. (1958). *British Medical Journal*, ii, 809.
3. WILSON, G. S. and MILES, A. A. (1964). p. 1148, *loc. cit.*
4. CHANOCK, R. M., HAYFLICK, L. and BARILE, M. F. (1962). *Proceedings of the National Academy of Science (Wash.)*, **48**, 41.
5. EATON, M. D., MEIKLEJOHN, G. and VAN HERICK, W. (1944). *Journal of Experimental Medicine*, **79**, 649.
6. LIU, C. (1957). *Ibid*, **106**, 455.

7. GOODBURN, G. M., MARMION, B. P. and KENDALL, E. J. C. (1963). *British Medical Journal*, i, 1266.
8. Leading Article (1967). *Lancet*, ii, 248.
9. DUTHIE, J. J. R. (1971). In *Modern Trends in Rheumatology*, 2, p. 78. Edited by A. G. S. Hill. London: Butterworths.
10. WILSON, G. S. and MILES, A. A. (1964). p. 1161, *loc. cit.*
11. COHEN, A. (1963). In *Mechanisms of Virus Infection*, p. 153. Edited by Wilson Smith. London and New York: Academic Press.
12. ISAACS, A. (1963). p. 191, *Ibid.*
13. SUMMERS, D. F. (1967). *New England Journal of Medicine*, **276**, 1016 and 1076.
14. FENNER, F. (1962). *British Medical Journal*, ii, 135.
15. BERRY, G. P. and DEDRICK, H. M. (1936). *Journal of Bacteriology*, **31**, 50.
16. ENDERS, J. F., WELLER, T. H. and ROBBINS, F. C. (1949). *Science*, **109**, 85.
17. GEY, G. O., COFFMAN, W. D. and KUBICEK, M. T. (1952). *Cancer Research*, **12**, 264.
18. HOORN, B. and TYRRELL, D. A. J. (1965). *British Journal of Experimental Pathology*, **46**, 109 and 514.
19. STOKER, M. G. P. (1957). *British Medical Journal*, i, 963.
20. WRIGHT, G. P. (1958). In *An Introduction to Pathology*, 3rd edn, p. 184. London: Longmans.
21. WARTHIN, A. S. (1931). *Archives of Pathology*, **11**, 864.
22. GORDON, H. and KNIGHTON, H. T. (1941). *American Journal of Pathology*, **17**, 165.
23. DOWNIE, A. W. (1963). In *Mechanisms of Virus Infections*, p. 101, *loc. cit.*
24. FENNER, F. (1948). *Lancet*, ii, 915.
25 BLANDFORD, G. and HEATH, R. B. (1970). In *Modern Trends in Medical Virology*, 2, p. 51. Edited by R. B. Heath and A. P. Waterson. London: Butterworths.
26. WESTWOOD, J. C. N. (1963). In *Mechanisms of Virus Infection*, p. 255, *loc. cit.*
27. GORDON SMITH, C. E. (1969). *Proceedings of the Royal Society of Medicine*, **62**, 292.
28. ANDREWES, C. H. (1929). *British Journal of Experimental Pathology*, **10**, 273.
29. REMINGTON, J. S. *et al.* (1964). *Journal of Clinical Investigation*, **43**, 1613.
30. BELLANTI, J. A., ARTENSTEIN, M. S. and BUESCHER, E. L. (1965). *Journal of Immunology*, **94**, 344.
31. BEARE, A. S. *et al.* (1968). *Lancet*, ii, 418.
32. EPSTEIN, L. B., CLINE, M. J. and MERIGAN, T. C. (1971). *Journal of Clinical Investigation*, **50**, 744.
33. FINTER, N. B. (1970). In *Modern Trends in Medical Virology*, 2, p. 262, *loc. cit.*
34. ISAACS, A. (1962). *British Medical Journal*, ii, 353.
35. KILBOURNE, E. D., SMART, K. M. and POKORNY, B. A. (1961). *Nature (London)*, **190**, 650.
36. RYTEL, M. W., SHOPE, R. E. and KILBOURNE, E. D. (1966). *Journal of Experimental Medicine*, **123**, 577.
37. KLEINSCHMIDT, W. J., CLINE, J. C. and MURPHY, E. B. (1964). *Proceedings of the National Academy of Sciences of the United States of America*, **52**, 741.
38. Interferon, A Ciba Foundation Symposium (1968). Edited by G. E. W. Wolstenholme and M. O'Connor, 271 pp. London: Churchill.
39. TYRRELL, D. A. J. (1969). *Proceedings of the Royal Society of Medicine*, **62**, 297.
40. HIRSCHMAN, S. Z. (1971). *American Journal of Medicine*, **51**, 699.
41. JUEL-JENSEN, B. E. (1970). *British Medical Journal*, ii, 154.
42. Leading Article (1967). *British Medical Journal*, i, 126.
43. McCORMACK, W. M. *et al.* (1973). *New England Journal of Medicine*, **288**, 78.
44. Leading Article (1973). *British Medical Journal*, i, 129.

Chapter 23. Virus Disease

II. VIRUS INFECTIONS OF HUMAN BEINGS

It is useful to consider some pathogenic viruses briefly with special reference to their mode of infectivity, their spread in the body, and methods that may be employed in producing active immunity against them.

THE ENTEROVIRUS INFECTIONS[1]

The enteroviruses are a group of small, spherical, RNA-containing viruses found particularly in the cells of the intestine. They are members of a larger group called the *picornaviruses* (pico = small+RNA), to which the foot-and-mouth disease virus of cattle and the rhinoviruses that cause the common cold also belong. The enteroviruses are especially associated with neurological diseases. There are three subgroups:

The polioviruses, of which there are three types. These cause poliomyelitis.

The Coxsackie viruses were first isolated in the town of Coxsackie in New York State in 1948. Some can be grown in tissue-culture systems. All are pathogenic to suckling mice and two groups are recognised by the lesions they produce. Group A (23 types) produce a fulminating myositis, while group B (6 types) attack the brown fatty tissue, the nervous system, and to a lesser extent muscle. Coxsackie A viruses are frequently found in the faeces of healthy children, but there are no normal carriers of Coxsackie B viruses.

Diseases caused by Coxsackie A viruses.

(*a*) *Herpangina*, a febrile disease of childhood in which the mouth and fauces are the seat of shallow greyish ulcers.

(*b*) *An upper respiratory, cold-like condition.* The virus responsible is the Coe virus (Coxsackie A21), so named after the first patient from whom it was isolated.[2]

(*c*) *Hand-foot-and-mouth disease*, caused by Coxsackie A16, usually occurring in children in whom bullae develop on the parts mentioned in the name, and a maculopapular eruption appears on the buttocks. Usually there is no fever. It is not to be confused with foot-and-mouth disease, which rarely affects man, and in which the bullae are larger and the constitutional disturbance is more severe.[3]

Other macular or maculopapular exanthemata are seen in outbreaks of both A and B strain viruses.

Diseases caused by Coxsackie B viruses.

(*a*) *Epidemic myalgia*, or *Bornholm disease*, so called because it was first described in the Danish island of Bornholm. It is characterised by fever and agonising pains in the chest and abdomen.

(*b*) *Neonatal myocarditis* and *pericarditis*, a fatal condition, transmitted to the fetus by the mother.[4] In adults *acute pericarditis* may occur.

(*c*) Cases of *lymphocytic meningitis* (aseptic meningitis) and *paralysis mimicking poliomyelitis* are caused by Coxsackie B and some A strains. They may occur in epidemics. Severe *necrotising encephalitis* is a rare event.[5]

The ECHO (Enteric, Cytopathogenic, Human, Orphan) viruses, of which there are about 36 types. They are found quite commonly in children's faeces, and for a long time they could not be associated with any disease, hence the name "orphan" (a virus in search of a disease). Many have now found their parents, and it is known that they can produce:

(*a*) *Aseptic meningitis* and *paralysis* similar to the Coxsackie viruses.

(*b*) *An epidemic febrile disease*, sometimes accompanied by meningoencephalitis. It is often associated with a diffuse maculopapular rash. The virus incriminated is ECHO type 9.[6]

(*c*) *Acute respiratory disease* of a cold-like nature.

(*d*) *Gastro-enteritis*. This association is not proven.

This group grows in monkey kidney cell culture, but is not pathogenic to mice.

Poliomyelitis is caused by the three types of polioviruses, of which type 1 produces the most severe disease. It is also the commonest of the three types of infection. The disease follows the ingestion of material that has been contaminated by virus-containing faeces, e.g. water from swimming-baths or for drinking, and also food exposed to house flies. Indirect contact with excretors, whose dirty hands contaminate fomites is another source of infection. The mode of transmission is similar to that of typhoid fever.

Spread in the body. The virus proliferates first in the cells of the pharynx and the lower part of the small bowel.

If it is not arrested at this stage, it enters the general circulation *via* the lymphatics, and it then multiplies in various extraneural sites like the spleen and kidneys. This marks the end of the incubation period, which usually lasts 7–14 days, but may extend up to 30 days. The viraemic phase is accompanied by a febrile reaction, and even at this stage the infection may be overcome.

If the condition proceeds, the virus settles finally in the central nervous system which it reaches by the blood stream.

It localises itself specifically in the anterior horn cells and their medullary counterparts, and paralysis ensues.

A second mode of spread is directly up the peripheral nerve endings of the bowel and especially the pharynx. Opinions vary about the importance of this method of spread; it probably accounts for the bulbar type of disease that sometimes follows tonsillectomy.

It is evident that much has still to be learned about the pathogenesis of the disease. One thing is clear: many people are infected with poliovirus, and either show no illness at all or else have a mild febrile reaction. Only a small unlucky minority develop paralysis. Poliomyelitis is an excellent example of an infection that tends to be subclinical.

Factors aggravating the disease. The incubation period is shortened, and the liability to nervous-system involvement increased by the following factors: heavy exercise and fatigue, pregnancy, operative procedures, and active immunisation. When the disease follows immunisation it is called *provocation poliomyelitis*; it is believed that alum and other adjuvants in the vaccines and toxoids are the important factors. The pathogenesis is unknown, but it has been suggested that the focus of inflammation acts as a nidus for proliferation of the virus during the period of viraemia. It might then travel up the local nerve to the spinal cord. The incidence of provocation poliomyelitis is about 1 per 37 000 inoculations.[7] Active immunisation procedures should be postponed during a poliomyelitis epidemic.

Excretion of virus. Faecal excretion of virus usually precedes the advent of symptoms by a few days, and it is usually present during the first two weeks of paralytic manifestations. After about 6 weeks only a quarter of patients still excrete the virus, and by 12 weeks excretion has usually ceased. Permanent carriage is unknown. The virus can be isolated from the throat just before and after the onset of symptoms. It cannot usually be isolated from the cerebro-spinal fluid.

Infectivity. Poliovirus is remarkable for its narrow range of host infectivity; only primates are readily susceptible. Fortunately the virus flourishes with consummate ease in the usual tissue-culture systems, and it is from these that effective vaccines have been developed. A consideration of poliomyelitis immunisation is valuable as a general exercise in comparing the relative merits of dead suspensions to those of live attenuated viruses.

Active immunisation.[8, 9] The first effective vaccine was devised by Salk, who used polioviruses grown in monkey kidney cells and subsequently inactivated by formolisation. At first a few fatal cases of poliomyelitis occurred following the use of inadequately inactivated virus suspensions, but since then the process has been so perfected that safety is assured and a potent vaccine produced. It is issued in trivalent form, and requires at least three intramuscular inoculations, the second a month after the first and the third about six months after the second. A fourth dose a year later is advisable. A high titre of circulating immunoglobulin should be produced, though often there is a disappointing

response to type-1 virus, the most dangerous of the three. Immunity depends on the presence of IgG antibody. The resistance of the small bowel to subsequent infection by polioviruses is not altered. The duration of immunity is not certain, and it is probable that revaccination will be required when an epidemic breaks out. An advantage of inactivated poliovaccine is that it can be combined with other vaccines and toxoids (see p. 171).

Later Sabin produced a vaccine consisting of living attenuated strains of poliovirus which had undergone mutation after passage through monkey-kidney cell cultures. These attenuated viruses are given orally, and the infection closely simulates the natural disease except that spread does not occur to the nervous system. The immunity produced depends not only on IgG but also on IgA present in the intestinal secretions, as has already been discussed. Two important drawbacks are (a) that the viruses might not enter the bowel cells. This might be due to one virus (notably type 2) interfering with the entry of the others, or to other enteroviruses or adenoviruses preventing the entry of all the attenuated viruses, or even more important to repeated attacks of infantile gastroenteritis preventing the virus settling in the small bowel. This last snag is of great moment in the tropics;[10] (b) that these viruses, which show a great tendency to undergo mutation in the alimentary tract, might revert to a virulent type, and after excretion infect other people in the vicinity with poliomyelitis. It has been proved that these excreted viruses may be more virulent to monkeys than the original vaccine.[11]

In practice it is found that any interfering tendency is obviated by giving several doses of trivalent vaccine. There is not doubt that any attenuated viruses and their variants, which are excreted in the faeces, will readily infect other people, but danger of disease is very slight. Vast populations in Russia and Czechoslovakia have been adventitiously immunised in this way. Not only has there been no outbreak of poliomyelitis in these countries following the introduction of the oral vaccine, but in fact there has been effective clearing of the people's alimentary tracts of wild polioviruses. On the other hand, isolated cases of paralytic poliomyelitis have rarely followed the use of attenuated virus; presumably it had retained some of its pathogenicity.[10]

The oral vaccine is recommended because it gives a better, long-lasting immunity and it acts more rapidly in a threatened epidemic than does the killed vaccine.[12] Despite its general safety it should not be given within three weeks of tonsillectomy or any immunisation procedure. It is a trivalent vaccine and is given in three doses at monthly intervals

A last consideration concerns the monkey kidney tissue on which the polioviruses are cultured. It has been known to harbour commensal simian viruses, and some of these are resistant even to formalin treatment. In the past, batches of Salk and Sabin vaccines have been contaminated with these simian viruses. Though no human disease has so far been attributed to these particular viruses, they must be regarded with concern when live vaccine is given; one at least is oncogenic to baby hamsters (see p. 384). The use of human cells would obviate this danger, but unfortunately these are more difficult to assemble in a large quantity, and they soon die out in repeated cultures. Exceptions are the strains of cancer cells, e.g. HeLa cells, but it would be unwise to use them for human vaccine production. At present diploid lines of human cells derived from fetal tissues are being investigated; some can undergo up to fifty subcultures before dying.[13]

THE POXVIRUS INFECTIONS[14]

The poxviruses are a group of large, brick-shaped DNA-containing viruses. The capsid has a complex symmetry (Fig. 23.1). This group produces vesicular skin lesions, and the affected cells contain large intracytoplasmic inclusion bodies. Many animals have their own variety of pox disease, e.g. *cow-pox*, *mouse-pox*, and *fowl-pox*. The important human disease is *smallpox*. *Molluscum contagiosum*, a skin

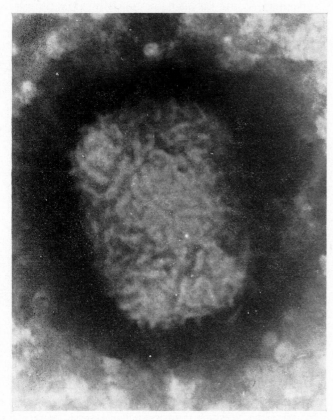

Figure 23.1
A poxvirus particle. This is vaccinia virus from a case of eczema vaccinatum. Note the complex symmetry of the capsid. Variola virus has a similar appearance. (Negatively stained with phospho-tungstate × 400 000). (*Photograph supplied by Dr. T. H. Flewett*)

condition consisting of pearly, elevated papules containing a curd-like material, is also included in the pox group.[15, 16]

Smallpox and vaccinia. There are two closely related viruses that cause smallpox, the classical *variola major* virus, and the virus causing the milder disease *alastrim*, or *variola minor*.

Smallpox is acquired by the inhalation of infected particles from a patient directly or from fomites indirectly. The bedding is particularly dangerous, and numerous instances are on record where laundry workers have contracted the disease from contaminated bedclothes.

Spread in the body. It is believed that a primary lesion may actually occur in the nasal mucosa, and that this is followed by systemic spread to the RE system. This is followed in turn by a phase of secondary viraemia, in the course of which the virus finally settles in the skin and produces the typical intra-epidermal vesicle. At an early stage Guarnieri bodies are present in the epidermal cells, and the characteristic elementary bodies (Paschen bodies) can be demonstrated in large numbers in the vesicles, pustules, and their crusts (Fig. 23.1). The incubation period is from 10 to 14 days, and virus can usually be demonstrated in the blood during the first two days of the prodromal period (which lasts 4 days). The patient is infectious only when the characteristic eruption appears, and remains so until desquamation is complete.

The viruses of variola major and alastrim are so similar that only painstaking tests can differentiate them, yet alastrim is a much milder disease with a mortality rate of under 1 per cent.

Variola virus produces characteristic pocks on the chorio-allantoic membranes of fertile eggs. Its host range is very narrow, for only primates develop typical smallpox lesions.

Active immunisation. The first really effective attempt at smallpox immunisation was performed by Edward Jenner, who discovered that the natural pox infection of bovine animals, *cow-pox*, could produce a similar lesion in human beings, and protect them against smallpox infection.

Since then a third virus has emerged, *vaccinia virus*. Its origin is obscure. It is believed to be a mutant of either variola or cow-pox viruses; probably most strains used nowadays were originally derived from cow-pox.[17] It resembles cow-pox virus closely, not only morphologically and antigenically (the differences between the two in these respects are infinitesimal), but also in the disease it produces and the immunity it affords against smallpox. Cow-pox vesicles are more bloodstained than those of vaccinia. In fact, the viruses of smallpox, vaccinia, and cow-pox are separate though closely related. The lesions they produce on the chorio-allantoic membrane of the fertile egg are quite distinct.

Vaccinia virus produces lesions in many animals, and the strains used prophylactically are passed through calves and rabbits. A sequence recommended is calf-rabbit-calf-child-calf-rabbit, etc.

The dangers of vaccination, apart from local bacterial infection, are:

(a) *Eczema vaccinatum.* This may vary from the presence of a few discrete lesions on the skin to a widely disseminated confluent eruption with a 30–40 per cent mortality rate. It occurs in subjects with a pre-existing skin disease, such as atopic dermatitis, and is one variety of *Kaposi's varicelliform eruption*, the other being *eczema herpeticum*, in which a herpes-simplex virus infection is superimposed on a pre-existing skin disease.

(b) *Generalised vaccinia.* In this condition multiple skin lesions occur as a result of blood-borne spread. It is self limiting and responds well to immune-globulin therapy.

(c) *Progressive vaccinia (vaccinia gangrenosa).* In this condition the lesion does not heal, but continues to spread until large areas of skin are involved (Fig. 23.2). It is par-

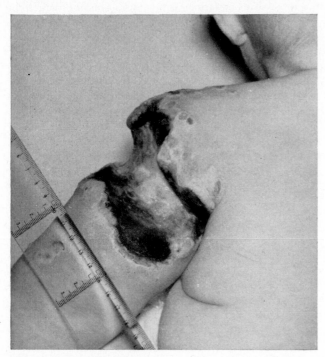

Figure 23.2
Vaccinia gangrenosa. This picture was taken 4½ months after the lesion first appeared. The extensive tissue destruction is apparent. *(From Hansson, O. and Vahlquist, B. (1963), Lancet, ii, 687)*

ticularly liable to occur in patients with T-lymphocyte deficiency. It is usually fatal after several months.

(d) *Postvaccinal encephalomyelitis.* This usually occurs 12–14 days after vaccination and has a 50 per cent death rate. There is marked demyelination around blood vessels. Opinions vary as to whether it is due to the virus (which cannot be isolated from the brain), or a second latent virus, or to allergy.

(e) *Vaccinial osteitis*, a rare complication, mimicking pyogenic osteomyelitis.[18]

(f) *Congenital vaccinia.* A fatal, generalised infection has occurred in fetuses whose mothers were vaccinated early in pregnancy. The first trimester is the dangerous period.[19, 20]

Though these complications are rare, it has become apparent that in many Western European countries the mortality due to them is greater than the indigenous smallpox mortality. It has therefore become the policy in Britain to dispense with the routine vaccination of infants and children, and reserve vaccination for those in immediate contact with a case of smallpox.[21, 22] Such vaccination of contacts within three days of exposure is usually effective. Of course, those whose occupation brings them into possible contact with the disease, e.g. doctors, nurses, and members of the armed forces, should be vaccinated regularly as long as they are at risk. Likewise, there are many foreign countries, entry into which necessitates prior vaccination.

The most important contra-indication to vaccination is the presence of any widespread skin disease, especially atopic dermatitis. Vaccination should also be avoided in patients with any immunological deficiency syndrome especially of cell-mediated immunity, and also in those who are pregnant or who are being treated with glucocorticosteroids (unless there is an emergency).[23]

Vaccinia immune human globulin and methisazone are used in the treatment of smallpox and vaccinia.[24]

VIRUSES AFFECTING THE RESPIRATORY TRACT[25]

The number of viruses incriminated in respiratory infections is legion. Many of the agents produce acute infections of the upper respiratory tract. The most important of these are the myxoviruses and paramyxoviruses (which include the influenza and para-influenza viruses), the adenoviruses, and some recently isolated viruses associated with the common cold.

Myxoviruses and Paramyxoviruses*

These are a group of medium-sized, filamentous, RNA-containing viruses. They have an affinity for mucins, hence their name. Most of them grow well in the amniotic cells of chick embryos. They have a conspicuous tendency to agglutinate the red cells of many species, e.g. fowls and guinea-pigs. They do this by their strong attachment to mucoprotein surface receptors on the red-cell envelopes, from which they act as bridges to other cells. Specific antisera inhibit this *haemagglutination*, thus aiding in typing the viruses.

Myxoviruses grow in tissue cultures of monkey kidney cells. If suspensions of guinea-pig red cells are introduced into the infected culture tubes, the cells are adsorbed on to the surface of the monkey kidney cells. This is called *haemadsorption*, and is useful in identifying the paramyxoviruses.

The important human myxovirus is the virus of influenza.

* These two groups are very similar, differing only in size (see p. 294).

The parainfluenza agents are paramyxoviruses, as is also the mumps virus. This is a disease of the salivary glands, and it sometimes affects the pancreas, gonads, and central nervous system.

Influenza.[26] The casual agents are three quite distinct types of influenza virus, A, B, and C, of which type A and its variants are by far the most important from an epidemiological point of view. Influenza is a disease predominantly of children and young adults. It is transmitted by inhalation just before and during the acute stage, but the possibility of transmission by healthy carriers has not been excluded. The incubation period is only one to two days. The disease is a systemic one, but the effects are predominantly respiratory, and there is much necrosis of the epithelium of the trachea and bronchi. The severe underlying acute inflammatory response accounts for the deep red congested appearance of the tracheal mucosa at necropsy. It is probable that even in severe pandemics the horrifying death rate is due to secondary pneumonias of bacterial origin rather than to the influenza.

Immunology. The most interesting feature of influenza A virus is its tendency to undergo frequent antigenic variation. The 1918 pandemic was probably caused by a mutant of the A virus, and since then new strains have emerged at about ten-year intervals. These have had different antigenic patterns from their predecessors, and have caused localised epidemics in the years 1932 and 1934. In 1946 a new strain emerged, and was so different from the standard A strains that it was classified as A¹ virus. This strain almost completely replaced the A strain, until it was in its turn superseded by the new A² virus that heralded the "Asian" influenza pandemic of 1957. The pandemic of 1968–69 was caused by yet another strain of the A² virus (the "Hong Kong strain"). As individuals grow older, they accumulate antibodies against different strains of influenza virus in their circulation, but they are still susceptible to new mutants. The swine influenza virus is closely related to the human A virus, and it has been suggested that the 1918 pandemic originated from pig-transmitted influenza viruses, and that perhaps animals provide a reservoir of infection between epidemics. This is unproven.

Influenza B virus is endemic and causes more circumscribed outbreaks, and has a much slower, less pronounced tendency to antigenic variation. Type C infection is rather uncommon, and the virus appears to exist as a single stable antigenic type.

It is obvious that effective immunisation against influenza is beset with difficulties. No one can forecast the nature of the next mutant that may cause a pandemic, and as the incubation period is so short, it is very difficult to immunise whole populations in time. International co-operation is essential in providing information about the origin and geography of spread of such a pandemic, so that distant communities can be immunised in time. At present killed and attenuated living vaccines are being tested for efficiency against known viruses in the hope of preparing a satisfactory

G.P.—10*

vaccine rapidly against a new mutant. Chemotherapy also promises to be of some use in the prevention of influenza. *Amantadine* and the interferon inducers, notably statolon, have been used (p. 280 and 281).

The para-influenza viruses[27] may be considered "little cousins" of the influenza group. These are associated in adults with mild upper respiratory-tract infections, and are one of the many possible agents causing cold-like infections. In children they cause acute tracheobronchitis. There are four types so far identified in human disease. One type causing acute laryngotracheobronchitis in children is called the "CA", or *croup associated virus*. The general biological features of these paramyxoviruses are similar to the influenza group, but they do not grow well in fertile eggs. They are differentiated on serological grounds.

Adenovirus Infections[28]

The adenoviruses are rather small, spherical, DNA-containing viruses which produce intranuclear inclusion bodies, and have a proclivity for the mucosa of the upper respiratory tract and the conjunctiva. There are 31 human serotypes, and also many that are specific for other animals, e.g. monkeys, dogs, cattle, and mice. A few human strains cause tumours in newborn hamsters. Adenoviruses are cultured on the usual tissue-culture systems consisting preferably of the cells of the animal species affected.

(*a*) Types 1, 2, and 5 infect the tonsils and adenoids in early childhood. They seldom produce ill-effects, and tend to lie *latent*. It is unknown whether they play any part in the common hyperplasia of tonsils and adenoids.[29]

(*b*) Types 3, 4, 7, 7a, and 14 produce explosive epidemics of *febrile pharyngitis* and other *acute respiratory diseases*. A primary atypical pneumonia syndrome may also occur. These infections occur most commonly in closed communities, and many epidemics have been described in military camps.

(*c*) These adenoviruses also have a strong proclivity for the conjunctiva[30] and may cause *acute follicular conjunctivitis* in the course of the upper respiratory disease.

(*d*) *Epidemic keratoconjunctivitis* is caused by the type-8 adenovirus, and is seen in factory workers whose corneas are liable to be abraded by particles of dust and metal.

(*e*) Adenoviruses are swallowed and can be isolated in the faeces. They have been incriminated in some cases of *gastroenteritis* in children, and are probably of importance in *mesenteric adenitis* occurring in children. The lymphoid hyperplasia of the bowel may be an important factor in some cases of *intussusception*.[31]

(*f*) Adenoviruses have been isolated from the urine, and type-11 has been associated with *acute haemorrhagic cystitis* in children.[32]

The Common Cold

The viruses that cause the common cold are called *rhinoviruses*. They are very small RNA-containing viruses, and are grouped among the picornaviruses.

The rhinoviruses are of interest in requiring a temperature of 33°C instead of 37°C for successful culture. Their habitat in the nose is probably related to this temperature requirement. They are cultured in human and monkey-embryo kidney tissue at a more acid pH than is usual.[33]

Cold-like diseases are also caused by some para-influenza viruses, ECHO viruses, the Coe virus, and also the *respiratory syncytial virus*, so called because it causes the cells in tissue-culture systems to coalesce into syncytial masses. A separate group of viruses that are associated with mild upper respiratory infections are the *REO* (*respiratory enteric orphan*) *viruses*. These are spherical RNA-containing viruses somewhat larger than the picornaviruses. Many of the above agents cause a type of pneumonia (see p. 227).

THE ARTHROPOD-BORNE VIRUS (ARBOVIRUS) INFECTIONS[34, 35]

Arboviruses are small (25–80 nm), RNA-containing viruses. They are distinctive in passing some part of their life-cycle in the tissues of an arthropod vector, where they actively multiply prior to being transmitted to a fresh host by the bite of the vector. The vector acquires the viruses from the blood of an animal host. Sometimes the life cycle is very complicated and implicates several vertebrate and invertebrate hosts. A wide range of animal infectivity is characteristic of this group. Of laboratory animals, the suckling mouse is the most susceptible, and is used diagnostically. Tissue cultures of chicken and mouse embryo cells are also useful.

The arthropod vectors are usually mosquitoes, but ticks and phlebotomus flies may also be implicated. It is not surprising that most of the diseases caused by these viruses have a distinctly tropical distribution. In human beings the chief arbovirus diseases are various types of *encephalitis, yellow fever, dengue fever, sandfly fever*, and a group of *virus haemorrhagic fevers*.

Arbovirus encephalitis is typically severe, and most types have a high mortality rate. The virus is widely disseminated throughout the central nervous system and affects the cerebral cortex particularly. There are different types of disease, which vary in geographical distribution. Eastern and Western Equine encephalitis occur especially in North America, whereas Japanese B, Murray Valley, and Russian spring-summer encephalitis are diseases endemic in Japan, Australia, and Russia respectively. St. Louis and West Nile encephalitis are other diseases of the same type occurring in the USA and the Middle East respectively. Most of these are mosquito-borne, but the Russian disease is transmitted by ticks.

Yellow fever is a disease primarily of monkeys, and is transmitted to them and to human victims by culicine *Aedes aegypti* mosquitoes. The disease is endemic in West Africa and Central America. Amongst the indigenous population subclinical infection is very common, though sometimes,

especially in Europeans, virulent yellow fever develops. It appears that after the virus has been injected into the skin by the mosquito's bite, it spreads to the local lymph nodes where it multiplies. It then invades the blood stream, and settles in the viscera producing necrotic lesions. The incubation period is only about 4 days. The typical lesion of yellow fever is a midzonal hepatic necrosis. Severe renal damage and a haemorrhagic tendency are also characteristic.

Nowadays yellow fever is rare in human beings, except in remote communities living in the tropics. Antimosquito measures and immunisation procedures have been responsible for this momentous eradication.

Active Immunisation. Active immunisation is mandatory for those travelling through endemic areas. It is performed by the subcutaneous or intramuscular injection of a suspension of living attenuated virus. This is the 17D strain, which was attenuated by passage through mice, and is now grown in chick embryos. These embryos are ground up and their juice is freeze-dried and placed in ampoules. The vaccine is reconstituted with normal saline immediately before use. The immunity is of a high degree, and lasts at least 6 years.

Diagnosis. The virus can be recovered from the blood during the first five days of illness, and when inoculated into suckling mice it leads to encephalitis. The mouse's brain is a good source of the virus, on which neutralisation tests can then be performed. The sera of convalescent patients contain high titres of complement-fixing and neutralising antibodies. These antibodies protect mice against the encephalitis caused by the virus. This is the basis of the *mouse protection test*, which has been employed in epidemiological surveys to ascertain the extent of subclinical yellow fever infection in a community.

Dengue fever occurs over a wide expanse of territory extending from the Levant to the Pacific Islands. The virus is transmitted by the *Aedes aegypti* mosquito, and is antigenically closely related to the yellow fever virus. The area of the mosquito bite is converted into a large red papule, which is the site of virus multiplication. The mode of dissemination is similar to that described in yellow fever, but the disease is quite different, consisting of a biphasic fever, severe headache and joint pains, and a variable maculopapular skin eruption. Pain in the acute phase is very severe, but death seldom occurs. The virus produces encephalitis in suckling mice, and can be neutralised by specific antibodies. Active artificial immunisation is possible but seldom performed.

Sandfly fever is an example of a short-term pyrexial illness accompanied by agonising muscular pains and headache, which is encountered quite frequently in countries around the Mediterranean and in Kenya. It is caused by a virus transmitted by the sandfly *Phlebotomus papatasi*. As with dengue fever a lesion appears locally, and after an incubation period of about 4 days the virus becomes systematised. It too is pathogenic for suckling mice.

Another arbovirus disease, **O'nyong-nyong**, has been reported in North Uganda.[36] It resembles dengue fever clinically, but it transmitted by *Anopheles* mosquitoes.

Virus haemorrhagic fevers[37] are a group of geographically widely-dispersed severe virus fevers in which a haemorrhagic tendency is prominent and the death rate high. Yellow fever itself comes into this category, but in addition there are other more distinctive arbovirus fevers of haemorrhagic nature. Arboviruses themselves are divided serologically into groups—group A arboviruses are called *alphaviruses*, and one of these, the Chikungunya virus, causes an African haemorrhagic fever. The group B arboviruses, called *flaviviruses* (because the yellow fever virus comes into this group) include some that cause haemorrhagic fevers in Siberia and India (Kyasanur forest fever). A Crimean haemorrhagic fever is caused by a new group of viruses called *Congo viruses*, because they have also been associated with febrile conditions in the Congo, and it is probable that the Congo viruses are also arboviruses.

There are other haemorrhagic fevers caused by another group of viruses called **arenoviruses**, which are not arboviruses. Lassa fever,[38] occurring in North East Nigeria and having a considerable mortality rate is an arenovirus infection, and there are others described in Bolivia and the Argentine (the Junin and Machupo viruses). The type specific arenovirus is that of lymphocytic choriomeningitis occurring in mice (see also page 294). The Tacaribe group of viruses are also arenoviruses.

VIRUS HEPATITIS[39]

There are two distinct diseases that come into this category, traditionally called infective hepatitis and serum hepatitis.

Infective hepatitis occurs endemically in institutions like schools and military camps, and its main incidence is among children and young adults. The agent is excreted in the faeces, and infects other individuals after the ingestion of contaminated food. During the preicteric and early icteric phases of the illness it is present also in the blood. Carriers harbour the agent in their faeces and in their blood. It therefore follows that this disease can be transmitted both by ingestion and inoculation. The agent has not yet been isolated, but it is tentatively called virus A.

The **serum hepatitis** agent is not generally present in the patient's faeces, but may be found in the blood for long periods. Subjects may carry the virus in their blood for over 5 years. The disease is exclusively human. It is transmitted not only by blood transfusion but also by the prick of a contaminated needle, for the amount of blood or serum necessary to convey the infection need be as little as 0·01 ml. In the past the disease was common in venereal disease clinics after arsenical injections, and during the 1939-45 war outbreaks followed yellow fever immunisation, because the vaccine was suspended in human serum at that time. Nowa-

days it is a major hazard among young drug-addicts, especially those who inject themselves intravenously ("mainliners"). People who handle blood or work in haemodialysis units are also at risk.[40] The agent, still not identified, is called virus B.

The diseases these two agents produce are pathologically very similar: a widespread focal necrosis which usually recovers by complete regeneration. Occasionally massive necrosis may follow, and the patient either dies or else is left with macronodular cirrhosis. Nevertheless, there are distinct clinical differences. Infective hepatitis has a much shorter incubation period than serum hepatitis (15–40 days as compared with 60–160 days), its onset is more abrupt, and it is accompanied by a sharper febrile reaction. Furthermore, its course is more benign, there being a far higher death rate and a much greater incidence of cirrhosis in serum hepatitis. Infective hepatitis occurs mostly in epidemics in young people, while serum hepatitis affects especially the adolescent drug-taker, the recipient of massive blood transfusions, and those who work in haemodialysis units. Prophylactic passive immunisation with γ-globulin is useful against infective hepatitis, but is of much less value against serum hepatitis.

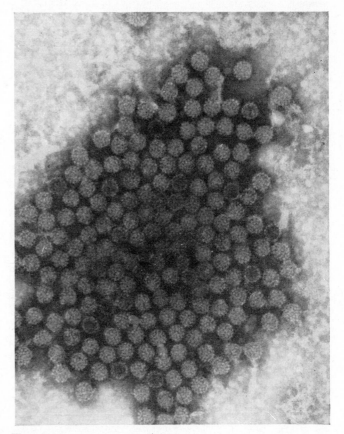

Figure 23.3
Hepatitis (Australia) antigen. Note the small round forms. (Negatively stained with phosphotungstate ×171 000). (*Photograph supplied by Dr. T. H. Flewett*)

There appears to be no cross-immunity between the two viruses.

An extremely important advance in our knowledge of virus hepatitis has followed the discovery of an antigen in the blood of some cases of serum hepatitis. It is of lipoprotein constitution, and was first noted in the serum of an Australian aborigine, in whom it was believed to be an unusual genetically determined plasma protein. Subsequently it was found in cases of leukaemia, Down's syndrome, and in those who had had a history of hepatitis, when its true association was elucidated. It is now called *Australia (Au) antigen* (alternative names are serum hepatitis (SH) antigen, hepatitis associated (HAA) antigen, and hepatitis-B antigen (HB ag)). Patients who have had many blood transfusions, e.g. haemophiliacs, and those who have recovered from serum hepatitis have a variable titre of antibodies against this antigen.

The nature of Australia antigen is still not properly understood.[41, 42] Under the electron microscope three types of particle can be seen: small round forms about 18 nm in diameter, long forms which are about 20 nm in diameter and of variable length, and a double-shelled form (the Dane particle) which is round and about 45 nm in total diameter, while the inner shell is about 20 nm in diameter (Figs. 23.3 and 23.4). This last form closely resembles a virion in configuration, but it does not appear to contain an appreciable amount of nucleic acid (traces of RNA have been reported, but substantiation is awaited).[43] Whether these particles are the infective agent, or the capsid of the agent, or indeed are a type of "slow virus" (see p. 293) is not known. Certainly the resistance of the agent of serum hepatitis to heat is quite unlike the lability of true viruses, and is more in keeping with the properties of a "slow" agent.

Antigenaemia develops in from 3 to 13 weeks after infection, and most cases subsequently develop hepatitis. Antibody builds up during the late incubation period, and occasionally immune-complex phenomena such as arthritis and arteritis precede the onset of hepatitis.[44] It is interesting that immunologically deficient people, e.g. lepromatous lepers, those on immuosuppressants, and especially those with chronic renal failure, carry the antigen for long periods. Such people do not appear to suffer from liver damage, but they are potent transmitters of the agent. Many cases of hepatitis have occurred in doctors and nurses working in renal dialysis units, and a disturbingly high mortality rate is characteristic of this type of infection. This latency of infection in immunlogically deficient hosts is clearly an exceptional state of affairs in virus disease, but it has its analogy in lymphocytic choriomeningitis in mice (see p. 279).

In the general population the carrier rate varies from about 0·1 per cent in the USA to over 10 per cent in some of the Pacific Islands. Perhaps primitive conditions, including tattooing, play a part in carrying infection around the community. Transmission by mosquito bite is another possibility, as these insects have been shown to carry Au antigen.[70]

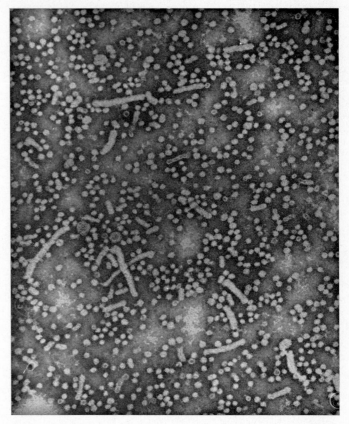

Figure 23.4
Hepatitis (Australia) antigen. This picture shows small round forms, long forms, and double-shelled forms. (Negatively stained with phosphotungstate ×142 000). *(Photograph supplied by T. H. Flewett.)*

It is apparent that there are two types of hepatitis, the Au-antigen-positive type and the Au-antigen-negative type. These are correlated with serum hepatitis and infective hepatitis respectively. It has been shown that Au-antigen-positive hepatitis can spread naturally from person to person and that serum containing antigen is infectious when given by mouth. Thus the old teaching that serum hepatitis could be transmitted only by injection is not absolutely true; nevertheless, the great majority of infections are acquired parenterally. We know little about the excretion of the antigen in the faeces and urine.

At any rate, the detection of Australia antigen in the serum of blood donors has been a most important advance in blood transfusion technique, for at last we have a means whereby recipients may be protected against a dangerous hazard. The antigen is demonstrated by immunological methods (gel diffusion, immunoeloctrophoresis, complement fixation, and other more complicated tests) using specific antibody obtained from haemophiliacs or from immunised animals. Electron microscopy may also be helpful. There is recent evidence that several strains of Au antigen exist. One, the ay strain, which is frequent in drug addicts, is more likely to cause liver damage than is the other common strain, called ad.[71]

We do not know how much cirrhosis and other chronic liver disease is due to Au-antigen-positive hepatitis, but quite a number of cases of macronodular cirrhosis show antigen in their serum. As regards active chronic hepatitis, primary billiary cirrhosis, and hepatoma the incidence varies, and is usually low.

HERPESVIRUS INFECTIONS

The herpesviruses are medium-sized, spherical, DNA-containing viruses. They produce large acidophilic, intranuclear inclusion bodies, and give rise to characteristic cytopathic effects in cells grown in tissue culture. The cells fuse into multinucleate giant forms.

The two most important herpesvirus infections of man are *herpes simplex* and *varicella-zoster*. This group of viruses does not possess a common antigen, and there is no cross-immunity between them.

Varicella and zoster.[45, 46] Though the well-known clinical features of these two infections are poles apart, there is good evidence that they are both caused by the same virus.

It has been recognized for a long time that children in contact with patients suffering from zoster tend to contract chickenpox, and this observation has been reproduced experimentally in susceptible children. The chickenpox so produced differs in no respect, either clinically or serologically, from chickenpox acquired from another child in the usual way, and the patient is subsequently rendered immune to chickenpox. A patient who already has had chickenpox will not acquire it after exposure to zoster.

Virus material derived from the vesicle fluids or crusts of chickenpox and zoster lesions produces identical cytopathic effects in tissue cultures of human amnion cells, and there is no antigenic difference between the two. The histology of zoster and chickenpox vesicles is also similar: the formation of multinucleate giant epithelial cells containing intranuclear inclusion bodies. There is no growth on the chorio-allantoic membrane of fertile eggs.

It is believed that after an attack of chickenpox the virus lies latent in the sensory ganglia of the nevous system, and is subsequently reactivated by some intercurrent episode, e.g. physical disease or psychological trauma.[47] It produces lesions specifically in the posterior root ganglia of the spinal, trigeminal, or facial nerves, and from there infection spreads down the nerve fibres to the skin of the dermatome, and also sometimes upwards to the posterior columns of the spinal cord. Occasionally infection may spread to the anterior horn cells and produce permanent paralysis. A rare complication is encephalitis.

Herpes simplex.[48] The virus of herpes simplex is one of the most widely distributed viruses in human beings. It is estimated that from 60–80 per cent of the population are affected. Of these only 10 per cent exhibit primary childhood lesions, such as *gingivo-stomatitis*, *keratoconjunctivitis*, and *vulvovaginitis*. *Eczema herpeticum* is described on p. 286. In some cases the virus may invade the internal organs and produce *meningo-encephalitis*. Worst of all is *generalised visceral herpes simplex*, a fatal condition of the newborn, in which white, necrotic lesions are present in many organs.[49]

Abrasions of the skin predispose to primary herpetic infection (*traumatic* or *inoculation herpes simplex*). A good example of this is the very painful *herpetic whitlow*,[50] which is seen in people who come into contact with naso-bronchial secretions. About 30 per cent of young adults lack antibodies to herpes simplex, and are susceptible to infection. The herpetic whitlow is therefore usually seen in anaesthetists and young doctors and nurses who care for patients with a tracheostomy. It also occurs in dentists

Usually, however, the primary infection remains sub-clinical, and the virus remains latent in the cells of the host. This symbiosis tends to be disturbed by intercurrent infections, e.g. the common cold, pneumonia, and malaria, and even, in very susceptible victims, by menstruation, emotional strain, and exposure to sunlight. There then develop typical *herpetic vesicles*, especially around the mucocutaneous junction of the lips and face. The skin of the genitalia is sometimes affected (*herpes genitalis*), and also occasionally the conjunctiva and cornea. Ocular involvement is serious because the keratitis leads to *dendritic ulceration*; scarring and impairment of vision may follow. Uveitis is an occasional complication. Herpes infections are common in T-lymphocyte deficiency, where they tend to assume a generalised, visceral character and are often fatal.

The virus is easily grown on the usual tissue culture systems, and is pathogenic to suckling mice, in which a fatal encephalitis is produced. On the chorio-allantoic membrane of fertile eggs characteristic pocks are produced. The virus is present in large amounts in the fluid of herpetic vesicles, the epithelial cells of which contain large intranuclear inclusion bodies similar to those of zoster and varicella.

It has been discovered that there are two antigenically distinct types of herpes simplex, called 1 and 2. *Herpesvirus hominis type 1* causes typical herpes febrilis of the face, mouth, pharynx, and cornea, and is also responsible for eczema herpeticum and herpes meningo-encephalitis. *Herpesvirus hominis type 2* causes herpes genitalis and vulvovaginitis, and also neonatal herpes.[51]

5-iodo-2'-deoxyuridine is used in the theraphy of herpes-simplex infections (p. 281).

Cytomegalic inclusion disease. This is another herpesvirus infection, and it is caused by the *cytomegalovirus*. It occurs most often in newborn infants to whom it is transmitted transplacentally.

Cytomegalic inclusion disease may develop as a fulminating lethal infection in the newborn, and at necropsy the parenchymatous cells of many organs, e.g. salivary glands, pancreas, liver, kidneys, and bronchial epithelium, are found to be distended by large intranuclear inclusion bodies (see Fig. 22.6, p. 275). The neonatal infection is not always fatal, but survivors are usually mentally retarded and microcephalic. A primary infection is not uncommon in young children below the age of five years, and they may excrete the virus for long periods in the throat and urine. Such children are often symptomless, but may show evidence of liver damage from which they eventually recover, and there may also be protracted respiratory illnesses.

In older children and adults infection is usually subclinical, but a few develop a condition resembling infectious mononucleosis with a negative Paul-Bunnell reaction. Finally cytomegalic inclusion disease is an important opportunistic infection in patients on immunosuppressive therapy. It is evident that the clinical presentation of the disease closely mimics that of toxoplasmosis. The condition is widespread, though clinical manifestations are rather uncommon; many adults have complement-fixing antibodies in their serum.[52-54]

The virus, strains of which infect many different animals, grows on tissue-culture growths of fibroblasts derived from the same animal species.

Epstein-Barr Virus. This herpesvirus, which has important associations with Burkitt's tumour, nasopharyngeal carcinoma, and infectious mononucleosis, is discussed further in Chapters 29 and 50.

MEASLES

Measles is probably the most infectious of all diseases, and it is transmitted by patients during the prodromal period, which is characterised by catarrhal inflammation of many mucous surfaces. The infected secretion is inspired by the next victim, and the virus appears to multiply in the lymphoid tissue of the respiratory tract for some time before it breaks out to produce a viraemia, which marks the beginning of the prodromal period lasting 3–4 days. Once the eruption appears, the patient rapidly becomes less infective. A characteristic feature of measles is the appearance of typical giant cells in the hyperplastic lymphoid follicles. *Giant-cell pneumonia of infants*, in which similar cells are found in the interstitial tissue of the lungs, is a manifestation of measles, and the virus can be cultured from the lungs.[55]

The virus contains RNA and is related antigenically to the viruses of canine distemper and rinderpest. It grows in tissue culture systems of human kidney and embryonic lung, and from these it can be adapted on to the more usual cell systems. It produces a typical cytopathic effect in which large giant cells are formed, similar to the Warthin-Finkeldey cells seen in the lymphoid follicles.

Measles, though rarely fatal in civilised countries, is still a serious disease, for apart from pneumonic complications and otitis media it may cause neurological complications such as encephalitis. The rare *subacute sclerosing panencephalitis* is due to the recrudesence of activity of measles virus lying latent in the brain.[56] Measles vaccines are licensed for human use. The administration of live, attenuated, Edmonston strain vaccine produces good immunity, but is sometimes followed by a febrile illness which appears to be a mild attack of measles. This may be avoided by the simultaneous administration of vaccine with measles immune globulin in a separate syringe at another site. Alternatively, the further attenuated Schwartz strain vaccine can be used, but in either event the immune response is less satisfactory. Vaccination should not be carried out in pregnant women, in cases of tuberculosis, and in patients with leukaemia or other disease in which immunity is impaired.

An injection of measles immune globulin will prevent an attack of measles in an exposed individual if given within 5 days. A small dose of the globulin will result in a mild attack, and this may be preferable since active immunity will then follow.

RUBELLA

German measles is a comparatively trivial acute infectious fever in children associated with an evanescent macular eruption. The virus contains RNA but its morphology is still imperfectly known. It produces rather feeble cytopathic effects in cell systems. Amongst other animals only monkeys are susceptible to a mild degree.

The importance of rubella is that women who contract it in the first trimester of pregnancy sometimes bear congenitally deformed infants. The incidence of deformed children is about 25 per cent, and the first month of pregnancy is the most dangerous period. The usual abnormalities are heart lesions,[57] cataract, and deafness; mental deficiency is not common. Some of these infants are born with the congenital rubella syndrome consisting of thrombocytopenic purpura, hepatosplenomegaly, jaundice, and osteochondritis, and sometimes the typical eruption. Virus may be excreted from the nasopharynx and urine for over four months after birth, and doctors and nurses may be infected.[58]

Pregnant women exposed to rubella during the first trimester should be examined to assess their immune status. If rubella antibodies are present, infection of the fetus is unlikely. If antibodies are absent, the test should be repeated in one month's time. If there has been a rise in antibody titre, recent infection can be inferred and termination of pregnancy should be considered, the decision made depending upon the patient's moral and religious convictions. Human immune serum is available, but its value in prophylaxis is debatable.

Attenuated rubella vaccine is available, and it is recommended for children aged 5–10 yrs. It should not be given to pregnant women, nor to girls if there is any risk of them becoming pregnant.

INFECTIOUS WARTS AND PAPOVAVIRUS INFECTIONS

The common wart *verruca vulgaris* appears as a sessile, discrete papillary mass on the skin, commonly that of the hands and feet. Other variants are the flattened *plantar wart* on the soles of the feet, the fungating *condyloma acuminatum* on the labia and the penile sulcus, and also the *laryngeal papilloma* of children. The epidermis is thickened (acanthosis) and thrown into papillary folds. Vacuolation of the superficial cells in the stratum granulosum is characteristic.

These lesions may persist for many months, and then disappear as rapidly as they arose. Genital warts (condylomata acuminata) may rarely become malignant.

The causal agents of viral papillomata in man and animals, e.g. the Shope papilloma, form an important group of the *papovaviruses*. These are small, spherical DNA-containing viruses. In some warts inclusion bodies are prominent in the nucleus and virus is easily demonstrable in them by electron microscopy; cultivation of the virus in human embryonic skin has been reported[59, 60], but not substantiated. In those warts without nuclear inclusion bodies no virus has yet been isolated, a fact which suggests that there are at least two distinct agents. Warts have been transmitted to volunteers using filtrates of wart tissue; the incubation period varies from six weeks to eight months.

Papovaviruses are also responsible for other important animal tumours, notably the polyoma lesions mentioned on p. 384. The SV 40 virus, alluded to on p. 285, which has been isolated from batches of monkey kidney used in tissue cultures, is a papovavirus (of the polyoma group). It is oncogenic, and produces a typical vacuolation of the cells in culture, hence its alternative name *vacuolating agent*. It is the first two letters of these three viruses that have been put together to form the name papovavirus (*PA*pilloma, *PO*lyoma, and *VA*cuolating agent).

Recently it has been discovered that a rare demyelinating disease of the central nervous system, *progressive multifocal leucoencephalopathy*,[61, 62] which is seen most often as a complication of lymphomata, is due to opportunistic infection by polyomaviruses of undetermined type. Some resemble the SV 40 virus. It is possible that these viruses lie latent in the tissues and are activated by states of immunosuppression, especially involving T lymphocytes. A polyomavirus has been isolated from the urine of an immunosuppressed patient with a renal homograft.[61] Progressive multifocal leucoencephalopathy is a rapidly fatal disease in which the white matter softens and disintegrates into a pulpy mass.

SLOW VIRUSES

Sheep and goats are prone to a degenerative neurological disease called *scrapie*, the main features of which are severe pruritus, incoordination, paralysis, and death in a few weeks. The incubation period is several years, hence the name "slow" virus. The disease can be transmitted to other animals (and also mice) from infected material, but the agent is so resistant to sterilising and other destructive procedures that it appears not to be a virus at all, for a nucleic acid or nucleoprotein could not withstand these procedures.[63, 64] At present the nature of the scrapie agent is under investigation. An interesting speculation is that it is a substance which complements an incompetent or incomplete virus which is present in, or part of, the normal cell.

There is a neurological disorder that affects certain remote tribes living in the highlands of New Guinea. It is called *kuru*, and its pathology resembles that of scrapie. The disease has been reproduced in chimpanzees inoculated with human brain material, and the incubation period is several years. It is suspected that cannibalism is responsible for transmitting the disease to each succeeding generation.[65]

A rare encephalopathy of man, *Creutzfeldt-Jakob disease*, the main features of which are ataxia, dementia, abnormal movements, stupor, and death in a few months (as in kuru), can also be transmitted to species of laboratory primates, and it would appear that both conditions are slow virus infections.[66]

Animal Viruses Transmissable Directly to Human Beings

Amongst virus diseases in this category are *cow-pox* and *contagious pustular dermatitis of sheep* (*orf*) which produce characteristic lesions on the skin of farm-workers; *Newcastle disease of fowls*, a paramyxovirus infection, which produces severe conjunctivitis in laboratory workers and fowl-keepers; *Virus B infection of monkeys*, a herpesvirus which produces a fatal encephalitis in animal-house keepers who are bitten by monkeys; *lymphocytic choriomeningitis*, a disease endemic in mice and which causes a lymphocytic meningitis when the secretions of these animals are inhaled; arboviruses and *yellow fever*; *rabies*.

Rabies[67] virus is transmitted to human beings by the bite of a rabid animal, usually a dog or cat. Sometimes wolves, jackals, badgers, opossums, and vampire bats may be responsible, and of these only the bat harbours the virus in a latent form. Foxes and skunks are the main wildlife reservoirs in North America. The virus multiplies locally, and then travels up the damaged nerve fibres to reach the brain and spinal cord. The incubation period is prolonged, sometimes lasting several months, but an almost invariably fatal encephalitis follows (a recovered case has recently been reported[68]).

The virus spreads from the brain along the nerves to the secreting glands and the cornea, and the condition can be diagnosed during life by making corneal impressions and performing fluorescent antibody staining on them.[69] A similar technique can be used on post-mortem brain smears. In addition, Negri bodies are present in the neurones, especially of the hippocampus. The diagnosis is confirmed by mouse transmission.

People bitten by a potentially rabid animal should be immunised. Hyperimmune antirabies serum (horse) should be given, and a quantity of it may be infiltrated around the wound. Active immunisation must then be started if there is the slightest suspicion that the animal was rabid. At least

14 daily injections of vaccine are given subcutaneously into the abdomen at different sites to prevent local reactions. The duck-embryo vaccine is recommended. Semple's nervous-tissue vaccine prepared from rabbit brain and inactivated by phenol may be used, but is occasionally responsible for the development of allergic peripheral neuritis or the more serious encephalomyelitis (pp. 171 and 207).

Dogs, cats, and cattle in endemic areas should be immunised by the Flury strain of living, attenuated, egg-adapted virus. It is not licensed for human use.

CLASSIFICATION OF VIRUSES

There is as yet no completely accepted classification of viruses, but a scheme based on nucleic acid, capsid symmetry, and the presence or absence of outer envelope is now being tentatively used.

RNA-containing Viruses

Picornaviruses. These are small (20–35 nm in size), the capsid has a cubical symmetry, and there is no outer envelope. Important members are the enteroviruses and rhinoviruses.

Reoviruses. These are about 70 nm in size, the capsid has a cubical symmetry, and there is no outer envelope. Their pathogenicity for man is by no means proven, but they are possibly the cause of mild upper-respiratory-tract infections and also diarrhoea in children.

Myxoviruses. These vary in size from 80 nm to 120 nm, the capsid has a helical symmetry, and there is an outer envelope. These are the viruses of influenza.

Paramyxoviruses. These differ from the myxoviruses in being larger (150–220 nm) and having a capsid with a wider diameter, but they are closely related. The viruses of mumps and Newcastle disease of fowls, and the para-influenza viruses come into this group.

Arboviruses. These are small (20–100 nm), and the capsid symmetry is cubical in some viruses—which are then called *togaviruses*—and helical in others. There is an outer envelope. The important viruses are those of encephalitis,

yellow fever, dengue, and sandfly fever, all of which are togaviruses. Most of the viruses causing haemorrhagic fevers are also togaviruses.

Rhabdoviruses. The name, derived from the Greek *rhabdos*, a rod, applies to a group of short cylindrical viruses with one end rounded and the other truncated. They are from 150–180 nm in size, the capsid has a helical symmetry, and there is an outer envelope. The important rhabdovirus infection of man is rabies.

Other RNA viruses. There are a number of RNA viruses whose systematic position still awaits elucidation. The viruses of measles, dog distemper, and rinderpest closely resemble paramyxoviruses morphologically, as does also the respiratory syncytial virus, but it has large surface projections. The name *coronavirus* has been suggested for this virus and those of mouse hepatitis and avian infectious bronchitis. Then there are the *arenoviruses* noted on p. 289; the name is derived from the sandy granules seen in the virus particles under electron microscopy.

DNA-containing Viruses

Adenoviruses. These vary in size from 60–90 nm, the capsid has a cubical symmetry, and there is no outer membrane. They cause upper-respiratory-tract infections and keratoconjunctivitis.

Papovaviruses. These are about 50 nm in size, the capsid has cubical symmetry, and there is no outer envelope. They cause verrucae in man and more definitely neoplastic lesions in other animals.

Herpesviruses. These are about 150 nm in diameter, the capsid has a cubical symmetry, and there is an outer envelope. They cause herpes simplex, varicella-zoster, cytomegalic inclusion disease, and infectious mononucleosis.

Poxviruses. These are large, varying in size from 200 nm to 300 nm, the capsid has a complex symmetry, and there are outer envelopes. They cause smallpox, vaccinia, and molluscum contagiosum in man. There are specific pox diseases in animals, and also orf in sheep and myxomatosis in rabbits.

REFERENCES

1. STUART-HARRIS, C. H. (1962). *British Medical Journal*, i, 1779.
2. LENNETTE, E. H. *et al.* (1958). *American Journal of Hygiene*, **68**, 272.
3. Leading Article (1967). *British Medical Journal*, iv, 503.
4. JAVETT, S. N. *et al.* (1956). *Journal of Pediatrics*, **48**, 1.
5. HEATHFIELD, K. W. G. *et al.* (1967). *Quarterly Journal of Medicine*, **36**, 579.
6. Leading Article (1968). *British Medical Journal*, i, 722.
7. Medical Research Council Report (1956). *Lancet*, ii, 1223.
8. STUART-HARRIS, C. H. (1964). *Proceedings of the Royal Society of Medicine*, **57**, 459.
9. DANE, D. S. (1964). *Ibid.*, 462.
10. Leading Article (1971). *British Medical Journal*, i, 686.
11. DANE, D. S. *et al.* (1961). *British Medical Journal*, ii, 269.
12. DANE, D. S., DICK. G. W. A. and BRIGGS, E. M. (1963). *Lancet*, i, 940.
13. HAYFLICK, L. *et al.* (1962). *American Journal of Hygiene*, **75**, 240.
14. WILSON, G. S. and MILES, A. A. (1964). In *Topley and Wilson's Principles of Bacteriology and Immunity*, 5th edn, p. 2268. London: Arnold.
15. OVERFIELD, T. M. and BRODY, J. A. (1966). *Journal of Pediatrics*, **69**, 640.

16. POSTLETHWAITE, R. *et al.* (1967). *Journal of Hygiene (London)*, **65**, 281.
17. FENNER, F. and BURNET, F. M. (1957). *Virology*, **4**, 305.
18. COCHRAN, W., CONNOLLY, J. H. and THOMPSON, I. D. (1963). *British Medical Journal*, ii, 285.
19. ENTWISTLE, D. M., BRAY, P. T. and LAURENCE, K. M. (1962). *British Medical Journal*, ii, 238.
20. TUCKER, S. M. and SIBSON, D. E. (1962). *Ibid.*, 237.
21. DICK, G. (1971). *British Medical Journal*, iii, 163.
22. Leading Article (1971). *British Medical Journal*, iii, 129 and 323.
23. Leading Article (1967). *British Medical Journal*, iv, 253.
24. BAUER, D. J. (1967). In *Modern Trends in Medical Virology*, I. Edited by R. B. Heath and A. P. Waterson, p. 49. London: Butterworths.
25. STUART-HARRIS, C. H. (1962). *British Medical Journal*, ii, 869.
26. Ibid. (1959). *British Medical Bulletin*, **15**, 216.
27. BEALE, A. J. *et al.* (1958). *British Medical Journal*, i, 302.
28. PEREIRA, H. G. (1959). *British Medical Bulletin*, **15**, 225.
29. ISRAEL, M. S. (1962). *Journal of Pathology and Bacteriology*, **84**, 169.
30. JONES, B. R. (1962). *Transactions of the Ophthalmological Society of the United Kindgom*, **82**, 621.
31. POTTER, C. W. (1967). In *Modern Trends in Medical Virology*, p. 162. *loc. cit.*
32. NUMAZAKI, Y. *et al.* (1968). *New England Journal of Medicine*, **278**, 700.
33. TYRRELL, D. A. J. and PARSONS, R. (1960). *Lancet*, i, 239.
34. WILSON, G. S. and MILES, A. A. (1964). p. 2332, *loc. cit.*
35. GORDON SMITH, C. E. (1959). *British Medical Bulletin*, **15**, 235.
36. WALKER, G. M. *et al.* (1962). *Transactions of the Royal Society of Tropical Medicine and Hygiene*, **56**, 496.
37. Leading Article (1971). *Lancet*, ii, 858.
38. Leading Article (1972). *British Medical Journal*, iv, 253 and *Lancet*, i, 576.
39. Various Authors (1972). *British Medical Bulletin*, **28**, No. 2.
40. Leading Article (1970). *British Medical Journal*, iv, 255.
41. COSSART, V. E. (1971). *Journal of Clinical Pathology*, **24**, 394.
42. Various Authors (1971). *Proceedings of the Royal Society of Medicine*, **64**, 273.
43. Leading Article (1971). *Lancet*, ii, 1242.
44. Leading Article (1971). *Lancet*, ii, 805.
45. WILSON, G. S. and MILES, A. A. (1964). p. 2302, *loc. cit.*
46. DOWNIE, A. W. (1959). *British Medical Bulletin*, **15**, 197.
47. BAMFORD, J. A. C. and BOUNDY, C. A. P. (1968). *Medical Journal of Australia*, **1**, 524 and 528.
48. WILSON, G. S. and MILES, A. A. (1964). p. 2296, *loc. cit.*
49. BIRD, T. *et al.* (1963). *Journal of Clinical Pathology*, 16, 423.
50. Leading Article (1971). *British Medical Journal*, iv, 444.
51. DUDGEON, J. A. (1970). In *Modern Trends in Medical Virology*, 2, p. 78. Edited by R. B. Heath and A. P. Waterson. London: Butterworths.
52. HANSHAW, J. B. (1966). *New England Journal of Medicine*, **275**, 476.
53. CANGIR, A. *et al.* (1967). *Journal of the American Medical Association*, **201**, 612.
54. Leading Article (1971). *British Medical Journal*, i, 687.
55. ENDERS, J. F. *et al.* (1959). *New England Journal of Medicine*, **261**, 875.
56. Leading Article (1972). *Lancet*, ii, 263.
57. CAMPBELL, M. (1961). *British Medical Journal*, i, 691.
58. DUDGEON, J. A. (1967). In *Modern Trends in Medical Virology*, p. 111. *loc. cit.*
59. OROSZLAN, S. and RICH, M. A. (1964). *Science*, **146**, 531.
60. NOYES, W. F. (1965). *Virology*, **25**, 358.
61. Leading Article (1972). *Lancet*, i, 826.
62. FLEWETT, T. H. (1972). *British Medical Journal*, i, 667.
63. GIBBONS, R. A. and HUNTER, G. D. (1967). *Nature (London)*, **215**, 1041.
64. Leading Article (1967). *Lancet*, ii, 705.
65. MATHEWS, J. D., GLASSE, R. and LINDENBAUM, S. (1968). *Lancet*, ii, 449.
66. Leading Article (1972). *Lancet*, i, 418.
67. Various Authors (1971). *Proceedings of the Royal Society of Medicine*, **64**, 225.
68. HATTWICK, M. A. W. *et al.* (1972). *Annals of Internal Medicine*, **76**, 931.
69. Leading Article (1971). *British Medical Journal*, ii, 483.
70. PRINCE, A. M. *et al.* (1972). *Lancet*, ii, 247.
71. Leading Article (1973). *British Medical Journal*, i, 127.

Chapter 24. Disorders of Growth ✓

Most organs of the body possess a considerable reserve of tissue which can be brought into play whenever additional work is demanded of them. At rest the inactive cells are maintained by an intermittent blood flow through their supplying capillaries. This mechanism results in an economical use of the circulation, and explains why noxious substances spread by the blood stream may nevertheless produce patchy effects. When more work has to be peformed, the shut-down vessels dilate and the organ shows active hyperaemia. This is well illustrated by the tremendous increase in blood flow through the salivary glands which occurs during periods of active secretion.

Growth Potentiality of Cells

In addition to this reserve mechanism, organs or tissues subjected to prolonged excessive strain respond by increasing their bulk. This may be done by either increasing the size of each constituent cell, or increasing the total cell number; which of these occurs depends upon the growth potentiality of the cells involved. Usually both occur together. Three classes of cells are described:[1, 2]

Labile Cells. These undergo frequent division throughout life to replace those lost through differentiation and subsequent desquamation.

The cells of lymph nodes, bone marrow, and most of the covering or protective epithelia (skin, endometrium, alimentary, respiratory, and urinary mucosa) come into this category.

Stable cells. These cells likewise show a definite pattern of replication with cells lost by wear and tear being replaced by the mitotic activity of others. Since the life span of each cell is long, the term stable is appropriate. DNA synthesis, when it takes place, occurs at a rate similar to that of other cells. It is the interval between mitoses which is long, and therefore very few mitotic figures are seen in a section of tissue from a normal adult. However, the cells never lose the ability to divide and can do so with great rapidity if suitably stimulated. This group includes most of the secretory epithelial structures (liver, kidney, pancreas, and endocrine glands).

Permanent cells. These non-replicating cells lose the ability to divide either at birth or shortly thereafter. Neurones and, to a lesser extent, muscle cells, striated, smooth, and cardiac, provide the important examples. Although mitoses are not seen in these cells, DNA synthesis and renewal can occur.[3] Striated, and especially smooth, muscle has a decided power of regeneration (see p. 120), but this cannot be compared with that of stable cells.

The factors which control the growth and differentiation of cells are largely unknown. Nevertheless, abnormalities of these two functions are frequent, forming an important part of many disease processes. They may be considered under three headings:

1. *Abnormalities of cellular growth*, which are either *excesses* (hypertrophy and hyperplasia) or *decreases*, either developmental (agenesis and hypoplasia) or acquired after full development (atrophy and aplasia).

2. *Abnormalities of cellular differentiation*, which comprise metaplasia and certain other dysplasias.

3. *Neoplasia*, a completely abnormal cellular growth considered in the chapters that follow.

Quantitative Abnormalities of Cellular Growth

Excessive growth. Tissues composed of labile or stable cells respond to an increased demand for work primarily by multiplication, but may also show some increase in size. Permanent cells either show no morphological change (neurones), or else only an increase in size (muscle). An increase in the cell number is called *hyperplasia*, and an increase in individual cell size is *hypertrophy*. It therefore follows that both conditions can occur in the presence of a stimulus; which occurs depends on whether the individual cells are capable of enlargement, multiplication, or both combined.

Both hyperplasia and hypertrophy are usually related to a tangible stimulus, which is often a basically physiological one acting to excess. The most important stimulus is an *increased demand for function*. As will be seen, this may take the form of increased muscular work in response to an abnormal load, an increased production of blood cells in response to hypoxia or infection, a thickening of protective epithelium in response to external trauma, or an increased secretion of a gland in response to some external need.

Some hyperplasias are related to an increased secretion of hormones, either physiologically during puberty or pregnancy or else pathologically as when the hormone is secreted by a tumour.

Finally, hyperplasia may be idiopathic. Many of the commonest glandular hyperplasias come into this category, e.g. senile prostatic hyperplasia, cystic hyperplasia of the breast, and primary hyperthyroidism (which is often associated with an autoantibody in the serum, p. 297).

HYPERPLASIA

Definition. Hyperplasia is the increase in size of an organ or tissue due to an increase in the number of its specialised constituent cells. Enlargements due to congestion, oedema, inflammation, amyloid infiltration, or tumour formation must be distinguished from hyperplasia.

It is important to note that those hyperplasias due to a specific stimulus persist only for so long as that stimulus is applied. When it is removed, the tissue tends to revert to its normal size. In this respect hyperplasia differs from neoplasia, for neoplastic tissue continues to grow even when the stimulus is withdrawn.

While the concept of hyperplasia is traditionally a morphological one, it must never be forgotten that the increase in size of the organ is accompanied by a corresponding increase in function. Nowhere is this more apparent than in hyperplasia of the endocrine glands.

Hyperplasia in the Endocrine Glands[4]

In the endocrine glands hyperplasia may be either diffuse or focal. Often it starts by causing diffuse enlargement of the gland (or glands, as the case may be), but later one or more focal, circumscribed, discrete nodules appear. These are often called adenomata, but it is unlikely that they are neoplastic; nodular hyperplasia is a better term. Malignancy seldom supervenes.

Parathyroids. In osteitis fibrosa cystica (von Recklinghausen's disease) the parathyroids are enlarged, usually as the result of diffuse hyperplasia, but sometimes a localised nodule ("adenoma") is present. The stimulus for this is not known.

In chronic renal failure there is a retention of phosphate with a rise in its blood level. The associated fall in serum calcium acts as a stimulus for parathyroid hyperplasia. The secondary hyperparathyroidism may give rise to the bony changes of "renal rickets" (see Chapter 42).

Thyroid. (*a*) A degree of thyroid hyperplasia occurs in girls at puberty and particularly during pregnancy. Presumably there is an increased demand for thyroxine at these periods. The maintenance of thyroid function is governed by the continuous secretion of thyrotrophic hormone from the pituitary, and presumably in these cases the secretion is increased.

(*b*) On the other hand the output of thyrotrophic hormone is itself regulated by the thyroid secretion. This "feed-back" mechanism can be interrupted by drugs of the thiouracil type which block the synthesis of thyroxine, and by a low-iodine diet which prevents its formation. The pituitary secretes large quantities of thyrotrophic hormone, which in turn leads to thyroid hyperplasia (Figs. 24.1 and 24.2).

(*c*) Marked thyroid hyperplasia occurs in primary thyrotoxicosis, or Graves's disease. There is also lymphoid hyperplasia, seen not only in the thyroid, but also in the lymph nodes, thymus, and spleen. There are accumulations of lymphocytes in the muscles ("lymphorrhages"), and these

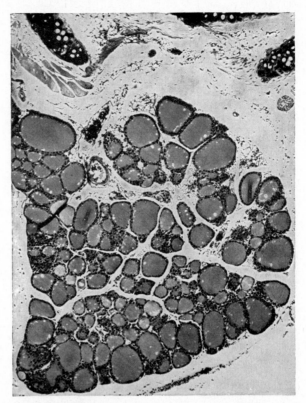

Figure 24.1

Normal mouse thyroid. Note the evenly disposed acini of fairly uniform size filled with colloid. The epithelium lining the acini is of low columnar type. This pattern is basically similar to that of the human thyroid. ×90. (*From Israel, M. S. and Ellis, I. R.* (1960), Brit. J. Cancer, **14**, 206)

contribute to the swelling of the ocular muscles that plays an important part in the exophthalmos often present in the disease. A thyroid stimulating factor has been isolated from the sera of about half the cases.[5] It differs from thyrotrophic hormone in having a much longer stimulating effect on the thyroid. It is called LATS (long-acting thyroid stimulator), and it is associated with the IgG fraction of the plasma. At present it is believed that LATS is an autoantibody, but how it acts and the nature of the corresponding antigen are still not clear. Since it is often absent, and is most pronounced in cases where there is localised, or pretibial, myxoedema, it is a matter of debate whether LATS causes the thyrotoxicosis or is merely a product of the disease.[5]

In all these conditions the hyperplastic acini are empty or filled with palely-staining colloid. The epithelium is columnar and often so exuberant that it invaginates into the collapsed acini.

Some of the greatest thyroid enlargements are found in colloid and nodular goitres, where in addition to hyperplasia there are also areas in which the acini are distended with thyroglobulin, which gives rise to the translucent appearance seen macroscopically. The cells of these acini are flattened

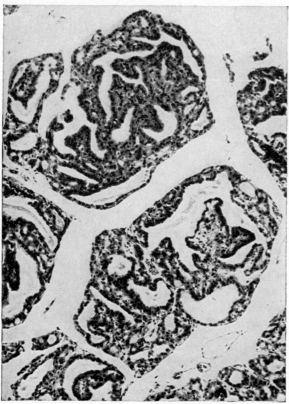

Figure 24.2
Thyroid of a mouse to which thiouracil has been administered. The gland is the seat of nodular hyperplasia. Two nodules are included in the section. They consist of irregular, elongated acini which are distorted by the papillary invagination of an exuberant columnar epithelium. The acini are empty. ×120. *(From Israel, M. S. and Ellis, I. R. (1960), Brit. J. Cancer, 14, 206)*

and inactive. This accumulation of "colloid" is due to phases of involution, and the hyperplasia to bouts of hyperactivity. In due course a grossly nodular pattern is produced, which is sometimes described as adenoma formation, but it is better to class it as hyperplasia. The usual cause of a nodular goitre is an absolute or relative iodine deficiency acting intermittently over many years. In such lesions, although the cause may be removed, return to normal is impossible owing to secondary degenerative changes, e.g. cyst formation, haemorrhage, and calcification.

Adrenal Cortex. Hyperplasia of the adrenal cortex occurs after trauma (see p. 430), and also after the therapeutic administration of ACTH. Most adrenal hyperplasia is, however, idiopathic; a pituitary or hypothalamic causation is possible but unproven. As with the thyroid gland, the hyperplasia is often nodular.

Hyperplasia, unaccompanied by evidence of overfunction, is a frequent incidental finding in routine *post-mortem* examinations. When there is evidence of oversecretion, the syndromes which result depend upon the particular hormones involved. The latter can be divided into three groups, and therefore three main syndromes are produced; mixed cases also occur.

Hydrocortisone (or cortisol)—Cushing's syndrome.

Sex hormones (mostly androgens)—adrenogenital syndrome (adrenal virilism).

Salt-regulating hormone (aldosterone)—Conn's syndrome.

Cushing's Syndrome.[6, 7] This is characterised by abdominal striae, polycythaemia, hypertension, glycosuria, osteoporosis, and in women hypertrichosis and amenorrhoea. There is a striking redistribution of fat, which results in obesity confined to the trunk, neck, and face. The characteristic moon face is partly attributable to this, but there is also fluid retention (see p. 495). All the signs and symptoms of Cushing's syndrome can be reproduced by prolonged excessive administration of glucocorticosteroids or ACTH.

The adrenal glands may be the seat of a simple adenoma, carcinoma, or bilateral hyperplasia.[8, 9] The cause of the last is undecided. Excessive ACTH production by the pituitary, perhaps as a result of hypothalamic overactivity, has been postulated, but remains unproven. The usual pituitary change in Cushing's syndrome is hyalinisation of the basophil cells. It may be that the adrenals are unduly sensitive to the effects of a normal amount of ACTH. Sometimes a pituitary tumour, either basophil or chromophobe, is present or becomes apparent at a later period after adrenalectomy. Its further overactivity can lead to marked hyperpigmentation due to ACTH or MSH overproduction.

Adrenogenital syndrome.[10] This is characterised by masculinisation in the female and precocious puberty in the male. When the condition commences *in utero*, the syndrome is made manifest at or shortly after birth. In the female pseudohermaphroditism may occur, and is later followed by masculinisation. It is usually due to bilateral cortical hyperplasia.

In cases of later onset an adenoma or carcinoma is the usual cause. With a carcinoma the picture may be a complex one and include Cushing's syndrome, glycosuria, and virilism. In adult males feminisation occasionally occurs.

The administration of glucocorticosteroids to cases of the adrenogenital syndrome due to adrenal hyperplasia leads to a remarkable amelioration of symptoms. This is mediated by depression of the pituitary. In the female progressive feminisation occurs, and the urinary output of 17-oxosteroids drops. When the virilism is due to an adrenal tumour, these agents are without effect. This provides an excellent example of the difference between hyperplasia and neoplasia: hyperplasia is in this case under the control of the pituitary, while neoplasia is not.

Conn's syndrome[11] (primary hyperaldosteronism). It is usually due to a tumour. There is hypertension, sodium retention, and excessive potassium loss, which may lead to periodic attacks of muscular weakness. There is no oedema.

Congenital adrenal hyperplasia is described on p. 39.

Pituitary. The feed-back mechanism that controls

thyrotrophic hormone secretion has already been mentioned. In myxoedema there is a considerable hyperplasia of the pituitary "thyrotrophs", which are numbered among the basophil cells.[12, 13]

Likewise after castration there is hyperplasia of the pituitary "gonadotrophs", which are also basophil cells. Oestrogen, like thyroxine, acts against its related trophic hormone (in this case the gonadotrophic hormones).

An idiopathic hyperplasia (or a true adenoma) of the acidophil cells leads to gigantism before the epiphyses have fused, and acromegaly in older patients. Acromegaly is an extreme example of generalised hyperplasia due to an excess of a hormone (growth hormone); there is an increase in size of all the viscera (splanchnomegaly) as well as the soft tissue and the bones, especially those of the acral, or distal, parts (the jaw, hands, and feet). Other effects are glycosuria, kyphosis, and hypertension.

Basophil hyperplasia may rarely be associated with Cushing's syndrome.

Proliferations of the chromophobe cells do not have a primary secretory function; they act by interfering with the pituitary and hypothalamic areas.

Islets of Langerhans.[14, 15] Islet-cell hyperplasia occurs in the child of a diabetic mother. Treatment of this rare condition is life-saving. The infant is subjected to a high

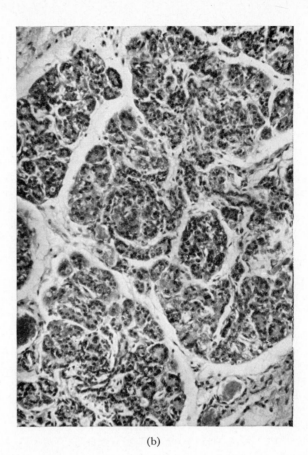

(b)

Figure 24.3
Hyperplasia of the islets of Langerhans. (*a*) This is a section of the pancreas of a newborn infant, whose mother was a diabetic. The greatly increased size of the islet of Langerhans is very obvious when compared with an islet of a normal newborn child, which is quite inconspicuous amid the acinar tissue (*b*). The enlargement is due to a proliferation of the constituent cells. × 150.

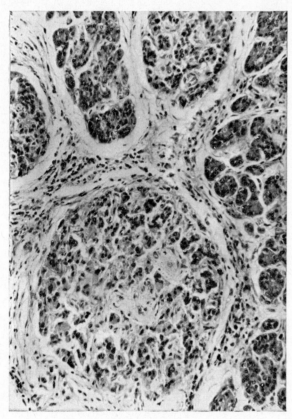

Figure 24.3 (a)

blood sugar level while *in utero*, and its islet cells respond by hyperplasia (Fig. 24.3). At birth these continue to secrete excess insulin, and therefore severe hypoglycaemia rapidly develops unless glucose is given. This hyperplasia occurs even in the children of prediabetic women. Its true nature is more obscure than would appear at first sight.

Interstitial cells of the testis. Hyperplasia may be induced by oestrogen administration in animals, but is rare in man.

Hyperplasia in the Target Organs of the Endocrine Glands

Breasts. Hyperplasia of the epithelial tissue and surrounding specialised connective tissue is a normal feature of the female breast at puberty, during pregnancy and lactation, and to a lesser extent towards the end of each menstrual cycle. These changes are brought about by oestrogens, progesterone, and the pituitary mammotrophic hormone. Gross enlargement ("hypertrophy") of the female breast, which occasionally occurs at puberty, is generally due to an excessive accumulation of fat rather than hyperplasia of specialised breast tissue.

An important idiopathic hyperplasia of the breast is the condition alternatively called chronic mastitis, *mammary dysplasia*, and *cystic hyperplasia*. The first name is a poor one as there is no chronic inflammation except as an occasional secondary event, and the noncommital term dysplasia is to be preferred since cyst formation is not invariable. In the early stages there is overgrowth of connective tissue and some dilatation of the ducts. In the next stage there is epithelial overgrowth so that the ducts become filled with cells (*epitheliosis*), or contain papillary ingrowths. New formation of glandular tissue produces the picture described as *adenosis*. In the most advanced stage the ducts form large cysts, and they are often lined by thin atrophic epithelium. This is the classical cystic disease of the breast; the blue-domed cyst is an extreme example. The condition is believed to be due to imbalance of ovarian hormones, probably excess oestrogen and too little progesterone. It is not precancerous.

The administration of oestrogen to the male (e.g. stilboestrol therapy in prostatic cancer) leads to a marked enlargement of the breasts. This is called *gynaecomastia*. It is also seen in advanced liver disease (p. 539) and rarely in carcinoma of the lung (p. 344).

Prostate. Senile enlargement of the prostate is due to epithelial hyperplasia as well as an increase in the fibro-muscular element. The condition is common over the age of 60 years, and is confusingly called "benign prostatic hypertrophy" or "adenomatosis of the prostate". The enlargement is confined to the lateral lobes and the middle lobe; the latter often projects over the urethral orifice and acts like a ball-valve. The atypical proliferation that occurs in the posterior lobes of old men is described in Chapter 25 under "latent cancer".

Endometrium. The endometrium is capable of marked hyperplasia as a response to the stimulation of prolonged oestrogen secretion. It may reach a thickness of over 1 cm, and be difficult to distinguish histologically from carcinoma. Such hyperplasia is seen in connexion with granulosa-cell tumour of the ovary, and more commonly in women given large doses of oestrogen therapeutically for menopausal symptoms.

An idiopathic endometrial hyperplasia is seen in metropathia haemorrhagica. There is an increased secretion of oestrogen, and the cause is probably ovarian dysfunction.

Changes of Puberty. The increase in size of the gonads and the secondary sexual organs may all be regarded as examples of physiological hyperplasia.

Covering Epithelia

The covering epithelia of the skin, mouth, alimentary tract, and respiratory passages are apt to undergo hyperplasia when confronted with any persistent traumatising agent ("chronic irritant"). The skin shows epidermal hyperplasia under the

mechanical trauma of an ill-fitting shoe when a corn develops. Likewise an ill-fitting denture leads to hyperplasia of the underlying gingiva.

Chronic inflammatory lesions lead to considerable hyperplasia of the involved epithelium. In the skin hyperplasia is a feature of many intrinsic diseases such as psoriasis, chronic dermatitis, and lichen planus. It is feature of some virus infections, being evanescent in chickenpox and prolonged in verruca vulgaris. The most extreme example of such epithelial hyperplasia is called pseudoepitheliomatous

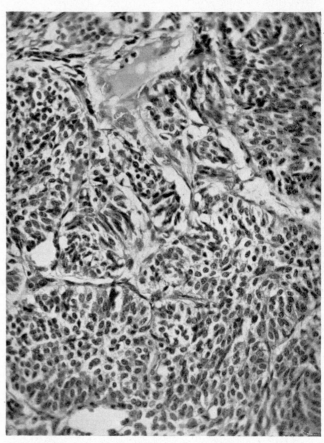

Figure 24.4
"Tumourlet" of lung composed of regular, evenly staining cells. The appearances resemble those of a bronchial "adenoma", but the lesions are multiple, self-limiting, and hyperplastic in nature. ×230. (*From Cunningham, G. J., Nassau, E. and Walter, J. B.* (1958), *Thorax,* **13,** 64)

hyperplasia and is described on p. 301. The "tumourlets" found in fibrotic lung bear some resemblance to bronchial carcinoid or carcinoma, but they are of small size, the cells are regular, and mitoses absent (Fig. 24.4). Likewise in cholecystitis glandularis proliferans seen in chronic cholecystitis, the excellent differentiation together with an awareness of the existence of the condition prevent a mistaken diagnosis of carcinoma.

Kidney

Removal of one kidney results in a compensatory enlargement of the other; although sometimes called hypertrophy, this is best considered as regeneration (see p. 124).

Bone Marrow

Pronounced hyperplasia is seen in the haematopoietic tissue when there is a demand for more blood cells. The erythroid series of cells proliferate in all types of anaemia except that due to primary bone-marrow aplasia. The cellular marrow extends into the long bones of the adult (normally filled with fatty marrow), while in childhood extramedullary foci of erythropoiesis may occur in the liver, spleen, and other organs. An extreme example of this is seen in erythroblastosis fetalis.

Erythroid hyperplasia producing secondary polycythaemia occurs in hypoxic states, e.g. living at a high altitude, in pulmonary disease, and in congenital cyanotic heart disease.

In infection it is the white-cell precursors which are affected.

RE System and Lymphoid Tissue

Both undergo hyperplasia in chronic infection and following antigenic stimulation. This is well-illustrated by the splenomegaly of malaria, kala-azar, and subacute infective endocarditis (see Chapter 30).

Liver

Following liver necrosis mitotic activity results in rapid replacement of the lost tissue. This is regeneration. It is doubtful whether true hyperplasia of the liver cells ever occurs. In cirrhosis of the liver there is, however, frequently considerable bile-duct hyperplasia (see p. 122).

PSEUDONEOPLASTIC HYPERPLASIA

Reference has been made to the difficulties in distinguishing nodular hyperplasia from benign neoplasia, particularly in the endocrine glands, the prostate, and the breast. From a practical point of view the distinction is unimportant since both processes are benign. There are, however, many examples of hyperplasia in which the mass of cells produced closely resembles a malignant tumour. Experience has taught that they are benign, since they either resolve spontaneously or respond to simple treatment. Their importance lies in their recognition, for a mistaken diagnosis can result in grave therapeutic errors. Almost any tissue can show such lesions and for their detailed descriptions special texts should be consulted.

Pseudomalignant Connective Tissue Hyperplasia

Pseudolymphoma. Pseudolymphoma of the skin[16] (Spiegler-Fendt sarcoid) appears as nodules of lymphoid tissue containing prominent follicles of large cells giving a histological picture which closely resembles that of the nodular type of lymphocytic lymphoma as seen in lymph nodes (see p. 402). Unlike the latter, however, the cutaneous lesions never become systematised nor develop into an overtly malignant disease. A somewhat similar lesion is the pseudolymphoma of the orbit, which closely resembles lymphocytic lymphoma (diffuse or nodular) histologically,[17] but again the behaviour is not one of malignancy. A similar benign lymphomatous lesion occurs in the rectum[18] and in the mediastinum.[19]

Pseudosarcoma in fibrous tissue. Examples of this are described on p. 321.

Pseudomalignant Epithelial Hyperplasia

Skin. Epidermal downgrowth and an appearance of dermal invasion by squamous cells is seen from time to time in a great variety of chronic ulcerating skin lesions ranging from blastomycosis and insect bites to basal-cell carcinoma. At times differentiation of these lesions from squamous-cell carcinoma is not possible, especially when small biopsy specimens alone are available for study.

A particularly good example of pseudoepitheliomatous hyperplasia is seen in *keratoacanthoma* (*molluscum sebaceum*).[20, 21] This lesion usually appears on the exposed parts, generally the face, grows for several months, and then involutes spontaneously. It consists of a central crater containing keratin surrounded by dysplastic squamous epithelium which closely resembles a squamous-cell carcinoma. The downgrowing epithelium extends to the level of the sebaceous glands and excites a surrounding inflammatory reaction. The nature of the process is debatable, but the most probable explanation is an exuberant epithelial hyperplasia to an irritant agent.

Pseudoepitheliomatous hyperplasia is also seen over a *myoblastoma*, a somewhat controversial lesion found most often on the tongue and occasionally in the skin. It is composed of very large polygonal and strap-shaped cells, the cytoplasm of which contains coarse eosinophilic granules. Some of these lesions are probably merely foci of degenerate muscle cells damaged during the wear and tear of mastication. But others are true tumours and may occasionally metastasise. The cell of origin of the lesion is disputed; by some it is thought to be the Schwann cell rather than muscle. The cause of the overlying epithelial hyperplasia is unknown.

There is little doubt that in the past pseudoepitheliomatous hyperplasia has often been confused with squamous-cell carcinoma, and that the good prognosis encountered in some series of carcinomata of the skin and lip was due to the inclusion of many non-neoplastic lesions.

Pseudoepitheliomatous hyperplasia is also described in other epithelial-covered surfaces, e.g. the mouth and the stomach adjacent to chronic ulcers.

HYPERTROPHY

Definition. Hypertrophy is the increase in size of an organ or tissue due to increase in size of its constituent specialised cells. Pure hypertrophy without accompanying hyperplasia occurs only in muscle, and the stimulus is almost always a mechanical one.

Smooth Muscle

Any obstruction to the outflow of the contents of a hollow muscular viscus results in hypertrophy of its muscle coat. The following may be listed as examples.

Bladder. Prostatic enlargement.
Urethral stricture.

The bladder wall is greatly thickened, and shows trabeculation due to the arrangement of its muscle fibres.

Alimentary tract.

Oesophagus Achalasia of the cardia.
Carcinoma.
Simple stricture.
Stomach Pyloric stenosis due to peptic ulcer or carcinoma.
Intestine Stricture following tuberculous enteritis or Crohn's disease.
Colon Carcinoma.

Hypertrophy is also seen in hollow organs when the wall is rigid and resists muscular contraction. This occurs in chronic inflammation, e.g. Crohn's disease, and in neoplastic infiltration. The hypertrophy in ulcerative colitis is not easily explained (p. 133).

Uterus. The myometrium shows the greatest hypertrophy known, and at a remarkably rapid rate. In pregnancy the muscle fibres eventually become ten times as long and five times as broad as those in the resting organ. The stimulus is partly mechanical and partly the effect of oestrogen.

Arteries. Muscular arteries show hypertrophy in hypertension.

Cardiac Muscle

Although the heart of a newborn child weighs only 30 g, it is believed that no further muscle cells are ever produced. The fibres increase in size seven-fold by the time adult life is reached. Any demand for increased work leads to hypertrophy of the fibres of the chambers affected. The stimulus is probably the stretching which results from the additional strain, and the ability of the heart to respond in this way constitutes part of the cardiac reserve (see Chapter 40).

Hypertrophy is best seen in the left ventricle (Fig. 24.5). Systemic hypertension, aortic valvular disease, and mitral regurgitation are common causes of enlargement. The biggest heart of all is the *cor bovinum*. This occurs when a heart with good coronary blood supply is subjected to overwork over a long period. Combined aortic and mitral regurgitation is the commonest cause.

Right ventricular hypertrophy occurs in left-to-right shunts (due to congenital heart disease), pulmonary and mitral valve lesions, pulmonary hypertension, and in chronic lung disease like emphysema and silicosis.

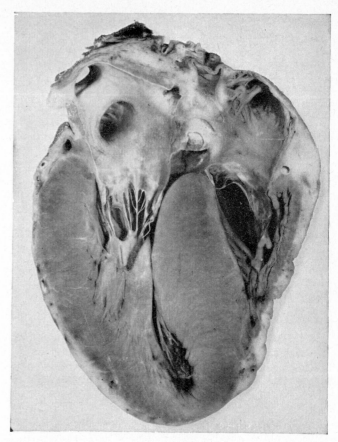

Figure 24.5
Hypertrophy of the heart. The wall of the left ventricle is greatly thickened due to hypertrophy of its muscle. *(C 20a.3, Reproduced by permission of the President and Council of the R.C.S. Eng.)*

Hypertrophy of individual fibres is also seen in areas of myocardial fibrosis.

Microscopically the muscle fibres are increased in width from the normal $14\,\mu$m up to $25\,\mu$m. The nuclei are characteristically square-shaped. It is claimed that one capillary supplies approximately one fibre. In hypertrophy no new vessels are formed, with the result that the contractile tissue tends to be separated from its blood supply. The ischaemia may cause anginal pain, and on a morphological level muscle necrosis with replacement fibrosis.

Skeletal Muscle

The village blacksmith's brawny arms provide a simple illustration of hypertrophy due to a mechanical stimulus. When he retires from work, his muscles return to a normal size.

Muscular dystrophy. A number of clinical syndromes exist in which specific groups of muscles undergo enlargement. Although in the early stages the muscle fibres become swollen, this is probably a degenerative change, because later on the fibres degenerate and are replaced by fibrous tissue. Much of the enlargement of the muscles is due to an increased deposition of fat, and is therefore not true hypertrophy. The syndromes are indeed characterised by muscular weakness. The common varieties are pseudohypertrophic muscular dystrophy (Duchenne type) and the facio-scapulo-humeral dystrophy of Landouzy and Dejerine.

Hypertrophy and hyperplasia compared. Both are cellular responses to an increased demand for work. The cells either enlarge or divide depending upon their growth potentialities. The stimulus for this is usually mechanical in hypertrophy, and chemical or hormonal in hyperplasia. When the stimulus is withdrawn, the condition regresses and the tissue reverts to normal. However, secondary structural alterations in the general architecture due to an accompanying degeneration may render a complete return to normal impossible.

DIMINISHED GROWTH

Nomenclature. A diminution in size may be of *developmental* origin due to a deficiency of growth, or it may be *acquired* after a period of normal growth.

Developmental diminutions of growth. These are usually present at birth, and the most extreme malformation of this type is *agenesis*, the complete failure of development of a part, which is therefore absent. A less severe condition is *hypoplasia*, in which there is a failure of development to a full, mature size. Such an organ (e.g. kidney) or tissue (e.g. enamel) is small in size or amount. Some hypoplastic kidneys are represented by only a fibrous nodule. Hypoplasia may become evident during childhood. Thus a testis which fails to mature at puberty is termed hypoplastic. These conditions are also noted on p. 346.

Acquired diminutions in growth. *Atrophy* is an acquired diminution in size of a part due to a diminution in the number or size of its constituent elements. It is the antithesis of hyperplasia and hypertrophy combined. Only in muscle is a decrease in size the all-important feature; in all other instances there is also a decrease in the number of cells. This is brought about by the slow, periodic destruction (necrosis) of cells, but the process is so insidious that necrotic elements are not conspicuous. Where the necrosis affects a large number of cells together and is microscopically evident, the condition should not be called atrophy; for instance, acute yellow "atrophy" of the liver is really massive necrosis.

Another term sometimes used is *aplasia*. It has been used to describe extreme hypoplasia, but it is redundant in such a context. It is commonly used by haematologists to describe a condition of the bone marrow caused by the damaging effects of ionising radiation and certain drugs, in which the blood-cell precursors stop dividing and undergo destruction, and there is little or not regeneration. As no mature cells enter the blood, pancytopenia ensues (see p. 608). Clearly the destructive process is related to necrosis (especially if it

is rapid) and to atrophy (if it is slow and sporadic). The term aplasia is preferably reserved for this usage.

ATROPHY

PHYSIOLOGICAL CAUSES

There are numerous examples of structures which are well developed at a certain period of life, but which subsequently undergo atrophy. The term *involution* is sometimes used synonymously with physiological atrophy. They may conveniently be considered under three age groups.

In the fetus, many structures form during embryonic development, and subsequently undergo regression. The branchial clefts, notochord, and thyroglossal duct are good examples.

In infancy, the ductus arteriosus and umbilical vessels either disappear or remain as fibrous cords. Soon after birth the fetal layer of the adrenal cortex undergoes involution.[22]

Later life. From adolescence onwards the lymphoid tissue undergoes a reduction in size. As a rule it is replaced by fibrous tissue: on occasions, however, fat is also laid down. This is particularly well-marked in atrophic lymph nodes, and is also seen in the thymus and appendix. Lymph nodes in the adult are frequently found to be composed of a nodule of fat with a thin surrounding demilune of lymphoid tissue. Atrophy is also seen in the uterus after parturition and the breasts after lactation.

After the menopause and in old age there is atrophy of the gonads themselves. Indeed, as age advances most tissues take part in the process, but this may be due in some measure to ischaemia.

PATHOLOGICAL ATROPHY

This may be generalised or local.

Generalised Atrophy

Starvation atrophy. During starvation the carbohydrate and fat stores are first used up. Later the proteins are metabolised, those of the brain and heart being the last to be removed. Generalised atrophy, seen in the cachexia of malignant disease, is probably largely dependent upon an inadequate food intake.

In extreme starvation the heart may be reduced from its normal 250–350 g to 100 g, the epicardial fat is replaced by pale, translucent material ("serous atrophy"), and the vessels are tortuous. Lipofuscins present in the small muscle fibres impart a brown colour, from which the name *brown atrophy of the heart* is coined. Starvation atrophy is a condition rarely seen in civilised countries. Occasional examples are encountered in neglected patients, and those dying of carcinoma of the oesophagus or stomach. It was also seen amongst the emaciated inmates of Belsen concentration camp in Germany

Senile atrophy. This is a marked accentuation of the process of physiological atrophy that has already been described as occurring in old age. Brown atrophy of the heart is especially prominent in senility, and other organs, e.g. the liver and brain, may also show a lipofuscin accumulation in their cells. It is not known how much ischaemia (due to cerebral arterial atheroma) contributes to the brain atrophy of old people.

Endocrine atrophy. Hypopituitarism leads to an atrophy of the thyroid, adrenal cortex, and gonads. In the most severe cases the whole body may become stunted, and the appearance of premature senility, or *progeria*, develops. This cachectic stage is in fact rare, but was described by Simmonds, and is called *Simmonds's disease*, a term now often used synonymously with hypopituitarism.

Usually in fact there is no wasting, and the patient develops myxoedema due to a predominant hypothyroidism. Other common features are hypoglycaemia, adrenocortical insufficiency, and loss of secondary sex characteristics. A well-known cause of hypopituitarism is *post-partum* infarction of the gland, which occasionally complicates severe haemorrhages occurring during labour. Hypopituitarism following obstetric accidents is known as *Sheehan's syndrome*.[23]

Osteoporosis[24-27]

Osteoporosis is a condition of bone atrophy. It has been aptly defined as a lesion in which the volume of bone tissue per unit volume of anatomical bone is reduced.[28] The generalised disorder is considered here; localised bone atrophy is mentioned in connexion with the effects of pressure and disuse. The essential feature of osteoporosis is a reduction in amount of the osteoid matrix, which, however, remains normally mineralised. It must be distinguished from osteomalacia, in which osteoid is present in abundance but is poorly calcified. In osteoporosis the bony trabeculae are greatly thinned, and the bone as a whole is weakened and liable to fracture. The radiological appearance is a reduction of bone density. But it must be remembered that this can be detected in routine films with certainty only when the content of calcium is reduced by at least half. Refined techniques may be more sensitive.[29]

Although bone is a rigid structure, it is constantly being remodelled; bone resorption and bone formation are continuously in progress even in the adult. Osteoporosis is brought about in one of two ways. There is either excessive bone destruction by osteoclastic activity, or else there is a failure in bone formation by the osteoblasts. Frequently the imbalance which results in the development of osteoporosis is of minor degree, and the period of calcium loss from the body extends over many months. By the time the patient is seen, a steady balanced state has been reached and there is no evidence of excessive calcium loss. The blood levels of calcium and phosphorus are usually within the normal limits, as is also the phosphatase level.

Causes of generalised osteoporosis. No satisfactory aetiological classification of osteoporosis is available. In the great majority of cases it is probable that many factors contribute to the final outcome: these include hormones, nutrition (including calcium), physical stress and its lack, and the blood supply. For descriptive purposes osteoporosis will be considered under the following headings:

Prolonged Recumbency.
Failure in Collagen Formation:
　Protein deficiency.
　Glucocorticosteroid excess.
　Scurvy.
Other Endocrine Disorders.
Senile and post-menopausal osteoporosis, including the idiopathic variety.

Prolonged recumbency. The effects of immobilisation have been studied in healthy volunteers placed in plaster casts from the waist to the toes.[30] There is a slow steady loss of calcium, tending to increase up to about 0·3 g per day. During the 6–7 weeks of the experiment 9–24 g of calcium were lost, but as this represents only 1–2 per cent of the total body calcium (about 1 kg), no effects were detectable on x-ray examination.

Hypercalcuria occurs during immobilisation, and this may be a factor in stone formation. It is more marked in children and in patients with active Paget's disease.[31, 32]

Albright and Reifenstein attribute the osteoporosis of disuse to a failure of formation of new bone, for they believe that osteoblastic activity requires the stimulus of stress and strain produced by movement.[31] However, more recent work suggests that immobilised limbs have a normal or even increased rate of bone formation, and that the osteoporosis is due to increased osteoclastic resorption.[33, 34]

Failure in collagen formation. Osteoporosis may occur in starvation and the malabsorption syndrome, and the bone lesions are sometimes complicated by osteomalacia due to vitamin-D deficiency. Osteoporosis has also been reported in children with chronic liver disease,[35] and is probably due to hypoproteinaemia.

Scurvy. In adults generalised osteoporosis occurs, while in infantile scurvy (Barlow's disease) osteogenesis at the epiphyses is affected.

Corticosteroid Excess. Severe osteoporosis is typical of Cushing's syndrome; an unusual feature is that the skull is involved. Prolonged administration of glucocorticosteroids, e.g. for asthma or rheumatoid arthritis, may likewise produce a disabling osteoporosis.

In these three conditions the inability to form collagen fibres results in a cessation of osteoid formation. Abnormalities in the ground substance (osseomucin) may also play a part. There is no evidence of excessive osteoclastic activity.

Other endocrine disorders. Osteoporosis is not uncommon in severe *thyrotoxicosis*, and, as in the osteoporosis of immobilisation, it is due to increased resorption rather than inadequate formation.[25] Hypercalcuria is a manifestation of this. There may rarely be fractures.[36] The osteoporosis of *acromegaly* may have a similar pathogenesis.

Senile and post-menopausal osteoporosis. Senile osteoporosis is common in the elderly, and is to be regarded as an exaggeration of the atrophy which is part and parcel of the ageing process. A similar condition is not uncommon among women of a younger age-group, and is then called *post-menopausal osteoporosis*. When the condition afflicts individuals of either sex at an earlier age, it is called *idiopathic osteoporosis*.

The mechanism involved is obscure; neither bone formation nor resorption seems to be impaired, but, as already noted, the trouble may have occurred at some time in the past and a state of balance achieved at the time of diagnosis. Anabolic steroids, both oestrogens and androgens, cause symptomatic amelioration, but their mode of action is unknown. Deficiency of either male or female sex hormones has been incriminated as the cause of senile and post-menopausal osteoporosis, but proof is lacking. Long-term dietary deficiency of calcium can produce osteoporosis in rats,[37] and it may play a subsidiary part in human senile osteoporosis.[38] It would seem that the best protection against excessive senile osteoporosis is the presence of a large skeletal mass in early adult life.

Effects of osteoporosis. Symptoms are generally referable to the spine and pelvis which are the parts of the skeleton most severely affected in generalised osteoporosis. Chronic backache and kyphosis are common, and collapse of the vertebrae may produce episodes of acute pain. Diminution in height is characteristic, and as much as 4–8 inches may be lost before being noticed by the patient. Fractures may complicate osteoporosis; the most important are those of the lower forearm in middle-aged and elderly women, the proximal femur in both sexes over 70 years old, and crush fracture of the vertebrae, especially in old women.[38]

Radiographs show diminution in bone density; enlargement of the intervertebral disc-spaces produces the "codfish-spine" appearance. The ribs and to a lesser extent the long bones show rarefaction.

Conditions Simulating Osteoporosis

Osteogenesis imperfecta (Fragilitas ossium).[39] This is characterised by a defect in osteoid formation which causes the bones to be very thin and extremely fragile. In some cases multiple fractures are present at birth, but in others the disease first appears during infancy or rarely during adolescence. The sclera may be abnormally transparent, thereby allowing the underlying choroid to give it a blue colour. Otosclerosis is also common. The condition is inherited as an autosomal dominant character.

Hyperparathyroidism. The lesion here is an excessive osteoclastic activity which may be so great as to produce tumour-like masses and large cysts. There is also much fibrous repair and the laying down of new bone. The condition, called osteitis fibrosa cystica, is described on p. 572.

These conditions have been mentioned as they may produce radiological appearances indistinguishable from osteoporosis. But the underlying pathology is different. In osteogenesis imperfecta there is a hypoplasia of osteoid, and in osteitis fibrosa cystica there is a gross destruction of bone by hyperactive osteoclasts with evidence of reparative osteogenesis. This leads to a characteristic rise in the level of alkaline phosphatase in the serum, which, as already noted, does not occur in osteoporosis.

Local Atrophy

Ischaemic atrophy. This is simply a local form of tissue malnutrition in which hypoxia is predominant. With gradual vascular obstruction the parenchyma of many tissues undergoes atrophy, which is followed by fibrous (or glial) replacement. This is a feature of cerebral arterial atheroma. In the case of coronary arterial disease atrophy of the heart is not a usual feature; there is overt necrosis, and the process merges into one of infarction.

Pressure atrophy. This is a variant of ischaemic atrophy. It is caused by pressure on a solid organ, the vessels of which are progressively occluded by compression. It is the capillaries that suffer most, and damage is caused both by malnutrition and hypoxia. In this way the capsule around a benign tumour or a cyst is formed (see Chapter 26).

Some of the best examples are provided by bone; cartilage, being avascular, is much less severely affected. This is well illustrated by the way epiphyseal cartilage is spared by an expanding simple bone cyst, and by the scalloped appearance produced by the protruding intervertebral discs following the atrophy of the spinal column caused by an aneurysm of the thoracic aorta. A meningioma growing from the dura mater and hollowing the underlying brain is another good example of pressure atrophy. So also is the atrophic kidney that forms a cap on an expanding hydronephrosis which develops as a result of partial or intermittent obstruction of a ureter.

Disuse atrophy. The best examples are seen in the locomotor system and in the exocrine glands. The atrophy of bone (local osteoporosis), ligaments, and muscles that follows joint immobilisation must always be borne in mind when limbs are encased in plaster. Atrophy may occur in bone adjacent to an inflammatory process. It also occurs when joints are ankylosed, or if movement is prevented by pain; the atrophy around rheumatoid and tuberculous arthritis is particularly marked.

Sudeck's acute bone atrophy is perhaps due to this.[40] It follows quite trivial trauma to the hands, and more rarely the feet, and is associated with marked pain and swelling. There is radiological evidence of patchy osteoporosis. The pain is usually out of all proportion to the extent of the injury, and in one series of cases abnormalities were found in the median nerve as it passed under the carpal tunnel.[41] The most likely explanation of both the osteoporosis and the oedema is disuse consequent on the pain; an alternative suggestion of "neuropathic" bone atrophy is less convincing.

When the duct of a secreting gland is suddenly and completely blocked, the parenchyma undergoes atrophy, e.g. after total obstruction of a ureter, a salivary duct, and the pancreatic duct. It is interesting to recall that it was this method of producing pancreatic atrophy which was employed by Banting and Best in the isolation of insulin.

Neuropathic atrophy. This term is sometimes applied to the pronounced wasting of paralysed limbs—particularly after lower motor neurone lesions, e.g. poliomyelitis, motor neurone disease, and syringomyelia, or following nerve section. It is doubtful whether it exists as an entity. It is certain that in the event of paralysis disuse atrophy ensues, affecting the muscles and the other tissues. Whether sensory denervation also plays a part is not known. Direct damage due to unnoticed trauma may sometimes be an additional factor as, for example, in syringomyelia, leprosy, and tabes dorsalis. Whether there is a specific "neuropathic" cause for the "succulent hand" of syringomyelia or for Sudeck's acute bone atrophy is not known.

Idiopathic atrophy. There are examples of atrophy where no cause is evident. The myopathies, progressive muscular atrophy (motor neurone disease), sterility due to testicular atrophy, thyroid atrophy in myxoedema, and Addison's disease due to adrenal atrophy are good examples. In some, an autoimmune basis has been suggested but as yet unconfirmed; in others, an inherited defect is indicated (Huntington's chorea and dystrophia myotonica), while in others the atrophy appears to be a presenile one, as in Alzheimer's disease.

ABNORMALITIES OF CELLULAR DIFFERENTIATION

As described in Chapter 4, cells which are subjected to abnormal influences can change their structure and function. The best defined of these changes, which can be recognised on light microscopy, is metaplasia.

Metaplasia

Metaplasia is a condition in which there is a change of one type of differentiated tissue to another type of similarly differentiated tissue. The importance of the word differentiated should be noted, because its use excludes tumour formation as a form of metaplasia. The persistence of a similar differentiated tissue implies that tissues do not radically change their character: thus one type of epithelium changes to another type of epithelium, and similarly connective tissue changes to connective tissue. However, as we shall see, epithelium and connective tissue are more interchangeable than was at one time thought.

TYPES

Epithelial Metaplasia

Squamous metaplasia. Many types of epithelium are capable of changing to a stratified squamous variety which may undergo keratinisation. It often appears to be the result of persistent trauma ("chronic irritation"). The following examples may be cited:

(*a*) Gall-bladder (simple columnar epithelium) in chronic cholecystitis, especially if accompanied by stones. The condition is pre-cancerous in some cases.

(*b*) Renal pelvis and bladder (transitional epithelium) in chronic infection. It is more common if stones are present.

(*c*) Uterus (simple columnar epithelium). Squamous metaplasia of the endometrium is an occasional senile change, and occurs in the rare condition of chronic inversion of the uterus. The glands of the cervix frequently undergo squamous metaplasia in chronic cervicitis, and the change may mimic early squamous-cell carcinoma. This metaplasia is especially common during pregnancy.

(*d*) Bronchi (pseudostratified columnar ciliated epithelium) (Fig. 24.6). Squamous metaplasia is common, and there is no evidence that it is precancerous. It is seen in chronic

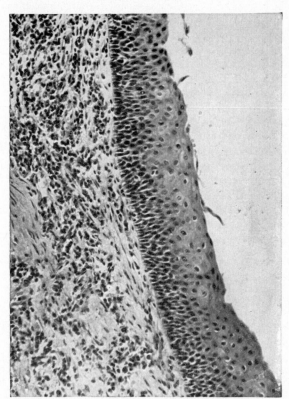

Figure 24.6
Squamous metaplasia of bronchial epithelium. The normal pseudostratified columnar ciliated respiratory epithelium of the bronchus has been replaced by a stratified squamous type of epithelium. ×200.

bronchitis, bronchiectasis, in epithelialised abscess cavities, and in bronchi draining tuberculous cavities. The almost constant occurrence of squamous metaplasia overlying a bronchial "adenoma" is of some practical importance. A superficial biopsy may lead to the mistaken diagnosis of squamous-cell carcinoma, and the true nature of the tumour be missed.

(*e*) Prostate (simple columnar epithelium). Squamous metaplasia is seen in the ducts in patients treated with oestrogen.

Although in many of these examples "chronic irritation" appears to be the cause of the metaplasia, there is one condition in which squamous metaplasia is common, but in which irritation plays no part. This is hypovitaminosis A. Squamous epithelia show hyperkeratinisation, which is manifested in the "toad-skin" appearance of the exposed parts of the skin and the conjunctival hyperkeratosis of xerophthalmia. Squamous metaplasia is widespread, being found in the nose, bronchi, and urinary tract. The explanation of these changes is not known, but Fell's work done on tissue cultures of chick embryo skin has shown that vitamin A is intimately concerned with the function of epithelium. If the medium used contains an excess of vitamin A, the epidermis changes to a ciliated, mucus-secreting epithelium. This metaplasia is reversible when the vitamin A concentration is reduced.[42, 43]

Columnar metaplasia. Squamous epithelium rarely changes to a columnar type. Cervical erosion is often cited as an example. In this condition the vaginal portion of the cervix is covered by columnar epithelium instead of the normal squamous type. This may arise in one of two ways. The cervix is covered by columnar epithelium during development and normally this changes to a squamous type, probably under the influence of oestrogenic stimulation. If columnar epithelium persists during childhood, the condition is termed a *congenital erosion*. The second type of erosion occurs in adults and usually follows childbirth. There is a pouting of the endocervical mucosa so that this becomes visible on the vaginal aspect. Subsequent squamous metaplasia may occur, and blockage of the mucous glands results in the production of retention cysts. These are the familiar Nabothian cysts. It is unlikely that columnar epithelium ever replaces a previously squamous-covered surface either by metaplasia or by growth over an ulcerated area.

Specialised columnar epithelia may change to a more simple type. The conversion of the pseudostratified columnar ciliated respiratory epithelium to a simple mucus-secreting columnar type is commonly seen in chronic bronchitis and bronchiectasis, and may well play an important part in predisposing patients with these conditions to broncho-pneumonia (see p. 88).

The occurrence of patches of an intestinal type of epithelium with villi in the stomach is not infrequent, and some authorities regard these areas as being particularly liable to malignant change.[44] Intestinal metaplasia also often occurs in a healed chronic gastric ulcer (see p. 121). The epithelium also functions like intestinal epithelium, and its absorptive capacity might provide an explanation of how carcinogens gain entrance to the gastric wall.[45]

The eosinophilic columnar epithelium, called "pale" or "pink" epithelium, often found lining some of the cysts in cystic hyperplasia of the breast, is another fine example of columnar metaplasia.[46] It closely resembles the epithelium of the normal apocrine glands found in the axilla, and serves as a reminder that the mammary glands are developmentally closely related both to these and to ordinary sweat glands.

Connective Tissue Metaplasia

Osseous metaplasia. The question as to whether fibroblasts can produce osteoid tissue or not is largely a matter of definition of fibroblasts and osteoblasts. They certainly exhibit morphological identity, and before the appearance of the intercellular substance, whether fibrous tissue or osteoid, they cannot be distinguished. "Fibroblasts" do not normally produce osteoid, but under some conditions they may be regarded as undergoing metaplasia to "osteoblasts". Bone then makes its appearance. An alternative explanation is that the osteoblasts are derived from primitive stem cells (see p. 397). Marrow is often found in the metaplastic bone. It could either be the result of metaplasia of the local mesenchymal cells or else follow the deposition of primitive haematopoietic cells from the blood stream. The relationship between fibroblasts, chondroblasts, and osteoblasts is discussed on pp. 118–119 in relation to fracture healing.

Osseous metaplasia occurs as an ageing process in cartilage, e.g. the hyoid and thyroid cartilages. A rare, interesting lesion is *tracheopathia osteoplastica*,[47] where cartilaginous and bony masses develop in the submucosa of the trachea and larger bronchi. Some of these foci apparently develop directly from the cartilage rings and bars, but others arise from the connective tissue by metaplasia.

Osseous metaplasia is also seen in soft tissue, e.g. in scars[48] and areas of dystrophic calcification such as old goitres, caseous foci, tonsils, and Mönckeberg's sclerosis. The ossification of such calcareous foci depends on the osteogenic potentiality of the adjacent fibroblasts; it is surprising how often ossification does not occur.

Foci of ossification are sometimes found in muscle. It is probable that local trauma is a predisposing factor. The muscles most often involved are the gluteus maximus and the adductors of the thigh. Ossification in muscle and tendon has been reported after tetanus,[49] and it is also a complication of paralytic poliomyelitis in which bone may develop in the wasted muscles. The reason for this is unknown. The most important example of metaplastic ossification in muscle, or *localised myositis ossificans* as it is often called, is seen in the bend of the elbow after a supracondylar fracture of the humerus. The bony mass forms in the insertion of the brachialis muscle. It would appear that traumatic myositis ossificans is due to the organisation and subsequent ossification of a haematoma. When this occurs in proximity to bone it may be that osteoblasts are drawn in from the periosteum.[50]

There are two rare but interesting conditions, both inherited as dominant characteristics, in which widespread osseous metaplasia occurs. In *fibrodysplasia ossificans progressiva*[51, 52] there is progressive laying-down of bone in aponeuroses, tendons, and fascia, so that the body eventually may become completely rigid. The disease is also called "myositis ossificans progressiva", but in fact the muscles are only secondarily involved in this ossification, the nature of which is obscure. In the early stages painful swellings develop in the tissues, and these subsequently ossify. An associated feature is microdactyly (with monophanangy of the big toe as a usual concomitant). In *pseudohypoparathyroidism*, which is mentioned on page 530, the body is unresponsive to parathormone. In addition, there are skeletal deformities, mental retardation, and a tendency to widespread subcutaneous calcification and ossification.[53] Osteoma cutis is quite common, and is not localised as after trauma or acne vulgaris.[54] In *pseudo-pseudohypoparathyroidism* similar skeletal deformities and subcutaneous ossification may occur, but there is normal responsiveness to parathormone and therefore no disturbance in calcium and phosphate metabolism. It is probable that this condition is merely an incompletely expressed form of a genetically determined abnormality of which pseudohypoparathyroidism represents the complete clinical syndrome. It is suggested that the syndrome be called *Albright's hereditary osteodystrophy*.[53, 54]

Changes in mesothelium. Squamous metaplasia may occur both in the pleura[55] and peritoneum,[56] and it can be produced in rabbits after the intrapleural injection of a mixture of Sudan III and sodium cholate in olive oil.[57] The authors have encountered a patch of keratinising stratified squamous epithelium overlying a pulmonary infarct. Some rare cases of squamous-cell carcinoma appear to arise from the pleura; it might be that they are derived from such an area of squamous metaplasia, but a tumour arising from an underlying bronchiole is very difficult to exclude as an alternative possibility.

Under other circumstances pleural mesothelium may become columnar, and even form tubules (Fig. 24.7). Endometriosis may represent a similar condition in the peritoneum,[58] although other explanations are available. The potentialities of the mesothelial cells covering the ovary should also be remembered; they can form germinal follicles and epithelial-lined cysts, as well as give rise to frankly epithelial tumours. Synovial cells may also closely resemble columnar epithelium,[59] and a synovioma may occasionally present the appearance of an adenocarcinoma.

It is apparent that mesothelium can form various cell types: herein lies one of the pitfalls in examining pleural or peritoneal exudates for malignant cells. Groups of cells arranged in the form of an acinus are not necessarily malignant.

Other cytological characteristics must be taken into account before a diagnosis of adenocarcinoma is made.

Finally, it should be noted that the metaplasia which can occur in mesothelium indicates that the division between connective tissue and epithelium is not as definite as is sometimes assumed. A striking example of this occurs in the

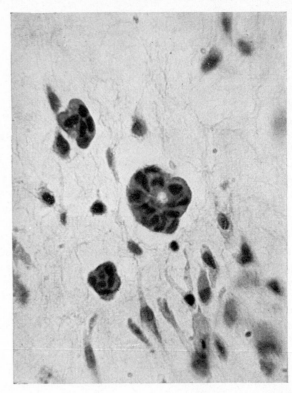

Figure 24.7
Metaplasia in mesothelium. Section of thickened pleura shows groups of altered mesothelial cells. It is understandable that such groups of cells might become detached and appear in a pleural effusion. × 700.

lens of the eye. In some examples of cataract the epithelial cells of the anterior aspect of the lens undergo metaplasia and form fibrous tissue.

Tumour Metaplasia

The occurrence of mixed adenocarcinoma and squamous-cell carcinoma (adenoacanthoma) is not an uncommon event, and may be explained on the basis of tumour metaplasia (Fig. 24.8). The assumption is that the tumour commences as an adenocarcinoma, but that a change occurs in some of its cells leading to squamous differentiation. It should be noted that this change is not "metaplasia" in the strict sense, because a tumour cannot be regarded as a completely differentiated tissue. It is therefore preferably called "tumour metaplasia", and is believed to be quite common in cancer of the lung. About a fifth of lung adenocarcinomata show squamous elements.[60] Indeed, tumour metaplasia may

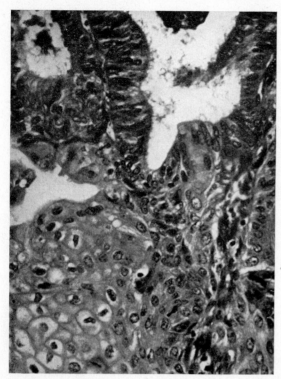

Figure 24.8
Squamous tumour metaplasia. This is a section of well-differentiated adenocarcinoma of the body of the uterus. Part of the columnar-cell lining of the malignant acinus is replaced by stratified squamous epithelium. × 320.

explain the origin of all squamous-cell carcinomata of lung if it is assumed that the squamous cells can outgrow and completely obliterate the adenocarcinomatous element. Another explanation may be that the tumours arise in areas of squamous metaplasia. These possibilities are shown diagrammatically in Fig. 24.9.

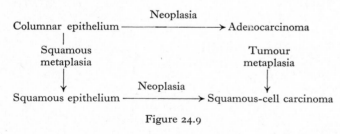

Figure 24.9

Tumour metaplasia of squamous type is also seen in carcinoma of the gall-bladder, in endometrial adenocarcinoma, and transitional-cell carcinoma of urinary tract. It is occasionally seen in pleomorphic salivary gland tumours, carcinoma of the breast, and more rarely in adenocarcinomata of other sites.

Mucoid metaplasia is occasionally seen in adenocarcinomata of the breast.

The stroma of a tumour can also undergo metaplasia, e.g. osseous metaplasia is common in fibro-adenomata of the canine breast.

The question arises whether, in general, epithelial metaplasia, particularly the squamous type, is a precancerous condition. It is impossible to give a dogmatic answer. There is no doubt that squamous-cell carcinomata can arise from the bronchus, the urinary passages, and the gall-bladder, but it is less certain whether they start on an area of metaplastic epithelium, or whether the tumour epithelium subsequently undergoes squamous change. The consensus of opinion is that the change succeeds neoplasia much more often than preceding it.

OTHER CELLULAR DYSTROPHIES

Dystrophy* may be defined as a disorder, usually congenital, of the structure or function of an organ or tissue due to its perverted nutrition. In its widest sense it includes agenesis, atrophy, hypertrophy, hyperplasia, and metaplasia, but in practice the term is usually applied to those disorders which do not readily fit into any of these other categories. The alternative term *dysplasia** may also be used for such an abnormal development of tissue, although strictly it should be applied to developmental disorders only. *Dyscrasia** literally means a bad mixture (of the four humours), and is now used only by haematologists to describe any blood disorder of uncertain aetiology.

One of the best examples of a dystrophy is the lesion found in pernicious anaemia. Although the abnormal nuclear maturation found in the red-cell precursors in this disease led Ehrlich to describe them as megaloblasts, it was not realised at that time that other cells showed similar changes. Examination of the cells of the gastric, buccal, nasal, vaginal, and other mucosae has revealed nuclear abnormalities presumably caused by vitamin-B_{12} deficiency. The changes include pleomorphism, giant nuclei, and large nucleoli.[61] These observations have an important application: the exfoliative cytologist must avoid mistaking these cells for malignant cells in sputum, gastric washings, urine, etc.[62] The premature greying of the hair and the degeneration of the spinal cord indicate that pernicious anaemia is more than merely a haematological disorder.[63]

Another interesting dystrophy is seen in the skin, sometimes following a burn, or superimposed on some existing lesion, such as a solar keratosis or a seborrhoeic keratosis. The abnormal squamous epithelium produces excessive keratin which adheres to produce a cutaneous horn (Fig. 24.10).

Many special dystrophies involving muscle, bone, cornea,

* The Greek derivation of these words is as follows:
  Dys—bad or difficult.
  Krasis—a mingling.
  Plasis—a forming.
  Trophe—nourishment.

310   *General Pathology*

Figure 24.10
Cutaneous horn. This amazing horny excrescence was
removed from the skin of the arm of a man who had been
severely burnt 20 years before. A skin graft had been
applied, and healing was excellent. Twenty years later
this truncated keratin horn developed at the site of the
burn after a minor injury to the part. On excision it was
found that the mass was not attached to the deeper
structures, and recovery was complete after another skin
graft had been applied.

Before the horn was excised, the patient's wife was
wont to saw off pieces with a hacksaw. The specimen
comprises the complete horn including the sawn-off
portions. (I 18a.4, *Reproduced by permission of the
President and Council of the R.C.S. Eng.)*

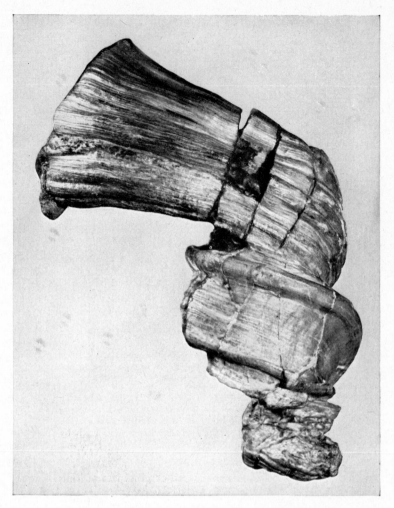

retina, etc., have been described, but these are outside the
scope of general pathology.

It must be reiterated that the term dystrophy has no specific
intrinsic meaning, but like dysplasia is used to describe a
lesion whose nature is not understood and for which the
author can find no other more appropriate name. In recent
years dysplasia has acquired a specific meaning when
applied to epithelium—most commonly that of the cervix
uteri. It is used to describe a type of hyperplasia which is
thought to progress to *carcinoma-in-situ* in some cases and

later to invasive cancer (p. 386). But dysplasia is also used in
other instances, e.g. fibrous dysplasia of bone and mammary
dysplasia, in which there is no suggestion of incipient neoplastic change.

In this chapter many different perversions of cell growth
have been described. With few exceptions, the one thing
they all have in common is that they are self-limiting and
reversible if the stimulus is removed. In the following
chapters neoplasia is considered. Here the perversion of cell
growth persists even when the stimulus is eradicated.

REFERENCES
1. Bizzozero, G. (1894). *British Medical Journal*, i, 728.
2. Post, J. and Hoffman, J. (1968). *New England Journal of Medicine*, **279**, 248.
3. Pelc, S. R. (1963). *Experimental Cell Research*, **29**, 194.
4. Doniach, I. (1960). In *Recent Advances in Pathology*, 7th edn, pp. 197–270. Edited by C. V. Harrison. London: Churchill.
5. Munro, D. S. (1972). *Journal of the Royal College of Physicians (London)*, **6**, 309.
6. Soffer, L. J. *et al.* (1955). *Ciba Foundation Colloquia on Endocrinology*, **8**, 487. London: Churchill.
7. Browne, J. S. L. *et al.* (1955). *Ciba Foundation Colloquia on Endocrinology*, **8**, 505. London: Churchill.
8. Ashworth, C. T. and Garvey, R. F. (1958). *American Journal of Pathology*, **34**, 1161.
9. Symington, T. *et al.* (1958). *Ciba Foundation Colloquia on Endocrinology*, **12**, 102. London: Churchill.
10. Wilkins, L. *et al.* (1955). *Ciba Foundation Colloquia on Endocrinology*, **8**, 460. London: Churchill.

11. CONN, J. W. (1963). *Journal of the American Medical Association*, **183**, 775 and 871.
12. RUSSFIELD, A. B. (1955). *Journal of Clinical Endocrinology*, **15**, 1393.
13. ISRAEL, M. S. and ELLIS, I. R. (1961). *British Journal of Cancer*, **15**, 763.
14. CARDELL, B. S. (1953). *Journal of Pathology and Bacteriology*, **66**, 335.
15. DRISCOLL, S. G., BENIRSCHKE, K. and CURTIS, G. W. (1960). *American Journal of Diseases in Childhood*, **100**, 818.
16. LEVER, W. F. (1967). *Histopathology of the Skin*, 4th edn, p. 761. Philadelphia and Toronto: Lippincott.
17. HOGAN, M. J. and ZIMMERMAN, L. E. (1962). *Ophthalmic Pathology*, 2nd edn, p. 765. Philadelphia and London: Saunder.
18. HARRISON, C. V. (1966). In *Recent Advances in Pathology*, 8th edn, p. 216. London: Churchill.
19. ANAGNOSTOU, D. and HARRISON, C. V. (1972). *Journal of Clinical Pathology*, **25**, 306.
20. MacCORMAC, H. and SCARFF, R. W. (1936). *British Journal of Dermatology*, **48**, 624.
21. CALNAN, C. D. and HABER, H. (1955). *Journal of Pathology and Bacteriology*, **69**, 61.
22. BAAR, H. S. (1954). *Lancet*, i, 670.
23. SHEEHAN, H. L. and SUMMERS, V. K. (1949). *Quarterly Journal of Medicine*, **18**, 319.
24. BARTTER, F. C. (1957). *American Journal of Medicine*, **22**, 797.
25. BALL, J. (1960). In *Recent Advances in Pathology*, 7th edn, p. 301, *loc. cit.*
26. FRASER, R. (1962). *Journal of Bone and Joint Surgery*, **44B**, 485.
27. BARZEL, U. S. (1970). *Osteoporosis*, 290 pp. New York and London: Grune and Stratton.
28. Leading Article (1971). *British Medical Journal*, i, 566.
29. MEEMA, H. E., HARRIS, C. K. and PORRETT, R. E. (1964). *Radiology*, **82**, 986.
30. DEITRICK, J. E., WHEDON, G. D. and SHORR, E. (1948). *American Journal of Medicine*, **4**, 3.
31. ALBRIGHT, F. and REIFENSTEIN, E. C. (1948). *The Parathyroid Glands and Metabolic Bone Disease*, p. 147. London: Baillière, Tindall and Cox.
32. Editorial (1942). *Annals of Internal Medicine*, **16**, 176.
33. HEANEY, R. P. (1962). *American Journal of Medicine*, **33**, 188.
34. Annotation (1963). *Lancet*, i, 150.
35. TENG, C. T. *et al.* (1961). *Journal of Pediatrics*, **59**, 684.
36. FRASER, S. A. *et al.* (1971). *Lancet*, i, 981.
37. GERSHON-COHEN, J. and JOWSEY, J. (1964). *Metabolism*, **13**, 221.
38. NORDIN, B. E. C. (1971). *British Medical Journal*, i, 571.
39. McKUSICK, V. A. (1966). *Heritable Disorders of Connective Tissue*, 3rd edn, p. 230. St. Louis: Mosby.
40. PLEWES, L. W. (1956). *Journal of Bone and Joint Surgery*, **38B**, 195.
41. STEIN, A. H. (1962). *Surgery, Gynecology and Obstetrics*, **115**, 713.
42. FELL, H. B. and MELLANBY, E. (1953). *Journal of Physiology (London)*, **119**, 470.
43. LASNITZKI, I. (1963). *Journal of Experimental Medicine*, **118**, 1.
44. MORSON, B. C. (1955). *British Journal of Cancer*, **9**, 365 and 377.
45. RUBIN, W. *et al.* (1967). *Laboratory Investigation*, **16**, 813.
46. HAAGENSEN, C. D. (1971). *Diseases of the Breast*, 2nd edn, pp. 165 and 282. *Philadelphia*: Saunders.
47. Leading Article (1968). *British Medical Journal*, ii, 4.
48. CLASSEN, K. L., WEIDERANDERS, R. E. and HERRINGTON, J. L. (1960). *Surgery*, **47**, 918.
49. GUNN, D. R. and YOUNG, W. B. (1959). *Journal of Bone and Joint Surgery*, **41B**, 535.
50. FLYNN, J. E. and GRAHAM, J. H. (1964). *Surgery, Gynecology and Obstetrics*, **118**, 1001.
51. LUTWAK, L. (1964). *American Journal of Medicine*, **37**, 269.
52. McKUSICK, V. A. (1966). *loc. cit.* p. 400.
53. MANN, J. B., ALTERMAN, S. and HILLS, A. G. (1962). *Annals of Internal Medicine*, **56**, 315.
54. BROOK, C. G. D. and VALMAN, H. B. (1971). *British Journal of Dermatology*, **85**, 471.
55. DUNNILL, M. S. (1959). *Journal of Pathology and Bacteriology*, **77**, 299.
56. CROME, L. (1950). *Journal of Pathology and Bacteriology*, **62**, 61.
57. YOUNG, J. S. (1928). *Journal of Pathology and Bacteriology*, **31**, 265.
58. MADDING, G. F. and KENNEDY, P. A. (1963). *Journal of the American Medical Association*, **183**, 686.
59. FISK, G. R. (1952). *Annals of the Royal College of Surgeons of England*, **11**, 157.
60. WALTER, J. B. and PRYCE, D. M. (1955). *Thorax*, **10**, 107.
61. RUBIN, C. E. and MASSEY, B. W. (1953). *Journal of Laboratory and Clinical Medicine*, **42**, 942.
62. BODDINGTON, M. M. and SPRIGGS, A. I. (1959). *Journal of Clinical Pathology*, **12**, 228.
63. MALLARMÉ, J. (1948). *Blood*, **3**, 103.

Chapter 25. Tumours: Introduction and Classification

It must be acknowledged that no completely satisfactory definition of a tumour exists. Since the exact nature and cause of tumour growth is unknown, the only existing definitions are in fact descriptions, and like most descriptions some are better than others.

To Powell White we owe the concept that "a tumour proper is a mass of cells, tissues or organs resembling those normally present, but arranged atypically. It grows at the expense of the organism without at the same time subserving any useful function". The cells of the tumour are sometimes arranged so atypically that their resemblance to the normal is difficult to recognise. Indeed, they may resemble those found during development rather than those present in post-uterine life. On the other hand, some tumour cells may so closely resemble the normal that a morphological distinction is scarcely possible. Thus the appearance of the cells is not of overriding importance.

Abnormal behaviour, on the other hand, is of greater significance than abnormal appearance. The continued growth at the expense of the host has been emphasised by such a trite definition of tumours as "autonomous parasites". Autonomy means self-government, and it is obvious that no tumour is entirely independent of the surrounding tissues; without a blood supply it would soon undergo necrosis. Benign tumours may show only limited autonomy, because growth often ceases when the tumour has attained a certain size. Some malignant tumours also, far from being completely autonomous, are known to be under definite hormonal control. The fetus is quite as autonomous as any tumour. It is a true parasite, but its natural history entails only a limited stay within its parent.

Nevertheless, it is probably true to say that a characteristic of all tumours is that the cells are behaving in an abnormal way, which indicates that they are escaping from some, if not all, the normal mechanisms which control cell growth and anatomical arrangement. Unfortunately we are ignorant even about these normal mechanisms.

This process of escape is often manifested by the production of a space-occupying mass or tumour, but this is not always the case. Sometimes the migration of cells outside the normal confining limits outweighs the abnormal proliferation; in this case no "tumour" as such exists. An excellent example of this is the diffuse infiltrating carcinoma of the stomach ("linitis plastica").

A term which is therefore more suitable is *neoplasia*; it indicates an abnormal type of new growth which not only may be evident in the intact animal, but which can also be seen and studied in tissue culture. Neoplasia differs from hyperplasia in several important respects:

(*a*) Neoplasia usually appears to arise spontaneously, but in those cases where the stimulus is known, it is abnormal, e.g. ionising radiation, chemical carcinogen, or virus infection. Hyperplasia, on the other hand, is usually produced by the excessive action of a normal stimulus, e.g. a hormone. Nevertheless, this is not an absolute distinction because hyperplasia can also be induced by agents similar to those which produce tumours. Epidermal hyperplasia is a marked feature in molluscum contagiosum and the common wart, both of which are caused by viruses. Epidermal hyperplasia is also seen in the skin's response to chemical irritants.

(*b*) The growth in hyperplasia is directly related to the degree of stimulation, while neoplasia, once it starts, proceeds irrespective of the stimulus.

(*c*) Once the stimulus is removed, hyperplasia regresses. Neoplasia, on the other hand, proceeds unabated.

The definition given by Willis embodies this concept: "*a tumour is an abnormal mass of tissue, the growth of which exceeds and is uncoordinated with that of the normal tissues, and persists in the same excessive manner after cessation of the stimuli which evoked the change*".

To this extent the tumour cells may be said to be autonomous and beyond normal growth control. It certainly seems that their continued growth is quite useless, and the neoplastic response to a stimulus appears to have no survival value in the evolutionary process. When it is remembered that most tumours occur during the post-reproductive years, this is not altogether surprising.

CLASSIFICATION

The difficulties encountered in the classification of neoplasias are those which are inherent in the classification of any condition of unknown aetiology. No single classification is wholly satisfactory; by examining tumours from different aspects various subdivisions are possible. While some classifications are more useful than others, none is more "correct" than another. Some classifications are dependent on a microscopical examination of the tumour, while others are related to the naked-eye appearance or behaviour. The following bases for classification may be recognised:

1. Naked-eye appearance including the organ of origin.

2. Histogenetic classification (including embryological considerations).
3. Histological.
4. Behavioural.
5. Aetiological.

Naked-eye Appearances and Regional Classification

When the patient is first seen clinically the organ of origin is the most striking feature of many tumours. There is a complaint of a lump or the effect of a lump in an organ. Although tumours of widely differing behaviour and origin can arise in one particular organ, this classification is nevertheless of some importance. A tumour of the brain or its meninges is invariably more serious than a tumour of a finger: it produces a characteristic clinical picture, and whatever its nature, demands early treatment if life is to be saved.

A naked-eye examination of tumours frequently reveals characteristics which by experience are known to coincide with other properties. For example, the terms "annular" and "fungating" (cauliflower) growth are often applied to gut tumours, and are self-explanatory. The former produces constriction, while the latter ulcerates and bleeds. "Scirrhous" tumours are hard, a feature due to the large amount of fibrous tissue present in the stroma. "Encephaloid" or "medullary" tumours are soft and brain-like due to the sparse stromal reaction. Mucoid tumours form another characteristic group.

Histogenetic Classification

The cell-type of origin forms an important feature of our present classification. The body has by convention been divided into epithelium and connective tissue, although the distinction between the two is by no means as clear-cut as is sometimes imagined. Two groups of tumours are therefore recognised:

Tumours of epithelial origin
Tumours of connective-tissue origin

Six main difficulties are apparent in this classification:

1. *The Nature of Endothelium, Mesothelium, and Synovium.* The flattened lining cells of the serous spaces present a problem. The endothelial or mesothelial cells, although generally classified as connective tissue, may on occasions give rise to tumours which resemble those of frankly epithelial origin. Thus, a mesothelioma of the pleura may closely resemble an adenocarcinoma, and indeed it has been maintained that many tumours so labelled are in fact secondary lung cancers and not primary tumours at all. It is now accepted, however, that genuine mesotheliomata do occur, for some are composed of spindle-shaped cells of connective tissue type, while in others both types of cells are present.[1, 2]

In the peritoneum the same types of difficulty arise. Many suspected mesotheliomata are in fact secondary carcinomata. Nevertheless, it is generally accepted that the cells covering the ovary can give rise to frankly epithelial tumours. Perhaps the same is true of other sites. In joints the synovium may

give rise to tumours which closely resemble adenocarcinomata. It is apparent that, although convention dictates that epithelial and connective tissue cells are quite distinct, the conversion of one type to another is not outside the realm of possibility. The subject is further discussed in relation to metaplasia (see p. 308).

2. *Undifferentiated Tumours.* A second difficulty in a histogenetic classification is the occurrence of tumours so poorly differentiated that they defy recognition, i.e. the parent tissue is very poorly reproduced.

3. *Tumour Metaplasia.* The occurrence of tumour metaplasia may further confuse the issue. For instance, a tumour of the lung may be undifferentiated, and yet have areas of prickle-cell formation and keratinisation. The supposition is that the tumour is a poorly-differentiated growth of columnar bronchial epithelium, and should therefore be called a polygonal-cell carcinoma with squamous metaplasia. Regardless of the true origin of a tumour it must be admitted that the label given to a particular growth is frequently a matter of personal prejudice on the part of the pathologist. An anaplastic squamous-cell carcinoma to one authority may be called a transitional-cell carcinoma, an anaplastic carcinoma, a reticulum-cell sarcoma, or merely an undifferentiated malignant tumour by other pathologists. The differences do not lie in the tumour, but in the observers.

4. *Debatable Origin of a Tissue.* Another difficulty is the histogenetic classification of tumours arising from cells whose precise origin has been disputed. The best example of this is the melanocyte of the skin. Those who favour the neural origin of Masson (see p. 355) might call malignant tumours of melanocytes melanotic sarcomata. Those who favour an epithelial origin (now an outdated hypothesis) would support the name naevocarcinoma.

5. *Origin from highly specialised tissues.* A fifth difficulty arises with certain very specialised tissues which produce tumours that are distinctive and unlike those found elsewhere. For example, the nervous system, excluding the ependyma, and the haematopoietic tissues, although included in the broad group of connective tissue, are so different from other connective tissues that some authorities prefer to separate them from the others when classifying the tissues from which tumours may take origin. This serves to point out the distinctive features of malignant lymphoma, leukaemia, phaeochromocytoma, the gliomata, etc., but it must be appreciated that the number of basic tissues recognised is an arbitrary affair. Bichat in fact recognised over thirty, and indeed if each type of epithelium and connective tissue is regarded as separate the number could greatly exceed this.

6. *Origin from placental and embryonic tissues.* Finally, certain tumours arise from cells which are not normally present in the adult body. Two groups can be recognised:

(*a*) Those of placental origin like the hydatidiform mole and choriocarcinoma. Both are derived from chorionic tissue, and are of fetal origin.

(*b*) Tumours of embryonic origin. These include some teratomata, and such tumours of infancy as the nephroblastoma, neuroblastoma, and medulloblastoma (see Chapter 27).

Teratomata arise from *totipotential cells*, i.e. cells capable of differentiating into any of the tissues of the body. This has given rise to the belief that representatives of each of the three germ-layers must be present before a teratoma can be diagnosed. In fact, in most of these tumours one particular tissue, usually skin, outgrows all the others, so that it would be difficult or even impossible to find all the other tissues in a teratoma. As will be shown, the concept of germ-layers is unhelpful in the classification of most tumours, and can be discarded without great loss.

The embryonic tumours of infancy arise from specific organs or areas of tissue during their development to a mature size, e.g. the pole of a kidney, the retina, or the area around the fourth ventricle. Some of the tumours consist only of the primitive cells pertaining to the part (e.g. retinoblastoma, medulloblastoma, and neuroblastoma), but others contain muscle fibres in addition (e.g. the Wilms tumour). Such tumours that consist of more than one element are called "mixed tumours". The teratoma is an extreme example of a mixed tumour. A cell capable of giving rise to several tissues is called *pluripotential*. It is obvious that these embryonic tumours of infancy and the teratomata are best explained on a developmental or embryological basis.

A further extension of an embryological classification was attempted, and finally abandoned as unsatisfactory.[3] Each tumour was described as *lepidic* if of epithelial origin or *hyalic* if from pulp or connective tissue. To this was prefixed either *epi-*, *meso-*, or *hypo-*, according to the germ-layer involved. Innocent tumours were designated *typical* while malignant tumours were regarded as *atypical*. Thus a squamous-cell carcinoma of the labium majus was called an atypical epilepidoma, while a similar tumour of the vagina was an atypical hypolepidoma. Such a cumbersome classification has little to recommend it. It is evident that the germ-layer of origin of tumour cells is of little importance in respect of tumour structure or behaviour. It should incidentally be noted that mesoderm can form epithelium as well as connective tissue, a fact which is not always appreciated. Renal tubules, ovary, testis, adrenal cortex, and endometrium are all mesodermal. Furthermore, ectoderm can form connective tissue: the muscle of the iris is ectodermal as is also the neuroglia.

Histological Classification

It sometimes happens that a malignant tumour consists merely of a diffuse mass of irregular cells which do not resemble any normal tissue. Such complete undifferentiation is called *anaplasia*. In this case the actual appearance of the neoplastic cells may be used as a basis for classification. A histological classification is used under the following circumstances:

When the tumour is so undifferentiated as to defy recognition of its site of origin. A tumour of glandular tissue which shows no evidence of glandular formation can be described only as polygonal-cell, spheroidal-cell, or anaplastic. The term actually used is frequently a matter of convention. A spheroidal-cell carcinoma at one hospital may be a polygonal-cell carcinoma at another. "Carcinoma simplex" is another term frequently used to describe this type of tumour. Sometimes the anaplasia is so great that it is uncertain whether the tumour has arisen from connective tissue or epithelium. One of the best examples of this difficulty is seen in the lung tumour now known as oat-cell (or small-cell in North America) carcinoma. Before 1926 it was labelled oat-cell sarcoma of the mediastinum.[4]

Small-cell, large-cell, pleomorphic-cell, giant-cell, spindle-cell, etc., are all self-explanatory terms when applied to tumours.

The occurrence of tumour metaplasia. Again pure description has to be used. The term "squamous-cell carcinoma" is used to describe a tumour of lung with a squamous differentiation, rather than to indicate a tumour arising from a stratified squamous epithelium (see p. 308).

The histological grading of tumours is based upon the degree of differentiation, and sometimes also the degree of irregularity, number of mitoses, etc. (see pp. 327, 329, and 339).

Classification According to Behaviour

Although the classical division of tumours into the two main groups, benign and malignant, is of great practical importance, it must be appreciated that intermediate types of behaviour exist which do not fall properly into either of these categories. The characteristics of the two groups must first be considered.

Benign or innocent tumours. The cells which constitute this type of growth show no tendency to invade the surrounding tissues. The excessive accumulation of cells produces an expanding lesion which causes pressure atrophy of the surrounding tissues. The stroma which remains forms the capsule which is a characteristic feature of benign tumours situated in a solid organ or tissue.

Benign tumours proliferate slowly, and usually show few mitoses. The arrangement of the cells closely resembles that of the parent tissue—they are *well-differentiated*. It must be realised that a benign tumour is one which behaves in a characteristic way, rather than one which has a particular microscopical appearance. Other characteristics of benign tumours are considered on pp. 323 and 343.

Malignant tumours. A malignant tumour always invades the surrounding tissues. It eventually enters channels like the lymphatics and blood vessels, and groups of cells are carried to other parts, where they set up secondary growths, or metastases. *Local invasion* and *embolic spread* are the two characteristics of malignant tumours. Both are probably related to the reduced cell adhesion which is a fundamental characteristic of cancer grown in tissue culture; the cells growing out of the explant do not resist mechanical separation as well as those of normal tissue.[5] The power to invade and spread combined with the capacity for progressive growth make the term "malignant" particularly suitable for this type of tumour. Death is inevitable in untreated cases although the rate of progression varies markedly from one case to the next (but see below).

Microscopically, malignant tumours tend to show less accurate reproduction of the parent tissue than do their benign counterparts. Other features of malignant tumours like irregularity, pleomorphism, etc., are described elsewhere (see p. 340).

In addition to the classical benign and malignant tumours there are other types which show noteworthy patterns of behaviour and fit into neither group.

Intermediate tumours. This category, named by Morehead,[6] includes tumours which are locally invasive, and therefore not benign, but which either show little or no tendency to metastasise (*locally malignant tumours* such as basal-cell carcinoma and ameloblastoma) or else sometimes give rise to metastases which progress slowly and usually cause little constitutional disturbance to the patient. These are the *tumours of erratic behaviour* which include pleomorphic tumour of the salivary glands, "adenoma" of the bronchus, and carcinoid tumours of the intestine. These are described in the next chapter.

Latent cancer. This is the name given to a proliferation of cells that has all the histological characteristics of carcinoma, including sometimes lymphatic and blood vessel invasion, and yet which remains clinically silent and does not metastasise. The most convincing examples of this condition have been described in the prostates of elderly men.[7] It is the outer zone that contains these lesions, and not the middle zone that is affected in benign hyperplasia and removed during partial prostatectomy. The nature of the condition is obscure. In some instances it may indeed be a carcinoma which is not progressing because the environment (e.g. hormonal) is not suitable, but most of the lesions are probably atypical epithelial hyperplasias associated with old age. The tendency for excessive epithelial hyperplasia to form pseudocarcinomatous downgrowths into the connective tissue has been noted on p. 301.

Carcinoma-in-situ. This is a pre-invasive proliferation of the epithelium which has the cytological features of malignancy. It is considered on p. 386.

Spontaneous Regressions.[8, 9, 10, 11] These are amongst the most fascinating phenomena of malignancy. There is now a considerable literature of cases of cancer which have suddenly regressed spontaneously and permanently. This rare occurrence is most often seen in cases of malignant melanoma, hypernephroma, neuroblastoma, and choriocarcinoma. The Burkitt tumour may sometimes regress, apparently permanently, after a single dose of a cytotoxic agent too small in amount to account for the result in terms of its known action.[12, 13] The mechanism of these regressions

is not known. It may be hormonal, thus relating it to the hormone-dependent tumours, or it may be immunological. The serum of cases of malignant melanoma that have regressed spontaneously has been noted to affect the course of malignant melanomata when administered to patients with this disease.[14, 15] Sometimes the removal of a primary tumour leads to the regression of its metastases, a phenomenon most often seen in choriocarcinoma and malignant melanoma. Incomplete resection of an inoperable tumour, even one as malignant as an oat-cell carcinoma invading the left atrium, has been known to end in a complete cure of the condition.[16]

Another mechanism involved in the remission of a tumour is a maturation of its cells to a benign or non-neoplastic form. This event is best documented in some cases of neuroblastoma and teratoma of the testis.[18]

Dormant cancer.[17] This is the late appearance of metastases after the primary tumour has been successfully removed. Its implications are considered on p. 371.

Aetiological Classification

Since the cause of most human tumours is unknown, this is at present an impractical basis for classification. Furthermore, there is no indication at the present time that such a classification is likely to be very useful. Tumours induced by radiations, chemical carcinogens, etc., can all look alike, and behave in the same way. Likewise a single agent, e.g. ionising radiations, can induce carcinoma of the skin, osteosarcoma, and leukaemia. It seems that the type of tumour growth is independent of the initiating cause.

Classification Currently Used

The tissue of origin and the behaviour pattern form the basis of the present classification (see tables on pp. 316–317). This is supplemented by a histological description. The suffix -*oma*, is used to denote a neoplasm. Unfortunately it is also used in connexion with some non-neoplastic swellings, e.g. haematoma, granuloma, and hamartoma.

It will be seen that benign tumours of surface epithelia are called papillomata. Benign tumours of solid epithelia are adenomata. These may be cystic (cystadenoma), and into these cysts papillary ingrowths may occur (papillary cystadenoma).

The malignant epithelial tumours are all carcinomata, and a histological description is appended.

In the connective tissues the benign tumours are named after the tissue of origin, e.g. fibroma and osteoma, while the malignant tumours are sarcomata, e.g. fibrosarcoma and osteosarcoma. The term spindle-cell sarcoma is used to describe a sarcoma in which the tissue of origin cannot be recognised. Certain tumours of specialised cells have characteristics which have led to them being given names which do not conform to these rules. Thus the clear-cell carcinoma of the kidney is commonly called a hypernephroma, and a tumour derived from the argentaffin cells a carcinoid. Finally, it should be noted that the term neoplasia is applied in any

Classification of tumours

Tissue of origin	Behaviour		
	Benign	*Intermediate*	*Malignant*
Epithelium.			
1. *Covering and Protective Epithelium.*			
(*a*) Squamous.	Squamous-cell papilloma.		Squamous-cell carcinoma.
(*b*) Transitional.	Transitional-cell papilloma.		Transitional-cell carcinoma.
(*c*) Columnar.	Columnar-cell papilloma.		Adenocarcinoma.
2. *Compact Secreting Epithelium.*	Adenoma. If cystic, cystadenoma or papillary cystadenoma.		Adenocarcinoma. If cystic, cystadenocarcinoma.
3. *Other Epithelial Tumours include.*		Basal-cell carcinoma. Salivary and mucous gland tumours. Carcinoid tumours (argentaffinoma).	
Connective tissue.			
Fibrous tissue.	Fibroma.		Fibrosarcoma.
Nerve sheath.	Neurofibroma.		Neurofibrosarcoma.
Fat.	Lipoma.		Liposarcoma.
Smooth muscle.	Leiomyoma.		Leiomyosarcoma
Striated muscle.	Rhabdomyoma.		Rhabdomyosarcoma.
Synovium.	Synovioma.		Malignant synovioma.
Cartilage.	Chondroma.		Chondrosarcoma.
Bone.			
Osteoblast.	Osteoma.	Giant-cell tumour.	Osteosarcoma.
Mesothelium.	Benign mesothelioma.		Malignant mesothelioma.
Blood vessels and lymphatics.	? Benign haemangioma and lymphangioma.		Angiosarcoma.
Meninges.	Meningioma.		Malignant meningioma.
Specialised connective tissue.			
Neuroglia and Ependyma		Astrocytoma; Oligodendroglioma Ependymoma.*	
Chromaffin tissue.	Carotid body tumour.		Malignant carotid body tumour.
Lymphoid and Haematopoietic tissue.	Benign lymphoma e.g. of rectum and skin.		Lymphocytic lymphoma. Reticulum-cell sarcoma. Hodgkin's disease. Multiple myeloma.
		Myeloproliferative disorders†	Leukaemias.
Melanocytes.			Malignant melanoma.
Fetal trophoblast.	Hydatidiform mole.		Choriocarcinoma.
Embryonic tissue.			
Totipotential cell.	Benign teratoma.		Malignant teratoma.

* These tumours are difficult to classify. The common types are locally malignant, but some also metastasise within the central nervous system. Rarely, and most often in children, they appear to be benign.

† These include polycythaemia vera, haemorrhagic thrombocythaemia, and myelosclerosis (see p. 611).

Classification of tumours—*continued*

Tissue of origin	Behaviour		
	Benign	*Intermediate*	*Malignant*
Pluripotential cell.			
Kidney.			Nephroblastoma.
Liver.			Hepatoblastoma.
Unipotential cell.			
Retina.			Retinoblastoma.
Hind-brain.			Medulloblastoma.
Sympathetic ganglia and	Ganglioneuroma.		Neuroblastoma.
adrenal medulla.			
Pelvic organs.			Rhabdomyosarcoma (sarcoma botryoides).
Embryonic vestiges.			
Notochord.			Chordoma.
Enamel organ.		Ameloblastoma.	
Parapituitary residues.		Craniopharyngioma.	
Branchial cyst.			Branchiogenic carcinoma.
Hamartoma.			
Melanotic.	? Benign melanoma.		Malignant melanoma.
Angiomatous.	? Benign angioma.		Angiosarcoma.
"Exostoses" and			
"Ecchondroses".			Chondrosarcoma.
Neurofibromatosis.	Neurofibroma.		Neurofibrosarcoma.
Tuberous sclerosis.	Glioma.		Malignant glioma.

type of tumour growth whether benign or malignant, while cancer is a colloquial term used to describe any type of malignant tumour whether carcinoma or sarcoma. However, in medical literature it is commonly used synonymously with carcinoma.

In conclusion it must be admitted that our present classification of tumours is far from satisfactory. The accepted division into benign and malignant is confounded by the existence of the group of intermediate tumours. When one adds the occasional instance of spontaneous regression of cancer and latent cancer, and the phenomenon of dormancy to the known unpredictable behaviour of cancer in any individual, it is obvious that there is still much to be learned about the behaviour and classification of tumours.

GENERAL READING

RAVEN, R. W. (1957–63). Edr. *Cancer*, 8 vols. London: Butterworths.
WILLIS, R. A. (1952). *The Spread of Tumours in the Human Body*, 2nd edn 447 pp. London: Butterworths.
WILLIS, R. A. (1967). *The Pathology of Tumours*, 4th edn, 1019 pp. London: Butterworths.
WILLIS, R. A. (1962). *The Borderland of Embryology and Pathology*, 2nd edn, 641 pp. London: Butterworths.

REFERENCES

1. GODWIN, M. C. (1957). *Cancer (Philadelphia)*, **10**, 298.
2. WINSLOW, D. J. and TAYLOR, H. B. (1960). *Cancer (Philadelphia)*, **13**, 127.
3. ADAMI, J. G. (1909). *Principles of Pathology*. London: Oxford University Press
4. BARNARD, W. G. (1926). *Journal of Pathology and Bacteriology*, **29**, 241.
5. ABERCROMBIE, M. and AMBROSE, E. J. (1962). *Cancer Research*, **22**, 525.
6. MOREHEAD, R. P. (1965). In *Human Pathology*, p. 181. New York: McGraw-Hill.
7. FRANKS, L. M. (1954). *Annals of the Royal College of Surgeons of England*, **15**, 236.
8. EVERSON, T. C. and COLE, W. H. (1956). *Annals of Surgery*, **144**, 366.
9. BRUNSCHWIG, A. (1963). *Surgery*, **53**, 423.
10. BOYD, W. (1966). *The Spontaneous Regression of Cancer*, 99 pp. Springfield, Illinois: Thomas.
11. EVERSON, T. C. (1964). *Annals of the New York Academy of Sciences*, **114**, 721.

12. BURKITT, D., HUTT, M. S .R. and WRIGHT, D. H. (1965). *Cancer (Philadelphia)*, **18**, 399.
13. DAVID, J. and BURKITT, D. (1968). *British Medical Journal*, iv, 288.
14. SUMNER, W. C. and FORAKER, A. G. (1960). *Cancer (Philadelphia)*, **13**, 79.
15. NATHANSON, L., HALL, T. C. and FARBER, S. (1967). *Cancer (Philadelphia)*, **20**, 650.
16. SMITH, R. A. (1971). *British Medical Journal*, ii, 563.
17. HADFIELD, G. (1954). *British Medical Journal*, ii, 607.
18. SMITHERS, D. W. (1969). *Lancet*, ii, 949.

Chapter 26. Structure and Effects of Some Common Tumours

BENIGN EPITHELIAL TUMOURS

Epithelial tumours may grow in one of two ways: either as sheets of neoplastic cells covering a surface (*papilloma*), or as solid masses of cells separated into groups by stromal connective tissue (*adenoma*). A tumour may show both types of growth. As in normal tissue the epithelial cells tend to adhere firmly to each other and be distinctly separate from the connective tissue. Epithelial cells are soft, therefore the consistency of their tumours depends upon the quantity and type of the supporting stroma; when this is abundant and collagenous the tumour is hard, but when it is scanty or cellular the tumour is soft.

Papillomata

Benign tumours of surface epithelia appear as warty or papillary overgrowths. Some papillomata are sessile, but most are pedunculated, and these are loosely called *polyps*, a morphological term applied to any pedunculated mass attached to a surface, and not necessarily neoplastic. Sometimes the papilloma is composed of many delicate finger-like processes, or fronds, and it is then called a *villous papilloma*.* These tumours are supplied by a core of connective-tissue stroma containing blood vessels, lymphatics, and nerves. The stroma is an integral part of the tumour and its growth is subservient to that of the epithelium. The stroma is therefore not considered to be primarily involved in the neoplastic process, and these tumours are not regarded as mixed. There is seldom any evidence of an inflammatory reaction in the stroma of a benign tumour, unless there is infection, ulceration, or necrosis.

The tumour is covered by a profuse neoplastic epithelium, which is regularly arranged and shows little evidence of mitotic activity. The basement membrane is always intact, but frequently in histological preparations the complex frond-like structure gives a false impression of invasion; the presence of inflammation due to trauma or infection may disrupt the basement membrane, and further add to the illusion of malignancy. Three main types of papilloma are described according to the nature of the epithelium involved:

Stratified squamous-cell papilloma. This tumour is found on the skin and other stratified squamous epithelial surfaces, e.g. tongue, larynx, and anus. There is invariably an increase in thickness of the prickle cell layer (acanthosis), an increase in the amount of adherent keratin (hyperkera-

* For reasons which are obscure the villous papilloma of the rectum is known as a villous adenoma in North America.

tosis), and retention of the nuclei of the desquamating keratinised cells in some areas (parakeratosis).

Papillary lesions of the skin in fact form a heterogeneous group and it is impossible to state which of them are truly neoplastic. Some indeed are of developmental origin (*epithelial naevus* or *naevus verrucosus*), while others are caused by a virus—the common wart *verruca vulgaris* being the usual lesion. Papillary lesions on the exposed parts are not uncommon in elderly people (*solar keratoses*), and are important because the epithelium often shows dysplasia and the lesions can progress to *in-situ* or invasive carcinoma. Similar lesions are found in those people who have ingested inorganic arsenic. These *arsenical keratoses* occur on the palms, soles, and trunk, and are premalignant and often multiple. A very common papillary lesion of the skin in elderly people is the basal-cell papilloma, or *seborrhoeic keratosis*. The proliferating cells tend to retain their basal-cell morphology. The lesion appears to be growing on the skin surface, there is no invasion of the dermis, and malignancy is almost unknown.

Transitional-cell papilloma. This occurs throughout the urinary passages, most frequently in the bladder. Multiple growths are characteristic. The villous character of the tumour is often so pronounced that it resembles a sea-anemone. The delicate fronds are easily torn, and haematuria is a common symptom. After these tumours are removed recurrence commonly takes place, and from a practical point of view they are best regarded as malignant. Since there is a poor correlation between the histological appearance of the biopsied material and the clinical behaviour of the lesion, some pathologists report all transitional-cell papillomatous lesions as carcinoma regardless of whether or not there is any cellular anaplasia or tissue invasion.

Columnar-cell papilloma. This occurs on any surface covered by columnar epithelium; in the colon the surface mucus-secreting epithelium may occasionally produce a villous papilloma, but this is an uncommon tumour and should not be confused with the pedunculated adenoma (see below).

Papillomata are also found in cystic adenomata (papillary cystadenoma), in the breast ducts, and occasionally in the gall-bladder and bronchi (Fig. 26.1).

Adenomata

A simple tumour of a solid glandular tissue is called an *adenoma*. It consists of dense masses of acini lined by exu-

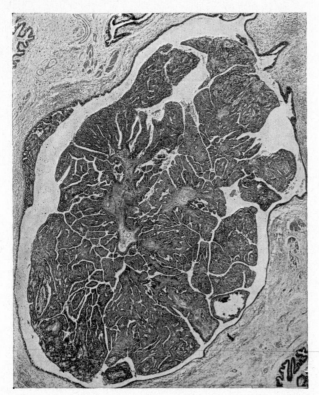

Figure 26.1
Duct papilloma of breast. The dilated duct contains a complex columnar-cell papilloma. The central stromal core is prolonged into an extensive framework which is surmounted by neoplastic epithelium. The stalk connecting this polypoid mass to the duct wall has not been included in the section, but the area of thickened epithelium from which it arose is apparent. There is no evidence of invasion. × 26.

berant epithelium which may be columnar or cuboidal in shape. Adenomata of endocrine glands often show no acini, but are merely composed of uniform polygonal or spheroidal cells arranged in solid groups.

Adenomata arising in glands opening directly on a surface often become pedunculated and form polyps. This is particularly common in the large intestine, and the tumours are frequently multiple. In the hereditary condition of *polyposis coli* thousands of tumours are present, and they may involve the rectum also. The exuberant epithelium of the tumours closely resembles that of the normal, except that the cells are usually larger and the nuclei more hyperchromatic. Any marked degree of irregularity should be viewed with suspicion, as malignant change is quite common.

If an adenoma arises at a distance from a surface it assumes the form of a spherical nodule with a capsule. This is produced as the result of pressure atrophy on the surrounding parenchyma: the more resistant connective tissue remains and condenses to produce a capsule. Adenomata may be found in any glandular organ; the breast, prostate, and endocrine glands are the most common sites, but they are also found in the secreting glands of the skin and bronchi. In the thyroid, adrenal cortex, and prostate the tumours are frequently multiple, and it is difficult to decide whether the condition is neoplastic or merely a nodular hyperplasia (see p.297).

Two variants of adenoma should be noted:

Cystadenoma. Sometimes adenomata form elaborate cystic spaces into which papillary ingrowths of neoplastic epithelium protrude. These papillary cystadenomata are most common in the ovary. Two types are found—one in which the epithelium secretes a serous fluid (serous cystadenoma) and the other in which mucin is produced (mucinous cystadenoma). Cystadenomata are also found in the pancreas, salivary glands, and kidney.

Fibro-adenoma. In the breast the specialised connective tissue surrounding the glandular epithelium is almost invariably involved when an adenoma develops. This overgrowth is more than an excessive stromal reaction, and is probably a true connective tissue neoplasia, because under rare conditions in which malignancy supervenes, a sarcoma, and not a carcinoma, is produced. The tumour is probably a truly "mixed" one.

Two types are described although mixed examples occur, and in practice the distinction is seldom made. In the *hard pericanalicular type* the ducts are small and are surrounded by dense connective tissue, whereas in the *soft intracanalicular type* the ducts are elongated and slit-like, because they are impinged on by looser connective tissue. In this variety the connective tissue sometimes shows such rapid growth that the overlying stretched skin may ulcerate. This is called *Brodie's tumour* (giant fibro-adenoma), and may be mistaken clinically for carcinoma, and histologically for a sarcoma. It is interesting that during pregnancy and lactation, not only does the normal breast epithelium undergo hyperplasia, but similar changes also occur in the epithelial element of a fibro-adenoma. The tumour is thus subject to hormonal influence. It undergoes atrophy and fibrosis after the menopause.

BENIGN CONNECTIVE TISSUE TUMOURS

On the whole this group is rather less important than the epithelial one. Nevertheless the commonest of all tumours belongs to this category, the uterine myoma.

The structure of these tumours is easily predictable in terms of the constituent tissue. There is merely a neoplastic overgrowth of the tissue (bone, muscle, etc.), and the individual cells are separated from each other by intercellular substance which they themselves have produced. The consistency of the tumour depends upon the nature and quantity of this substance rather than that of the stroma (cf. epithelial tumours). Thus a chondroma is harder than a fibroma. The stroma consists of blood vessels and perhaps some surrounding connective tissue. It tends to merge with the neoplastic tissue, particularly so in fibromata. A poorly delineated stroma is, however, a characteristic of all connective-tissue tumours.

Fibroma. Fibromata are not common tumours. They consist of circumscribed collections of fibroblasts between which there is a variable amount of collagen. "Hard" fibromata have much collagen, whereas the "soft" variety are predominantly cellular. They are found in many sites, e.g. skin, stomach, ovary, etc.

An unusual type is the *desmoid tumour*,* also known as the *recurring fibroma of Paget*. This is a tumour of musculoaponeurotic origin, arising most commonly from the rectus sheath of parous women. It is not encapsulated and invades the surrounding muscles, recurring if not completely excised, but it is well differentiated and does not metastasise. It is best regarded as an intermediate tumour of fibrous tissue. Similar tumours are known to occur in other sites and have been given unnecessarily complicated names, e.g. recurring dermatofibroma of Darier and dermatofibrosarcoma protuberans of the skin.

There are, in fact, a number of curious proliferative conditions of fibrous tissue, sometimes grouped as the *fibromatoses*, in which histological assessment of malignancy is difficult.[1, 2] In *nodular fasciitis*, which affects the subcutaneous tissues and deep fascia, there is the rapid growth of a highly vascular mass which diffusely infiltrates the surrounding tissues; in spite of the malignant microscopic appearance the lesion is quite benign. Similar benign lesions are *juvenile fibromatosis* and *pseudosarcomatous dermatofibroma* of the skin. *Palmar (Dupuytren's contracture) and plantar fibromatosis* are in a similar category, for they are ill-defined fibromatous overgrowths which may appear malignant microscopically, but which never behave so clinically. *Idiopathic mediastinal fibrosis*, which causes superior-venacaval obstruction, and *retroperitoneal fibrosis*, which frequently obstructs the ureters, may both fall into this same group. It is of interest that the latter appears to be caused by the ingestion of the drug methysergide used in the prophylaxis of migraine.[3] The association of Dupuytren's contracture with hepatic dysfunction, as in chronic alcoholism, may be a further indication that a chemical agent can cause a localised fibromatous overgrowth.

Myxomatous change may be found in some fibromata. Such a tumour is then called a *myxofibroma*, or if the change is marked, a *myxoma*.

Myoma. Tumours of muscle are of two types:

Leiomyoma. This is the commonest of all tumours, being found in the uteri of about 20 per cent of women over 30 years of age. Leiomyomata of the skin, stomach, and intestine are also not uncommon. These tumours are often multiple. A leiomyoma is composed of whorls of smooth muscle cells, interspersed among which there is a variable amount of fibrous tissue. In due course the muscle element may be replaced by the fibrous tissue, and a fibroleiomyoma (or "fibroid") is produced. Such a tumour may undergo cystic change or else become densely calcified. On section the

* The word is derived from the Greek *desmos*, a band or tendon, and alludes to the tendon-like consistency of the tumour.

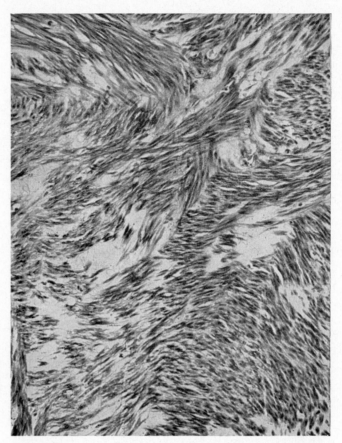

Figure 26.2
Leiomyoma. This uterine tumour consists of sheaves of elongated, spindle-shaped smooth muscle cells. There is a patchy replacement of the muscular element by hyaline fibrous tissue. It is this process that gives rise to the name fibroid. × 200.

whorled interlacing pattern of glistening, white bundles resembling watered-silk is characteristic.

Rhabdomyoma. A tumour of striated muscle is very uncommon. Most examples are malignant rhabdomyosarcomata occurring in young children (see Chapter 27). Rhabdomyomata of the heart are described, but most of these are malformations occurring in tuberous sclerosis.

Tumours of Nerve Sheath Origin[4]

The literature on this subject is confusing because of the uncertainty regarding the parent cell of origin. Two types of lesion can be recognised, but it is not known whether they are distinct entities or merely variations of a single process.

Neurofibroma. This tumour is now thought to arise from Schwann cells rather than fibroblasts. It causes a diffuse fusiform enlargement of a nerve, and is composed of spindle cells arranged in flowing streams with a varying amount of intervening reticulin and collagen. Nerve fibres pass through the tumour, and myxomatous change is not infrequently present. The tumours may be solitary, and can occur on a spinal nerve root or a peripheral nerve. Often they are multiple, and their presence constitutes a major feature of von Recklinghausen's disease. Whether all the nodules in this disease are true neoplasms is debatable—it might be more reasonable to regard them as hamartomatous or areas of dysplasia. Nevertheless, meningiomata, schwannomata, and even gliomata can also be found in this disease, and these are classified as tumours. Malignant change is not uncommon especially in patients with multiple lesions. Another lesion on the borderline of neoplasia is the *plexiform neuroma*, a diffuse overgrowth of the connective tissue of a nerve which produces great thickening, coiling, and distortion of the nerve. When occurring in a limb there may be other developmental anomalies, e.g. local gigantism. This too may occur as part of von Recklinghausen's disease.

Schwannoma. This tumour is usually solitary and may arise from any cranial or peripheral nerve. It is encapsulated and appears to arise focally on a nerve trunk, so that the nerve itself is stretched over the tumour rather than running through it as in the neurofibroma. A common site for schwannomata is the auditory nerve, and they may be bilateral. The tumour may occur on spinal nerve roots and indeed on any large nerve trunk. A mediastinal location is not uncommon. Apart from arising on large nerve trunks these tumours may appear in relation to a small peripheral nerve of the skin or an internal viscus, e.g. stomach.

Macroscopically and microscopically the tumour is very similar to a leiomyoma, the whorled arrangement of spindle cells being common to both. Sometimes these spindle cells have a palisaded, or regimented, appearance, all the nuclei being aligned in one strip, and the clear cytoplasm of the cells in an adjacent strip (Fig. 26.3). This appearance may be seen in leiomyomata, but it can be distinguished by phosphotungstic-acid haematoxylin staining, which is taken up by muscle cells.

As the name suggests, the schwannoma is thought to arise from the Schwann cells of the nerve sheath. Neurilemoma is an alternative name, but is falling into disuse on the objection that the neurilemma signifies the sheath or basement membrane of the Schwann cells rather than the cells themselves. The schwannoma can produce collagen, and on electron microscopy the neoplastic cells have a basement membrane, thereby resembling adult Schwann cells.[5] The same cell type is seen in neurofibromata, and this argues against them being fibroblasts, which have no surrounding basement membrane. Both neurofibromata and schwannomata therefore arise from this cell type, and it is not surprising that both types of lesion may occur in the same patient or even in the same tumour mass.

Meningioma. This is a tumour of the arachnoid cells that lie on the deep surface of the dura and on the arachnoid granulations. Meningiomata are usually situated in relation to the superior sagittal sinus, the transverse sinus, and the falx cerebri, and by pressure on the underlying brain a

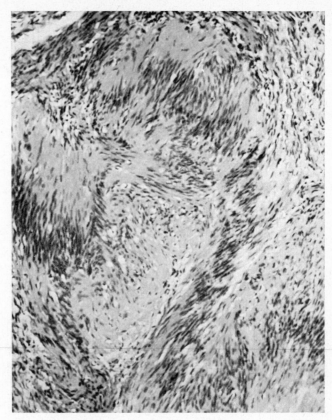

Figure 26.3
Schwannoma. Note the palisaded, or regimented, appearance of the long, spindle-shaped cells; their nuclei form a continuous sinuous column, and on each side there is a similar column composed of clear cytoplasm. × 200.

hollow is formed. Sometimes the calvaria is implicated by the tumour, and excessive bone formation results. In structure these tumours consist of plump epithelial-like clumps of arachnoid cells, usually arranged in a whorled pattern. There is a variable fibrous stroma, and sometimes a vascular element is prominent. Spherules of calcification are common in the arachnoid cell clumps (psammoma bodies), and this brain "sand" is alluded to in the alternative name "psammoma" which is applied to these tumours (Fig. 26.4).

Lipoma. This common tumour is composed of adult adipose tissue. It is usually subcutaneous, but may be retroperitoneal or subserosal.

Giant-cell tumour of bone. This is composed of fusiform fibroblastic cells and numerous giant cells, some of which have enormous numbers of nuclei (Fig. 26.5). These giant cells are believed to be neoplastic osteoclasts, but as some authorities dispute this, the alternative name "osteoclastoma" is best avoided. It is usually found at the metaphysis of the long bone. It produces pressure atrophy of the bone. It occurs in young adults up to about the age of 30 years. It frequently undergoes central cystic change, and

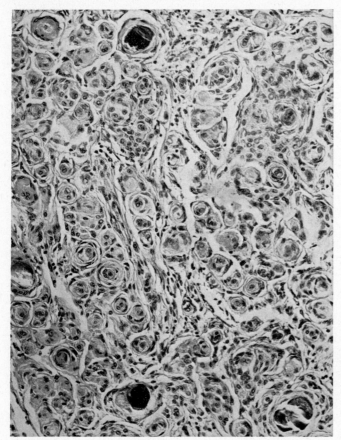

Figure 26.4
Meningioma. It is composed of circumscribed, whorled aggregations of plump, epithelial-like cells surrounded by a vascular stroma. A few darkly-staining, calcareous spherules (psammoma bodies) are present amid the cellular clumps. × 150.

appears radiologically as an osteolytic tumour in which a few bony trabeculae are still recognisable. Macroscopically it is an expansive haemorrhagic cyst with an egg-shell covering of bone. Although this tumour is generally classified as benign, some examples are locally malignant and a small percentage metastasise.

In hyperparathyroidism tumour-like lesions may develop in the bones, and they closely resemble giant-cell tumours. These *brown tumours*, as they are termed, are usually multiple but can occasionally occur as a solitary lesion. Hence recurrence after treatment should always lead to an investigation of calcium metabolism.

Chondroma. A benign chondroma is comparatively uncommon, for most examples are really skeletal malformations involving the epiphyseal cartilage. One type involves the hands, and by its expanding nature leads to great deformity. It consists of mature cartilage with regular chondrocytes.

Osteoma. Many osteomata, e.g. the common exostoses, are malformations, but now and again solitary tumours of this

type are encountered, especially in the skull. They may consist of compact bone (hard or ivory osteomata) or of spongy bone (cancellous osteomata).

Characteristics of Benign Tumours

Benign tumours are usually circumscribed, and apart from surface growths like papillomata, they usually possess a capsule. Their shape is usually round, but they tend to be moulded by surrounding structures. Thus a particular arrangement of fascia may make them oval. On the other hand, a neurofibroma of a posterior nerve root tends to expand into the spinal canal in one direction, and into the thoracic cavity in the other: the result is a dumb-bell shaped tumour.

Size. Although *benign tumours are usually smaller* than malignant ones, they may at times attain enormous proportions. Some of the largest tumours reported are ovarian cystadenomata and uterine fibroids, and the largest tumour in the museum of the Royal College of Surgeons of England is a fibroma of the kidney weighing 82 pounds (37 kg). A

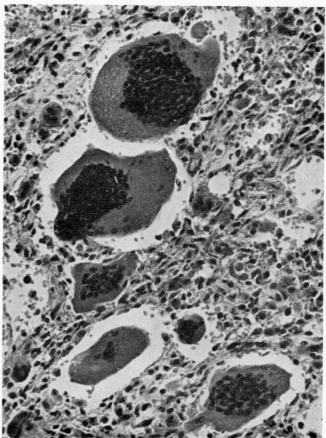

Figure 26.5
Giant-cell tumour of bone. It is composed of many large giant cells, interspersed among which there are smaller, spindle-shaped fibroblastic cells. × 200.

malignant tumour would have killed the patient long before reaching this size.

Ulceration and haemorrhage are rare except in surface tumours, e.g. papillomata and submucous fibroids, and even in these they are infinitely less severe than in their malignant counterparts.

The rate of growth of benign tumours is generally slow. It is often erratic, and usually tends to cease after a period.

Both structurally and functionally the tumour cells tend to copy the parent tissue. The cells themselves are regular, and mitotic figures are few. Tumours of the endocrine glands, in addition, may secrete an excess of hormone which can have serious and sometimes even fatal results. While both benign and malignant tumours can produce hormones, the most marked effects are usually seen in adenomata:

(i) An adenoma of the β cells of the *pancreatic islets* secretes insulin, and the hyperinsulinism may lead to severe attacks of hypoglycaemia. A non-β-cell islet tumour (often a carcinoma) may produce the *Zollinger-Ellison syndrome*,[6, 7] in which there is hypersecretion of gastric hydrochloric acid and intractable peptic ulceration. Gastrin has been isolated from these tumours.[8] There may also be intractable diarrhoea with severe hypokalaemia, and the condition is then called the *Verner-Morrison syndrome*. The cause of the diarrhoea is not understood; when there is hyperchlorhydria it could be that the very acid gastric juice interferes with the digestive enzymes of the pancreas, which require an alkaline pH in which to function. But in some cases there is achlorhydria.[9] Steatorrhoea has also been described.

(ii) Tumours of the adrenal medulla (*phaeochromocytomata*) secrete noradrenaline and adrenaline; a classical paroxysmal hypertension may be produced, which tends later to become sustained. There is an increased excretion of catecholamines in the urine in these patients. This is a useful diagnostic aid. If the tumour secretes adrenaline there may also be hyperglycaemia (noradrenaline does not have this effect).

(iii) Tumours of the *adrenal cortex* produce a wide range of steroid hormones. The following syndromes may be produced by such tumours: (*a*) the adrenogenital syndrome, (*b*) Cushing's syndrome, (*c*) Conn's syndrome (see p. 298).

(iv) *Pituitary tumours* produce several different syndromes: (*a*) *Gigantism* in children and *acromegaly* in adults due to acidophil adenomata, (*b*) *Cushing's syndrome* due to basophil adenomata (see p. 298).

(v) *Parathyroid tumours* are associated with osteitis fibrosa cystica (von Recklinghausen's disease of bone).

(vi) *Thyroid adenomata* and carcinomata rarely produce hyperthyroidism.

(vii) In the ovary *granulosa-cell tumours* are oestrogen producers and lead to endometrial hyperplasia with uterine bleeding, while the *arrhenoblastoma* is androgenic and causes virilisation. The *choriocarcinoma* and *hydatidiform mole* produce large quantities of placental gonadotrophic hormone.

(viii) The *interstitial-cell adenoma* of the testis may secrete either androgens or oestrogens. When it occurs in boys there may be premature puberty; others develop gynaecomastia.

(ix) *Carcinoid tumours* produce a specific syndrome, see p. 336.

(x) Not infrequently multiple endocrine adenomata occur together in a patient. The commonest combination involves the parathyroids, pituitary (chromophobe or acidophil), and pancreatic islets; less often the adrenals and thyroid are also affected. This syndrome of *multiple endocrine adenomatosis* is often associated with peptic ulcer, and not infrequently the Zollinger-Ellison syndrome is present. The syndrome is often hereditary, being inherited as a dominant trait with variable penetrance and expressivity.[10, 11] Isolated familial parathyroid adenomatosis with hyperparathyroidism has also been reported on several occasions; it may be an incomplete manifestation of the larger syndrome.[12]

Benign tumours may also produce serious mechanical effects by virtue of their position. In this way intracranial and spinal tumours like meningiomata and neurofibromata are dangerous. Natural passages may be blocked, and extensive damage results. Thus obstruction to a bronchus leads to bronchiectasis, while an occluded ureter produces a hydronephrosis with secondary infection. Tumours of the gut, e.g. polypoid adenomata and lipomata, may produce intestinal obstruction by precipitating an intussusception. Occasionally the heart's action is impaired by a benign growth. These effects are, of course, also produced by malignant tumours.

Finally, *benign tumours never metastasise.*

MALIGNANT EPITHELIAL TUMOURS—CARCINOMATA

The carcinomata are the commonest of all malignant tumours, probably because epithelium is a continuously dividing (labile) tissue. Some carcinomata involve covering non-secreting epithelium, and are called squamous-cell or transitional-cell carcinomata. Carcinoma of secretory epithelium is called adenocarcinoma provided it is sufficiently well differentiated to show glandular structure.

Three main types are recognised as with the papillomata:

Squamous-cell Carcinomata

These tumours arise at any site normally covered by stratified squamous epithelium—skin, mouth, oesophagus, anus, ectocervix, etc. At other sites they may occur as a result of tumour metaplasia, or possibly neoplasia in an area of squamous metaplasia (see p. 308), e.g. lung, urinary tract, gall-bladder, etc.

Macroscopic types. Two are usually described:

The papillary carcinoma appears as a warty outgrowth with an infiltrating base; this type may arise in a papilloma.

The nodular type produces a hard, nodular mass beneath the surface, and shows more rapid infiltration and dissemination. Both types usually ulcerate to form a typical *carcinomatous ulcer*. This has a raised, craggy, rolled edge which is fixed to surrounding skin and deeper structures. The base is composed of white necrotic tumour, which is usually friable and bleeds easily.

Histological type. In considering the histological structure of a squamous-cell carcinoma it is necessary first to understand its formation (Fig. 26.6).

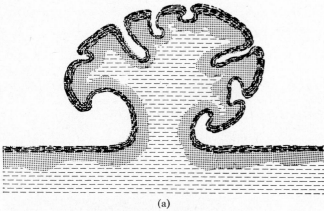

(a)

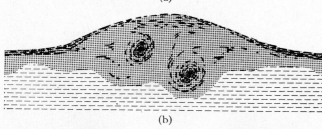

(b)

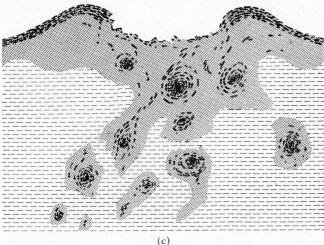

(c)

Figure 26.6
Three types of neoplasia of a keratinising squamous stratified epithelium.
(a) Benign neoplasia results in an excessive production of regular epithelium, which in order to be accommodated is thrown into a complicated folded structure. This is a papilloma.
(b) In *carcinoma-in-situ* the epithelial overgrowth is irregular; the cells are bizarre and lose their polarity. The epithelium is thickened and contains areas of keratinisation within its depths. The basement membrane is intact and there is no invasion.
(c) In carcinoma the basement membrane is destroyed, and atypical cells invade the underlying tissues.

Formation. When epithelium shows malignant propensities, there is a progressive proliferation of the prickle-cell layer. This is sometimes so irregular that, even before it actually breaks through the basement membrane, it may give the microscopical impression of malignancy. To this condition the name *carcinoma-in-situ*, or *intraepithelial carcinoma*, is applied. Whether all such "carcinomata" do in fact proceed to frank invasive malignancy is questionable, and the subject is considered in detail in Chapter 29.

The criterion of truly invasive carcinoma is the destruction of the basement membrane by masses of malignant cells, which then spread down into the deeper connective tissue and muscle. As they proceed, they tend to break up into separate groups or columns. These clumps may comprise hundreds of cancer cells, or else only a few. In the most anaplastic tumours there may be no attempt at any splitting up, and the tumour cells proceed in one diffuse mass.

As the tumour infiltrates, it destroys the tissue with which it comes in contact, and this is replaced by a fibrous stroma which may be dense and acellular as in scirrhous cancers, or else loose and vascular, and infiltrated with lymphocytes, plasma cells, and even polymorphs and eosinophils. Nearly all malignant tumours excite an inflammatory reaction around them, of which the lymphocytic component is very

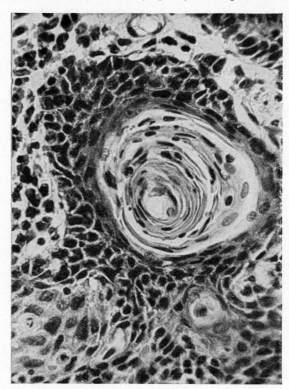

Figure 26.7
A cell nest or epithelial pearl. This is a group of cells from a well-differentiated squamous-cell carcinoma. In the centre of the group the cells have differentiated so well that they resemble stratum granulosum and corneum with keratin in the midst. × 380.

important, because cell-meditaed immunity is especially involved in checking the spread of malignant tumours. Lymphocytes are present around tumours of low-grade malignancy and during the early stages of malignant change (see p. 359). Once ulceration of the surface occurs, there is a more acute type of response due to secondary bacterial infection.

In those carcinomata which break up into discrete columns, each individual clump may then differentiate partly or completely to resemble the normal epithelium from which it has arisen.

Differentiation. Squamous-cell carcinomata vary considerably in the degree of differentiation which they show. When differentiation is good, *epithelial pearls* (also called *keratin pearls, horn pearls,* or *cell nests*) are formed. These are groups of cells, which by differentiating produce a central whorl of keratin (Fig. 26.7). Surrounding this there are prickle cells, and occasionally a stratum granulosum is recognisable. A basal-cell layer is not well formed. In this way there is a fairly accurate reproduction of the upper layers of normal stratified squamous keratinising epithelium. The cells are usually fairly uniform in size and shape, their nuclei are evenly staining, and mitoses are scanty. On the whole spread is slow. The skin is the commonest site, but

sometimes well-differentiated cancers occur in the oral cavity and bronchus.

The more undifferentiated tumours contain no keratin, but groups of prickle cells may still be recognisable (Fig. 26.8).

Highly undifferentiated, or anaplastic, tumours show no attempt at prickle-cell formation. There is a diffuse sheet of neoplastic cells supported by a scanty, vascular stroma with no separation into groups. The cells themselves show great variation in size and shape, their nuclei are darkly-staining and irregular in morphology, and mitotic figures abound (some of these are bizarre). Tumour giant cells may be present (Fig. 26.9). It may be impossible to distinguish the tumour from a connective tissue neoplasm. This type of tumour is found usually in the mouth, bronchus, and cervix.

Variations of Squamous-cell Carcinoma

"Transitional-cell" papillary carcinoma. Some squamous-cell carcinomata of the nasopharynx and lung have a papillary

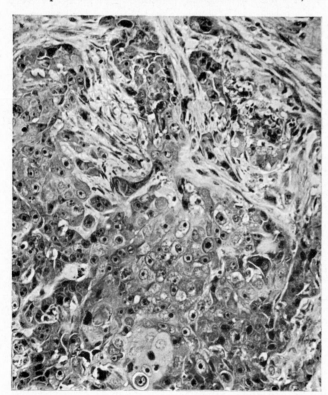

Figure 26.8
Poorly-differentiated squamous-cell carcinoma. In this section there are well-formed clumps of squamous cells which show considerable pleomorphism. There is no attempt at keratin formation. ×200.

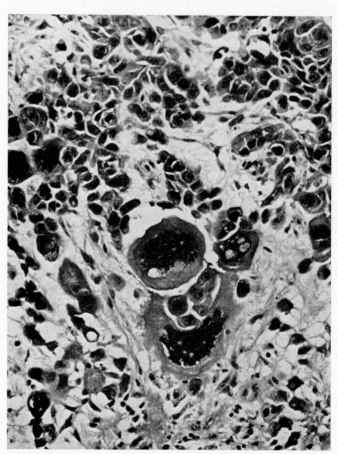

Figure 26.9
Anaplasia. This is part of an anaplastic squamous-cell carcinoma from the maxillary antrum. The cells are arranged in irregular sheets surrounded by a vascular stroma. Cellular pleomorphism is very marked. In the centre of the field there are two tumour giant cells. Elsewhere there is much variation in cell size and shape and in nuclear size and staining intensity. ×240

structure, and are composed of a transitional type of epithelium similar to that of the urinary passages. It is better not to
call this type of tumour transitional-celled, as it simply
causes confusion.

Verrucous Carcinoma.[47] This papillomatous, well-differentiated tumour occurs in the mouth, larynx, and genital
region. Histological evidence of invasion is sometimes
difficult to find, particularly in biopsy material. The
tumour is noteworthy for its very good prognosis.

Lymphoepithelioma. Anaplastic tumours of epithelium overlying lymphoid tissue sometimes contain sheets of undifferentiated cells copiously intermingled with lymphocytes.

The histological distinction from reticulum-cell sarcoma
may be extremely difficult. This type of neoplasm usually
occurs in the pharynx, especially in connexion with the
tonsils. It is of high-grade malignancy, and often the first
sign of disease is the appearance of large metastases in the
cervical lymph nodes; at this stage the primary may be so
small that it is missed.

Spindle-cell squamous-cell carcinoma. Occasionally the cells
of a squamous-cell carcinoma are fusiform or spindle-
shaped. This is a very undifferentiated type of tumour, and it
may be impossible to distinguish from a sarcoma or an
amelanotic melanoma.

Grading. Histological grading as described by Broders is
of some slight help in assessing prognosis. Four grades are
recognised, according to the degree of differentiation.[13]

Grade I   More than 75 per cent cell-differentiation.
Grade II   50–75 per cent cell-differentiation.

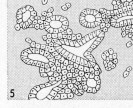
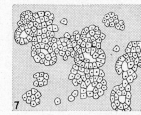
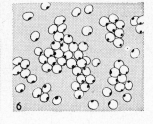
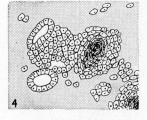
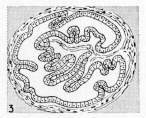
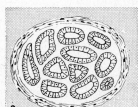
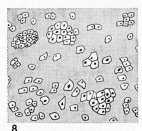
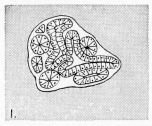
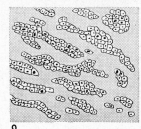
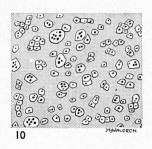

Figure 26.10
Tumours derived from glandular epithelium.
The normal gland (1) is contained within a
sheath of connective tissue. Benign neoplasia
results in the formation of an adenoma (2)
with well-differentiated structure and encapsulation. Cystic dilatation of acini and complicated infolding of the epithelium produce
a cystadenoma (3). The remainder of the
tumours are malignant. The adenocarcinomata show some tubular differentiation which
may be good (5) or poor (7). Lack of differentiation results in a carcinoma simplex
(9). The most anaplastic tumours form a sheet
of loosely attached cells (8). Giant-cell forms
may predominate (10). These anaplastic
tumours may be indistinguishable from
sarcomata, melanomata, and tumours of
squamous epithelial origin. Abnormal differentiation results in squamous metaplasia
(4) or the formation of signet-ring cell
carcinoma (6).

Grade III   25–50 per cent cell-differentiation.
Grade IV   Less than 25 per cent cell-differentiation.

Accurate grading on a numerical basis is seldom used, because (*a*) it is time-consuming and difficult, and there is bound to be a difference of opinion among pathologists as to what constitutes a differentiated cell; most pathologists would agree about grades I and IV, but not about grades II and III, and (*b*) to be done accurately, the whole tumour should be serially sectioned. This is impossible in practice. It not infrequently happens that one area of a tumour is better differentiated than another. The same often applies to metastases of the tumour. It is obvious that the painstaking grading of a few sections is quite inadequate. (*c*) Prognosis is not infallibly related to the grade. The relationship is only approximate.

It is therefore more reasonable to define three grades—well-differentiated, poorly-differentiated, and undifferentiated. On the whole, the higher the grade, the worse is the prognosis, but the greater is the degree of radiosensitivity.

Some authorities are not convinced that grading is of any great help in the individual case, because many exceptions are found. Certainly the site of the tumour is of great importance. A grade-I squamous-cell carcinoma of the skin has an excellent prognosis, while in the lung the outlook is poor. Similarly, a grade-IV tumour of the cervix has a much better prognosis than a similar tumour of the lung or pharynx. The prognosis can also be related to the cause of a tumour, for instance the prognosis of squamous-cell carcinomata of the skin arising in actinic keratoses is much better than that of similar tumours arising *de novo* or in Bowen's disease.[14]

Carcinomata of Glandular Epithelium

These tumours arise from surface, secreting epithelia as well as from underlying glands. They may on occasions arise from columnar-cell papillomata and adenomata.

The pattern of invasion of neoplastic epithelium beneath the basement membrane into the deeper tissue is similar to that already described; in this case the groups of cancer cells, instead of producing keratin, tend to arrange themselves into acinar structures containing a central lumen into which secretion pours. The cells surrounding this lumen may be columnar, cuboidal, polygonal, or spheroidal (Fig. 26.10). The best differentiated cancers show excellent acinus formation, which may mimic normal glandular structure. These tumours are called adenocarcinomata (Fig. 26.11).

In less well differentiated tumours there are merely clumps of cells surrounded by a stroma. There is no attempt at central

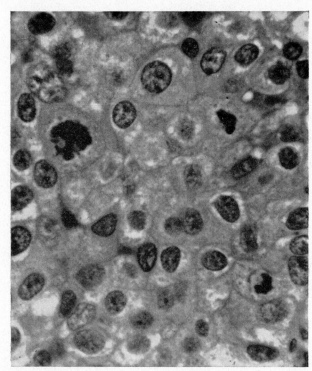

Figure 26.12
Poorly-differentiated tumour of lung. This is in fact a section of an adenocarcinoma of the lung; in some parts it contained tubules and in others mucus-secreting cells. In this field there is complete undifferentiation—the cells are pleomorphic and there are three abnormal mitotic figures. If the whole tumour were of this type of cell, it would be termed a polygonal-cell carcinoma. ×910.
(*From Walter, J. B. and Pryce, D. M.* (1955), Thorax, **10**, 107)

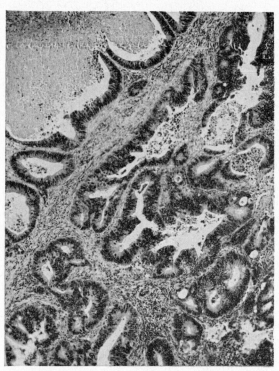

Figure 26.11
Columnar-cell adenocarcinoma. This is a well-differentiated adenocarcinoma of the colon. It consists of large, well-formed acini containing secretion, and is lined by exuberant columnar cells. It is infiltrating the muscle diffusely. ×80.

cavitation to produce acini. To this type of cancer the name *carcinoma simplex* is applied. It is seen most commonly in the breast, where the cancer clumps are often surrounded by a dense fibrous stroma. There may be acinus formation elsewhere in the tumour (Fig. 26.12).

The most undifferentiated examples cannot be distinguished from other anaplastic tumours.

Mucoid cancer. Sometimes the cells of a carcinoma simplex contain demonstrable mucus. This is evidence of glandular function, and it is not unreasonable to call such a tumour an adenocarcinoma even if there is no evidence of acinus formation. However, most pathologists restrict the term adenocarcinoma to tumours showing structural glandular differentiation. Sometimes there is so large an accumulation of mucus in the cytoplasm that the nucleus is compressed on to the cell wall. This type of cell is called a *signet-ring cell*, and it bears a morphological resemblance to an adult fat cell. If mucus secretion is marked, the tumour is called a *mucoid cancer*.

In some adenocarcinomata so much mucus is formed that it infiltrates into the stroma, which appears as a basophilic

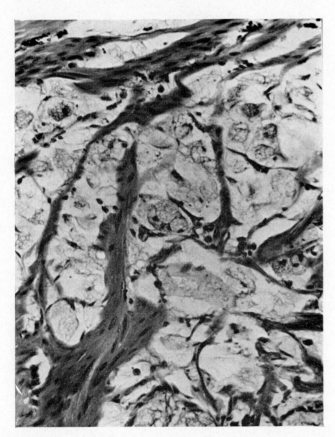

Figure 26.13
Mucoid cancer. This is a mucus-secreting carcinoma infiltrating the muscular coat of the stomach. Most of the space between the muscle fibres consists of lakes of mucus, in the midst of which the distintegrating cancer cells are still recognisable. × 300.

lake, in the midst of which lies disintegrating tumour tissue (Fig. 26.13). This forms another type of mucus-secreting, or mucoid, carcinoma, and both types may be found in the stomach, large bowel, lung, and rarely in the breast. Mucoid breast cancer is an example of mucus-secreting tumour metaplasia of neoplastic breast epithelium; mucous glands are not normally found in the breast.

Mucoid cancers are commonly miscalled "colloid" cancers; this is a bad term because it carries the false association of thyroid tissue.

Mucoid cancer presents a characteristic naked-eye appearance of a bulky, gelatinous, mucoid mass. The mucus tends to stimulate a considerable fibrous tissue reaction in its vicinity. Mucoid cancers are notorious for the ease with which they spread locally, and their prognosis is worse than that of other adenocarcinomata.

Grading of glandular carcinomata on a system similar to that of Broders has been used to assess malignancy. In cancer of the breast a system based upon that first described by Greenough in the USA has proved of some value.[15] Three features were taken into account when grading a tumour:

(*a*) Tubule formation.
(*b*) Regularity in size, shape, and staining of nuclei.
(*c*) Number of mitoses.

The prognosis in relation to stage (see p. 371) and grade of tumour is shown in Fig. 16.14.

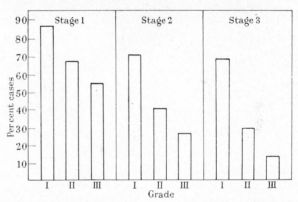

Figure 26.14
Stage, grade, and prognosis in cancer of the breast. Percentage of cases alive at 5 years (all treatments). *(From Bloom, H. J. G.* (1950), *"Prognosis in carcinoma of the breast",* Brit. J. Cancer, **4,** 259*)*

Stromal reaction. The reaction of the invaded tissue to the carcinoma cells varies; it may be so stimulated to grow that a fibrotic, hard (*scirrhous*) type of tumour is produced. Most breast cancers are of this type (Fig. 26.15). The dense fibrosis appears to be associated with a contracting tendency, which is ill understood. In the breast there is an accompanying retraction of the nipple and dimpling of the skin. Eventually a stony fixation to the chest wall ensues.

Scirrhous tumours are also commonly found in the alimentary tract. In the stomach a pyloric cancer may cause

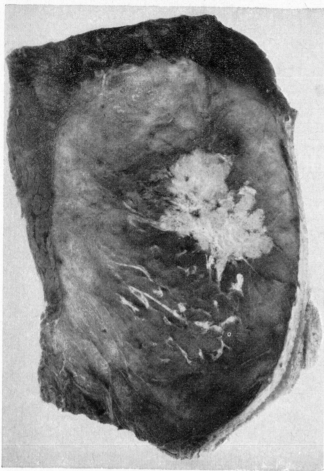

Figure 26.15
Carcinoma of the breast. The section through the breast shows a typical scirrhous carcinoma. Its outline is irregular and ill-defined, for it spreads sinuously into the surrounding fibro-fatty tissue. *(EB 10.1, Reproduced by permission of the President and Council of the R.C.S. Eng.)*

thickening of the wall and obstruction. In the diffuse infiltrating form of gastric cancer (linitis plastica) the fibrous tissue response is so marked that a careless histologist may miss the scanty carcinoma cells scattered throughout. The annular, or purse-string, type of cancer of the colon is another example of a scirrhous cancer, and it too causes obstruction. It should be noted that, although the fibrosis seen in scirrhous tumours gives the impression of an attempt by the host to strangle the tumour cells, this does not appear to be the case in practice. The prognosis of scirrhous cancer is quite as poor as that of the encephaloid type. The metastases of scirrhous cancer also tend to have the same dense fibrous stroma.

When the tumour has little stroma in relation to the cell bulk, the growth is soft and is described as medullary, or *encephaloid*. Some breast cancers, e.g. during lactation, and the "cauliflower" cancer of large bowel, e.g. caecum, are of this type.

Transitional-cell Carcinoma

These tumours occur in the renal pelvis, ureter, and bladder. They are often papillomatous in appearance. Microscopically the tumours vary from well-differentiated columns of transitional epithelial cells to highly anaplastic tumour differing in no way from other undifferentiated neoplasms. Squamous metaplasia is common.

Special Types of Carcinoma

It is useful at this stage to consider the structure of a few special carcinomata in greater detail.

Carcinoma of kidney. This common tumour has a characteristic naked-eye appearance: situated usually at one pole of a kidney (most commonly the upper) it has a variegated appearance due to areas of orange colour interspersed amid white stroma with contrasting red areas of haemorrhage (Fig. 26.16).

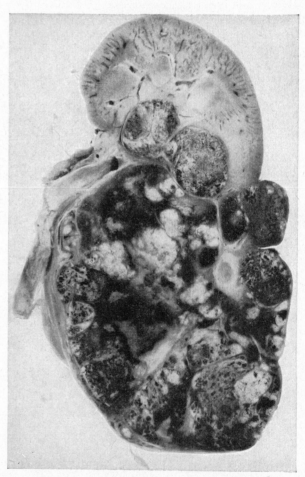

Figure 26.16
Hypernephroma. The lower pole of the kidney has been replaced by an encephaloid tumour, which is infiltrating into the upper pole and is occluding the ureter. The substance of the mass has a typical variegated appearance. *(EU 30.1, Reproduced by permission of the President and Council of the R.C.S. Eng.)*

Microscopically it is composed of large, polygonal, clear cells arranged in groups, and sometimes disposed in tubules. The resemblance of these cells to those of the adrenal cortex led to the belief that these tumours arose from the ectopic adrenal rests which are found quite frequently on the surface of the kidney. The widely-used name "hypernephroma" is a relic of this erroneous hypothesis. The tumour is certainly renal in origin. Small adenomata of the kidney are not uncommon, and in many of these similar clear cells are found. Furthermore, "hypernephromata" are not found outside the kidney in the other sites where adrenal rests are known to occur.

The clear appearance of the cells is due to their high content of glycogen and lipid, which tend to be removed

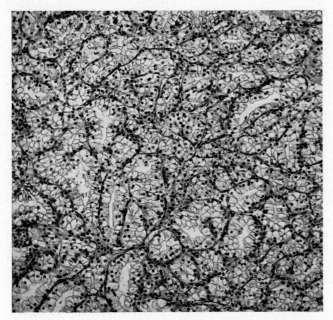

Figure 26.17
Clear-cell carcinoma of the kidney (hypernephroma). The tumour consists of collections of round and polygonal cells with darkly-staining nuclei and clear cytoplasm. The tumour is fairly well-differentiated, for many of the cell groups are arranged in acini. × 130.

during histological preparation. The orange colour of the tumour is due to the lipochrome content of these cells. The best name is *clear-cell carcinoma of the kidney.**

Lung carcinoma. Tumours may arise from the large bronchi (central) or small bronchioles (peripheral). Peripheral cancer is thought by some (including the authors)[16]

* Clear-cell tumours are typical of the adrenal cortex and para-thyroid also. Occasionally adenocarcinomata of other organs, and even squamous-cell carcinomata, consist of clear cells. It is apparently related to glycogen content in these cases. Although the name "hypernephroma" is to be deprecated on theoretical grounds, it is so firmly entrenched in British nomenclature that its use has been retained in this book.

to be the commoner type, but the classical view is that central growths are the more frequent. Four histological types are usually recognised.[17]

(1) The *adenocarcinoma*, which tends to occur peripherally, is more frequent in women, and apart from a tendency towards squamous metaplasia does not differ from similar tumours elsewhere. A mucoid variant occasionally occurs.

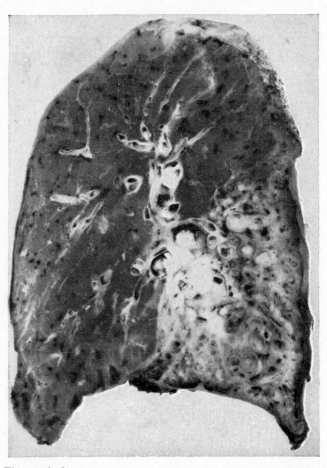

Figure 26.18
Carcinoma of the lung. This tumour has arisen from the left lower lobe main bronchus. Not only has it infiltrated into the lower lobe extensively, but it has also led to distal bronchiectasis. The hilar lymph nodes are also involved in the tumour. The tumour proved to be a squamous-cell carcinoma. (R 45.1, *Reproduced by permission of the President and Council of the R.C.S. Eng.)*

"Alveolar-cell carcinoma." This uncommon type of lung cancer presents a characteristic radiological and naked-eye appearance. Both lungs show numerous small discrete foci of growth, which radiologically give a "snow-storm" effect. The tumour appears to arise multifocally, but inhalation metastasis from a small localised primary tumour cannot be absolutely excluded.

Microscopically the tumour is a well-differentiated adenocarcinoma; tumour cells may be seen lining the alveoli,

Figure 26.19
Carcinoma of the lung. The tumour has arisen from the right main bronchus, and has infiltrated extensively into all the lobes. The hilar lymph nodes are enlarged and invaded by the tumour. The tumour was proved to be an oat-cell carcinoma. *(R 45.3, Reproduced by permission of the President and Council of the R.C.S. Eng.)*

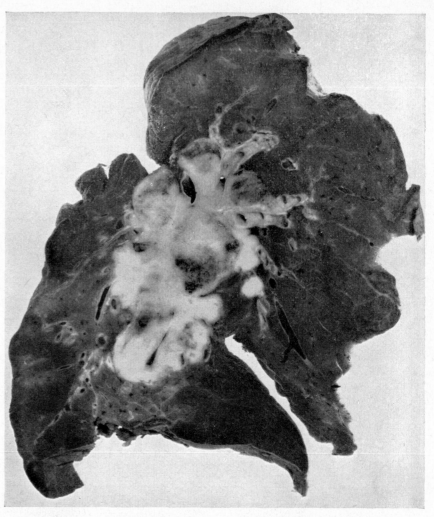

but there is no evidence to suggest that it arises from the alveolar cells themselves. In fact, it does not differ microscopically from many localised well-differentiated lung adenocarcinomata, and it therefore presumably arises from bronchiolar epithelium.

It is important to note that many fair examples of "alveolar-cell carcinoma" are in fact secondary deposits from adenocarcinomata arising elsewhere, e.g. thyroid, ovary, or pancreas. Indeed, it is important to exclude secondary tumours before diagnosing primary lung cancer, even when there is a solitary mass.

(2) The *squamous-cell carcinoma* affects the larger bronchi more frequently, but even in this type peripheral growths are common.

(3) *Oat-cell carcinoma.* The commonest type is variously called the small-cell (USA) or oat-cell carcinoma (Britain). The naked-eye appearance is often characteristic in advanced cases: masses of fleshy white tumour are seen invading the lung and the lymphatics around the blood vessels and bronchi. The lymph nodes of the mediastinum are massively involved,

which accounts for the misconception that the tumour was a mediastinal sarcoma. Microscopically the growth is composed of sheets of small, basophilic cells with hyperchromatic nuclei, which are either round, oval, or "oat-shaped". The cytoplasm is scanty, and superficially the cells resemble lymphocytes. Rosettes or tubular structures are not infrequently present amid the diffuse sheets, and these are evidence of the epithelial origin of the tumour.

Oat-cell carcinoma appears to be a distinct tumour, and is probably derived from neurosecretory cells of the bronchial mucosa akin to the argentaffin cells of the intestine. In this respect it shares a common origin with the carcinoid type of bronchial adenoma.[18] It is found predominantly in men, and is highly malignant and equally highly radiosensitive.

(4) *Polygonal-cell carcinoma (large-cell carcinoma).* This type of tumour is undifferentiated, and consists of sheets and groups of large, eosinophilic polygonal cells (Fig. 26.12).

Carcinoma of the testis. The commonest testicular cancer is derived from the seminiferous epithelium, and is called a *seminoma.* It is found in middle-aged and elderly

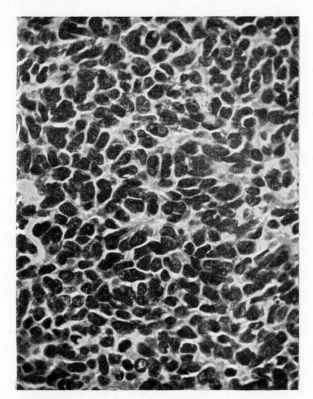

Figure 26.20
Oat-cell carcinoma of lung. The tumour is composed of a sheet of uniform, small, darkly-staining cells. Their fusiform shape gives rise to the descriptive term "oat cell". × 500.

men. It has a very typical microscopical appearance: columns of large spheroidal cells with prominent round, darkly-staining nuclei and scanty cytoplasm. These cells are clearly neoplastic spermatocytes (Fig. 26.21). The columns are separated by thin fibrous trabeculae in which there are often many lymphocytes. Macroscopically it is a white encephaloid tumour which tends to spread up the spermatic cord to the regional lymph nodes.

The *teratoma* occurs usually in a somewhat younger age-group, and is considered in Chapter 27.

Carcinoma of the skin. The common skin cancer is a *squamous-cell carcinoma*, which is usually well differentiated. It usually ulcerates early and becomes secondarily infected. Spread is slow, and as the tumour is very radiosensitive, cure may be achieved with comparatively little cosmetic disturbance (see also p. 328).

The other important skin cancer is the *basal-cell carcinoma* described below.

Adenocarcinomata of the accessory skin appendages (sweat and sebaceous glands) are occasionally encountered. Some sweat-gland tumours behave like pleomorphic salivary adenomata which are described below.

The *malignant melanoma* is usually found in the skin. It is considered in Chapter 27.

Intermediate Epithelial Tumours

Some tumours, although locally invasive, very seldom show distant metastases; these are the locally malignant tumours, of which the basal-cell carcinoma is the typical example. Another group of tumours is characterised by a more erratic type of behaviour, some being benign, some locally malignant, and others frankly malignant.

Locally malignant tumours. *Basal-cell carcinoma*, or *rodent ulcer*, occurs most frequently on the skin of the face of fair-skinned people exposed excessively to the sun.

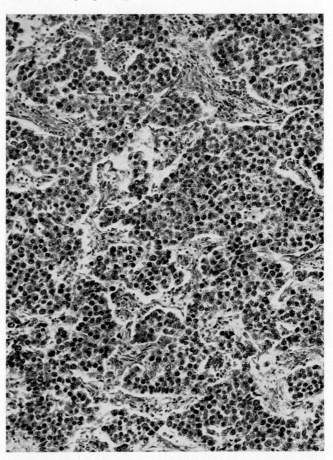

Figure 26.21
Seminoma. The tumour is composed of columns of large, round cells which are neoplastic spermatocytes. These columns are separated by thin fibrous trabeculae containing lymphocytes. × 150.

Microscopically the dermis is infiltrated by groups of small, basophilic, fusiform cells with prominent darkly-staining nuclei (Figs. 26.22 and 26.23). These cells resemble "oat cells", and there is often considerable mitotic activity in their midst, yet the prognosis of the lesion is excellent. The layer of cells at the edge of each clump is usually arranged in the form of a "palisade", perpendicular to the surrounding connective tissue. It resembles the germinative layer of the epidermis very closely, and is not found in squamous-cell

Figure 26.22
Basal-cell carcinoma. Separated from the epidermis
there is a well-defined group of basal-cell carcinoma
cells. In this section the peripheral palisading of
the cells perpendicular to the dermal stroma is well
shown. ×200.

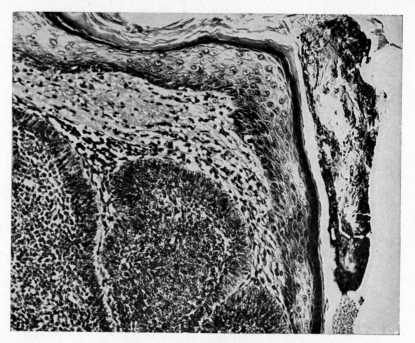

carcinoma. Degenerative changes within the clump may produce central cystic spaces (Fig. 26.23).

The origin of the tumour is debatable. The appearance of tongues of growth protruding downwards from the surface epithelium has given rise to the concept that it is a "basal-cell carcinoma". The continuity of the basal germinal cells with the outer palisaded tumour cells confirms this. It seems inevitable, however, that squamous-cell carcinomata must also ultimately arise from the basal cells. An alternative and more attractive theory is that the basal-cell carcinoma is derived from basal cells tending towards differentiation into hair follicles, sweat glands, and sebaceous glands. When it is remembered that the adnexae are formed as buds of epithelial cells into the dermis, a close similarity between their genesis and that of the basal-cell carcinoma is apparent. Furthermore, in these tumours foci of keratinisation may sometimes be found; these might well represent hairs (less commonly differentiation into glandular structures is seen). Whatever the histogenesis of this tumour, there is no doubt that it is distinct from the squamous-cell carcinoma in behaviour. Even though it may show squamous metaplasia and marked mitotic activity, the basal-cell carcinoma very rarely metastasises. It may, however, invade local structures relentlessly, and cause extensive damage and ultimate death. As it progresses it destroys the nose and eyes, and eventually erodes through the skull and leads to meningitis.

Cylindroma. This tumour has a structure which resembles that of a basal-cell carcinoma but in spite of this it is almost invariably benign. It is composed of small darkly-staining cells arranged in clumps. Outer palisading around each clump is a well marked feature, and external to this there is a conspicuous hyaline sheath. This consists of the basement membrane proper and an associated layer of collagen fibres. Occasional tubule formation is present and thought to indicate apocrine differentiation. Cylindromata usually occur on the face or scalp. They are sometimes multiple and inherited as an autosomal dominant characteristic (turban tumours). The name cylindroma is unsatisfactory because it refers merely to the microscopic appearance of the groups or cylinders of cells. Cylindroma has also been applied to some pleomorphic salivary gland tumours and bronchial adenomata, and a similar appearance can be seen in basal-cell carcinoma and even oat-cell carcinoma of lung.

Trichoepithelioma. Like the cylindroma this tumour is usually benign and also occurs on the face or scalp. If multiple it is inherited as a dominant trait. Both types of tumour may co-exist. Trichoepithelioma consists of groups of cells not unlike basal-cell carcinoma, but the centre of each clump is occupied by a well-marked whorl of keratin. This gives the tumour a cystic appearance and an alternative name is *epithelioma adenoides cysticum.*

It should be noted that the term epithelioma is often used as a synonym of squamous-cell carcinoma in Britain. However, in the North American continent it has no such malignant connotation, and is used to include other epithelial tumours of the skin, benign as well as malignant, e.g. benign calcifying epithelioma. The term should therefore never be used without qualification.

Ameloblastoma. This is a tumour derived from the enamel organ, and is considered in Chapter 27. It too has considerable powers of local destructive spread, but seldom metastasises. A peculiar tumour of the tibia, also called an ameloblastoma, is described. Like the dental tumour it bears some histological resemblance to a basal-cell carcinoma, but unlike

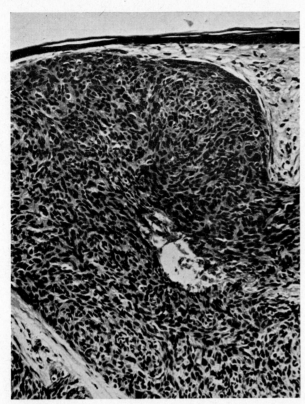

Figure 26.23
Basal-cell carcinoma. A collection of basal-cell carcinoma cells underneath the thinned epidermis is present in this section. The cells are small and fusiform, and have a scanty cytoplasm and relatively large, darkly-staining nuclei. In this section peripheral palisading is not well marked. A central cystic area due to degeneration is present. × 160.

it there is a tendency to lung metastasis. Whether it is an atypical synovioma or an aberrant epithelial tumour is not known.

Tumours of erratic behaviour. *Pleomorphic salivary gland tumours.* These tumours, found most commonly in the parotid, tend to behave for the most part like adenomata. They consist of acini, cords, and thin strands of epithelial cells suspended in a stroma which often has a myxomatous appearance (Fig. 26.24). This was once regarded as true cartilage, and the tumour was called a "mixed salivary tumour". It is now realised that the mucoid appearance is due to a sero-mucous secretion from the tumour acini into the stroma. True cartilage is very rarely found, and when present, it is due to chondral metaplasia of the altered stroma. The epithelium itself often shows squamous metaplasia.

The tumour may appear encapsulated, but the capsule is often infiltrated by lateral extensions of growth. Simple enucleation is likely to be followed by recurrence. Furthermore, local invasion may sometimes occur. Occasionally distant blood-borne metastases are encountered, even in tumours which in one area "look benign". There are all

degrees of transition from adenoma to frank carcinoma in this type of neoplasm.

Other pleomorphic adenomata. Tumours of similar type are found in the palate, nasopharynx, and bronchi, and are derived from mucous glands. Pleomorphic lacrimal gland tumours are recognised, and finally some sweat-gland tumours of the skin have a similar appearance. In them the mucoid stromal change is less in evidence. Many of these tumours have a cylindromatous appearance in some parts,

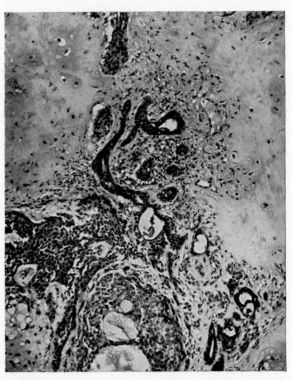

Figure 26.24
Pleomorphic salivary gland tumour ("adenoma"). The structure consists of masses of epithelial cells, some of which are disposed in well-formed ductules. The stroma is copious and dense, and much of it has a cartilaginous appearance. × 110.

and a more frankly adenomatous one elsewhere. Their behaviour is very similar to that of the salivary variety. In the trachea and bronchi they invariably exhibit local invasion, while in the skin they are usually benign.

Bronchial "adenoma". This term, which now serves no useful purpose and should be dropped, has been applied to a group of bronchial tumours which forms about 1 per cent of all pulmonary neoplasms.[19] Four distinct entities are included. The rarest is a mucous-gland adenoma of the bronchus. The other three are best classified as tumours of intermediate type since they tend to grow slowly, invade locally, sometimes spread to the regional lymph nodes, and rarely disseminate by the blood stream. The carcinoid tumour is the most common and arises from neurosecretory cells. Occasionally it gives rise to hormonal effects like its highly malignant counterpart, the oat-cell carcinoma. The two other types are the cylindroma (also called adenoid cystic carcinoma) and the mucoepidermoid carcinoma, which histologically resemble similar tumours occurring in the salivary gland. These tumours may occur peripherally, but more commonly they are central and involve one of the major bronchi. They bulge into the lumen and produce obstruction, and invade the bronchial wall between the cartilage rings, leading to an "iceberg" effect. Endoscopic removal is therefore unlikely to be curative.

Carcinoid tumour (*argentaffinoma*). This is found most commonly in the bowel, especially in the appendix, and rather

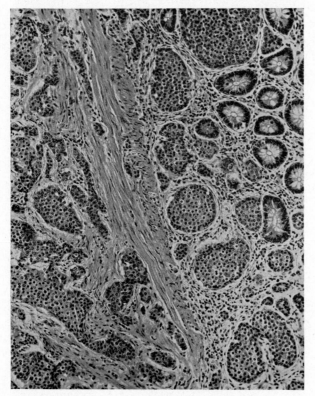

Figure 26.25
Argentaffin tumour of colon. There is an infiltration of the sub-mucosa and muscular coat of the colon by groups of tumour cells. These are small, spherical and uniform in appearance, and are arranged in cylinders and elongated trabeculae. To the right of the section some normal mucous glands are present. × 120.

less frequently in the terminal ileum and the large intestine. But it has also been described in the stomach, and it forms one type of bronchial "adenoma". It arises from the argentaffin cells of Kultschitzky. It has a characteristic yellow colour, and tends to stimulate a scirrhous reaction so that a stricture forms around the bowel.

The small, round, darkly-staining cells are arranged in solid clumps or cylinders; acinar differentiation is unusual.

If the cells are fixed freshly in formalin, special granules can be demonstrated with silver stains. The tumour is locally invasive, and may metastasise to the regional lymph nodes and the liver, especially in lesions of the small and large bowel. Despite multiple metastases the patient may survive for many years in comparatively good health.

In about 1 per cent of all cases and in 20 per cent of those with metastases an endocrine syndrome, the *carcinoid syndrome*,[20] develops. It consists of paroxysmal facial flushing, diarrhoea, bronchospasm with dyspnoea, and sometimes organic heart disease—usually pulmonary stenosis or tricuspid regurgitation. The tumour produces large amounts of 5-hydroxytryptamine (5-HT), which is excreted in the urine mostly as 5-hydroxyindoleacetic acid (5-HIAA). The 5-HT is not the main cause of symptoms, for an intravenous injection of it does not produce them. Adrenaline, on the other hand, does induce an attack in these patients, and it appears that catecholamines act as a trigger while the actual mediator is a kinin, probably bradykinin.[21] Alcohol can also induce an attack, perhaps by leading to the release of catecholamines.[21] The most recent evidence suggests that 5-HT plays a subsidiary part, especially in the diarrhoea, and 5-HT antagonists are very useful in relieving it. Some gastric carcinoids produce 5-hydroxytryptophane, and these also show a relief of gastrointestinal symptoms when treated with antagonistic drugs. Carcinoids of the stomach and bronchus sometimes also secrete histamine, in which case there is a tendency to peptic ulceration.

Medullary carcinoma of the thyroid. This uncommon tumour consists of solid sheets and cords of uniform cells in a hyaline stroma rich in amyloid material. Despite its anaplastic appearance the tumour behaves very similarly to the carcinoid tumour, often causing death many years after metastases have developed. It arises from the parafollicular (C) cells of the thyroid, and is quite distinct from other thyroid carcinomata. These cells secrete calcitonin (see p. 571), but so far no case of hypocalcaemia has been reported in association with the tumour. On the other hand, a carcinoid syndrome has been noted, and the tumour may elaborate 5-HT, a kinin-forming enzyme, and prostaglandins. The presence of stromal amyloid is not understood.[22, 23]

TUMOURS OF CHORION-EPITHELIUM

Choriocarcinoma (*chorion-epithelioma*) is a distinctive tumour of fetal origin, being derived from the trophoblast. It may be considered together with the carcinomata, for it has much in common with highly malignant tumours of other epithelia.

The well-known *hydatidiform mole* is the benign counterpart of this tumour: the characteristic grape-like clusters that are expelled from the uterus consist of oedematous placental villi surmounted by proliferating chorion-epithelium.

Sometimes there are foci in which the cells are extremely pleomorphic, and these may invade the wall extensively. This is called an *invasive mole* (*chorio-adenoma destruens*), but in spite of its appearance it rarely metastasises. It is important in this respect to realise that even normal chorionic tissue invades the uterine veins, and fragments are found in the lungs in pregnancy and especially during parturition.

In the rare *choriocarcinoma* there is an anaplastic proliferation of chorionic cells which are large and irregular. Many fuse to form syncytial masses, which are in fact a type of tumour giant cell. The tumour actively invades blood vessels and therefore bleeds easily; massive haemorrhage is a notable feature of the condition. Metastases occur early, and the lung is usually the first site of secondary deposits. These tumours are interesting in that they secrete a large amount of gonadotrophic hormone (of placental type). This produces bilateral theca-lutein ovarian cysts. The pregnancy tests are strongly positive. Very rarely a similar type of tumour is found in a testicular teratoma. It should be noted that other anaplastic neoplasms may produce a histological appearance of pleomorphic giant cells which is very similar to that of a choriocarcinoma.

MALIGNANT TUMOURS OF CONNECTIVE TISSUE—SARCOMATA

Sarcomata are much less common than carcinomata, and unlike them, they occur at all ages. While the cells in a carcinoma tend to be arranged in discrete cellular clumps surrounded by a variable stroma (this does not apply to the most anaplastic of them), those in a sarcoma are disposed in diffuse sheets, in which the neoplastic cells merge inseparably into the stroma.

On the whole, sarcomata spread more rapidly than carcinomata, and the prognosis is correspondingly more grave. Early blood-borne metastases are the rule, and the lungs are often riddled with secondary deposits. Radical resection affords the best hope of cure, for these tumours are very radioresistant. Even when complete removal of a sarcoma is possible, e.g. osteosarcoma and malignant synovioma of an extremity, later pulmonary metastases are the rule.

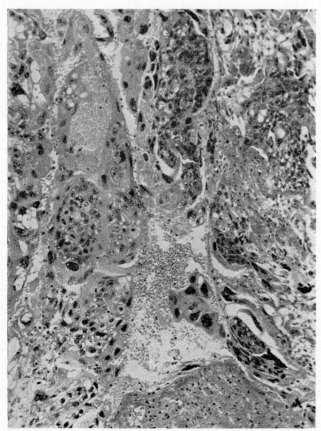

Figure 26.26
Choriocarcinoma. This section shows the large, pleomorphic cells with darkly-staining nuclei that are the neoplastic element of the tumour. In the centre of the field there is a large vascular space which contains tumour tissue arranged in extensive syncytial masses. × 100.

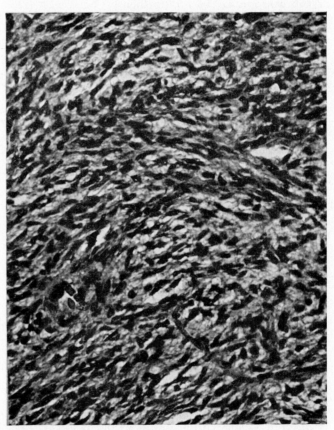

Figure 26.27
Fibrosarcoma. The tumour is composed of sheets of large spindle-shaped cells with a minimal amount of intervening stroma. There is some pleomorphism and nuclear irregularity. × 400.

TABLE 26.1   A comparison of malignant epithelial tumours (carcinomata) and connective tissue tumours (sarcomata, excluding the lymphomata)

Carcinoma	Sarcoma
Age incidence Commonest in middle and old age. A very common tumour.	Occurs at all times of life; common in young people. A much less common tumour.
Structure (*a*) Typically arranged in groups and columns, except in the most anaplastic tumours. (*b*) Stroma often well-formed. Haemorrhage and necrosis less extensive, except in anaplastic tumours.	(*a*) Arranged in diffuse sheets intimately related to the stroma. (*b*) Stroma nearly always poorly-formed and inadequate for the growth of the tumour. Haemorrhage and necrosis extensive.
Growth pattern Often somewhat slowly-growing.	Growth usually very rapid.
Metastases (*a*) Early lymphatic metastases. (*b*) Blood-borne metastases usually evident a little later. (*c*) Commonest seat of blood-borne metastasis is the liver. Other organs often involved are the lungs, brain, bones, kidneys, and adrenals.	(*a*) Lymphatic spread rare. (*b*) Blood-borne metastases appear very early. (*c*) Commonest seat of metastasis is the lung. Other organs may also be involved. Skeletal deposits are rare.
Radiosensitivity Many are highly radiosensitive.	Much more radioresistant.

Fibrosarcoma. This is the malignant counterpart of the fibroma. It differs from the benign tumour in that it infiltrates the surrounding tissues and metastasises. Although it is not encapsulated, in practice it is very difficult to assess infiltration until the tumour is quite large. An important diagnostic feature that distinguishes a fibrosarcoma from a cellular fibroma is the irregular, pleomorphic appearance of the individual cells. There is always evidence of mitotic activity, but it is often difficult to arrive at a decision which is of the utmost importance from the patient's point of view.

The more malignant varieties of fibrosarcoma show greater cellular pleomorphism, nuclear hyperchromatism, and mitotic activity; giant cells are quite common. Collagen formation is scanty (Fig. 26.27).

The most anaplastic tumours show no collagen, and the cells are either spindle-shaped (*spindle-cell sarcoma*) or plumper, and are then scarcely distinguishable from anaplastic carcinomata. Haemorrhage and necrosis are common features of most sarcomata, because the stroma is delicate and the vascular supply inadequate to meet the demands of the tumour.

Osteosarcoma. This is one of the common forms of sarcoma. It tends to occur in later childhood, and is notoriously malignant. It may also occur as a complication of Paget's disease in older patients. The cell of its origin is the osteoblast. As in other sarcomata the tumour cells are very pleomorphic, and giant cells are often numerous. If the tumour is well differentiated there is osteoid formation which may or may not calcify to produce bone (Fig. 26.28). Sometimes islets of cartilage are formed, but the osteosarcoma should be distinguished from the chondrosarcoma, in which neoplastic cartilage is laid down in large amounts. It is a less malignant tumour.

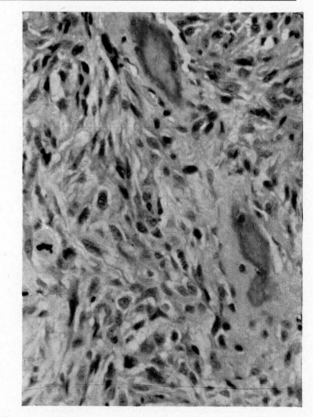

Figure 26.28
Osteosarcoma. The section consists of sheets of spindle-shaped cells intimately connected with the intervening stroma. In their midst there are two spicules of osteoid. There is a conspicuous mitotic figure at the left side of the section. × 350. (*Photograph supplied by Dr. A. D. Thomson*)

As an osteosarcoma grows (it usually starts at the metaphysis of a long bone), it tends to elevate the periosteum. A fusiform swelling is produced, and bone forms under the periosteum and around the stretched-out periosteal vessels. In this way the characteristic sun-ray appearance of bony spicules is produced. It is interesting that the epiphyseal cartilage forms a barrier to the spread of the tumour, and that most osteosarcomata do not invade joints (Fig. 26.29).

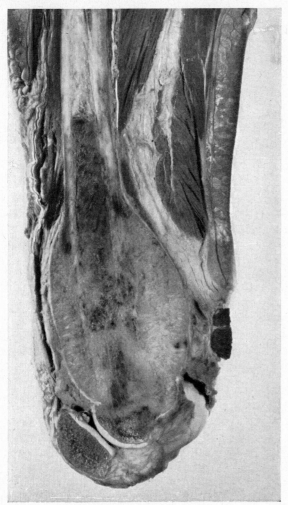

Figure 26.29
Osteosarcoma. The lower end of the femur has been destroyed by an osteosarcoma which has spread almost as far as the knee joint. The tendency for the tumour to lift up the periosteum and assume a fusiform shape is well shown in this specimen. *(S 72a.5, Reproduced by permission of the President and Council of the R.C.S. Eng.)*

THE LYMPHOMATA

These tumours together with the leukaemias constitute the commonest type of malignancy after the carcinomata. It is the "labile" lymphoid and haematopoietic tissues which

are involved. It is better not to class them with the sarcomata, as their behaviour and radiosensitivity are quite distinctive (see Chapter 30).

THE GLIOMATA

Four main types are recognised:

1. *Medulloblastoma.* This is an embryonic tumour which is considered in Chapter 27.
2. *Oligodendroglioma.*
3. *Ependymoma.*
4. *Astrocytoma.*

The astrocytoma is the commonest glioma. The differentiated tumours are composed of cells which closely resemble astrocytes with abundant glial processes. Although only locally invasive, their situation renders them very lethal tumours. In the more anaplastic tumours the cells have fewer glial processes and show the pleomorphism and mitotic activity characteristic of malignant tumours. The old name glioblastoma multiforme emphasises this feature. At one time it was thought that the tumour cells resembled the spongioblasts present during embryonic development, and it has also been called a spongioblastoma. It is now believed that this is a purely fortuitous feature of anaplasia, and in reality the tumour is derived from adult astrocytes. There is, however, a school of thought that still classes the glioblastoma multiforme as a distinct tumour.

Astrocytomata are generally classified according to their degree of differentiation and described as being well-differentiated, poorly-differentiated, or undifferentiated (Fig. 26.31).[24]

The oligodendroglioma consists of uniform sheets of rectangular, box-like cells with a clear cytoplasm and darkly-staining nuclei. Malignancy is, as usual, indicated by pleomorphism and mitotic activity.

The ependymoma consists of irregular spaces lined by exuberant ependymal cells similar to those seen in the walls of the ventricles and the central canal of the spinal cord.

Both oligodendrogliomata and ependymomata are rare tumours, and their growth potentiality resembles that of the astrocytoma.

Dystrophic calcification is prominent in these brain tumours (especially the oligodendroglioma), and is useful in radiological diagnosis.

CHARACTERISTICS OF MALIGNANT TUMOURS

The criterion of malignancy is *invasiveness*. The tumour edge is therefore ill-defined, contrasting with the encapsulation of benign tumours. It is this infiltrative capacity which gives the name "cancer" (the crab). Some rapidly-growing tumours may indeed show evidence of expansile growth,

Figure 26.30
Malignant glioma. The left cerebral hemisphere contains a large haemorrhagic tumour. It is poorly demarcated, and the swelling it has occasioned has partly occluded the lateral ventricle which is pushed over to the opposite side. (N 33.5, *Reproduced by permission of the President and Council of the R.C.S. Eng.*)

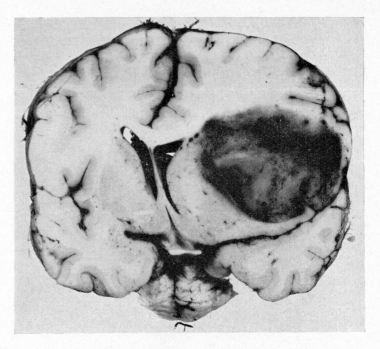

and a false appearance of encapsulation may be produced. Hypernephromata, for instance, may appear to be well circumscribed: microscopy, however, reveals invasion.

Excluding the locally malignant group, all malignant

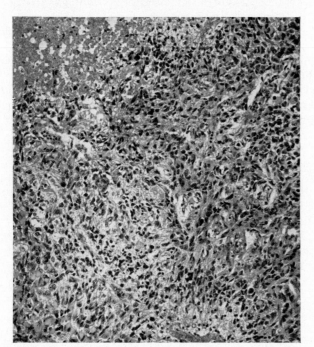

Figure 26.31
Malignant astrocytoma. This poorly-differentiated tumour is composed of fairly uniform, plump, spindle-shaped cells with little intervening glial tissue. In one corner there is an area of necrosis. × 170.

tumours *metastasise*. The spread of tumours is considered in detail in Chapter 28.

Malignant tumours usually undergo a *rapid increase in size*. Therefore, unless death occurs very early in the course of the condition, a greater size is attained than with benign tumours. Enormous size is, however, uncommon.

Microscopical Features

Microscopically several important features should be noted. The tumour tissue may resemble the parent tissue to a considerable extent, but the similarity is not as great as in benign tumours. Differentiation is not so well developed, and recognition of the tissue of origin is sometimes difficult or impossible. It is the estimation of the degree of differentiation which forms the basis of tumour grading. At one time it was thought that normal differentiated cells could undergo neoplasia and revert to a more primitive state and appearance. This process of "dedifferentiation" is nowadays discredited. Primitive cell-forms are now ascribed to a basically primitive cell-origin with a subsequent failure of normal differentiation. Neoplastic cells do differentiate, but frequently the differentiation is abnormal and does not conform to that found normally in the tissue. To describe a tumour as poorly differentiated is probably inaccurate, but it is a common practice and means that to the observer the neoplastic cells are making little attempt to resemble the structure of those found normally in the tissue.

Malignant tumours usually show much mitotic activity. The buildup of DNA prior to division results in nuclear enlargement and hyperchromatism. This factor together with the formation of aneuploid and polyploid cells accounts for the irregularity in size, shape, and staining which is so characteristic of malignant tumours. Mitoses are not only numerous, but are also sometimes abnormal. The number of chromosomes formed during division often diverges from the normal 46. Such aneuploid cells usually contain an excess of chromosomes, some perhaps with abnormal forms. A histogram of the DNA content of malignant cells therefore shows a wider scatter than normal. With the exception of the Philadelphia chromosome there is no single constant change in chromosomal form or number that is characteristic of malignancy. Triradiate mitoses with the formation of three daughter cells is particularly characteristic of malignancy, but the authors have also noted it in *carcinoma-in-situ* such as may occur in actinic keratoses.

Anaplasia. This term was introduced by Hansemann to describe new cells which deviated from the normal and resembled those of embryonic tissue. The term is generally restricted to the abnormalities seen in tumours and can be applied widely to all the variations that occur. One may therefore have architectural anaplasia when the cells produce an abnormal structure, such as when smooth muscle cells produce an irregular interwoven myoma rather than an orderly sheet of smooth muscle. Likewise when applied to individual cells the term may be used to indicate the structural and functional aberrations ranging from the degree of differentiation and the cellular pleomorphism to the production of an abnormal hormone. Nevertheless, in practice the term anaplasia is used in respect of the microscopic cellular changes of neoplasia. An anaplastic tumour is one which has little or no normal differentiation and which exhibits the cellular changes depicted in Fig. 26.32.

Giant cells. Giant cells may occur in malignant tumours under a variety of circumstances:

1. They are seen in some tumours as a regular occurrence due to the nature of the growth, e.g. giant-cell tumour of bone, osteosarcoma, Hodgkin's disease, and choriocarcinoma.

2. They occur as a feature of anaplasia in any malignant tumour. Giant-cell variants of many neoplasms are known, e.g. carcinoma of the lung and thyroid.

3. Giant cells may form in a tumour which is growing under adverse conditions, e.g. a tongue of lung cancer growing into the lumen of a bronchus.

4. Finally, foreign-body giant cells may form in relationship to necrotic tissue, cholesterol, keratin, etc.

Malignant tumours are thus characterised by a failure of the cells to differentiate normally, by their irregular disposition, by the number of mitoses, by prominent nucleoli, and finally by abnormalities in cell shape, size, and staining. These features are frequently relied upon in the clinical diagnosis of cancer. When small biopsies are taken, the arrangement of a few groups of cells may be sufficient to establish a diagnosis; in exfoliative cytology a few abnormal cells may suffice. Although in practised hands diagnoses based upon these cellular changes may be reliable, it must never be

forgotten that the only absolute criterion is tumour behaviour. *It is only by the detection of spread that cancer can be diagnosed with absolute certainty*. In clinical practice the tumour is often inoperable by the time this stage is reached. Morphological changes may be extremely useful in early diagnosis, but they are never an absolute indication of malignancy. For example,

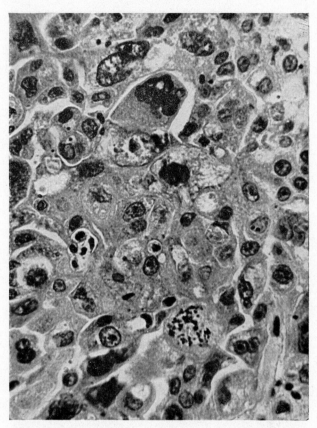

Figure 26.32
Anaplastic tumour of lung. This section shows the main features of malignant cells—pleomorphism, nuclear irregularity in size and staining capacity, giant cells, and a bizarre mitotic figure. ×570.

mitoses may be seen in hyperplastic lesions and some benign tumours, and abnormal cell-forms can occur in irradiated tissue.

The clinician and the patient are anxious to know the behavioural characteristics of a particular tumour. The pathologist has to rely on the morphological appearance of the tumour and the accumulated wisdom of past experience. A pathological diagnosis of malignancy is generally substantiated clinically unless effective treatment is available. Exceptions occur, but it is remarkable that these are so infrequent considering our ignorance about the basic nature of malignancy. There is indeed no reason for complacency, because the prognosis for an individual patient with a tumour, especially a "malignant" one, is always in doubt.

Effects of Malignant Tumours

Malignant tumours produce their ill-effects in a large number of ways:

Like benign tumours by causing mechanical pressure and obstruction. The obstruction produced by a malignant tumour is more pronounced and complete than

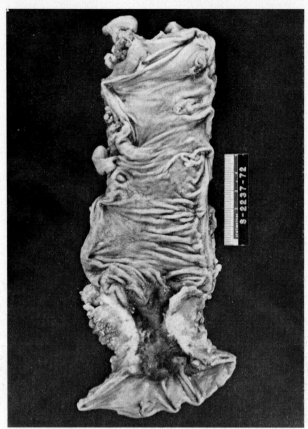

Figure 26.33
Carcinoma of colon. This resection specimen from a man aged 66 years shows an adenocarcinoma at the recto-sigmoid junction. The tumour involves the whole circumference of the gut, and has produced stenosis. The pericolic fat has been invaded, and several regional lymph nodes contained metastatic carcinoma. *(Photograph supplied by Dr. J. B. Cullen).*

that of a benign tumour, e.g. a carcinoma of the colon soon leads to intestinal obstruction, and a bronchial carcinoma may rapidly cause collapse of a lobe. Pressure is also greater, and vessels may be occluded at an early stage.

Destruction of tissue. In addition, malignant tumours infiltrate and destroy vital structures. Their metastases similarly destroy vital organs. This is the usual mode of death in cancer. A carcinoma of the cervix eventually implicates the ureters and leads to uraemia; a breast cancer metastasises to the spinal column and damages the cord; a prostatic cancer metastasises to the bones and causes marrow destruction leading to anaemia, etc. It is this de-

structive character of cancer that is the root of the havoc wreaked by the disease. In addition, there are other subsidiary factors.

Haemorrhage. Carcinomata of surface epithelia eventually ulcerate and bleed. Usually the haemorrhage is occult, e.g. in gastro-intestinal tumours, but large arteries may be eroded. This leads to a final fatal bleed.

Secondary infection. All ulcerative cancers undergo secondary bacterial infection, and this aggravates the clinical condition. The element of obstruction already mentioned is also complicated by infection, e.g. bronchopneumonia and bronchiectasis distal to a bronchial cancer, pyelonephritis and cystitis in prostatic cancer, etc. Cancer of the mouth interferes so much with deglutition that in due course food and saliva are inspired into the respiratory passages. It is not surprising that suppurative bronchopneumonia is the commonest cause of death in this condition.

Starvation. In cancers of the mouth, oesophagus, and stomach there may be a directly nutritional effect due to a failure of intake. In cancer of the colon there may be diarrhoea, and if there are intestinal fistulae, there will be a severe malabsorption syndrome.

Pain. In advanced malignancy pain may be severe. It occasions anxiety, and leads to insomnia.

Haematological changes. *Anaemia* is common in cancer. Apart from such obvious causes as haemorrhage, malabsorption, and bone-marrow replacement, it is not infrequently due to increased red-cell destruction. This haemolytic anaemia may be accompanied by autoantibodies in the serum, especially in the lymphomata, but usually these are not present.

There is commonly a *neutrophil leucocytosis* in progressive cancer, and occasionally an eosinophilia also.

Cachexia. Most patients with advanced cancer are emaciated and have an earthy skin pigmentation, but some remain obese to the end. The generalised body atrophy of malignant disease is attributable to secondary factors, such as infection, starvation, malabsorption, liver involvement, and serous effusions, as well as anxiety, pain, and insomnia. The possibility that neoplastic tissue liberates a toxic product has not been confirmed. The basal metabolic rate is raised in advanced cancer, and there is often moderate *pyrexia* irrespective of secondary infection. The cause of this is unknown.

Immunological effects. On the whole there is not much impairment in the immune response in cancer except perhaps terminally. Lymphomata, however, do depress the immune response—Hodgkin's disease the cell-mediated part, multiple myeloma the immunoglobulins, and chronic lymphatic leukaemia sometimes both. An occasional occurrence is *amyloidosis*, especially in Hodgkin's disease and renal carcinoma; more frequently it complicates multiple myeloma.

Cases of the *nephrotic syndrome* have been found in association with cancer.[25],[26] Effective treatment of the tumour has led to a reversal of the renal condition, and in some cases deposits of IgG and IgM have been demonstrated on the glomerular basement membrane. The lumpy appearance of these deposits is that of non-specific antigen-antibody complexes, and on one occasion the antigen eluted from the glomeruli was found to be similar to that extracted from the lung tumour.[26] It is surprising that this nephrotic syndrome does not occur more often.

CARCINOMATOUS SYNDROMES

A variety of syndromes have been reported in association with neoplasms which are not explicable in terms of infiltration either by the primary tumour or its metastases.

Neuropathic effects.[27] Some cancers, especially those of the lung, stomach, breast, and ovary, may be accompanied by progressive destruction of neurones throughout the central nervous system. This occurs in the absence of metastases in the brain and cord, and the nature of the degenerative process is unknown. Sometimes the clinical picture is one of a cerebellar degeneration and at other times it resembles peripheral neuritis. Encephalomyelitic forms are also described.

Myopathic effects. Some tumours, especially oat-cell lung cancer and cancer of the breast and colon, may produce a *myopathy* involving the limb girdles and proximal limb muscles. Sometimes, especially in lung cancer, there are also features of *myasthenia gravis*. Another occasional complication of visceral cancer is *dermatomyositis*, which is considered in Chapter 16. The possibility of these intriguing neurological and myopathic manifestations being due to an im-munological mechanism is suggested by some authorities.

Dermatological effects.[28-30] Sometimes an internal neoplasm first makes its existence known by the production of a widespread skin lesion. A good example is the condition of *acanthosis nigricans*, in which profuse, black, warty lesions develop in the axillae and groins in the course of an adenocarcinoma of the stomach, pancreas, lung, or other internal organ. Sometimes a figurate erythematous eruption with elaborate gyrate lesions may herald the clinical onset of malignancy, as may also urticaria, erythema multiforme, and bullous pemphigoid. Recurrent attacks of *zoster* are not uncommon in patients with a lymphoma, and are no doubt an expression of impaired cell-mediated immunity. Heavy *pigmentation* of the skin has been ascribed to the secretion of melanocyte stimulating hormone by the tumour—particularly carcinoma of the pancreas.

Thrombotic complications. *Thrombophlebitis migrans* (see p. 462) in an occasional concomitant of deep-seated cancer, usually of the pancreas, lung, and stomach.[31] It may affect superficial or deep veins in any part of the body, and though the tumour is usually inoperable, cases have been reported in which removal of the cancer has been followed by relief of the phlebitis. Another occasional thombotic complication of visceral cancer is *non-bacterial thrombotic endocarditis*. This type of endocarditis is also found at necropsy in patients dying of many other diseases,[32] but it does seem to be unusually common in cases of cancer, especially the mucoid variety.[33]

The onset of Raynaud's syndrome and ischaemic necrosis of fingers may be the first sign of occult carcinoma.[34]

Afibrinogenaemia. This is a rare occurrence in visceral

TABLE 26.2 A comparison of the main features of benign and malignant tumours

Benign	Malignant
1. Growth. (a) Slowly-growing. (b) Expansive type of growth. (c) The progress of growth is erratic with a tendency to cease.	(a) Rapidly-growing. (b) Invasive type of growth. (c) The progress is usually relentless until death occurs.
2. Metastases never occur.	Metastases frequent.
3. Size. Usually of small size, but occasionally enormous.	Usually of large size.
4. Histological structure. (a) Well-differentiated. (b) Well-formed stroma with little tendency to haemorrhage and necrosis. (c) Cells regular. Few mitoses.	(a) Less well-differentiated and sometimes completely anaplastic. (b) Stroma often poorly formed. Haemorrhage and necrosis common. (c) Cells are often pleomorphic. Mitosis often numerous.
5. Cause of death. Usually not fatal. If death occurs, it is due to mechanical pressure and obstructive effects. Endocrine adenomata may have hormonal effects.	Almost invariably fatal if untreated. Cause of death a combination of mechanical and destructive effects, together with blood loss, secondary infection, starvation, etc.

cancer, usually of the prostate.[35] This organ normally secretes a fibrinolysin, and occasionally in metastatic prostatic carcinoma there occurs a bleeding syndrome due to fibrinolysis (see p. 623).

Hormonal effects. These come into two categories: (*a*) tumours of endocrine tissue secreting their own hormones, a topic considered on p. 324, and (*b*) tumours of non-endocrine origin producing a hormonal effect.[36, 37] The most important of these are *Cushing's syndrome* often with pronounced hypokalaemic alkalosis (usually with oat-cell lung cancer and thymoma, and sometimes with carcinoid tumours and medullary carcinoma of the thyroid[38]), *hypoglycaemia* (usually with mesothelioma and liver cancer), *hypercalcaemia*[39, 40] (usually with squamous-cell lung cancer and carcinoma of the kidney), and water retention with *hyponatraemia* (with oat-cell lung cancer).

Two other hormonal effects worth noting are *polycythaemia* associated with renal carcinoma and a few other lesions mentioned on p. 596 and *hyperthyroidism* associated with hydatidiform mole and choriocarcinoma. This is produced by a specific thyrotrophic hormone secreted by molar tissue; it differs from pituitary TSH, chorionic TSH secreted normally during pregnancy, and the LATS of Graves's disease.[41]

The mechanism of these curious syndromes appears to be the production by the tumours of a hormone or hormone-like substance. The hyponatraemia seems to be due to the production of antidiuretic hormone, and the hypercalcaemia to parathormone. The Cushing syndrome is probably caused by the secretion of ACTH, for adrenocortical hyperplasia is usually present, and the hypoglycaemia may be due to the inappropriate secretion of insulin. An increasing number of syndromes are being described, for it seems that almost any tumour can produce any hormone. Cancer of the lung seems to be particularly adept at this perverted behaviour, for in addition to the syndromes already noted, the occurrence of *gynaecomastia* has been described due to the production of a gonadotrophin. The tumour is usually anaplastic with many giant cells.[42] It has been noted that ACTH-secreting lung tumours have a particularly bad prognosis, due apparently to the immunosuppressive action of the cortisol the ACTH releases.[43] By contrast, ADH-secreting lung tumours do not have a worse prognosis than that of tumours not secreting hormones.[43]

Apart from the amines produced by the carcinoid type of tumour (p. 336), all these hormones are of polypeptide nature, and it is evident that their production by tumours is a functional aspect of anaplasia. Presumably all cells have the genetic information necessary for the manufacture of these hormones, but it is normally repressed except in the appropriate endocrine gland.[44]

The production of polypeptides with biological activity is possibly an explanation for the death of some patients with cancer in whom the extent of the tumour seems too limited to be lethal.[43] Such a polypeptide might interfere with a vital biological process by inhibiting other active peptides or by altering the protein binding of biologically active substances. Thus cases of lung cancer have been known which have had all the clinical features of Addison's disase and yet the plasma cortisol level has been very high. It would seem that the cortisol has been largely bound to peptides secreted by the tumour, and free, biologically-active cortisol almost absent. There is thus physiological adrenal insufficiency despite an excess of cortisol. The administration of a glucocorticosteroid with low protein binding, e.g. prednisolone, relieves the adrenal symptoms without, of course, altering the ultimate prognosis of the tumour.[43]

Pulmonary osteoarthropathy.[45] This is seen in lung cancer and also in fibrous mesothelioma of the pleura and chronic suppurative lung disease (bronchiectasis and empyema). There is marked finger clubbing with pain and swelling of the wrists and ankles, sometimes sufficient to simulate rheumatoid arthritis. There is subperiosteal new-bone formation and often mild synovitis. In cases due to lung cancer the tumour is often small and peripheral, and its resection causes rapid amelioration of the arthropathy. In inoperable cases cervical vagotomy similarly relieves the condition, suggesting that it is mediated through the afferent fibres of the vagus.[46] The condition has not been found in association with oat-cell cancer.

Our knowledge about the effects of malignancy is increasing, yet our understanding of the fundamental process of neoplasia is as inadequate as ever.

REFERENCES

1. ACKERMAN, L. V. and BUTCHER, H. R. (1964). *Surgical Pathology*, 3rd edn, p. 960. Saint Louis: Mosby.
2. MACKENZIE, D. H. (1972). *British Medical Journal*, iv, 277.
3. GRAHAM, J. R. et al. (1966). *New England Journal of Medicine*, **274**, 359.
4. RUSSELL, D. S. and RUBENSTEIN, L. J. (1963). *Pathology of Tumours of the Nervous System*, 2nd edn, p. 242. London: Arnold.
5. FISHER, E. R. and VUZEVSKI, V. D. (1968). *American Journal of Clinical Pathology*, **49**, 141.
6. ZOLLINGER, R. M. and ELLISON, E. H. (1955). *Annals of Surgery*, **142**, 709.
7. ZOLLINGER, R. M. et al. (1962). *Annals of Surgery*, **156**, 570.
8. GREGORY, R. A. et al. (1960). *Lancet*, i, 1045.
9. ZOLLINGER, R. M. et al. (1968). *Annals of Surgery*, **168**, 502.
10. BALLARD, H. S., FRAME, B. and HARTSOCK, R. J. (1964). *Medicine (Baltimore)*, **43**, 481.
11. JOHNSON, G. J. et al. (1967). *New England Journal of Medicine*, **277**, 1379.
12. MARSDEN, P. et al. (1971). *British Medical Journal*, iii, 87.

13. BRODERS, A. C. (1921). *Annals of Surgery*, **73**, 141.
14. LEVER, W. F. (1967). *Histopathology of the Skin*, 4th edn, p. 505. Philadelphia: Lippincott.
15. GREENOUGH, R. B. (1925). *Journal of Cancer Research*, **9**, 453.
16. WALTER, J. B. and PRYCE, D. M. (1955). *Thorax*, **10**, 107 and 117.
17. KREYBERG, L., LIEBOW, A. A. and UEHLINGER, E. A. (1967). *Histological Typing of Lung Tumours*, International Histological Classification of Tumours, No. 1. Geneva: W.H.O.
18. BENSCH, K. G. *et al.* (1968). *Cancer (Philadelphia)*, **22**, 1163.
19. Leading Article (1972). *Lancet*, i, 1322.
20. Leading Article (1966). *Lancet*, ii, 1013 and (1968). *Lancet*, i, 404.
21. ADAMSON, A. R. *et al.* (1969). *Lancet*, ii, 293.
22. WILLIAMS, E. D., BROWN, C. L. and DONIACH, I. (1966). *Journal of Clinical Pathology*, **19**, 103.
23. WILLIAMS, E. D. (1966). *Journal of Clinical Pathology*, **19**, 114.
24. KERNOHAN, J. W. *et al.* (1949). *Proceedings of Staff Meetings of the Mayo Clinic*, **24**, 71.
25. LOUGHRIDGE, L. W. and LEWIS, M. G. (1971). *Lancet*, i, 256.
26. LEWIS, M. G., LOUGHRIDGE, L. W. and PHILLIPS, T. M. (1971). *Lancet*, ii, 134.
27. BRAIN, R. (1963). *Lancet*, i, 179.
28. SNEDDON, I. B. (1963). *British Medical Journal*, ii, 405.
29. WHEELER, C. E., ABELE, D. C. and BRIGGAMAN, R. A. (1967). *Postgraduate Medicine*, **41**, 494.
30. NEWBOLD, P. C. H. (1970). *Archives of Dermatology*, **102**, 680.
31. LIEBERMAN, J. S. *et al.* (1961). *Journal of the American Medical Association*, **177**, 542.
32. Leading Article (1967). *British Medical Journal*, iii, 812.
33. Leading Article (1971). *British Medical Journal*, iii, 5.
34. HAWLEY, P. R., JOHNSTON, A. W. and RANKIN, J. T. (1967). *British Medical Journal*, iii, 208.
35. TAGNON, H. J. *et al.* (1953). *American Journal of Medicine*, **15**, 875.
36. HOBBS, C. B. and MILLER, A. L. (1966). *Journal of Clinical Pathology*, **19**, 119.
37. BOWER, B. F. and GORDON, G. S. (1965). *Annual Review of Medicine*, **16**, 83.
38. WILLIAMS, E. D., MORALES, A. M. and HORN, R. C. (1968). *Journal of Clinical Pathology*, **21**, 129.
39. MELICK, R. A., MARTIN, T. J. and HICKS, J. D. (1972). *British Medical Journal*, ii, 204.
40. OMENN, G. S., ROTH, S. I. and BAKER, W. H. (1969). *Cancer (Philadelphia)*, **24**, 1004.
41. Leading Article (1971). *British Medical Journal*, ii, 606.
42. NEVILLE, A. M. (1972). *Proceedings of the Royal Society of Medicine*, **65**, 55.
43. ROSS, E. J. (1972). *Proceedings of the Royal Society of Medicine*, **65**, 59.
44. Leading Article (1967). *Lancet*, i, 86.
45. HOLLING, H. E. and BRODEY, R. S. (1961). *Journal of the American Medical Association*, **178**, 977.
46. YACOUB, M. H. (1965). *British Journal of Diseases of the Chest*, **59**, 28; and *Thorax*, **20**, 537.
47. LUCAS, R. B. (1972). In *Pathology of Tumours of the Oral Tissues*, 2nd edn., p. 133. London: Churchill.

Chapter 27. Developmental Tumours and Tumour-Like Conditions

INTRODUCTION

It is remarkable that in the course of a few months a single cell, the fertilised ovum, can proliferate and differentiate into the complex system of organs and tissues that characterises the mature organism. The science of embryology has revealed in great detail how these tissues originate, and has thrown suggestive sidelights on the mode of production of the various malformations that may blight the development of the growing embryo. A *malformation* is essentially an anatomical error arising during the development of an organism to its final adult proportions. Most malformations are manifest when the fetus is born, but quite a number first make their presence obvious during the actively growing period of childhood and adolescence. In such cases it must be assumed that the fundamental defect was already present at birth, but that it was of such a nature that it first became apparent during post-natal life. Sometimes the malformation is concealed in the depths of the tissues, and comes to light only in later life as the result of some secondary change in it, e.g. a chordoma developing from the notochordal remnants, or a branchial cyst appearing as the result of excessive secretion of the cells of the residual branchial vestige.

Malformations may take many forms. There may be complete failure of development of a part (*agenesis*), or the part may never attain a full, mature size and remain rudimentary (*hypoplasia*). Sometimes there may be a *failure of fusion* of parts (e.g. cleft palate and spina bifida), and sometimes there may be a *failure of separation* (e.g. webbed digits) *or of canalisation* (e.g. imperforate anus and vaginal atresia).

Some malformations may consist of a simple overgrowth (e.g. an enlarged digit or limb in neurofibromatosis), and this is often rather dubiously called "hypertrophy" or "hyperplasia". It should be called *local gigantism* because the organ has never been normal in relation to the remainder of the body. In true hyperplasia the part is initially normal in size, and subsequently undergoes enlargement (see Chapter 24). Sometimes there is a superfluity of parts resulting in the production of *supernumerary organs* (e.g. double ureter, polydactyly, and accessory spleens or spleniculi).

Sometimes organs and tissues are found in abnormal sites. This is called *ectopia*, *heterotopia*, or *aberrance*. It may come about in one of three ways: (*a*) *Persistence* or growth of a tissue which normally atrophies or remains vestigial. In this way thyroid tissue may be found at the upper end of the thyroglossal duct. Patent ductus arteriosus, Meckel's diverticulum, and branchial cysts are further examples. (b) *Dislocation* of part or all of a developing organ. Thus an ectopic testis may be found in the perineum or the pelvis. (c) *Heteroplasia*. This is the anomalous differentiation of tissue. A well-known example is the presence of gastric mucosa in a Meckel's diverticulum or in part of the oesophagus. Heteroplasia must be distinguished from metaplasia, in which the alteration of tissue occurs after it has already differentiated normally. In heteroplasia the abnormal differentiation is a primary affair. It is of interest in illustrating the varied growth potentialities of a particular tissue. Thus there are many examples of cysts or masses in the region of the bladder, alimentary tract, or bronchi in which a wide variety of tissues is present. Willis describes a cystic facial mass which contained intestinal, gastric, and respiratory epithelium together with differentiated liver and pancreatic tissue.[1] Such a mass could be derived by heteroplasia in a portion of displaced endoderm. The term *choristoma* is applied to these non-neoplastic, tumour-like masses of developmental origin in which there are found tissues foreign to the part.

A more common lesion is the *hamartoma*; it consists of a tumour-like mass composed of a haphazard mixture of the tissues normally found in the part. Finally, the malformed tissues may assume the independent proliferative activity of a true tumour. It is these last two varieties of malformation, the *developmental tumours* and the hamartomata, that this chapter discusses in greatest detail.

Before leaving the subject of malformation it is worth completing the list by including those many malformations which manifest themselves primarily at a *cellular* or even a *biochemical level*. An inherited defect in an amino-acid sequence of the globin moiety of the haemoglobin molecule may lead to a sickle-cell or target-cell malformation of the erythrocytes (see p. 585), and a failure in the tubular reabsorption of phosphate may lead to a variety of osteomalacia (see p. 529).

All malformations are either congenital or else arise in the early years of life. Some are also hereditary, e.g. cleidocranial dysostosis and hereditary haemorrhagic telangiectasia, but the majority show no particularly familial tendency.

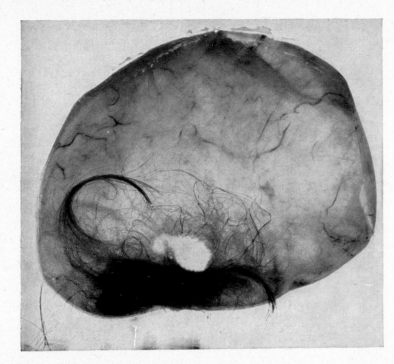

Figure 27.1
Ovarian teratoma. This cystic mass has a thin wall. At the base of the tumour there is a prominent umbo from which a mass of dark hair sprouts. *(EF 13.1, Reproduced by permission of the President and Council of the R.C.S. Eng.)*

THE DEVELOPMENTAL TUMOURS

Our knowledge about the histogenesis of developmental tumours is far from adequate, and the student of pathology is constantly disconcerted to read conflicting accounts about the origin of teratomata and related tumours in various authoritative text-books. It is best at the outset to admit our ignorance, and assess the matter with cool detachment.

TERATOMATA

A *teratoma* is a tumour consisting of multiple tissues foreign to the part from which it arises. This definition, derived from Willis, is subject to the rider that it is most aptly applicable to well-differentiated benign teratomata. Some, e.g. the testicular variety, may be so undifferentiated that their bulk is composed of bizarre anaplastic cells, which cannot be said to be forming any recognisable tissues at all. A careful inspection may be necessary to find elements that are recognisably foreign to the testis. In the so-called "embryonal carcinoma" of the testis the tumour cells are so anaplastic that it is impossible to be certain whether they are derived from a teratoma or some adult testicular component.

The vast majority of teratomata occur in the gonads, the ovary being much more often affected than the testis.

Ovarian teratomata are usually well-differentiated and benign. They are encountered chiefly in young and middle-aged women, and they constitute a variety of "ovarian cyst". In structure they usually comprise a thin-walled cystic mass which is filled with sebaceous, keratinous debris and matted hair. In one portion of the wall there is an eminence, or *umbo*,

which may bear teeth and a tongue-like structure, and contain bone and cartilage (Figs. 27.1 and 27.2). Histologically the cyst is lined in most cases by stratified squamous epithe-

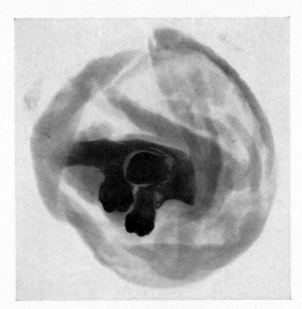

Figure 27.2
Ovarian teratoma. The patient was a woman of 32 years who was admitted to hospital with pain in the right iliac fossa. X-rays showed an ovarian cyst containing teeth.

The cyst was x-rayed after excision; it shows an irregular plate of bone bearing three teeth embedded in the projecting ridge. *(F 13.1, Reproduced by permission of the President and Council of the R.C.S. Eng.)*

348 General Pathology

lium, and skin appendages are prominent in the wall. This appearance has given rise to the erroneous name of "dermoid cyst", but unlike a true dermoid cyst other tissues are also present, especially in the area of the umbo. Here various types of epithelium may be identified (e.g. intestinal and respiratory), bone and cartilage abound, and foci of nervous tissue can often be distinguished. Rarely the entire teratoma may be composed of one such tissue, e.g. the *struma ovarii*, which consists of mature thyroid tissue. These teratomata are true tumours: they grow and gradually destroy the surrounding ovary. Malignant change is uncommon, and when it occurs it usually takes the form of a squamous-cell carcinoma. A much less common solid teratoma is also described, and this is usually malignant.

Testicular teratomata afflict young and middle-aged men, in whom they are almost invariably malignant by the time they manifest themselves. They are usually solid, though

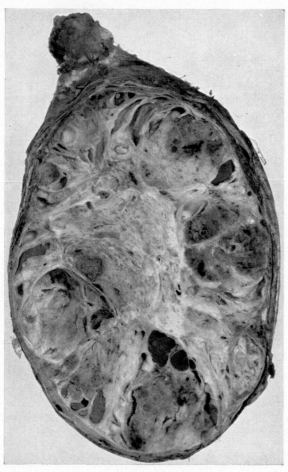

Figure 27.3
Teratoma of testis. The substance of the testis is replaced by a large fleshy mass consisting of areas of bone, cartilage, fibrous tissue, and many cysts. Some of these contain blood and others a mucous fluid. (M 12.2, *Reproduced by permission of the President and Council of the R.C.S. Eng.*

often there are cystic spaces amid the solid matrix (Fig. 27.3). Histologically a testicular teratoma usually consists of irregularly dilated gland-like spaces lined by atypical cells which tend to resemble squamous, respiratory, and intestinal epithelium in different places. There are often interspersed masses of bone, cartilage, and muscle, and the whole is supported by a primitive mesenchymal type of stroma. Sometimes the entire teratoma is composed of large anaplastic cells arranged in sheets, and rarely there is an authentic choriocarcinomatous differentiation, the tumour then consisting of enormous polyhedral cells and syncytial masses amid a haemorrhagic background. In such cases there may be an excretion of chorionic gonadotrophins in the urine in sufficient quantity to give a positive pregnancy test, and there may also be gynaecomastia.

Testicular teratomata metastasise rapidly, both by the lymphatics and the blood stream, and their deposits are usually as complex in structure as the primary lesion.

Much less frequently teratomata are found in the *anterior mediastinum, the retroperitoneal tissues,* and *intracranially.* These are usually benign, but carcinomatous change may supervene. *Sacrococcygeal teratomata* appear as enormous masses in the newborn, and they often contain at least one malignant component. Another rare neonatal teratoma is the large *epignathus* which arises from the base of the skull and protrudes from the mouth. It is usually well differentiated, but it soon kills because of mechanical interference with the functions of this part of the body.

The origin of teratomata. The histogenesis of teratomata has given rise to much speculation, and there is remarkable fluidity in current opinion. It is important to distinguish between attached parasitic twins and teratomata. The presence of a spinal axis is the prerequisite for diagnosing the fetiformity of any such mass, and no teratoma has been known to possess a vertebral axis. Neither are the tissues of even the best differentiated teratomata arranged into composite organs, e.g. there may be teeth and even a tongue but there is no mouth. However, it must be admitted that an attached parasitic twin might become so reduced and amorphous as to be indistinguishable from a benign teratoma, and it is conceivable that some sacrococcygeal teratomata and epignathi might arise in this way. The term "embryoma" has been used synonymously with teratoma (and also with Wilms's nephroblastoma); it should be discarded until there is good evidence that teratomata arise from embryos.

The most popular theory, championed especially by Willis, is that teratomata arise from foci of totipotential embryonic cells that escape the influence of the primary organiser during embryonic development. He believes that the disturbance takes place especially in the area of the primitive streak and head process, as most teratomata occur in the median or paramedian regions of the body. Such totipotential cells are capable of producing all the tissues of the body.

Gonadal and mediastinal teratomata usually occur in adults.

Admittedly the ovarian and mediastinal ones might have been present since infancy, and been unsuspected until later life because of the capaciousness of the surrounding tissues, but it is hard to believe that a testicular lesion could lie undiscovered for so long. A more reasonable explanation is that a small "embryonic rest" was always present, but became neoplastic only in adult life. In fact no such rests have yet been found.

The fact that the vast majority of teratomata are gonadal suggests a third possible explanation: an abnormal development of one or more germ cells leading to a perverted type of parthenogenesis. It is interesting that teratomata in women always have a female nuclear sex, while those in men sometimes have a male nuclear configuration, and sometimes are female.[2] Indeed, they have been known to contain a mosaic of male and female tissues.[3] Tumours generally have the same nuclear sex as their victims, but there may be aberrations in anaplastic lesions. It is also interesting that testicular teratomata have been produced in cocks as a result of the local injection of zinc salts.[4] This suggests that the presence of cell rests is not necessary for the development of a teratoma.

The question of the origin of teratomata has been considered in some detail in order to emphasise a very important principle in pathology: there are often several possible modes of production of a single morbid condition. The way to ascertain which of these is operative in any one instance is to trace the development of the condition from its initiation. Mere argument is futile.

THE EMBRYONIC TUMOURS OF INFANCY

Unlike the teratomata which contain a wide assortment of the body's tissues, this group of tumours consists only of those elements present in a particular part of the body, e.g. the kidney, retina, liver, and brain. It would appear that during the development of these particular areas a perversion of organogenesis occurs. A part of the developing organ undergoes neoplastic transformation, and a tumour, usually highly malignant, may result. Some of these lesions are present at birth, but most develop within the first five years of life at a time when the tissues are continuing their development. Very rarely authentic cases have been reported in adults, and it must be assumed that the lesion has remained latent until later life in such instances, or that it has developed from a "cell rest".

Nephroblastoma (Wilms's Tumour)

This tumour manifests itself as an abdominal mass in infancy and early childhood. It is very malignant, metastasising both by the lymphatics and the blood stream. Macroscopically it is a large, pinkish-white, soft tumour that replaces most of the kidney.

The neoplastic tissue is composed of both epithelial and connective tissue elements. The epithelium may form tubules, and also be arranged in the form of primitive glomeruli (proglomeruli). In fact, the tumour usually contains easily recognisable renal elements, such as would be expected in the kidney of a normal four to five months old fetus. The tumour may contain bone, cartilage, or adipose tissue, and of greater interest, striated muscle fibres. Sometimes striated muscle cannot be demonstrated, and at other times it forms the bulk of the tumour. Some tumours are undifferentiated, and are composed of small darkly-staining cells with little or no attempt at tubular differentiation.

There is no doubt that this is a tumour of the renal blastema, but the origin of the striated muscle has aroused some controversy. It is generally believed to be due to a simple heteroplasia of the tissue of the blastema (comparable with the bone and cartilage which may also be present). Such a blastema would then be truly *pluripotential*, and responsible for the development of the "mixed tumour". It is not impossible, of course, that the muscle is derived from an adjacent myotome.

Neuroblastoma

This tumour arises almost invariably from the adrenal medulla or one of the sympathetic ganglia. It is doubtful whether it ever develops from the central nervous system. It often appears as an abdominal swelling in infancy, but its most characteristic feature is its capacity to metastasise to predictable sites. If the liver is extensively involved (and this may occur as the result of direct extension from a tumour of the right adrenal), hepatomegaly accounts for much of the abdominal swelling (*Pepper's syndrome*). Sometimes osseous metastases predominate, and a characteristic feature is the presence of enormous deposits in the skull especially around the orbits. Exophthalmos and bruising around the eyelids are early signs of this tendency (*Hutchison's syndrome*). Lymphatic metastases are also frequent.

Histologically the neoplasm consists of tightly-packed masses of darkly-staining round cells easily mistaken for lymphocytes. Sometimes these cells are disposed in rosette-like clusters, and if differentiation is particularly good, it may be possible to recognise tiny fibrils in the centres of the rosettes. These represent primitive nerve fibres, and the rosettes themselves resemble those seen in the normally developing sympathetic ganglia of a four to five months old fetus. Sometimes the round cells become pear-shaped and may actually develop into young nerve cells, in which case the fibres extrude from them like axons. If all the tumour cells differentiate into neurones, the tumour regresses; cure has been known to follow vitamin B_{12} therapy or to occur spontaneously.

True *ganglioneuromata* are often silent, or else they may manifest themselves in later childhood and during adult life. They consist entirely of mature nerve fibres and cells which closely resemble normal ganglion cells, even to the extent of containing brown pigment in their cytoplasm. The fibres may form interlacing bundles which may be provided with

plentiful Schwann cells (Fig. 27.4). These tumours are benign, and once again demonstrate that as differentiation
proceeds, so malignancy recedes. Many neuroblastomata
contain well-formed ganglioneuromatous tissue in their
midst. It is generally believed that all ganglioneuromata
arise from primitive neuroblasts, because it does not seem

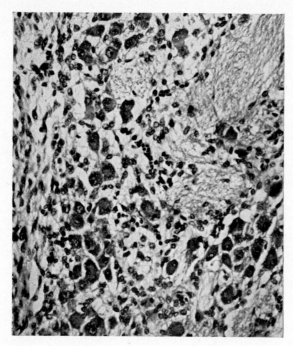

Figure 27.4
Ganglioneuroma. The tumour consists of aggregations of mature
ganglion cells interspersed among which there are well-formed
nerve fibres. × 260.

likely that mature nerve cells would start proliferating to
form a tumour. It is sometimes possible to diagnose these
tumours biochemically, for there may be an increased
secretion of catecholamines, e.g. dopamine, noradrenaline,
and vanilmandelic acid, in the urine.[5]

Medulloblastoma

This highly malignant brain tumour is found in the region
of the fourth ventricle near the cerebellum. It occurs predominantly in young children, but it has been reported
occasionally in adults. Like other malignant cerebral
neoplasms it does not metastasise outside the central nervous
system, but intrathecal seedlings right down the spinal cord
are quite common. The histological appearance is very
similar to that of a poorly-differentiated neuroblastoma:
sheets of small dark cells, round or elongated in shape, and
arranged in clumps or rosettes. Some appear to be differentiating into neuroglial cells such as oligodendrocytes and
astrocytes, but there is no evidence of nerve-cell formation.
This tumour is therefore classified with the gliomata. Some

authorities, however, believe that the "medulloblast" is
capable of forming nerve cells as well as neuroglial cells,
and that the medulloblastoma is derived from the granular
layer of the fetal cerebellum. In fact the neuroblastic
differentiation of the medulloblast is still unproven, and it is
more truthful to admit that the derivation of this tumour is
not known.

Retinoblastoma

This developmental tumour has the distinction of exhibiting a definite hereditary incidence. It is usually sporadic, but
when familial it is transmitted as a dominant characteristic
with variable penetrance, for the condition may be transmitted through apparently unaffected people. About a third
of cases are bilateral, and this tragedy is most likely to occur
in the hereditary group. There is a relationship between
retinoblastoma and a deletion of the long arm of a D chromosome, and some of these cases also show mental deficiency
and a tendency to develop other tumours, especially osteosarcoma.[6, 7]

It is a disease of infancy and early childhood. If enucleation
is not performed expeditiously, widespread lymphatic and
blood-borne metastases ensue. Histologically the rosette
pattern of the neuroblastoma and medulloblastoma group is
reproduced (Fig. 27.5). The centre of the rosette may be
demarcated by a distinct membrane. Rod-shaped processes
from the inner margins of the cells may project into the

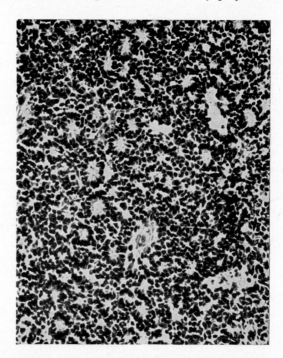

Figure 27.5
Retinoblastoma. The tumour consists of small, darkly-staining
fusiform cells which tend to be arranged in rosettes. Some of the
rosettes enclose a well-formed central cavity. × 150.

central cavity in a manner exactly reminiscent of the rod and cone cells and the external limiting membrane of the normal retina.

Hepatoblastoma

This is a very rare developmental tumour which like the nephroblastoma (and unlike the other three described) is truly "mixed". It consists of primitive liver-cell parenchyma, and often there is an admixture of connective tissue elements including bone, cartilage, and striated muscle. Whether the latter is derived from the septum transversum (which eventually forms the diaphragm), or whether it develops as a result of heteroplasia from the hepatic blastema, is not certain.

A mixed tumour similar to the hepatoblastoma occurs in the lung. This pulmonary blastoma is very rare.[47]

Embryonic Sarcomata

A rare group of rhabdomyosarcomata usually involving the vagina, urethra, bladder, prostate, or orbit is well recognised. These highly malignant tumours occur in young children, and are due to a neoplastic proliferation of mesenchymal connective tissue. There is often a non-neoplastic proliferation of the surface epithelium, with the result that these tumours have a polypoid or grape-like appearance (hence the name *sarcoma botryoides*). Histologically the picture is one of a spindle-cell or pleomorphic-cell sarcoma in a myxomatous type of stroma. Striated rhabdomyoblasts are usually easily demonstrable, especially if an iron-haematoxylin stain is used to demonstrate their stripes. Very undifferentiated tumours may show no evidence of muscle fibres at all. It is probable that this rhabdomyosarcomatous differentiation is due to heteroplasia, though once again the alternative possibility of derivation of primitive rhabdomyoblasts from a neighbouring myotome cannot be discounted.

THE HAMARTOMATA

A *hamartoma* is a tumour-like malformation in which the tissues of a particular part of the body are arranged haphazardly, usually with an excess of one or more of its components. The term was coined by Albrecht in 1904,[8]* and the concept it embodies is of great importance, for a large number of common lesions fall into the general category of hamartomata.

A typical example of a hamartoma is the isolated cartilaginous mass not infrequently found in the substance of a lung. This is usually 2–3 cm in diameter and has a white, pearly appearance and a hard consistency. On section it is found to be composed of mature hyaline cartilage, similar to that present in the bronchi. In the substance of the cartilage there are clefts lined by respiratory epithelium, and surrounding the cartilaginous masses there is connective tissue

* It is derived from the Greek, *hamartanein* to err, in that the body has made an error in the formation of some of its tissues.

and smooth muscle. There is no true capsule between the lesion and the surrounding lung parenchyma. It is evident that this lesion contains several different elements (i.e. it is "mixed"), but that all of these are normally found in the lung. It seems likely that it is a malformation derived from a developing bronchus, for all the tissues of a bronchus are present in it, though they are grossly misaligned, and there is an excess of cartilage (Figs. 27.6 and 27.7).

It is very important to distinguish this type of lesion from a teratoma.

(*a*) The tissues present are those specific to the part from which it arises.

(*b*) The lesion has no tendency towards excessive growth. Its growth is co-ordinated with that of the surrounding tissues, and it stops after adolescence. There is no capsule

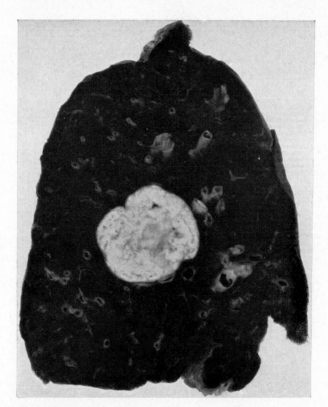

Figure 27.6
Hamartoma of lung. In the centre of the upper lobe there is a circumscribed, pearly-white, round mass. It consists predominantly of mature hyaline cartilage, and there is no obvious capsule around it. (ER 22.1, *Reproduced by permission of the President and Council of the R.C.S. Eng.*)

around a hamartoma; as its growth proceeds *pari passu* with that of its surroundings, there is no pressure atrophy and therefore no connective tissue condensation. Hamartomata are not tumours, but it is possible for a tumour to develop in a hamartoma. In the pulmonary lesion just described this does not happen.

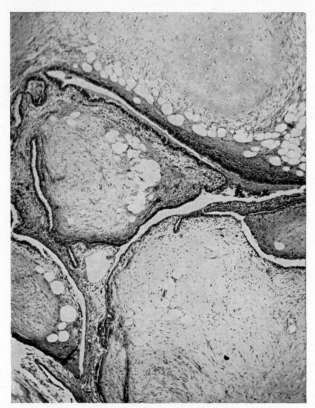

Figure 27.7
Hamartoma of lung. This specimen consists mostly of masses of compact connective tissue containing deep clefts lined by respiratory epithelium. Foci of adipose tissue are also conspicuous, and at the top there is a mass of hyaline cartilage. × 55.

It should be noted that many hamartomata are given "tumour-sounding" names. These are so much part and parcel of pathological nomenclature that they are bound to persist, e.g. angioma, benign melanoma, and chondroma of the lung.

Most hamartomata are present at birth or in the early years of childhood, but only those on exposed areas like the skin and mouth will be recognised as early as this. The cartilaginous hamartoma of the lung is always described in adults, though no doubt the original nidus was present at birth, and thereafter underwent steady growth to its final mature size. It is usually discovered during a routine radiological examination of the chest, and if misdiagnosed as carcinoma may be the cause of a completely unnecessary pneumonectomy.

Vascular Hamartomata

The very common *haemangioma* is a hamartomatous malformation and not a true tumour. It is usually present at birth or else appears soon afterwards, and though its growth is sometimes quite active in early childhood, it soon becomes quiescent, and may even undergo regression as the result of interference with its vascular supply. This is particularly true of the strawberry naevus, which starts as an inconspicuous lesion on an infant's face, grows rapidly to giant proportions, and then after a few years regresses and finally disappears leaving an area of scarring.[9]

The commonest type of haemangioma is seen on the skin where it forms a variety of *naevus*. This word is used to describe any type of developmental blemish of the skin (birthmark), e.g. hairy, melanotic, or sebaceous. Sometimes vascular naevi are small and spider-like, sometimes raised (strawberry naevi), and sometimes flattened and extensive, covering a considerable expanse of skin (*naevus flammeus*). Characteristically they blanch on pressure due to an emptying of their contained blood. Haemangiomata are also often found in the mouth and on the lips, and their frequency in solid organs like the liver, brain, bones (especially the vertebrae), and muscles is well recognised (Fig. 27.8).

Microscopically they consist of poorly-demarcated, non-encapsulated masses and leashes of vascular channels, most of which contain blood. Sometimes the channels are capacious and confluent like the erectile tissue of the penis (*cavernous haemangiomata*), sometimes they are narrow and well-formed (*capillary haemangiomata*), and sometimes they are provided with large tortuous arterioles and venules (*plexiform haemangiomata*). All three types may occur together. Sometimes there are extensive areas of endothelial cells arranged in uncanalised clumps. It is the subsequent canalisation of these areas that often gives the clinical impression of rapid growth of an angioma. Large haemangiomata occurring in infancy may rarely selectively trap circulating platelets, and lead to thrombocytopenic purpura[10] (see also Chapter 51). There are all degrees of angiomatous malformations from single small fiat naevi up to extensive cirsoid aneurysms (Fig. 27.9).

Some haemangiomata enlarge and undergo progressive fibrosis, probably as a result of repeated haemorrhage into their substance. These *sclerosing haemangiomata* contain much free haemosiderin pigment and also foci of foamy macrophages and giant cells reminiscent of a xanthoma. The final picture is indistinguishable from a dermatofibroma, a common lesion variously regarded as a benign neoplasm or a reaction to injury, such as an insect bite.

Angiomatous syndromes.[11] A very important feature of the haemangiomata is their tendency towards multiplicity. Some very characteristic syndromes are produced in this way, e.g. (*a*) *Hereditary haemorrhagic telangiectasia* (Rendu-Osler-Weber disease—see Chapter 51). (*b*) *Sturge-Weber syndrome,* in which there is a combined naevus flammeus over one half of the face and a haemangioma of the ipsilateral cerebral hemisphere.[12] (*c*) Haemangiomatosis of the retina and central nervous system (*von Hippel-Lindau disease*).[13]

There are sometimes other malformations present as well, e.g. *Kast's* or *Maffucci's syndrome*, in which there is enchondromatosis of the bones as well as multiple cutaneous haemangiomatosis.[11]

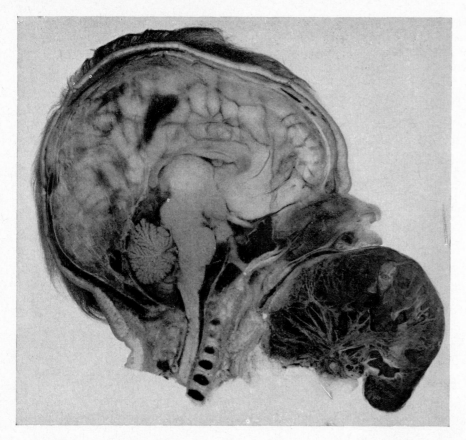

Figure 27.8
Haemangioma of tongue. This specimen of the sagittal section of skull comes from a child who survived 4 days. The tongue is enormously enlarged, and protrudes from the mouth as a purplish mass. It is almost completely replaced by cavernous vascular tissue. *(A 7.2, Reproduced by permission of the President and Council of the R.C.S. Eng.)*

Angioblastic tumours. The question often arises as to whether there are true tumours of the blood vessels, or whether all angiomata are malformations. The answer is that true angioblastic neoplasms do exist, but that they are very uncommon except in the Negro.

(a) *Haemangiosarcoma* may arise either spontaneously,[14] or very rarely in a congenital angioma. When an angioma undergoes malignant change, the endothelial cells show variations in size and shape and numerous mitotic figures. To diagnose a haemangiosarcoma it is necessary to establish

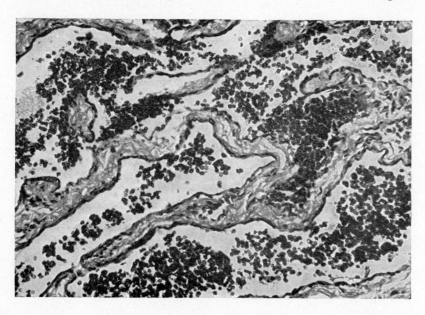

Figure 27.9
Haemangioma. This is a typical cavernous haemangioma. It consists of loose strands of connective tissue lined by endothelium enclosing extensive vascular spaces. It resembles normal erectile tissue. × 200.

the vasoformative nature of the tumour, for many undifferentiated tumours with an abundant sinusoidal vasculature can mimic it. In haemangiosarcoma (and lymphangiosarcoma) a reticulin stain demonstrates that the proliferating tumour cells lie within the reticulin sheaths. This also distinguishes the tumour from a haemangiopericytoma, in which the neoplastic cells lie external to the silver-impregnated endothelial basement membrane.

There are two interesting tumours that come into the category of haemangiosarcoma: (1) *Post-mastectomy angiosarcoma*, which is a remote complication of breast cancer. These cases first develop severe lymphoedema of the arm due to the occlusion of the axillary lymphatics following their permeation by cancer cells and their further obliteration by radiotherapy. Several years later multiple angio-

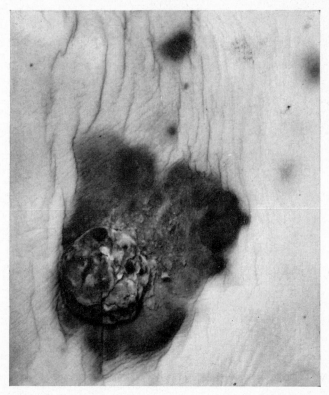

Figure 27.10
Post-mastectomy angiosarcoma of skin of arm. The patient had had a radical mastectomy 5 years before. Immediately after operation her arm became oedematous, and there was also a severe reaction over the neck and shoulder following radiotherapy. The swelling of the arm persisted, and about 2 years later a red spot was noticed on the inner aspect of the arm. It continued to enlarge and became pedunculated at one point. Biopsy revealed an angiomatous tumour resembling Kaposi's sarcoma, and a forequarter amputation was performed. The specimen consists of a portion of the skin of the inner aspect of the arm. The main lesion is an irregular dusky area 7.5 cm in diameter, projecting from the surface of which there is an ulcerated, pedunculated mass about 2.5 cm in diameter. (I 27.1, *Reproduced by permission of the President and Council of the R.S.C. Eng.)*

sarcomata develop in the skin of the arm, and these may metastasise to the lungs. The condition is called the *Stewart-Treves syndrome*,[15] and it has a combined haemangiomatous and lymphangiomatous element (Fig. 27.10).

Some authorities doubt the existence of the post-mastectomy angiosarcoma, and attribute the tumour to a metastasis of the original breast cancer.[16, 17] However, authentic angiosarcoma has also been reported arising in chronic congenital and idiopathic lymphoedema where there has been no question of coincidental carcinoma.[18] The Stewart-Treves syndrome is a definite entity, but a reticulin stain is essential to confirm the diagnosis.

(2) *Kaposi's sarcoma.*[19, 20] This consists histologically of proliferating plump spindle cells and angiomatous tissue. It has been described as an "idiopathic haemorrhagic sarcoma" and is often classified with the angiosarcomata, but the histogenesis of the neoplastic spindle cells is not known. The tumour is seen in Eastern Europeans, but its area of maximum prevalence is Eastern and Southern Africa where it is one of the commonest types of cancer. The disease runs a variable course, but sometimes it is fulminating and associated with visceral lesions. In European cases there is not infrequently an association with neoplasms of the lymphoreticular system, but in Africans this is exceptional.

(*b*) A completely different tumour is the *glomangioma*, or glomus tumour, which is benign. It usually occurs on the skin of the extremities where it gives rise to paroxysms of severe pain. It is a tumour of the arteriolar-venous anastomosis, or glomus, which contains a thick layer of cuboidal cells in its wall. These cells are of myoneural origin, and their ultrastructure resembles that of the smooth muscle cell.[21] Glomangiomata consist of irregular vascular spaces which are surrounded by many layers of characteristic cuboidal glomus cells.

Another type of vascular hamartoma is the *lymphangioma*. It differs in no important respect from the commoner haemangioma, except that it contains no blood. A well-known extensive lymphangioma of infancy is the *cystic hygroma of the neck*. It infiltrates the vital surrounding structures so intimately that complete removal is seldom possible.

Melanotic Hamartomata (Naevocellular Naevus*)

The common *naevocellular naevus* of the skin is another important example of a hamartomatous malformation, which, unlike the angioma, shows a more definite tendency towards malignant change. The parent cell, the melanocyte (the melanin-producing cell of the body, see Chapter 46), is believed to originate in the region of the neural crest and to

---

* Many terms are used to describe this lesion: benign melanoma, pigmented mole, pigmented naevus, naevocellular naevus, etc. The last is perhaps the most precise. The word melanoma should never be used unqualified, because to many people it has a malignant connotation. The term naevus may be used alone provided it is the naevocellular variety which is being described (e.g. compound naevus).

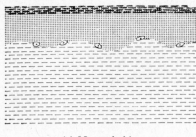

(a) Normal skin.

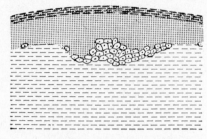

(b) Junctional naevus with activity.

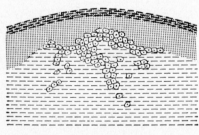

(c) Developing compound naevus.

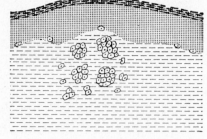

(d) Quiescent intradermal naevus.

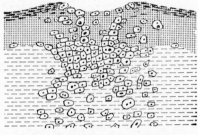

(e) Malignant melanoma.

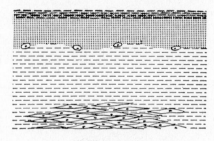

(f) Blue naevus.

Figure 27.11
Sketches to show the various types of melanotic naevi: the only cells drawn are melanocytes and naevus cells. In the normal skin melanocytes are present only in the basal layer of the epidermis. A focal proliferation of these cells produces a junctional naevus (b) which may be regarded as a stage in the development of a compound and intradermal naevus. Such junctional activity is of little importance in a young person, but in an adult is to be regarded as dangerous; (c) shows the formation of a compound naevus by the invasion of the dermis by melanocytes. When the junctional activity regresses, the naevus cells remain in the dermis as an intradermal naevus (d); (e) shows a malignant melanoma which in addition to junctional activity, shows invasion of the epidermis as well as the dermis and deeper structures. Atypicality of the cells serves as a further distinguishing feature from the compound naevus, which an early malignant melanoma may resemble. (f) The strap-like naevus cells situated deep in the dermis impart the colour to the blue naevus.

migrate to the epidermis with the peripheral nerves. This is Masson's hypothesis,[22] and it has now gained general acceptance.

By the time of birth there are moderate numbers of melanocytes in the basal layer of the epidermis, though in fair-skinned individuals the DOPA reaction may be necessary to reveal them. There is surely not a single individual who does not have a number of pigmented "moles", or melanotic naevi, on his skin either at the time of his birth, or else shortly afterwards. These are simply accumulations of excess melanocytes which have developed during fetal and neonatal life. They may be associated with malformations of the epidermis, hair follicles, and sebaceous glands, so that large, papillomatous, hairy naevi are sometimes present as well as the flatter, darker lesions that are composed only of *naevus cells*, as the altered melanocytes of a pigmented mole are usually called.

The focal proliferation and accumulation of melanocytes, usually containing much melanin, at the junction of the epidermis and dermis is invariable in infancy, and the lesion so formed is called a *junctional naevus*. It is flat and deeply pigmented. As the child grows older, there is a tendency for the naevus cells to be shed from the basal layer of the epidermis into the dense connective tissue of the dermis, where they lie characteristically in inert clumps which are completely unencapsulated. The cells are cuboidal in shape, and have a somewhat basophilic cytoplasm which usually contains little or no melanin pigment. The appearance of these cells "invading" the dermis is disconcerting, but must be regarded as a normal event in the evolution of the naevus.

By the time adult life is reached, all the naevus cells in many naevi have left the epidermis and are sequestrated in the underlying dermis. The flesh-coloured papule so produced is described as an *intradermal naevus*, and is believed to be perfectly harmless (Fig. 27.12). The naevus cells often become spindle shaped, especially in the deeper part of the lesion, and this is interpreted as differentiation into Schwann cells. Indeed, old naevi may contain areas resembling a

Figure 27.12
Intradermal naevus. There is an extensive
accumulation of naevus cells in the deeper layer
of the dermis, but they are well separated from
the overlying epidermis. × 130.

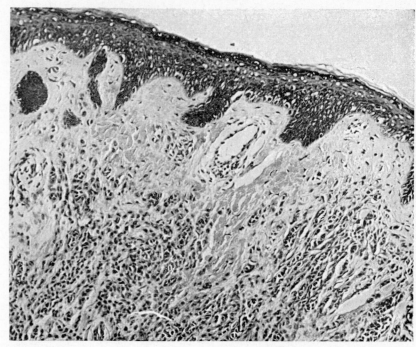

neurofibroma. In some naevi, some or even all the naevus cells retain their attachment to the epidermis, so that the naevus is either partly intradermal and partly junctional (*compound naevus*), or else it remains completely junctional.[23]

Junctional activity. It is the junctional component of a naevus which is potentially dangerous, because it is these cells which are liable to undergo proliferation from time to time. During childhood a naevus often manifests signs of active growth of a degree rather greater than would be expected of a truly hamartomatous lesion, and histologically such a naevus may show quite an alarming degree of active proliferation of its junctional component, even with mitotic figures and general pleomorphism. This is called *junctional activity*. Experience has taught us that such junctional activity is quite common and should not arouse undue alarm. When, however, similar activity occurs in a naevus of a

Figure 27.13
Junctional activity in a compound naevus. The
aggregation of naevus cells is not only in contact
with the epidermis, but through proliferation
has impinged on it and led to a degree of thin-
ning. Such an appearance in an adult must be
regarded with grave suspicion. × 130.

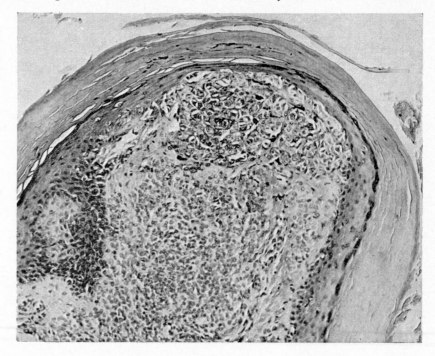

person over the age of 30 years, the matter is much more serious, for it may indeed be the first indication of malignancy (Fig. 27.13). Even in adult life, however, junctional activity is sometimes a phasic affair, and does not necessarily terminate in malignancy.

Juvenile melanoma.[24] This is a type of compound naevus which generally occurs in young people and because of its rapid growth mimics a malignant melanoma. Histologically the predominant cell type is usually spindle shaped, and the presence of mitoses can easily lead to a diagnosis of malignancy. Nevertheless, the lesion is entirely benign.

Regression of naevi.[25, 26] Occasionally one or more naevi undergo spontaneous regression and are surrounded by a zone of depigmentation. Such a lesion is called a *halo*, or *Sutton's*, *naevus.* Histologically there is a chronic inflammatory infiltrate, and this must not be misinterpreted as evidence of malignancy in a naevus (see p. 359). The halo phenomenon can also be seen in malignant melanoma and is generally interpreted as evidence of an autoimmune reaction.

MALIGNANT MELANOMA OF THE SKIN AND MUCOUS MEMBRANES

This is a malignant tumour derived from melanocytes and may arise *de novo* or else in some pre-existing lesion, such as a naevus or an *in-situ* melanoma. Estimates of the number that arise from naevi vary considerably, due in part to the fact that most patients are poor historians and in part to the varying criteria used by pathologists in recognising malignant change in a naevocellular naevus.

Some put the figure at about 40 per cent,[27] while others regard it as occurring in less than 10 per cent.[28] Nevertheless, malignant change in a naevus should be suspected if any of the following changes occur: increase in size; change in colour whether darker, lighter, or mottled; bleeding;

ulceration; crusting. When any of these changes occur, excisional biopsy is recommended before radical treatment is considered, since clinical misdiagnosis is common.

Aetiology. It is doubtful whether trauma or hormonal changes, such as occur in pregnancy, are important. *Ultraviolet light* is however important.[29] Malignant melanoma is common in fair-skinned people living in the northern parts of Australia and in the southern states of the USA.[30] It is also common in Negroes, in whom the plantar region is most often affected. This is an area which is normally feebly pigmented, and it seems that pre-existing plantar naevi form the basis for these tumours. *Areas of ectopic pigmentation*, e.g. of the soles, mouth, and nose, are particularly vulnerable to melanomatous change in Negroes.[31] The subungual melanoma is usually malignant by the time it is diagnosed. There is also a *hereditary element* in some cases of malignant melanoma; these tend to be multiple, and they occur at an earlier age than that at which sporadic melanomata develop (which is about 50 years).[32, 33] There is one type of naevus which is definitely precancerous: the *giant*, or *bathing-trunk*, *naevus*, which is truly congenital and of massive proportions. It may be associated with meningeal melanosis, and malignant melanoma develops in up to 25 per cent of cases.[26]

Two other rare but definitely premalignant conditions should be noted; both may be regarded as examples of *in-situ* melanoma.

Conjunctival melanosis.[34] This consists of the appearance of a diffuse brown patch on the conjunctiva, usually in middle-aged people whose conjunctivae were previously normal. This patch spreads and may implicate the surrounding skin. Histologically it is a proliferation of atypical melanocytes in the epithelium, and invasive melanoma tends to supervene, though this often takes many years to occur.

Lentigo maligna, or *Hutchinson's freckle*,[35] is a similar

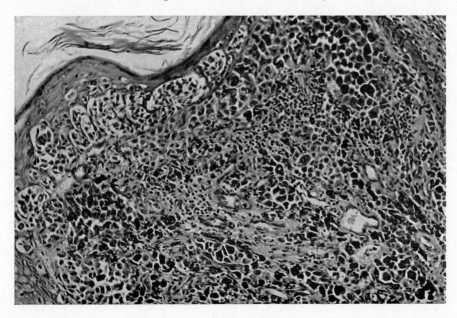

Figure 27.14
Malignant melanoma. The dermis is diffusely infiltrated with pleomorphic tumour cells, some of which are heavily pigmented. The epidermis is also involved, and the deeper layers have been destroyed. Elsewhere there was ulceration. × 130.

Figure 27.15
Malignant melanoma. This is the
lentigo maligna type, and has the best
prognosis. *(Photograph supplied by Dr.
Wallace J. Clark, Jr.)*

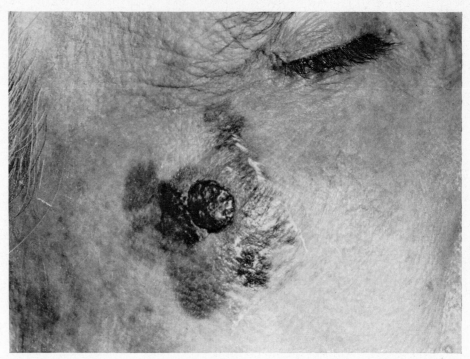

condition and is generally seen on the face of elderly individuals. There is marked junctional activity with proliferation of bizarre atypical melanocytes and disorganisation of
the deeper layers of the epidermis but no dermal invasion.
Invasion and metastasis can occur, often after 10 years or
even longer.

Types of melanoma. The unpredictable behaviour of
malignant melanoma has led to many attempts at classification. These have been designed to relate macroscopic and
histological features to prognosis. The classification of
Clark and his colleagues is currently favoured.[28, 36] Three
types are recognised:

(a) *Lentigo-maligna melanoma.* This tumour develops
slowly at the site of a previous Hutchinson's freckle. It has a
relatively good prognosis (Fig. 27.15).

(b) *Superficial spreading melanoma.* This is a flat lesion
which can occur on any area of the skin and histologically
shows a wide area of proliferation of atypical melanoblasts at
the dermo-epidermal junction. Dermal invasion occurs later,
and nodular lesions can then develop (Fig. 27.16).

(c) *Nodular melanoma.* Early dermal invasion produces a
nodular lesion, and there is no flanking junctional component
as is seen in the superficial spreading variety. The prognosis
is worst in this type (Fig. 27.17).

Any of these three types of melanoma may show different
types of cells. These may be of epithelial appearance (some-

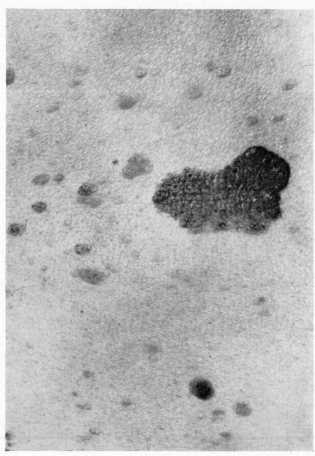

Figure 27.16
Malignant melanoma. This is the superficial spreading type and is
an extensive flat lesion. *(Photograph supplied by Dr. Wallace H.
Clark, Jr.)*

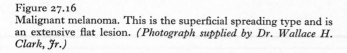

times exhibiting considerable pleomorphism with giant forms), spindle shaped, or small. It is the occurrence of the small cells together with the presence of junctional proliferation in the superficial spreading melanoma that makes it difficult to recognise the pre-existence of a benign naevus in an established malignant melanoma.

The detection of malignancy in a pre-existing naevus is often a matter of great difficulty. The presence of atypical, pleomorphic cells, mitoses, and epidermal invasion leading to ulceration are points in favour of diagnosing such a change (Fig. 27.14). So also is a dermal inflammatory reaction, but it must be remembered that inflammation is not uncommon in response to trauma, an infected hair follicle, or the regressive changes seen in a halo naevus.

When a malignant melanoma enters into an aggressive phase, there is a rapid invasion of local lymphatics which may sometimes show black streaking due to melanomatous permation. Early lymph-node and blood-borne metastases are the rule, and the condition is a fearful one. Metastases may occur in unusual sites, e.g. bowel, heart, and spleen. Often both

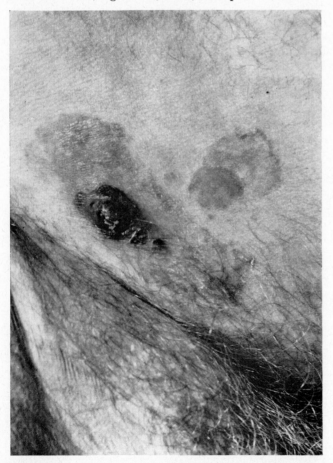

Figure 27.17
Malignant melanoma. This is the nodular type. It has the worst prognosis of the three. *(Photograph supplied by Dr. Wallace H. Clark, Jr.)*

the primary tumour and its metastases are well-pigmented, but sometimes they contain very little pigment. Such an amelanotic melanoma is difficult to distinguish from an anaplastic carcinoma or sarcoma; the DOPA reaction may help in the diagnosis, but to be of value the tissue must be processed after a short period of fixation. In practice, some melanin can be found in routine sections provided an adequate amount of tumour is available for examination.

It is important to be aware that not all skin tumours pigmented with melanin are malignant melanomata. Apart from naevocellular and blue naevi, basal-cell carcinomata and seborrhoeic keratoses often show heavy melanin pigmentation due either to hyperactivity or to hyperplasia of the melanocytes. This is much less common in squamous-cell tumours and Bowen's disease.

The blue naevus.[26] This is a special type of melanotic naevus which is intradermal from the start, and blue in colour because its melanocytes are deeply situated in the skin. They are elongated, strap-shaped dendritic cells scattered in the deep layers of the dermis. The epidermis itself is normal. This is the one type of naevus which may undergo malignant change in its intradermal portion. Nevertheless malignant change is very rare. The cells of the blue naevus are derived from a dermal pigmentary system in addition to the epidermal system of melanocytes, that is normally present in other mammals and especially the higher apes. It is usually vestigial in man. Collections of such cells are to be found normally only in the sacral area at birth, especially in the Mongolian and Negro races, and are called the *mongolian spot*. This usually involutes completely at puberty, but sometimes there are heterotopic collections of dermal melanocytes, and these may give rise to blue naevi, which are not truly congenital. The commonest sites for a blue naevus are the face, dorsum of the hand and foot, and the buttock. The histogenesis of the dermal melanocyte is uncertain; it may either be neural in origin or else develop locally.

Mucosal melanomata. Malignant melanomata may rarely occur in the nasal cavity, mouth, oesophagus, rectum, vagina, and vulva. These lesions are extremely malignant. It is not certain whether they arise in pre-existing naevi or whether they develop on normal epithelium.

Uveal melanoma. Malignant melanoma is one of the most common intraocular tumours. It usually arises in the choroid, but it may affect any part of the uveal tract. It is much commoner in Europeans than Africans, in whom it is a rare tumour.[31] The melanoma may arise from pre-existing melanotic hamartomata in the choroid and iris, but it often develops spontaneously. Some tumours are composed of large spindle-shaped cells which are usually heavily pigmented, and this type has a better prognosis than the tumours which are composed of plump epithelial-type cells ("epithelioid"). A characteristic feature is late metastasis, especially to the liver; this is a classical example of dormant cancer (see p. 371). It is generally accepted that the choroidal melanocytes are neural in origin. It is of interest that malignant melanoma of the iris has a particularly good prognosis, and often responds well to local excision in spite of its malignant histological appearance.

Other melanomata. Melanocytes are present in the *pia arachnoid* especially around the base of the brain, and from these a diffuse melanomatous infiltration may envelop the brain.[37] Similarly the *adrenal medulla* contains melanocytes which may give rise to a malignant melanoma.

Skeletal Hamartomata

The common *solitary exostosis* which grows out from the epiphyseal cartilage of a long bone is a good example of a cartilaginous hamartoma. It stops growing after puberty, when it becomes completely ossified. The rarer condition of multiple exostoses is a generalised hamartomatous disorder of the same nature, and it involves most of the bones derived from cartilage. In addition to the exostoses there is a general failure of bone remodelling, and the name *diaphysial aclasis*[38] is aptly applied. These lesions may sometimes undergo chondrosarcomatous change (this applies to a solitary exostosis also).[39] Diaphysial aclasis is inherited as an autosomal dominant characteristic.

Generalised Hamartomatous Dysplasias
Neurofibromatosis (von Recklinghausen's Disease).

In this condition there is a widespread hamartomatous overgrowth of nerve-sheath tissue. It is characterised by neurofibromatous masses surrounding the peripheral nerves of the limbs and the skin. Histologically the masses of nerve-sheath tissue are much more diffuse in extent and arrangement than those found in solitary neurofibromata. Palisading is usually very poorly developed (see p. 322). Other interesting features are *regional gigantism* due to a congenital overgrowth of tissues, and the rather frequent *café-au-lait spots* on the skin. The disease is inherited as an autosomal dominant characteristic.

Typical schwannomata of the auditory nerves commonly complicate neurofibromatosis. Of even greater importance is the tendency for neurogenic sarcomata to arise in the hamartomatous lesions involving the larger peripheral nerves of the limbs. Histologically these tumours resemble fibrosarcomata, and pulmonary metastases may occur.

Tuberous sclerosis (epiloia). This is another familial hamartomatous condition inherited as a dominant trait. There are focal overgrowths of the glial tissues in the central nervous system and the retina. On the face multiple papules due to focal fibroangiomatous overgrowth are characteristic.* Sub-ungual "fibromata" also occur. A similar focal overgrowth of fibrous tissue occurs in the kidneys (forming large tumour-like masses) and the lungs (leading to fibrosis

---

* These lesions are often erroneously referred to as "adenoma sebaceum". In fact, there is atrophy of the sebaceous glands, and the lesions are not related to the true sebaceous adenoma, which is a benign tumour of sebaceous glands.

and cystic change with a danger of spontaneous pneumothorax). Areas of malformed myocardium (so-called "rhabdomyomata"), the fibres of which are rich in a type of glycogen, are also characteristic of this disease. Occasionally the renal lesions become sarcomatous, and gliomata may develop in the central nervous system on the basis of a pre-existing glial hamartoma.

Cysts Developing on the Basis of Pre-existing Malformations

A **cyst** (derived from the Greek *kustis*, a bladder) is a pathological fluid-filled sac bounded by a wall. The fluid may be secreted by cells lining the wall or it may be derived from the tissue fluid of the area. It is often clear and colourless, but it may be thick and turbid, or contain shimmering crystals of cholesterol. If it contains pus or blood, the lesion is preferably called an abscess or a haematoma as the case may be, but, of course, a cyst may be the seat of secondary infection or haemorrhage.

Where the cyst wall is lined by an epithelium, this may be derived from developmental residues such as the epithelial rests of Malassez in the periodontal ligament or epithelial residues lying in planes of embryonic fusion. On the other hand, it may arise from a normal anatomical structure, such as the cells lining the ducts and acini of an exocrine gland. Usually the stimulus that evokes the epithelial proliferation is not known, but sometimes chronic inflammation is a factor, as in the development of the dental cyst. Here the chronic inflammation in the periapical tissues around a dead tooth stimulates the epithelial rests of Malassez to proliferate and line the liquefied apical granuloma, thus forming part of the wall of the dental cyst, the contents of which are turbid and characteristically contain cholesterol crystals, which are a product of tissue breakdown.

A classification of cysts is difficult, but the most practical one is based on the pathogenesis of the lesion.

(a) *Developmental.* These are described below.

(b) *Inflammatory*, e.g. the dental cyst, encysted pleural effusions, and pancreatic "pseudocysts" following acute pancreatitis.

(c) *Degenerative*, e.g. cystic change in goitres, in solid tumours like the uterine leiomyoma, and in other pathological lesions like fibrous dysplasia of bone. The precipitating factor is necrosis, nearly always ischaemic in origin, with liquefaction of the necrotic debris. The ischaemia may be due to general vascular disease, as in brain cysts following infarction, or to a locally inadequate blood supply in a tumour or other lesion.

(d) *Retention*, e.g. mucous cysts of the mouth. The ranula, a cystic dilatation in the submandibular or sublingual gland, is believed to form as a result of obstruction of the duct (the Latin *ranula*, a little frog, alludes to the shape of the swelling produced).

(e) *Implantation.* This is the epidermoid cyst mentioned on pp. 112 and 361.

(f) Parasitic, e.g. the hydatid cyst, found especially in the liver and lungs, is due to the proliferation and growth of the larval form of the canine tapeworm *Echinococcus granulosus*. The germinative layer secretes the "hydatid fluid".

(g) Hyperplastic, e.g. mammary dysplasia (blue-domed cyst of the breast).

(h) Neoplastic, e.g. the cystadenoma and the cystic teratoma.

Developmental cysts arise in several different ways.

(a) The persistence of normally vestigial remnants. Examples of this type of cyst are the branchial and thyroglossal cysts. A branchial cyst[40] is due to the persistence of a portion of the cervical sinus, and it is lined by stratified squamous epithelium which is heavily invested in lymphoid tissue. It contains turbid material which is rich in cholesterol crystals. Some cysts of dental origin (e.g. primordial and dentigerous cysts) are due to changes in the enamel organ during the development of a tooth. The juxta-testicular vestiges, e.g the appendix testis and paradidymis, sometimes undergo cystic dilatation in old men.

(b) Ectopia of various tissues. Ectopia is frequently due to the dislocation of a tissue into a neighbouring area where it tends to form a cyst. A good example of this is the *dermoid cyst*, which is due to the sequestration of a piece of skin beneath one of the lines of fusion of the various embryonic body processes. Such cysts occur most commonly in the subcutaneous tissue of the face, usually near one of the angles of the orbit. Sometimes they are intracranial, in which case it appears that the dislocation of the skin must have occurred before the bony skull was laid down. A dermoid cyst is lined by stratified squamous epithelium, and in its wall there are hair follicles, sebaceous glands, and sweat glands. It contains sebaceous debris and matted hairs. Unlike a teratoma it does not include any other tissues in its wall.

An *epidermoid cyst* is also lined by a layer of stratified squamous epithelium, but external to this there is only connective tissue. Skin appendages are not present, and its cavity contains only keratin. Some epidermoid cysts are due to the implantation of a piece of epidermis into the deeper layers of the skin and subcutaneous tissue as the result of trauma or acne vulgaris, and a few are probably true congenital ectopias of epidermis. Most epidermoid cysts are, however, derived from plugged pilo-sebaceous follicles, and form the common variety of "sebaceous cyst".

Enterogenous cysts are the result of an ectopia of the intestinal mucosa. They occur not only in the bowel wall, but also in the mesentery and the retroperitoneal tissues.

(c) A failure of connexion of tubular elements. Polycystic kidney is probably due to a failure of fusion of the metanephric tubules with the collecting tubules.[41] Another widely-held view is that it is due to the persistence of earlier generations of nephric tubules (pronephros and mesonephros). Polycystic disease often affects the liver and pancreas as well as the kidneys, and it is probably due to a malformation of the biliary and pancreatic ducts in an early stage of development.

The same explanation is probably true of congenital cystic lung, in which there appears to be severe bronchiolar maldevelopment.

(d) As a hamartomatous process. Cystic dilatations may occur in haemangiomata and lymphangiomata. The cystic hygroma of the neck and the lymphatic cysts occasionally found in the greater omentum are good examples.

TUMOURS DEVELOPING IN PRE-EXISTING MALFORMATIONS

I. Tumours Developing in Hamartomata

This topic has already been mentioned (see table on p. 317).

II. Tumours Arising from Vestigial Remnants

Chordoma. Vestiges of the embryonic notochord may be found throughout the vertebral axis, and are commonest in the spheno–occipital area of the skull and the sacrococcygeal region. Occasionally a recognisable button-like remnant, or "ecchordosis", may be found under the dura mater of the dorsum sellae in the course of a necropsy. The chordoma is a rare tumour derived from these remnants, and is found most frequently in the two sites already mentioned. It is a pale pink, soft, gelatinous tumour which infiltrates the bone and surrounding soft tissues. Histologically it consists of groups of polyhedral cells, the larger ones of which contain large vacuoles in their cytoplasm. These are called *physaliferous cells* (i.e. bubble-bearing cells), and they may coalesce to produce a blurred vacuolated syncytium. The gelatinous consistency of the tumour is due to its mucoid nature (Fig. 27.18).

A chordoma is a slowly-growing malignant tumour which metastasises rather late by the blood stream. It is commonest in middle-aged and elderly people. By virtue of its situation it can seldom be eradicated surgically, nor is it very sensitive to x-rays.

Ameloblastoma (adamantinoma). This is a yellowish, cystic tumour of the jaws, which is slowly-growing and only locally malignant. Both in behaviour and in structure it resembles the common basal-cell carcinoma quite closely. It usually occurs in the mandible, and is commonest in young adults. It consists of angular clumps of small epithelial cells, and in the centres of these aggregations there is often an open meshwork resembling the "stellate reticulum" of the enamel organ (Fig. 27.19). In between the cells there may be accumulations of fluid, which give rise to the cystic appearance so typical of this tumour. Despite its name the tumour does not form enamel. It probably arises from remnants of the dental lamina and the enamel organ.

Craniopharyngioma. Foci of epithelium (usually squamous) derived from Rathke's pouch are often found in the body of the sphenoid bone and around the pituitary

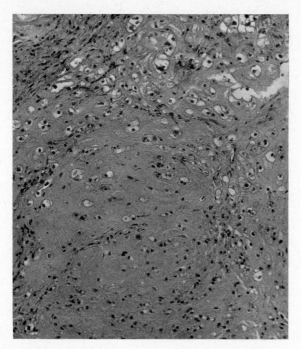

Figure 27.18
Chordoma. The tumour is composed of polygonal cells arranged in a dense stroma which is heavily infiltrated by a mucopolysaccharide secreted by the cells themselves. The empty, vacuolated cytoplasm of many of the cells is quite conspicuous; these are the physaliferous cells. The over-all appearance resembles that of a tumour of cartilage, both because of the mucoid nature of the stroma and the vacuolated tumour cells. × 110.

Figure 27.19
Ameloblastoma. The tumour consists of aggregations of small epithelial cells, the outer layers of which form a palisade as is found in the basal-cell carcinoma. In the midst of the central clump, there is an open meshwork reminiscent of the stellate reticulum of the developing tooth germ ("enamel organ"). The other clumps have undergone cystic change, and surrounding the cysts the cells show squamous metaplasia. × 150.

itself. These epithelial residues may occasionally give rise to cysts and also to slowly-growing, locally malignant tumours called craniopharyngiomata. These usually have the structure of ameloblastomata, but sometimes they resemble squamous-cell carcinomata. Extensive foci of ossification are characteristic of these tumours, and cystic change is also conspicuous.

Branchiogenic carcinoma. This is a highly malignant squamous-cell carcinoma developing in the tissues of the front of the neck. The majority of reported tumours are probably secondary lymph-node metastases from undetected primary pulmonary or oropharyngeal carcinomata, but it is possible that very occasionally a carcinoma may develop on the basis of a branchial cyst.[42]

Urachal tumours. The urachus is the intra-abdominal part of the allantois, and it extends from the vertex of the bladder to the umbilicus. Occasionally vestiges persist, and these may give rise to cysts and also to papillary and mucus-secreting adenocarcinomata.

III. Tumours Arising from Ectopic Organs and Tissues

Squamous-cell carcinomata very occasionally arise in dermoid cysts, and enterogenous cysts occasionally form the sites of origin of adenocarcinomata, usually of a mucus-secreting type.

Cryptorchidism is due either to the imperfect descent of a testis or to its malposition in neighbouring areas (ectopia). In either event these testes are notoriously liable to undergo

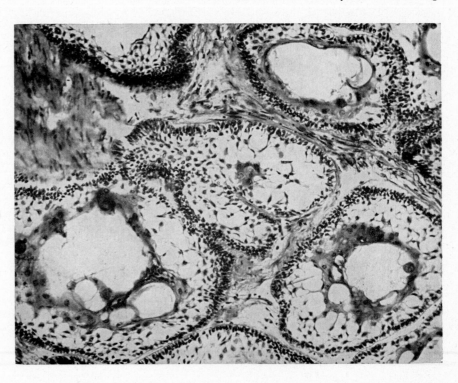

malignant change, both of a seminomatous and a teratomatous nature. It appears that there is some fundamental abnormality in such testes which predisposes them to neoplasia.

CONCLUSION

A study of perverted embryogenesis is one of the most fascinating facets of pathology, and an enthusiast may well be tempted to attribute many morbid processes to a fundamental developmental defect. As it is often impossible to deny the possibility of such a pathogenesis in respect of many lesions appearing in adults, a type of reasoning may easily be fostered in which all morbid processes are believed to be basically developmental in origin. This approach gave rise to Cohnheim's "cell rest" theory of the origin of tumours, which is mentioned in Chapter 29.

It is a challenging thought that some diseases of adult life may have their basis in a defect that first arose during the course of embryogenesis. Such a defect may come about in a variety of ways.

Malformations may be due to *genetic factors*. These may vary from gross *chromosomal abnormalities*, e.g. the syndromes of Down, Turner, and Klinefelter, to *single point mutations* involving biochemical mechanisms. For example, galactosaemia leads to abnormalities of liver, kidney, brain, and eye. In many hereditary diseases the actual defect is unknown, e.g. in achondroplasia. Sometimes the malformation becomes evident only in adult life, e.g. hereditary haemorrhagic telangiectasia.

Most malformations, however, are not genetic in origin, but are due apparently to external factors. Many of these are unknown, but among the important *teratogenic agents* are the following:

Drugs.[43] The most notorious is the sedative *thalidomide* which leads to the absence of limbs (amelus) or parts of limbs, haemangiomatosis of the upper lip and nose, and severe malformations of the alimentary tract, heart, and genito-urinary system.[44] *Cytotoxic agents* also produce malformations, and the use of large doses of *progesterone* can produce genital deformities in female infants. *Cortisol* given to pregnant mice leads to cleft palate in the offspring in certain strains but not in others. This is yet another example of how genetic and environmental factors can interact. *Lysergic acid diethylamide (LSD)* can cause chromosomal damage, abortion, and malformation in rats, and may well do so in man.[45] The anticonvulsant drug phenytoin may also be added to the list of teratogenic drugs.[48]

The effects of these agents depends upon two factors:

(*a*) The specific action of the agent itself.

(*b*) The susceptibility of the organ or tissue of the fetus. Organs are particularly vulnerable during the period of rapid growth and differentiation. Thus the human fetus is most sensitive to thalidomide 20 to 40 days after conception, while the heart is liable to be affected during the short period 40 to 45 days after conception.

Ionising radiations.

Infections of the fetus in utero, e.g. toxoplasmosis, syphilis and certain virus diseases, notably rubella.[46]

Rhesus incompatibility, i.e. erythroblastosis fetalis.

It is in this group of acquired defects that success is most likely to attend measures designed to reduce the incidence of congenital malformations.

REFERENCES

1. WILLIS, R. A. (1968). *British Medical Journal*, iii, 267.
2. LENNOX, B. (1960). In *Recent Advances in Pathology*, 7th edn, p. 278. Edited by C. V. Harrison. London: Churchill.
3. MYERS, L. M. (1959). *Journal of Pathology and Bacteriology*, **78**, 43.
4. CARLETON, R. L., FRIEDMAN, N. B. and BOMZE, E. J. (1953). *Cancer (Philadelphia)*, **6**, 464.
5. WALTERS, G. (1968). In *Recent Advances in Clinical Pathology*, Series Five, p. 337. Edited by S. C. Dyke. London: Churchill.
6. Leading Article (1971). *Lancet*, ii, 1016.
7. JENSEN, R. D. and MILLER, R. W. (1971). *New England Journal of Medicine*, **285**, 307.
8. ALBRECHT, E. (1904). *Verhandlungen der Deutschen Pathologischen Gesellschaft*, **7**, 153.
9. WALSH, T. S. and TOMPKINS, V. N. (1956). *Cancer (Philadelphia)*, **9**, 869.
10. JAMES, D. H. and TUTTLE, A. H. (1961). *Journal of Pediatrics*, **59**, 234.
11. BEAN, W. B. (1958). *Vascular Spiders and Related Lesions of the Skin*, p. 166. Oxford: Blackwell.
12. NUSSEY, A. M. and MILLER, H. H. (1939). *British Medical Journal*, i, 822.
13. LINDAU, A. (1931). *Proceedings of the Royal Society of Medicine*, **24**, 363.
14. KESSLER, E. and KOZENITZKY, I. L. (1971). *Journal of Clinical Pathology*, **24**, 530.
15. STEWART, F. W. and TREVES, N. (1948). *Cancer (Philadelphia)*, **1**, 64.
16. SALM, R. (1963). *Journal of Pathology and Bacteriology*, **85**, 445.
17. WILLIS, R. A. (1967). In *Pathology of Tumours*, 4th edn, p. 244. London: Butterworths.
18. MACKENZIE, D. H. (1971). *Journal of Clinical Pathology*, **24**, 524.
19. Symposium on Kaposi's Sarcoma (1962). *Acta Unio Internationalis contra Cancrum*, **18**, 322–511.
20. Leading Article (1967). *Lancet*, ii, 1290.
21. HARRIS, M. (1971). *Journal of Clinical Pathology*, **24**, 520.
22. MASSON, P. (1951). *Cancer (Philadelphia)*, **4**, 9.
23. ALLEN, A. C. (1949). *Cancer (Philadelphia)*, **2**, 28.
24. SPITZ, S. (1948). *American Journal of Pathology*, **24**, 591.
25. WAYTE, D. M. and HELWIG, E. B. (1968). *Cancer*, **22**, 69.
26. LEVENE, A. (1972). *Proceedings of the Royal Society of Medicine*, **65**, 137.

27. Leading Article (1967). *British Medical Journal*, ii, 129.
28. CLARK, W. H. *et al.* (1969). *Cancer Research*, **29**, 705.
29. Leading Article (1971). *Lancet*, i, 172.
30. Leading Article (1972). *British Medical Journal*, i, 130.
31. Leading Article (1968). *Lancet*, i, 76.
32. ANDERSON, D. E., SMITH, J. L. and McBRIDE, C. M. (1967). *Journal of the American Medical Association*, **200**, 741.
33. Leading Article (1967). *British Medical Journal*, iii, 191.
34. JAY, B. (1964). *Proceedings of the Royal Society of Medicine*, **57**, 497.
35. LEVER, W. F. (1967). *Histopathology of Skin*, 4th edn, p. 700 *et seq.* Philadelphia and Toronto: Lippincott.
36. MIHM, M. C., CLARK, W. H. and FROM, L. (1971). *New England Journal of Medicine*, **284**, 1078.
37. GIBSON, J. B., BURROWS, D. and WEIR, W. P. (1957). *Journal of Pathology and Bacteriology*, **74**, 419.
38. FAIRBANK, H. A. T. (1935). *Proceedings of the Royal Society of Medicine*, **28**, 1611.
39. JAFFE, H. L. (1943). *Archives of Pathology*, **36**, 335.
40. WILSON, C. P. (1955). *Annals of the Royal College of Surgeons of England*, **17**, 1.
41. OSATHANONDH, V. and POTTER, E. L. (1964). *Archives of Pathology*, **77**, 459.
42. COLLINS, N. P. and EDGERTON, M. T. (1959). *Cancer (Philadelphia)*, **12**, 235.
43. SMITHELLS, R. W. (1966). *Advances in Tetrology*, **1**, 250.
44. Leading Article (1962). *Lancet*, i, 307; and ii, 336.
45. Leading Article (1967). *British Medical Journal*, iv, 124.
46. BROWN, G. C. (1966). *Advances in Tetrology*, **1**, 55.
47. MINKEN, S. L., CRAVER, W. L. and ADAMS, J. T. (1968). *Archives of Pathology*, **86**, 442.
48. LOUGHNAN, P. M., GOLD, H. and VANCE, J. C. (1973). *Lancet*, i, 70.

Chapter 28.   Spread of Malignant Tumours

The mode of spread of cancer cells has given rise to much speculation, but there is still little understanding of the process. The reduction in cell adhesiveness (see p. 13) may play a part, and furthermore some tumour cells are feebly motile in tissue culture. It has been suggested that tumours may secrete toxins or enzymes that facilitate spread in the tissues; hyaluronidase is favoured by some workers, but the evidence is far from convincing. Others stress the importance of fibrin in providing a network on which the tumour cells grow, and they claim that fibrinolysins may inhibit the spread of the tumour.[1] Be this as it may, infiltration into the surrounding tissues is the salient feature of all malignant tumours. The invading cells penetrate various natural passages which afford an easy route for further spread. The most important of these are the lymphatics and blood vessels, and in both the malignant cells may become detached as emboli which are carried to distant sites. If the cells survive and multiply a secondary isolated mass of tumour is produced

This is a *metastasis*. *Direct invasion* and *embolisation* are thus the two main methods of spread.

DIRECT SPREAD

Local spread. The direct infiltration of the surrounding tissues common to all malignant tumours means that the microscopic extent of a tumour exceeds what is macroscopically apparent. For this reason any excision which aims at removing all the neoplastic cells must incorporate a wide extent of the surrounding tissue. The invading cells tend to follow natural clefts or tissue planes, and to move in the line of least resistance. Dense fascial sheaths may confine malignant cells for some time. This is well shown in osteosarcoma of a long bone: the tumour reaches the periosteum, but is there held up; it invades in the subperiosteal plane to produce a fusiform swelling. Cartilage is resistant to tumour infiltration; osteosarcoma seldom destroys the epiphyseal

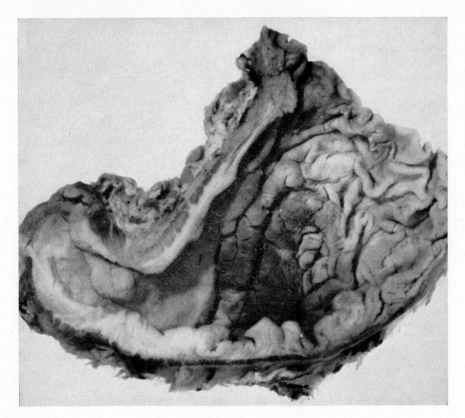

Figure 28.1
Infiltrating carcinoma of the stomach. The pyloric portion is greatly thickened, and the wall is diffusely infiltrated by pale tumour tissue. There is extensive invasion of the septa between muscle fibres by the tumour. This is most pronounced in the wall of the lower part of the lesser curvature, where segmentation is evident. *(EA. 42.1, Reproduced by permission of the President and Council of the R.C.S. Eng.)*

cartilage until late in its course. Likewise, secondary cancer and myeloma in a vertebra do not invade the intervertebral disc.

The tendency of carcinoma cells to invade along tissue septa is demonstrated in the breast; particularly characteristic is the appearance of a column of cells in single file invading between collagen bundles. Infiltration often occurs in the ligaments of Astley Cooper, causing the tumour to become attached both to the dermis and the deep fascia. The fibrous reaction caused by the scirrhous tumour leads to the contraction which is responsible for the skin dimpling seen clinically. Why this contraction should occur is not easily explained. In cancers of the stomach and colon the invasion of the septa between the muscle fibres produces the characteristic appearance of *segmentation* of the muscle layer (Fig. 28.1).

Infiltration can also occur into individual cells. Thus squamous-cell cancers of the cervical lymph nodes may infiltrate into the fibres of the adjacent striated muscles.

Infiltration can also proceed into the epidermis from a nearby duct which is the seat of neoplasia. Paget's disease of the nipple has been explained in this way, but it is probably a primary intra-epithelial lesion (p. 387). Epidermal invasion is important in malignant melanoma and is also seen in malignant lymphoma of skin. Its detection is a useful diagnostic feature of mycosis fungoides (p. 405), and the collections of lymphoma cells within the epidermis are known as Pautrier micro-abscesses.*

Evidence of local invasion is an important sign, for its detection is tantamount to a diagnosis of malignancy. The basal-cell carcinoma is the prototype of a group of tumours the spread of which is entirely local.

Invasion of lymphatics. Carcinoma shows a particular tendency to invade the local lymphatics at an early stage. Sarcomata only occasionally spread *via* the lymphatics.

Sampson Handley drew attention to the spread which may occur along these vessels in breast cancer. The tumour cells grow progressively within the lumen of the lymphatics as a solid cord which extends in all directions to involve an ever-widening area of tissue. This process is called *permeation* (Fig. 28.2). The central area of the malignant cord may undergo necrosis and even disappear while the advancing end proliferates. Eventually the cord of cells reaches the draining lymph nodes. By blocking the main ducts, the lymph is diverted to adjacent channels, and in this way there may be retrograde deviation of tumour cells. It is not surprising that numerous outlying nodules of tumour may be found in the skin of such a breast. In extreme cases the entire skin of the chest wall may be the seat of confluent carcinoma, producing *cancer en cuirasse*. Lymphatic permeation also causes the local dermal oedema which produces the *peau d'orange* appearance seen in breast cancer.

In the lung the major lymphatics run with the bronchi and

* This is an unfortunate misuse of the term abscess, but being time honoured, is likely to persist.

the main pulmonary vessels. If they are infiltrated with cancer, these other structures may be cuffed with the tumour; oat-cell cancer is the usual cause of this. Extensive invasion of the pulmonary lymphatics produces the condition sometimes known as "lymphangitis carcinomatosa". The tumour-filled vessels give the lung a reticulated appearance both macroscopically and radiologically. This

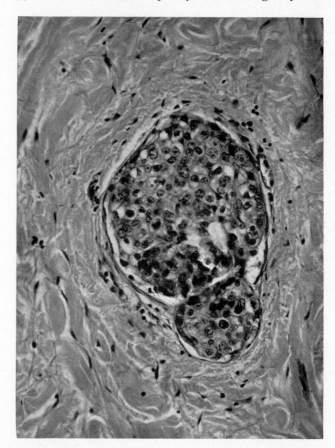

Figure 28.2
Lymphatic permeation. This is a section of a spheroidal-cell carcinoma of the breast. A lymphatic channel has been completely occluded by a solid cord of cancer cells. × 200.

almost always denotes a secondary carcinoma arising from the breast, and is curiously uncommon in primary lung cancer. Malignant melanoma is also liable to invade lymph vessels, which may appear clinically as black streaks emerging from the primary tumour. In some cases of cancer of the lung and colon permeation of the subpleural and subperitoneal lymphatics is so marked that these distended vessels are easily visible to the naked eye.

Perineural invasion and spread. This is seen in many types of carcinoma, and is a useful diagnostic feature when the possibly malignant nature of a lesion is being assessed, e.g. in a section of prostate or pancreas. It is usually attributed to lymphatic spread, but it is doubtful whether there are any perineural lymphatics. The appearance of malignant cells lying in a space is often taken to indicate lymphatic invasion, but unless a clear endothelial lining is present, one cannot be sure that the cells are not lying in a tissue space.

Venous invasion. The invasion of large veins is seen most frequently in lung cancer because of the large number of vessels available. The tumour becomes covered by thrombus, and this venous extension is easily missed.

Hypernephroma is another tumour in which venous invasion is common. A solid mass of growth may be found in the renal vein, and cases have been described in which this has extended into the vena cava and up to the right atrium. Occasionally a left-sided varicocele is the first indication of a hypernephroma of the left kidney which has spread into the renal vein. As the left spermatic vein drains into the renal vein (the right drains directly into the inferior vena cava), it is to be expected that there would be a back-pressure effect.

Arterial invasion. It is generally stated that the thick elastic wall of large arteries effectively prevents tumour ingrowth. In the lung, however, careful examination not infrequently reveals invasion of the pulmonary arteries.[2] Arterial obstruction may be responsible for tumour necrosis as well as infarction of the adjacent lung.

Small vessels. It is probably true to say that small vessels are invaded in every case of malignant disease. This is particularly noticeable in sarcomata, since the tumour cells may actually line the vascular spaces. An extreme example of this is found in angiosarcomata. Choriocarcinoma is another tumour notorious for the ease with which it invades blood vessels; the tumours are typically haemorrhagic and necrotic.

Serous spaces. Tumours reaching a serous surface like the visceral pleura tend to erode the mesothelium. Fibrinous adhesions may then form to the parietal surface. Tumour cells can thus traverse the space; in this way some peripheral lung cancers invade the chest wall directly.

SPREAD BY METASTASIS

Lymphatic Spread

The detachment of groups of tumour cells in an invaded lymphatic leads to the production of emboli, which become lodged in the subcapsular sinus of the regional lymph node. If the cells survive and grow, the node soon becomes replaced by the tumour, and further spread occurs to the next group of glands by way of the efferent channel. This is a familiar event in carcinoma and melanoma, but is rare in sarcoma. The extent of the lymphatic involvement is important in assessing the prognosis and is one of the factors taken into consideration in the staging of tumours.

Retrograde embolism is a term used to denote spread in a reverse direction to the usual flow. If a lymphatic is blocked (nearly always due to permeation), the flow of lymph may be reversed, and subsequent embolism produces metastases in unusual sites. The importance of the phenomenon has been greatly exaggerated. A well-known example is the involvement of the left cervical lymph nodes (Virchow's node) in gastric cancer (Troisier's sign). This is probably due to blockage of the thoracic duct near its entry into the left subclavian vein.

Some carcinomata, e.g. of the breast and lung, appear to spread very rapidly to the regional nodes, whereas those of the skin and lip do so at a late stage. Tongue carcinoma, on the other hand, is usually attended by early cervical-node involvement. This has been attributed to the mobility of the tongue, and the massaging of cancer cells into the lymphatics during speech and mastication. In fact, the spreading tendency of malignant tumours is probably an inherent property of the cancer itself, and for some reason at present unknown cancers of the mouth are generally more malignant in their course than are those of the skin and lip.

Blood Spread

The occurrence of blood-spread metastasis is the feature of malignant disease which is responsible for death in most cases. It is also the factor which limits the surgical and radiotherapeutic treatment of cancer.

At first sight the mode of production of secondary tumours is easy to understand. Malignant cells invade small vessels or veins, become detached, and are then carried by the blood stream to some distant site where they reach a capillary network. There the emboli become impacted, proliferate, and develop into secondary tumours. A second method of blood-borne metastasis is by way of the lymphatics. Eventually all the lymph drains into the venous circulation, and the first capillary network the tumour cells meet is in the lung. It is difficult to assess how much blood spread is due to primary venous invasion, and how much is secondary to lymphatic involvement. In the sarcomata, which spread into the blood stream at a very early stage, there is no doubt that invasion is primarily venous, as lymphatic spread is most uncommon. In the carcinomata blood spread usually manifests itself some time after lymphatic involvement, and it is quite possible that much of the blood stream invasion is secondary to regional lymphatic spread. It is often said that sarcomata spread by the blood stream and carcinomata by the lymphatics; this is a half-truth, because carcinomata also spread by the blood stream, although the first metastases usually appear in the lymph nodes.

As would be expected, one of the commonest sites for secondaries from most tumours is the lung. Likewise, primary tumours arising from the area of tissue drained by the portal vein regularly metastasise to the liver. Purely anatomical factors would appear to account for this distribution, but closer examination makes such an explantion inadequate.

Many tumours, e.g. of the breast and kidney, give rise to secondaries not only in the lungs, but also in the liver, bones, and other organs. Systemic metastases sometimes occur in the absence of apparent lung deposits. It is possible that these are really present, but have been missed because of an inadequate *post-mortem* examination by the pathologist. Alternatively the cells may be able to pass through the lung capillaries, and become arrested elsewhere. Another explanation is the possibility of a direct venous communication between the primary and secondary sites.*

The distribution of secondary tumours might be expected to be related to the blood supply, but this is not the case. Cardiac and skeletal muscle have an abundant blood supply, and yet are rarely the site of metastasis. The spleen likewise is not usually involved. The liver, on the other hand, is

certain sites are particularly favoured. The "seed" may be widespread, but only where the "soil" is suitable does growth occur. Some examples of this *selective metastasis* must now be examined.

(*a*) The commonest organ in which blood-borne metastases occur is the *liver*. Not only do gastro-intestinal cancers regularly metastasise there, but also carcinomata of the genito-urinary system, lungs, and breast, melanomata, and sarcomata. Apparently the liver affords an excellent nutritional medium for tumour cells. It may even be the seat of transplacental metastases, as shown in Fig. 28.3.

Figure 28.3
Transplacental metastasis of malignant melanoma. In this remarkable case a woman suffering from extensive malignant melanomatosis gave birth to a child shortly before her death. The placenta was massively involved in the tumour. The infant progressed well at first, but at about 9 months developed marasmus, hepatomegaly, and secondary infection. It soon died, and at necropsy the liver was found to contain metastases of malignant melanoma. *(A 110.1, Reproduced by permission of the President and Council of the R.C.S. Eng.)*

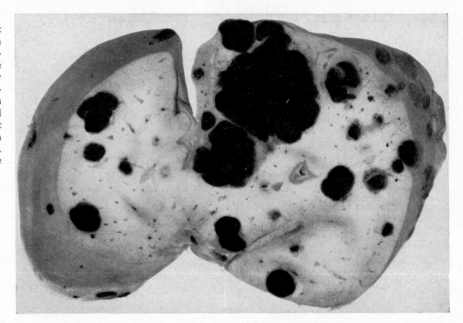

frequently the site of secondary tumours regardless of the site of the primary.

It has been found that tumour cells are present in the blood stream in cases of malignant disease,[3–5] but the frequency of this event is undecided. The cells are not plentiful, and many techniques for concentrating them have been devised. Considerable difficulty is experienced in distinguishing immature blood cells from malignant cells, and different investigators report widely divergent results. Thus, the reported incidence in known cases of cancer has varied from 100 per cent to 0 per cent. Perhaps 10 per cent is a realistic figure.[6] There is no general agreement as to the significance of finding cells in the blood, for it does not seem to be related to prognosis. It is probable that many of the cells die. Only the selected few are able to take root to grow into secondary deposits. What factors govern this are not known, but it appears likely that

(*b*) The next most common site for metastases is the *lung*; it is especially frequently involved in sarcomata, and carcinomata of the thyroid, breast, and kidney. Testicular tumours and choriocarcinomata also favour the lungs (Fig. 28.4).

(*c*) *Bone Metastases.*[7, 8] After the liver and lungs, the bones are the most frequent sites of secondary deposits.[9] The primary tumour is usually a carcinoma of lung, breast, prostate, kidney (hypernephroma), or thyroid. The neuroblastoma also spreads in this way (see Hutchison's syndrome, p. 349). Of the lung cancers it is the oat-cell carcinoma that is particularly liable to metastasise to the skeleton;[10] by contrast the squamous-cell carcinoma, adenocarcinoma, and undifferentiated carcinoma only occasionally produce skeletal deposits. It is the follicular carcinoma of the thyroid that produces metastases in bone most commonly;[11] the papillary carcinoma rarely spreads this way, and the anaplastic carcinoma only occasionally. These distinctive patterns of metastasis indicate the biological individuality of different cancers arising from a single organ.

Secondaries from prostatic cancer are particularly liable to occur in the pelvic bones and vertebrae. The communica-

---

* In cases where there is extensive venous invasion, e.g. in hypernephroma, there may be retrograde venous embolism comparable with that described in regard to the lymphatics. This accounts for the occasional metastases in the left spermatic cord, vulva, and vagina in the course of a hypernephroma of the left kidney.

tions between the prostatic venous plexus and the various vertebral plexuses are believed by some to account for this, since often there is no evidence of pulmonary involvement, but selective metastasis would seem a more likely explanation.

Osseous metastases may be osteoplastic (osteosclerotic) or osteolytic. In the former there is much new bone laid down,

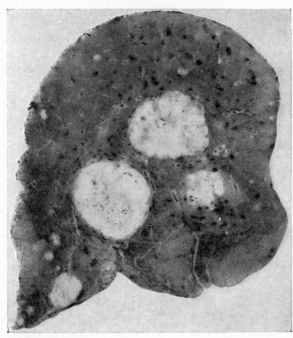

Figure 28.4
Metastatic carcinoma in lung. Note the circumscribed white deposits, apparently encapsulated from the parenchyma. Primary lung cancer infiltrates into the surrounding tissue much more obviously. The primary site in this case was the breast. *(*R 47.3, *Reproduced by permission of the President and Council of the R.C.S. Eng.)*

and as a result the secondaries are hard and radio-opaque. The osteogenesis is reflected in a raised level of serum alkaline phosphatase, while the serum calcium and phosphate levels remain normal. Most osteoplastic secondaries are due to prostatic cancer, when there is usually a raised level of serum acid phosphatase as well. Both the primary lesion and the widespread skeletal metastases produce this enzyme, which may possibly be responsible for the characteristic osteosclerosis of prostatic cancer.

Occasionally other secondary tumours, e.g. neuroblastoma and carcinoma of the breast or colon, cause new bone to be produced, but much more frequently they, and the other tumours mentioned, cause osteolysis. This is seen radiologically as an area of translucency in the bone, and it may lead to spontaneous fracture. The serum alkaline phosphatase level is normal, but sometimes there may be sufficient demineralisation to lead to severe hypercalcaemia and renal failure (see Chapter 47).

If much of the bone marrow is replaced by tumour tissue leuco-erythroblastic anaemia may result.

(*d*) The *brain* is sometimes a site for secondary tumours, and here the usual primary source is the lung. Whenever a middle-aged or elderly man suddenly develops neurological or psychiatric symptoms, it is most important to x-ray his chest before proceeding with other investigations. Carcinomata of the breast and melanomata sometimes also spread to the brain. It has been postulated that there is a direct communication between the bronchial veins and the vertebral plexus, but the importance of this has not been proven.[12]

(*e*) Of the *endocrine glands* the adrenal is the one which most frequently contains metastases; usually the medulla is involved, but discrete cortical deposits are not uncommon. Lung cancer, especially the oat-cell variety, frequently metastasises to this site, and some authorities believe that the route of spread may be lymphatic rather than haematogenous in some instances. It is estimated that about a third of all fatal lung cancers show adrenal deposits. Cancer of the breast also often spreads to the adrenals, as is noted after bilateral adrenalectomy (see p. 383). The ovaries also often harbour metastases in this condition.

The other endocrine glands are less often involved in metastases. The thyroid may harbour secondary tumours of various types, and it is interesting that a goitrous gland is more vulnerable than a healthy one. It may be that the vascular arrangement in a goitre is more prone to entrap emboli than that of a normal gland.

(*f*) The *skin* is occasionally the site of metastases, which tend to erupt as discrete nodules. The primary source is usually the lung or the breast. Multiple cutaneous deposits are also characteristic of malignant melanoma.

(*g*) Occasionally metastases occur within *benign tumours*. Widespread cancer of the breast may rarely metastasise to uterine fibroids, and occasionally a deposit of oat-cell lung cancer is found in association with a colonic adenoma.

The metastasising powers of tumours vary widely. Amongst those with the greatest tendency are carcinomata of the breast and lungs. The lethal effects of breast cancer are attributable almost entirely to its widespread blood-borne metastases which are found especially in the lungs, liver, and vertebral column. Cancer of the lung, especially the oat-cell variety, is also notorious for the speed with which it metastasises. In addition to the common sites, e.g. liver, adrenals, and bones, it may spread in a more bizarre way. Sometimes whole organs, e.g. pancreas, gonads, and thyroid, are replaced by the tumour, while the usually affected organs remain free. The spleen and bowel are also occasionally implicated. When a lung tumour metastasises to the brain there is often little evidence of other blood-borne deposits; perhaps the cerebral lesion kills too rapidly for these to develop.

Sarcomata metastasise early, and the lung is by far the most heavily implicated organ. The liver and brain are also frequently affected, but bone deposits are uncommon.

Malignant brain tumours rarely metastasise outside the cranial cavity. The absence of lymphatic metastases is attributable to the lack of a lymphatic drainage in the brain. The absence of blood-borne deposits may be related to the raised intracranial pressure occluding the adjacent cerebral veins; the larger venous sinuses are so well separated from the brain that the tumour kills the patient before it can spread to invade them. Extracerebral metastases may occasionally follow surgical procedures, especially decompression operations leaving large gaps in the dura and skull so that the tumour comes into direct contact with the surrounding soft tissues. Shunting operations for obstructive hydrocephalus, in which the cerebrospinal fluid is drained into the right atrium, may also lead to such metastases.[13, 14] The very rare glioma arising in an ovarian teratoma may also metastasise.

Although tumour emboli are very common, most of them, after impaction in a small vessel, become covered by thrombus and die. The vascular occlusion may itself produce damage; thus right-sided heart failure may follow the obliteration of many lung vessels.[15]

Occasionally a large vein is invaded by growth; this may break off to produce a large embolus. In cancer of the lung a large piece of tumour growing in a pulmonary vein has been known to break off and produce a massive systemic embolus.[16] Similarly massive tumour pulmonary embolism may occur in limb sarcoma, testicular teratoma, and hypernephroma, tumours which tend to invade the large systemic veins.[17, 18]

Secondary tumours are usually multiple; the solitary, cannon–ball lung metastases sometimes seen in hypernephroma and seminoma are obvious exceptions. Metastases in liver and lung frequently grow so rapidly that expansion exceeds local infiltration. The growths then give the impression of being sharply demarcated.

Transcoelomic Spread

When a tumour invades the serosal layer of a viscus, it excites a local inflammatory response with a small effusion into the serous cavity. Malignant cells become incorporated into the local fibrinous exudate, and are then detached. They are swept into the effusion, and carried by it into the cavity. They settle widely on its wall, proliferate, and set up innumerable "seedlings". These excite the formation of more inflammatory exudate, and in due course the space may contain a great deal of fluid. Sometimes the exudate is more fibrinous, and the viscera are bound together by dense adhesions.

The commonest example of transcoelomic spread is seen in the peritoneal cavity in cases of primary gastric, colonic, and ovarian carcinomata. The greater omentum may be so massively infiltrated that it is converted into a thick, spongy, gelatinous mass of tumour (omental cake). Metastases are common in the pouch of Douglas, doubtless due to a gravitational effect.

In gastric and colonic cancer there may also be trans-peritoneal spread to the ovaries. The best-known example of this is the *Krukenberg tumour*. This is usually bilateral: both ovaries are enlarged, their surfaces are smooth and thickened, and their substance is completely replaced by a mass of mucoid carcinoma. There is usually a primary mucoid cancer elsewhere, most often in the stomach or colon, but occasionally in the breast. The mode of metastasis has caused much speculation. Some authorities attribute it to retrograde lymphatic spread, because the surfaces of the ovaries are smooth and free of seedling deposits. However, some cases may be true examples of transcoelomic spread. It is known that mucoid cancer penetrates very easily, and it is therefore possible that the cells deposited on the surface invade the ovary without destroying the tunica albuginea. Mucoid cancer tends to stimulate a dense stromal reaction, and this may account for the thickened surface. In those cases secondary to breast cancer a haematogenous metastasis is the most likely explanation, but in the gastric and colonic cases there is often little evidence of extensive blood-borne or lymphatic deposits elsewhere. Occasionally a Krukenberg tumour appears to be a primary ovarian carcinoma.

Transpleural spread occurs in some cases of lung and breast cancer, and in both these examples there may also be pericardial involvement. Secondary tumours in the lung can spread likewise.

A related type of spread is the metastasis of primary cerebral tumours down the subarachnoid space to the spinal theca. Seedlings of this type are characteristic of medulloblastoma, oligodendroglioma, and ependymoma.[14] They may be seen in anaplastic astrocytomata and also in secondary tumours involving the brain.

It is important to note that peritoneal effusions are not confined to malignant tumours. A benign tumour in close proximity to a serous surface can also excite an inflammatory reaction. A good example of this is the ovarian fibroma, which sometimes gives rise to a considerable ascites. If there is also a pleural effusion, the condition is called *Meigs's syndrome* The mechanism of this pleural effusion is still not understood.

An even more spectacular condition is *pseudomyxoma peritonei*, in which a mucus-secreting lesion, usually of the appendix or the ovary, ruptures and discharges its contents into the peritoneal cavity. The secreting cells take root, and secrete large amounts of mucinous material which produces a chronic peritonitis. In most cases the initial lesion is a low-grade adenocarcinoma, but the cells in the peritoneal cavity show no tendency to invade the deeper tissues. If the material is removed and the primary lesion extirpated, life may be preserved for many years.[19]

Spread Along Epithelial-lined Spaces

It is common in papillary tumours of the renal pelvis to find other similar tumours scattered along the ureter and even in the bladder. Likewise it is sometimes noted that a cancer on the lower lip may be associated with a cancer on the opposing upper lip. At one time this was attributed to the transfer of malignant cells from one surface to another. It seems very unlikely that tumour cells can penetrate intact epithelia in this way. Although the possibility of epithelial implantation cannot entirely be excluded, these tumours are best explained as examples of multicentric neoplasia on a preconditioned field of growth (see Chapter 29).

A different type of spread by implantation can occur during an operation on a tumour-bearing area. Clumsy surgical technique may allow the implantation of cancer cells on to the adjacent incised tissues, from which a new tumour may subsequently develop.

STAGING OF MALIGNANT TUMOURS

Staging is an important method of documenting the spread of a tumour, which can then be related to the prognosis.[20] A well-known scheme is that used in breast cancer:

STAGE I Tumour confined to the breast including the skin immediately over it.

STAGE II The tumour involves the axillary lymph nodes on the same side, but both breast and nodes are mobile.

STAGE III Spread to the chest wall or the supraclavicular nodes of the same side.

STAGE IV Further spread than Stage III including blood-borne metastases.

A very important staging of rectal cancer is that devised by Dukes:[21]

STAGE A Tumour confined to the muscular coat of the wall of the rectum.

STAGE B Tumour invading the pararectal tissues, but without lymph-node metastases.

STAGE C Involvement of lymph nodes.

The prognosis after abdomino-perineal resection has been related to the three stages:[22]

STAGE A 80–90 per cent survive for 5 years.

STAGE B 60–70 per cent survive for 5 years.

STAGE C Less than 25 per cent survive for 5 years.

This example shows how the prognosis of a tumour can be predicted by assessing its degree of spread. But it does not necessarily follow that a Stage I tumour is always an "early" one. It might be of long standing, but of such low-grade malignancy that it progresses very slowly and does not metastasise. Likewise a Stage IV tumour is not necessarily a "late" one. It might be one of high-grade malignancy which metastasises widely before it producs a conspicuous local lesion. Though nobody would advocate delay in treating cancer, it must be remembered that the most important factor in the prognosis is the intrinsic malignancy of the tumour. The degree of spread is an external manifestation of this. The good prognosis that follows the resection of a Stage I cancer is probably due more to its low-grade char-

acter than to the speed of detection. If left alone it might remain at this stage for a considerable time, causing the patient little trouble. But, of course, it might also advance to Stages II, III, and IV, and it is this possibility which makes immediate treatment necessary. This consideration is relevant when the results of operative treatment are assessed in relation to the stage of the tumour, especially when radical resections are advocated for Stage I lesions.

Dormant cancer.[23] This is the appearance of metastases many years after the primary tumour has been successfully removed. The phenomenon of dormancy is seen most often in carcinoma of the breast and kidney and malignant melanoma (especially of the uveal tract), when some 10–35 years after the resection of the organ affected the patient may suddenly develop metastases (usually in the bones following breast and kidney carcinoma, and in the liver following uveal melanoma). In these cases there is no local recurrence, and the patient is quite well during the dormant period. The eruption of metastases is usually unheralded, but it sometimes follows a severe intercurrent illness, an operation, or an accident. Psychological trauma is another precipitating factor.

Once the metastases appear they develop rapidly, and if not treated will lead to the patient's death. It is evident that for reasons not yet understood the tumour cells have lain dormant in distant sites. Perhaps the hormonal environment was not suitable or else the patient's immunological state prevented the growth of metastases. At any rate it must be assumed that at a certain time the environment becomes propitious for the growth of tumour cells, and then metastases develop.

The phenomenon of dormancy is obviously of importance when the prognosis of a tumour is being considered. A 5-year survival rate, a fair measure of cure in many types of malignancy treated by radical surgery, is of much less use in the cancers mentioned above. Indeed, no woman who has had a mastectomy for breast cancer can ever be certified as cured;[24] metastases have been known to develop 32 years after resection.[25] The natural history of cancer is still poorly understood, and until it is studied with care and dispassion, many erroneous assumptions will be made about the efficacy of various forms of treatment.

SURGICAL TREATMENT IN RELATION TO SPREAD OF TUMOUR

The surgical treatment of cancer is based on the following time-honoured assumptions:

1. That cancer commences as a local disease and remains so in many cases, even though the tumour has progressed sufficiently to produce clinical signs or symptoms.
2. That the common carcinomata spread first *via* the lymphatics and later by the blood stream.

3. That cure is attained by removing all malignant cells, and that with suitably designed operations this is possible in many cases.

As lymphatic routes of spread were mapped out, so the magnitude of the operations increased. This is well illustrated by the super-radical mastectomy which is practised by some surgeons for cancer of the breast. Another approach to improving the results of treatment was to attempt to detect cancer at an early stage; the earlier the disease is diagnosed and treated the greater should be the chance of cure.

There is now considerable evidence that these views are an oversimplification of the situation.[26] Thus, in cancer of the stomach, some series show that the relationship between the prognosis and the duration of symptoms is the reverse of what would be expected: the longer the history, the greater the survival-rate.[27, 28] In cancer of the breast it has been found that early diagnosis has not appreciably altered the death-rate.[29] Nor are the results of various forms of treatment greatly different. Furthermore, in view of the fact that blood-borne metastases may lie dormant for long periods, it can no longer be accepted as proven that blood spread occurs after lymphatic involvement. All that is known is that lymphatic metastases are usually apparent before those derived from blood-borne emboli. It is evident that in cancer of the breast, occult haematogenous spread presents a hazard which can neither be totally assessed nor guarded against. Bony metastases can now be looked for by radioactive-strontium scan before major surgery is performed in cases of lung and breast cancer.

The factors determining whether a particular tumour will progress or not are its intrinsic malignancy[30] and the host's immunity. Unfortunately, neither can be measured with precision. Histological grading gives some indication of the malignancy of a particular tumour, but is in general unreliable. A lymphocytic infiltration around the tumour is associated with a better prognosis in some instances, e.g. breast and stomach,[31, 32] but in other tumours an admixture of lymphocytes does not appear to be particularly favourable prognostically, e.g. in carcinoma of the pharynx and seminoma. The presence of tumour immunoglobulins has been claimed to indicate immunity in malignant melanoma, but this principle has not been extended to other tumours. Hormonal environment is important in certain tumours. The phenomena of dormancy and spontaneous regression emphasise this defence mechanism.

In cancer of the breast the phenomenon of dormancy indicates that the seeds of the secondary deposits were already sown at the time of operation, and that, in this event, radical surgery can offer no more in terms of survival than less mutilating procedures designed to remove the local tumour, including its field of growth. It is not known how frequent "occult metastases" are when the patient is first seen, nor is it known what forces hold them in check. Until this information is available, therapy can be based only on information obtained by observing the results of different forms of treatment. Unfortunately there are so many variables to consider in assessing these results that no satisfactory conclusion can yet be reached.[35] Commonly a course of treatment which appears to be superior to another in one centre is found by others to offer no advantage.[33, 34]

The treatment of many cancers is based largely on the concepts derived from the study of breast cancer. It is apparent that the subject of surgery in relation to the treatment of malignant disease needs a fresh appraisal.

GENERAL READING

WILLIS, R. A. (1952). *The Spread of Tumours in the Human Body*, 2nd edn, 447p. London: Butterworths.

REFERENCES

1. Leading Article (1971). *British Medical Journal*, iv, 641.
2. PRYCE, D. M. and WALTER, J. B. (1960). *Journal of Pathology and Bacteriology*, **79**, 141.
3. NEDELKOFF, B., CHRISTOPHERSON, W. M. and HARTER, J. S. (1962). *Acta Cytologica (Philadelphia)*, **6**, 319.
4. FLEMING, J. A. (1963). *Proceedings of the Royal Society Medicine*, **56**, 497.
5. GOLDBLATT, S. A. and NADEL, E. M. (1963). In *Cancer, Progress Volume 1963*, pp. 119–40. Edited by R. W. Raven. London: Butterworths.
6. Leading Article (1967). *Lancet*, ii, 84.
7. SKELTON, M. O. (1959). *Journal of Clinical Pathology*, **12**, 70.
8. DRURY, R. A. B., PALMER, P. H. and HIGHMAN, W. J. (1964). *Journal of Clinical Pathology*, **17**, 448.
9. WILLIS, R. A. (1941). *Medical Journal of Australia*, **2**, 258.
10. HANSEN, H. H., MUGGIA, F. M. and SELAWRY, O. S. (1971). *Lancet*, ii, 443.
11. FRANSSILA, K. (1971). *Acta Pathologica et Microbiologica Scandinavia*, A, Supplement No. 225.
12. BATSON, O. V. (1942). *Annals of Internal Medicine*, **16**, 38.
13. RUSSELL, D. S. and RUBINSTEIN, L. J. (1963). *Pathology of Tumours of the Nervous System*, 2nd edn, pp. 216–220. London: Arnold.
14. EADE, O. E. and URICH, H. (1971). *Journal of Pathology*, **103**, 245.
15. STORSTEIN, O. (1951). *Circulation*, **4**, 913.
16. PROBERT, W. R. (1956). *British Medical Journal*, i, 435.
17. MASSON, A. H. B. and BRANWOOD, A. W. (1955). *British Medical Journal*, i, 1514.
18. DeLAND, F. H. and BENNETT, W. A. (1957). *Archives of Pathology*, 63, 13.

19. LITTLE, J. M., HALLIDAY, J. P. and GLENN, D. C. (1969). *Lancet*, ii, 659.
20. HARMER, M. (1958). In *Cancer*, Volume 4, p. 1, and *Cancer Progress* (1960) p. 128. Edited by R. W. Raven. London: Butterworths.
21. DUKES, C. E. (1940). *Journal of Pathology and Bacteriology*, **50,** 527.
22. DUKES, C. E. (1958). In *Cancer*, Volume 2, p. 136. Edited by R. W. Raven. London: Butterworths.
23. HADFIELD, G. (1954). *British Medical Journal*, ii, 607.
24. TRUSCOTT, B. M. (1947). *British Journal of Cancer*, **1,** 129.
25. GORDON-TAYLOR, G. (1959). *British Medical Journal*, i, 455.
26. Leading Article (1954). *Lancet*, i, 714.
27. SWYNNERTON, B. F. and TRUELOVE, S. C. (1952). *British Medical Journal*, i, 287.
28. SHAHON, D. B., HOROWITZ, S. and KELLY, W. D. (1956). *Surgery*, **39,** 204.
29. McKINNON, N. E. (1954). *Lancet*, i, 251.
30. BLOOM, H. J. G. (1965). *British Journal of Cancer*, **19,** 228.
31. PAILE, A. (1971). *Annales chirurgiae et gynaecologiae Fenniae*, **60,** Supplement No. 175.
32. Leading Article (1971). *British Medical Journal*, iv, 67.
33. ATKINS, H. J. B. *et al.* (1960). *Lancet*, i, 1148
34. MACDONALD, I. (1962). *Surgery, Gynecology and Obstetrics*, **115,** 215.
35. Leading Article (1972). *British Medical Journal*, ii, 417

Chapter 29. The Aetiology and Incidence of Tumours

Research into the aetiology of cancer has both a clinical and an experimental approach. It has been recognised for a long time that some types of malignancy are particularly common in certain occupations, while on a more individual level, certain families have been known to bear the trait of rare neoplastic diseases. More recently it has been noted that local environmental factors predispose large groups of people to the risk of cancer. Now that medicine is moving from the field of treatment to that of prevention, social and industrial medicine are assuming ever-increasing importance in cancer prophylaxis. The result has been the recognition of many exogenous carcinogenic agents. Furthermore, precancerous lesions are being detected with greater frequency.

The experimental side of cancer research concerns the artificial production of tumours in animals. At first only substances carcinogenic to man were used, but now their range is much greater than this. They include innumerable chemical agents, radiations of various types, hormones, and viruses. The object of this work is to elucidate the nature of the change that heralds malignancy in a cell. Furthermore, it is hoped that the results may eventually be applied to human beings, in respect of the prevention not only of occupational and environmental tumours but also those which seem to bear no relationship to these factors.

THE ORIGIN OF TUMOURS

The mode of origin of a tumour is still not completely understood. An early theory introduced by Cohnheim in 1875 was that tumours arose from "cell rests" sequestrated during embryonic life, which underwent neoplastic change many years later. While this theory may explain the development of the embryonic tumours of infancy, there is no evidence that the common adult tumours arise from cell rests, the very existence of which has not been proved.

At present the two rival theories of tumour development are that the neoplasm derives from a *single cell* that undergoes a change, and that a whole area of tissue becomes predisposed to neoplasia; such an area is called a *field of growth*. The best example of the first type of development is the group of monoclonal gammopathies that are described in Chapter 45. In multiple myeloma, for example, it appears that one clone of plasma cells becomes malignant, and by metastatic spread as well as local proliferation crowds out the many normal clones of immunoglobulin-forming cells. These neoplastic cells produce only one type of immunoglobluin and so can be easily identified. It is possible that the lymphomata and the tumours of haematopoietic tissue develop similarly.

The field of growth theory is based on the frequent tendency for multiple tumours to arise on a restricted area of tissue, and also for apparently recurrent tumours to develop near the site of removal of a primary tumour. It is exceptional for a whole field of tissue to undergo neoplastic

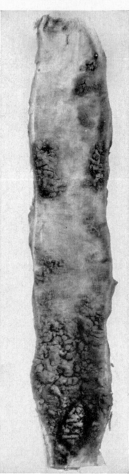

Figure 29.1

Multiple papillomata of the ureter. The ureter shows extensive areas of sessile papillomata. This is a good example of multiple tumours on a field of growth. (U 49.2, *Reproduced by permission of the President and Council of R.C.S. Eng.)*

change; much more usually there are circumscribed foci of change in it, presumably arising from a change in the cells, or even a cell, in each focus. There are numerous examples of *multiple primary tumours* arising in a particular field:

(*a*) Transitional-cell tumours of the urinary tract, from the pelvis and ureter to the bladder (Fig. 29.1).

(*b*) Polyposis coli (see p. 380). In ulcerative colitis multiple malignancy is also the rule.

(*c*) Squamous-cell and basal-cell carcinomata of the skin in those exposed to sunlight and in xeroderma pigmentosum.

(*d*) Uterine leiomyomata.

(*e*) Breast cancer is bilateral in about 9 per cent of cases. Sometimes there are multiple fibro-adenomata of the breast.

(*f*) Hepatoma developing on cirrhosis of the liver is often multicentric.

(*g*) Sometimes there is widespread malignancy in an expanse of epithelium with a common embryological derivation, e.g. carcinoma involving the gall-bladder, bile ducts (intrahepatic as well as extrahepatic), and pancreatic ducts in a continuous wave. Another example is cloacogenic cancer[1], in which multiple tumours arise in epithelium that derived from the primitive cloaca, e.g. vagina, vulva, and anus.

The origin of some types of *recurrence* can also be explained in terms of a preconditioned field of growth. Thus it is not uncommon to find an area of early basal-cell or squamous-cell carcinomatous change close to an excised rodent ulcer or squamous-cell cancer of the skin or mouth, as the case may be, but separated from it by a variable extent of healthy epidermis. (Fig. 29.2). It is such unnoticed areas of early neoplasia that probably provide the basis for a later recurrence, but, of course, some recurrences are due to an inadequate resection of the primary tumour. Whatever the origin of local recurrences, there is no doubt that the field is better removed at the time of resection of the tumour. This is often impossible, as in the case of cancer of the exposed areas of skin, but in such a localised area as a burn or varicose ulcer from which a carcinoma has arisen, that whole site must be excised, if the tumour is not to recur. This may necessitate an amputation. The pleomorphic salivary tumour also tends to recur after enucleation, but whether this is due to local infiltration or to seedling tumours in the capsule is undecided. The right treatment is subtotal parotidectomy.

Factors Producing a Field of Growth

If one accepts that much neoplasia develops in an area of tissue which has been previously conditioned, one must consider the factors responsible for this malevolent predisposition. This is in fact the *precancerous state*. A field of growth may bear a recognisable lesion, but often it appears completely healthy until at some stage of the individual's life a succession of tumours arise on it.

Most cancers in adults arise spontaneously in response to an unknown stimulus, but a few can be attributed with

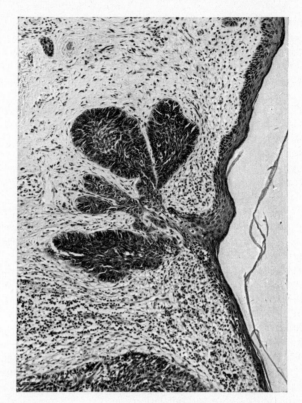

Figure 29.2
Multifocal origin of basal-cell carcinoma. The mode of origin of the tumour as a downgrowth from the basal-cell layer is apparent, and its resemblance to an embryonic hair follicle is quite marked. The surrounding epidermis is normal, but at the edge of the section there is part of a much larger basal-cell carcinoma. × 100.

certainty to some tangible preceding cause. The three factors generally recognised as causes of human neoplasia are:

Extrinsic physical and chemical agents.
Hereditary predisposition.
Chronic disease, usually of an inflammatory nature.

Two additional factors have to be considered: *hormones* and *viruses*.

EXTRINSIC CARCINOGENIC AGENTS[2, 3]

These can be divided into chemical and physical carcinogens.

Chemical

The first chemical agents to be incriminated in human cancer were derived from soot, coal tar, and mineral oils. The first occupational cancer to be carefully documented was *chimney-sweep's cancer* of the scrotum which was described by Percivall Pott in 1775. Later on the high temperature destructive distillation of coal yielded coal tar, which produced cancer of the skin of the head, neck, and arms of exposed workers. The crude distillation products of mineral oils, particularly shale-oil mined in Scotland, led to *shale-oil cancer* of the hands and arms. When this oil was used as a lubricant in the Lancashire cotton-spinning industry, *mule-spinner's cancer** of the abdominal wall and scrotum occurred due to seepage of the splashed oil through the workers' clothing. Scrotal cancer[4] also occurs in road workers and coal-gas and coke makers, who are exposed to coal tar, and in automatic lathe operators and chain makers, whose clothes may be penetrated by the low-viscosity cutting oils used in these trades. Manufacturers of coal-tar dyes may be similarly endangered. All these types of cancer are due to certain polycyclic aromatic hydrocarbons which have been the source of much experimental work.

In 1895 bladder cancer was first described amongst manufacturers of synthetic dyestuffs, and it was subsequently discovered that certain aromatic amines were responsible.

It was also found that workers using arsenic were prone to develop cancers of the skin of the limbs and face. This follows the ingestion of the arsenic, and people who took the inorganic form of the metal medicinally as Fowler's solution have been similarly endangered. Furthermore there is evidence that it may cause lung cancer.[5]

Cancer of the lung is also seen in those whose occupation brings them into contact with hot tar fumes, chromium, nickel, and asbestos, all of which presumably produce a local reaction following inhalation.

A recently discovered occupational hazard is adenocarcinoma of the nasal sinuses occurring in woodworkers in the furniture industry.[6] This incidence has reached a considerable height in the High Wycombe area of Buckinghamshire. Apparently it is the inhaled dust that contains the carcinogenic factor, but its nature is obscure.

Physical

The important physical agents associated with neoplasia are ionising and ultraviolet radiations.

The relationship between *ionising radiations* and cancer is considered in detail in Chapter 31. It will suffice at this stage to note that pioneer x-ray workers, radiotherapists, patients who have been treated with radioactive materials or x-rays, and the victims of nuclear fall-out have all developed malignant conditions.

Ultraviolet radiations exert their harmful effects in the strong sunlight continually acting on the exposed skin of fair-complexioned people. Farmers in Australia and South Africa, sailors, and others habitually exposed to the elements tend in later life to develop keratotic papillomata on their faces and hands (senile, actinic, or solar keratoses), and these may develop into multiple squamous-cell carcinomata. Basal-cell cancers are also frequently encountered in this group of people. Cancer of the lip, typically seen in elderly agricultural workers, is probably also related to prolonged

* A "mule" is a spinning machine used in the Lancashire cotton industry.

exposure of the face to sunlight. Exposure to sunlight also predisposes to malignant melanoma.

It is questionable whether *thermal radiation* acting alone is ever adequate to produce neoplasia. It probably acts as a "promoter" of cancer in an area that has already been "initiated" by carcinogenic agents like ultraviolet light or the tar products from burning coals or tobacco. This would account for the increased incidence of lip cancer in pipe-smokers, and also for the cancers of the abdominal skin seen in the Kangri basket-carriers.

The latent period. An important factor notable in all the occupational and environmental cancers mentioned above is the long latent period that elapses from the time of application of the agent to the time of first appearance of the neoplasm. It varied from about 20 years in chimney-sweeps and 10 years in pioneer x-ray workers to about 5 years in those developing leukaemia as the result of whole-body irradiation. There is ample time for the initiating stimulus to be completely forgotten by the patient. This is of great importance both in research work and in the question of the workman's compensation.

Experimental Carcinogenesis

This is best considered in the light of occupational cancer. Carcinogenic substances are given to animals in order to produce tumours, but two basic pitfalls must be remembered.

Firstly, there is a tendency for many animals to develop spontaneous tumours. Of the laboratory animals mice tend to develop tumours of the breast, lungs, and lymphoid tissue, whereas rats are prone to mammary fibro-adenomata, bone and skin sarcoma, lymphocytic lymphoma, and thymic tumours. The tumour incidence in mice may vary according to the strain: C_3H mice have a high incidence of breast cancer but a low one of leukaemia, whereas Ak mice have a high leukaemia incidence but seldom get breast cancer.

Secondly, animals react specifically to carcinogenic stimuli. Many fruitless years were spent trying to induce coal-tar cancers in rats and dogs, animals which are almost completely resistant. Likewise β-naphthylamine induces bladder tumours in dogs and man, but is without effect in rats and rabbits. The necessity for the most scrupulous controls in animal experiments is obvious. It is interesting in this respect that arsenic is carcinogenic only to man.

The most important chemicals employed in experimental work are the *polycyclic hydrocarbons* responsible for soot, tar, and oil-induced tumours, the *aromatic amines* used in the aniline-dye industry, and the *azo-compounds* which are used to colour foods.

The aromatic polycyclic hydrocarbons. Credit is due to the Japanese workers Yamagiwa and Ichikawa who, in the second decade of this century, first produced skin cancers in rabbits by painting their ears with tar. It was then found that mice were also susceptible to such treatment.

The next step was the isolation of the actual substances in

the tar which were responsible for carcinogenesis. It was found that these were present in the higher-boiling fractions obtained during distillation, and that the fluorescent spectra of these fractions resembled that of the polycyclic hydrocarbon 1 : 2 benzanthracene.

This substance itself is only feebly carcinogenic, but Kennaway experimented with allied hydrocarbons, and found that *1 : 2 : 5 : 6-dibenzanthracene* was powerfully carcinogenic. This discovery in 1930 is of historical importance, as it was the first of a long list of chemical carcinogens to be isolated in a pure form. In fact it is not an actual constituent of tar.

Since then many more potent hydrocarbon carcinogens have been isolated,[7] the most important of which are *9 : 10-dimethyl-1 : 2-benzanthracene*, the most powerful of them all; *methylcholanthrene*, which is related chemically to the bile acids; and **3 : 4 benzpyrene**, which is certainly the most important carcinogenic constituent of coal tar and the most significant hydrocarbon carcinogen to man. The following structural formulae indicate how the carcinogenic potency of these polycyclic hydrocarbons is increased by substitution groups at the positions 10, 9, 6, and 5 of the benzanthracene complex.

substances are workers in the aniline-dye industry. More recently bladder tumours have been noted unusually frequently in those working in the rubber and cable industries.[9] This has been attributed to the addition of an antioxidant to the rubber to prevent it perishing. Before 1949 this antioxidant contained a trace of β-naphthylamine, so that workers with rubber and cables (which contain rubber) exposed before that date are endangered.

Bladder tumours can also be produced in dogs fed on β-naphthylamine, yet the local application of this substance to a dog's bladder mucosa produces no effect. An intermediary metabolic product, *2-amino-1-naphthol*, is the carcinogenic agent. It is produced in the liver, where it is at once detoxified by conjugation with glucuronic acid. The resulting 2-amino-1-naphthyl glucuronide is harmless when excreted in the urine, but unforunately the bladder mucosa of human beings and dogs secretes the enzyme β-glucuronidase which splits the compound and releases free carcinogen. Saccharolactone inhibits this enzyme, and can protect dogs against bladder cancer. It has also been used in exposed workers. Induction of bladder tumours by the aromatic amines is a good example of *remote carcinogenesis*, for the agent is taken by mouth yet produces its effects on the bladder.

1:2-BENZANTHRACENE

1:2:5:6-DIBENZANTHRACENE

9:10-DIMETHYL-1:2-
BENZANTHRACENE

3:4-BENZPYRENE

METHYLCHOLANTHRENE

The tumours these hydrocarbons produce generally appear at the site of application of the agent. Squamous-cell carcinoma follows application to the skin, while subcutaneous injections induce sarcoma formation. It has been found, however, that the agents may also be absorbed, and produce neoplasms in sites remote from the area of application. Tumours of the lung have followed surface applications of these agents in mice. It is also noteworthy that pure polycyclic hydrocarbons have a much more extensive species range than crude coal tar; dogs, rats, and even guinea-pigs may develop tumours after exposure.

The aromatic amines.[8] The important carcinogens of this category are *α-naphthylamine*, *β-naphthylamine*, and *benzidine*, and those most likely to come in contact with these

It may be that intermediary aminophenol substances produced during the metabolism of tryptophane are of importance in the aetiology of spontaneously occurring bladder tumours.[8]

Another important aromatic amine that has been used extensively in experimental work is *2-acetylaminofluorene*,[10] which was nearly marketed as an insecticide. Fortunately its powerful carcinogenic activity was discovered in time. It too is a remote carcinogen, but unlike the naphthylamines it produces a wide range of cancers in different animals. Tumours of the liver, breast, lung, bladder, and intestines are produced in mice, rats, dogs, and rabbits, and a rather surprising addition is carcinoma of the external auditory meatus. Once again some unidentified intermediary product apparently produces tumours at its sites of excretion. The structural formulae of some of these chemicals are given below.

great potency and closely related in intermediate metabolism to cycasin.

2−NAPHTHYLAMINE

2−AMINO−1−NAPHTHOL

2−AMINO−1−NAPHTHYL GLUCURONIDE

BENZIDINE

2−ACETYLAMINOFLUORENE

The azo-compounds.[11] Azo-dyes like *scarlet red* (which contains in its molecule 2′ : 3-dimethyl-4-aminoazobenzene) and *butter yellow* (4-dimethylaminoazobenzene), when fed to rats, produce different varieties of liver tumours, e.g. hepatomata and cholangiomata, usually without the supervention of previous necrosis or cirrhosis. Mice are much less susceptible. This is yet another example of remote carcinogenesis. Azo-dye carcinogenesis is greatly facilitated by a diet deficient in riboflavin. Some of these azo-compounds have been used commercially as dyes for leather and in foodstuffs, but there is no definite evidence that human cancer has been caused by these compounds.

IMMUNOLOGICAL ASPECTS OF CARCINOGENESIS[14–16]

Tumours can differ antigenically from their host and therefore may excite an immune response.

Loss of antigen. Some tumours lose tissue-specific antigens because of their poor differentiation, but the transplantation antigens are retained.

Development of new antigen. The development of new transplantation antigens on the surface of tumour cells is an important feature of neoplasia. In virus-induced tumours the new antigen is a tumour-specific transplanta-

Butter yellow
4−DIMETHYLAMINOAZOBENZENE

Scarlet red

CARCINOGENS OF NATURAL ORIGIN[12]

Certain natural foodstuffs also carry a carcinogenic hazard, indicating that a return to a "natural" way of living advocated by enthusiasts need not necessarily eliminate cancer. Two important carcinogens are:

Aflatoxin. This is the toxic principle of the mould *Aspergillus flaveus* which may contaminate foodstuffs such as ground-nut meal. Aflatoxin is a powerful liver carcinogen, and it may well be that some of the human liver cancer so prevalent in Africa and elsewhere is due to it rather than to the effects of malnutrition.

Cycasin. This is a glycoside isolated from a palm-like tree *Cycas circinalis*, which grows in certain areas of the Far East. Cycasin is a general carcinogen producing neoplasms at various sites in different animals; liver cancer is frequently produced.

Both aflatoxin and cycasin act by interference with DNA synthesis, an effect they share in common with the **nitrosamines,**[13] a recently discovered chemical carcinogen of

tion antigen, and is the same in all tumours produced by the particular virus. It is quite distinct from the antigens of the mature virions. In carcinogen-induced tumours the new transplantation antigen is weak and is individual for the particular tumour; it is different from antigens present in other tumours produced by the particular carcinogen.[17, 18] Radiation-induced tumours likewise are individual.

Tumours may also produce antigens which are not transplantation antigens. Thus distinctive antigens have been found with some human tumours, e.g. the Burkitt tumour antigen and the carcino-embryonic antigen (see p. 379). Specific antiviral antibodies are found in animal virus-induced tumours.

The effects of antigenic difference between host and its tumour may be immunological or non-immunological.

IMMUNOLOGICAL EFFECTS

Immunoglobulin formation may be associated with enhancement of tumour growth or tumour rejection. Immune cells can cause tumour destruction. Finally there may be no antibody production due to the induction of tolerance.

In animal tumours transplanted to genetically non-identical recipients there is a homograft reaction and the tumour is promptly rejected, unless a privileged site is used.

It is noteworthy that immunologically tolerant animals, for example newborn mice, and especially those that are thymectomised, develop most virus-induced tumours much more rapidly than do adult animals. An exception is the group of oncogenic viruses that proliferate in the lymphocyte before causing tumour formation, e.g. the Bittner factor and the mouse leukaemia virus, in which neonatal thymectomy decreases the incidence of tumours by causing severe lymphocytic depletion.

The part played by the immune response in the restraint and rejection of human tumours is much less certain, although the graft rejection phenomenon is explained teleologically as a homeostatic mechanism devised to recognise and destroy aberrant mutant cells that develop transplantation antigens unnatural to the individual. This function is called *immunological surveillance*. The findings supporting an immunological restraint on tumours are:

(*a*) The increased incidence of tumours in the immunological deficiency syndromes (see p. 171) and after immunosuppression for homografts. Most of these tumours are lymphomata.

(*b*) The heavy lymphocytic infiltration around tumours of low-grade malignancy. Indeed, the evidence points to the great importance of cell-mediated immunity in solid tumours, and lymphocytes from such patients are destructive to tumour cells grown in tissue culture.

(*c*) Circulating immunoglobulins have been demonstrated against some tumours. The difficulty here lies in the assessment of the specificity of the tumour antigen; as yet none has been proved to be specific for the tumour. One antigen that has aroused much attention is found in some colonic carcinoma cells. Both antigen and corresponding antibody have been found in patients' serum. Though the antigen is not found in normal intestinal epithelium, it is present in fetal tissues, and has therefore been called *carcino-embryonic antigen (CEA)*.[19, 20, 135] It is present in the sera of pregnant women as well as in many patients with primary gastro-intestinal tumours. Smaller amounts of CEA are found in sera of patients with other tumours and occasionally in non-neoplastic diseases. Some other fetal antigens have been reported in human tumours, but these too are non-specific. It would seem that the numerous antibodies to tumours that patients may have in their sera are autoantibodies to normal adult or fetal components that are exposed or are in greater concentration than in normal tissue.

The antibodies probably play no part in the control of tumour growth. Nevertheless, since both antibody and antigen (e.g. CEA) can be present in the blood, it is possible that antigen-antibody complexes can lead to a type of immune-complex disease.[21] This may be the explanation of weight loss, fever, raised ESR, nephrotic syndrome, arthralgia, skin eruptions, and other obscure features of human malignant disease.

There are, however, a few tumours in which immunological mechanisms do appear to be very important.[22, 23] In Burkitt's tumour autoantibodies to the tumour cells are invariable, and they appear to react against antigens associated with the EB virus (see p. 385). In this tumour many apparently permanent cures have followed the administration of totally inadequate doses (even one) of cyclophosphamide. It would seem that when the main bulk of the tumour is killed, the immunoglobulins can destroy the remainder. A similar situation may occur in chorio-carcinoma treated with methotrexate. Specific anti-tumour immunoglobulins are found in the early stages of malignant melanoma, but these tend to disappear as the tumour metastasises.[24]

It should be noted that some immunoglobulins formed against tumours actually enhance the growth of the neoplasm, presumably by inhibiting the immune response in its afferent arc or preventing cytotoxic antibody (whether immunoglobulin or lymphocyte) acting in the efferent arc (see p. 152). Thus at least two types of immunoglobulin are produced: a deleterious enhancing one and a beneficial cytotoxic one that activates complement. Perhaps there is also an unblocking antibody to reverse the enhancement of the first immunoglobulin mentioned. Serum from patients who have recovered from malignant melanoma and hypernephroma has occasionally helped other victims of these tumours.

There is evidence in both animal and human tumour victims that cell-mediated immunity develops against specific tumour antigens. The lymphocytotoxic effect can be blocked by serum factors—probably complexes of tumour antigen and immunoglobulin.[136] Unblocking antibodies have also been identified.[137]

The status of immunotherapy is slight at present. It is agreed that the bulk of the tumour must first be destroyed by conventional methods, so that only a small residuum of tumour cells is left.[138] Non-specific stimulation of the RE system with BCG is worth trying. Mathé has combined this with immunisation using irradiated leukaemic cells, and has achieved noteworthy remissions in acute leukaemia (he already used conventional treatment on these patients). Specifically stimulated lymphoid cells are not very satisfactory, and the casual use of antisera may well enhance the growth rather than destroy it.

NON-IMMUNOLOGICAL MECHANISM IN TUMOUR CONTROL[25, 26]

If allogeneic cells are made to grow in close proximity to each other in tissue culture, each type of cell inhibits the growth of the other. This is called *allogeneic inhibition*, and appears not to be immunological because the phenomenon can be demonstrated using immunologically incompetent cells. Tumour cells which lack antigens can be shown to be at a disadvantage when in company with normal cells. This can be demonstrated by injecting tumour cells into a histo-compatible host and *in vitro*. The inhibitory effect can be swamped if a large inoculum is used. The reaction seems to be well adapted to the destruction of small groups of tumour cells.

HEREDITARY PREDISPOSITION[27]

There is little significant hereditary predisposition to most of the common types of cancer, and statistical surveys amongst relations of cancer patients have not yielded convincing evidence of an increased incidence of tumours in them. Cancer of the breast, however, is somewhat commoner in the relatives of affected women than in the population at large.

There are nevertheless a number of uncommon neoplastic diseases which are inherited, and the affected tissue could be considered a field of growth predisposed to cancer from the time of its conception, though the lethal tendency may manifest itself only in adult life.

The three important examples of such a tendency are polyposis coli, xeroderma pigmentosum, and retinoblastoma (see p. 350).

The trait of *polyposis coli* is transmitted as an autosomal dominant.[28] The condition is not present at birth, but usually first manifests itself at puberty with the passage of blood and mucus in the faeces. The colon and rectum are studded with innumerable adenomata (Fig. 29.3), and by about the age of thirty years multiple carcinomata develop. Total resection of colon and rectum will alone ensure cure. In a related condition, *Gardner's syndrome*, colonic polyposis is found in association with sebaceous cysts, osteomata of the face and skull, desmoid tumours, and multiple fibromata. This too is inherited as a dominant trait and terminates in colonic cancer.[29]

Xeroderma pigmentosum is inherited as an autosomal recessive trait.[30] In this condition the skin is abnormally susceptible to the effects of sunlight. Within the first few years of life exposed areas show blotchy pigmentation which is followed by atrophy of the skin and telangiectasia. Multiple basal-cell and squamous-cell carcinomata then develop, and unless the patient is protected from sunlight by covering up all the exposed parts, death occurs within the first decade.

Figure 29.3
Polyposis coli. These are portions of the descending colon and rectum resected from a patient with polyposis coli. The mucosa is studded with innumerable polyps, some of which are pedunculated and others sessile. There is no evidence of carcinomatous change in any of the polyps. (A 74.4, *Reproduced by permission of the President and Council of the R.C.S. Eng.)*

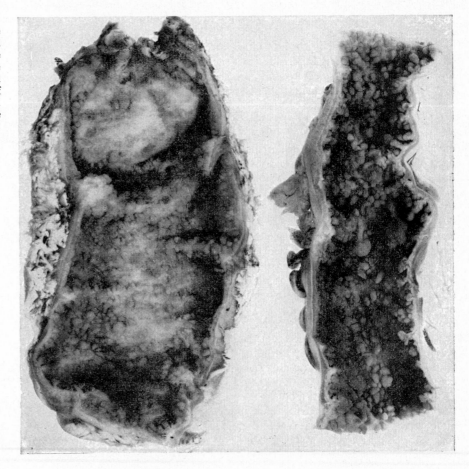

The mechanism of xeroderma pigmentosum has now been elucidated.[31] Ultraviolet light gives rise to dimer formation between neighbouring thymidine radicles in DNA, and when such DNA replicates, the dimer causes a mutation. In normal cells there are enzymes that can cut out the dimer and replace it by the correct nitrogen bases. In xeroderma pigmentosum one such enzyme is lacking, and the disease is an inborn error of metabolism. This mechanism also explains actinic skin cancer; without DNA-repairing enzymes the frequency of skin cancer among fair-skinned people would be extremely high even in youth.

Some varieties of basal–cell carcinoma also show a hereditary pattern. In the *naevoid basal-cell carcinoma syndrome*[32] multiple carcinomata occur on the exposed parts at a very early age, and there is often an association with cysts of the jaws, malformations of the skull, spine, ribs, and extremities, and calcification of the falx cerebri. The condition is inherited as an autosomal dominant trait, as are also two adnexal skin tumours (in some patients). These are the *trichoepithelioma* and the *cylindroma*. Multiple tumours are present, on the face with trichoepithelioma and on the scalp with cylindroma (turban tumour).[33] Both tumours may occur in the same patient. Hereditary aspects of *malignant melanoma* and *multiple endocrine adenomatosis* are mentioned on pp. 357 and 324.

CANCER FOLLOWING CHRONIC DISEASE

Virchow believed that cancer was the result of prolonged stimulation of the tissues through "chronic irritation". The concept of chronic irritation is too vague now that a large number of specific carcinogenic agents have been isolated. It is doubtful whether physical irritation acting alone can ever produce cancer, though it may certainly "promote" a tumour in a field already "initiated" by a carcinogenic substance. Corns on the toes of those who wear ill-fitting shoes and callosities on the fingers of string instrumentalists do not become malignant, nor does cancer tend to supervene on a hyperplasia of a gum subjected to the friction of a jagged tooth or an ill-fitting denture. These are true examples of hyperplasia of protective epithelium in response to trauma, and once the stimulus is removed, regression may be expected. Nevertheless, there are a number of chronic diseases which may from time to time be complicated by malignancy, and these must be included in the list of precancerous lesions.

Chronic Inflammatory Conditions of Surface Epithelia

Chronic varicose ulcers, the sinuses of chronic osteomyelitis particularly of the tibia, and *old burn scars* occasionally give rise to squamous-cell cancers. These are nowadays collectively called *Marjolin's ulcer*, though the name should properly be reserved for cancer developing in a chronic leg ulcer. *Tropical ulcers* (non-specific chronic skin ulcers found in Africans, the cause of which is obscure) may also

become malignant. The degree of malignancy in Marjolin's ulcer is greater than in the actinic skin cancers[34] (Fig. 29.4).

Tertiary syphilis of the mouth was said to have been frequently complicated by leucoplakia and carcinoma, but there may have been other factors acting also.

Gastric ulcers may occasionally be the site of origin of cancer of the stomach. Probably less than 4 per cent of ulcers are complicated by cancer,[35] and only 6 per cent of cancers

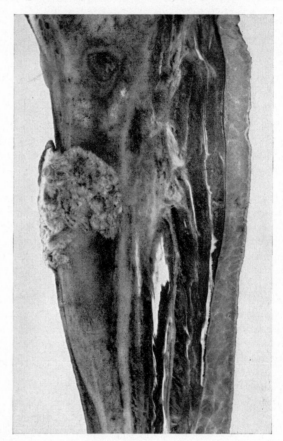

Figure 29.4
Carcinoma of chronic osteomyelitis sinus. There is chronic osteomyelitis of the upper part of the tibia; the bone is sclerotic, and there is an abscess cavity in its neck. At the site of a sinus there is an extensive squamous-cell carcinoma, which has infiltrated completely through the shaft of the bone. (I 19.10, *Reproduction by permission of the President and Council of the R.C.S. Eng.*)

arise in pre-existing ulcers,[36] and the opinion generally held is that there is no significant causal relationship between the two. Duodenal ulcers are never complicated by cancer, which is in keeping with the mysterious resistance of the duodenum to carcinoma, except when involved in neoplasia of the ampulla of Vater.

Ulcerative colitis is an important precancerous condition.[37] About 4 per cent of all cases undergo neoplasia, but it is those with repeated relapses that are most at risk; at least a third of all cases lasting 12 years develop cancer, usually multifocally.

The incidence is greatest when the disease starts before the age of 25 years and when the entire large bowel is affected.

Gall-stones are found in about three-quarters of cases of cancer of the gall-bladder.[38, 39] Nevertheless, carcinoma is a rare complication of this very common condition.

Cancer of the renal pelvis is occasionally associated with calculi, but these may have arisen secondarily to the tumour.

Schistosomiasis may be a predisposing factor to bladder cancer in areas of heavy infestation, e.g. Egypt, for the age incidence is lower than usual and the lesion is nearly always squamous-celled and not transitional-celled. Nevertheless the association is not proven, for there is still no evidence of a higher incidence of bladder cancer in Egypt than elsewhere.[40]

Metabolic and Deficiency Disease

About 90 per cent of primary liver-cell cancer in man is superimposed on a previous cirrhosis; in the bile-duct type of liver cancer the figure is only 25 per cent.[41] Liver-cell cancer is prevalent in African races in whom there is usually a preceding cirrhosis considered nutritional in origin, though the possibility of aflatoxin is now being suggested as an alternative. The incidence of liver cancer is very much less in American Negroes, proving that exogenous factors rather than racial constitution are important in causing the disease. Europeans with cirrhosis likewise have a high incidence of liver cancer; the fine, "Morocco-leather" cirrhosis of haemochromatosis is complicated by cancer in at least 10 per cent of cases.[42]

Thyroid cancer is traditionally associated with the goitre of iodine definciency, and it was common in Switzerland, where goitre was very rife; a survey in the USA revealed a higher incidence in a goitre-belt than elsewhere.[43, 44] Nevertheless, the current view is that cancer arises independently of previous thyroid disease. Though found in goitrous glands, it occurs more frequently in glands that are otherwise normal.[45] Indeed, considering the frequency of goitre, cancer is a rare complication. Furthermore, it is possible that in some cases the tumour lay latent and masqueraded as a nodular goitre.

Post-cricoid carinoma may be associated with an iron-deficiency anaemia, characteristically in middle-aged women, in whom there is also glossitis and dysphagia. This is the *Plummer-Vinson syndrome.** The pathological basis is obscure: atrophic changes in the mucosa and underlying muscle of the mouth and pharynx are described, with later web formation and strictures. Malignancy commonly ensues.[46]

In Paget's disease of bone osteosarcoma is an occasional complication, occurring in about 1 per cent of cases. More rarely a giant-cell tumour develops.

Chronic lymphatic oedema is occasionally complicated by an angiosarcoma of the skin (see p. 354).

---

* This syndrome was first described in 1906 by Paterson, and soon afterwards by Kelly; both were laryngologists. It should rightly be called the Paterson-Kelly syndrome.

Harmartomatous Malformations

There are a number of localised and generalised hamartomatous lesions which occasionally become malignant (see Chapter 27). A congenitally abnormal organ, e.g. an imperfectly descended testis, is more liable to malignacy than a normal one.

Benign Tumours

There is no doubt that an apparently benign tumour, e.g. a uterine myoma or a bladder papilloma, which has been quiescent may suddenly assume malignant potentialities. The question arises whether the tumour was malignant from the start, but in a latent phase, or whether there is indeed true malignant transformation. At present there is no definite solution to this problem.

HORMONES AND NEOPLASIA

The relationship between hormones and neoplasia has become greatly clarified in recent years.[47, 48]

Earlier workers had noted that ovariectomised mice seldom developed breast cancer, and in 1932 Lacassagne successfully produced mammary cancers in mice of both sexes by administering large doses of *oestrogen*. This was hailed as an epoch-making discovery, as it was the first example of neoplasia due to an endogenous agent, which incidentally was closely related to the carcinogenic hydrocarbons in its chemical structure.

Since then it has been discovered that mice can be divided into low-cancer and high-cancer strains. The latter develop cancer of the breast at a comparatively early age due to the presence of a virus first described by Bittner in 1936, and called the *milk factor*. It is transmitted to the young in the mother's milk, and is not effective after the first few days of life. If the suckling mice are fed by foster-mothers of a low-cancer strain, they do not become infected with the tumour-inducing virus, and do not develop cancer. It is in mice of a high-cancer strain that oestrogen induces mammary tumours while in low-cancer strains cystic hyperplasia of the breast alone ensues. Conversely, castration serves to decrease the liability of a high-cancer strain mouse to mammary neoplasia. The hormone merely "promotes" a tumour in a breast already "initiated" by a tumour virus. Certain polycyclic hydrocarbons can similarly initiate a mouse's breast to malignancy, which may then be promoted by oestrogen.

Large doses of oestrogen in mice also lead to hyperplasia of the endometrium, interstitial cells of the testis, and the pituitary acidophils, and if the stimulus is continued indefinitely, true adenomata may develop. Occasionally endometrial carcinoma may supervene.

The *pituitary hormones* have also been the subject of much experimental work. A classical method of subjecting a mouse to an excess of *gonadotrophic hormone* is to remove one ovary and transplant the other into its spleen. The ovarian hormones are inactivated by the liver, and can no longer inhibit the secretion of pituitary gonadotrophins, which are then free to act on the transplanted ovary. Ovarian cancer may sometimes be produced in this way.

Similarly rats and mice can be subjected to large doses of *thyrotrophic hormone* if they are given thiouracil derivatives and fed on a low-iodine diet. Thyroxine formation is curtailed, and once again the inhibitory effect on the pituitary is lost. The excess thyrotrophic hormone produces great thyroid hyperplasia which is often accompanied by discrete adenomata. Occasionally thyroid cancer supervenes.[49]

Castrated animals develop marked hyperplasia of the pituitary basophil "gonadotrophic cells", and thyroidectomised animals develop a comparable hyperplasia of the pituitary "thyrotrophs". Large adenomata composed of these cells are frequently produced if the animal lives long enough.[50] The pituitary acidophil tumours induced by oestrogen are mammotrophic in effect. It is doubtful whether any of these pituitary tumours ever becomes malignant.

It would therefore appear that animal tumours are produced only after massive doses of hormones administered over a long period of time. The effect is one of hyperplasia merging imperceptibly into circumscribed adenomatous formations in the affected organs. Malignancy may occur, but its supervention is not common. In man hormones are not usually an important factor in causing cancer. There are a few exceptions: (*a*) granulosa-cell tumour of the ovary, which produces large amounts of oestrogen, leads to great endometrial hyperplasia which may occasionally proceed to carcinoma of the body of the uterus. (*b*) Men who have undergone artificial sex change and have taken large doses of oestrogen in order to produce breast enlargement occasionally develop breast cancer.[51] (*c*) A remarkable clustering of vaginal adenocarcinoma has recently come to light in seven young women, aged 15 to 22 years. This tumour is rare at any age, and it was found that in each case the mother of the patient had been given diethylstilboestrol during the first trimester of that pregnancy.[52, 53] It appears that fetal tissue is more sensitive to this carcinogen than is the adult and that transplacental transfer of drugs is a factor to be reckoned with in carcinogenesis. Many more cases have since been reported.[139]

Hormone Dependency

While hormones play only a small role in the aetiology of human cancer, they are of great importance in maintaining the growth of some tumours. These are called *hormone dependent tumours*. Such neoplasms depend on specific hormones for their continued growth, and if deprived of them undergo regression, only to recur when the hormone is restored. It seems that during a stage in the development of certain tumours a propitious hormonal *milieu* is essential for their continued growth. This is a transient phase, however, for these tumours eventually progress to complete hormone independence. Nevertheless, a patient suffering from such a cancer may enjoy some years of amelioration of symptoms if the responsible hormone is eradicated from the body. Both in this respect and from the further light that is shed on the nature of carcinogenesis, hormone dependence is worth careful study.

Prostate. Prostatic cancer was the first neoplasm of man to be successfully repressed by hormonal therapy. It is often androgen dependent, and following castration there is dramatic relief with regression of the tumour and its metastases and a fall in the acid phosphatase level of the plasma. Nowadays large doses of stilboestrol are given, either as an adjunct to orchidectomy or else alone. Unfortunately such large doses may lead to cardiovascular complications, so that although the tumour may regress for a considerable time, the patient's life is sometimes not substantially prolonged by the therapy.[54]

Breast. Breast cancer manifests hormone dependency in less than half the affected patients. The hormones on which it may depend are oestrogens, progestins, and prolactin (the pituitary mammotrophic hormone).[55]

In pre-menopausal women oophorectomy often produces a remission usually lasting about 6 months, but occasionally up to several years. It removes the major source of oestrogens and progestins. Bilateral adrenalectomy is sometimes performed at the same time to eliminate the other source of these hormones. In this respect it is noteworthy that breast cancer is particularly lethal during pregnancy and lactation.

If a relapse follows oophorectomy, hypophysectomy may be performed. This is the most radical endocrine operation for breast cancer, and a further remission lasting up to 18 months may follow. Probably the tumour depends more on prolactin than on the ovarian hormones.

In post-menopausal women hypophysectomy is sometimes recommended. There is an interesting variation of response to hormone therapy amongst these cases. Some respond well to large doses of oestrogens, some to progestins, and some to androgens. In some these hormones cause remissions of 6–12 months, while in others they lead to sudden exacerbations and rapid death. Corticosteroids also sometimes have an ameliorative effect, probably in part by inhibiting the adrenals.

Since most cases of breast cancer are hormone independent from the start, much research has been undertaken to determine which patients are most likely to respond to hormone therapy. This consists of assays of steroids in the urine. The results are inconclusive, and treatment is still a matter of trial and error.

Thyroid. Some cancers of the thyroid, usually the well-differentiated ones, are under the control of pituitary thyrotrophic hormone. Treatment of the tumour by excision or with ^{131}I may cause excessive pituitary secretion and so stimulate any remaining growth to activity. The administration of thyroid hormone, on the other hand, can cause a remission due to its inhibitory effect on the pituitary.[56–58]

Other tumours.[59] Progestins sometimes produce remissions in metastatic endometrial carcinoma and renal carcinoma. Hypernephroma seems sometimes to be under definite hormonal control, and may respond to oestrogen also.

A somewhat different type of dependence is seen with the amino acid L-asparagine. Normal cells do not require an external source, while some neoplastic cells cannot grow without it in tissue culture. The systemic administration of L-asparaginase (derived from *Esch. coli*) has been tried as a treatment for malignant disease, in particular leukaemia.[60]

Pregnancy and Tumours

Some tumours may increase in size in pregnancy, and may even show an increased tendency to become malignant. The melanotic hamartoma tends to darken during pregnancy, an effect probably related to an increased secretion of melanocyte stimulating hormone. It is commonly held that malignancy is especially liable to occur at this period, though detailed studies have not substantiated this view.[61, 62] Nevertheless, metastases occurring during pregnancy have been known to regress after its termination.[63] Neurofibromatosis is another hamartomatous disorder in which the lesions tend to grow during pregnancy, and during which sarcomatous change may occasionally supervene. The bad effect of pregnancy on breast cancer has already been noted, and the same is true of cancer of the cervix.

VIRUSES AND NEOPLASIA[64–66, 140]

Tumour-producing (oncogenic) viruses are of great importance not only in the aetiology of some animal tumours but also because some human tumours are associated, if not actually caused, by viruses. The first virus-induced animal tumour to be discovered was fowl leukaemia (Ellerman and Bang, 1908), and it was followed by fowl sarcoma (Rous, 1911),* rabbit papilloma (Shope, 1932), renal adenocarcinoma in frogs (Lucké, 1934), and mammary cancer in mice (Bittner, 1936).

Gross (1951) isolated the virus of mouse leukaemia by transmitting the disease from an animal of a high-incidence strain, Ak, to the newborn of a low-incidence strain, C3H. In 1953 a second, unrelated virus was found in Gross's material—this produced tumours in mice, rats, hamsters, and many other animals. The salivary glands were especially vulnerable, but tumours of the connective tissues, breasts, and kidneys were also encountered. This agent is now called polyoma virus.

One of the many viruses present in a latent form in monkey kidneys is oncogenic to newborn hamsters. This agent, simian virus (SV) 40, has been adventitiously inoculated into human beings who were given poliomyelitis vaccines (see

---

* It is an interesting but sad reflection of the remarkable resistance of contemporary medicine to new ideas, that had Rous not lived to be an octogenarian he would not have received the Nobel Prize for Medicine in 1966.

---

p. 285). A number of human and animal adenoviruses are also oncogenic to baby hamsters. Two more recently proved animal tumours are cat lymphosarcoma and Marek's disease of chickens (a lymphoma).[67]

The factors involved in the induction of tumours by these viruses are complex.[65] The agents concerned in mammary cancer and leukaemia in mice are infinitely more pathogenic to newborn animals than to adults. The strain of animal is also important; thus although the Bittner virus can cause mammary cancer in low incidence strains when introduced early in life, the virus becomes less potent in successive generations and ultimately dies out. The hormonal environment is also important: oestrogen accelerates tumour production, as already explained. Mouse leukaemia can be induced both by the virus and by ionising radiations (radiation-induced leukaemias in mice have been shown to yield a leukaemia-producing virus which was apparently latent).[68] When both factors act together the incidence of leukaemia is much increased. The Shope papilloma virus assumes malignant propensities much more rapidly when the ears of the rabbits have been tarred beforehand.[69] The polyoma virus is widely distributed in nature, apparently lying latent in many mice. When grown in tissue culture (as was done with Gross's material) it acquires greatly enhanced virulence.

In order to establish the virus aetiology of a tumour, it is necessary to transmit the lesion by means of bacteriologically sterile, cell-free filtrates to other animals. It has also been found that some of these viruses, notably polyoma[70] and SV 40,[71] induce changes in cells grown in tissue culture. This phenomenon, *cell transformation*, is indicated by a rapid, unruly proliferation of the cells with copious, irregular mitotic activity, and when they are transplanted into animals they exhibit malignant propensities.

It is important to realise that the mere presence of a virus in a cancer is no indication of its causal role. Cancers frequently harbour "passenger viruses"; these lie latent there, because neoplastic cells produce less interferon than normal ones.[65] Some of these passengers may be quite dangerous pathogens, but in respect of the tumour they are irrelevant. Conversely, in some virus-induced tumours the agent itself cannot be demonstrated—this applies especially to transplanted tumours caused originally by the Shope papilloma, polyoma, and SV 40 viruses. The Rous virus, on the other hand, is usually recoverable from its sarcomata. Even when the virus which induced the tumour cannot be isolated from a transplanted tumour, it is often possible to demonstrate antibodies against the virus in question. Furthermore, if an animal is first inoculated with the virus, and then has the corresponding tumour transplanted into it, it tends to reject the tumour due to the immunity already acquired.[71, 72]

With the DNA-containing viruses (SV 40, Shope papilloma, and polyoma viruses) the infected cells undergo transformation, and infective virus can no longer be detected. It is thought that the viral DNA becomes incorporated in the cell's genome and replicates with it.[73, 74] The finding of mRNA of viral type in these tumours supports this hypothesis.[75] The situation is not unlike that of lysogeny in bacteria, when bacteriophage may remain latent in the organismal DNA during a temperate phase, but so far it has not been possible to induce the tumour viruses to multiply excessively and kill the host cell as occurs with bacteriophage in a virulent phase. Perhaps this takes place when tumours regress spontaneously or as a result of x-ray therapy; there is, however, no evidence for it.

A RNA tumour virus can transform a normal cell into a genetically stable cancer cell because of the presence of *RNA-dependent (or directed) DNA polymerase*, also called *reverse transcriptase*.[76, 77] This enzyme has been found in six different RNA tumour viruses. The enzyme transcribes the viral RNA into DNA provirus, which is then integrated with the DNA of the chromosomes of the host cell. This process is of great theoretical interest in being a reversal of the usual sequence of DNA control of RNA and protein formation in the cell (see pp. 18–19).

It is not certain whether oncogenic viruses merely initiate the cells, which then pursue an independent course of neoplasia (as with chemical agents), or whether the presence of the virus (perhaps in an unrecognized form) is necessary for the continued propagation of the tumour. It is certain that Koch's postulates (Appendix II) have to be modified in respect to establishing the virus aetiology of tumours, inasmuch as it is common to find no virus at all in such a tumour, at least by currently available methods.

At present much research is being done in investigating a virus aetiology for certain human tumours. The essential criterion, the inoculation of suspected viruses into human beings, is clearly impracticable. Instead, a train of circumstantial evidence is necessary:

(a) The isolation and titration of virus or viral nucleic acid in human tumours.
(b) Its effect on cells grown in tissue culture with special reference to transformation. This applies to the DNA viruses; the RNA viruses do not cause transformation.
(c) Its oncogenic effect in animals.
(d) The presence of antibodies in the affected individual and in the population in general.
(e) The epidemiology of the lesion.
(f) The prophylactic effect of a vaccine against the virus in reducing the incidence of the tumour.

Of human tumours, four seem to have an association with viruses. (a) *Burkitt's tumour*, which is described on p. 403, is associated with a herpesvirus called the EB virus, after the two workers Epstein and Barr who first isolated it in 1964. This virus has been cultured from the neoplastic lymphocytes of the tumour, and all patients have high-titre antibodies to the virus. The picture is, however, complicated by the fact that antibodies are present in lower titre in many normal controls, and that the virus is established as the cause of infectious mononucleosis with a positive Paul-Bunnell reaction. It is therefore impossible to incriminate EB virus as the cause of Burkitt's tumour without serious reservations. It might be merely a passenger. Another possibility is that it produces infectious mononucleosis in healthy people, but in children with chronic infections that have already caused RE and lymphocytic hyperplasia, the added assault of the EB virus leads to lymphocytic neoplasia. This suggestion would explain the geographical distribution of the tumour—it is found where there is a high incidence of endemic malaria. There is experimental evidence that mice given *Plasmodium berghei yoelii* malaria suffer immunological suppression, and are particularly susceptible to a lymphoma from Maloney leukaemogenic virus.[78] Immunosuppression has also been reported in children with malaria.[79]

(b) *Nasopharyngeal carcinoma*.[80] Some patients with this tumour have a high titre of antibodies to the EB virus, but as with the Burkitt tumour the precise relationship between the virus and the tumour is complex and poorly defined.

(c) Virus particles identical electron microscopically with the Bittner factor have been found in human *breast cancer* cells.[81–83] Of even greater significance, the milk of women with a close family history of cancer of the breast contains similar virus particles much more frequently (60 per cent) than does the milk of normal women (5 per cent). In the Parsi community of Bombay there is a very high incidence of breast cancer, much greater than in the Hindu and Moslem population, and once again virus particles have been frequently found in the milk of Parsi women (39 per cent).[82]

The murine (Bittner) RNA virus contains RNA-dependent DNA polymerase which catalyses the synthesis of DNA. This DNA has a base sequence which is complementery to that of the viral RNA and will hybridise with it. Thus the DNA may be used as a specific agent for detecting viral RNA. It has been found by Spiegelman that DNA synthesised under the influence of murine virus will hybridise *in vitro* with RNA extracted from human mammary cancers (67 per cent), but not with extracts from normal breasts or benign tumours.[141, 142] This is very strong evidence that human tumours contain an oncogenic RNA virus very similar to the Bittner factor, but nevertheless its precise relationship to the tumour remains to be determined. The technique of detecting molecular hybridisation of RNA from human tumours with DNA formed by known animal oncogenic RNA viruses is being extended. Thus human sarcomata[143] and lymphomata[144] contain RNA related to mouse leukaemia virus.

(d) Women with *carcinoma of the cervix*[84, 145] have a higher incidence of antibodies to herpes simplex virus type 2 than do normal women. There is a close relationship between cervical cancer and sexual intercourse. The tumour is almost unknown in nuns and is commonest in prostitutes.

Summary

It is apparent from the above discussion that most tumours arising in adult life have no known cause. Some, however, can be related to occupational and environmental factors, some are associated with pre–existent disease of a particular area of tissue, and finally there is a group of rare conditions in which there is an hereditary predisposition to tumour formation at a particular site. Hormones do not appear to play a very significant role in causing cancer, but are of great importance in the life-history of some tumours that depend on them for their survival. The role of viruses in human cancer is still problematic.

THE PRECANCEROUS STATE: INITIATION AND PROMOTION[85]

It was already noted in the early years of experimental coal-tar carcinogenesis that when the skin of a mouse had been painted with tar it was peculiarly prone to develop tumours at the site of any wound inflicted on the painted area. In the decade 1940-1950 there was enough evidence to indicate that carcinogenesis was a multiple stage phenomenon. When the skins of mice or rabbits were treated with carcinogenic hydrocarbons and later with croton oil, many tumours developed on that area. The concept arose that a sub-threshold dose of carcinogen had *initiated* a group of cells, so that they became "latent" tumour cells which were finally *promoted* to overt cancerous activity by a non-specific traumatising agent like croton oil. The interesting hypothesis of initiation and promotion has received much support from the work of Berenblum and his colleagues,[86] who found that after painting an area of mouse skin with one application of a carcinogen and then subjecting it to numerous applications of croton oil, a latent period elapsed, after which a specific number of tumours appeared. If the croton oil treatment was delayed, the development of tumours was equally delayed, but the final number that developed was the same as when the croton oil had been applied at once. Initiating agents have a dose-dependent, irreversible, and additive effect which is transmissable to the cell's progeny. Cell proliferation is next needed, and after a number of divisions, the cancer cell emerges. Injury, such as that produced by the action of a promoting agent, speeds up this process. Promoting agents are therefore non-specific and act slowly. It is postulated that carcinogens, or their activated products, alter DNA either by binding to it directly or by modifying RNA-dependent DNA polymerase.[87] When the concept of initiation and promotion is applied to occupational cancer, the long latent period between leaving employment and developing the tumour becomes readily understandable.

In fact the processes of initiation and promotion are less clearly divisible than has been described above.[88] No pure chemical promoter has yet been isolated, for even croton oil has a mildly carcinogenic action on mouse skin. Nearly all initiators are also promoters, but urethane is said to be a pure initiator for mouse skin. As most local carcinogens, even the polycyclic hydrocarbons, tend to be absorbed, they are capable of initiating a wider area of tissue than would be expected at first sight. Nowadays the concept of *cocarcinogenesis*, the collaboration of a number of different factors in the production of cancer, is often used instead of initiation and promotion.[89]

Thus a whole field of tissue could be so altered by an initiating agent, that when subjected to non-specific promoting agents, like croton oil, heat, or physical trauma, it tends towards multicentric malignancy. During the phase of initiation the tissue shows no changes to indicate a cancerous transformation. It is normal microscopically. Only later promotion indicates its latent malignant potentiality.

There is a similar two-stage mode of carcinogenesis in respect of remotely-acting agents. Croton oil promotes cancer in skin initiated with oral 2-acetylaminofluorene.[90] Likewise, oestrogen will promote cancer in mouse breasts initiated by hydrocarbons or the Bittner virus.[91]

EARLY MALIGNANT LESIONS

In the early days of experimental tar carcinogenesis it was noted that areas of hyperplasia and even discrete papillomata appeared at the sites of treatment, but that they tended to disappear if the agent was discontinued in time. They recurred rapidly, however, if the agent was reapplied. The nature of these lesions is obscure.

In man the question of early malignant change is of great importance, for it is at this stage that complete eradication is easiest. In recent years a number of interesting lesions involving epithelial surfaces have been recognised. In these areas the epithelium is undergoing atypical proliferation. The cells vary in size and shape, have large, darkly-staining nuclei, and show an increased amount of mitotic activity. The term *dysplasia* is applied to this change. When it is severe, the cells appear anaplastic, tend to lose their polarity, and lie haphazardly in relationship to one another. They have the microscopic changes usually associated with malignancy, and since there is no invasion of the underlying connective tissue, the terms *carcinoma-in-situ* or *intraepithelial carcinoma* are used. In stratified squamous epithelium there may be foci of abnormal keratinisation within the area of cell proliferation, and this is called *malignant dyskeratosis* (Fig. 29.5).

The natural history of these premalignant changes is not known for certain. Dysplasia may progress to *carcinoma-in-situ* and ultimately invasive tumour. The progression from one stage to the next is often slow, and the possibility exists that some lesions regress.

Carcinoma-in-situ has been described in most epithelia, and it is encountered most typically in the stratified squamous covering epithelium of the skin, mouth, and cervix. Some clinical examples are worth noting:

Bowen's disease of the skin. This occurs in the middle-aged and elderly, and appears as discrete, red plaques which are sometimes mistaken for superficial basal-cell carcinoma, or resistant chronic dermatitis or psoriasis. Any area of the carcinoma is found to co-exist. For this reason all erosions should be examined cytologically.

Similar changes may be encountered in adenomatous polyps of the uterus and colon that are undergoing early cancerous transformation. The gastric and bronchial epithelia may also be affected.

Paget's disease of the skin.[92] This has its greatest incidence on the nipple, but may also occur on the vulva, anus, axilla, and other areas of the skin. Clinically there is an eczematous lesion which consists histologically of large, round Paget cells with pale, clear cytoplasm (often containing much mucoprotein) and large, vesicular nuclei with prominent nucleoli infiltrating the lower part of the epidermis (Fig. 29.6). In many instances, especially in the mammary and anal lesions, there is an underlying adenocarcinoma which may be contiguous with the skin lesion, and it was originally suggested that this was the result of intra-epithelial invasion of the deeper cancer. However, in many cases elsewhere in the skin there is no underlying malignancy, and the

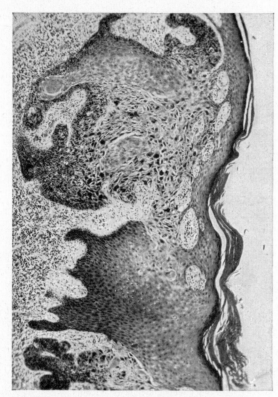

Figure 29.5
Malignant dyskeratosis. This was a biopsy from a case of Bowen's disease. The typical pleomorphic appearance of *carcinoma-in-situ* is evident in the proliferating epithelial mass, and in its advancing edge there is an epithelial pearl. Although in places there is an appearance of invasion, serial sections of the block did not confirm this. Note the heavy dermal lymphocyte infiltration, which may represent an immune response to the incipient malignancy. ×83

skin may be implicated. Invasive carcinoma may finally ensue, sometimes after many years.

Senile or solar keratoses. All gradations of change are seen varying from mild atypicality of the epithelial cells to *carcinoma-in-situ* and on occasions invasive squamous-cell carcinoma. This rarely metastasises, but it is advisable to treat all senile keratoses.

Erythroplasia of Queyrat. This is a rare condition almost always involving the penis, and it manifests itself as a red, velvety plaque.

Leukoplakia. This appears as dead-white shiny plaques on a mucous membrane. The mouth and tongue are commonly affected, and the vulva is another favourite site. Microscopically the epithelium shows hyperplasia and all degrees of cellular atypicality ranging from mild dysplasia to *carcinoma-in-situ*. Invasive squamous-cell carcinoma may develop, especially in the vulva. The oral lesions of lichen planus should not be confused with leukoplakia, for they are quite distinctive histologically and are not premalignant.

Cervical erosions. Most of these are quite benign, but occasionally *carcinoma-in-situ* and even an early invasive

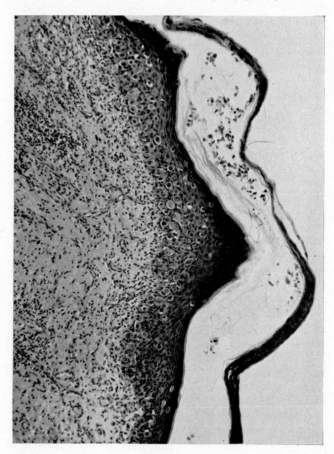

Figure 29.6
Paget's disease of nipple. The prickle-cell layer of the epidermis contains numerous large, palely-staining, round cells with prominent vesicular nuclei. These are typical Paget cells. The stratum corneum has become detached. In the dermis there is an inflammatory reaction. ×90.

breast tumour itself is sometimes too deep to be in contact with the skin lesion. It is now widely held that Paget's disease is an example of *carcinoma-in-situ*, and that where there is an underlying tumour, it is to be regarded as a second primary neoplasm in a field of growth.

Whenever *carcinoma-in-situ* is encountered histologically, it is important to examine multiple sections of the tissue in order to exclude the possibility of invasive cancer in an adjacent area.

EXFOLIATIVE CYTOLOGY[93, 94]

When cancer involves a lining epithelium, some of the neoplastic cells are shed on to the surrounding surface. If the surface is internal, these cells are trapped in the secretion of the part, and ultimately discharged to the exterior. Bronchial carcinoma cells may be coughed up in the sputum, gastric carcinoma cells may be aspirated in the gastric juice, and cervical carcinoma cells may be shed into the vaginal secretions. In recent years much progress has been made in recognising clumps of cancer cells in such secretions, and sometimes this allows for an early diagnosis of malignant disease. The technique of exfoliative cytology has its greatest value in the diagnosis of cervical cancer, where an area of early carcinoma may be so small that it is missed in a routine examination of the part.

Cancer of the Cervix Uteri

Papanicolaou and his colleagues first described the use of vaginal and cervical smears in the diagnosis of uterine cancer, and they have shown that malignancy can be diagnosed by the recognition of abnormal exfoliated cells. In addition to obvious cancer cells, other abnormal forms are sometimes found. These cellular abnormalities have been called *dyskaryosis* by Papanicolaou, because the principal changes are found in the nucleus. The nuclei are enlarged and show variation in size and shape. Hyperchromatism is present, and the nucleoli are enlarged. A careful comparison of the smears with subsequent biopsy specimens has confirmed that the morphology of the cells accurately reflects the changes in the cervical mucosa. The varying degrees of dysplasia, *carcinoma-in-situ*, and invasive carcinoma may therefore be diagnosed by the exfoliative cytologist.

The significance of these cervical lesions is at present under review, but there is convincing statistical evidence from the USA that many cases of epithelial dysplasia progress to *carcinoma-in-situ* and finally invasive cancer. In the cervix at least, cancer appears to develop over a period of many years, and the appearance of invasive tumour heralds the final act of a long drama which commences with mild atypia and progresses through dysplasia and *carcinoma-in-situ*. Extensive projects are now under way in which whole populations are being routinely screened for cervical disease, and the treatment of these early lesions already appears to be reducing the incidence of invasive cancer. Before such campaigns are

started, there are two prerequisites: firstly, there must be an adequate number of trained diagnostic cytologists, and secondly, the surgeons must be aware of the nature of the lesions which they will be called upon to treat. The finding of dyskaryotic or cancer cells calls for a biopsy to exclude obvious invasive cancer, and if this is negative, it is followed by a cold cone biopsy to identify the source of the abnormal cells. The final treatment calls for fine judgement; some of the patients are young and anxious to have children. Careful

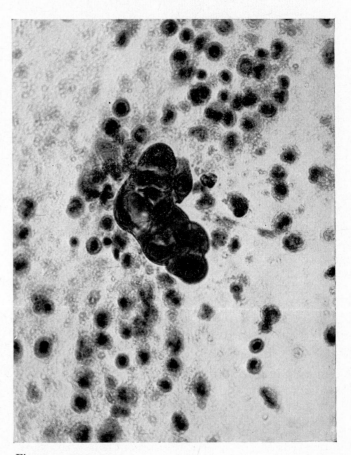

Figure 29.7
Cancer cells in the sputum. In this smear there is a clump of darkly-staining cancer cells amid a mass of pus cells. Note the size and irregularity of the cells. This patient was later proven to have an adenocarcinoma. × 550. (*Photograph supplied by the late Dr. J. Bamforth*)

follow-ups with repeated cell studies should be undertaken; some patients have had children without mishap. It is evident that much has yet to be learned about the treatment of these conditions, so that the dangerous lesions are removed before invasion occurs, and, on the other hand, unnecessary radical surgery is not performed on lesions which are not progressive.

Sputum, gastric contents, urine, and the fluid obtained by prostatic massage can all be examined for malignant cells. A similar technique can be used to investigate pleural and peritoneal effusions. Those secondary to cancer may contain numbers of neoplastic cells, and the method is useful both diagnostically and prognostically. Care must be taken not to mistake metaplastic serosal cells for malignant cells.

THE INCIDENCE OF TUMOURS

Incidence of tumours in plants.[95] True tumours are described in plants and form a fascinating subject. The best known is *crown gall* caused by the bacterium *Phytomonas tumefaciens*; the organism is present in the primary but not in the secondary growths. Mushrooms develop tumours when treated with tar, and in clover tumours can be induced by a virus acting after injury.

Incidence of tumours in animals.[95] Tumours have been described in most species which have been studied. Thus melanoma and lymphoma occur in *Drosophila*. So far as vertebrates are concerned, the best-known tumours occur in species valued as pets, or used for food or experimental purposes. The following may be cited:

DOGS: Mammary fibro-adenoma, interstitial-cell tumours of testis, carcinoma of skin, tonsil, and breast. Boston and Scottish terriers have a high incidence of mast-cell tumours.

PARAKEETS AND BUDGERIGARS: Pituitary tumours.

HORSES: Teratoma of testis, melanoma of skin, carcinoma of skin, mouth, and nasal sinuses.

BOVINE ANIMALS: Carcinoma of skin, adrenal cortical tumours.

PIGS: Nephroblastoma.

Incidence of Tumours in Man

Age. In European children the incidence of malignancy is small, the commonest tumours being acute leukaemia and the rather uncommon embryonic tumours mentioned in Chapter 27. Nevertheless, cancer is one of the most important causes of childhood mortality in civilised countries now that infections have been so well combated. In adolescence and early adult life malignancy is also uncommon, the most frequent tumours being osteosarcoma, leukaemia, and Hodgkin's disease. At this age carcinoma occurs sporadically, but its incidence does not become significant until the fifth decade is reached, when it rapidly assumes its lethal role especially between the ages of 60 and 75 years. The Registrar-General's figures for England and Wales for the year 1969 reveal that 62 584 males and 53 471 females died as the result of tumours (including leukaemia), and that about 80 per cent of the victims were over the age of 60 years. The question repeatedly arises as to whether there is an actual increase in the incidence of tumours in the world's population as a whole, or in the population of any country in particular. It is extremely difficult to give a straight answer to this. In only the most civilised countries are the statistics of tumour incidence of any value, and even in such areas many fatal tumours are not confirmed by histological examination. It is amongst civilised communities that the medical services are the most adequate, and many tumours are revealed in them which would remain undiagnosed in primitive, under-privileged groups. On the other hand, as cancer incidence increases with age, it is the civilised groups who, by living longer, are more prone to develop neoplasms. Cancer is widespread in many primitive communities, in whom the age of onset is often earlier than in Europeans. As will be seen, the pattern of tumours is different. The age expectancy of such groups is also less due to the effects of poverty. It will be interesting to see whether this tumour pattern will approximate more closely to the European one when the fundamental causes of disease have been removed by education and economic progress.

Sex. Apart from the malignancy of those organs peculiar to each sex it seems that most neoplasms are commoner in men than in women. According to the Registrar-General's Statistics for 1969 fatal cancer of the oral cavity, tongue, and bladder was about twice as common in men as in women, while cancer of the respiratory tract five times more common in the male sex: in the kidney, pancreas, stomach, and rectum there was a slight male predominance. A few noteworthy exceptions to this rule were cancers of the breast, gall-bladder, and thyroid. Breast cancer was 150 times commoner in women than in men, and it accounted for about a fifth of all fatal neoplasia in women. Cancer of the biliary passages and thyroid cancer were two to three times as common in women as in men. Hypopharyngeal carcinoma was the one malignancy in the oropharyngeal region which was commoner in women than in men, and much of it is associated with a pre-existing Plummer-Vinson syndrome. Cancer of the colon, excluding the rectum, was distinctly more common in the female sex (5 915 fatal cases in women as opposed to 3 980 in men). The commonest fatal neoplasm in women was cancer of the breast (10 622 cases), and in men cancer of the lung (24 651 cases).

Over the age of 80 years there was a moderate decrease in the incidence of malignancy, a tendency more marked in men than in women. In extreme old age cancer was distinctly commoner in the female sex, a trend accentuated by the greater longevity of women as compared with men.

Social class. Apart from specific occupational factors already discussed there is statistical evidence that cancer of the skin, penis, mouth, oesophagus, and stomach is commoner in the "lower" social groups, whereas cancer of the breast is decidedly more prevalent in women of the "higher" social groups.

Heredity. This has already been discussed.

The Incidence of Specific Tumours

It is by investigating the incidence of specific tumours in a community that aetiological factors are most likely to be discovered. Detailed surveys have now established that lung cancer is much commoner in heavy smokers than in those who smoke moderately or not at all. Likewise the danger of leukaemia has been proved to be much greater in those who have been exposed to large doses of ionising radiation than in the population at large. The data of geographical pathology have thrown much light on the incidence of tumours in different countries.[96-98] For instance, the commonest malignancies in Europeans affect the lung, breast, stomach, and colon, whereas in Africans these types of cancer (other than the breast) are generally not at all common, while cancer of the skin, penis, cervix, and liver predominate. But even this statement is too vague—there are millions of Africans, and in even one country the incidence of tumours may vary according to locality. A survey in Uganda[99] showed inexplicable concentrations of penile, gastric, oesophageal, and skin cancers in various localities; where one tumour was common another was hardly ever seen. It was particularly interesting that the incidence of penile cancer varied tremendously despite the fact that nearly all the men were uncircumcised. Similarly Kaposi's tumour, generally regarded as one of the commonest neoplasms in Africans, shows great regional variations, and is much commoner in East and Southern Africa than in West Africa. Nasopharyngeal cancer is very common in South-East Asians, especially those of Chinese origin, and is also frequent in some East Africans. It must be admitted that there is no explanation of these facts.

In order to rationalise the knowledge about the geographical incidence of tumours, the following factors may be cited:

External environment. This may be of some importance in stomach cancer, for in Britain there is an excess of cases in North Wales and the Fen District of East Anglia,[100] and the high peat content of the soil has been incriminated.[101] The actual effect of this is unknown. Actinic skin cancer is another example.

Nutrition. Liver cancer in Africans and Asians has been attributed to nutritional cirrhosis. Aflatoxin is another possibility.

Occupation. This has already been discussed.

Cultural and religious customs. The rarity of penile cancer in those groups who practise ritual circumcision, and the liability to oral cancer of those South-East Asians who chew betel quid are good examples of regional variations of tumours due to national habits.

Racial constitution. A good example is the virtual immunity of the dark-skinned races to the carcinogenic action of sunlight on the skin. Carcinoma of the testis is almost unknown in the Negro, and carcinoma of the prostate and chronic lymphatic leukaemia are very uncommon in the Japanese and Chinese.[102] By contrast chronic lymphatic leukaemia is common in Israeli Jews.[102] The explanation of these findings is not known. It seems probable that in all tumours genetic factors must play some part even when there is overwhelming evidence of an exogenous cause.

It will be useful to conclude this discussion of the aetiology of tumours by briefly considering some factors that are of importance in the incidence of various neoplasms.

Cancer of the skin. *Geographical factors*. Actinic skin cancer is discussed on p. 376. Regional examples of skin cancer are the *Kangri cancer* of Kashmir and the *Kang cancer* of North-West China. The Kangri is a charcoal heater carried close to the abdomen, and following its continual use carcinoma of the abdominal skin may develop.[103, 104]

Figure 29.8
Kang cancer. A portion of skin removed from the trochanteric region of the thigh. There is an extensive area of fungating squamous-cell carcinoma. *(I 19.6, Reproduced by permission of the President and Council of the R.C.S. Eng.)*

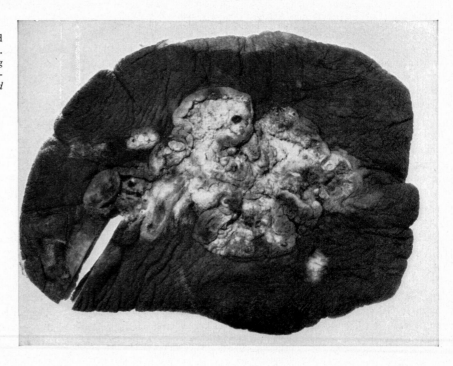

The Kang is a hollow bed heated from below by burning coals. People who sleep on such a bed may develop cancer of the skin of the thigh and leg.[105] It is probable that carcinogenic agents in the soot initiate the tumour, and the heat of the burner merely acts as a promoting agent. Melanoma of the feet is common in Negroes as is also Kaposi's tumour.

Occupational factors. Ionising radiations and the application of hydrocarbons may produce squamous-cell cancers of the skin. Ingested arsenic is also carcinogenic, and may lead to cutaneous cancer many years after exposure has ceased. Keratoses on the palms are characteristic, and these may show malignant change. Multiple superficial basal-cell carcinomata, Bowen's disease, and invasive squamous-cell carcinomata are also common.[106]

Genetic factors. Xeroderma pigmentosum has already been mentioned. Another condition inherited as a recessive character which is liable to be complicated by skin cancer is albinism (p. 560).

Chronic skin lesions, e.g. varicose ulcers and old osteomyelitis sinuses, have already been described as precursors of squamous-cell cancer.

Cancer of the penis. Penile cancer is almost unknown in Jews, who practise circumcision soon after birth, and uncommon in Moslems, who perform it later in childhood. However, it is an uncommon form of cancer in uncircumcised Europeans, especially of the higher social groups, and even in uncircumcised Africans its incidence varies greatly according to locality (see p. 390). It is probable that the smegma acts as a solvent for carcinogenic agents in the environment. The cancer is commonest in those whose standard of personal hygiene is low, and is probably always preceded by chronic balanitis.

Cancer of the lip. This is commonest in elderly pipe-smoking agricultural workers. The sunlight probably initiates the tumour, and the heat of the pipe promotes it to activity.

Cancer of the mouth. *Geographical factors.* Oral cancer is very common amongst some communities in South-East Asia who indulge in the habit of betel chewing.[107] The quid, which is kept in the mouth for long periods of time, consists of betel nut, spices, tobacco, lime, and buyo leaves. The carcinogenic principle probably resides in the betel nut.[108] The buccal aspect of the cheek and lower jaw is the usual site, but the tongue may also be involved. Another peculiar habit associated with oral cancer is reverse-cigar smoking, which is practised in parts of India, Sardinia, and Latin America. The lighted end of the cigar is held in the mouth which is burned in consequence. Cancer of the palate may ensue.[109]

Chronic disease. There is little evidence that hot food, alcohol, or chronic dental disease predispose to oral cancer, but tobacco smoking is of importance. Women with the Plummer-Vinson syndrome show an increased incidence of oral cancer.

Cancer of the oesophagus. *Geographical factors.* The interesting feature of the epidemiology of oesophageal cancer is its tendency to occur in almost epidemic proportions in circumscribed areas, while elsewhere it is quite uncommon.[102] Areas of high incidence include the Transkei in the Eastern Cape Province of South Africa, the area of Bulawayo in Rhodesia, that part of the USSR around the Caspian sea, Northern Iran, and around the Kenyan coast of Lake Victoria. The reason for these local areas of high incidence is not known. A carcinogen in the maize used for the preparation of beer is suspected.

Genetic factors. There is an interesting association between a type of congenital tylosis (thickening of the epidermis of the palms and soles) and oesophageal cancer.[110]

Chronic disease. There is an association with tobacco smoking. Long-standing achalasia of the cardia is sometimes complicated by cancer.[111] The relation of the Plummer-Vinson syndrome to postcricoid and upper oesophageal cancer has already been noted.

Cancer of the stomach. *Geographical factors.* Cancer of the stomach is most prevalent in the Japanese, and is also common in parts of Siberia. Its incidence falls through Eastern Europe to the West, and it is low in the white-skinned community of the USA, South Africa, and Australasia. Japanese and African groups conform to the white-skinned population's incidence of stomach cancer in Hawaii and the USA respectively.[102] There is no known dietary association with the condition. The possibility that soil conditions may be important has been noted, but at present the evidence is unimpressive.

Genetic factors. There is an increased incidence of blood group A in cases of gastric cancer.

Chronic disease. As already noted, there is no causal relationship between peptic ulceration and cancer. On the other hand, it is accepted that pernicious anaemia (Chapter 49) may predispose to malignancy, for the incidence of cancer is three times that found in normal stomachs.[112] In one series it was found that 10 per cent of patients with pernicious anaemia eventually developed gastric cancer.[113] Gastric adenomata sometimes become malignant. There is no positive proof that alcohol, hot food, or imperfectly masticated material are important factors in the aetiology of gastric cancer.

Cancer of the colon. *Geographical factors.* These are not as definite as in gastric or oesophageal cancer, but the tumour is common throughout Western Europe, North America, and Australasia.[102] Its relative uncommonness in Africans may be due to the high-fibre diets they take. Colonic cancer is seven times commoner in people on a low-fibre diet, and this may be due to the effect of constipation in allowing carcinogens in the diet to remain for a longer period in contact with the colonic mucosa than would be the case in those with regular bowel actions.[114]

Genetic factors. The classical example of polyposis coli has already been discussed.

Chronic disease. The relationship between ulcerative colitis and cancer has already been mentioned. Solitary and multiple benign polyps (papillary adenomata and villous papillomata) also tend to become malignant. In some there is a familial tendency.[115]

Cancer of the lung. *Geographical factors.* Lung cancer has its maximum incidence in Britain, especially Scotland. It is common in Western Europe, especially Finland and Germany, but is not nearly so common in the USA, Canada, Australia, and South Africa despite the large number of cigarettes smoked in these countries. It is very common in the Maoris and Hawaiians.[102]

Occupational factors are of importance in the aetiology of the disease.[2] The peculiar pulmonary malady that afflicted the miners of Schneeberg and Joachimstal for so long has now been diagnosed as lung cancer, and it is generally attributed to radioactive substances, like radon, rather than metallic ores present in the inhaled dust. Nickel workers are prone to cancer of the nasal passages and the lungs, and there is evidence that chromium may have a similar effect. Arsenical sheep-dip workers are also predisposed to lung cancer.

Some of the pneumoconioses predispose to cancer; *asbestosis* is by far the most important, the tumour being either a squamous-cell carcinoma or else a diffusely spreading pleural lesion described as a mesothelioma.[116] Similar lesions of the peritoneum have also been found. It is the crocidolite fibre that is the most dangerous, and at present a considerable number of cases of mesothelioma are occurring in workers who have been unwittingly exposed to the dust.[117] There is some tendency for haematite-worker's lung (sidero-silicosis) to undergo malignant change,[118] but uncomplicated silicosis and coal-miner's pneumoconiosis are not precancerous.[119]

There can be little doubt that *heavy tobacco smoking* predisposes to lung cancer, and that the danger is greater in cigarette users than in pipe smokers.[120, 121] The malignancy is usually of squamous-cell or oat-cell type. At present no adequate cause has been found to explain the dangerous effects of tobacco smoking. Another factor of undetermined importance is atmospheric pollution with soot and smoke: it probably acts in concert with tobacco smoking in producing lung cancer. Since the incidence of lung cancer drops even if smoking is discontinued late in life, it may be that the tobacco acts more as a promoter than an initiator.

There is no evidence that chronic inflammatory disease, such as tuberculosis, bronchiectasis, or fungous disease, is precancerous. Bronchitis is, however, commoner in patients with cancer.[122] This is no doubt attributable to smoking (see p. 515).

Cancer of the liver. The importance of preceding cirrhosis has already been mentioned. Other inflammatory diseases of the liver, such as schistosomiasis and syphilis, do not appear to be precancerous. However, cancer of the larger intrahepatic bile ducts (malignant cholangioma) is very common in the Far East, and is attributable to infestation of the bile ducts with liver flukes.

Cancer of the breast. The incidence of breast cancer is greatest in the USA and Canada and in Western Europe. It decreases in Eastern Europe and the USSR and is uncommon

in Central Asia and Japan—indeed, its incidence is the reverse of that of gastric cancer. While not very common in the African Negro, it is as common in the American Negro as in the white-skinned population of the USA. It is traditionally held that childlessness and inadequate lactation are important predisposing causes of breast cancer, but more recent investigations have not substantiated this theory. Perhaps there is a dietary factor involved.[102] Cystic hyperplasia of the breast (mammary dysplasia) is not in itself precancerous.

Cancer of the uterus. The relationship between cervical cancer and coitus has already been noted. The tumour is generally a common one, but is rare in Jewesses.[102] The circumcision of the Jewish husband may be an important factor. Cancer of the body of the uterus is much less common than cervical cancer; it has a fair incidence in Canada and the USA. The relationship between ovarian granulosa-cell tumour and endometrial cancer has been mentioned.

Cancer of the bladder. The relation to aromatic amines has been noted. Tobacco smoking predisposes to bladder cancer, particularly in the male.[123]

Cancer of the thyroid. Its relationship to goitre has already been noted. It has also followed the exposure of the area to ionising radiation (see p. 414).

Testicular tumours. A considerable increase in the incidence of testicular tumours has taken place recently in Denmark, and probably also elsewhere.[124] The reason for this is unknown.

Osteosarcoma. Radioactive elements that are stored in the bones are possible agents in producing osteosarcomata. The case of the girls who swallowed radium and mesothorium in the luminous paint used for painting watch-dials is mentioned on p. 413. A more current hazard is the pollution of the atmosphere with radioactive strontium following nuclear explosions. Strontium, like radium and calcium, is stored in the bones. The relationship of Paget's disease to osteosarcoma has already been noted.

THE NATURE OF CANCER

Neoplasia is generally assumed to be related to the uncontrolled growth of cells. Whether the change is in the cells themselves or in the local tissue environment is not known. Thus it is possible that carcinoma is due not to a change in the involved epithelial cells but to a disturbance of the epithelial-connective tissue arrangement. Such interaction is well known in embryogenesis,[125] and there is some evidence that the same is true in neoplasia. When skin is treated with methylcholanthrene, an early change is fragmentation and reduplication of the basement membrane and destruction of the superficial connective tissue.[126] Such changes are not seen in skin treated with non-carcinogenic irritants.[127] Furthermore, polyoma virus will produce tumours in the submandibular gland tissue in embryo mice only if epithelial and connective tissue are both present.[128]

In spite of these interesting observations it is currently believed that the events responsible for the development of malignancy reside in the affected neoplastic cells, and it is convenient at this point to summarise the known properties of malignant cells. The variations from the normal which they exhibit have been extensively studied in the hope that this would explain the fundamental nature of the malignant process itself, and provide the basis for rational treatment.

Changes in Appearance

The pleomorphism and bizarre appearances of malignant cells have already been considered in detail, as have also the nuclear changes, chromosomal abnormalities, and variations in DNA content (see p. 340). There is, however, no constant variation characteristic of all tumour cells.

Changes in Chemical Content

Nucleic acid. Whether the change in DNA content noted above is a reflection of an abnormality in the molecular structure is not known, i.e. there is no definite evidence of a mutation. The incorporation of viral DNA or virus-produced DNA has been described. The RNA content of malignant cells tends to be as high as in any actively growing tissue. The endoplasmic reticulum is usually poorly formed.

Enzymatic activity.[129] The early studies on tumour metabolism *in vitro* led Warburg to conclude that tumour cells obtained their energy by glycolysis, even in the presence of oxygen. Exceptions to the rule have since been found, and furthermore some normal tissues, e.g. retina, have a similar type of metabolism. Extensive investigations into the enzyme contents of cancer cells have shown that tumour cells tend to contain the same enzymes as the parent tissue, but that the quantity is usually reduced. Numerous quantitative biochemical abnormalities have been described in cancer cells and in patients also. So far no reliable tests have materialised, though many have been tried. Thus, an increase of β-glucuronidase activity has been found in the vaginal secretions of women with cervical carcinoma, but the test is unreliable.[130]

Antigens. This has already been discussed (p. 378).

Changes in Behaviour

In vivo. Progressive growth is the characteristic of neoplasia; malignant tumours invade and metastasise. Even so, the phenomena of dormancy and regression indicate that some tumours undergo phases of retrenchment.

Inappropriate secretion.[131] This is a common phenomenon. Epidermal cells can produce mucus, as in Paget's disease, and respiratory epithelial tumours can form keratin (see metaplasia p. 308). The inappropriate secretion of hormones is described on page 344. Tumour cells may revert to activities normally seen only in their parents during embryonic life. The formation of carcino-embryonic antigen has been noted on p. 379. Another example of considerable practical importance is seen in cancer of the liver. a_1-*fetoglobulin* is a globulin which normally forms about 50 per cent of the total plasma proteins of the fetus. Its formation ceases in the third trimester, and it is therefore absent from the serum at birth. In 50–79 per cent of cases of hepatoma a_1-fetoglobulin reappears in the plasma, and its presence has proved to be a useful diagnostic test. It is occasionally found in cases of testicular embryonal carcinoma.

In vitro. Malignant cells do not, on the whole, grow nearly so well as cells from normal tissues. However, a few lines of cancer cells have so adapted themselves to cell culture that they are now well established and grown in many laboratories; the HeLa cell is a good example. Such cells lack the alignment of normal cells grown in tissue culture, and tend to heap up into several layers. Normal cells (with the exception of lymphocytes and haematopoietic cells) form monolayers, and will grow only on a firm surface such as glass or solid agar: they are described as *anchorage dependent*. Growth ceases if the concentration of cells becomes too high, a phenomenon described as *contact inhibition of growth*. Normal cells also need an unidentified factor present in normal serum for their growth. Virus-transformed malignant cells are less anchorage dependent, and will grow in soft agar. They show less contact inhibition of growth and require little or no serum factor. Finally, normal cells seem to have a finite life-span, while some neoplastic cells have acquired the property of indefinite life provided suitable growth facilities are provided either in tissue culture or in a host animal.[132]

This brief survey of the properties of the cancer cell is sufficient to indicate that although there are often many points of difference from the normal, there is no single characteristic by which it can be recognised. Perhaps it is wrong to expect that this should be so. The well-documented morphological features of cancer cells are of great importance to the cytologist, but researches into cell metabolism have been essentially sterile both as regards a reliable cancer test and the elaboration of an effective chemotherapeutic agent. Studies of the antigenic composition and the *in-vitro* behaviour of tumour cells may perhaps yield more fruitful results.

CONCLUSION

It is humiliating to reflect that the vast majority of tumours arising in adults have no apparent cause, and appear to develop spontaneously. While some geographical factors are suggestive and a few occupational hazards have been successfully unmasked and controlled, there is still no indication as to the cause of cancer or the nature of its perverted growth. At present all that can be hoped for in the treatment of cancer is a radical removal using surgical resection or radiotherapy. These measures are only effective when the tumour is localised, but there is much evidence that cancer is not a local disease. Even if removal of the entire field of growth is feasible, the presence of secondary deposits presents an unknown hazard. Since these may remain dormant for many years, it is evident that the assessment of the effects of local treatment is very difficult. When the disease is clinically generalised, the cytotoxic agents may be used as the means of attack. Hormone therapy may produce some alleviation of symptoms.

The most successful approach to the control of cancer at the present time lies in its prevention.[133] The many known physical and chemical carcinogenic agents have already been described, and their avoidance can appreciably reduce the incidence of cancer. Each tumour must be considered separately, e.g. a reduction in the amount of cigarette smoking and atmospheric pollution would undoubtedly reduce the incidence of lung cancer, while the control of malnutrition might diminish that of liver cancer. The careful screening of drugs for carcinogenic activity in animals is an important aspect of public health.[134] It is impossible to foretell the carcinogenicity of a substance from its chemical formula alone.

A second method of cancer prophylaxis is the treatment of known precancerous lesions. In the previous chapters a point of view has been expressed that cancer must be defined and diagnosed in terms of its invasive behaviour. The observations on the development of uterine cancer indicate that invasive tumour is the final development of a sequence of precancerous lesions. These are sometimes reflected in the abnormal appearance of the cells, and in the cervix can be detected and treated with relative ease. Cancer of the cervix uteri is therefore a preventable disease. It is probable that all invasive cancers commence in a similar manner, but in the vital organs treatment is not so easy. Thus in the case of the lung, *carcinoma-in-situ* can be diagnosed and located with the aid of the exfoliative cytologist, but even if it is practicable to excise the lesion, it is impossible to remove the whole field of growth, i.e. both lungs. The avoidance of carcinogens is obviously a more practical method of controlling the tumour. So far, no effective methods have been devised to control the common gastric, colonic, and mammary cancers.

The failure of workers in basic cancer research to produce any results which can be translated into action in the treatment of human disease has encouraged clinicians to adopt a more experimental approach to cancer therapy. The ritual of applying standard treatment to cases where the outlook is hopeless is being augmented or replaced, in well-controlled series, by other methods—for instance those based on an immunological concept.

REFERENCES

1. STERN, B. D. and KAPLAN, L. (1969). *American Journal of Obstetrics and Gynecology*, **104**, 255.
2. HUEPER, W. C. (1954). *Archives of Pathology*, **58**, 360, 475, and 645.
3. GOLDBLATT, M. W. (1958). *British Medical Bulletin*, **14**, 136.
4. Leading Article (1972). *British Medical Journal*, iv, 3.
5. ROBSON, A. O. and JELLIFFE, A. M. (1963). *British Medical Journal*, ii, 207.
6. HADFIELD, E. H. (1970). *Annals of the Royal College of Surgeons of England*, **46**, 301.
7. CLAYSON, D. B. (1962). *Chemical Carcinogenesis*, 467 pp. London: Churchill.
8. BOYLAND, E. (1958). *British Medical Bulletin*, **14**, 153.
9. CASE, R. A. M. (1966). *Annals of the Royal College of Surgeons of England*, **39**, 213.
10. WEISBURGER, E. K. and WEISBURGER, J. H. (1958). *Advances in Cancer Research*, **5**, 331. New York: Academic Press.
11. MILLER, J. A. and MILLER, E. C. (1953). *Advances in Cancer Research*, **1**, 339. Ibid.
12. BONSER, G. M. (1967). *British Medical Journal*, ii, 655.
13. Leading Article (1968). *Lancet*, i, 1071.
14. HAUGHTON, G. and AMOS, D. B. (1968). *Cancer Research*, **28**, 1839.
15. HUMPHREY, J. H. and WHITE, R. G. (1970). In *Immunology for Students of Medicine*. 3rd edn, pp. 580–599. Oxford: Blackwell.
16. FAIRLEY, G. H. (1971). *British Journal of Hospital Medicine*, **6**, 633.
17. KLEIN, G. (1968). *Cancer Research*, **28**, 625 and 1354.
18. PREHN, R. T. (1968). *Cancer Research*, **28**, 1326.
19. COLLINS, J. J. and BLACK, P. H. (1971). *New England Journal of Medicine*, **285**, 175.
20. Leading Article (1971). *Lancet*, ii, 645.
21. SMITH, R. T. and ADLER, W. H. (1970). *New England Journal of Medicine*, **282**, 1320.
22. Leading Article (1971). *Lancet*, ii, 753.
23. Leading Article (1971). *British Medical Journal*, iv, 505.
24. LEWIS, M. G. et al. (1969). *British Medical Journal*, iii, 547.
25. HELLSTRÖM, I. and HELLSTRÖM, K. E. (1966). *Annals of the New York Academy of Sciences*, **129**, 724.
26. MÖLLER, G. and MÖLLER, E. (1966). *Annals of the New York Academy of Sciences*, **129**, 735.
27. LYNCH, H. T. (1969). *Medical Clinics of North America*, **53**, 923.
28. DUKES, C. E. (1952). *Annals of Eugenics (London)*, **17**, 1.
29. LOCKHART-MUMMERY, H. E. (1967). *Proceedings of the Royal Society of Medicine*, **60**, 381.
30. COPELAND, M. M. and MARTIN, H. E. (1932). *American Journal of Cancer*, **16**, 1337.
31. SWANBECK, G. (1971). *British Journal of Dermatology*, **85**, 394.
32. ANDERSON, D. E. et al. (1967). *American Journal of Human Genetics*, **19**, 12.
33. RONCHESE, F. (1933). *American Journal of Cancer*, **18**, 875.
34. CRUIKSHANK, A. H., McCONNELL, E. M. and MILLER, D. G. (1963). *Journal of Clinical Pathology*, **16**, 573.
35. NEWCOMB, W. D. (1932). *British Journal of Surgery*, **20**, 279.
36. DIBLE, J. H. (1925). *British Journal of Surgery*, **12**, 666.

37. HINTON, J. M. (1966). *Gut*, **7**, 427.
38. KIRSHBAUM, J. D. and KOZOLL, D. D. (1941). *Surgery, Gynecology and Obstetrics*, **73**, 740.
39. COOPER, W. A. (1937). *Archives of Surgery*, **35**, 431.
40. WYNDER, E. L., ONDERDONK, J. and MANTEL, N. (1963). *Cancer (Philadelphia)*, **16**, 1388.
41. EDMONDSON, H. A. and STEINER, P. E. (1954). *Cancer (Philadelphia)*, **7**, 462.
42. WARREN, S. and DRAKE, W. L. (1951). *American Journal of Pathology*, **27**, 573.
43. MORTENSEN, J. D., WOOLNER, L. B. and BENNETT, W. A. (1955). *Journal of Clinical Endocrinology*, **15**, 1270.
44. HURXTHAL, L. M. and HEINEMAN, A. C. (1958). *New England Journal of Medicine*, **258**, 457.
45. SLOAN, L. W. (1954). *Journal of Clinical Endocrinology*, **14**, 1309.
46. WYNDER, E. L. and FRYER, J. H. (1958). *Annals of Internal Medicine*, **49**, 1106.
47. BIELSCHOWSKY, F. and HORNING, E. S. (1958). *British Medical Bulletin*, **14**, 106.
48. BONSER, G. M. and JULL, J. W. (1960). In *Recent Advances in Pathology*, 7th edn, p. 415. Edited by C. V. Harrison. London: Churchill.
49. ISRAEL, M. S. and ELLIS, I. R. (1960). *British Journal of Cancer*, **14**, 206.
50. FURTH, J. and CLIFTON, K. H. (1958). *Ciba Foundation Colloquium on Endocrinology*, **12**, 3. London: Churchill.
51. SYMMERS, W. StC. (1968). *British Medical Journal*, ii, 83.
52. HERBST, A. L. and SCULLY, R. E. (1970). *Cancer (New York)*, **25**, 745.
53. HERBST, A. L., ULFELDER, H. and POSKANZER, D. C. (1971). *New England Journal of Medicine*, **284**, 878.
54. Veterans Administration Co-operative Urological Research Group (1967). *Surgery, Gynecology and Obstetrics*, **124**, 1011.
55. Leading Article (1969). *British Medical Journal*, i, 265.
56. CRILE, G. (1957). *Cancer (Philadelphia)*, **10**, 1119.
57. CRILE, G. (1960). *American Journal of Surgery*, **99**, 533.
58. SMITHERS, D. W. (1959). *Journal of the Faculty of Radiology (London)*, **10**, 3.
59. Leading Article (1971). *British Medical Journal*, i, 360.
60. Leading Article (1969). *British Medical Journal*, ii, 465.
61. GEORGE, P. A., FORTNER, J. G. and PACK, G. T. (1960). *Cancer (Philadelphia)*, **13**, 854.
62. WHITE, L. P. *et al.* (1961). *Journal of the American Medical Association*, **177**, 235.
63. ALLEN, E. P. (1955). *British Medical Journal*, ii, 1067.
64. GROSS, L. (1963). *Annals of the Royal College of Surgeons of England*, **33**, 67.
65. ANDREWES, C. (1964). *British Medical Journal*, i, 653.
66. EPSTEIN, M. A. (1971). *Lancet*, i, 1344.
67. Leading Article (1969). *Lancet*, i, 610.
68. FURTH, J. YOROKO, K. and TAKEMOTO, H. (1962). In *Ciba Foundation Symposium on Tumour Viruses of Murine Origin*, p. 138. Edited by G. E. W. Wolstenholme and M. O'Connor. London: Churchill.
69. VOGT, M. and DULBECCO, R. (1960). *Proceedings of the National Academy of Science. (Washington)*, **46**, 365.
70. KOPROWSKI, H. *et al.* (1962). *Journal of Cellular and Comparative Physiology*, **59**, 281.
71. HABEL, K. (1961). *Proceedings of the Society for Experimental Biology and Medicine*, **106**, 722.
72. HUEBNER, R. J. *et al.* (1963). *Proceedings of the National Academy of Science. (Washington)*, **50**, 379.
73. BURDETTE, W. J. (1966). Editor. *Viruses Including Cancer*, 498 pp. Salt Lake City: University of Utah Press.
74. DULBECCO, R. (1965). *American Journal of Medicine*, **38**, 669.
75. FUJINAGA, K. and GREEN, M. (1966). *Proceedings of the National Academy of Science (Washington)*, **55**, 1567.
76. Editorial (1970). *Nature (London)*, **226**, 1198.
77. CRICK, F. (1970). *Nature (London)*, **227**, 561.
78. WEDDERBURN, N. (1970). *Lancet*, ii, 1114.
79. GREENWOOD, B. M. *et al.* (1972). *Lancet*, i, 169.
80. Leading Article (1971). *Lancet*, i, 218.
81. MOORE, D. H. *et al.* (1971). *Nature (London)*, **229**, 611.
82. Leading Article (1971). *Lancet*, i, 741.
83. Leading Article (1972). *Lancet*, i, 359.
84. Leading Article (1972). *British Medical Journal*, i, 264.
85. BONSER, G. M. and JULL, J. W. (1960). In *Recent Advances in Pathology*, 7th edn, p. 384. Edited by C. V. Harrison. London: Churchill.
86. BERENBLUM, I. and SHUBIK, P. (1947). *British Journal of Cancer*, **1**, 379 and 383.
87. RYSER, H. J-P. (1971). *New England Journal of Medicine*, **285**, 721.
88. ROE, F. J. C. (1956). *British Journal of Cancer*, **10**, 61 and 72.
89. SALAMAN, M. H. and ROE, F. J. C. (1964). *British Medical Bulletin*, **20**, 139.
90. RITCHIE, A. C. and SAFFIOTTI, U. (1955). *Cancer Research*, **15**, 84.
91. JULL, J. W. (1954). *Journal of Pathology and Bacteriology*, **68**, 547.
92. Leading Article (1972). *British Medical Journal*, i, 707.
93. WAY, S. (1963). *The Diagnosis of Early Carcinoma of the Cervix*. London: Churchill.
94. KOSS, L. G. (1968). *Diagnostic Cytology and its Histopathologic Bases*, 2nd edn. Philadelphia: Lippincott.
95. McMANUS, J. F. A. (1966). *General Pathology*, p. 64 *et seq.* Chicago: Year Book Medical Publishers.
96. DAVIES, J. N. P. *et al.* (1964). *British Medical Journal*, i, 259 and 336.
97. BARUAH, B. D. (1964). *Cancer (Philadelphia)*, **17**, 413.
98. FARAGO, C. (1963). *Cancer (Philadelphia)*, **16**, 670.
99. HUTT, M. S. R. and BURKITT, D. (1965). *British Medical Journal*, ii, 719.
100. LEGON, C. D. (1951). *British Journal of Cancer*, **5**, 175.

101. Stocks, P. and Davies, R. I. (1960). *British Journal of Cancer*, **14**, 8.
102. Doll, R. (1972). *Proceedings of the Royal Society of Medicine*, **65**, 49.
103. Neve, E. F. (1923). *British Medical Journal*, ii, 1255.
104. Vaughan, K. (1925). *British Medical Journal*, ii, 495.
105. Laycock, H. T. (1948). *British Medical Journal*, i, 982.
106. Leading Article (1968). *British Medical Journal*, ii, 191.
107. Orr, I. M. (1933). *Lancet*, ii, 575.
108. Suri, K., Goldman, H. M. and Wells, H. (1971). *Nature*, **230**, 383.
109. Kini, M. G. (1944). *Indian Medical Gazette*, **79**, 572.
110. Clarke, C. A., Howel-Evans, A. W. and McConnell, R. B. (1957). *British Medical Journal*, i, 945.
111. Peyman, M. A. (1959). *British Medical Journal*, i, 23.
112. Kaplan, H. S. and Rigler, L. G. (1945). *American Journal of Medical Science*, **209**, 339.
113. Zamcheck, N. *et al.* (1955). *New England Journal of Medicine*, **252**, 1103.
114. Burkitt, D. P. (1971). *Cancer (Philadelphia)*, **28**, 3.
115. Morson, B. C. (1971). *Proceedings of the Royal Society of Medicine*, **64**, 959.
116. Hourihane, D. O. (1964). *Thorax*, **19**, 268.
117. Leading Article (1967). *British Medical Journal*, iii, 62.
118. Faulds, J. S. and Stewart, M. J. (1956). *Journal of Pathology and Bacteriology*, **72**, 353.
119. Kennaway, E. L. and Kennaway, N. M. (1947). *British Journal of Cancer*, **1**, 260.
120. Doll, R. and Hill, A. B. (1950). *British Medical Journal*, ii, 739.
121. Doll, R. and Hill, A. B. (1964). *British Medical Journal*, i, 1399 and 1460.
122. Leading Article (1963). *British Medical Journal*, ii, 1144.
123. Leading Articles (1971). *Lancet*, i, 635 and (1972). *British Medical Journal*, i, 763.
124. Annotation (1968). *Lancet*, ii, 164.
125. Fleischmajer, R. and Billingham, R. E. (1968). Editors. *Epithelial-Mesenchymal Interactions*, p. 326. Baltimore: Williams and Wilkins.
126. Tarin, D. (1967). *International Journal of Cancer*, **2**, 195.
127. Tarin, D. (1968). *International Journal of Cancer*, **3**, 734.
128. Dawe, C. J., Morgan, W. D. and Slatick, M. S. (1966). *International Journal of Cancer*, **1**, 419.
129. Greenstein, J. P. (1954). *Biochemistry of Cancer*, pp. 327–506. New York: Academic Press.
130. Nixon, W. C. W., Bonham, D. G. and Gibbs, D. F. (1961). *Annual Reports of the British Empire Cancer Campaign*, **39**, 277.
131. Smith, J. B. (1970). *Medical Clinics of North America*, **54**, 797.
132. Stoker, M. (1970). *British Medical Journal*, iii, 541.
133. Raven, R. W. and Roe, F. J. C. (1967). *The Prevention of Cancer*. London: Butterworths.
134. Bonser, G. M. (1967). *British Medical Journal*, iv, 129.
135. Zamcheck, N. *et al.* (1972). *New England Journal of Medicine*, **286**, 83.
136. Hellström, K. E. and Hellström, I. (1972). *Triangle*, **11**, 23.
137. Bansal, S. C. and Sjögren, H. O. (1972). *International Journal of Cancer*, **9**, 490.
138. Leading Article (1972). *Lancet*, i, 523.
139. Herbst, A. L. *et al.* (1972). *New England Journal of Medicine*, **287**, 1259.
140. Allen, D. W. and Cole, P. (1972). *New England Journal of Medicine*, **286**, 70.
141. Leading Article (1972). *Lancet*, i, 359.
142. Axel, R., Schlom, J. and Spiegelman, S. (1972). *Nature*, **235**, 32.
143. Kufe, D., Hehlmann, R. and Spiegelman, S. (1972). *Science*, **175**, 182.
144. Hehlmann, R., Kufe, D. and Spiegelman, S. (1972). *Proceeding of the National Academy of Sciences of the United States of America*, **69**, 1727.
145. Leading Article. (1972). *British Medical Journal*, ii, 548.

Chapter 30. The Stem Cell and the Reticulo-Endothelial System: Their Pathological Associations

The connective tissues of the body, apart from those of the central nervous system, differentiate from mesenchyme. This embryonic connective tissue consists of stellate cells embedded in a gelatinous ground substance in which there are reticulin fibres. While mesenchyme, as thus defined, is found only in the fetus, there are nevertheless primitive connective tissue elements that persist throughout life, and are capable of proliferation and differentiation as the necessity arises. These elements exist as large cells with a pale, basophilic cytoplasm and a round or indented nucleus containing prominent nucleoli. They are multipotential and are called *stem cells*. Though probably scattered throughout all the tissues, they are found in greatest number in the lymph nodes, spleen, and bone marrow, where they are closely associated with the reticulin framework of the organs. It is indeed probable that some of these cells have differentiated sufficiently to produce the fibres. They have therefore also been called *reticulum cells* (or *reticular cells*), a name often used synonymously with the stem cell. Though this is theoretically wrong, it is very difficult to distinguish between stem cells and reticulum cells. Indeed, some authorities do not recognise the existence of reticulum cells as such, and speak of undifferentiated "stem cells" and differentiated "histiocytes",[1] but in this book the term reticulum cell will be used as described above, and the histiocyte reserved for the resting connective tissue macrophage.

It is now considered that morphologically a stem cell can be a small lymphocyte.[2] The precise morphology of bone-marrow stem cells is less clear[3] (see p. 582). Allogeneic small lymphocytes labelled with tritiated thymidine have been seen to enlarge and undergo mitosis when administered to an animal,[4, 5] and in irradiated animals lymphocytes not only repopulate the lymph nodes but also provide fresh lymphoid tissue.[6] It should be noted that, although the immunologically competent cell is also a lymphocyte, it does not follow that every lymphocyte is immunologically competent. The body's content of lymphocytes probably includes a number of different types of cell, each with a similar appearance but of dissimilar function. The immunologically competent cell may be regarded as a lymphocyte that has differentiated towards an immunological function.

The stem cell is capable of giving rise to the following cells:

The reticulo-endothelial system, which is endowed with phagocytic powers.

The haematopoietic cells.[37]

Connective tissue cells, i.e. fibroblasts, chondroblasts, osteoblasts, and synovial cells. A stem cell which is differentiating in this direction first starts to lay down reticulin fibres, and is called a reticulum cell. Stem cells may also give rise to fat cells and mast cells.

Vascular endothelial cells, at least during embryonic development. The newly formed blood vessels so prominent in granulation tissue are believed to be derived from the proliferation of adjacent endothelial cells.

Smooth muscle cells. It is possible that the muscle forming the wall of arterioles which develop in a healing wound is derived from the local fibroblastic elements which have assumed an embryonic multipotentiality during the repair process. This may be the basis of connective tissue metaplasia, when fibroblasts assume an osteoblastic or synovial potentiality.[7]

The stem cells of the adult are found predominantly in the spleen, liver, bone marrow, and lymph nodes, where they give rise to the lymphoid, haematopoietic, and reticulo-endothelial cells of these organs. They also lay down the reticulin framework. The development of the blood cells is described in Chapters 49, 50, and 51, while the connective tissue elements are discussed in Chapter 5. At this stage it is therefore necessary to consider the reticulo-endothelial system.

THE RETICULO-ENDOTHELIAL SYSTEM

The term *reticulo-endothelial system* was coined by Aschoff in 1924 to delineate a large collection of cells that shared a common origin, morphology, and phagocytic function. The characteristic phagocytic functions he regarded as essential for grouping these cells into a single system were the uptake of a vital dye, e.g. trypan blue, and the scavenging of a particulate marker e.g. colloidal carbon. In fact neither of these two functions provides an acid test, for poorly phagocytic cells, like reticulum cells, endothelial cells, and fibroblasts, can also become labelled by pinocytosis, and if the markers are released from strongly phagocytic cells, e.g. when these cells die, they can be taken up by other more feebly phagocytic cells. The cells that have been included in Aschoff's reticulo-endothelial system are the reticulum cells of the spleen and lymph nodes, the cells lining the lymphatic and blood sinuses, e.g. of the lymph nodes, spleen, and liver (where they are called Kupffer cells), the monocytes of the blood, and the tissue histiocytes. The name reticulo-endothelium was derived from the close relationship of some of these cells to the reticulin framework that intersects the lymph nodes and spleen, and their endothelium-like appearance when lining sinuses in these organs. But the cells of this system are very different both morphologically and functionally from both endothelial cells and reticulum cells, and the name reticulo-endothelial (RE) system is inappropriate. It is retained in this book because it is in general use by pathologists.

At a conference held in Leiden in 1969 a group of workers proposed a new classification of this system of cells, which they call the *mononuclear phagocyte system*.[8] They propose that the following cells form part of this system:

Precursor cells from the bone marrow.

Promonocytes from the bone marrow.

Monocytes from the bone marrow and the blood.

Macrophages, which include the connective-tissue histiocytes, the liver Kupffer cells, the alveolar macrophages of the lung, the sinus-lining cells and free macrophages of the spleen and lymph nodes, the pleural and peritoneal macrophages and those of the bone marrow, and probably also the osteoclast which is believed to arise by coalescence of monocytes. The microglial cell of the central nervous system is also regarded as a probable candidate for membership of this system.

The functional criteria for including the macrophages, monocytes, and promonocytes in a single system are avid phagocytosis and pinocytosis (especially phagocytosis), and the ability to attach firmly to a glass surface. Monocytes and macrophages have receptor sites for immunoglobulins and complement at the cell surface. They are to be regarded as "professional" phagocytes as opposed to such "facultative" phagocytes as the fibroblast, endothelial cell, and reticulum cell, which can ingest particles at a low rate independent of immunoglobulins or complement, and probably have no receptors for these components.[8]

Morphologically these cells tend to vary considerably. Thus macrophages have many more lysosomes and mitochondria than do monocytes. But they are fairly large cells, 10–25 μm in diameter with kidney-shaped or oval nuclei which are single and contain nucleoli. Sometimes they are difficult to distinguish from lymphocytes, which, of course, differ in function, life span, and origin. A lymphocyte should not be called a phagocytic mononuclear cell.

The cells of the mononuclear phagocyte system originate from precursor cells in the bone marrow, are transported in the blood as monocytes, and eventually become tissue macrophages. This sequence is described on page 128 in respect of chronic inflammation. There is no evidence that mononuclear phagocytes are derived from lymphocytes. The most immature member of the system that can be recognised in the bone marrow is the promonocyte, but presumably there is an even more immature precursor cell. The monocytes are a pool of relatively immature cells in the blood, and when conditions are favourable for phagocytosis, these cells become macrophages and develop the necessary equipment for digesting phagocytosed material. Thus the monocyte is the origin of the macrophage populations in the various organs mentioned above. Whether the fixed macrophages of the spleen, lymph nodes, and bone marrow (the sinus-lining cells) are also derived from monocytes is not certain, but the probability is that they are. In the spleen and lymph nodes both free and fixed macrophages lie in close association with the reticulin fibres—the free ones lie in the interstices of the framework formed by reticulum cells, while the fixed ones

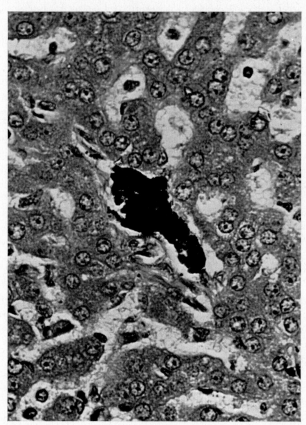

Figure 30.1
Sinus-lining cell of liver (Kupffer cell). It is particularly prominent because it has phagocytosed a great deal of malarial pigment. × 550.

are attached to cytoplasmic extensions of the reticulum cells, but unlike these cells, the fixed macrophages do not form reticulin fibres.[8]

While the RE (or mononuclear phagocyte) system is widely dispersed throughout the tissues of the body, most of its content is present in the liver, bone marrow, lymph nodes, and spleen. They are sometimes called the *reticulo-endothelial organs* on this account. They are also sometimes described as the *lymphoreticular tissues* because of their reticulin framework and the predominance of lymphocytes, though in the marrow the granulocytic and normoblastic elements far outnumber the lymphocytic ones.

FUNCTIONS OF THE RETICULO-ENDOTHELIAL SYSTEM

Phagocytosis

LOCAL. The appearance of large phagocytic cells is characteristic of the demolition phase that follows acute inflammation. It is seen during the stage of resolution, and also in the early phases of repair by granulation tissue (Fig. 30.2). These macrophages ingest cell debris, broken-down

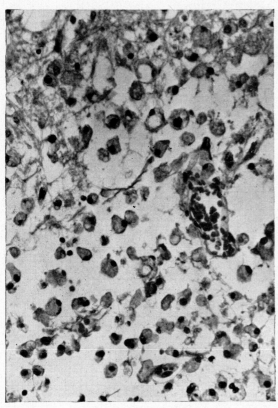

Figure 30.2
Microglial reaction in an area of cerebral softening. There is almost complete disintegration of brain substance, and an infiltration of round, swollen macrophages. These are phagocytosing the debris, and the granular appearance of their cytoplasm is due to its content of fat and haemosiderin. These cells are called compound granular corpuscles. × 330.

red cells, fibrin, and organisms, e.g. *S. typhi*, *Myco. tuberculosis*, *Myco. leprae*, and many of the fungous and protozoan pathogens. Macrophages are the predominant cells of foreign-body reactions.

GENERAL. Once an organism gains access to the lymphatics and blood stream, the sinus-lining cells of the lymph nodes, liver, spleen, and bone marrow provide an effective defence. In bacteraemia these last three organs are able to eliminate the offending organism quite rapidly, but in septicaemia they are inadequate (see Chapter 8).

On some occasions the organisms are engulfed by the RE cells, and enter into a state of virtual symbiosis. This occurs in histoplasmosis and leishmaniasis. Inevitably some damage is produced by the organism, but the disease runs a very protracted course. Either the patient or the organism may finally win the battle.

The Immune Response

The relationship between the RE system, the lymphocyte, and the formation of antibodies is described in detail in Chapter 12.

Red-Cell Destruction and Iron Metabolism

Effete red cells are broken down by the RE cells, especially in the spleen, after fragmentation in the circulation (see Chapter 49). The haem moiety of the haemoglobin is divested of its iron, which is stored in the RE cell. It is combined there with apoferritin to form *ferritin*, which consists of about 23 per cent ferric iron. Where there is massive blood breakdown, e.g. following a local extravasation, the iron-binding protein is supersaturated with ferric iron (over 35 per cent) to form *haemosiderin*. The tetrapyrrolic ring structure of the haem is broken up, and eventually bilirubin is formed.

Storage

The RE system stores excess amounts of lipids and mucoproteins, and the cells become swollen. In the event of cholesterol storage the cytoplasm assumes a foamy appearance in paraffin sections (Fig. 30.3).

PROLIFERATIVE LESIONS OF THE STEM CELL AND ITS DERIVATIVES

Proliferation of the stem cell and its derivatives is a very common condition, and, when generalised, it is manifested clinically by an enlargement of the liver, spleen, and lymph nodes. Such a proliferation may be an apparently purposeful response to some stimulus, e.g. infection, when it comes into the category of hyperplasia, or else it may entail the purposeless progressive multiplication of neoplasia. These proliferations have in the past been assembled under a single heading of "reticulosis", but fortunately this term and the unwieldy classifications that were derived from it are no longer in vogue.

Hyperplasia

INFECTIVE ("REACTIVE") HYPERPLASIA. This very common condition is seen to its best advantage in the lymph nodes. Proliferation involves not only the reticulo-endothelial elements but also the cells involved in the immune response. When immunoglobulin production is evoked, the lymphoid follicles are enlarged and increased in number, and in their midst there are large pale germinal centres. Coincidentally many plasma cells are formed in the medulla. Hyperplasia occurs in the paracortical zone when cell-mediated immunity is stimulated. The reticulo-endothelial hyperplasia is evidenced by proliferation of the sinus-lining cells, producing accumulations of macrophages in the dilated sinuses ("sinus catarrh").

Reactive hyperplasia may produce such marked distortion of lymph-node structure that lymphoma is sometimes closely simulated. This has been described in *toxoplasmosis*,[9] *infectious mononucleosis*,[9] in the lymph nodes draining a site of vaccination (*post-vaccinal lymphadenitis*),[10] and in epileptic patients who take *anti-convulsant drugs* such as dilantin[11] and mesantoin,[12] and develop a morbilliform eruption, arthropathy, hepato-splenomegaly, and lymphadenopathy.

In chronic widespread pruritic skin diseases there is often a marked regional lymphadenopathy. The characteristic feature is a dense accumulation of RE cells (and reticulum cells) especially in the periphery of the nodes. Some of these cells contain droplets of fat and granules of melanin. This condition of *dermatopathic lymphadenitis* (*lipomelanic reticulosis*) is merely a florid variation of reactive hyperplasia.

Sometimes the RE cells play a very active part in the response against the agent: in sarcoidosis, tuberculosis, cat-scratch disease, and the deep-seated mycoses there are dense focal accumulations of altered macrophages (epithelioid cells), which tend to be arranged in discrete follicles.

The most exuberant examples of infective hyperplasia of the RE system are met with in the systematised (disseminated) conditions of visceral leishmaniasis and histoplasmosis, where there are vast accumulations of parasitised macrophages in many organs.

In chronic infective hyperplasia of a lymph node there is an ever-increasing thickening of the reticulin framework, and in due course this is converted into dense collagen fibre. Once again the versatility of the proliferating stem cell is demonstrated. In this instance it is giving rise to reticulum cells and fibroblasts.

HAEMATOPOIETIC HYPERPLASIA. In conditions which demand an increased formation of one of the elements of the blood, there is a hyperplasia of its precursor cells in the bone marrow, e.g. *normoblastic hyperplasia* of the marrow after severe haemorrhage or in people who live at high altitudes, and *leucoblastic (myeloid) hyperplasia* in acute pyogenic infections. If all the marrow space is occupied (as in children in whom there is no reserve of fatty marrow), or if it is replaced by fibrous tissue (as in myelosclerosis), foci of haematopoiesis will be found in extramedullary sites like the spleen, liver, and lymph nodes. This myeloid differentiation is yet another example of the ease with which the multipotential stem cell diverts its development towards one particular line in response to a specific stimulus.

STORAGE HYPERPLASIA. This is of greatest importance in conditions of lipid excess; the RE cells proliferate to accommodate the load. Generalised disorders of lipid storage are called the *lipidoses*. The following are important:

Hyperlipoproteinaemia. Following prolonged hyperlipo-

proteinaemia there may be sufficient RE cell hyperplasia to cause moderate splenomegaly. Focal accumulations of fat-laden macrophages with occasional Touton giant cells may also be seen in the skin, and are called *xanthomata* (Fig. 30.3). These yellow-orange lesions are not tumours. They are found particularly on the extensor aspects of the limbs and

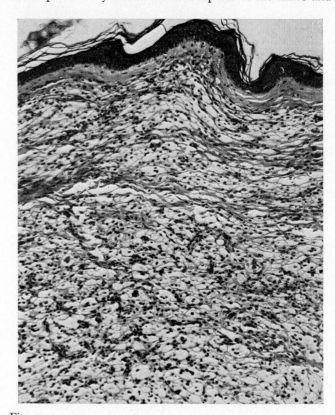

Figure 30.3
Xanthoma of skin. In the dermis there is an extensive accumulation of "foam cells". These are macrophages filled with lipid material (mostly cholesterol). In the histological process of clearing in chloroform, the fat is dissolved out of the cells, and this accounts for the appearance of clear cytoplasm surrounding the central nuclei. × 90.

on the eyelids. Plaques of xanthomata on the eyelids of elderly people are called *xanthelasma*; this common lesion may be encountered also in people who have normal plasma lipid levels.

Hypercholesterolaemia with splenomegaly is seen as a rare complication of diabetes mellitus (untreated) and prolonged obstructive jaundice. In addition, there are various types of *familial hyperlipoproteinaemia* which are described in Chapter 45. Xanthomata are common, and in some types there is splenomegaly and hepatomegaly due to the accumulation of lipid-laden macrophages.

In the other lipidoses, Gaucher's disease and Niemann-Pick disease, the RE cells are filled with abnormal lipids. Both conditions are usually inherited as autosomal recessive characteristics, and both are found most frequently in Jewish people.

Gaucher's disease.[13] In the common *adult form* of this disease, which runs a protracted course, there is a particularly massive accumulation of macrophages in the spleen which is enormously enlarged, and may lead to secondary hypersplenism (Fig. 30.4). The liver is also enlarged and the bone marrow is extensively involved, but the lymph nodes show much milder changes. Gaucher's disease is accompanied

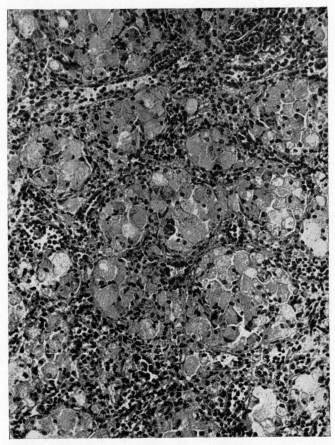

Figure 30.4
Gaucher's disease. In this section of spleen the red pulp contains large numbers of swollen macrophages. Their cytoplasm is full of abnormal lipid which produces a pale, reticulated appearance in histological section. × 160.

by a generalised haemosiderosis which gives rise to a brown pigmentation of the skin. A characteristic feature of the disease is the presence of wedge-shaped pingueculae (pigmented scleral thickenings) on each side of the corneae, and these too contain the characteristic cells. The *Gaucher cell* is a grossly enlarged macrophage about 50 μm in diameter with a pale fibrillary cytoplasm somewhat reminiscent of a spider's web. It is not vacuolated, and the usual fat stains are negative, but it is PAS-positive. The lipid contained in the Gaucher cell is a glucocerebroside, and it accumulates because of a deficiency

of glucocerebrosidase. Glucocerebroside is probably derived from effete white and red cells in the RES, and it is not surprising that it is here that the main accumulation of lipid is found. In the brain glucocerebroside is derived from gangliosides, which have a rapid turnover in infancy. It follows that central nervous involvement with severe mental retardation and death is a feature of the *acute neuropathic (infantile)* and *subacute neuropathic (juvenile)* forms of Gaucher's disease. Each type is probably determined by a separate recessive gene.

Niemann-Pick disease.[13] This is a more severe condition, which is usually fatal in infancy. The spleen, liver, lymph nodes, and bone marrow are all extensively infiltrated with lipid-laden macrophages, and the parenchymatous cells of the endocrine glands, lungs, bowel, and brain are also affected. Mental retardation is usually present, and about a quarter of the cases present the features of *amaurotic familial idiocy* (including the pathognomonic cherry-red spot in the macula of the retina).*

The cells are somewhat smaller than those of Gaucher's disease, and their cytoplasm is not wrinkled, but instead contains foamy droplets which stain positively with Sudan III and other fat stains. The lipids consist of cholesterol and its esters and a phosphatide called sphingomyelin. Haemosiderosis is not a feature of this disease.

Both Gaucher's disease and Niemann-Pick disease are examples of inherited disturbances of lipid metabolism associated with a specific enzyme defect. Variants of each probably exist, and there are many other rare lipid storage diseases known, some affecting only the central nervous system.*

Mucopolysaccharide storage. There are a number of rare diseases in which mucopolysaccharide accumulates in phagocytic cells as well as parenchymal tissue. The best known is Hurler's syndrome (gargoylism) (see p. 60).

HISTIOCYTOSIS-X. This non-committal title describes a triad of diseases, Letterer-Siwe disease, Hand-Schüller-Christian disease, and eosinophilic granuloma of bone, in which there are focal accumulations of large macrophages in various organs. These cells often contain cholesterol, especially in the more chronic forms of the condition, but this is apparently secondary and not a storage effect. The condition is normocholesterolaemic, and it is not an example of lipid-storage disease.

The most severe of the three disorders is *Letterer-Siwe disease*, which is usually a rapidly fatal malady of infancy. Destructive accumulations of RE cells are found in many organs, especially the spleen, bone marrow, liver, lymph nodes, intestinal mucosa, skin, and lungs. The cells are large

* *Amaurotic familial idiocy* is itself a fatal disease characterised by blindness, paralysis, and dementia. Only the nervous system is affected, and the ganglion cells show ballooning with ganglioside. In the infantile form (*Tay-Sachs disease*), which is confined to Jewish families, there is a characteristic cherry-red spot in the macula. Late infantile, juvenile, and adult forms are also recognised, and these are genetically and biochemically distinct.

and pale, and contain phagocytosed debris. There is usually a mild infiltration of neutrophil and eosinophil polymorphs among these active macrophages.

Hand-Schüller-Christian disease affects a somewhat older age group, and the histiocytic lesions are usually confined to the bones, especially those of the skull. A classical triad of manifestations is produced: defects in the membranous bones of the skull, exophthalmos, and diabetes insipidus. The mandible is often affected, and loosening of the teeth is a common symptom. Occasionally diffuse pulmonary involvement leads to the condition of cystic lung which may be complicated by a spontaneous pneumothorax. Involvement of the liver, spleen, and lymph nodes may also occur, but is much less conspicuous than in Letterer-Siwe disease.

Eosinophilic granuloma of bone is the most benign of the three diseases. It usually affects older children and young adults, and it is typically confined to one bone. It produces a painful bony swelling, which is seen radiologically as an area of destruction.

Histologically, in these last two diseases there are focal accumulations of foamy macrophages and giant cells with a variable admixture of eosinophils and polymorphs. The eosinophilia is particularly marked in eosinophilic granuloma of bone. The histiocytic lesions of Hand-Schüller-Christian disease are more proliferative than those of eosinophilic granuloma of bone. As the lesions heal, there is much dense fibrosis replacing the fat-laden macrophages.

The nature of the process underlying these three diseases is obscure. Although Letterer-Siwe disease has many of the features of a highly malignant neoplasm, its histology is rather like that of a chronic inflammatory lesion, and it sometimes merges into the Hand-Schüller-Christian syndrome, which is not clinically reminiscent of a tumour.

Neoplasia of the Stem Cell and its Derivatives[9, 14]

The neoplastic lesions of these cells are the *lymphomata* and the *tumours of the haemopoietic tissues*.

LYMPHOMATA.

These are all malignant, and since they vary considerably in their clinical course, many attempts have been made to classify them so that behaviour may be correlated with histological type. There is no agreed classification, and the nomenclature is confusing. Hence it is often impossible to compare the results of treatment in one centre with those in another.

The recommended classification is based on two features. The first is the type of cell involved in the neoplastic process, whether lymphocytic or reticulum cell. Hodgkin's disease is given a separate status because of special features which will be described later. The second important feature is whether the neoplastic cells are disposed in distinct nodules or whether they are arranged in a diffuse manner.[15] The nodular lymphomata have a better prognosis than that of their diffuse counterparts and were at one time grouped together as *giant follicular lymphomata*, or Brill-Symmers's disease, terms

which are not now in use. The nodular lymphomata may become diffuse as the disease progresses, but the diffuse ones never become nodular. The lesions therefore always tend to become more malignant.

The following lymphomata are described:[14, 15]
Reticulum-cell sarcoma—nodular or diffuse.
Lymphocytic lymphoma—nodular or diffuse. Each may be poorly, moderately, or well differentiated.
Lymphoma, mixed cell type—nodular or diffuse.
Hodgkin's disease. The subdivisions are described later.
Reticulum-cell sarcoma, also called reticulosarcoma and histiocytic lymphoma, is a disease predominantly of later life. It usually commences in one particular group of lymph nodes, but sometimes the tonsils or the small bowel are the sites of the primary lesion. It soon becomes systematised with splenic, hepatic, and bone-marrow infiltration. Deposits in the lungs, heart, and kidneys are not infrequent. The spread of this group of tumours to the lymph nodes and viscera is probably due both to lymphatic and blood-borne metastasis and to the development of new tumours in a field of growth that includes all the lymphoid tissues. Histologically there is complete obliteration of the normal architecture of the affected lymph nodes, which are massively infiltrated by large, pale reticulum cells. On the whole these are uniform in size and shape, but mitotic activity is usually pronounced. Foci of necrosis are usually present, and capsular invasion is a conspicuous feature. Sometimes the reticulum cells are pleomorphic with many giant cells among them, so that there may be a resemblance to Hodgkin's disease. It is sometimes difficult to distinguish between a reticulum-cell sarcoma and an anaplastic carcinoma. In some tumours the cells appear primitive and resemble stem cells. Pleomorphism is not marked and the tumour is called a *stem-cell sarcoma*.

Lymphocytic lymphoma. This tumour is commonly called a *lymphosarcoma*, a term which is deprecated by many experts in the field, but which may yet retain its place by virtue of common usage. The neoplastic cells can vary in differentiation and resemble mature lymphocytes (lymphocytic lymphosarcoma) or immature lymphoblasts (lymphoblastic lymphosarcoma). An intermediate group can also be recognised. The nodular variants of these tumours form the common type of the tumour previously called the *giant follicular lymphoma*.* See Fig. 30.7, p. 404.

Lymphocytic lymphoma is about twice as common as reticulum-cell sarcoma. It too affects an older age group predominantly, and its mode of presentation is similar to that of reticulum-cell sarcoma. Histologically the architecture of the lymph node is destroyed by sheets or nodules of fairly uniform lymphocytes, either well or poorly differentiated. Mitotic activity and capsular invasion are both important features. This condition is clearly very similar to reticulum-

* This has also been called "reticular lymphoma" in the past. This is a source of confusion because the reticular type of Hodgkin's disease described by Lukes is a tumour with a poor prognosis, see pp. 404–405.

cell sarcoma, and differs only in so far as the stem cell has differentiated into a neoplastic lymphocytic cell.

The histological appearance of the lymph nodes in chronic lymphatic leukaemia is indistinguishable from that of well-differentiated lymphocytic lymphoma. It is sometimes stated that mitotic activity is uncommon in leukaemia, and that capsular invasion is infrequent, but both these features are unreliable. The distinction between the two conditions rests entirely on an examination of the peripheral blood. In lymphoma the white-cell count should be within the normal range, whereas in chronic lymphatic leukaemia there is a great excess of circulating mature lymphocytes (see Chapter 50). A case of lymphoma occasionally develops the blood picture of chronic lymphatic leukaemia.

The *Burkitt tumour*[16] is a type of lymphocytic lymphoma found almost exclusively in children aged from 2–14 years. It has two distinctive features: (a) the lesions affect the jaws, ovaries, retroperitoneal lymph nodes, kidneys, and thyroid gland particularly, while the superficial nodes, liver, and spleen are much less severely affected, and (b) there is a great preponderance in low-lying, moist tropical areas. It was first described in Central Africa, and indeed its greatest incidence is in tropical Africa, but it is also found in New Guinea and Colombia, and is met with from time to time in Europe and North America in areas that are temperate or even cold.[17] Histologically it resembles other diffuse lymphocytic lymphomata; there are numerous palely-staining histiocytes amongst the lymphocytic cells producing a "starry-sky" appearance (Fig. 30.5), but this is seen in some cases of lymphomata that do not fall into the category of Burkitt's tumour, and so is not diagnostic.[18] The aetiology of the condition is discussed on p. 385. It is interesting that in endemic areas of Africa the incidence of acute childhood leukaemia is much less than in Europe. There seems to be a reciprocal relationship between Burkitt's tumour and acute leukaemia.

Lymphoma, mixed-cell type. The lymph-node architecture is destroyed by neoplastic lymphoblasts and reticulum cells. The reticulum cells are not markedly phagocytic, a point which helps to distinguish the lesion histologically from extreme degrees of reactive hyperplasia. Sternberg-Reed cells are absent, and the lesion does not have the pleomorphism so commonly seen in Hodgkin's disease.

Hodgkin's disease. This is the commonest of this group of neoplasms, occurring at all ages, especially amongst young and middle-aged adults. It usually starts in a single group of lymph nodes, often the cervical or mediastinal ones, and after a variable time it becomes generalised to implicate the lymphoreticular tissues of the body including the spleen, liver, and bone marrow. There may be little constitutional disturbance at first, but later cachexia occurs and there may be considerable pyrexia. A more acute variety affects the abdominal nodes and spleen primarily, and manifests itself as a "pyrexia of unknown origin", which is characteristically intermittent, the *Pel-Ebstein fever*. Abdominal Hodgkin's

disease runs a rapid course and is usually fatal within six months.

Other noteworthy features of Hodgkin's disease are a distressing generalised pruritus, sometimes accompanied by skin infiltrations of a type resembling mycosis fungoides. In some cases the ingestion of alcohol causes severe pain in the lesions, especially in the bones. There is no satisfactory explanation for this effect, which is also encountered in other types of cancer but much less often.[19]

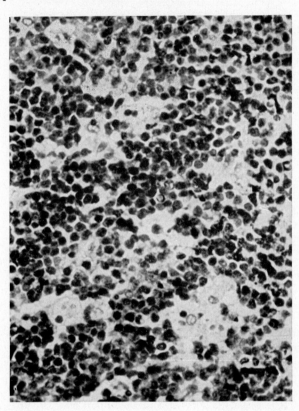

Figure 30.5
Burkitt's tumour. Note the uniform lymphocytes, interspersed among which there are large histiocytes. This is the "starry-sky appearance" stressed in Burkitt's tumour, though seen in other lymphocytic lymphomata also. × 400.

Histologically the normal structure of the lymph node is replaced by a pleomorphic mass of cells that comprises (a) reticulum cells, (b) lymphocytes, (c) histiocytes, (d) neutrophil and eosinophil polymorphs, and (e) plasma cells. Of these the most important is the reticulum cell, for it is the essential neoplastic element. Many of these cells vary in size and shape, and there is mitotic activity among them. Bizarre giant forms are present, including the pathognomonic *Sternberg-Reed cell*, a giant neoplastic reticulum cell with double mirror-image nuclei having vesicular chromatin and a prominent nucleolus (Fig. 30.6). There is often a considerable excess of mature lymphocytes, especially in the early stages and in those types which are least malignant. In progressive

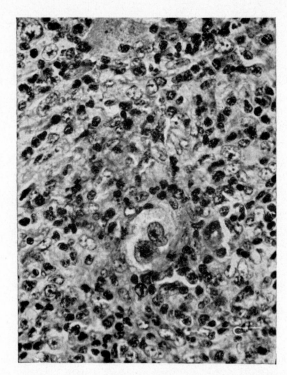

Figure 30.6
Hodgkin's disease. In the centre of the field there is a binucleate Sternberg-Reed cell. It is surrounded by reticulum cells and lymphocytes. × 350.

disease the lymphocytic element is crowded out by reticulum cells, and this may account for the impaired cell-mediated immunity seen in the condition. This impairs delayed-type hypersensitivity and homograft rejection. The lymphocytic depletion is important in causing death, for these patients are very susceptible to opportunistic infection. Thus lymphocytic depletion is associated with a poor prognosis.

There is usually a variable infiltration of plasma cells and polymorphs, amongst which eosinophils are often prominent. Sometimes there is extensive necrosis, and often there is fibrosis. Capsular invasion may occur, and considerable infiltration is seen in the abdominal type of disease where the retroperitoneal tissues may be diffusely involved.

Classification of Hodgkin's disease.[20-23] The important current histopathological classification was devised by Lukes,[20, 21] and later simplified into four categories at a conference held at Rye, New York in 1965:[24]

(*a*) *Lymphocytic and histiocytic predominance* (Lukes). In this group either lymphocytes or histiocytes may predominate or there may be an equal mixture. Of each type there are nodular and diffuse variants. There are few plasma cells or eosinophils and typical Sternberg-Reed cells are scanty. There is no fibrosis or necrosis. The diffuse lymphocyte-predominating type corresponds to the old "paragranuloma".[25, 26] This whole group is classified by the Rye conference as "Hodgkin's disease, lymphocytic predominance", but there

seems to be some virtue in retaining Lukes's subdivision, since the nodular variants have an appreciably better prognosis than do the diffuse types. The remaining four headings are those of the Rye conference:

(*b*) *Nodular sclerosis.* Collagenous bands circumscribe nodules of lymphomatous tissue containing Sternberg-Reed cells. There is either a lymphocytic or a mixed lymphocyte-histiocyte predominance. In advanced disease eosinophils and neutrophils are present, and fibrosis increases.

(*c*) *Mixed cellularity type.* Histiocytes, neutrophils, eosinophils, plasma cells, and a variable number of lymphocytes are present. There are numerous Sternberg-Reed cells, a moderate degree of fibrosis, and sometimes a little necrosis. This is the classical picture of Hodgkin's disease and was previously described as "Hodgkin's granuloma".

(*d*) *Lymphocytic depletion type.* This group is divided into two types by Lukes. In the *diffuse fibrosis type* there is diffuse fibrosis with necrosis and very few cells, those remaining being nearly all Sternberg-Reed cells. It represents the final stage of the disease. In the second type, described as

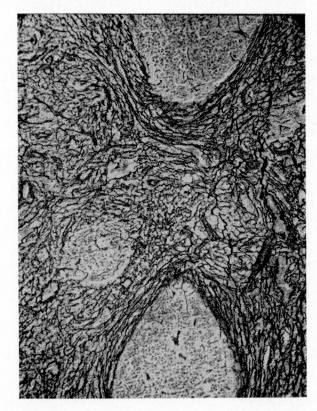

Figure 30.7
Nodular type of lymphocytic lymphoma. The lymph node has been stained by a silver impregnation method to demonstrate its pattern of reticulin fibres. The abnormal follicles are surrounded by compressed reticulin fibres, but do not themselves contain any. Normal germinal centres are not surrounded by compressed reticulin. × 55. *(From Stewart, P. D. (1963), J. roy. Army med. Cps., 109, 22)*

reticular by Lukes, there is a heavy infiltration of Sternberg-Reed cells, with or without other cells, but always with few lymphocytes. If the Sternberg-Reed cells are pleomorphic and atypical this group corresponds to the "Hodgkin's sarcoma" of the Jackson and Parker classification.[25] This term, together with granuloma, and paragranuloma of the same classification are all now obsolete.

The prognosis is best in the lymphocytic predominance grade, in which Lukes found a 43·5 per cent 15-year survival rate in nodular disposition and 27·5 in diffuse disposition. The nodular sclerosis grade had a 15·4 per cent 15-year survival rate, mixed cellularity 10·3 per cent, and lymphocytic depletion less than 5 per cent.

It is evident that Hodgkin's disease is a tumour of the reticulum cell, which differentiates towards fibre formation. As the disease progresses lymphocytic depletion intensifies, and the later grades are the most malignant. The nodular sclerosing type seems to be particularly common in the mediastinal lymph nodes, while the lymphocytic predominance and mixed cellularity types do not usually affect the chest markedly.[27] The granulocytic, histiocytic, and plasma cell reactions are apparently secondary phenomena.

Course

A clinical staging based on the Rye conference is used in Hodgkin's disease:[28]

> Stage I. Disease limited to a single lymph-node group.
> Stage II. Disease limited to two or more lymph-node groups either above or below the diaphragm.
> Stage III. Disease limited to lymph nodes but affecting groups both above and below the diaphragm.
> Stage IV. Multiple or disseminated foci of involvement of one or more extranodal organs or tissues with or without lymph-node involvement.

These stagings were originally established following the introduction of lymphangiography as a means of diagnosing nodal involvement. Laparotomies were also often performed, and the spleen removed and examined. Cases in which there is involvement of the spleen but not any other extranodal organ are now included in group III and given a subscript (IIIs). Each stage may usefully be subdivided into two groups, either A or B depending upon the absence or presence respectively of systemic manifestations (fever, night sweats, or pruritus).

In stage I disease there is a 40 per cent 15-year remission rate following adequate radiotherapy. Lymphangiography is an important investigation in assessing the extent of the disease. Once the condition becomes generalised the prognosis is very bad; eventually the disease becomes unresponsive to radiotherapy and cytotoxic drugs, and death occurs.

The lymphocytic predominance and nodular sclerosing types of Hodgkin's disease have the best prognosis. Follicular lymphocytic lymphoma also has a fair prognosis, over half the cases surviving for 5 years.

Localised types of "lymphoma" can involve such single organs as the bowel, stomach, lungs, and bones.* These lesions may have the histological features of any one of the three neoplasms mentioned above. They are important conditions to be aware of, because the prognosis is surprisingly good if the affected parts are resected and the areas then treated with radiotherapy. The follicular "lymphoma" of the rectum appears to be completely benign, and may be regarded as reactive rather than neoplastic.[31]

The uncommon dermatological condition *mycosis fungoides*[32] has also been alluded to. It usually starts as an extensive intractable pruritic dermatitis which is followed by the appearance of many soft, necrotic tumours on the affected skin. Sometimes the tumours appear without prior dermatitis. The condition responds well to radiotherapy, but in due course systematisation usually occurs. It is a lymphoma primarily affecting the skin. Some cases are clearly related to Hodgkin's disease.

The morbid anatomy of these four conditions is basically similar. In lymphosarcoma and reticulum-cell sarcoma the affected lymph nodes are replaced by white, soft tumour which infiltrates into the surrounding tissues. Similar deposits are found in the spleen, liver, and other organs. In Hodgkin's disease the lymph nodes are firmer and have a pinkish-yellow coloration. Deposits of Hodgkin's disease are sometimes rather diffuse in distribution. The spleen may be uniformly seeded with yellowish-white deposits, a few millimetres in diameter, and the appearance of the cut surface may closely resemble that of "hardbake" (almond toffee). Nevertheless, *hardbake spleen* is an exceptional appearance in Hodgkin's disease, and usually the deposits occur as large discrete masses indistinguishable from the other diseases of this type.

In practice it is not possible to distinguish between these conditions without the aid of the microscope, and considerable specialised knowledge is often needed to arrive at a correct diagnosis. The most difficult problem is to distinguish between reactive hyperplasia and one of these neoplastic conditions. From the patient's point of view the decision is one of life and death. The most important deciding factors in such cases are an assessment of the general structure of the lymph node and a detailed study of the proliferating reticulum cells.

Destruction of the normal architecture, such as loss of sinus structure or loss of definition between cortex and medulla, is an important feature of lymphoma and may affect a focal area or be diffuse and affect the whole node. In the nodular lymphomata, the nodules tend to be uniform in size, poorly delineated, and to occupy all parts of the node.

---

* A peculiar round-cell tumour of bone is *Ewing's tumour*. It is not osteogenic. It causes a raising-up of the periosteum. Its nature is obscure; some examples may be reticulum-cell sarcomata of bone or else metastases of an adrenal neuroblastoma or anaplastic carcinoma. It tends to spread to many bones, and is accompanied by marked fever.[29] [30]

Normal germinal centres, on the other hand, are situated in the cortex, are sharply outlined by lymphocytes, and do not compress the surrounding reticulin framework (see Fig. 30.7). Invasion of the capsule and the pericapsular fat points to lymphoma, but some infiltration by normal small lymphocytes is often seen in reactive hyperplasia. It is evident that it can be extremely difficult to interpret the histological features of some lymph nodes, and close clinico-pathological correlation is necessary (see also p. 301). Sometimes it is best to admit one's inadequacy and await events. In practice such lymph nodes are sent to experts in the field, and it is by the detailed follow-up of these cases that our knowledge of the natural history of these diseases becomes broadened. The recently acquired information about the more benign types of Hodgkin's disease is a triumph of this type.

Furthermore other new entities have been recognised. *Sinus histiocytosis with lymphadenopathy*[33] is a benign condition with fever and lymphadenopathy in which massive proliferation of sinus histiocytes can mimic a lymphoma histologically. "*Chronic pseudolymphomatous lymphadenopathy*"[34] associated with lymphadenopathy, hepatosplenomegaly, Coombs-positive anaemia, hypergammaglobulinaemia, and thrombocytopenia in childhood may likewise mimic lymphoma histologically, although its clinical course is benign.

Neoplasms of the Haematopoietic System

The commonest neoplasms of this group involve the white-cell precursors and are called *leukaemias*. Sometimes the neoplastic process affects the most primitive white cells, e.g. the myeloblasts, lymphoblasts, or even the haemocytoblast itself, and the marrow is crowded out with these cells. This condition is called acute leukaemia. On the other hand, the proliferation may affect the intermediate myelocytic cells, when chronic myeloid leukaemia will ensue. The relationship between lymphocytic lymphoma and chronic lymphatic leukaemia has already been mentioned.

Sometimes the neoplastic process is focused primarily on the erythroblastic series, and *polycythaemia vera* results. Rarely, a type of leukaemia occurs (erythroblastic leukaemia, or Di Guglielmo's disease). A similar megakaryocytic neoplasia leads to the rare *haemorrhagic thrombocythaemia*. All these conditions are considered in detail in the chapters devoted to disorders of the blood. They are all manifested by haematological abnormalities, but in some of the acute ("aleukaemic") leukaemias abnormal cells may be very scanty in the peripheral blood.

Haematological abnormalities may certainly occur in Hodgkin's disease and allied disorders, but they are never primary. If they occur, they are due to secondary processes, e.g. hypersplenism causing haemolytic anaemia, or bone-marrow involvement leading to leuco-erythroblastic anaemia.

Multiple myeloma is a neoplasm of the bone marrow affecting the plasma cells primarily. Only rarely do these neoplastic myeloma cells enter the general circulation.

The following table summarises the main proliferative processes of the stem cell and its derivatives.

Cell	Hyperplasia	Neoplasia
Reticulum Cell.	Infection.	Reticulum-cell sarcoma. Hodgkin's disease.
Lymphocyte.	Infection.	Lymphocytic lymphoma and chronic lymphatic leukaemia.
RE Cell.	Infection. Storage. Idiopathic histiocytosis.	
Blood-forming Cells.	Leucoblastic hyperplasia in infection.	Leukaemia. Polycythaemia vera.
	Normoblastic hyperplasia in hypoxia.	Haemorrhagic thrombocythaemia.
Plasma Cell.	Infection.	Multiple myeloma.

Other lymphomata. Although the majority of conditions in which there is a malignant proliferation of the stem cell and its derivatives can be placed in one of the categories already described, there are a number of rare diseases which appear to be separate entities. For these the concept of malignant reticulosis can be retained. *Waldenström's macroglobulinaemia* is one such example, for there is a widespread infiltration of the bone marrow, lymph nodes, spleen, and liver by cells which resemble lymphocytes but which bear some of the features of plasma cells, and the disease does not closely resemble multiple myeloma. (see p. 552). Another example is the rare *histiocytic medullary reticulosis*.[35] Clinically this is characterised by an acute onset of fever, lymphadenopathy, hepato-splenomegaly, and jaundice. The course is relentless and death occurs within a few months. Severe anaemia, leucopenia, and thrombocytopenia are other features. Histologically, there is a widespread proliferation of atypical histiocytes in the liver, spleen, lymph nodes, and elsewhere. The cells infiltrate the tissues but do not destroy the parenchyma, as is seen in Hodgkin's disease. A characteristic of the cells is that they actively phagocytose red cells (erythrophagocytosis). A benign varient has also been described.[36]

Incidence

The Registrar-General's figures for England and Wales reveal that 3 716 men and 3 189 women died of neoplastic diseases of the lymphatic and haematopoietic tissues in 1969. Of this about a fifth was due to lymphocytic lymphoma and reticulum-cell sarcoma, and a seventh to Hodgkin's disease.

A quarter of the deaths were attributed to acute leukaemia, and a little over a sixth each to chronic leukaemia and multiple myeloma.

There was a slight male predominance, except in multiple myeloma, where there was a slight preponderance of women.

The brunt was borne by the older age groups (from 45 years onwards), except in the case of (*a*) acute leukaemia, which was remarkably evenly distributed over all age groups; it killed 343 children under the age of 10 years, and (*b*) Hodgkin's disease, which was evenly distributed over all groups over the age of 20 years.

Apart from the carcinomata, these neoplasms cause most of the mortality from malignant disease. They are also the most responsive to ionising radiations and cytotoxic drugs.

REFERENCES

1. GALL, E. A. (1958). *Annals of the New York Academy of Sciences*, **73**, 120.
2. YOFFEY, J. M. and COURTICE, F. C. (1956). In *Lymphatics, Lymph and Lymphoid Tissue*, 2nd edn, p. 404. London: Arnold.
3. Leading Article (1973). *Lancet*, i, 139.
4. GOWANS, J. L., GESNER, B. M. and McGREGOR, D. D. (1961). In *Biological Activity of the Leucocyte*, p. 32. Ciba Foundation Study Group, No. 10. London: Churchill.
5. PORTER, K. A. and COOPER, E. H. (1962). *Lancet*, ii, 317.
6. FORD, C. E., MICKLEM, H. S. and OGDEN, D. A. (1968). *Lancet*, i, 621.
7. WILLIS, R. A. (1962). *The Borderland of Embryology and Pathology*, 2nd edn, p. 577. London: Butterworths.
8. VAN FURTH, R. *et al.* (1972). *Bulletin of the World Health Organisation*, **46**, 845.
9. HARRISON, C. V. (1966). In *Recent Advances in Pathology*, 8th edn, p. 207. London: Churchill.
10. HARTSOCK, R. J. (1968). *Cancer (Philadelphia)*, **21**, 632.
11. LEVAN, P. and BIERMAN, S. M. (1962). *Archives of Dermatology*, **86**, 254.
12. LINDQVIST, T. (1957). *Acta Medica Scandinavica*, **158**, 131.
13. STANBURY, J. B., WYNGAARDEN, J. B. and FREDRICKSON, D. S. (1972). Editors. *The Metabolic Basis of Inherited Disease*, 3rd edn, p. 730 *et seq.* New York: McGraw-Hill.
14. ANDERSON, W. A. D. (1971). Editor. *Pathology*, 6th edn, vol. 2, p. 1336 *et seq.* St. Louis: Mosby.
15. RAPPAPORT, H., WINTER, W. J. and HICKS, E. B. (1956). *Cancer (Philadelphia)*, **9**, 792.
16. HARRIS, R. J. C. (1964). *British Medical Bulletin*, **20**, 149.
17. Leading Article (1965). *Lancet*, ii, 1225.
18. Editorial (1963). *New England Journal of Medicine*, **269**, 982.
19. JAMES, A. H. (1960). *Quarterly Journal of Medicine*, **29**, 47.
20. LUKES, R. J. (1963). *American Journal of Roentgenology*, **90**, 944.
21. LUKES, R. J. and BUTLER, J. J. (1966). *Cancer Research*, **26**, 1063.
22. LUKES, R. J., BUTLER, J. J. and HICKS, E. B. (1966). *Cancer (Philadelphia)*, **19**, 317.
23. Leading Article (1969). *British Medical Journal*, i, 138.
24. LUKES, R. J. (1966). *Cancer Research*, **26**, 1311.
25. JACKSON, H. and PARKER, F. (1944). *New England Journal of Medicine*, **230**, 1; and **231**, 35 and 639.
26. DAWSON, P. J. and HARRISON, C. V. (1961). *Journal of Clinical Pathology*, **14**, 219.
27. KAPLAN, H. S. (1972). *Proceedings of the Royal Society of Medicine*, **65**, 62.
28. AISENBERG, A. C. (1973). *New England Journal of Medicine*, **288**, 883.
29. BAIRD, R. J. and KRAUSE, V. W. (1963). *Canadian Journal of Surgery*, **6**, 136.
30. MARSDEN, H. B. and STEWARD, J. K. (1964). *Journal of Clinical Pathology*, **17**, 411.
31. HARRISON, C. V. (1966). In *Recent Advances in Pathology*, 8th edn, p. 216, *loc. cit.*
32. EPSTEIN, H. E. *et al.* (1972). *Medicine (Baltimore)*, **51**, 61.
33. ROSAI, J. and DORFMAN, R. F. (1969). *Archives of Pathology*, **87**, 63.
34. CANALE, V. C. and SMITH, C. H. (1967). *Journal of Pediatrics*, **70**, 891.
35. GREENBERG, E. *et al.* (1962). *Proceedings of Staff Meetings of the Mayo Clinic*, **37**, 271.
36. Leading Article (1973). *Lancet*, i, 139.
37. Leading Article (1971). *Lancet*, ii, 304.

Chapter 31. The Effect of Ionising Radiation

The ever-increasing use of radioactive substances both in industry and medicine has made the study of radiation damage of great practical importance. On the human body its effects vary from local tissue necrosis to genetic damage, cancer, and death. With such a perplexing array of effects, it is little wonder that the ionising radiations are regarded with fear and amazement. As their physical nature is so well understood, it might be expected that the mechanisms involved in the damage which they produce would be equally explicable. It is important to understand why this is not so.

The ionising radiations produce changes in the structure of the atoms through which they pass. These subatomic lesions produce effects at a chemical level. If these chemicals are part of a living cell, a "biochemical lesion" similar in nature to that described in Chapter 4 is produced. The morphological and biochemical sequelae will be recognised as *radiation damage*, while the sum-total of the damage to all the cells and tissues will amount to the effects of *total body irradiation*. It is therefore understandable that with so many steps there are many gaps in our knowledge of the mechanism of radiation damage.

It is, however, no more of a mystery than is the damage produced by other agents. Formaldehyde causes mutations, staphylococci produce tissue necrosis, and arsenic initiates cancer. These changes are as mysterious as those of radiation damage, and differ only in that the exciting agents are more tangible.

Radiation damage will therefore firstly be described at a physical level; the chemical changes which it induces will then be examined. The effects on the living cell should be analysed in the light of this knowledge: the result of total body radiation represents the summation of damage to each cell and tissue.

Physical Considerations

In order to understand the primary effect of ionising radiations, the nature of the rays and the atoms through which they pass must be understood: these are considered in Appendix III.

The energy absorbed by the tissue appears partly as heat, but this is of negligible quantity. The *ions* and *free radicals* are of much greater importance, and are presumed to be responsible for much of the radiation damage. Another effect which has been less studied is the *excitation of molecules*: this change renders the molecule unstable.

Chemical Considerations

There are two ways in which a chemical change may be induced in a molecule by radiation. The absorbed energy in the molecule itself may produce either ionisation or excitation, which then results in a chemical change. This is *direct action*. Alternatively a chemical change may occur due to the action of free radicals or ions produced in other adjacent molecules, e.g. OH˙ from water. This is *indirect action*. Which of these actions is the more important in biological systems is of some significance. With indirect action chemical protection against radiation damage is possible, because the free radicals or ions could be intercepted before they attack vital molecules. With direct action protection is much less likely; it is, however, still theoretically possible, because a molecule could transmit its energy to the protector and thereby avoid any change within itself.

Both direct and indirect actions have been shown to affect viruses and many enzymes, but, whereas viruses are more easily killed by direct action, the indirect effect is more important in the inactivation of enzymes.

Effect of Radiation on Chemicals of Biological Importance

Enzymes. Although there is no doubt that ionising radiations can inactivate enzymes *in vitro*, the dose necessary is generally in excess of that needed to damage a cell. Some enzymes which depend upon a sulphydryl group, —SH, are oxidised to the inactive disulphide form, (—S—S—):

$$-SH + HS- + 2OH˙ = -S-S- + 2H_2O$$

However, there seems no reason why this should not be reduced back to an active form in the body, for the addition of cellular material protects a solution of an enzyme from radiation inactivation.

Many enzymatic changes have been observed in irradiated cells, but it appears that they are the effect of cell damage rather than its cause. Thus, although a biochemical lesion may be postulated, we are quite ignorant of its nature.

DNA. The viscous solution of DNA is liquefied by radiation, and a direct effect is thought to be the most important factor; the changes produced are complex, and do not seem to be related to the observed cell damage. Thus, densely ionising rays, like α-particles, are very effective in producing cell damage, but less so in degrading DNA.

Effects Upon the Cell[1]

Although it would be desirable to explain the cellular damage in terms of the known physico-chemical changes, it must be admitted that this is not yet possible. The effect of ionising radiation on cell cultures has been studied extensively. Suitable cell-lines can be plated in a Petri dish so that each cell produces a clone which is visible to the naked eye. If the culture has been irradiated previously, the effect on the reproductive activity of the cells can be assessed. Cells actually in mitosis tend to be less adherent to glass and may be separated from the remainder. By this and other techniques it is possible to obtain cultures in which the majority of the cells are at the same stage in the mitotic cycle. Hence the effect of irradiation at different stages of the cycle can be studied.

The effects of irradiation on cells may be summarised:

1. Immediate death of the cell occurs with very heavy dosage, i.e. 10 000 r or more. This effect occurs regardless of the stage of mitosis and is called *interphase death*. It is also seen in very sensitive cells, e.g. small lymphocytes, with moderate dosage.

2. DNA synthesis is inhibited.

3. Mitosis is delayed, usually due to a prolongation of the G_2 phase.

4. DNA synthesis may occur unrelated to mitosis, so that giant-cell forms are produced.

5. When mitosis does occur in irradiated cells, abnormalities such as chromosome breaks may occur. At this stage the cell may die. Nevertheless, a cell may go through several mitotic cycles before death finally occurs.

6. The growth rate may be slowed down even in sublethally irradiated cells.

7. Fractionated doses of radiation do not produce a strictly cumulative effect. Hence there appear to exist intracellular mechanisms whereby radiation damage can be reversed or "repaired".

8. The sensitivity of cells to damage varies according to the stage in the mitotic cycle when the radiation is given. Maximum sensitivity occurs in most cell-types during mitosis itself. They are relatively resistant during most of the G_1 phase, but radiosensitivity returns during the late G_1 and early synthetic (S) phases. They are most resistant during the late S and early G_2 phases (see pp. 26–7).

Two main theories have been put forward to explain cellular damage.

The target theory supposes that the injury is due to damage at some specific sensitive spot in the cell. This may be caused either by direct or indirect action. If the action is assumed to be direct, and if one ionisation is assumed to cause damage, the size of the target can be calculated. In respect of virus inactivation the calculated target size and the observed size of the organisms tally remarkably well. In larger cells, however, the evidence for there being a sensitive target is much less convincing. Attractive as it may be to visualise a chromo-some or centromere as a target, there is little to support the theory.

The poison theory proposes that the ionisation leads to the production of poisonous substances—usually powerful oxidising agents, which then cause the damage. Such substances are known to appear. For instance, with α-particles the closely adjacent OH· radicals unite to form H_2O_2. Alpha-radiation has thus been likened to multiple jets of hydrogen peroxide.

Effect on intracellular barriers. It has been suggested that ionising radiation may upset the highly complex system of barriers in the cytoplasm. In this way enzymes may be released (presumably from lysosomes), and cause cell damage.

Effect on mitosis. As noted above mitosis is delayed, and in tissue-culture systems even a dose as small as 35 r will produce this effect.

When mitosis does occur, there may be various abnormalities. The chromosomes may appear to be "sticky", and abnormalities in spindle-formation occur. A very characteristic effect is the production of breaks in the chromosomes or chromatids. Figure 31.1 represents a break in two chromatids. The small fragments unite to form a small nuclear

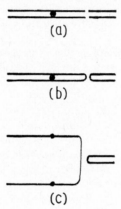

(a)

(b)

(c)

Figure 31.1
Diagram to show the effects of a break in two chromatids. The broken ends unite as shown in (b), and at anaphase (c) a bridge is produced when the centromere divides and the chromatids attempt to separate.

body, which, not being attached to the spindle, persists as a separate unit. A micronucleus formed in this way is very characteristic of irradiated tissue. The larger fragments may unite and form a bridge which interferes with the separation of chromatids at anaphase.

Although the chromosome abnormalities are striking, their significance is not clear. In some of the cells the abnormality is severe enough to cause death. Although at first sight the breaks would seem to indicate a visible change which might coincide with a genetic mutation, this is in fact unlikely. Thus, for the same total dose the number of chromosomal abnormalities increases with the dose rate; on the other hand, dose rate does not influence the number of genetic mutations.

Relative sensitivity of cells. *The law of Bergonié and Tribondeau*:* "The sensitivity of cells to irradiation is in direct proportion to their reproductive activity, and inversely proportional to their degree of differentiation." This "law" states in general terms the observed sensitivity of the various cells of the body—it does not explain the difference in sensitivity. The germinal cells of the ovary are most sensitive. Then follow the spermatogonia, lymphocytes, the erythropoietic and myeloid marrow cells, and the intestinal epithelium. Least sensitive are the neurones and muscle cells.

The differences in the sensitivity of various species are not understood. Thus, the LD_{50} for paramoecium is about 300 000 r, for amoebae 100 000 r, *Esch. coli* 5 000 r, frogs 700 r, mice 400–650 r, pigs 275 r, and man 450–500 r.

Effect of oxygen tension.[2] In the absence of oxygen the effect of x-rays and γ-rays is diminished by a factor of 2–3. The hypoxia must be present during the period of irradiation. The effect is invariable, i.e. it protects against all radiation effects in all species. This is strong evidence in favour of the importance of the indirect effect on biological systems: the formation of $HO_2^{\cdot}$ is described in Appendix III.

This oxygen effect is of great importance when considering radiotherapy for cancer. The centre of a nodule of tumour is almost certainly hypoxic and its cells are therefore protected.

One way of overcoming this is to allow the patient to breathe oxygen under pressure. The results of this type of treatment are encouraging with some tumours, e.g. carcinoma of the nose and mouth, but few well-controlled series have been reported and the possible benefit of hyperbaric oxygen and radiotherapy is still under review.[3] One of the main difficulties is the technical problem of giving oxygen under pressure. Thus the patient must be given a general anaesthetic, and the dose–fractionation scheme has to be modified. An alternative approach would be to render the whole body hypoxic (possibly under hypothermia) and then give a larger dose of radiation. The oxygen effect is not nearly so marked with the densely ionising α-particles and neutrons.

Effect Upon Cells and Tissues in the Intact Animal

This most important aspect of radiology is also the most difficult. A feature which is outstanding is the remarkable *delay* in the appearance of radiation damage. The initial damage caused by radiation must be almost instantaneous, and yet the effect may not be apparent for days, weeks, or even months. Thus, if a single dose of 5 500 r is applied to a small circular area of guinea-pig skin, erythema does not appear until about the tenth day, and necrosis not until after the third week.[4]

Experiments with amphibians help to explain this phenomenon. Frogs can be given a dose of radiation which will kill

* Translated by Spear, F. G. (1953), "Radiation and living Cells". London: Chapman and Hall.

them within six weeks. If the irradiated animals are kept at 5°C, they remain alive for several months, but on being warmed up, die within six weeks like the control animals kept at normal temperature.[5] These and similar experiments on hibernating animals indicate that radiation damage is manifest only when cells are active. This lends strong support to the concept that a biochemical lesion is produced. Such a lesion is not in itself harmful, but produces effects when cellular activity commences. Unfortunately, we are ignorant of the nature of this biochemical lesion even assuming that it exists. The fact that radiation damage is manifested only after cellular activity helps to explain the differing radiosensitivities of various tissues.

It may also explain why several phases of damage sometimes occur, inasmuch as different tissues have different rates of division and metabolic activity.[4] Irradiated tissue therefore shows changes which persist for many weeks or even months and have the characteristics of chronic inflammation even after a single exposure.

Effect of irradiation on skin. Following a single exposure to x-rays, an erythema may appear after 24 hours but is fleeting and may be missed. It reappears after about 10 days, and there are all the features of acute inflammation. Pigmentation is increased, giving the skin a red, dusky hue. With heavy dosage, necrosis of tissue occurs, collagen becomes "fibrinoid", vessels thrombose, ulceration results, and subsequent healing is slow. Before necrosis occurs the epidermis shows degenerative changes, including the formation of giant cells and micronuclei (Fig. 31.2). Even when healed, ulceration may recur after trivial injury.

With lower dosage a smouldering chronic inflammation occurs. There is a proliferation of fibroblasts often with the production of *bizarre giant forms*. These are presumably produced by the failure of cell division to keep pace with DNA synthesis. Both the newly-formed and the original collagen becomes hyalinised, and the blood vessels show endarteritis obliterans. Although the tissue becomes devascularised, thin-walled telangiectases may develop. The epithelium becomes atrophic and lacks the normal rete ridges. The hair follicles and accessory glands are much more sensitive to radiation than is the less active surface epithelium. With a dosage above 700 r these structures undergo necrosis, and do not regenerate. In chronic radiodermatitis the skin appendages are therefore absent.

Thus ionising radiation produces a type of chronic inflammatory reaction with ensuing dense fibrosis. In healing wounds radiation *delays* the growth of granulation tissue. Even doses as low as 500 r retard the growth in a rabbit ear-chamber. The delaying effect on wound contraction is described on p. 105.

One remarkable effect is that the adjacent normal skin has a protective action. Thus in experimental irradiation the ulcer produced by 5 500 r is not as large as the area treated. The explanation is not known, but advantage is taken of this in clinical radiotherapy. The use of a grid helps prevent

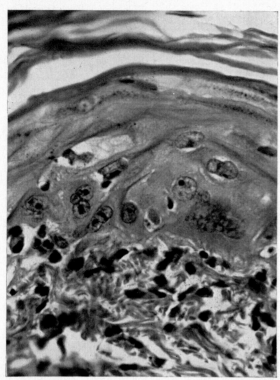

Figure 31.2
Abnormal changes in epithelium following x-irradiation. This section was taken from a guinea-pig 16 days after a heavy irradiation. A multinucleate mass of epithelial cells is shown. On the left there is a cell with two nuclei and a micronucleus in between them. ×480. *(From Mellett, P. G., Walter, J. B. and Houghton, L. E. (1960), Brit. J. exp. Path., **41**, 160)*

skin damage, and enables a larger tumour-dose to be given than would otherwise be possible (see p. 415).

Effect of irradiation on other tissues. This has been less intensively studied. In the *testis* the seminiferous tubules undergo atrophy following the destruction of their spermatogonia. Mature sperms are not affected, so that sterility does not develop immediately. Irradiation of the *lungs* produces inflammatory changes which culminate in fibrosis:[6] this is sometimes seen as a complication of radiotherapy for breast cancer. The condition is characterised clinically by marked dyspnoea. The *kidney* shows a progressive glomerular fibrosis, and malignant hypertension may develop. Irradiation of *bone* produces changes which may persist for years, and are punctuated by episodes of painful "radionecrosis". Doses of over 1 000 r inhibit growth at the epiphysis, an effect which should be remembered when using radiotherapy in children. The *intestine*, both large and small, is readily damaged by radiation, and ulceration, haemorrhage, perforation, and the late formation of fistulae, adhesions, and strictures are well-recognised complications of radiotherapy for cancer of the cervix uteri. If the *spinal cord* is irradiated, damage, probably due to ischaemia, may develop 2–4 years later; it can lead to quadriplegia.

An unusual complication of radiotherapy is anuria due to the *blockage of the renal tubules* by uric-acid crystals. This follows the treatment of a large, highly sensitive tumour, and is due to the release of nucleoprotein following necrosis of the tumour cells.

When considering the action of radiation on any tissue, two main effects must be borne in mind. These have been called "direct" and "indirect", but the terms are best avoided, as they have already been used in another connexion (see p. 408). The *primary effect* is directly due to the irradiation of the tissue concerned; the *secondary effect* is due to damage to an adjacent tissue. For instance, epidermis irradiated on its own is more resistant than as part of the intact skin. Presumably therefore the epithelial damage is partly secondary to dermal injury. It seems likely that this damage is due to vascular occlusion;[5] indeed, some authorities attribute much of the beneficial effect of radiotherapy in cancer to this mechanism.

TOTAL BODY IRRADIATION[7]

During the last decade the applications of atomic science in both civilian and military fields have brought to the fore the hazards of total body irradiation in man. A mass of data is available about the effects on animals, but since few human beings have been subjected to total body irradiation, our knowledge about its effects in man is scanty. Many of the Japanese survivors of the Hiroshima and Nagasaki explosions were subjected to total body irradiation, but the exact dosage was unknown, and their exposure was probably uneven due to the shielding effects of buildings, etc. Furthermore, the presence of burns and other injuries complicated the clinical picture.[8]

In the H-bomb fall-out on the Marshall Islands the situation was complicated by β-radiation damage to the skin, and in the various civilian accidents the victims have usually been subjected to both γ-ray and neutron bombardment.[9]

Our information is therefore extremely incomplete, and it is hardly surprising that even the LD_{50} dose is not known with any degree of certainty; 450 r is the figure generally quoted, but the actual level obviously depends upon many factors, the type of radiation being not the least important.

It is convenient to describe the effect of total body irradiation under two headings—those occurring during the first two months (immediate), and those occurring later.

Immediate Effects

These depend largely upon the dose received. Although no hard-and-fast rules can be given, three groups of cases may be recognised:

Very high dosage (over 5 000 r single exposure). The first effects of high dosage are nausea and vomiting, which occur early and are subsequently followed by a state of shock and prostration. There is an initial rise in temperature which later drops, tremors and convulsions occur, and within a day or two death ensues. These symptoms are classified as the *cerebral syndrome*, because they occur not only with a very high single total body exposure, but also as a result of irradiation of the head alone. Only one human case has been recorded; animal experiments have proved that the cerebral syndrome is invariably fatal. Even if life is prolonged for a few days, gastrointestinal damage soon leads to death.

Moderate dosage (800–5 000 r single exposure). Anorexia, nausea, and vomiting develop soon after irradiation for reasons which are not clear. These symptoms may persist, but are more likely to abate, only to recur after 2 or 3 days with intractable severity. This later episode of vomiting is accompanied by severe diarrhoea, and is due to necrosis of the gastrointestinal epithelium. This clinical picture is called the *gastrointestinal syndrome* and results in severe dehydration, haemoconcentration, and shock. Death may be averted by vigorous supportive measures, and the gastrointestinal epithelium regenerates in about 10 days. Nevertheless, 2 to 3 weeks later the effects of marrow aplasia appear, and death occurs.

Lower dosage (under 800 r single exposure). Initial nausea and vomiting are less severe, and the patient may then appear to make a complete recovery. Two to three weeks later the results of bone-marrow aplasia become apparent. The serious effects of irradiation at this stage are due to damage to the haematopoietic tissues. White cells, platelets, and red cells are all affected, and their deficiency explains the clinical picture seen during this *haematological phase*. Epilation may also occur, but regrowth of hair is usual in those who survive.

Blood Changes Following Irradiation

Lymphocytes. Lymphopenia is the earliest blood change of total body irradiation, and is most marked after a day or two. In those who survive the count remains low, and does not return to normal for months or even years. The lymphocyte count is therefore no useful guide to prognosis.

Granulocytes. The granulocyte count may increase initially, but during the ensuing weeks it shows a marked decline. With heavy dosage neutropenia becomes severe by the end of the second week, while with smaller doses the lowest count occurs around the fifth or sixth week. The count may take a year or more to return to normal.

Platelets. There is an initial rise, but within a few days the number of platelets drops. In severe cases they are virtually completely absent after about four weeks.

The red cells. Because primitive erythroblastic cells are highly radiosensitive and the mature red cells resistant, the effect of marrow aplasia on the peripheral count is delayed, being manifested as an anaemia of gradual onset. The actual red-cell count may, however, be influenced by the effects of haemoconcentration during the gastrointestinal phase, and haemorrhage occurring later.

Although the changes in the white-cell and platelet counts commence shortly after irradiation, their effects on the patient do not become apparent for at least 2–3 weeks. The two most important manifestations are infection and haemorrhage.

Infection. Many factors play a part in this manifestation of marrow aplasia, the neutropenia and diminished phagocytic power of the polymorphs probably being the most important. The RE system is damaged, and although phagocytosis is not impaired, and may even be enhanced, the phagocytes are less capable of destroying bacteria.[10] In addition, antibody production is impaired (p. 142). Organisms may gain access to the tissues through the denuded intestine, the mouth, and the respiratory tract. Treatment with antibiotics is worth trying, although experiments with germ-free animals given a lethal dose are reported to show that the avoidance of infection merely delays death.

Haemorrhage. The thrombocytopenia leads to a haemorrhagic tendency, which may manifest itself either as trivial petechial haemorrhages into the skin and other organs, or as severe intestinal and pulmonary bleeding. Death is not infrequently due to massive haemorrhage, and treatment with fresh blood or platelet transfusions may be of value.

Late Effects of Total Body Irradiation

Those exposed to a sublethal dose may show the following after–effects:

Premature aging. Following one large sublethal dose, mice are found to die sooner than normal, but this effect does not seem to occur after slow continuous exposure (e.g. 5 r per week). No data are available for man.

Cataract. In man the development of cataract may occasionally follow a large dose especially after neutron irradiation.

Sterility. The sterility which occurs in those who survive total body irradiation is not permanent: in the male complete recovery is usual, but in the female the result is less predictable. Permanent sterility occurs only when the gonads have received a dose which would cause death if applied to the whole body.

Fetal abnormalities. Although the effects in man are not known, mice irradiated *in utero* during early pregnancy have been shown to develop abnormalities.

Malignant disease (see p. 413).

Genetic effect (see p. 414).

PROTECTION FROM RADIATION DAMAGE

Marrow protection or replacement. One of the best ways of reducing the effects of radiation is to shield a part of the body which has a haematopoietic function, e.g. the bone marrow, or in some animals the spleen. This is because the destroyed marrow is repopulated by unaffected haematopoietic cells.

The use of high-energy x- and γ-radiation in radiotherapy reduces the bone dosage relative to that received by the soft tissues. Thus for a given soft tissue dose of 250 kV x-rays, the bones will receive about three times that received using a 2–4 MeV beam.

Animals exposed to moderate total body irradiation may be

saved if injected with autologous, homologous, or even heterologous marrow cells. This method has been tried in man, but the results were inconclusive, as it is debatable whether the homologous cells survived.[9] Radiation chimeras are further described on page 196.

The oxygen effect has already been described.

Chemical protection.[11] A large number of chemicals are known which protect against radiation; curiously enough, not only do they protect a wide range of living matter against the lethal effects of radiation, but some also preserve solutions of polymers, like polymethylmethacrylate, against degradation. The various test systems do not, however, always give the same quantitative results. Amongst known chemical agents, those which have been shown to afford protection are cyanides, nitrites, 5-hydroxytryptamine, and adrenaline. They probably act by producing tissue hypoxia, and are too toxic for animal use. So far the most effective compounds are derivatives of cysteine.

Cysteine itself (HS—CH$_2$—CH$\overset{\displaystyle NH_2}{\underset{\displaystyle COOH}{\Big\langle}}$)

is an effective protector whether given by mouth or injection. Some of its derivatives are even more powerful and suitable for animal administration. Cysteamine, HS—CH$_2$CH$_2$NH$_2$,

and cystamine, $\overset{\displaystyle S—CH_2CH_2NH_2}{\underset{\displaystyle S—CH_2CH_2NH_2}{|}}$,

which is converted into cysteamine *in vivo*, have been used, and reduce the effect of x-rays by about 50 per cent. One of the most promising derivatives is AET.* Glutathione, a tripeptide containing one molecule of cysteine, is another related protector, but is only effective by injection.

The following features should be noted:

(1) All substances must be given before exposure to radiation; they are quite ineffective if administered afterwards, and therefore cannot be considered a curative form of treatment once radiation damage has been sustained.

(2) They are not very effective against high density ionising particles, e.g. α-particles.

(3) They are less effective under hypoxic conditions.

(4) Their action is almost universal. They protect a wide range of animals, infusoria, bacteria, and tissue cultures.

Although it is tempting to think that the —SH group is important, not all substances containing it are active. Reducing power may also be a factor, but not all protective substances are reducing agents. Ascorbic acid is a powerful reducing substance, but has little protective activity. Some compounds may act by producing hypoxia, but it seems unlikely that all chemicals protect in the same way. The following alternatives have been suggested:

(a) The protecting chemicals compete for the free radicals, e.g. OH˙ and HO$_2$˙. As the powerfully oxidising HO$_2$˙ is

* S-β-Aminoethyl*iso*thiouronium bromide hydrobromide.

found only in the presence of oxygen, this theory would explain why the effects of hypoxia and chemicals overlap.

(b) The protector may convert the altered chemical, e.g. an enzyme, back to its normal state, e.g. by its —SH groupings.

(c) Protectors may combine with receptor groups of important molecules, and render them non-reactive to free radicals.

(d) Even if the effect of radiation is *direct*, the protector may prevent the transfer of energy from one part of a macromolecule to another part.

It is not yet possible to state which of these four is the most important. Topical applications of AET or DMSO (dimethylsulphoxide) have been shown to provide some degree of protection against local irradiation in animals.[12]

Most of the work done on chemical protection has been based on the lethal action of total body irradiation, and it is not known whether this applies to the other effects of ionising radiation, e.g. the carcinogenic and genetic hazards.

CARCINOGENIC EFFECT

It has been realised since the beginning of this century that tumours may develop after the application of ionising radiation. The first case, a carcinoma of the skin, was reported in 1902, and subsequently cancers of the skin of the hands have been frequently seen in x-ray workers.

In animals it has been found possible to produce tumours by the local irradiation of both normal and inflamed tissues. In this way skin cancers, subcutaneous sarcomata, and osteosarcomata have been produced, frequently after a latent interval of many months.

Irradiation as a Cause of Human Malignant Disease

Skin. Irradiation of the skin, whether accidental as in the early radium workers, or therapeutic for some other condition, may be followed years later by the development of squamous-cell carcinoma (Fig. 31.3). Irradiated lupus vulgaris frequently underwent malignancy.

Bone. Osteosarcoma may develop following local irradiation. It usually appears several years after the treatment of either a benign tumour or an inflammatory lesion, like tuberculosis. Radiation-induced osteosarcoma more commonly follows the deposition of long-lived radioactive elements in the bone itself (internal irradiation). Certain metals, e.g. radium, mesothorium, and strontium, are treated like calcium, and become deposited in bone, where the long-continued radiation causes neoplasia. A classical instance of this occurred in 1928 when some girls, who were employed in painting the dials of watches with a luminous paint containing radium and mesothorium, sucked the tips of the brushes, and swallowed quantities of the radioactive elements.[13, 14] Tumours developed 1 to 5 years after exposure to the carcinogen. More recently anxiety has been expressed because the ^{90}Sr released from nuclear devices is taken up by

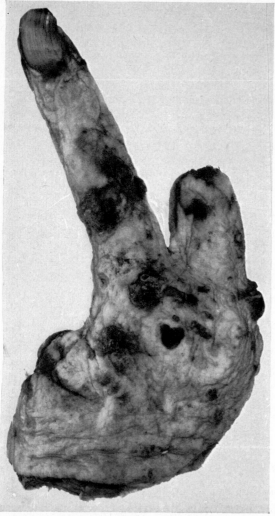

Figure 31.3
X-ray neoplasia of the skin. This specimen demonstrates many of
the changes that the hands of pioneer radiologists underwent. The
skin is scarred and the nail deformed. On the atrophic skin of the
finger there are several large papillomata as well as many smaller
ones. The neighbouring finger has already been amputated. (I 2.6,
*Reproduced by permission of the President and Council of the
R.C.S. Eng.*)

the grass, and finally reaches human bones *via* ingested
cows' milk. This may obviously lead to osteosarcoma and
leukaemia, but it is probable that ⁹⁰Sr is eliminated more
rapidly than was originally thought, and that the risk is not as
great as was at one time feared.

Leukaemia. The steady increase in the incidence of
leukaemia over the last thirty years has led to the investigation
of ionising radiation of the bone marrow as a causative factor.
An increased incidence has been noted in the survivors of the
Nagasaki and Hiroshima atomic bomb attacks,[15] and a
statistically significant risk has been shown to attend treatment of ankylosing spondylitis with x-rays.[16] Leukaemia was

also more common in radiologists before strict protective
standards were introduced.[17, 18] Statistical evidence suggests that irradiation of the abdomen for pelvimetry during
pregnancy increases the incidence of leukaemia in the
child.[19–21] However, not all investigators have confirmed this
finding.[22] Diagnostic radiology in the adult also increases the
incidence of leukaemia.[23]

The latent period between irradiation and disease is seldom
less than two years and usually five to eight. After ten years
the risk appears to diminish. The type of leukaemia induced
is predominantly acute. Chronic myeloid leukaemia occurs
much less commonly, and chronic lymphatic leukaemia is
very rare. The increased incidence of the last disease is
therefore unlikely to be due to the radiation hazard. Whether,
in fact, the observed increase of acute leukaemia is due to the
effects of irradiation is not known, but it is certain that the
population is now exposed to more radiation than ever before.
Diagnostic radiology constitutes the greatest hazard, but
luminous watches, fluorescent shoe-fitting machines, radiotherapy, and bomb fall-out all contribute to the general
increase. It would seem prudent to limit the exposure of all
individuals to x-rays, especially if they are young or pregnant.
It should, however, be borne in mind that the risk of leukaemia is very small. Common surgical operations, even
under the best conditions, have a greater mortality risk than
the complication of radiotherapy for spondylitis. The
negligible risk of diagnostic radiography should therefore be
seen in proper perspective.

Thyroid. Irradiation of the adult thyroid is not usually
followed by malignancy, although a few cases have been
reported. It was, however, the fashion at one time, in the
USA especially, to treat children suffering from "thymic
asthma" with radiotherapy. The thyroid gland received
considerable radiation, and some three to eighteen years
later cancer was found to develop in a number of these
patients.[24]

Liver. Thorotrast, a preparation of thorium dioxide, was
at one time used as a contrast medium in angiography. It
accumulates in the liver and spleen and there causes tumours,
the most common of which is an angiosarcoma of the liver.[25]
Other liver tumours may arise, as may also leukaemia.

Other organs. Cancer of the pharynx has been described
following irradiation. Cancer of the lung in the Schneeberg
miners is mentioned on page 392.

GENETIC EFFECT OF IONISING RADIATION

The ability of ionising rays to increase the rate of mutation
is well established in micro-organisms, plants, and animals.
In somatic cells this effect is probably not important, but in
the germ cells it is of potential significance, since the new
factor may have a profound effect, and is handed down to
subsequent generations. It is generally believed that the *type*
of mutation is not influenced by radiation—it is only the *rate*
which is changed. Within wide limits it is thought that the

number of mutations is related to the total dose received by the gonads regardless of the rate at which it is given. However, with very low dosage it is probable that the genetic effect is much less than the calculations from the cumulative dose would lead one to postulate. In man the genetic hazard is difficult to assess, since most of the abnormal genes produced are likely to be recessive, and may therefore remain hidden for generations. It is generally agreed that most mutations are harmful, although it should not be forgotten that in the heterozygous state "harmful" genes may confer some advantage upon the individual, e.g. sickle-cell trait in relation to malaria. Furthermore, if the improvement of species and the process of evolution itself are dependent upon the occurrence of mutations, then an increase in their frequency might in the long run be of benefit.

THE PERMISSIBLE DOSE[26]

It is probable that ionising radiation produces some effect on living matter, however small the dose. Whether the damage is of any consequence depends upon many factors, including dosage-rate and age. Evidence is accumulating to show that with slow dosage-rates damage is considerably lessened. The increased liability of children to ill-effects after irradiation is well known to radiotherapists, and was borne out by the experiences of those exposed to fall-out on the Marshall Islands in 1954. The problem of whether a threshold dose* exists is therefore complex: it depends not only upon factors like type of radiation, area of body exposed, dosage-rate, etc., but also upon our ability to detect damage in exposed individuals or experimental animals. The permissible dose for x-ray workers is therefore chosen arbitrarily as a dose unlikely to cause appreciable damage to the worker, and at the same time which allows the work to be pursued.

The present trend has been to emphasise the importance of a cumulative dose. For radiation workers the maximum permissible dose to the gonads, the blood-forming organs, and the lens of the eye is 3 rem. in any period of 13 consecutive weeks. However, the maximum whole body radiation from the age of 18 to 65 is 235 rem. This corresponds to an over-all average of about 5 rem./year or 0·1 rem./week. Further details are available in the Medical Research Council's Second Report of 1960.

RADIOTHERAPY[27]

The destructive effects of ionising radiations on living cells, particularly those in an active state, have led to the widespread use of these radiations in the treatment of malignant disease. Nowadays radiotherapy plays an important part in the curative treatment of some primary cancers as well as in the palliation of those which have already metastasised and are beyond the scope of surgical excision.

* The term "threshold" is used in the sense that a dose below it produces no detectable effect.

Tumours differ widely in their reaction to radiotherapy, and it is only after treatment has been commenced that the response can be assessed. However, some guide to the probable local results of treatment may be given by a consideration of the following factors:

Tissue of origin. The relative sensitivities of normal tissues are often reflected in the radiosensitivities of the tumours derived from them. Thus, seminoma of the testis and tumours of the lymphoreticular system are generally very radiosensitive; sarcomata are usually resistant. On the other hand, there are some exceptions to this rule: carcinomata of the gastrointestinal tract do not usually respond well, and the medulloblastoma, although of neural origin, is highly radiosensitive.

Degree of differentiation and mitotic activity. It is generally taught that within any tumour group, the most undifferentiated tumours are also the most radiosensitive. As a generalisation this is true, but nevertheless it is found that the histological appearances of an individual tumour are no sure guide to the results obtained in practice. It is found, for instance, that well-differentiated squamous-cell carcinoma of the skin and tongue frequently responds very well.

The tumour bed. The nature of the tumour bed is thought to play an important role in the response of a tumour to ionising radiation. Several factors are probably involved. An avascular bed rendering the growth hypoxic may make the tumour more resistant due to the oxygen effect (see p. 410). Irradiation damage to the stromal blood vessels may lead to the destruction of the tumour by a process of infarction.

There are some authorities who maintain that the connective tissues have an even more important role. It is possible that the tumour bed with its inflammatory response has a restraining effect upon the growth which can lead to its destruction. If the bed is itself damaged by excessive irradiation, the results of treatment are said to be poor. This concept has led to the development of sieve therapy, whereby a grid or sieve is placed in the x-ray beam and only parts of the tumour and its stroma are irradiated.[28] Whatever may be the merits of this approach, there seems little doubt that the effects of ionising radiation on a tumour are due only partly to a primary destructive effect on the malignant cells. Some viable cells remain, and in those cases where clinical success is apparent it is probable that the body defences either destroy the remaining tumour or else induce it to enter into a dormant phase.

Recurrent tumour following previous irradiation generally responds poorly. This may be a result of selection whereby resistant cells survive, but the ischaemia which accompanies the radiation fibrosis may also play a part.

Nature of the individual tumour. Certain tumours respond well, e.g. most basal-cell and squamous-cell carcinomata of the skin. Some squamous-cell carcinomata of the cervix respond well, while others are resistant. Squamous-cell tumours of the lung respond poorly. It is evident that tumours of identical histological appearances in different organs react very differently to irradiation. The reason for this is not apparent.

The cure rate to be expected from radiotherapy must, as with surgical treatment, be considered in relation to the general properties of the tumour. Many malignant conditions, e.g. those of the lymphoreticular system, cannot be considered as local diseases, and although a tumour mass may respond remarkably well to treatment, the disease usually progresses sooner or later. Some carcinomata, e.g. oat-cell carcinoma of the lung, appear to spread so early that treatment of any sort directed to the primary growth does not greatly influence the course of the disease.

TABLE 31.1   Prognosis in treated carcinoma of the cervix uteri

Stage	5-year survivals %
I	71·2
II	52·8
III	25.2
IV	11·7
Total	43·8

The figures are quoted from Raven, R. W. (1959), "Cancer", vol. 5, p. 282. London: Butterworth. The classification of stages is the one recommended by W.H.O. (*see* Raven, R. W. (1958). "Cancer", vol. 4, p. 4, London: Butterworth).

When the growth is localised, excellent results may be obtained, e.g. with basal-cell carcinoma of the skin. The results of treatment of cancer of the cervix illustrate the ability of ionising radiation to eradicate local disease.

Radiotherapy is often useful as an effective palliative treatment. It can reduce the size of tumour masses and thereby produce great clinical relief; this is well seen in mediastinal tumours producing obstruction of the great vessels. It can control haemorrhage from a bleeding carcinoma of the bladder, and help to clear up fungating tumours, e.g. a carcinoma of the breast. Pain due to metastases in bone may be alleviated, and combined with surgery, radiotherapy can relieve compression of the spinal cord, thereby delaying the onset of paraplegia. Slowly-growing tumours, like carcinoma of the breast and Hodgkin's disease, can sometimes be held in check, and at times a tumour which appears hopelessly advanced may respond dramatically, thereby giving the patient several years of useful life. It may well be that radiotherapy and surgery are both forms of palliation which allow the body to retard the growth of the tumour. Depending on whether the remaining malignant cells stay dormant for a short or a long period, one may speak of a "5-year cure", a "10-year cure", etc. It is doubtful, however, whether any of our present treatments of cancer can be regarded as producing a "cure", if by this is meant the complete eradication of all malignant cells.

GENERAL READING

ALEXANDER, P. (1957). *Atomic Radiation and Life*, 239 pp. Harmondsworth: Penguin Books Ltd. A simple account of ionising radiations and their effects.

BACQ, Z. M. and ALEXANDER, P. (1961). *Fundamentals of Radiobiology*, 2nd edn, 555 pp. Oxford: Pergamon Press. Both this and the first edition (1955, London: Butterworths) should be consulted for details on specific aspects of radiobiology.

CRONKITE, E. P. and BOND, V. P. (1960). *Radiation Injury in Man*, 200 pp. Springfield, Illinois: Thomas.

GLASSER, O., QUIMBY, E. H., TAYLOR, L. S., WEATHERWAX, J. L. and MORGAN, R. H. (1961). *Pyhsical Foundations of Radiology*, 3rd edn, 503 pp. London: Pitman Medical.

MOLE, R. H. (1960). *The Toxicity of Radiation*, in Recent Advances in Pathology, edited by C. V. Harrison, 7th edn., pp. 339–383. London: Churchill.

WARREN, S. (1961). *The Pathology of Ionising Radiation*, 42 pp. Springfield, Illinois: Thomas.

REFERENCES

1. LITTLE, J. B. (1968). *New England Journal of Medicine*, **278**, 308 and 369.
2. GRAY, L. H. (1957–58). *Lectures on the Scientific Basis of Medicine*, **7**, 314. London: Athlone Press.
3. Leading Article (1972). *British Medical Journal*, **2**, 368.
4. MELLETT, P. G., WALTER, J. B. and HOUGHTON, L. E. (1960). *British Journal of Experimental Pathology*, **41**, 160.
5. PATT, H. M. and SWIFT, M. N. (1948). *American Journal of Physiology*, **155**, 388.
6. SMITH, J. C. (1963). *American Review of Respiratory Diseases*, **87**, 647.
7. MOLE, R. H. (1959). In *Modern Trends in Pathology*, edited by D. H. Collins, p. 91. London: Butterworths.
8. LIEBOW, A. A., WARREN, S. and DeCOURSEY, E. (1949). *American Journal of Pathology*, **25**, 853.
9. ANDREWS, G. A. (1962). *Journal of the American Medical Association*, **179**, 191.
10. GORDON, L. E., COOPER, D. B. and MILLER, C. P. (1955). *Proceedings of the Society of Experimental Biology and Medicine*, **89**, 577.
11. BACQ, Z. M. (1961). *Triangle*, **5**, 2.
12. Annotation (1969). *Lancet*, i, 1039.
13. MARTLAND, H. S. (1931). *American Journal of Cancer*, **15**, 2435.
14. DAVIS, C., BROWN, R. G. and ALEXANDER, R. W. (1963). *Archives of Surgery*, **86**, 190.
15. HEYSSEL, R. *et al.* (1960). *Blood*, **15**, 313.
16. COURT BROWN, W. M. and ABBATT, J. D. (1955). *Lancet*, i, 1283.
17. MARCH, H. C. (1950). *American Journal of Medical Science*, **220**, 282.
18. COURT BROWN, W. M. and DOLL, R. (1958). *British Medical Journal*, ii, 181.

19. STEWART, A. *et al.* (1956). *Lancet*, ii, 447.
20. Leading Article (1963). *Lancet*, i, 255.
21. MACMAHON, B. (1962). *Journal of the National Cancer Institute*, **28**, 1173.
22. Leading Article (1960). *Lancet*, ii, 1383.
23. STEWART, A., PENNYBACKER, W. and BARBER, R. (1962). *British Medical Journal*, ii, 882.
24. WILSON, G. M. *et al.* (1958). *British Medical Journal*, ii, 929.
25. DA SILVA HORTA, J. *et al.* (1965). *Lancet*, ii, 201.
26. BARNES, D. E. and TAYLOR, D. (1963). *Radiation Hazards and Protection*, 2nd edn. London: Newnes.
27. Various Authors (1959). *Cancer*, vol. 5, edited by R. W. Raven. London: Butterworths.
28. JOLLES, B. (1953). *X-ray Sieve Therapy in Cancer*. London: Lewis.

Chapter 32. The General Reaction to Trauma: Haemorrhage and Shock

Following major trauma there ensues a complex series of changes from which scarcely any tissue of the body escapes. The nervous system responds promptly with an increased outflow of autonomic impulses. An outpouring of catecholamines from the adrenal medulla causes a breakdown of hepatic glycogen and an increase in the level of blood glucose. The other endocrine glands respond more slowly: stimulation of the hypothalamus leads to an increase in the secretion of ACTH from the pituitary, and this results in adrenocortical overactivity. These changes are presumably designed to assist the injured animal to withstand trauma; in fact, there is little doubt that the adrenalectomised animal is less able to withstand infection and trauma. Continued stress in the intact animal leads to adrenal hyperplasia and an excessive secretion of its hormones. It has been suggested that this might lead to disease,[1] and sometimes it does seem that stress, either physical or psychological, precipitates an illness, e.g. Graves's disease. Nevertheless, there is little evidence that continued stress is a major cause of the "collagen diseases", a group in which this pathogenesis was at one time favoured.[1]

One very obvious effect of trauma is on the circulatory system. When the trauma is severe, these events culminate in the production of a state from which recovery may or may not occur; this is called *shock*, and is characterised by inadequate perfusion of the tissues, hypotension, and depression of general metabolic activity.

If the patient survives, metabolic changes occur which result in complete recovery. This is called the period of convalescence.

For descriptive purposes therefore it is convenient to consider the response to injury under three headings:

The Immediate Circulatory Changes.

Shock.

Convalescence.

The changes in the circulation are seen to their best advantage following acute haemorrhage; this will therefore be described first.

HAEMORRHAGE

Haemorrhage is the most dramatic of the circulatory disorders. The bleeding may occur externally or into the body tissues, usually a hollow viscus or one of the serous cavities. The blood loss may be large and sudden, or small bleeds may occur repeatedly. The changes which follow differ markedly in these two instances; chronic blood loss produces an iron-deficiency anaemia (see p. 589), while acute haemorrhage, which may be arterial or venous, leads to more serious immediate consequences.

Causes of Acute Haemorrhage

Trauma. Penetrating wounds involving the heart or large vessels may result in the very rapid loss of large quantities of blood. Bleeding from the large vascular spaces exposed during labour can be of frightening severity.

Abnormalities of the blood-vessel wall. *Inflammatory lesions* may cause weakening of a vessel wall, usually arterial, with subsequent rupture. Aneurysmal dilatation may occur before the final rupture. Bleeding from a chronic peptic ulcer, typhoid ulcers, Rasmussen's aneurysm traversing a tuberculous cavity in the lung, and syphilitic aortic aneurysm are well-known examples. The inflammation need not always be infective, e.g. polyarteritis nodosa.

Neoplastic invasion. Haemorrhage is a frequent terminal event in carcinoma of the tongue, and is due to rupture of the lingual artery. Infection is probably a major factor in the weakening of the wall.

Other vascular diseases. Atheroma, either with or without aneurysmal dilatation, is the most common cause. Aneurysms due to trauma or persistent friction, e.g. subclavian aneurysm due to cervical rib, also fall into this category.

High pressure within the vessels. Systemic hypertension may precipitate haemorrhage at sites of arterial weakness. Raised venous pressure with varicose-vein formation, e.g. in the legs or oesophagus, is another important cause of severe haemorrhage.

Effects of Acute Haemorrhage[2]

These depend mainly upon two factors:

1. The amount of blood lost.

2. The speed with which the loss occurs.

The general effects are slight when less than 20 per cent of the blood volume is lost. A sudden loss of 33 per cent may cause death, but it the bleeding extends over a period of twenty-four hours, a loss of over 50 per cent of blood volume is not necessarily fatal. However, with losses of over 50 per cent the effects are always serious. Individuals, both human and animal, show a considerable variation in their response to blood loss, even though the amount and rate are constant. It is therefore impossible to assess accurately the magnitude of any haemorrhage on purely clinical grounds.

The body response to acute haemorrhage may be divided into three phases:

PHASE I

The early changes. During the first few hours the manifestations are mostly due to nervous mechanisms. An immediate syncope may occur, and this is followed by important vascular changes which result in the redistribution of the remaining blood, the volume of which is considerably depleted.

Immediate syncope ("Primary Shock"). The vasovagal attack, or faint, is seen only in man, and may perhaps represent an escape mechanism. It commences with yawning, sighing respiration, nausea, and vomiting. This is followed by loss of consciousness, but the attack rarely lasts for more than a few minutes. The condition is characterised by a fall in blood pressure, a slow pulse, and pallor and coldness of the extremities. The cardiac output remains unchanged,[2, 3] but there is a widespread dilatation of the arteries of the muscles which results in a dramatic fall in blood pressure and a reduction in the cerebral blood flow.[4, 5] This leads to a loss of consciousness.

Emotional stress has been shown to lead to vasodilatation of muscular vessels in normal individuals, and an overaction of this mechanism in sensitive individuals can lead to fainting.[6, 7] Thus, although syncope is more common after large haemorrhages than small ones, psychological factors such as fear and anxiety also play a large part. Healthy people may faint when only a few ml of blood are withdrawn, and even the sight of blood may be sufficient. Pain is also an important factor. It is possible that the fainting reflex helps to divert blood to the brain by causing the patient to fall to the ground. When the horizontal position is assumed recovery soon occurs.

The Phase of Redistribution of Available Blood to Vital Centres.[5, 8] The changes are summarised in Fig. 32.1. Following haemorrhage the venous return to the heart falls; cardiac catheterisation confirms that the right atrial pressure is low.[3] In this way the cardiac output is reduced, and the blood pressure tends to fall.[2] The tonic inhibitory impulses arising from the aortic and carotid sinuses are therefore reduced. Baroreceptors are also present in the atria. The increased activity of the vasomotor centre results in an increased peripheral resistance, and the *blood pressure is maintained*. The blood vessels of the brain are not affected by this generalised vasoconstriction, whilst the coronary vessels actually dilate. There is also *tachycardia*. Normally impulses from the carotid and aortic sinuses stimulate the cardiac centre which is responsible for slowing the heart *via* the vagus. If the impulses drop, vagal activity is reduced.

Contraction of the spleen occurs in animals, and the reserve of blood injected into the circulation helps maintain the blood volume. This is of little importance in man. The venous

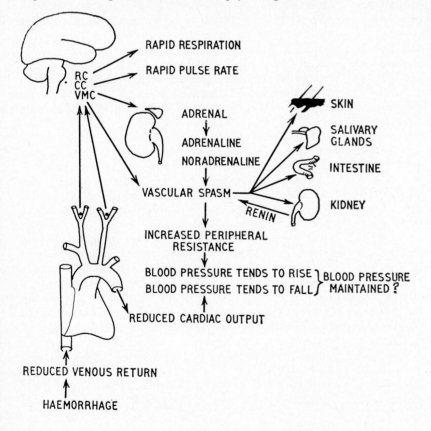

Figure 32.1
The cardiovascular effects of sudden haemorrhage.
RC: Respiratory Centre. CC: Cardiac Centre.
VMC: Vasomotor Centre.

reservoir is of greater significance. In man 60–70 per cent of the blood volume is contained in the veins and venules. Constriction of these vessels can readily increase the venous return to the heart; following a 10 per cent blood loss, contraction of the venous reservoir can prevent any change occurring in the cardiac output and blood pressure.[8]

The arteriolar constriction is selective: the blood flow to the skin, salivary glands, intestines, liver, spleen, and kidneys is reduced. The skin becomes pale, clammy, and cold. Salivary secretion stops, the mouth becomes dry, and thirst results. The intestine manifests impaired digestion, and water is not well absorbed—a point to remember when treating patients.

The blood flow to essential organs is, however, maintained. These include the brain, heart, diaphragm, intercostal muscles, and skeletal muscles generally. Although this selective vasoconstriction is mediated mainly by autonomic nerves, two additional mechanisms play some part:

(*a*) The *adrenal medulla* secretes excess adrenaline and noradrenaline.[9] Both are general vasoconstrictors, but adrenaline dilates skeletal muscular arteries while noradrenaline dilates the coronary vessels.

(*b*) There is also an increased secretion of *renin* by the kidneys, due to a decreased renal arterial pulse pressure (see Chapter 42).

These mechanisms tend to restore the blood pressure, and divert blood from the less essential organs to those of immediate importance, namely the heart and brain. With a blood loss of less than 30 per cent the blood pressure tends to remain almost unchanged. Blood pressure measurements are therefore not an accurate guide to the severity of the bleeding. If the blood loss is of such a magnitude that these compensatory mechanisms are unable to maintain an effective blood pressure, *haemorrhagic shock* ensues.

Occasionally *hypertension* occurs soon after a haemorrhage, but this is usually a transient phase, and is presumably due to the overaction of the compensatory nervous adjustments already described. The pulse rate is either normal or slow, and the blood volume not reduced below 80 per cent.

Changes in respiration.[8] The pulmonary blood flow is reduced *pari passu* with the cardiac output. There is an increase in the physiological dead-space due to the underperfusion of the upper parts of the lungs. The increase in dead-space ventilation in part explains the hyperpnoea which characteristically occurs after haemorrhage. The major factor causing this air hunger, however, is a fall in arterial blood pH due to metabolic acidosis.

Blood supply to the brain.[10] The blood flow through the brain can be measured experimentally by the use of radioactive krypton. A quantity of the gas, dissolved in saline, is injected into the arterial supply, and on reaching the brain there is equilibration between blood and tissue. The ^{85}Kr which passes through into the venous blood is nearly all excreted in the lungs, and there is very little recirculation. The dissolved gas in the brain tissue is measured by an end-window Geiger-Muller tube, and its rate of disappearance is a measure of the cerebral blood flow in that area.[11]

The blood flow to the brain is determined by the systemic blood pressure and the resistance of the cerebral vasculature. When the blood flow to the brain is reduced as a result of hypotension, the Po_2 of the brain tissue is reduced and the Pco_2 rises. These changes cause vasodilatation and a corresponding increase in blood flow. Thus, the cerebral blood flow is maintained at the expense of the other tissues. Any marked reduction of arterial Pco_2 due to hyperpnoea tends to impair the cerebral circulation, because the cerebral vessels are very sensitive to changes in CO_2 tension.[12] The administration of morphine under these circumstances will so depress respiration that the arterial Pco_2 rises, the cerebral vessels dilate, and the blood flow to the brain is improved.[13] When the flow falls below a critical level for any length of time, the cortical neurones undergo necrosis. The neurones of the brain-stem appear to be less susceptible to hypoxia, and remain unaffected even in the presence of cortical damage. Blindness may occasionally follow acute haemorrhage, especially gastro-intestinal. The mechanism involved is not well understood; spasm of the retinal arteries may be a factor.[14, 15]

Blood supply to the heart. The coronary blood flow is related to the systemic blood pressure and the duration of ventricular diastole. Tachycardia and hypotension both tend to produce myocardial ischaemia. Heart failure may therefore occur (see later).

Renal blood flow. There is intense renal vasoconstriction which leads to oliguria and even anuria (see Chapter 42). Prolonged ischaemia can cause severe damage to the kidneys.[16] Antidiuretic hormone (ADH) secretion contributes to the oliguria. Moderate ischaemia can interfere with tubular function such that there is an inability to concentrate urine. Hence there may be an increased excretion of a dilute urine. This effect is ADH resistant.

Blood changes. A haemorrhage should be viewed in the same light as an amputation of any organ. Immediately after the trauma the remainder of the organ is unchanged. In other words, the haemoglobin level and the red-cell count are both normal immediately after haemorrhage. It is useless to use these estimations as immediate guides to the amount of blood lost.

The *platelet count* rapidly rises after haemorrhage, and may be 1 000 000 per μl within an hour. The *coagulation time* decreases within a few minutes and the *fibrinolytic system* is activated.[17] It is an old observation by William Hewson, a friend of the Hunters, that when animals are killed by bleeding, "the blood which issued last coagulated first."[18] In one experiment with rabbits, a 15·4 per cent blood loss reduced the coagulation time from 2·5 to 1·75 minutes, while a 30·9 per cent loss reduced it to 1 minute.[19] The accelerated clotting and increased fibrinolysis are transient phenomena which are soon succeeded by other important changes.[17] Aggregation of red cells (sludging) is described as occurring within a few hours of injury, and this impedes the flow of blood in the small vessels.[20] Small clumps of platelets and fibrin further obstruct the circulation,[21] and multiple microthrombi have been described in the lungs following haemorrhage, shock, and operations involving the use of an extracorporeal circulation.[22] These changes last for 2–3 days. The blood fibrinogen level rises and with it the ESR; a peak is reached in 2–3 days, and this is followed by a slow return to normal.[23]

The *white-cell count* rises within 2–5 hours, and may reach 35 000 per μl. The excess cells are neutrophil leucocytes released from the stores in the bone marrow. Many of the cells are young, and occasional myelocytes appear.

PHASE II

The restoration of blood volume. During this phase fluid is withdrawn from the tissue spaces into the blood stream. The mechanism is as follows: the arteriolar spasm results in a lowering of the capillary pressure. On Starling's hypothesis fluid therefore passes into the vessels, and this continues until the reduction in plasma osmotic pressure due to the dilution of the plasma proteins is sufficiently great to offset the forces tending to draw fluid into the blood. The lost plasma proteins are replaced within 2–3 days. As the blood volume is restored, the vasospasm passes off, and the capillary pressure rises. Thus, extracellular fluid passes into the blood until the forces governing the interchange of fluid across the capillary wall are balanced. During this phase there is progressive haemodilution, rapid at first and complete by about two days (see Fig. 32.2).[24]

Haemoglobin estimations are now of value, because they reflect the magnitude of the original blood loss. The importance of knowing the haemoglobin level immediately after the haemorrhage is apparent, for it provides a baseline from which subsequent changes can be assessed.

PHASE III

The replacement of lost red cells. *During the dilution phase anaemia becomes apparent, and is of a normochromic, normocytic type.* The dilute blood is an inefficient oxygenator of the tissues, and therefore more oxygen is extracted from it. The total amount of oxygen supplied to the tissues may be adequate, but the oxygen tension of tissue and venous blood is low. Sometimes the quantity of oxygen supplied to the tissues is insufficient; the anaemic hypoxia so engendered leads to anaerobic cell metabolism, resulting in the release of lactic acid. A metabolic acidosis follows, and is accompanied by hyperpnoea.

Within 4–7 days the *reticulocyte count* reaches 5–15 per cent, indicating active red-cell formation. The bone marrow shows normoblastic hyperplasia, the stimulus for which is probably erythropoietin (see p. 587). Generally the anaemia remains normochromic and normocytic; macrocytosis may develop due to the large number of reticulocytes. Hypochromic, microcytic anaemia does not generally occur, unless the patient is already suffering from iron deficiency due, for example, to previous haemorrhage. The reticulocytosis should abate after 10–14 days; failure to do so suggests recurrent haemorrhage. The white-cell count should return to normal after 3–4 days.

The rate of recovery of the red cells is dependent upon the severity of the anaemia. At first red cells are produced rapidly, e.g. 2 per cent increase in haemoglobin each day, but as the count approaches normal, the rate slows down. Complete

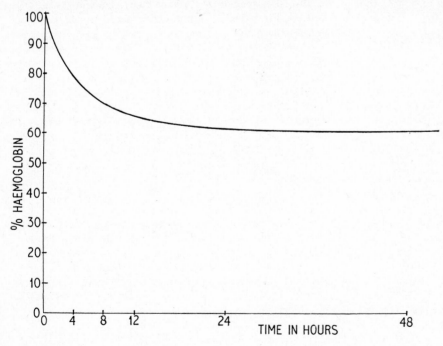

Figure 32.2
Haemoglobin levels after haemorrhage involving loss of 40 per cent of blood volume.

recovery takes about six weeks regardless of the severity of the original haemorrhage. Of course, in practice the process is accelerated by blood transfusions.

SHOCK

Shock is the name given to a clinical state in which the patient has a tachycardia, and is pale, ashen, and sweating. The transient *primary shock*, or vasovagal attack, which follows immediately after injury has already been described (see p. 419). Though the vasovagal attack is transient and benign, death has been attributed to it following certain surgical procedures, e.g. "obstetric shock" following manual removal of the placenta, and "pleural shock" after paracentesis. It has been reported that syncope occurring during the induction of anaesthesia may be fatal if the anaesthetic is administered with the patient in the upright position, e.g. in a dental chair.[25] The remainder of this section will be devoted to the much more important *secondary shock*.

The patient presents a characteristic appearance. He lies still and apathetic, his temperature is subnormal, his skin cold and clammy, and his face ashen-grey. Obvious cyanosis may be present. The blood pressure is low, and the pulse rapid and thready. Little or no urine is passed. This has been appropriately called the "ebb phase" following trauma, in contrast with the "flow" of catabolic hyperactivity which follows it in those who survive.[26]

The clinical picture of shock may occur in many conditions, and these have been included in the general classification of "shock":

> *Loss of blood* (haemorrhagic shock).
> *Overwhelming infection*, e.g. anthrax septicaemia and gas-gangrene.
> *Loss of plasma*, e.g. burns.
> *Loss of fluid and electrolytes*, e.g. diabetic coma, sodium and water depletion, etc.
> *Cardiogenic shock*, e.g. myocardial infarction.
> *Anaphylactic shock*, see Chapter 14.

The inclusion of so many divergent syndromes under this one heading has tended to obscure our understanding of the condition. They all produce a similar clinical picture which is described as shock, but it is hardly to be expected that the mechanisms involved would be the same in each case. It should also be remembered that a state of shock frequently precedes death regardless of the cause, e.g. electrocution, overdose of drugs, drowning, or following massive total body irradiation (p. 411). To attempt to understand "shock" it is necessary to consider each condition separately.

Methods of Investigating Haemorrhagic and Traumatic Shock

Attempts to produce a standard response to injury in animals have not been very successful. Many variable factors are involved, including the age and nutrition of the animal,

temperature, etc. These often result in great variations in response even after a standard injury. The situation in fact is similar to that encountered in injured patients. The following standard injuries have been used:

1. Rats are placed in a drum, which on rotation throws the animals against fixed projections.[27] The injury can be varied by altering the number of revolutions, but the use of this method on unanaesthetised animals is to be deprecated.
2. Bleeding.
3. Scalding.[28]
4. Occluding the blood supply to a limb (tourniquet shock, see p. 425). [29, 30]

The simplest and most intensively studied is haemorrhagic shock.

Haemorrhagic Shock

The loss of blood volume and the reduction of cardiac output tend to lower the blood pressure. If the compensatory mechanisms described on page 419 are effective, the blood pressure is maintained and no "shock" develops. This end-result of haemorrhage is familiar to any blood donor.

If the compensatory mechanisms fail to maintain the blood pressure, either as a result of their own inefficiency or the excessive load placed upon them by a large haemorrhage, the patient enters into a state of *shock*. Recovery may occur spontaneously or as a result of efficient treatment, e.g. transfusion; such shock is therefore said to be *reversible*. It sometimes happens that in spite of vigorous and efficient treatment the blood pressure continues to fall, the patient's clinical condition deteriorates, and death ensues. This is *irreversible shock* (Fig. 32.3).

The phenomenon can be demonstrated experimentally. If an animal is bled to the extent that its blood pressure is considerably reduced, immediate replacement of the blood restores the blood pressure to its previous level—the shock is reversible. If the experiment is repeated, but on this occasion the animal is allowed to remain in a hypotensive state ("shock") for some period before reinfusing the lost blood, it is found that the blood pressure is not restored to normal, but continues to fall. The animal is in a state of irreversible shock, and dies in spite of a full restoration of blood volume. Some other mechanism must be involved. This is one of the main problems which has to be solved before the cause of the irreversibility of shock can be explained.

Traumatic Shock

In spite of the considerable amount of research which has been done on the changes that follow trauma, no comprehensive account can yet be given.

The *circulatory changes* which occur resemble those already described following acute haemorrhage. In man fainting may occur. This is related to many factors amongst which may be mentioned age, sex, extent of the injury, amount of blood loss, and pain.

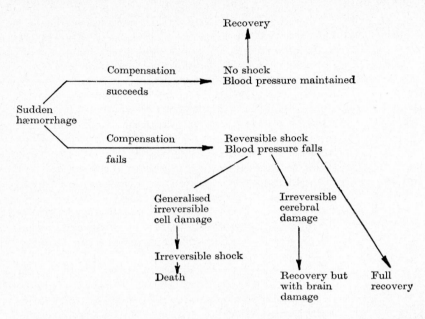

Figure 32.3
The possible end-results of a sudden haemorrhage.

Following this the various nervous mechanisms come into play to help maintain the blood pressure. If these are unsuccessful, a state of shock develops. The possible causes of this more dangerous secondary shock must now be considered.

Loss of blood.[31] In the past it has not been fully recognised that there is considerable loss of blood from the circulation in all but the most trivial injuries. In closed injuries of the limbs an estimate of this blood loss may be made by measuring the extent of the swelling. Actual measurements of the blood volume following fractures have shown the magnitude of this blood loss. Thus, in simple closed fractures of the tibia and fibula $\frac{1}{2}$–1 litre is usually lost, but it may exceed 3 litres in severe cases. An average closed fracture of the shaft of the femur loses about 2 litres into the surrounding tissues.[31]

A practical rule which is a guide in traumatic surgery is to relate blood loss to wound size as measured in terms of a clenched fist.[32]

		% Blood Volume Lost
Small Wounds:	Less than 1 hand	20
Moderate Wounds:	1–3 hands	20–40
Large Wounds:	3–5 hands	40
Very Large Wounds:	Over 5 hands	50

Blood loss during operations is often quite considerable, and in all major surgery reliable methods must be employed to measure it. The amount on swabs can be estimated by weighing, or by extracting the haemoglobin and measuring it colorimetrically.[33] Blood-volume measurements can now be made more easily (see p. 428).

It is evident therefore that the circulatory changes which follow physical trauma could be due largely to haemorrhage.

Toxins from the damaged area. Many toxic substances have been isolated from damaged tissue, but none has been proved to be the cause of the shock. Potassium is liberated from damaged cells, especially muscle, and it exerts a noxious influence upon the cardiac muscle. This has not, however, been shown to be of any great practical importance. Other substances which have been isolated are histamine and adenosine triphosphate (ATP). On intravenous injection these substances produce a state of shock, but it has never been shown that they are of any great clinical importance.

Increase in vascular permeability to proteins. It has been postulated that loss of circulating plasma results from a generalised increase in vascular permeability. This has never been substantiated, although some loss must obviously occur into the wound itself due to the formation of an acute inflammatory exudate. Fluid loss into the injured area is thought to be a major factor in the production of tourniquet shock.[30]

Infection of the wound. There is little doubt that the powerful exotoxins of the pathogenic clostridia exert a profound effect on the circulation. Gas-gangrene, even in the absence of substantial traumatic damage, causes a shock-like condition which may terminate in death. It is equally probable that the toxins of other organisms contribute to shock: staphylococcal α-toxin may be cited as an example.

Experiments designed to show that damaged tissues liberate "toxin" are often invalidated by the fact that normal tissues may be contaminated with bacteria. In the dog, for example, the muscles frequently contain *Clostridium welchii*.[34] Furthermore, wounds in experimental animals frequently become infected from external sources.

Endotoxic factor in shock[35, 36] (Sanarelli phenomenon[37]). It has been shown that bacterial endotoxins are capable of producing shock by some type of sensitisation. Experimentally it is known that an intravenous injection of a suspension of certain organisms, e.g. *V. cholerae*, meningococci, and many members of the coli-typhoid group, will induce a state of "sensitisation", such that if the injection is repeated intravenously *24 hours later*, a shock-like condition results.[38] The reaction is most easily elicited in rabbits, and frequently results in death after a few hours. Many small vessels are blocked by fibrin,[39, 40] and bilateral cortical necrosis of the kidney is a characteristic *post-mortem* finding in animals dying at about 24 hours (Fig. 32.4).

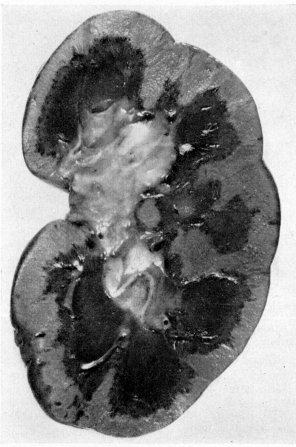

Figure 32.4
Cortical necrosis of kidney. This kidney came from a patient who died of bilateral symmetrical cortical necrosis following abruptio placentae. The outer two thirds of the cortex is pale and infarcted, while the inner part of the kidney is very congested. A similar appearance is seen in the rabbit kidney as a result of the Sanarelli phenomenon.

Some important features should be noted:

(*a*) Lipoprotein extracts ("endotoxins") can be used instead of whole organisms.

(*b*) The reaction is completely non-specific, i.e. the same organism need not be used for both injections.

(*c*) The state of sensitivity is of temporary duration; it remains for 1–2 days only, and is in no way connected with antibody production.

No certain explanation of this remarkable phenomenon is known. Probably a temporary blockade of the RE system is an important factor, and perhaps this defect, combined with the excessive formation of fibrin, is responsible for the production of intravascular fibrin plugs which are characteristic of the lesions seen in endotoxic shock. Such a pathogenesis would explain why the prior administration of heparin inhibits the reaction. Intravascular coagulation is probably initiated by the release of platelet factors which occurs when platelets interact with endotoxin.[41] Rendering animals thrombocytopenic protects them against the Sanarelli phenomenon, as does the administration of aspirin, which interferes with the platelet release reaction (p. 613). Complement is also involved, for the injection of venom from the cobra *Naja naja* is also protective, presumably by depleting the terminal components of complement *via* activation of the alternate pathway[42] (p. 163).

The original observations were made by Sanarelli at the end of the last century and a somewhat similar non-specific local sensitisation was later described by Shwartzman.[43] For this reason the generalised response is sometimes known as the "generalised Shwartzman phenomenon".

It has been suggested that organisms of the coliform group normally pass from the gut into the portal blood stream and then to the liver. It is therefore possible that such continuous intravenous injections of organisms or their endotoxins could produce a Shwartzman-like state, if one postulates that the liver's normal function is to remove these, and that in shock this mechanism is impaired.[44] It has been shown that the blood from a dog in shock contains a toxic substance which has the properties of bacterial endotoxin.[44] Furthermore, oral antibiotics can markedly influence the severity of shock produced by bleeding.[45, 46] There is thus some evidence that toxic substances in the intestine are concerned in the production of shock. However, some investigators have found that oral antibiotics are without protective effect on haemorrhagic shock.[47] Furthermore, it has been shown that shock can be produced just as easily in germ-free rats as in normal ones.[48] At first sight this argues against the importance of the bacterial factor. Nevertheless, bacterial products present in the food might be absorbed and produce a toxic effect.[35, 45, 48] Whether bacterial endotoxin plays any part in the production of haemorrhagic or traumatic shock in man has yet to be determined.[49]

It should be noted that most of the experiments designed to illustrate the importance of the endotoxic factor in haemorrhagic or traumatic shock have been performed on the dog or the rabbit. Both exhibit certain peculiarities: thus, the rabbit is particularly susceptible to the Sanarelli phenomenon, and the dog's intestine is very sensitive to ischaemia. Dogs dying of haemorrhagic shock show striking necrosis of the small intestine, and it is not surprising that toxic substances are absorbed.[8, 46]

Endotoxic shock in man. Sudden collapse may occur during a variety of infections, commonly those of the urinary tract.[50, 51] Usually the condition is precipitated by some manipulation or operation on the urethra or bladder. It is ascribed to the sudden entry into the blood of Gram-negative bacilli, and a positive blood culture may be obtained. An alternative name is therefore *bacteraemic shock*. The condition may also occur in cirrhosis of the liver, as a consequence of the portal-systemic venous shunts, and in patients on immunosuppressive therapy. Energetic steroid and antibiotic treatment may be life-saving.

Damage to the gastrointestinal tract. In man ischaemia of the gastrointestinal tract after shock is less striking than in the dog. Acute *stress ulcers* of the stomach or duodenum may occur after any injury, but are best known in association with severe burns (Curling's ulcer).[117] These acute ulcers may bleed profusely. Ischaemia of the intestine can lead to focal areas of mucosal infarction in both the small and large intestine.[52] The ensuing ulceration causes loss of blood and fluid which adds to the patient's plight.

Liver damage. Quite apart from the effect on the RE cells causing undue susceptibility to bacterial endotoxin[45] it has been suggested that the poor blood flow to the liver has other results. Impaired liver function may be detected by suitable clinical tests, and at necropsy focal necrosis, usually centrilobular, may be noted.

It has been claimed that the liver releases a vasodepressor material (VDM, which is reduced ferritin) which causes vasodilatation, and makes vessels unresponsive to adrenaline. The consensus of opinion is that this is not an important factor in shock.[53] The release of lysosomal enzymes from the liver has also been postulated as a factor in the pathogenesis of shock. The effect of glucocorticosteroids on stabilising the lysosomes could explain how this drug protects rabbits against endotoxic shock.[54]

Lung damage. Pulmonary congestion and oedema are common in patients dying of shock and are also seen following cardio-pulmonary bypass procedures. The sequestration of polymorphs in the lung capillaries and the release of their lysosomal enzymes is one suggested mechanism in this "shock-lung syndrome".[55]

Fat embolism. An occasional feature of shock in man is the occurrence of fat embolism. It has been shown experimentally in animals that the deliberate introduction of fat emboli into the circulation does not have any effect upon the degree of shock that is produced by trauma.[56] This factor therefore can be discounted as an important cause of shock.

Conclusion. Although the causes of shock following mechanical trauma are poorly understood, the most important factor in the early stages is loss of blood. Local inflammation and the effects of infection may later aggravate this, but their relative importance probably varies from case to case.

Shock in Bacterial Infections

In addition to Gram-negative endotoxic shock described above, a shock-like state followed by death has been described in many infections, including those produced by Gram-positive organisms. The pathogenesis is not necessarily the same in the two types.[57, 58] It occurs in diphtheria and gas-gangrene, and can be produced experimentally by injecting animals with the respective exotoxins. In overwhelming infections with an invasive organism various factors play a part. In *B. anthracis* septicaemia in guinea-pigs it has been shown that a toxin is produced, and that the rapid formation of oedema leads to hypovolaemic shock.[57] In *Yersinia pestis* infections, on the other hand, oligaemia does not occur, and the shock appears to be due to a pooling of the blood in the splanchnic area. The mechanisms whereby shock is produced are complex, and probably vary in different infections. The possibility that bacterial toxins damage specific organs must also be considered: thus diphtheria toxin damages the heart and kidneys. Another example is acute adrenal haemorrhage. This occurs in the *Waterhouse-Friderichsen syndrome*, which is characterised by bilateral adrenal haemorrhages and confluent purpura occurring in patients with septicaemia (usually meningococcal) dying rapidly in a state of shock. Death has been ascribed to acute adrenal insufficiency, but this is most improbable. The normal levels of serum electrolytes, the rapid course of the syndrome, and the inconstancy of the adrenal haemorrhages all point to the conclusion that the cause of death is the infection itself, while the haemorrhages are secondary.[59, 60] They are believed to be due to a defibrination syndrome (p. 623).

Shock due to Loss of Plasma

Rapid loss of plasma from the circulation occurs whenever an acute inflammatory reaction involves a large area of the body. This is seen experimentally in *tourniquet shock*.[29, 30] The blood supply to a limb is occluded by means of a rubber band for 5 hours, and when this is released the animal subsequently goes into a state of shock and dies. This is due to a leakage of plasma into the infarcted limb. A similar condition is seen in man in the crush syndrome, following extensive burns, and when there is the rapid accumulation of an exudate, e.g. ascites. Generalised loss of plasma from the circulation is a factor in the shock of anaphylaxis and in the rare, but remarkable, case of cyclical oedema noted on p. 495.

Burn Shock[61, 62]

The shock produced by extensive burning is very similar to that of haemorrhage. There are, however, certain differences. The early clinical picture is often misleading. A patient admitted with a 40 per cent burn may appear to be in excellent condition 1–2 hours after the accident. Ten hours later, however, he may be in a state of irreversible shock. In general, the severity of the shock is proportional to the extent of the skin burned. Thus in children, if the area of burning exceeds 10 per cent of the surface area, or in adults 15 per cent, the patient is likely to need intravenous therapy.[63] The area burned may be estimated by the simple *rule of nines*. This is shown diagrammatically in Fig. 32.5.

The effect of heat on tissues has been studied experimentally. A temperature of 50°C leads to vasodilatation with an additional formation of protein-poor extravascular fluid. A temperature of 55°C causes, in addition, an increase in vascular permeability. This leads to the formation of a protein-rich exudate. Temperatures of 100°C or more simply coagulate the tissue, and cause complete cessation of blood

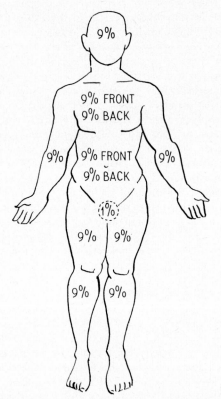

Figure 32.5
The rule of nines. The body surface of an adult may be divided into eleven areas each comprising 9 per cent approximately. (*After Wallace, A. B.* (1951), Lancet, i, 501)

flow. An important feature of burns therefore is the loss of fluid from the circulation, and much of that which exudes from the burned area has a composition similar to plasma.[61] It has been shown in animals that the volume of fluid lost in a 50 per cent burn is equal to the entire circulating plasma volume.[64] This fluid loss results in a low blood volume. In burns, unlike haemorrhage, the viscosity of the blood is increased; haemoconcentration occurs instead of dilution. Although the loss of plasma from the circulating blood is important in the causation of burn shock, other factors may also play a part and contribute to the overall picture observed clinically:

Vomiting is not uncommon, and leads to dehydration.
Infection may occur in the wound.

Red cells may be damaged in the burned area. This results in a haemolytic anaemia, especially after extensive burning. Haemoglobinuria occasionally occurs.
Sludging of the blood is a prominent feature.
Anaesthetics may potentiate the shock.
Liver damage: this was usually seen following the application of tannic acid to the burns.
Gastro-intestinal ulceration and bleeding: (see p. 425).
Cerebral damage:[65, 66] burns may be followed, particularly in children, by psychiatric and neurological complications. These are often fatal, and those patients who survive may suffer permanent cerebral damage. The cause of these phenomena is not known, but cerebral oedema and hypoxia have been suggested.

Shock from Fluid Loss

Shock may be induced in animals by subjecting them to prolonged unnatural postures. If an anaesthetised dog is suspended with its feet hanging down it passes into a state of shock, especially if a small quantity of blood is removed at the same time.[67] Haemoconcentration develops due to the loss of fluid through the vessels in the dependent parts.

Subcutaneous injections of hypertonic solutions, e.g. 40 per cent glucose, will also lead to the withdrawal of fluid from the circulating blood, thereby producing a shock-like state with haemoconcentration.[19] In man shock may result from dehydration due to inadequate fluid intake or excessive loss, such as may follow excessive sweating, vomiting, or diarrhoea. Infants are particularly vulnerable because they cannot secrete as concentrated a urine as can adults. Diarrhoea is therefore a serious condition in this age group. Dehydration is also a feature of diabetic coma.

It appears that the most important causative factor in the types of shock so far considered is the loss of circulating blood volume. A convenient term is therefore *hypovolaemic shock*. It is due to loss of blood, plasma, or fluid.

In other types of shock the blood volume is not primarily or greatly altered, and some other mechanisms must be invoked. These are not clearly defined at the present time; four aspects should be considered:

Cardiogenic shock.
Peripheral vascular failure.
The metabolic upset.
Poor capillary circulation due to sludging.

Cardiogenic Shock[68]

Myocardial infarction may sometimes produce a clinical state of shock which resembles that of hypovolaemic shock. The cardiac output is reduced, and the poor perfusion of tissues is responsible for a metabolic acidosis.[69] This acidosis can lead to peripheral vasodilatation with pooling of blood and subsequent transudation; the loss of fluid tends to lower the blood volume and accentuate the shock. Cardiogenic shock is also seen in a number of other conditions: myo-carditis, acute valvular dysfunction such as occurs following the rupture of a papillary muscle (itself often the result of infarction), serious cardiac arrhythmias, cardiac tamponade, and tension pneumothorax with marked mediastinal shift.

Heart failure may be an important additional factor in the pathogenesis of hypovolaemic shock. In experiments with dogs,[70] a state of haemorrhagic shock can be induced such that replacement of the lost blood does not save the animals. Further transfusion causes a rise in central venous pressure and a fall in cardiac output—a sure indication that the heart is failing. The administration of digitalis improves the state of the animals. Thus, heart failure may be an important factor in experimental irreversible shock.[71]

In man, focal microscopic or massive myocardial infarcts are sometimes found at necropsy in patients dying in shock, and in these cases heart failure appears to have been the immediate cause of death. Nevertheless, there is little evidence that heart failure contributes significantly to most cases of haemorrhagic, traumatic, or endotoxic shock, and digitalis is without beneficial effect.

Peripheral Vascular Failure

The concept of peripheral vascular failure embodies the idea that the circulation is impaired, not by a decrease in the blood volume, but by an increase in the capacity of the vascular system. This might occur in various ways. Blood could be *sequestrated*, and in this way lost from a functional point of view. Thus, if rabbits are suspended erect they become unconscious in 20–120 minutes, and may die in a shock-like state within 24 hours.[72] They show a low blood pressure, oliguria, and a metabolic acidosis. Haemoconcentration does not occur, and the condition is due to the pooling of the blood in the splanchnic area, with the result that the supply of oxygen to the vital organs is impaired. The fainting of guardsmen on parade is due to a similar mechanism—the blood becomes sequestrated in the leg veins—but the condition is not serious, for the automatic assumption of the horizontal position effects a cure!

The contraction of arterioles and veins is an important compensatory reaction in hypotension, and a failure in this mechanism could be an additional factor in shock due initially to other causes. Furthermore, if the venous constriction is maintained whilst the arterioles relax, blood becomes sequestrated or pooled in the capillary bed. This has been described in the shock of myocardial infarction[69] in some types of bacterial shock, e.g. in septicaemic plague, and as a complication of metabolic acidosis.[73]

Metabolic Upset During Shock[74]

There is another important feature of shock yet to be examined. This is the *lowering of body temperature*. The skin is cool, and its blood flow reduced. There is no evidence of increased heat loss; the hypothermia is therefore due to decreased heat production. In shock the carbohydrate stores are rapidly utilised, and there is a profound depression in energy production. The patient remains still and apathetic.

In shock there are important alterations in carbohydrate metabolism:[75] the glycogen stores in the muscles are depleted and there is an increase in liver glycogen. Deamination is impaired and the blood amino–acid level therefore rises.[76] The blood sugar tends to rise during the early phase of shock, but in spite of this its utilisation is blocked. It has been found that glucose 6-phosphate accumulates in the tissues, which suggests a hold-up at this point.

In shock, although there is abundant evidence of an upset in carbohydrate metabolism and diminished energy production, the exact nature of the changes remains a mystery. The secretions of the adrenal medulla and cortex are probably important,[74] and these are considered further on in relation to the other metabolic disturbances.

Another important metabolic upset that develops during shock is *metabolic acidosis*. The cause is tissue hypoxia with resulting anaerobic glycolysis and the release of pyruvate and lactate into the circulation. Metabolic acidosis is very well marked in haemorrhagic shock,[77] but is also seen in any condition in which there is *underperfusion of the tissues* with blood. Thus, it occurs in many types of shock, and is a well-recognised complication of inadequate blood flow in the extracorporeal cardio-pulmonary by-pass.[78]

Sludging[23, 79, 80]

"Shock is not merely a problem of blood volume, blood pressure, and anaemia, but essentially a problem of flow".[20] The concept has arisen since techniques have been devised to study the flow of blood in vessels of microscopic size. In shock it has been observed that the flow is poor and that the red cells are clumped together. That such clumping can occur *in vivo* is no new observation,[81] but it is largely due to the work of Knisely and his associates that the phenomenon is now being more widely recognised.[82–87] Working with malaria-infected monkeys they described thick, glassy precipitates between and around the blood cells, binding the red cells together in wads and masses, thus converting the "circulating blood into a thick muck-like sludge". The red cells are adherent to each other to form aggregates, more irregular than the "pile of plates" appearance of rouleaux, but differing from true agglutination in that the masses can be broken up again. Some degree of aggregation occurs normally in the post-capillary venules when the flow is slow, and indeed some observers have regarded sludging as a result of stasis rather than its cause.[88] However, there seems little doubt that under certain conditions a solid aggregation of red cells occurs, not only in the venules but also in the arterioles.[23] In this way the blood-flow through the tissues is impaired and the tissue suffers accordingly. Micro-infarcts have been described.[89]

Sludging occurs after trauma, especially burns, haemorrhage, and in shock. It is seen in many infections and also to a minor extent in pregnancy. It is a feature of the generalised

Shwartzman phenomenon, and is a complicating factor in the use of extracorporeal circulation techniques.

The suspension stability of the red cells is determined by the composition of the plasma. An increase in the proportion of high-molecular-weight substances results in sludging; in practice a rise in fibrinogen is the most important factor. Administration of high-molecular-weight dextrans has a similar effect.

Low-molecular-weight substances, e.g. albumin and dextran, inhibit or reverse sludging.[90] A low-molecular-weight dextran preparation* is now available for intravenous administration and its value is being assessed. In shock it appears to diminish the amount of sludging and improve the circulation of blood through the small vessels.[91, 92]

Quite apart from impeding the circulation, sludging has been suggested as a cause of the anaemia of injury. The clumps of red cells may be trapped in the vessels and thereby become sequestrated from the general circulation.[93]

IRREVERSIBLE SHOCK[45]

The reasons why shock becomes irreversible are poorly understood. Irreversibility means that the blood pressure continues to fall despite the compensatory mechanisms and also treatment. The patient's condition steadily deteriorates, and death ensues.

The present concept of shock is that the major abnormality is the underperfusion of certain vital organs.[94] If this ischaemia persists, irreparable damage is done and death becomes inevitable. In the dog the organ most obviously affected is the intestine, and haemorrhagic infarction results. In man the situation is less clear, but renal, cardiac, pulmonary, hepatic, and intestinal damage may all ensue. Death from shock may occur for one of many reasons, either directly related to a particular organ (e.g. myocardial infarction) or as an indirect consequence of organ damage, e.g. metabolic acidosis or electrolyte imbalance. From a practical point of view the efficiency of treatment is of overriding importance, because many of the potentially lethal effects of shock can be counter-acted. Irreversible shock may be regarded as being almost always due to inefficient treatment.

The types of treatment will therefore be summarised:

Restoration of Blood Volume

The importance of restoring the blood volume as soon as possible in hypovolaemic shock is widely recognised. So long as the cardiac output is low, there is compensatory peripheral vasoconstriction. This has the effect of maintaining the blood pressure. At first this is advantageous, but if it persists it may lead ultimately to damage in vital organs.[95]

1. **Blood transfusion.** In severe haemorrhage it is often not appreciated that blood must be given rapidly. Several

---

* This is known as *Rheomacrodex*(R), and has an average molecular weight of about 40 000.

pints must be administered by the fastest means available. Some workers have used intra-arterial transfusions, and it is claimed that these give better results, as the blood is immediately available to support the coronary and cerebral circulations. The use of slow intravenous transfusions after a severe haemorrhage merely leads to a false sense of security in both patient and doctor. One of the curious features of human traumatic shock is the response to treatment by transfusion. In wartime this was found to be very effective both in preventing and treating shock. In civilian life, however, the results of such treatment are not nearly so dramatic or effective. This may be related to the fact that in wartime the casualties are usually young healthy people, while in civilian practice it is the elderly and sick who are most frequently affected. It is known that shock tends to be more severe in such subjects.[8, 96]

2. **Administration of fluid and electrolytes.** Although some workers have found "irreversible shock" to be quite unresponsive to fluid therapy,[97] others have been more successful. Thus, hypertonic saline has been reported to be beneficial in severe haemorrhagic shock in dogs,[98, 99] and vigorous fluid replacement is of value in experimental shock due to burns, haemorrhage, and trauma.[28] It is often taught that the body is defenceless against an overdosage of sodium in shock, but this is by no means universally accepted.[100, 101] In the management of patients, the measurement of the blood volume is of much greater value than that of blood pressure. The *Volemetron*,[102] a machine using an isotope dilution technique and incorporating a built-in computer, is invaluable in this respect.

Unfortunately the measurement of blood volume in a shocked patient produces a value which is not easy to interpret. The capacity of the venous reservoir is dependent on the venous tone (p. 420), and furthermore large quantities of blood can be sequestrated in the splanchnic area and to all intents and purposes be lost so far as the maintenance of an efficient circulation is concerned. Hence the measurement of the *central venous pressure* is a useful guide to the quantity of fluid which can be administered intravenously to fill up the vascular system, without at the same time causing pulmonary oedema.[103]

Maintenance of Renal Function

The administration of adequate fluids can do much to maintain the urine output, and some authorities advocate the intravenous administration of an osmotic diuretic, e.g. mannitol. This appears to increase glomerular filtration by causing vasodilatation.[104] Renal damage is a potent cause of death if shock is prolonged.[16] The tubules are most severely affected, and the damage is generally attributable to ischaemia.[101] This, however, is not accepted by all authorities.[105]

Reversal of Sludging

Adequate fluid administration and intravenous Rheomacrodex(R) can do much to reverse the sludging in shock.

Correction of Metabolic Acidosis

Sodium bicarbonate can be given intravenously in sufficient quantity to correct the acidosis.

Maintenance of Adequate Pulmonary Ventilation

Because of the increase in dead-space ventilation, any interference with the hyperpnoea may cause arterial desaturation and respiratory acidosis. Avoidance of airways obstruction is life-saving, and the inhalation of 30 per cent oxygen is helpful.

The Administration of Drugs

It is worth remembering that in any form of shock drugs administered by the intramuscular or subcutaneous routes are slowly absorbed owing to the poor state of the circulation. Failure to get a satisfactory clinical response may necessitate a repetition of the dose. In this way a large depot, e.g. of morphine, may accumulate in the tissues, only to be absorbed later; poisoning then results.

Patients in shock are particularly sensitive to depressant drugs like barbiturates and anaesthetic agents. Furthermore, they decrease venous tone[106] and their injudicious use may be detrimental. Halothane is especially dangerous.[107] The place of morphine in shock is very limited. It is useful in alleviating severe pain, and it may allay the apprehension that follows severe haemorrhage, e.g. haematemesis, but on the whole it is best avoided.

Vasoactive drugs.[108, 109] The administration of adrenergic drugs with a predominant α-receptor stimulating effect,* e.g. noradrenaline and metaraminol (aramine), raises the blood pressure in shock, but far from being beneficial tends to worsen the prognosis, because the vasoconstriction which is induced further compromises the already inadequate blood supply to various vital organs, e.g. the kidneys and intestine. An alternative approach, stressed by Lillehei,[47, 94] is therefore to administer vasodilator drugs, e.g. phenoxybenzamine (dibenyline) which has a powerful α-adrenergic blocking action. Experimentally it counters traumatic, haemorrhagic, and endotoxic shock as well as the shock which follows the administration of toxic doses of adrenaline. Drugs with a β-adrenergic receptor stimulating effect, such as isoprenaline (isoproterenol), have also been used. Pharmacological or massive doses of glucocorticosteroids have also been advocated in the treatment of shock, and there is experimental evidence that they protect against endotoxic shock. The mode of action is not clear, but one suggestion is that in pharmacological doses (e.g. 15–30 mg per kg of hydrocortisone every 24 hours) they block the action of adrenaline. The logical drug treatment of shock is therefore to administer agents which produce vasodilatation in the vital organs, and

---

* The α-adrenergic receptor stimulating effects are vasoconstriction and mydriasis. The β effects are vasodilatation, increased force and rate of cardiac contraction, and bronchial relaxation. Adrenaline has both α and β effects, while noradrenaline is predominantly α.

at the same time to give adequate intravenous fluids to guard against the development of dangerous hypotension.

Temperature

If the patient is actively warmed, the skin vessels dilate and the effective circulating blood volume is further diminished. The administration of alcohol has a similar effect, and both of these time-honoured treatments of shock should be avoided.

Treatment of Infection

Although obvious enough in diseases like gas-gangrene or diphtheria, infection may sometimes pass unnoticed and untreated.

Treatment of Mechanical Complications

The development of raised intracranial pressure, pneumothorax, haemopericardium, etc. may cause a rapid deterioration of the patient's condition, which is liable to be misdiagnosed as shock and left untreated.

Even with efficient treatment the blood pressure may continue to fall, and the patient dies. This is seen under the following circumstances:

(*a*) With very severe injuries.
(*b*) When the shock has been present for some time.
(*c*) In patients already ill with some disease.
(*d*) In the presence of severe infection.

It is evident that the treatment of shock is often complicated and costly. The more intensive the treatment, the less likely is the patient to die. "Irreversible shock" should not be accepted as a diagnosis except *post mortem*: there are some surgeons who feel that the term "shock" itself should be abandoned, as its use tends to result in remediable conditions being overlooked. Nevertheless, there can be little doubt that the condition of shock does exist, and that in spite of even the best treatment some patients die. This may be as a result of the initial injury involving some vital organ, or else through damage sustained during the period of shock. As pointed out previously, there is considerable uncertainty as to which organ is most affected: the intestine, heart, kidney, liver, and brain have all been suggested.[45] Undoubtedly under particular circumstances failure of one of these organs can cause death, and it is naïve to expect the pathogenesis of all types of shock to be identical.

CONVALESCENCE

Assuming that the patient survives the initial shock, there ensues a period of metabolic upset characterised by excessive protein breakdown and a negative nitrogen balance. This catabolic phase is later followed by an anabolic period during which the body's stores are replenished. These important metabolic changes have been widely studied both in animals and man.

CHANGES IN METABOLISM

Protein Metabolism[26, 110, 111]

The average daily consumption of protein is 60–100 g, or 10–15 g expressed as nitrogen (6·25 g of dry protein = 1 g of nitrogen). After injury patients lose protein in a number of ways:

1. By blood loss and in exudates. Infection aggravates this loss.
2. By tissue loss, e.g. in burns.
3. As the result of disuse atrophy following immobilisation.
4. As an inevitable result of the process of convalescence itself. This is the early catabolic phase which follows injury. It is this aspect of protein metabolism which must now be considered.

At least twenty grams of nitrogen (as urea) may be lost daily, though the loss seldom exceeds 10 g. Its duration varies with the extent of the trauma. After a simple herniorraphy it may last only a day or two, but with severe burns it can continue for 10 days or more. Fractures cause more disturbance than might be supposed from the clinical condition. Chronic suppuration may prolong the catabolic state for weeks. The following points should be noted.

1. The nitrogen loss cannot be abolished by increasing the protein intake. If extra protein is given in the diet it is broken down, and the extra nitrogen is excreted. There is therefore no point in forcing patients to ingest protein during this phase.
2. Carbohydrate administration does reduce the nitrogen loss very considerably.
3. Protein starvation prior to injury depletes the protein reserve of the body, and virtually abolishes the nitrogen loss.
4. Patients with Addison's disease and adrenalectomised animals do not show post-traumatic nitrogen loss.

Source of the lost protein. The effect of starvation (see above) indicates that it is the labile reserves which are used. These are generally assumed to be in the liver and especially the muscles, but their nature is not known. Proteins are broken down to amino acids, and subsequently deaminated in the liver. The blood amino-acid level is therefore high.

Mechanism of the Protein Loss

1. The metabolic effects of injury are closely simulated by glucocorticosteroids.
2. The adrenal glands are known to enlarge following injury.
3. There is an increased secretion of adrenal cortical hormones following trauma.
4. Adrenalectomised animals do not show this nitrogen loss.

It would therefore be not unreasonable to assume that excessive adrenal function explains the loss, but that this is not so is shown by the finding that adrenalectomised animals[112] (and man[113,114]) on a constant maintenance dose of cortisone, still show the same negative nitrogen balance when subjected to trauma. Adrenal hormones are thus necessary for this metabolic change, but apparently they do not directly produce it. Possibly some other mechanism renders the body more sensitive to the action of these hormones.[115]

Anabolic phase. During the latter part of convalescence, nitrogen is retained and the body's protein stores are built up. The amount of nitrogen retained each day is seldom more than 2 g, and therefore an excessive intake of protein is of no value.

Sodium and Water Metabolism[110]

During the early period after trauma the urine volume diminishes owing to a secretion of ADH, and sodium is retained by the kidneys as a result of aldosterone secretion. This phase of sodium retention is a little shorter than the catabolic protein phase; it has been held that this is obligatory, and that the body is defenceless against overdosage, because it cannot excrete sodium and water[5, 116] (see p. 452). However, this view has been disputed (see p. 428).

There is a later return of sodium to the urine; unless there was excessive administration during the oliguric phase, its excretion is not much increased.

Potassium Metabolism[110]

A negative potassium balance occurs during the initial phase, and is most marked on the first day. Because potassium is intracellular it is presumed to be liberated at the same time as protein is metabolised: the loss is 2·5–3·0 mEq per 1·0 g of nitrogen, and the total loss after a major operation, e.g. gastrectomy, is about 100 mEq.

The average daily intake is about 70 mEq, therefore there is little point in supplementing the diet during convalescence.

Mechanism of the Metabolic Response[110]

Although it is evident that these metabolic effects can be explained in terms of an increased secretion of adrenal cortical hormones, there is no irrefutable evidence that these are the operative agents. It is worth while considering some alternative factors that also come into action after injury.

Immobilisation. This has been studied in healthy volunteers placed in a plaster cast from the waist down. The main effect is a loss of calcium (see p. 304); the nitrogen loss is about 1 g each day, and there is a commensurate potassium loss. Sodium balance is unaffected.

Starvation. Its effects resemble those of trauma more closely, but (a) the nitrogen loss is remedied by food, (b) the potassium loss is not great initially, but it persists as starvation continues and is then of a high order, (c) the sodium retention becomes established only after 4–5 days.

Other Metabolic Changes

1. There is an increased urinary excretion of creatine (derived presumably from the muscles), phosphate, and

sulphur. This occurs *pari passu* with the nitrogenous and potassium excretion, and is due to cellular breakdown.

2. There is retention of vitamin C, which disappears from the urine. A scorbutic state may develop despite this careful guarding of the ascorbic-acid stores. Riboflavin, on the other hand, is excreted in excess.

3. The early effects on carbohydrate metabolism have already been noted; the most conspicuous change during the catabolic phase is moderate hyperglycaemia due to gluconeogenesis. There may occasionally be glycosuria.

During this catabolic phase there is a marked loss of weight. A moderate pyrexia is invariable, and is not due to concomitant infection.

The haematological changes are a moderate neutrophilia accompanied by lymphopenia and eosinopenia. A thrombocytosis also occurs (see p. 457). An interesting feature of severe trauma is the development of a progressive normochromic, normocytic anaemia. This is not due to iron deficiency; perhaps there is deficient haemoglobin synthesis during a period of general protein breakdown. Sludging may accentuate this anaemia (see p. 428). All these changes are reversed during the ensuing anabolic phase.

SUMMARY

The changes that occur in a wounded animal from the time of injury to return to complete health are thus highly complex.

During the first few hours the response is concerned largely with circulatory adjustments, the aim of which appears to be to maintain an adequate blood supply to the vital organs. It is only when these mechanisms fail to keep pace with the load placed upon them that the clinical state of shock occurs. During this phase there is reduced energy production due to a change in carbohydrate metabolism, the nature of which is poorly understood. The only obvious advantage that this confers would seem to be a reduction in the amount of food required during a phase when the injured animal is unlikely to be able to hunt.

Following the successful circulatory adjustment, the animal enters the state of *convalescence*. This consists of two phases:

A catabolic phase, in which protein breakdown is the most conspicuous feature, and is accompanied by sodium and water retention.

An anabolic phase, in which protein is laid down, weight is gained, and the electrolyte balance returns to normal.

It is difficult to explain these changes other than on a teleological basis. During the early phase, the retained sodium and water is required for the inflammatory exudate as well as to help maintain the circulation. A little later the body proteins are broken down and converted into amino acids and glucose. The purpose of this catabolism appears to be twofold. In the first place it provides a source of energy during the early phase of convalescence; for this reason glucose administration reduces the rate of protein breakdown. There is, however, a second reason: when healing commences, the products of protein breakdown provide the raw materials from which are built the new tissues required for repair and regeneration. In the formation of collagen, the sulphur-containing amino acids are essential, and it has been suggested that the catabolism of protein is largely designed to meet this local need in the wounded area. Vitamin C is also required, and this may explain why it also is so carefully conserved.

The duration of the catabolic phase is related to the severity of the injury, and rarely exceeds 10–14 days in the absence of further haemorrhage or secondary infection. Considerable loss of weight is to be expected during this phase. As convalescence proceeds and the wounded area heals, the animal becomes fit enough to resume its search for nourishment. Protein catabolism ceases, and energy is produced from ingested food; the depleted stores are replaced and health is restored.

It would be foolish to imagine that the above account explains the changes that occur in the wounded animal. It is, however, not unreasonable to assume that the complex reactions, while not designed to aid in the restoration of health, have nevertheless been evolved by a process of selection as a means of attaining that same end. John Hunter nearly two centuries ago appreciated this, for in his treatise on the blood, inflammation, and gun-shot wounds, which was published in 1794, a year after his death, he wrote: "There is a circumstance attending accidental injury which does not belong to disease, viz., that the injury done has in all cases a tendency to produce both the disposition and the means of cure."

REFERENCES

1. SELYE, H. (1954). *British Medical Journal*, i, 1167.
2. BARCROFT, H. *et al.* (1944). *Lancet*, i, 489.
3. WARREN, J. V. *et al.* (1945). *Journal of Clinical Investigation*, **24**, 337.
4. BARCROFT, H. and EDHOLM, O. G. (1945). *Journal of Physiology*, (*London*), **104**, 161.
5. DICKINSON, C. J. and PENTECOST, B. L. (1968). In *Clinical Physiology*, 3rd edn, p. 63. Edited by E. J. M. Campbell, C. J. Dickinson and J. D. H. Slater. Oxford: Blackwell.
6. BLAIR, D. A. *et al.* (1959). *Journal of Physiology*, (*London*), **148**, 633.
7. RODDIE, I. C. and SHEPHERD, J. T. (1963). *British Medical Bulletin*, **19**, 115.
8. FREEMAN, J. (1963). *Annals of the Royal College of Surgeons of England*, **33**, 138.
9. PEKKARINEN, A. (1960). In *Biochemical Response to Injury*: a C.I.O.M.S. Symposium. Edited by H. B. Stoner and C. J. Threlfall, p. 217. Oxford: Blackwell.

10. WYKE, B. D. (1965). *Principles of General Neurophysiology relating to Anaesthesia and Surgery*, 2nd edn. London: Butterworths.
11. HARPER, A. M. and BELL, G. (1966). In *Wound Healing*. Edited by C. Illingworth, p. 181. London: Churchill.
12. KETY, S. S. and SCHMIDT, C. F. (1948). *Journal of Clinical Investigation*, **27**, 484.
13. STONE, H. H. *et al.* (1954). *Surgery Forum*, **5**, 789.
14. Annotation (1960). *British Medical Journal*, ii, 1661.
15. PEARS, M. A. and PICKERING, G. W. (1960). *Quarterly Journal of Medicine*, **29**, 153.
16. BRUN, C. and MUNCK, O. (1957). *Lancet*, i, 603.
17. Leading Article (1964). *British Medical Journal*, i, 1328.
18. GULLIVER, G. (1846). Editor. *The Works of William Hewson*, F.R.S., p. 46. London: Sydenham Society.
19. ROBERTS, K. B. (1970). In *General Pathology*, 4th edn, p. 319. Edited by H. W. Florey. London: Lloyd Luke.
20. GELIN, L.-E. (1963). p. 6 in Reference 80.
21. ROBB, H. J. (1963). *Annals of Surgery*, **158**, 685.
22. Leading Article (1967). *Lancet*, i, 429.
23. WELLS, R. E. (1963). *Anesthesiology*, **24**, 828.
24. MOORE, F. D. (1959). In *Metabolic Care of the Surgical Patient*, p. 162. Philadelphia: Saunders.
25. Leading Article (1967). *British Medical Journal*, i, 447.
26. CUTHBERTSON, D. P. (1960). p. 193 in C.I.O.M.S. Symposium, *loc. cit.*
27. NOBLE, R. L. and COLLIP, J. B. (1942). *Quarterly Journal of Experimental Physiology*, **31**, 187.
28. ROSENTHAL, S. M. and TABOR, H. (1945). *Archives of Surgery*, **51**, 244.
29. KOLETSKY, S. and GUSTAFSON, G. E. (1946). *Journal of Clinical Investigation*, **25**, 744.
30. KOLETSKY, S. and KLEIN, D. E. (1955). *American Journal of Physiology*, **182**, 439.
31. CLARKE, R. *et al.* (1961). *Lancet*, ii, 381.
32. GRANT, R. T. and REEVE, E. B. (1951). *Special Report Series. Medical Research Council, London*, No. 277.
33. THORNTON, J. A. (1963). *Annals of the Royal College of Surgeons of England*, **33**, 164.
34. POPE, A. *et al.* (1945). *Journal of Clinical Investigation*, **24**, 856.
35. FINE, J. *et al.* (1960). p. 377 in C.I.O.M.S. Symposium, *loc. cit.*
36. LEE, L. and STETSON, C. A. (1965). In *The Inflammatory Process*, p. 791. Edited by B. W. Zweifach, L. Grant and R. T. McCluskey. New York and London: Academic Press.
37. SANARELLI, G. (1924). *Annals of the Institute Pasteur*, **38**, 11.
38. THOMAS, L. and GOOD, R. A. (1952). *Journal of Experimental Medicine*, **95**, 409 and **96**, 605.
39. McKAY, D. G. and SHAPIRO, S. S. (1958). *Journal of Experimental Medicine*, **107**, 353 and (with J. N. Shanberge) 369.
40. PAPPAS, G. D., ROSS, M. H. and THOMAS, L. (1958). *Journal of Experimental Medicine*, **107**, 333.
41. MUSTARD, J. F. and PACKHAM, M. A. (1970). *Canadian Medical Association Journal*, **103**, 859.
42. FONG, J. S. C. and GOOD, R. A. (1971). *Journal of Experimental Medicine*, **134**, 642.
43. ALECHINSKY, A. (1939). *Annals of the Institute Pasteur*, **63**, 41.
44. FINE, J. *et al.* (1959). *New England Journal of Medicine*, **260**, 214.
45. ZWEIFACH, B. W. (1958). *British Journal of Anaesthesia*, **30**, 466.
46. FINE, J. (1958). *British Journal of Anaesthesia*, **30**, 485.
47. LILLEHEI, R. C., LONGERBEAM, J. K. and ROSENBERG, J. C. (1962). In *Shock, Pathogenesis, and Therapy*, p. 106. Edited by K. D. Bock. Berlin Gottingen and Heidelberg: Springer-Verlag.
48. ZWEIFACH, B. W. *et al.* (1958). *Journal of Experimental Medicine*, **107**, 437.
49. Leading Article (1972). *Lancet*, i, 1377.
50. Leading Article (1964). *British Medical Journal*, i, 254.
51. SHUBIN, H. and WEIL, M. H. (1963). *Journal of the American Medical Association*, **185**, 850.
52. Leading Article (1971). *British Medical Journal*, iii, 132.
53. FUHRMAN, F. A. (1960). p. 418 in C.I.O.M.S. Symposium, *loc. cit.*
54. WEISSMANN, G. and THOMAS, L. (1962). *Journal of Experimental Medicine*, **116**, 433.
55. WILSON, J. W. (1972). *Surgery, Gynecology and Obstetrics*, **134**, 675.
56. GRANT, R. T. (1954). *British Medical Bulletin*, **10**, 17.
57. SMITH, H. (1960). p. 341 in C.I.O.M.S. Symposium, *loc. cit.*
58. KWAAN, H. M. and WEIL, M. H. (1969). *Surgery, Gynecology and Obstetrics*, **128**, 37.
59. Leading Article (1959). *British Medical Journal*, ii, 483.
60. BENSON, P. F. and BOYD, M. E. (1960). *Guy's Hospital Reports*, **109**, 219.
61. BULL, J. P. (1954). *British Medical Bulletin*, **10**, 9.
62. BLOCKER, T. G. and BLOCKER, V. (1963). *Progressive Surgery (Basel)*, **3**, 70.
63. BARCLAY, T. L. and WALLACE, A. B. (1954). *Lancet*, i, 98.
64. ROSSITER, R. J. (1943). *Bulletin of War Medicine*, **4**, 181.
65. Leading Article (1963). *British Medical Journal*, ii, 1350.
66. WARLOW, C. P. and HINTON, P. (1969). *Lancet*, ii, 978.
67. MAYERSON, H. S. (1944). *American Journal of Physiology*, **141**, 227.
68. Leading Article (1966). *British Medical Journal*, ii, 481.
69. MACKENZIE, G. T. *et al.* (1964). *Lancet*, ii, 825.
70. CROWELL, J. W. and GUYTON, A. C. (1962). *American Journal of Physiology*, **203**, 248.
71. WEALE, F. E. (1963). *Lancet*, i, 973.
72. COLE, W. H. *et al.* (1944). *American Journal of Physiology*, **141**, 165.
73. THROWER, W. B., DARBY, T. D. and ALDINGER, E. E. (1961). *Archives of Surgery*, **82**, 56.
74. STONER, H. B. and THRELFALL, C. J. (1960). p. 105 in C.I.O.M.S. Symposium, *loc. cit.*

75. GREEN, H. N. and STONER, H. B. (1954). *British Medical Bulletin*, **10**, 38.
76. ENGEL, F. L., HARRISON, H. C. and LONG, C. N. H. (1944). *Journal of Experimental Medicine*, **79**, 9.
77. WEIDNER, M. G. and SIMEONE, F. A. (1962). *Annals of Surgery*, **156**, 493.
78. MACKENZIE, G. J. *et al.* (1963). *Thorax*, **18**, 215.
79. FÅHRAEUS, R. (1960). p. 161 in C.I.O.M.S. Symposium, *loc cit.*
80. Various Authors (1963). *Proceedings of a Conference on the Evaluation of Low Molecular Weight Dextran in Shock: Pharmacology and Pertinent Rheology.* Edited by B. Eiseman and P. Bosomworth. Washington, D.C.: National Research Council Division of Medical Sciences.
81. NORRIS, R. (1869). *Proceedings of the Royal Society*, **17**, 429.
82. KNISELY, M. H., STRATMAN-THOMAS, W. K. and ELIOT, T. S. (1941). *Journal of the American Medical Association*, **116**, 2430.
83. KNISELY, M. H., STRATMAN-THOMAS, W. K. and ELIOT, T. S. (1941). *Anatomical Record.* Supplement, **79**, 90.
84. KNISELY, M. H. and BLOCH, E. H. (1942). *Anatomical Record*, **82**, 426.
85. KNISELY, M. H., ELIOT, T. S. and BLOCH, E. H. (1945). *Archives of Surgery*, **51**, 220.
86. BLOCH, E. H. (1945). *Journal of the National Malaria Society*, **4**, 287.
87. KNISELY, M. H. *et al.* (1947). *Science*, **106**, 431.
88. LUTZ, B. R. (1951). *Physiological Reviews*, **31**, 107.
89. LEE, W. H. (1963). p. 40 in Reference 80.
90. GELIN, L.-E. and SHOEMAKER, W. C. (1961). *Surgery*, **49**, 713.
91. LONG, D. M. *et al.* (1961). *Surgery*, **50**, 12.
92. LONG, D. M. (1963). p. 26 in Reference 80.
93. GELIN, L.-E. (1956). *Acta Chirurgia Scandinavia*, Supplement 210.
94. LILLEHEI, R. C. *et al.* (1964). *Annals of Surgery*, **160**, 682.
95. Leading Article (1963). *Lancet*, ii, 1365.
96. SMITH, L. L. and MOORE, F. D. (1962). *New England Journal of Medicine*, **267**, 733.
97. FRANK, H. A., SELIGMAN, A. M. and FINE, J. (1945). *Journal of Clinical Investigation*, **24**, 435.
98. BROOKS, D. K. *et al.* (1963). *Lancet*, **i**, 521.
99. Leading Article (1963). *Lancet*, i, 539.
100. SHIRES, T. and JACKSON, D. E. (1962). *Archives of Surgery*, **84**, 703.
101. BOBA, A. and LANDMESSER, C. M. (1961). *Anesthesiology*, **22**, 781.
102. WILLIAMS, J. A. and FINE, J. (1961). *New England Journal of Medicine*, **264**, 842.
103. SYKES, M. K. (1963). *Annals of the Royal College of Surgeons, England*, **33**, 185.
104. PETERS, G., BRUNNER, H. and SCHEER, P. (1963). *American Journal of Physiology*, **204**, 555.
105. BRUN, C. and MUNCK, O. (1964). *Progressive Surgery (Basel)*, **4**, 1.
106. SHARPEY-SCHAFER, E. P. (1963). *British Medical Bulletin*, **19**, 145.
107. WOLFSON. L. J. (1963). *Annals of the Royal College of Surgeons of England*, **33**, 158.
108. NICKERSON, M. (1962). In *Shock, Pathogenesis and Therapy*, p. 356, *loc. cit.*
109. Leading Article (1970). *British Medical Journal*, i, 3.
110. JAMIESON, R. A. and KAY, A. W. (1965). In *A Textbook of Surgical Physiology*, 2nd edn, p. 71. Edinburgh: Livingstone.
111. STONER, H. B. (1961). In *The Scientific Basis of Medicine Annual Reviews*, p. 172. London: Athlone Press.
112. INGLE, D. J., MEEKS, R. C. and THOMAS, K. E. (1951). *Endocrinology*, **49**, 703.
113. RANDALL, R. E. and PAPPER, S. (1958). *Journal of Clinical Investigation*, **37**, 1628.
114. GRABER, I. G. and BEACONSFIELD, P. (1955). *British Medical Journal*, ii, 704.
115. INGLE, D. J. (1952). In *Proceedings of the Society for Endocrinology, Journal of Endocrinology*, 8, p. xxiii in appendix.
116. HAYES, M. A., WILLIAMSON, R. J. and HEIDENREICH, W. F. (1957). *Surgery*, **41**, 353.
117. SKILLMAN, J. J. and SILEN, W. (1972). *Lancet*, ii, 1303.

One of the most important developments in the higher animal is the evolution of mechanisms whereby a constant environment is maintained for its constituent cells. This fixity of the internal environment has been well recognised since the time of Claude Bernard. Temperature regulation is an important aspect of homeostasis, which in man and other warm-blooded mammals has attained a high degree of efficiency. Cellular activity, involving as it does numerous chemical reactions largely dependent upon enzymatic activity, is very susceptible to changes in temperature. On the other hand, some of the energy produced during cell respiration is emitted as heat. Indeed, the temperature of highly active organs, like the brain and heart, would rise were it not for the cooling effect of the blood stream which carries away the excess heat and distributes it to those areas where it can be dissipated to the atmosphere, viz. the skin and the mucosa of the upper respiratory tract.

It is probable that the development of a reliable temperature-regulating mechanism has contributed considerably to the biological supremacy of the warm-blooded group of animals.

The Normal Body Temperature

It is curious that, although fever has been recognised since ancient times, actual measurements of body temperature were not made till comparatively recently. Reliable clinical thermometers became available in the seventeenth century, but it was not until the nineteenth century that they were used to any extent.

Body temperature is usually measured with the thermometer placed under the tongue, or else in the axilla, groin, or rectum. Of these, readings obtained from the axilla and groin show the widest variation, and are generally regarded as being least reliable. This is hardly surprising, since the surface skin temperature fluctuates widely, and may approximate to that of the external environment. The rectal temperature is highest, being about 0·3°C higher than the arterial temperature.[1, 2] Measuring the urine temperature has also been advocated, and it approximates to the rectal temperature.[3] The rectal temperature is said to be the least responsive to changes in the arterial temperature. Thus, if warm saline is infused into a vein, the rise in blood temperature is reflected in an elevation of the sublingual temperature but not that of the rectum. The sublingual temperature taken with the lips closed is therefore held to be the most reliable guide to the arterial temperature[4] (see p. 435).

The normal temperature taken in this way is 36·8°C with a range of 36·1°C–37·4°C (97–99·3°F). The maximum temperature is generally attained at about 6 p.m., while it is at its lowest at about 3 a.m. In women there is an elevation of the temperature during the middle of the menstrual cycle; its onset is thought to herald ovulation.

MECHANISM OF TEMPERATURE REGULATION[5, 6, 63]

The constancy of the body's temperature is attained by balancing the amount of heat gained with that lost.

Sources of Heat Gain

From the environment. Whenever the external temperature exceeds that of the body, heat will be gained by radiation, conduction, and convection. It is a remarkable fact that under such conditions the body's temperature can be maintained at its correct level. The regulating mechanisms are not, however, working under favourable conditions, and it is not surprising that they may break down under these circumstances (see heatstroke, p. 435).

From metabolic activity. The heat production under fasting conditions with the individual at complete mental and physical rest is called the Basal Metabolic Rate (BMR). This ranges from 1 400–1 800 calories per day, and appears to be more closely related to surface area than to weight. The BMR is increased by thyroxine; this effect is seen in individuals exposed to cold and in thyrotoxicosis. Fever also affects the BMR, a rise of 1°C in body temperature increasing it by about 13 per cent.

The metabolic rate of a normal active individual is the summation of the BMR and the additional metabolism needed to sustain exercise, strenuous degrees of which may increase the metabolic rate by as much as 15 times the resting level. Involuntary muscular activity, e.g. contraction of the arrector pili muscles and shivering, further increases heat production. The ingestion of food also increases the metabolic rate, the effect of protein being particularly marked (specific dynamic action of protein).

Sources of Heat Loss

Heat loss occurs in three main ways:

Heat required to warm inspired air and ingested food. In man the amount of heat lost in this way is to a large extent governed by factors beyond the control of the heat-regulating mechanism. The heat lost in the breath is dependent not only upon the temperature of the inspired air, but also upon the rate of breathing. In the dog the amount of heat lost can be increased by panting, but in man this is of little importance.

Heat lost by convection, conduction, and radiation from the body surface. The amount of heat lost depends on three factors:

(*a*) The temperature of the skin.
(*b*) The temperature of the environment.
(*c*) The movement of air over the skin.

The temperature of the skin is dependent on its blood supply, which is under the control of the autonomic nervous system. Heat is lost from the skin surface by conduction to the adjacent air, which is then carried away by convection currents. Clothing hinders the removal of this layer of warm air.

Heat loss by evaporation of water. There is a constant insensible water loss from the skin surface and the respiratory tract. In the respiratory passages the amount lost depends on the temperature and humidity of the air. This heat loss is obligatory, but can be increased in dogs by panting. It comes into its own during strenuous exercise.

In the skin there is also the sweating mechanism which is under control. In temperate climates the amount of sweat secreted is negligible, but in the tropics it is a very important source of water loss.

The Regulating Mechanisms

To maintain a constant body temperature heat loss must be adjusted to balance heat gain. The most important mechanism is the blood flow through the skin.

Vasodilatation increases heat loss, and is effected by the withdrawal of sympathetic vasoconstrictor activity. It also produces a subjective feeling of warmth and induces such voluntary actions as the removal of clothing and withdrawal from the sun's rays.

Vasoconstriction conserves heat, and by producing a chill induces appropriate voluntary action to be taken, e.g. putting on warm clothes and performing exercise.

If these regulating mechanisms do not suffice, heat loss is augmented by sweating. This furthermore stimulates vasodilatation through the mediation of bradykinin,[7, 8] which is released during sweating. On the other hand, the need for more heat stimulates shivering and contraction of the arrector pili muscles.

Control of the Regulating Mechanisms

The heat-sensitive receptors are situated both peripherally in the skin and within the central nervous system.

The central receptor.[9, 10] The exact site of the heat-regulating centre has not been defined, but it is probably hypothalamic; damage to this area in animals upsets the heat-regulating mechanism. The central receptor responds to changes in blood temperature, and its activity, as evidenced by the changes in heat loss, is closely related to the temperature of the blood perfusing the brain. For this reason a

thermometer in the mouth, which is near the hypothalamus, is a more useful guide to the body's temperature than one placed on the skin or in the rectum.

A change in blood temperature of as little as $0.2°C$ can activate the compensatory mechanisms. The intravenous injection of cold fluids leads to cutaneous vasoconstriction, while hot fluids cause vasodilatation.

The peripheral receptors—skin reflexes. If one arm is immersed in cold water, the other undergoes vasoconstriction within a few seconds. This occurs even if the circulation in the cooled arm is occluded, indicating that a nervous reflex rather than a change in blood temperature is involved. After a while this vasoconstriction wanes, but on restoring the circulation a more prolonged period of vasoconstriction ensues due to the action of the central mechanism.[11] There is evidence that the skin also contains warm receptors.[12]

It is evident that there are heat-sensitive receptors both in the skin and the hypothalamus; the latter are by far the more important. When stimulated they produce reflex activity of the autonomic nervous system, which controls skin blood flow, shivering, and sweat secretion.

FEVER

Fever, or pyrexia, may be defined as an elevation of the body's temperature consequent upon a disturbance of the regulating mechanism. When the temperature reaches or exceeds $40.5°C$ ($105°F$) the condition is called *hyperpyrexia*. Fever occurs under the following conditions:

Heatstroke.[13] Some rise in body temperature normally occurs during severe exercise when the heat-eliminating mechanisms cannot keep pace with the excessive heat production in the muscles. When the environment is hot and humid, even mild exercise may cause a marked rise in body temperature.* Sometimes the heat-regulating mechanism breaks down under these circumstances, and the temperature rises to $41°C$ or more. This is "heatstroke", or "sunstroke", and unless treated promptly the temperature may continue to rise, reaching $43°C$ or more, a level at which the patient becomes comatose. Cerebral, hepatic, and renal damage is prominent. Convulsions are common, and permanent brain damage may be evident if the patient survives.

Infection. Fever is a frequent accompaniment of infection by viruses, bacteria, and larger parasites. The pattern of the pyrexia is often characteristic of particular diseases, e.g. the intermittent fever of benign malaria and the relapsing course of brucellosis.

Infarction. This is particularly useful in the diagnosis of myocardial infarction.

Tumours. Some tumours are particularly liable to produce pyrexia, e.g. Ewing's tumour of bone and hypernephroma. The cyclical Pel-Ebstein fever is characteristic of deep-seated Hodgkin's disease.

* Heatstroke was the largest single cause of death amongst the pilgrims to Mecca in 1959 and 1960.

Haemorrhage. Fever may follow haemorrhage, especially into the gastrointestinal tract or coelomic cavities, e.g. after a ruptured ectopic pregnancy.

Brain damage. Cerebral haemorrhage, especially in the region of the pons, and other intracranial lesions may disturb the central regulating mechanism. This leads to a rise in temperature.

Following injury during the catabolic phase of convalescence.

In severe anaemia, and following acute haemolysis.

Miscellaneous conditions. Fever is a prominent feature of acute gout and some of the collagen diseases, e.g. acute rheumatic fever. A slight rise may occur in thyrotoxicosis (especially during a crisis) and in congestive heart failure.

Of all the causes of pyrexia infection is by far the most important. The development of fever in acute illnesses like lobar pneumonia or malaria has been the object of most study. Three stages are described:

The cold stage. At the onset of the illness there is a feeling of intense cold, peripheral vasoconstriction is manifested by pallor, and the patient starts to shiver. Chattering of the teeth completes this picture of the familiar rigor. Heat production is thereby increased, and heat loss reduced; the temperature rises, as does also the blood pressure. There is usually a rise in pulse rate of 18 beats per minute for each 1°C rise of temperature (10 per 1°F).

The hot stage. As the temperature approaches its peak, the peripheral vasoconstriction relaxes and the patient feels dry and warm. Heat loss now balances heat gain, and the temperature remains constant. The heat-regulating mechanism is still in control, but is geared to maintain the temperature at a level higher than normal. The extra heat produced is due to the raised metabolic rate caused by the fever. Should hyperpyrexia occur, this regulation may fail. During this phase the blood pressure falls. The RQ* is low, and there is a tendency to ketosis. Wasting of fat and muscle occurs together with an increased excretion of nitrogen in the urine.

The sweating phase. The temperature begins to fall, and the patient soon experiences a sensation of intense heat. Bedclothes are thrown off, sweating becomes profuse, and the temperature returns to normal. This is described as termination by *crisis*.

The Cause of Fever[14]

The fact that fever often accompanies necrosis, e.g. in tumours and infarcts, suggests that dead tissue contains a pyrogenic substance, and pyrogens similar to those of bacteria have been isolated.[15] The intravenous injection of pus has long been known to cause fever. Menkin claims that "pyrexin" found in inflammatory exudates is derived from dead tissue.[16, 17] This also produces fever on injection, but

---

* Respiratory quotient (RQ) is the ratio
$$\frac{\text{Volume of } CO_2 \text{ produced}}{\text{Volume of } O_2 \text{ consumed}}$$

its properties suggest that it is identical with the bacterial pyrogens (see below).

Intravenous injections of Gram-negative organisms produce a sharp rise in temperature. This appears to be due to lipopolysaccharide or polysaccharide substances which are called *bacterial pyrogens*. These have the following properties.[14, 18–21]

(a) On injection they produce fever after a latent period.

(b) Leucopenia also occurs.

(c) Repeated injections lead to a state of refractoriness. This tolerance is not due to antibody production. It can be abolished by the prior injection of thorotrast, and appears to be due to the heightened ability of the RE system to remove endotoxin.

These bacterial pyrogens are of importance because they can produce febrile reactions by polluting the fluids and apparatus used in intravenous therapy.

The pyrogens are thought to act indirectly. They cause the polymorphs to release an *endogenous pyrogen*, which acts on the central regulating mechanism.[22] In man there is evidence that a similar pyrogen can be released from monocytes as well as polymorphs. This helps to explain the pyrexia which occurs in infections with organisms that excite a mononuclear response and also the fever in patients with agranulocytosis.[23, 24] It has also been reported that a pyrogen is released by sensitised mononuclear cells when they react with specific antigen *in vitro*.[25] This may explain the fever of diseases in which there is a large autoimmune component, e.g. systemic lupus erythematosus.

This endogenous pyrogen differs from the bacterial pyrogens in several respects. The fever which it causes is more rapid in onset, but also more transient. There is no leucopenia, and tolerance does not develop. Animals made resistant to bacterial pyrogen remain sensitive to endogenous pyrogen.[14, 18–21] It appears therefore that fever is produced by an endogenous chemical mediator.

Certain *steroid hormones* can produce a rise of body temperature.[26, 27] Progesterone is an example, and is probably responsible for the temperature changes occurring during the menstrual cycle. Another steroid, *aetiocholanolone*, which arises from the metabolism of adrenocortical and gonadal hormones and is found in the oxosteroid fraction of the urine, causes a marked rise in temperature after injection.[27, 28] There is a latent period of 4–8 hours, and the fever abates after 18 hours.

Disturbances of the central nervous system also affect the body's temperature.[29] Emotion can raise it, and *periodic fever*,[30] a cyclical pyrexia of unknown origin, is perhaps related to cerebral dysfunction, but some authorities blame excessive aetiocholanolone production.[27, 31] General anaesthesia impairs the heat regulating mechanism—the fully anaesthetised patient is poikilothermic.

Fulminating, or malignant, hyperpyrexia:[32, 33] This newly recognised syndrome is characterised by a rapid rise in temperature during the administration of a general anaesthetic; in most cases either halothane or suxamethonium has been given. Tachypnoea, tachycardia, hypotension, cyanosis, and metabolic acidosis develop, and the pyrexia may go unrecognized until by chance the patient is noted to be very hot. The progress of the pyrexia is extremely rapid, and unless vigorous cooling is employed the temperature rises to very high levels, e.g. 43–44°C (110–112°F), and death occurs from cardiac arrest. In the majority of cases the skeletal muscles develop an increase in tone and show fasciculation. It is believed that this is responsible for the sudden increase in heat production, but in a minority of cases rigidity is absent and some other mechanism must be postulated. In some cases of malignant hyperpyrexia, particularly those which develop rigidity, an inherited abnormality has been suggested; in some families the predisposition towards malignant hyperpyrexia is inherited as an autosomal dominant trait. In some families a type of myopathy has been demonstrated, and if subclinical this may be detected by an elevation in the serum levels of creatine phosphokinase (CPK) and aldolase. A preoperative estimation of the CPK level will indeed help to prevent some cases of malignant hyperpyrexia.

Although recent work has shed some light on the mystery of fever, much has yet to be learned. It would be satisfying to believe that a rise in temperature in infection was a beneficial reaction designed to aid the body's defences. There is, however, little evidence that this is so. As yet we must regard the maintenance of body temperature as an important homeostatic mechanism for the proper functioning of the body. Any marked departure from the normal appears to be at the best, of no value, and at the worst, deleterious to well-being.

Attention has been drawn to the possibly beneficial effect of fever on virus infections. There is considerable evidence to indicate that viruses, especially those of poor virulence, stimulate the production of larger amounts of interferon at higher temperatures, e.g. up to 42°C (107·6°F). It may be that fever stimulates greater interferon production by the infected cells, and so limits the course of virus disease.[34]

HYPOTHERMIA

Hypothermia may be defined as a body temperature below 35°C (95°F). It is an important cause of death in cold climates especially at the extremes of life, and it has therapeutic implications.

Three grades of lowered body temperature can be recognised.[35]

(a) 37–32·2°C (98·4–90°F), in which the body reacts vigorously (maximally at 35°C or 95°F) against the chilling. There is violent shivering, cutaneous vasoconstriction, tachycardia, and a raised blood pressure. Breathing is increased, and a diuresis is common.

(b) 32·2–24°C (90–75°F), in which the tissue metabolism throughout the body is depressed. There is a progressive decrease in the pulse rate, respiration, and blood pressure. This is the range generally employed in surgery.

(c) Below 24°C (75°F), in which the temperature-regulating centre ceases to function, and heat is lost from the body as from an inanimate object.

THE BODY'S RESPONSE TO HYPOTHERMIA

Much experimental work has been done on the physiological response to hypothermia, but as this depends on such diverse factors as the species, age, and size of the animal used, the duration of chilling, the temperature reached, the season of the year, and the anaesthetic used, it is hardly surprising that a mass of conflicting data has accumulated, and complete correlation is not yet possible.

Effect on the Circulatory System[36]

There is general depression. The heart rate, cardiac output, and regional blood flow to the organs are decreased. The blood pressure falls despite an increased peripheral resistance—sometimes there is vasodilatation at very low temperatures. The renal blood flow is reduced due to vasoconstriction and the low blood pressure.

The effect on the blood volume varies according to the species, but in general there is haemoconcentration due to a shift of fluid to the interstitial tissues. The increased viscosity of the blood is an important factor in causing vascular stasis. Sludging is also a common finding.

A great danger is ventricular fibrillation. It is related to the degree of chilling and the anaesthetic used. Its cause is not known; hypoxia cannot usually be blamed, but it is possible that it is related to local electrolyte imbalance involving potassium, calcium, and hydrogen ions.

Effect on the Metabolism[37]

There is a reduced oxygen consumption. As already explained, less oxygen reaches the tissues due to circulatory depression and vasoconstriction, but in addition the oxygen requirements of the tissue drop almost proportionately to the decreased blood flow. Therefore there is little oxygen debt when the temperature is raised once more. This applies even to the brain (it is estimated that 8 minutes' occlusion of the cerebral circulation at 30°C (86°F) or 45 minutes' occlusion at 15°C (59°F) is safe). Oxygen dissociation is retarded as the temperature falls, and the curve shifts to the left (see p. 512).

As hypothermia proceeds, there is a mounting retention of CO_2, for although CO_2 production drops, there is an even greater impairment of ventilation. Furthermore, the solubility of CO_2 in plasma increases at lower temperatures. There is therefore a respiratory acidosis, which is easily reversed by controlled respiration. There is usually also a metabolic acidosis due to hypoxia during the stage of induction (associated with shivering and possibly hypovolaemic shock) causing anaerobic glycolysis. It is much reduced if these factors are corrected by proper technique.

Glucose consumption is reduced to a greater extent than oxygen consumption, and the RQ falls. Hepatic and renal function are severely depressed.

Effect on the Nervous System[38]

There is progressive depression of function. There is probably little interference with enzyme activity and synaptic conduction until 28°C (82·4°F). In mild hypothermia the nervous system may be hyper-reactive, and convulsions are not uncommon. Nervous tissue can tolerate severe cooling for limited periods of time.

Effect on the Endocrine Glands[39]

There is no clear-cut pattern, as the response depends on the species, age, and size of the animal. In general, the effect is explicable in terms of ischaemia secondary to vasoconstriction and sludging rather than to any primary effect on the glands themselves.

HYPOTHERMIA IN INFANCY

Newborn infants are particularly susceptible to cold because of the relatively high ratio of surface area to body mass, the paucity of subcutaneous fat, and the low production of heat by physical means because of the inability to take exercise or to shiver. Furthermore, the thermoregulatory mechanism is relatively inefficient at birth, at least for several hours.

The effects are somewhat offset by the action of the collection of *brown fat*.[40–43] This tissue is composed of special fat cells in which there are numerous small lipid droplets, as against the large droplet which characterises the common white-fat cell. A further difference is the presence of numerous mitochondria; indeed, the brown colour is due to the high concentration of iron-containing cytochromes, an essential part of the oxidising enzyme apparatus in the mitochondria. Brown fat is an important tissue in relation to heat production in the very young of some species, in animals during hibernation, and during cold adaptation. In the human infant it is present between the shoulder blades and around the neck, with smaller deposits behind the sternum and along the spinal column. Under the influence of noradrenaline released at the sympathetic nerve endings lipid turnover in the brown fat is increased, and the cells split triglyceride molecules into glycerol and fatty acids. The fatty acids are metabolised locally, and this triggers the cycle of heat production. In this way the brown fat helps to increase metabolism and heat production without shivering.

In the first few weeks of life infants need constant warmth, especially when ill. In cold countries there is a danger of neglect as coal fires go out and electric and gas heaters are extinguished because of power cuts. Open windows are another hazard. Lukewarm baths in cold surroundings are dangerous as is also the use of tight wrappings which restrict movement.

The early signs of cold injury are lethargy and difficulty in feeding. Indeed, the child has a still, serene appearance, and the cheeks, nose, and extremities have a flush that deludes the onlooker into believing that all is well. The cry is whimpering, and the body feels very cold. The rectal temperature may fall to 32·2°C (90°F). Later there is bradycardia and oedema of the eyelids and extremities.[44, 45] There may be hardening of the subcutaneous tissues in the worst cases.

Oliguria is a common accompaniment, and infection and haemorrhage from the respiratory tract are important complications. Indeed, diffuse pulmonary haemorrhage is an invariable *post-mortem* finding; its cause is obscure, for there is usually little bleeding elsewhere.

The infants should be gradually warmed up for a period of days in a hospital. Prophylaxis is important: the domiciliary midwife should be instructed, and clinical thermometers that record to 24°C (75°F) should be provided.

HYPOTHERMIA IN ADULTS

Hypothermia can occur in adults in a number of circumstances. *Immersion hypothermia* is one of the lethal factors in shipwreck.[46] Hypothermia is an important complication of severe *myxoedema* and *hypopituitarism*, and it occurs also in patients with *widespread eczema* and *generalised erythroderma*. In such skin diseases the passive diffusion of water through the epidermis is greatly increased, and heat is lost by evaporation.[47]

The most important example is the *spontaneous hypothermia* that occurs in old people, usually women, who live alone in poorly-heated rooms and are poorly clothed.[48] Undernutrition is sometimes an additional factor, for in both caloric and protein deficient states the basal metabolic rate is decreased.[49] There is often senile dementia, or else depressant drugs like alcohol and chlorpromazine have dulled the mind.[50] There is sometimes a severe precipitating infection such as pneumonia.

Patients in hypothermia look ill; there is a corpse-like chill of the body, and the rectal temperature may drop as low as 21°C (70°F). The skin is pale and the subcutaneous tissues are pliant and doughy. The limbs are still, the muscles rigid, and shivering is rare. The tendon reflexes are sluggish and delayed, and the pupils react sluggishly to light. There is bradycardia, often with atrial fibrillation, and characteristic ECG changes are seen.[51] Peripheral oedema and puffy eyelids are common, so that myxoedema may be simulated in euthyroid individuals. The blood pressure is low, and breathing slow with a prolonged expiratory phase.

Renal function is depressed, and oliguria is a common complication. Pancreatic damage is particularly frequent,[52] and raised serum amylase levels are often noted. Hyperglycaemia is common, and hypoglycaemia may occur as the condition improves. Hypoxia and CO_2 retention due to respiratory depression are other effects of hypothermia.[53] Death occurs from cardiac arrest.[54]

Post-mortem findings include micro-infarcts of many organs (bowel, heart, lung, spleen, kidney, and brain), due probably to stagnation of blood as a result of haemoconcentration and sludging. Pancreatitis and gastric erosions are also frequent findings. Their cause is unknown, but vascular occlusion is the most likely explanation.[35]

The patient should be immersed in warm water and returned expeditiously to a warm atmosphere while general supportive treatment is given.[54] The prognosis is, on the whole, bad. In one series of cases only seven out of twenty-three survived.[35] Death usually occurs at a temperature of about 25°C (77°F). It has been found that survivors do not respond to cold with as much increase in heat production and decrease in heat loss as would be expected in normal people. There may be a fundamental abnormality in temperature regulation in these people.[55]

INDUCED HYPOTHERMIA

Hypothermia has played an important part in the development of cardiac surgery, for at a low temperature the body's metabolism is so reduced that cardiac standstill can be tolerated for about an hour. In the early days surface cooling (by immersion in cold water) and venovenous cooling (by removing blood from the body, passing it through a cooling system, and returning it to the body) were used. These procedures are unsatisfactory because ventricular fibrillation occurs at a temperature of about 28°C (82·4°F).

The development of extracorporeal circulatory systems has allowed profound hypothermia to be used in open-heart surgery. In one method the blood is cooled rapidly by passage through a heat-exchanger, and the circulation maintained extracorporeally.[56] At a temperature of 13–15°C (55·4–59°F) this circulation is stopped, and the heart opened in a bloodless field. When the operation is finished, the blood is rewarmed, the heart defibrillated, and a normal circulation restored. Nowadays extracorporeal circulations are so efficient that hypothermia is not used at all or else merely as an adjunct during the period when the extracorporeal circulation is being discontinued and the patient's own circulation restored.

Experimental hypothermia in animals has revealed remarkable survival patterns.[57] Small animals, like mice, rats, and hamsters, can be cooled to temperatures below 0°C (32°F). They are first made to ingest propylene glycol, and are precooled to 15°C (59°F) under CO_2 narcosis. They are finally immersed in a refrigerant solution until the colonic temperature reaches −3°C (26·6°F) to −5°C (23°F). They can be kept in suspended animation for about an hour and then be re-animated by artificial respiration and microwave diathermy. Larger animals do not tolerate this treatment

so well. Although there may be initial survival, death invariably occurs within a few days: gastric haemorrhage and heart failure are common findings.

LOCAL HYPOTHERMIA

When the extremities are exposed to a low temperature there is intense vasoconstriction. Interestingly enough, this is often succeeded by vasodilatation. The blood flow passes through the arteriovenous anastomoses,[58] but the mechanism is still debated; it can occur even after sympathectomy, but is often abnormal in patients with digital vasospasm.[58] The response is best in those who are habitually exposed to the cold. The muscular vessels also dilate when the forearm is immersed in ice-cold water.[59]

Extreme examples of cold injury occur in explorers, soldiers, and mountaineers, in whom there is direct damage to the capillary bed. In severe cases the vascular occlusion leads to infarction and gangrene. This condition of "frostbite", or "trench-foot", is considered further on p. 481. It is important to note that local cold injury is due to vascular occlusion and not intracellular ice-crystal formation. This occurs only at extremely low temperatures. A milder cold injury is the common chilblain (*erythema pernio*). It is an inflammation of the subcutaneous fat, i.e. a panniculitis, and appears as a tender, red, pruritic swelling.

There are a number of pathological conditions aggravated by cold: (*a*) *Raynaud's phenomenon*,[60] where even minor degrees of cold can cause vascular spasm and digital ischaemia; (*b*) *cold-antibody syndromes* due to haemagglutinins or haemolysins leading to peripheral vascular occlusion or paroxysmal cold haemoglobinuria (p. 593); (*c*) *cryoglobulinaemia* causing vascular occlusion; (*d*) *cold urticaria*,[61] in which histamine is released from the skin following local or general exposure to the cold. It may cause severe shock. Some of these patients have a factor in their serum which will transfer the urticaria to a normal person. If the person is given an intradermal injection of the patient's serum, a localised urticarial lesion develops when the area is exposed to cold. The factor appears to be IgE. How the effect is produced and how common it is for such patients to have a transferable IgE in their serum are not known.[61]

Local hypothermia is also used therapeutically. Skin freezing with ethyl chloride spray is an old-fashioned method of local anaesthesia.

Extreme cold is being used in surgical practice (*cryosugery*).[62] Probes of various shapes refrigerated by liquid nitrogen and other liquefied gases, or by thermo-electric devices, are used. The applications include the destruction of tumours both benign and malignant, ophthalmological procedures, especially the fixation of detached retinae, and destructive intracranial surgery. Gastric hypothermia for controlling peptic ulceration has proved disappointing. At present, the use of cold in surgery is confined to specialist centres, and the late effects are still being assessed.

REFERENCES

1. EICHNA, L. W. *et al.* (1951). *Journal of Clinical Investigation*, **30,** 353.
2. COOPER, K. E. and KENYON, J. R. (1957). *British Journal of Surgery*, **44,** 616.
3. FOX, R. H. *et al.* (1971). *Lancet*, i, 424.
4. CRANSTON, W. I., GERBRANDY, J. and SNELL, E. S. (1954). *Journal of Physiology* (*London*), **126,** 347.
5. PICKERING, G. W. (1958). *Lancet*, i, 1 and 59.
6. HARDY, J. D. (1961). *Physiological Reviews*, **41,** 521.
7. SNELL, E. S. (1954). *Journal of Physiology* (*London*), **125,** 361.
8. FOX, R. H. and HILTON, S. M. (1958). *Journal of Physiology* (*London*), **142,** 219.
9. BENZINGER, T. H. (1961). *Scientific American*, **204,** No. 1, 134.
10. COOPER, K. E. (1966). *British Medical Bulletin*, **22,** 238.
11. PICKERING, G. W. (1932). *Heart*, **16,** 115.
12. COOPER, K. E. and KERSLAKE, D. M. (1953). *Journal of Physiology* (*London*), **119,** 18.
13. Leading Article (1968). *Lancet*, ii, 31.
14. ATKINS, E. (1960). *Physiological Reviews*, **40,** 580.
15. LANDY, M. and SHEAR, M. J. (1957). *Journal of Experimental Medicine*, **106,** 77.
16. MENKIN, V. (1945). *Archives of Pathology*, **39,** 28.
17. MENKIN, V. (1955). *Journal of Laboratory and Clinical Medicine*, **46,** 423.
18. WOOD, W. B. (1958). *Lancet*, ii, 53.
19. WOOD, W. B. (1958). *New England Journal of Medicine*, **258,** 1023.
20. BORNSTEIN, D. L., BREDENBERG, C. and WOOD, W. B. (1963). *Journal of Experimental Medicine*, **117,** 349.
21. KAISER, H. K. and WOOD, W. B. (1962). *Journal of Experimental Medicine*, **115,** 27.
22. BEESON, P. B. (1948). *Journal of Clinical Investigation*, **27,** 524.
23. BODEL, P. and ATKINS, E. (1967). *New England Journal of Medicine*, **276,** 1002.
24. Editorial (1967). *New England Journal of Medicine*, **276,** 1036.
25. ATKINS, E., BODEL, P. and FRANCIS, L. (1967). *Journal of Experimental Medicine*, **126,** 357.
26. Leading Article (1959). *British Medical Journal*, i, 492.
27. Leading Article (1961). *Lancet*, ii, 1240.
28. KAPPAS, A. *et al.* (1960). *Archives of Internal Medicine*, **105,** 701.
29. Leading Article (1960). *Lancet*, ii, 475.
30. REIMANN, H. A. (1948). *Journal of the American Medical Association*, **136,** 239.
31. BONDY, P. K. *et al.* (1958). *Yale Journal of Biology and Medicine*, **30,** 395.
32. Leading Article (1971). *British Medical Journal*, iii, 441.
33. KALOW, W. *et al.* (1970). *Lancet*, ii, 895.
34. ISAACS, A. (1962). *British Medical Journal*, ii, 353.
35. DUGUID, H. SIMPSON, R. G. and STOWERS, J. M. (1961). *Lancet*, ii, 1213.
36. COOPER, K. E. (1961). *British Medical Bulletin*, **17,** 48.
37. FAIRLEY, H. B. (1961). *Ibid.*, **17,** 52.
38. LOUGHEED, W. M. (1961). *Ibid.*, **17,** 61.
39. BIGELOW, W. G. and SIDLOFSKY, S. (1961). *Ibid.*, **17,** 56.
40. DAWKINS, M. J. R. and HULL, D. (1965). *Scientific American*, **213,** No. 2, 62.
41. DAWKINS, M. J. R. and SCOPES, J. W. (1965). *Nature* (*London*), **206,** 201.
42. LINDBERG, O. (1970). Editor. *Brown Adipose Tissue*, 337 pp. New York: Elsevier.
43. HOLLENBERG, C. H., ANGEL, A. and STEINER, G. (1970). *Canadian Medical Association Journal*, **103,** 843.
44. MANN, T. P. and ELLIOTT, R. I. K. (1957). *Lancet*, i, 229.
45. BOWER, B. D., JONES, L. F. and WEEKS, M. M. (1960). *British Medical Journal*, i, 303.
46. KEATINGE, W. R. (1965). *British Medical Journal*, ii, 1537.
47. GRICE, K. A. and BETTLEY, F. R. (1967). *British Medical Journal*, iv, 195.
48. Leading Article (1966). *British Medical Journal*, ii, 1471.
49. ABLETT, J. G. and McCANCE, R. A. (1971). *Lancet*, ii, 517.
50. PRESCOTT, L. F., PEARD, M. C. and WALLACE, I. R. (1962). *British Medical Journal*, ii, 1367.
51. EMSLIE-SMITH, D. (1958). *Lancet*, ii, 492.
52. READ, A. E. *et al.* (1961). *Lancet*, ii, 1219.
53. McNICOL, M. W. and SMITH, R. (1964). *British Medical Journal*, i, 19.
54. Leading Article (1972). *Lancet*, i, 237.
55. MACMILLAN, *et al.* (1967). *Lancet*, ii, 165.
56. DREW, C. E. (1961). *British Medical Bulletin*, **17,** 37.
57. KENYON, J. R. (1961). *Ibid.*, **17,** 43.
58. FOX, R. H. (1968). *Proceedings of the Royal Society of Medicine*, **61,** 785.
59. HELLON, R. F. (1963). *British Medical Bulletin*, **19,** 141.
60. BIRNSTINGL, M. (1968). *Proceedings of the Royal Society of Medicine*, **61,** 790.
61. HOUSER, D. D. *et al.* (1970). *American Journal of Medicine*, **49,** 23.
62. Leading Article (1968). *British Medical Journal*, iv, 342.
63. ATKINS, E. and BODEL, P. (1972). *New England Journal of Medicine*, **286,** 27.

Chapter 34. Disturbances in the Body's Fluid and Electrolyte Balance

Water is the principal constituent of the body. It forms the bulk of the cellular protoplasm, and is the vehicle of transport of essential metabolic factors to the cell and of waste products to the exterior. In this aqueous medium the electrolytes of the body are held in solution. Some of these, like potassium, calcium, and magnesium, are necessary for normal cell function, whereas others, like sodium and chloride, maintain an adequate osmotic pressure for the extracellular water. Cells can survive only within a very narrow range of hydrogen ion concentration, and the pH of the extracellular water is regulated to a great extent by the bicarbonate ion.

Any serious deficiency of water soon interferes with the circulation of the blood, and death rapidly ensues. This circulating fluid is sustained osmotically by those electrolytes which are normally present in the greatest concentration, namely sodium and chloride. A depletion of salt rapidly leads to circulatory failure. For this reason it is necessary always to relate disturbances in water metabolism to the state of salt balance in the body. In the clinical condition of "dehydration" there is usually a combined salt and water depletion, but even if there is a pure water deficiency, the ensuing manifestations are related to a secondary alteration in salt balance as well as to the primary water lack.

THE NORMAL DISTRIBUTION OF WATER AND ELECTROLYTES IN THE BODY WATER[1]

About two-thirds of the lean body weight consists of water. As the water content of adipose tissue is very low, the actual water content of the body is somewhat less than this; it is about 60 per cent in the normal adult male, and about 5 per cent less in the female. This water is contained in two compartments, an intracellular and an extracellular one. The extracellular compartment is further subdivided into an intravascular and extravascular (interstitial) space. There is a constant interchange of fluid between the intracellular and extracellular compartments, and the methods used to determine the body's fluid spaces depend on the principle of administering a known amount of a substance whose distribution is accurately confined to one or more spaces, and then determining its final concentration in the plasma. Thus, tritiated water or urea is used to measure the *total body water*, inulin or radioactive sodium the *extracellular fluid volume*, and dye-dilution techniques (using Evans blue) or radioiodinated plasma proteins the *plasma volume*.

The following figures provide a guide for the volumes in a normal adult man:

Total body water: 40–45 litres.

Intracellular water: 25 litres (55–60 per cent of total body water, or 36 per cent of the body's weight). It is obtained by subtracting the extracellular volume from the total body water.

Extracellular water: 15 litres (40 per cent of total body water, or 20–25 per cent of the body's weight). It has two components:

Interstitial water: 12 litres are present in the extracellular extravascular space. This is obtained by subtracting the plasma volume from the extracellular water.

Plasma volume: 3 litres.

Blood volume: 5 litres. This is obtained by adding the red-cell mass, as measured directly or calculated from the haematocrit reading, to the plasma volume.

In practice it is difficult to define the boundary between the extracellular and intracellular water, because some of the extracellular water is sequestrated in dense connective tissue, cartilage, and especially bone, and cannot equilibrate rapidly with the other portions of the extracellular fluid, viz. the plasma, interstitial fluid, and lymph. About 15 per cent of the body's water is present in dense connective tissue and bone, and is liable to be included in the intracellular moiety in equilibration measurements. Nevertheless, the concept of separate tissue spaces is helpful so long as the difficulties in absolute measurement are borne in mind.

Electrolytes[1]

The electrolyte composition of the intracellular and extracellular fluids is quite distinct:

(*a*) In the intracellular fluid the principal cations are *potassium* and *magnesium*, and the principal anions are *phosphate* and *protein*.

(*b*) In the extracellular fluid the predominant cation is *sodium*, and the principal anions are *chloride* and *bicarbonate*.

The electrolytes perform two main functions:

1. They are principal *solutes* in the body fluids, and therefore account for most of their osmotic pressure.

2. The concentration of individual *ions* influences the properties and behaviour of excitable membranes, e.g. of nerve cells, and the performance of many intracellular enzymes.

Electrolytes as solutes. The osmotic effect of substances in solution is determined by the number of particles, present, i.e. ions and unionised molecules. For dilute solutions, the osmotic activity is very nearly equal to the actual concentration of particles: a solute concentration of 1 millimole per litre has an osmotic activity of 1 milliosmole per litre. A millimole is one thousandth of a mole, or gram-molecular weight. Thus, one millimole of glucose (MW 180) is 180 mg, and one millimole of urea (MW 60) is 60 mg. The same terminology can be used for ions, so that one millimole of Na^+ is 23 mg, one millimole of Cl^- is 35·5 mg, and one millimole of Ca^{++} is 40 mg. The osmotic activity of electrolytes depends on the number of ions. Thus 58·5 mg NaCl in one litre of water becomes 23 mg Na^+ and 35·5 mg of Cl^-; the concentration of each ion is 1 millimole per litre, but the osmotic activity of the solution is due to both ions, and will be 2 milliosmoles per litre. Again, 111 mg of $CaCl_2$ in a litre of water becomes 40 mg of Ca^{++} and 71 mg of Cl^-; the concentration of Ca^{++} is one millimole per litre, that of Cl^- is 2 millimoles per litre, and the osmotic activity of the solution is 3 milliosmoles per litre.

The total osmotic activity of plasma (measured by depression of freezing point) is about 300 milliosmoles per kg water. Expressing each solute in the same terms (millimoles per litre), Na^+ (140) and Cl^- (100) are clearly the predominant contributors, followed by HCO_3^- (27), K^+, urea, and glucose (about 5 each), with much smaller contributions from Ca^{++}, protein, phosphate, Mg^{++}, etc. *The concentration of sodium is the best indication of the osmolality* of the plasma, i.e. the concentration of particles in solution.*

The osmotic pressure of the interstitial fluid (extravascular extracellular fluid) differs from that of plasma only by the small contribution of plasma protein. This is about 1·5 milliosmoles per litre, which corresponds to a hydrostatic pressure of 25 mm Hg.

The osmotic pressure of intracellular fluid is thought to be equal to that of interstitial fluid because measurements of the depression of freezing point show no difference. However, since the concentrations, and indeed the effective molecular weights, of many of the intracellular constituents are still unknown, one cannot draw up an exact table of their respective contributions to the total intracellular osmotic pressure. The principal solutes are K^+, Mg^{++}, protein, and organic phosphates.

Electrolytes as ions. Ions are charged particles, either atoms (e.g. Na^+ and Cl^-), or larger radicals (e.g. HCO_3^- and SO_4^{--}), or molecules (e.g. protein, which carries a net negative charge at the pH of body fluids). *Cations* are positively charged, and *anions* negatively charged. Any one positive charge is equivalent to any one negative charge. Thus, one Na (monovalent) ion is equivalent to one Cl (monovalent)

ion, but one Ca (divalent) ion is equivalent to two Cl ions. The equivalent weight of an ion is its atomic or molecular weight in grams divided by its valency, and a milliequivalent is one thousandth part of an equivalent. A milliequivalent of Na^+ (atomic weight 23) is 23 mg; of Cl^- 35·5 mg, and of Ca^{++} (atomic weight 40) 20 mg.

The biological effect of an electrolyte depends to a considerable extent on its equivalent concentration, i.e. the number of particles present and the number of charges carried by each. It is therefore appropriate to describe the concentration of electrolytes in milli-equivalents per litre.* Not only is this a more logical description of electrolytes than one in grams or milligrams per 100 ml, but it also allows the relative importance of each ion to be seen. Moreover, since any solution must contain the same concentration of cations as of anions, a balance can be struck between the two categories of electrolytes. This is shown in the following table of the composition of plasma:

Cations (in mEq per litre)		*Anions* (in mEq per litre)	
Na^+	142 (range 137–148)	Cl^-	103 (range 99–108)
K^+	5 (range 4·0–5·5)	HCO_3^-	27 (range 25–31)
Ca^{++}	5 (range 4·5–5·5)	Other	8 (includes HPO_4^{--}
Mg^{++}	2 (range 1·5–2·4)	anions	SO_4^{--}, and organic acids, e.g. keto acids)
		Protein	16 (range 15–20)
Total: 154		Total: 154	

It is clear from the table that sodium is all-important in sustaining the cationic level of the extracellular fluid, and that it is balanced on the anionic side by the combined concentrations of chloride and bicarbonate. This combined level is normally 10 mEq per litre less than that of sodium. In practice the level of plasma chloride follows the level of plasma sodium quite closely, provided the plasma bicarbonate level remains constant. An alteration of plasma bicarbonate in response to an acidosis or alkalosis is usually attended by a reciprocal alteration in the chloride level, and the combined concentration of the two anions remains fairly constant. If, however, the acidosis is due to an excess of keto acids, as in diabetic coma, the plasma bicarbonate falls, the chloride is unchanged, and the keto acids rise.

The mode of transport of water and electrolytes from one compartment to another is still imperfectly understood. It is generally accepted that the three compartments (see Fig. 34.1) are in osmotic equilibrium with one another, and that shifts from one to another are always secondary to

---

* *Osmolality* = solute concentration per kg water.
  Osmolarity = solute concentration per litre solution.
In most biological fluids the two are very similar, but the procedures used (determinations of freezing point and vapour pressure) measure osmolality (in millosmoles per kg water) rather than osmolarity.

* In order to convert concentrations of ions from mg per 100 ml to mEq per litre, a simple formula is used:

$$\left(\frac{\text{mg per 100 ml}}{\text{equivalent weight of element}}\right) \times 10$$

In practice the value in mg per 100 ml is divided by 2·3 for sodium, 3·9 for potassium, 2·24 for bicarbonate (as ml CO_2 per 100 ml), and 3·55 for chloride. To convert protein in g per 100 ml to mEq per litre, divide by 0·41.

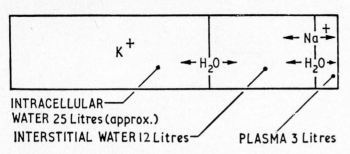

Figure 34.1
Diagrammatic representation of the three compartments in which the body's water is accommodated. An excess or deficiency of water, which is freely diffusible, produces the greatest effects in the largest compartment, the intracellular one, whereas changes in sodium affect mainly the volume of the interstitial fluid.

changes in electrolyte concentration, so that the movement of water in or out of compartments depends on the balance of ions on either side of the dividing membrane.

DISTURBANCES IN WATER AND SODIUM METABOLISM[1]

Normal Water Balance

The loss of water from the body is of two types: uncontrolled, or inevitable, as from the skin and lungs, and controlled as from the sweat glands and kidneys. The inevitable skin loss is due to diffusion of water from the deeper layers, which is evaporated from the surface. It is called transpiration and in temperate climates is from 300–500 ml per day. It is important in the regulation of the body's temperature, and can, if necessary, be supplemented by the active secretion of sweat. This is not pure water, like the fluid of transpiration, but contains actively secreted sodium chloride in a concentration rather less than half that of plasma. The secretion of sweat is normally less than 100 ml per day in temperate climates.

The loss of water from the lungs is about 700 ml per day, and is due to the humidification of air in the respiratory tract. About 200 ml of water are lost in the faeces each day; the remainder of the 8 litres secreted in the alimentary tract is reabsorbed. Finally there is the obligatory loss in the urine. This varies according to the fluid intake; the kidney can concentrate urine to 1 400 milliosmoles per kg (this represents a specific gravity of 1·035), and dilute it down to 30 milliosmoles per kg.

The precise fluid intake varies with the climate and personal habits of the individual. A minimum in temperate climates is from 500 to 1 000 ml per day. Some of this is consumed as food, for from 200 to 300 ml are provided from the water of oxidation of the food.

Normal Sodium Balance

The sodium content of a normal adult is about 4 000 mEq (90 g). Only about 3 per cent is present in the intracellular fluid. Forty per cent is stored in the bones, and the remainder circulates in the extracellular fluid. All the sodium present in the soft tissues is freely exchangeable, but only about 45 per cent of that in the bones is available for exchange. About 70 per cent of the total sodium is exchangeable.

The average daily intake of sodium in a temperate climate is probably 100–300 mEq (2·3–6·9 g). In hot climates, where sweating is profuse, it is much greater than this. An amount almost equal to the intake of sodium is excreted in the urine each day, and a much smaller quantity is lost in the faeces. The amount lost by sweating is negligible in temperate climates.

The balance of sodium (and chloride) is finely adjusted by the kidney. Two mechanisms are known:

The glomerular filtration rate. About 80 per cent of the sodium is normally reabsorbed by the proximal convoluted tubule. While some authorities believe that this is under hormonal control, the more important factor is the rate of glomerular filtration. If this is reduced, the amount of sodium reabsorbed is increased and sodium is retained. This occurs promptly whenever the cardiac output is decreased, e.g. following haemorrhage or the assumption of the erect posture. The afferent part of this reflex arc is believed to be the baroreceptors which are present on the venous side, e.g. in the left atrium, and on the arterial side, e.g. in the carotid sinus. These are susceptible to changes in blood volume. The efferent side of the reflex is probably *via* the vasomotor centre and the sympathetic outflow. In this way the renal blood flow is reduced whenever the blood volume is reduced; glomerular filtration is decreased and sodium is retained.

The completeness of reabsorption of sodium by the distal tubule. This is controlled by *aldosterone*, secreted by the zona glomerulosa of the adrenal cortex. It is the principal mineralocorticoid, and has an important influence on the exchanges of sodium, potassium, and hydrogen in the distal tubule. The secretion of aldosterone is related to the volume of the exrtacellular fluid and the concentration of sodium in it. The most important stimulator of aldosterone is angiotensin,[2] which itself is produced when the renal blood flow is decreased. Angiotensin also has a direct effect on sodium excretion by the kidney—slow infusions cause its retention and more rapid ones may lead to a diuresis of sodium and water.[1] ACTH has little effect on aldosterone secretion.

Cortisol has mild mineralocorticoid activity. It is important for the sustenance of a normal rate of glomerular filtration and the normal response to a water load (see p. 521).

It therefore follows that a reduction of blood volume, in addition to reducing the glomerular filtration rate, also leads to the secretion of aldosterone and the further retention of sodium (Fig. 34.2). Intravenous infusions of isotonic solutions, mechanical distension of the left atrium, and the assumption of a recumbent posture produce the reverse effect, causing sodium excretion and a diuresis.

Figure 34.2
Diagrammatic representation of the means whereby
the body retains sodium after a sudden reduction in
blood volume, e.g. following severe haemorrhage.

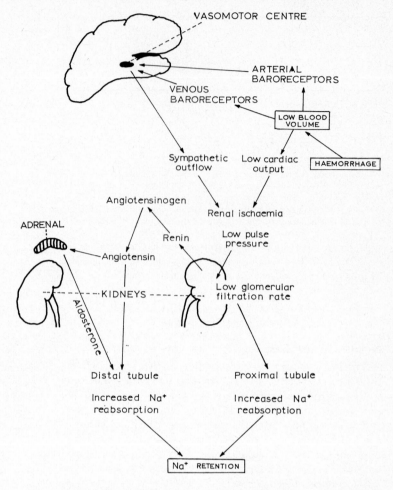

Fluid balance is controlled by three factors:

1. Indirectly by the mechanisms that regulate sodium balance. Sodium cannot be retained without water.

2. The mechanisms that regulate the output of water by the kidney—the antidiuretic hormone of the pituitary is important.

3. Regulation of water intake by the sensation of thirst.

Antidiuretic hormone (ADH), or *vasopressin*, is secreted by the posterior lobe of the pituitary, which is closely connected to the hypothalamus. It conserves water by increasing reabsorption from the distal tubules and collecting ducts (p. 521). Its secretion is regulated by the following factors:

The osmotic concentration of the extracellular fluid in the hypothalamus. If this is diluted, there is a diuresis of hypotonic urine, whereas if it is concentrated through fluid deprivation, a scanty hypertonic urine is secreted. This response is mediated by osmoreceptors, which lie close to the supraoptic nuclei of the hypothalamus.[3]

The baroreceptors sensitive to blood volume. A reduction of blood volume stimulates ADH secretion. On the other hand, left atrial distension simulates an increase in blood volume

and inhibits its secretion.[4] The baroreceptor effect on ADH secretion is less powerful than the osmoreceptor effect. Thus, the rapid ingestion of a litre of water so decreases the osmolality of the plasma and interstitial fluids that a diuresis ensues within 15–30 minutes, and the whole volume is excreted in a few hours. If the fluid is isotonic saline, the diuresis is much slower and more prolonged; 12–24 hours may elapse before the litre is eliminated. Thus a change in osmolality affects ADH secretion more rapidly than does an alteration in blood volume.

Pain, fear, and *certain pharmacological agents,* e.g. nicotine, anaesthetics, adrenaline, and histamine, all stimulate ADH secretion, while alcohol inhibits it and causes a diuresis.

Thirst.[5, 6] The sensation of dryness in the mouth and throat that accompanies thirst is of great importance in motivating fluid intake, but its mechanism is not well understood. It is experienced both after a reduction in extracellular fluid volume, e.g. haemorrhage, and when there is intracellular dehydration, e.g. after salt ingestion. Presumably impulses from the baroreceptors and osmoreceptors are integrated centrally in the hypothalamus, where fresh impulses control the secretions of the mouth and throat. However, the thirst is quenched long before the water is absorbed from the intestine. Perhaps a central mechanism receives afferent impulses directly from the oesophagus and stomach.

DISTURBANCES OF WATER AND SODIUM BALANCE[7]

Pure Water Deficiency

There is a direct deprivation or loss of water without a corresponding depletion of electrolytes. It is uncommon, but may occur under the following circumstances:

(*a*) Following deprivation of water, e.g. in people who cannot swallow because of oesophageal obstruction or coma, during enforced starvation, and after shipwreck.

(*b*) In diabetes insipidus, where there is defective reabsorption of water from the collecting tubules of the kidney.

Effects. There is an increased osmolality of the extracellular fluid. This leads to a transfer of intracellular water to the extracellular compartment and a consequent cellular dehydration. As the water leaves the cells, it is accompanied by potassium ions. The water excretion in the urine is reduced to a minimum (in diabetes insipidus there can be no spontaneous decrease in urinary volume) as a result of an increased secretion of ADH. Sodium excretion is unchanged at first, but later on, when there is a shrinkage of the extracellular fluid volume, aldosterone is secreted, and this reduces sodium excretion. This effect is accentuated in those cases where the water deprivation is part of a general starvation. Loss of potassium in the urine continues, and is indeed augmented by the increased secretion of aldosterone. This type of dehydration affects the intracellular fluid *par excellence*, and is associated especially with water and potassium loss.

Clinical and Biochemical Manifestations

Intense Thirst.

Oliguria. The urine is concentrated and of very high specific gravity. It contains much sodium chloride at first, but later on the level drops. In diabetes insipidus there is a continued polyuria.

Plasma changes. The plasma constituents, e.g. sodium and proteins, rise in concentration, but the haemoglobin concentration and packed cell volume are unchanged because of a loss of water from the red cells. The blood urea level rises early because of the increased urea reabsorption from the tubules, and not through renal failure.

Fever. This is important in infants.

Results. There are no immediate ill-effects, but eventually hypotension and coma occur due to intracellular dehydration of vital organs.

Treatment. Non-saline fluids are given orally or parenterally.

Combined Sodium and Water Deficiency

This is a combined deficiency, but sodium depletion often predominates. It is often called salt depletion, for sodium and chloride are usually lost in equal proportions. But in vomiting due to gastric disease and in the diuresis that follows the use of some diuretics, the chloride loss exceeds that of sodium. This does not affect the volume of the extracellular fluid appreciably, as the chloride is replaced by bicarbonate (see p. 442). Thus the level of chloride in the plasma or urine is an unsatisfactory index of sodium balance.

The deficiency is due to a loss of sodium and water:

From the gastro-intestinal tract. The commonest examples are encountered in gastro-intestinal disorders associated with severe vomiting or diarrhoea, e.g. intestinal obstruction, pyloric stenosis, acute dilatation of the stomach, ulcerative colitis, and cholera. Intestinal and biliary fistulae have a similar effect.

From the sweat. A single large sweat produces the picture of pure water depletion with severe thirst and oliguria, but repeated sweating leads to sodium depletion as well. If the water loss is remedied without giving adequate additional salt, the picture becomes one of predominant sodium deficiency, and the state of *heat exhaustion* follows.

From the urine. One of the commonest examples of severe sodium loss from the kidneys is seen in patients with chronic heart failure who are fed on a low-salt diet and given mercurial diuretics. Other conditions associated with increased sodium loss in the urine are Addison's disease, salt-losing nephritis, and diabetes mellitus with its osmotic diuresis. Acute pathological processes involving the brain, e.g. bulbar poliomyelitis, acute encephalitis, and cerebrovascular disease are sometimes accompanied by an increased excretion of salt in the urine and hyponatraemia, though occasionally the reverse condition of decreased urinary salt excretion and hypernatraemia is encountered. The mechanism is obscure: a nervous connexion between the brain and the kidneys is possibly destroyed by the disease. There are some authorities who deny the existence of a specific syndrome, and attribute the disturbances to the effects of starvation and dehydration.[8]

From the blood and plasma. Severe haemorrhage and the great plasma loss following extensive burns lead to sodium deficiency.

Effects. The effect of sodium deficiency is the undermining of the osmotic support of the extracellular fluid. Furthermore, the volume of the extracellular fluid is reduced as a result of water loss. In order to maintain its tonicity, the extracellular fluid transfers its water to the cells which become relatively overhydrated. In the early stage there may even be a similar tendency to excrete water in the urine, and oliguria is not necessarily an immediate manifestation, particularly when sodium depletion predominates. Rapidly, however, the volume of extracellular fluid becomes seriously reduced, and a state of shock follows. This is manifested particularly in the renal circulation, the arteries of which undergo vasoconstriction. This type of dehydration affects the extracellular fluid *par excellence*, and is associated with severe water and sodium loss.

Clinical and biochemical manifestations. *"Dehydration"*. The eyeballs are sunken, the skin wrinkled, the tongue dry, and the face haggard. Thirst is often absent. Despite a compensatory vasoconstriction, the blood pressure is low and the veins are poorly filled. There is tachycardia.

The urine contains very little sodium and chloride. Early on there may be no reduction in volume, and the concentrating power of the kidneys is good. Later there is severe oliguria due to renal failure.

Plasma changes. There is a reduced plasma volume evidenced by raised levels of proteins, packed cell volume, and haemoglobin. The viscosity of the blood is increased, and its specific gravity—normally 1·050 to 1·060—rises. The plasma sodium level drops as the condition progresses. A rising blood urea indicates renal failure.

Results. Death due to circulatory failure rapidly follows. In patients who survive there is a danger of subsequent renal tubular necrosis.

Treatment. Remedy the cause and administer saline solutions.

Pure Water Excess

This is called *water intoxication* and it is encountered under the following circumstances:

(*a*) In the early postoperative period when patients are given large infusions of glucose solution. This cannot be excreted rapidly because of the tendency to water and salt retention after traumatic incidents.

(*b*) The administration of water to patients suffering from sodium depletion, e.g. in cardiac disease being treated with diuretics and a low-sodium diet, in Addison's disease where there is an inability to excrete a water load as well as a salt deficiency, and in heatstroke.

(*c*) The administration of injudiciously large amounts of water in renal failure, especially the acute type.

(*d*) Where there is excessive secretion of ADH. This may occur in lesions near the supraoptic nuclei. ADH is produced in some cases of oat-cell lung cancer (see p. 344).

Effects. The extracellular compartment is distended and its osmolality is reduced. The excess water is diverted into the cells, and the resulting intracellular oedema causes damage. There may be an early diuresis, but soon the renal cells also are damaged, and oliguria or even anuria may follow.

Clinical and biochemical manifestations. *Nausea, Vomiting, Weakness, and Muscle Cramps in the Legs and Abdomen.*

Cerebral symptoms, e.g. headache, drowsiness, apathy, stupor, epileptiform convulsions, and coma.

Plasma changes. There is a reduction in the concentration of all the plasma electrolytes, and the plasma osmolality is decreased. The packed cell volume and plasma protein level are also reduced.

Results. Death due to widespread cellular damage occurs if the condition persists.

Treatment. Hypertonic saline is given intravenously.

Combined Sodium and Water Excess

This is an artificially-induced condition in which patients with defective renal function are given excessive amounts of saline solutions, e.g. during the early postoperative period or during the course of acute renal failure. The fluid is distributed evenly throughout the extracellular compartment which becomes expanded. There is no alteration in the level of plasma electrolytes, but the packed cell volume and plasma protein level is decreased. The manifestations are an increased venous pressure and systemic oedema. In due course pulmonary oedema and heart failure occur.

DISTURBANCES OF POTASSIUM BALANCE[1]

Normal Potassium Balance

The potassium content of a normal adult is about 133g (3 400 mEq). Over 95 per cent of it is intracellular, and less

TABLE 34.1   The main metabolic changes in the various types of sodium and water disturbance

	Plasma sodium	Blood urea	Plasma proteins	Packed Cell volume	Urine
Pure Water Deficiency.	Raised.	Raised.	Raised.	Normal.	Oliguria* (concentrated).
Salt and Water Deficiency.	Reduced.	Raised later.	Raised.	Raised.	Variable at first; soon severely reduced.
Water Excess.	Reduced.	Raised terminally.	Reduced.	Reduced.	Variable. Reduced terminally.

Water and Salt Excess—No specific changes apart from expansion of extracellular compartment. There is a lowering of plasma proteins and packed cell volume.

* This does not apply to diabetes insipidus.

than 5 per cent extracellular. About three-quarters of the intracellular potassium is present in the skeletal musculature.

The normal daily consumption of potassium is 2–3 g (52–78 mEq), and a similar amount is excreted in the urine, together with small quantities in the faeces and sweat. There is an active secretion of potassium from the colonic mucosa.[9, 10]

The concentration of potassium in the extracellular fluid is very low (4–5·5 mEq per litre); it is predominantly a cellular electrolyte, forming two-thirds of the intracellular cations. When it leaves the cells, it is rapidly excreted by the kidneys. A plasma level above 7·5 mEq per litre produces clinical symptoms, and one over 10 mEq per litre is rapidly fatal. The body possesses no means of intensive potassium retention comparable with those for sodium.

An unobtrusive loss of potassium from the cells into the plasma and then into the urine occurs under the following circumstances:

Whenever water is mobilised from the cells, e.g. during water deprivation.

Whenever cell protein is broken down, e.g. as a normal response to trauma or following starvation. It is estimated that 100–120 mg potassium are liberated with every gram of nitrogen (about 2·5–3·0 mEq per gram).

Conversely, the administration of glucose and insulin diverts the extracellular potassium into the cells where it aids in the deposition of glycogen.

Potassium is actively secreted by the distal tubules of the kidney, and this is potentiated by aldosterone, and to a lesser extent by cortisol and deoxycorticosterone.

The concentration of potassium in the plasma is an inadequate indication of potassium balance, because a high level may be merely an indication of its effective mobilisation from the cells prior to its excretion by the kidneys. Only in prolonged stages of potassium loss does the plasma concentration fall appreciably. In the same way a low concentration may be merely an indication of a diversion of potassium ions into the cells, as after glucose and insulin administration. In the commonest type of the rare disorder *familial periodic paralysis*[11, 12] there are paroxysms of generalised muscular weakness associated with a dramatic fall in the level of plasma potassium and a decrease in its urinary excretion. It appears that there is a shift of potassium to the intracellular phase, and that attacks may be precipitated by agencies that potentiate this shift, e.g. adrenaline, emotion, carbohydrate ingestion, and insulin. The condition is relieved by the administration of potassium salts.

Potassium Depletion

The loss of potassium will take place either in the gastro-intestinal secretions or in the urine.

From the gastro-intestinal tract. The gastric juice contains about twice the concentration of potassium of plasma, but severe vomiting is not an important cause of hypokalaemia unless there are secondary renal changes as in pyloric stenosis

(see p. 453). The faecal excretion of potassium is high (twice that of sodium), and chronic diarrhoea, as in ulcerative colities and the malabsorption syndrome, leads to serious potassium deficiency. Potassium-secreting villous adenomata of the colon have the same effect.[13] Obsessional purgative-users may develop extreme hypokalaemia.[14]

From the urine. The osmotic diuresis of diabetes mellitus is a potent cause of potassium loss. Diuretics, e.g. chlorothiazide, may have the same effect. Primary hyperaldosteronism (Conn's syndrome) leads to very severe potassium loss, and is easily mistaken for potassium-losing nephritis. Cushing's syndrome produces a milder effect, but the Cushing-like disorder associated with oat-cell lung cancers that secrete ACTH may lead to severe hypokalaemic alkalosis (see p. 344).

Finally, intrinsic renal disease may lead to serious potassium loss. This is uncommon, and is always associated with an impaired excretion of hydrogen ions by the distal tubules (see Chapter 42). Uretero-colic anastomosis leads to hypokalaemia by a combined colonic and renal loss.

Effects. Potassium deprivation impairs cellular function; muscular weakness is a feature of this. The kidneys are damaged by severe potassium depletion. Histologically there appears to be vacuolation of the cells of the proximal tubules, but in fact this is due to the accumulation of fluid outside the cells (p. 51). Potassium deficiency probably also predisposes the kidney to pyelonephritis.

Hypokalaemia leads to metabolic alkalosis. Hydrogen ions and sodium ions enter the intracellular fluid to replace the lost potassium ions.[15] Thus there is a cellular acidosis and sodium retention with an extracellular alkalosis and sodium depletion. In true potassium-losing nephritis there is severe acidosis because the primary defect is a failure of urine acidification.

Clinical manifestations. *Intense muscular asthenia.* This is not confined to the skeletal musculature, but affects the smooth muscle of the gut also, and may lead to paralytic ileus. Paradoxically enough, potassium depletion occasionally causes tetany.

Mental changes. Apathy, confusion, and amnesia may be prominent. Coma eventually follows.

Renal dysfunction is particularly important in chronic potassium deficiency. There is an early failure of concentration, for the tubules do not respond to antidiuretic hormone. Polyuria and nocturia are prominent symptoms, and later on clinical pyelonephritis may supervene. There may be a *paradoxical aciduria*, i.e. an acid urine in the presence of a metabolic alkalosis. This is due to the distal tubules secreting hydrogen ions in place of potassium. The condition is seen most frequently in pyloric stenosis.

Cardiac changes. These are particularly common in elderly people. There is irregularity of the heart rate, hypotension, and cardiac dilatation; the toxic effects of digitalis are potentiated. The electrocardiograph shows flattened T waves with ST segment depression.

Death is generally due to respiratory failure caused by weakness of the muscles of respiration, though it may also be attributable to cardiac failure and renal damage.

Potassium Excess

Hyperkalaemia is due to renal inadequacy in excreting potassium. The most important cause of severe potassium retention is acute renal failure with anuria. In the terminal uraemia of chronic renal failure there is also considerable potassium retention.

In Addison's disease there is moderate hyperkalaemia due to a deficiency of adrenal cortical hormones, but the raised potassium concentration in the plasma is seldom sufficient to produce ill-effects.

A third cause of hyperkalaemia is the rapid infusion of potassium salts in conditions of hypokalaemia. Sudden death has followed the injudicious parenteral administration of potassium salts.

The clinical manifestations of potassium retention are somewhat vague. Confusion, apathy, and sensory disturbances (paraesthesiae) are often present and, rather unexpectedly, there may also be severe muscular weakness as in potassium depletion. Indeed, there is a very rare form of familial periodic paralysis due to hyperkalaemia.[16] Cardiac dysfunction is important. There are characteristically high, peaked T waves on the electrocardiograph. Ventricular fibrillation may follow, and cause death.

DISTURBANCES IN MAGNESIUM BALANCE[1, 17, 18]

Magnesium is the second most important intracellular cation, forming a third of the cationic content of the cells. The daily intake is 0·2–0·6 g, of which 60–80 per cent is lost directly in the faeces, and the remainder absorbed. The blood level is low (1·5–1·8 mEq per litre). Magnesium is filtered, and some is reabsorbed in the renal tubules. In some respects its metabolism resembles that of potassium, and aldosterone promotes its excretion in the urine, but there is no active tubular secretion as is seen in connexion with potassium.

Magnesium excess. This occurs in chronic renal failure, especially if magnesium sulphate is given to the patient. There is drowsiness (at a blood level of 8 mEq per litre) and coma (at 14 mEq per litre). Peripheral vasodilatation, hypotension, and muscular flaccidity like that produced by curare are other features.

Magnesium depletion. When the magnesium level in the blood falls, there is renal conservation. It is difficult to produce hypomagnesaemia experimentally in man. It is seen clinically in renal tubular defects, chronic alcoholism, hyperaldosteronism, hepatic cirrhosis, and the malabsorption syndrome. It gives rise to severe psychotic symptoms (delirium, delusions, and hallucinations), tremor, muscular twitching, athetoid movements, and convulsions. There is,

however, often a poor correlation between blood levels and clinical effects. When it occurs in the malabsorption syndrome there is also hypocalcaemia, but hypomagnesaemia is sometimes found in hyperparathyroidism in association with hypercalcaemia; the magnesium level falls after parathyroidectomy due probably to its sequestration in bone.

ACID-BASE BALANCE—THE BICARBONATE ION[19-23]

During the course of normal metabolic activity various acids are produced, e.g. phosphoric, sulphuric, lactic, and hydrochloric acid. In addition, the keto acids β-hydroxybutyric and acetoacetic acid are formed in considerable quantities during starvation and especially in uncontrolled diabetes mellitus. The acid produced in the largest amount, however, is carbonic acid, for it is an inevitable product of aerobic tissue activity. Despite this acidifying tendency the pH of the blood remains constantly at about 7·4 in health, and this is due to the buffering capacity of the body and the disposal of acid from the body, which limit any change.

It is accepted that *an acid is a molecule or an ion which is capable of yielding a hydrogen ion (i.e. a proton), while a base is a molecule or an ion which is capable of taking up a hydrogen ion to form an acid.* This is called the *Bronsted-Lowry proposition.* The strength of an acid or a base depends on its ability to give up or receive a hydrogen ion. In the equation $HB \rightleftharpoons H^+ + B^-$, which symbolises the dissociation and formation of an acid, B^- is the base, and is called the *conjugate base* of the acid HB, just as HB is the *conjugate acid* of the base B^-. HB and B^- together are the *conjugate pair.* The more readily the acid gives up its hydrogen ion, the less readily does the conjugate base accept it, i.e. the stronger the acid, the weaker is its conjugate base. In the equation $HCl \rightleftharpoons H^+ + Cl^-$, the conjugate base Cl^- is very weak, because HCl is a very strong acid; on the other hand, in the equation $H_2CO_3 \rightleftharpoons H^+ + HCO_3^-$, the conjugate base HCO_3^- is strong, because H_2CO_3 is a weak acid. When sodium hydroxide is added to water, it contributes equal quantities of Na^+ ions (which are neither acidic nor basic) and OH^- ions, which are strongly basic. As the product $[H^+].[OH^-]$ has to remain constant, H^+ ions are removed from the solution by reacting with the OH^- ions, according to the equation $H^+ + OH^- \rightleftharpoons H_2O$. At 25°C the product of the molar concentrations of hydrogen and hydroxyl ions in pure water is 10^{-14}, i.e. $[H^+] = [OH^-] = 10^{-7}$. A pH* of 7 corresponds to neutrality. If H^+ ions are removed the pH rises, and if H^+ ions are added the pH falls. According to this the solution becomes alkaline or acid. In fact, a proton cannot exist free in aqueous solution, and it at once combines

* The pH is the negative logarithm of the hydrogen ion concentration of a solution. The form $[H^+]$ = hydrogen ion concentration. At 37°C the product $[H^+].[OH^-] = 10^{-13.6}$. This means that at body temperature a pH of 6·8 corresponds to neutrality.

with a molecule of water to form an OH_3^+ ion (hydroxonium ion), but by convention it is referred to as a hydrogen ion. Water itself can act both as a very weak acid, as in the equation $H_2O \rightleftharpoons H^+ + OH^-$, in which the conjugate base OH^- is extremely strong, and as a very weak base, as when it takes up a hydrogen ion to form the extremely strong acid OH_3^+.

Buffers

In order to limit the change in hydrogen ion concentration to the range (pH 6·8–8·0) within which survival is possible, the body is provided with certain *buffer* systems. These are capable of mopping up an excess of H^+ ions, and are also able to contribute H^+ ions if the pH rises too much. The essential feature of a buffer is that it consists of a strong base and a weak conjugate acid. In the dissociation equation of such a weak acid, $HB \rightleftharpoons H^+ + B^-$, it is found that if there is an excess of H^+ ions, these are removed from solution by combining with the strong base, B^-, to form more of the weak acid. On the other hand, if the pH rises too much, there is an increased dissociation of the acid with the production of more H^+ ions. In other words, the conjugate pairs take up H^+ ions when the pH falls, and supply them when the pH rises.

By far the most important buffer in extracellular fluid is the bicarbonate ion, the normal concentration of which in plasma is 25–31 mEq per litre. It is aided by two other bases, monohydrogen phosphate and the plasma proteins (which carry a negative charge at the pH of the blood). Intracellularly, haemoglobin is extremely important as a buffer, and so probably are the other cell proteins. The following equations illustrate the buffering of an acid in the circulation:

$$H^+ + HCO_3^- \rightarrow H_2CO_3$$
$$H^+ + HPO_4^{--} \rightarrow H_2PO_4^-$$
$$H^+ + Protein^{n-} \rightarrow H\,Protein^{(n-1)-}$$

The carbonic acid produced in the first reaction is removed by its diffusion as CO_2 into the alveolar air of the lungs. *The great importance of the bicarbonate ion lies not only in its buffering capacity, but also in the extreme volatility of carbonic acid and its ease of elimination by the lungs.*

The only other route whereby H^+ ions can be excreted from the body is in the urine. The cells of the tubules secrete H^+ ions which are buffered in the glomerular filtrate, partly by phosphate, but also by combination with ammonia to form ammonium ions. Filtered bicarbonate ions combine with secreted H^+ ions to form carbonic acid, which dissociates so that CO_2 diffuses back into the blood, where it can reform bicarbonate ions. The whole process amounts to a reabsorption of the filtered bicarbonate ions.

The handling of the carbonic acid produced during tissue activity is a supreme tribute to the red cells which contain both haemoglobin, the most important buffer in the blood after bicarbonate, and a high content of carbonic anhydrase, which accelerates the following reversible reaction:

$$CO_2 + H_2O \rightleftharpoons H_2CO_3$$

The carbonic acid then dissociates into bicarbonate and hydrogen ions:

$$H_2CO_3 \rightarrow HCO_3^- + H^+$$

The hydrogen ions are largely buffered by the haemoglobin:

$$H^+ + Hb^- \rightleftharpoons HHb$$

The excess bicarbonate ions then diffuse into the plasma in exchange for chloride ions, which diffuse into the red cells. This is called the *chloride shift*. In this way the bicarbonate level of the plasma rises. There is no cation exchange between the red cells and the plasma comparable with this shift of anions.

In the lungs, as CO_2 diffuses into the alveolar air, these reactions are reversed. The reversal is assisted by the oxygenation of the Hb, because oxyhaemoglobin is a stronger acid than reduced haemoglobin, i.e. it gives off H^+ ions more readily. The carbonic anhydrase converts carbonic acid into its anhydride, CO_2.

There is a second method of CO_2 transport in the blood: a direct reversible combination with Hb to form a carbamino compound.

In general the body copes with an influex of strong acid firstly by the effect of dilution with the copious tissue fluids, and secondly by buffering. Finally the pulmonary and renal mechanisms come into play to restore equilibrium once more. Of these the lungs act more immediately than do the kidneys.

The Maintenance of the pH of the Blood

According to the Henderson-Hasselbalch equation

$$pH = pK + \log \frac{[salt]}{[acid]},$$

where pK is the negative logarithm of the dissociation constant of an acid. The pK is equal to the pH of a dilute solution in which a weak acid is half neutralised, so that the concentrations of the acid and its conjugate base are equal. The stronger the acid, the smaller is its pK.

Applying this equation to the pH of the blood,

$$pH = pK + \log \frac{[conjugate\ base]}{[conjugate\ acid]},$$

it is found that the pK for carbonic acid is 6·1, the concentration of bicarbonate is about 27 mEq per litre, and the concentration of H_2CO_3 in solution, at a partial pressure of CO_2 of 40 mm Hg (the normal alveolar tension), is about 1·35 millimole per litre. Therefore

$$pH = 6·1 + \log \frac{27}{1·35} = 6·1 + \log 20 = 6·1 + 1·3 = 7·4.$$

The equation can also be written as follows:

$$pH = 6·1 + \log \frac{[HCO_3^-]}{\alpha.P_{CO_2}},$$

where α is the solubility coefficient per mm Hg, and P_{CO_2} is the partial pressure of CO_2 in mm Hg. This at once demonstrates that the pH of the plasma depends principally on two factors: (*a*) the concentration of bicarbonate, and (*b*) the partial pressure of CO_2, which determines the concentration of carbonic acid. If the pH is to be maintained at 7·4, the

ratio $\dfrac{[HCO_3^-]}{[H_2CO_3]}$ has to remain at 20.

ABNORMALITIES OF THE pH OF THE BLOOD

An increase in the hydrogen ion concentration of the blood (pH less than 7·36) is called an *acidaemia* and a decrease (pH over 7·44) an *alkalaemia* (or *basaemia*). The terms *acidosis* and *alkalosis* are sometimes used synonymously with acidaemia and alkalaemia, but it is preferable to restrict them to describing conditions in which there would be an appropriate change in pH were there no compensation.

Respiratory Acidosis and Alkalosis

If the P_{CO_2} changes, the pH moves in the opposite direction, whereas a change in the concentration of bicarbonate moves the pH in the same direction. The P_{CO_2} is closely dependent on the removal of CO_2 from the lungs. If ventilation is inadequate, P_{CO_2} rises. This is called *respiratory acidosis*, because the retained CO_2 forms carbonic acid, which is a source of H^+. $[HCO_3^-]$ rises too, but by a lesser amount; the ratio of $[HCO_3^-]$ to $[H_2CO_3]$ falls, as does the pH. In the opposite state of hyperventilation, P_{CO_2} falls. So does $[HCO_3^-]$, but by a lesser amount. The ratio of $[HCO_3^-]$ to $[H_2CO_3]$ rises, as does the pH. This is *respiratory alkalosis*.

It is evident that respiratory acidosis is directly related to underventilation of the lungs with a resulting rise in the arterial P_{CO_2}. Likewise in respiratory alkalosis there is overventilation with a drop in arterial P_{CO_2}. A measurement of the arterial P_{CO_2} is therefore an accurate and useful method of assessing the respiratory component of acid-base balance.

Respiratory acidosis. This is due to underventilation of the lungs leading to CO_2 retention and a rise in arterial P_{CO_2} (see Chapter 41). The blood pH falls and the plasma bicarbonate level rises. The standard bicarbonate remains normal (p. 451).

Clinical and biological effects. *There is peripheral vasodilatation*, which is the direct effect of raised P_{CO_2}. Such vasodilatation may raise the intracranial pressure. Other effects of acidosis are described under metabolic acidosis (see below).

Excretion of hydrogen ions and ammonia by the distal tubules of the kidney with a concomitant reabsorption of bicarbonate. In acute respiratory acidosis the renal excretion of sodium and potassium is decreased, while chloride is excreted in proportionately greater amounts.

The level of the plasma chloride drops in proportion to the rise in the plasma bicarbonate level. This is particularly marked in chronic respiratory acidosis.

Respiratory alkalosis. There is a rise in blood pH and a fall in the plasma bicarbonate level. It is due to hyperventilation removing so much carbon dioxide that its tension in the blood is reduced. Hyperventilation is ventilation in excess of that required to remove CO_2 as fast as it is produced. It is encountered:

During hysteria, working at high temperatures or at great altitudes, or following salicylate intoxication. Salicylates in toxic doses have a directly stimulating effect on the respiratory centre. The effects of salicylate poisoning are complex, because there is also a tendency towards metabolic acidosis.[24]

During anaesthesia, when muscular relaxants are being used and excessively vigorous artificial respiration is applied.

Clinical and biochemical effects. *Pallor* due to peripheral vasoconstriction, a direct effect of the low tension of CO_2 in the blood.

Tetany.

A tendency towards sudden respiratory arrest. This can be reversed by the inhalation of carbon dioxide.

The renal change described in metabolic alkalosis. There is a great bicarbonate excretion, whilst the secretion of hydrogen ions is much reduced.

A corresponding rise in the level of plasma chlorides.

Non-Respiratory, or Metabolic, Acidosis and Alkalosis

If there is an excess of H^+ ions in the blood as a result of the ingestion or production of acid substances, the bicarbonate of the plasma is replaced by chloride and other anions; the $[HCO_3^-]$ drops. There is a secondary fall in the P_{CO_2} to match this low concentration of bicarbonate, an effect produced by the low pH stimulating the respiratory centre and increasing ventilation. This is a *metabolic acidosis*. On the other hand, the ingestion of sodium bicarbonate leads to a rise of $[HCO_3^-]$ and pH of the plasma. There is little reduction in ventilation, however, and therefore little secondary rise of P_{CO_2} (see p. 451). This is a *metabolic alkalosis*.

Metabolic acidosis. There is a fall in both the pH of the blood and the bicarbonate level of the plasma. It is encountered in the following conditions:

In shock, when there is underperfusion of the tissues and subsequent anaerobic metabolism with the production of lactic acid (see p. 427).

In severe diarrhoea, where there is a greater loss of hydroxyl ions than hydrogen ions in the faeces. The same effect may occur with pancreatic and biliary fistulae.

In starvation, and especially in uncontrolled diabetes mellitus, where there is a ketosis. The acetoacetic and β-hydroxybutyric acids produce extra H^+ ions.

Following the administration of ammonium chloride. The ammonia is converted into urea by the liver, while hydrogen ions are left behind with chloride ions.

$$Cl^- + NH_4^+ \rightarrow HN_3 \text{ (removed)} + H^+ + Cl^-$$

In renal disease, due either to impaired filtration as in anuria and terminal uraemia, or else to a failure of acidification by the distal tubules as in renal tubular acidosis. In this type of condition H+ ions are retained and not secreted.

After uretero-colic anastomosis. This is described later.

Clinical and biochemical effects. *The classical symptom of air-hunger* (deep, sighing, rapid respiration). It is a compensatory mechanism because it lowers the P_{CO_2}, and thereby causes a respiratory alkalosis which tends to reverse the fall of the blood. It is believed that the lowered blood pH stimulates the respiratory centre.

Excretion of hydrogen ions and ammonia by the distal tubules of the kidney with a concomitant reabsorption of bicarbonate. This mechanism is impaired in an acidosis of renal origin.

As the plasma bicarbonate falls, there is a corresponding rise in some of the other plasma anions. The plasma chloride concentration often rises to produce a *hyperchloraemic acidosis*. In diabetic acidosis the keto acid level increases considerably.

Severe metabolic acidosis may cause various neurological symptoms culminating in coma and death. It impairs cardiac contraction, and a state of shock with low cardiac output and hypotension may result. Acidosis seems to potentiate the effects of trauma and haemorrhage, and has been considered an important cause of irreversible shock. Cardiac arrhythmias, cardiac arrest, and sudden death have also been attributed to severe acidosis even when there has been no preceding evidence of failure.

Metabolic alkalosis. There is a rise both in the blood pH and the bicarbonate level of the plasma. It is encountered in the following conditions:

Following the administration of an alkaline salt like sodium bicarbonate. Salts with organic anions, e.g. potassium citrate and sodium lactate, are also alkalinising, presumably because the anion is metabolised to form bicarbonate.

In a condition of persistent vomiting, e.g. pyloric stenosis. There is a loss of hydrogen ions in excess of hydroxyl ions.

In severe hypokalaemia as in primary hyperaldosteronism and Cushing's syndrome. The mechanism of the ensuing alkalosis has already been described.

Clinical and biological effects. *Depression of respiration,* which would, by causing retention of CO_2, tend to reverse the rise of pH of the blood, is inconspicuous. It is probably limited by the effect of hypoxia on the chemoreceptors.

Tetany may occur due to a decrease in the ionised fraction of plasma calcium as well as by a direct effect of the lowered H+ ion concentration.

There is an increased glomerular filtration rate with corresponding increase in the amount of bicarbonate in the filtrate. The tubules respond by reabsorbing less bicarbonate than normally. There is also a decreased secretion of hydrogen ions, and a tendency towards increased potassium secretion. There may be a diminished reabsorption of sodium.

There is a fall in the level of plasma chloride, corresponding to the rise in plasma bicarbonate.

Assessment of the Metabolic Component of Acid-Base Balance

The assessment of the metabolic, or non-respiratory, component of acid-base balance is a subject of considerable difficulty and controversy. Merely measuring the plasma bicarbonate is of limited value, for although the level is raised in metabolic alkalosis and reduced in metabolic acidosis, it is also influenced by respiratory function. Thus in respiratory alkalosis it is *reduced*, and in respiratory acidosis it is *raised*. Several methods can be used to eliminate this respiratory component.

The alkali reserve. This is the bicarbonate content of plasma after it has been separated from the blood cells and equilibrated at 38°C with a gas mixture containing CO_2 at a partial pressure of 40 mm Hg.

Standard bicarbonate. This is the bicarbonate content of plasma after a sample of *whole blood* has been equilibrated at P_{CO_2} of 40 mm Hg. at 38°C. It is thought to be more useful than the alkali reserve. It is raised in metabolic alkalosis and reduced in metabolic acidosis. The normal range is 22–26 mEq per litre.

Buffer base. This is the sum effect of the buffer anions in the blood. The normal range is 44–48 mEq per litre.

The most logical measurement of the metabolic component of the acid-base balance is probably the *standard bicarbonate*. The effect of any abnormality in P_{CO_2} in life is corrected by

TABLE 34.2 The main metabolic changes in different types of acidosis and alkalosis (uncompensated)

	Blood pH	Plasma bicarbonate	Plasma chloride	Urine
Metabolic Acidosis	Low	Low	Usually raised	Much hydrogen ions and ammonia. Little bicarbonate.
Respiratory Acidosis	Low	Raised	Low	As above.
Metabolic Alkalosis	High	Raised	Low	Much bicarbonate. Little ammonia and hydrogen ions.
Respiratory Alkalosis	High	Low	Raised	As above.

equilibrating the blood at P_{CO_2} 40 mm Hg *in vitro*. The hydrogen ion concentration is then related to the metabolic component and is expressed in the bicarbonate content. The buffer base determinations include other buffers, e.g. protein, also present in the plasma. However, these buffers are largely confined to the plasma, while bicarbonate is present in the extracellular, extravascular fluids as well—a volume about four times that of the plasma.

It must be stressed that isolated measurements of pH are of limited value. A low level may occur in either respiratory or metabolic acidosis, and furthermore a normal pH can occur in the presence of severe acid–base derangements. Thus a patient with severe respiratory failure and respiratory acidosis, by secreting excess hydrogen ions in the urine (perhaps aided by diuretics), may develop a compensating metabolic alkalosis, so that a normal pH results. It is indeed usual for an acidosis or alkalosis of one type to be adjusted by an appropriate metabolic or respiratory compensation. However, this does not always occur, for both components may work in the same direction, as is commonly seen in the postoperative period when respiratory complications cause respiratory acidosis and shock leads to an additional metabolic acidosis.

ABNORMALITIES IN ELECTROLYTE BALANCE IN VARIOUS CONDITIONS

It is instructive to conclude this discussion of electrolyte balance by briefly considering a few clinical conditions in which disturbances of the balance are important.

Postoperative Alterations in Electrolyte Balance[1]

From the time of operation until nearly a week afterwards there is a consistent alteration in electrolyte and water balance. The response described below is the classical account of electrolyte changes following trauma, but it can be altered by the use of intensive intravenous therapy, as mentioned in Chapter 32, where the changes in nitrogen metabolism are also considered (see pp. 428 and 429–431).

The main feature of the postoperative response is a marked oliguria which normally persists for 24–48 hours. During this period there is an almost complete retention of sodium and chloride ions. After the first two days the urinary volume gradually increases, until it reaches a full amount after the first week, by which time there is a normal excretion of sodium and chloride ions. Within 24 hours of operation there is an increased urinary excretion of potassium, which persists for about 4 days.

These changes are associated with an increased secretion of adrenal steroids. They can be explained teleologically in terms of the extensive inflammatory exudate that forms around any traumatised area. This exudate is rich in water, sodium chloride, and protein, all of which are necessary for the healing process. There is therefore a decreased loss of

water and sodium chloride in the urine. The protein (and also extra water) is derived from the protoplasmic breakdown of other body tissues, especially skeletal muscle, and in this process of catabolism there is a release of potassium ions which are excreted in the urine.

During the early postoperative period there may be a very slight rise in the levels of blood urea and potassium, because they are being produced in such great quantities that they may not be excreted by the kidneys with sufficient speed. This explains the paradox of increased blood level despite a negative metabolic balance.

On the other hand, the blood levels of sodium and chloride are low despite their retention in the body. This "sodium paradox" has been attributed to a dilution effect secondary to an even greater water retention, the water having been extracted from the cells during their breakdown. Another suggestion is the intracellular deviation of sodium and chloride following the extrusion of potassium, phosphate, and sulphate into the extracellular fluid.

The inability to secrete a water load is the result of an excessive secretion of ADH. This occurs postoperatively as a result of pain, trauma, and anaesthetic and analgesic drugs.

It is important to be aware of these minor changes in blood chemistry, lest patients be given intravenous fluids at a time when they cannot excrete an extra water and salt load in the urine.

Likewise the passage of a small volume of urine low in sodium and chloride content need occasion no alarm during the first few days after an operation. Such urine should, however, be highly concentrated. A low specific gravity of around 1·010 is ominous, and may be the first indication of tubular necrosis.

Conditions of Gastrointestinal Fluid Loss

The secretions of the gastrointestinal tract are not only copious in amount, but they also contain high concentrations of electrolytes. The intestinal juice, for example, has roughly the same concentrations of sodium, chloride, and bicarbonate as the plasma, but twice as much potassium. Normally about 3 000 ml are secreted each day. The gastric juice, the daily volume of which is about 2 500 ml, has only a third of the sodium concentration of the plasma, but twice as much potassium and one-and-a-half times as much chloride.[25] Being strongly acid it has a high concentration of hydrogen ions and no free bicarbonate.

The biliary secretion, normally 500 ml a day, resembles the plasma closely in its electrolyte content, though it has a slightly increased concentration of bicarbonate. The pancreatic juice, normally 700 ml a day, though similar in sodium and potassium concentration to plasma, has a lower chloride and a much higher bicarbonate concentration.

Normally all these secretions are reabsorbed, but when they are lost there are serious disturbances in the body's electrolyte balance.

Acute intestinal obstruction. In any *mechanical*

obstruction there is a dilatation of the loops of bowel proximal to it. These become distended with secretion, and the greater the distension, the greater the stimulus to further secretion. In addition there is also a loss of fluid into the wall of the bowel and into the peritoneal cavity. The higher up the obstruction, the more marked is the fluid loss and the earlier is the advent of severe vomiting. A high jejunal obstruction may lead to the loss of several litres of fluid in a day, whereas an obstruction involving the rectum may persist for several weeks and cause little fluid loss.

A high intestinal obstruction is always accompanied by great sodium and water depletion, and this rapidly produces severe dehydration. In the event of extensive strangulation there is also an extravasation of blood into the devitalised loop and its mesentery. As fluid is replaced by infusion, so more secretion enters the distended loops above an obstruction. It therefore follows that the obstruction should be relieved as soon as possible.

Ileus secondary to *generalised peritonitis* presents special problems. In addition to the secretion of much fluid into the distended loops of bowel, there is also a considerable plasma loss in the extensive inflammatory exudate filling the peritoneal cavity. The combined loss of fluid in the intestinal secretion and inflammatory exudate produces a characteristically intractable dehydration.

Severe shock is characteristic of acute peritonitis, and it may be unresponsive to intravenous infusions of blood and plasma as well as saline. There is an important bacteraemic element in this shock and also in that of acute intestinal obstruction, where intestinal organisms penetrate the devitalised bowel wall and enter the circulation.

Primary *paralytic ileus* presents a somewhat similar picture, but here the atony is due to an intrinsic impairment of muscular motility and co-ordination. There is some evidence that is may be precipitated by a fall in the concentration of blood potassium.[26] Another important cause is the use of ganglion-blocking agents.

Pyloric stenosis. Of all the disturbances of electrolyte balance pyloric stenosis is the most complex. Unlike acute intestinal obstruction it runs a more protracted course, so that there is time for a depletion of potassium and a disturbance of acid-base equilibrium to complicate the picture of sodium and water depletion.[27] It has already been noted that pure gastric juice has a high concentration of potassium and hydrogen ions, though the content of sodium is low. On the other hand, the intrinsic disease of the stomach responsible for the stenosis may alter this composition, e.g. gastric carcinoma is usually accompanied by an achlorhydria. The three common causes of pyloric stenosis are a cicatrising or oedematous peptic ulcer, pyloric cancer, and hypertrophy of the pyloric muscle in infants. In adults the picture is often complicated by a previous overdose of sodium bicarbonate.[28] The following sequence of events follows the persistent vomiting of pyloric stenosis:

(*a*) There is a primary depletion of sodium, chloride, and water which leads to a moderate degree of dehydration with oliguria.

(*b*) Soon the loss of hydrogen ions leads to a metabolic alkalosis. The kidney responds by secreting an alkaline urine rich in bicarbonate as well as sodium and potassium. This excellent renal function causes further sodium and potassium depletion, though it succeeds in depressing the raised concentration of plasma bicarbonate.

(*c*) By this time potassium depletion due to the vomiting and the renal loss becomes serious. It not only accentuates the metabolic alkalosis by diverting hydrogen ions in the cells, but it also impairs renal function by interfering with the normal concentration of the urine. Sometimes polyuria may develop, and this increases the dehydration.

(*d*) In due course the sodium loss may become very severe as a result of the vomiting and the renal loss. If both the sodium and potassium depletion become marked, the condition of "paradoxical aciduria" may occur. This remarkable state of affairs is brought about by the almost complete reabsorption of sodium by the distal tubule. As there is virtually no potassium to be excreted in exchange, the place of this cation is taken by hydrogen ions, which are then secreted into the urine.[29, 30, 31] The high concentration of hydrogen ions in the cells secondary to potassium depletion assists this process. It is the reverse of that occurring in renal tubular acidosis, where, because of an inability to secrete hydrogen ions, the distal tubule secretes excess potassium ions. In tubular acidosis the urine is almost alkaline despite a severe metabolic acidosis (see p. 530).

There is therefore no single pattern of electrolyte disturbance in pyloric stenosis. There may be oliguria or polyuria, and the urine may be alkaline or acid. A fall in plasma chloride level is inevitable, and with it there is a rise in the level of plasma bicarbonate. The plasma potassium level may be deceptively high due to its mobilisation from the cells prior to its loss in the vomitus and the urine. Despite the sodium depletion, the level of sodium in the plasma is often raised in the early stages due to a disproportionate loss of water in the vomitus. If much water is retained following the quenching of the thirst that is so troublesome, the plasma concentration of sodium will drop below normal. Sodium bicarbonate administration aggravates the alkalosis and all the effects accruing from it.

Uretero-Colic Anastomosis

Following the transplantation of both ureters into the colon, an operation that is performed after total cystectomy for carcinoma of the bladder, a complex derangement of electrolyte balance follows.[15, 32] It is due to the absorption of urea, hydrogen ions, and chloride from the colon, and it is manifested by a severe metabolic acidosis. In addition there is sometimes a serious depletion of potassium ions. The mechanism of the disturbance is as follows:

(*a*) There is an absorption of hydrogen ions. This produces a metabolic acidosis. There is also a concurrent absorption of chloride ions, which are absorbed from the bowel in excess of sodium ions. The result is a severe hyperchloraemic acidosis.

(*b*) Urea is absorbed, so that there is a corresponding rise in its blood concentration. In addition some of the urea is split up by the bacteria of the colon, and ammonia is produced. This combines with the hydrogen ions to form NH_4^+, and the ammonium chloride ultimately produced is absorbed. Ammonium chloride produces a metabolic acidosis as already described. The H^+ ions liberated in the body are equal in amount to those absorbed from the bowel. In essence this is simply another means whereby H^+ ions are absorbed into the circulation.

(*c*) There is a tendency towards potassium depletion. This is due mainly to an increased colonic loss, which is probably secondary to an ion exchange by the colon, which absorbs sodium ions in exchange for potassium ions.[9] In addition there may possibly be a renal basis for the potassium loss, as progressive pyelonephritis is inevitable.[33, 34] This is an example of potassium depletion due to a combined faecal and urinary loss.

(*d*) There is also sodium absorption which may occasionally be sufficient to lead to oedema. The plasma sodium concentration is sometimes slightly raised.

In due course the kidneys adapt themselves to the excretion of an extra load of urea, sodium chloride, hydrogen ions, and ammonia, and furthermore the absorption of sodium and chloride from the bowel becomes equalised. The acidosis is relieved, but there is an ever-present danger of pyelonephritis and ureteric occlusion. These two complications impair tubular function and lead to an accentuated acidosis and a loss of potassium.

The intricate pattern of electrolyte disturbance that complicates uretero-colic transplantation is a fine example of the baneful effects that may follow interference with a normal anatomical pathway. Both the renal and the alimentary systems are damaged, and both contribute their share to the ensuing metabolic disorder.

REFERENCES

1. SLATER, J. D. H. (1968). In *Clinical Physiology*, 3rd edn, p. 1. Edited by E. J. M. Campbell, C. J. Dickinson and J. D. H. Slater. Oxford: Blackwell.
2. DAVIS, J. O. (1961). *Progress in Cardiovascular Disease*, **4,** 27.
3. VERNEY, E. B. (1954). *Irish Journal of Medical Science*, **345,** 377.
4. GAUER, O. H., HENRY, J. P. and SIEKER, H. O. (1961). *Progress in Cardiovascular Disease*, **4,** 1.
5. GILMAN, A. (1937). *American Journal of Physiology*, **120,** 323.
6. KLEEMAN, C. R. and FICHMAN, M. P. (1967). *New England Journal of Medicine*, **277,** 1300.
7. MARRIOTT, H. L. (1947). *British Medical Journal*, i, 245, 285 and 328.
8. Leading Article (1962). *Lancet*, ii, 438.
9. D'AGOSTINO, A., LEADBETTER, W. F. and SCHWARTZ, W. B. (1953). *Journal of Clinical Investigation*, **32,** 444.
10. BLACK, D. A. K. (1964). In *The Scientific Basis of Medicine Annual Reviews*, p. 291. London: Athlone Press.
11. ALLOTT, E. N. and McARDLE, B. (1938). *Clinical Science*, **3,** 229.
12. McARDLE, B. (1956). *British Medical Bulletin*, **12,** 226.
13. ROY, A. D. and ELLIS, H. (1959). *Lancet*, i, 759.
14. LITCHFIELD, J. A. (1959). *Gastroenterology*, **37,** 483.
15. COOKE, R. E. *et al.* (1952). *Journal of Clinical Investigation*, **31,** 798.
16. FRENCH, F. F. and SOLER, N. G. (1968). *British Medical Journal*, ii, 472.
17. MacINTYRE, I. (1963). In *The Scientific Basis of Medicine Annual Reviews*, p. 216. London: Athlone Press.
18. Leading Article (1967). *British Medical Journal*, ii, 195.
19. ROBINSON, J. R. (1967). *Fundamentals of Acid-Base Regulation*, 3rd edn, 109 pp. Oxford: Blackwell.
20. CAMPBELL, E. J. M. (1968). In *Clinical Physiology*, p. 198, *loc. cit.*
21. NUNN, J. F. (1965). In *General Anaesthesia*, p. 300, Volume 1, 2nd edn, edited by F. T. Evans and T. C. Gray. London: Butterworths.
22. SIGGAARD-ANDERSON, O. (1965). *The Acid-Base Status of the Blood*, 3rd edn, 134 pp. Baltimore: Williams and Wilkins. Also (1963). *Scandinavian Journal of Clinical Laboratory Investigation*, **15,** Supplement 70.
23. SIGGAARD-ANDERSON, O. (1967). In *Modern Trends in Anaesthesia*, p. 99, 3. Edited by F. T. Evans and T. C. Gray. London: Butterworths.
24. GHOSE, R. R. and JOEKES, A. M. (1964). *Lancet*, i, 1409.
25. DAVENPORT, H. W. (1966). *Physiology of the Digestive Tract*, 2nd edn, pp. 100–101. Chicago: Year Book Medical Publishers.
26. STREETEN, D. H. P. and WARD-McQUAID, J. N. (1952). *British Medical Journal*, ii, 587.
27. BURNETT, C. H. *et al.* (1950). *Journal of Clinical Investigation*, **29,** 169 and 175.
28. COPE, C. L. (1936). *British Medical Journal*, ii, 914.
29. KENNEDY, T. J., WINKLEY, J. H. and DUNNING, M. F. (1949). *American Journal of Medicine*, **6,** 790.
30. BERLINER, R. W., KENNEDY, T. J. and ORLOFF, J. (1951). *American Journal of Medicine*, **11,** 274.
31. RELMAN, A. S., ETSTEIN, B. and SCHWARTZ, W. B. (1953). *Journal of Clinical Investigation*, **32,** 972.
32. PARSONS, F. M. *et al.* (1952). *British Journal of Urology*, **24,** 317.
33. POOL, T. L. and COOK, E. N. (1950). *British Journal of Urology*, **63,** 228.
34. GRAVES, R. C. and BUDDINGTON, W. T. (1950). *British Journal of Urology*, **63,** 261.

Chapter 35.   General Features of Thrombosis and its Occurrence in the Venous System

Two obvious prerequisites of any circulation are the presence of fluid and a means whereby this can be retained in the vessels should they be damaged. In the blood vascular system the clotting mechanism guards against the danger of haemorrhage, while vascular damage is remedied by the deposition of platelets and fibrin on the vessel wall. If this deposition becomes excessive, the circulation is progressively obstructed and eventually completely occluded by *thrombus*. It is evident that there must be a balance between platelet deposition and clotting on the one hand and the fluidity of blood on the other. This homeostatic mechanism guards the body against the two hazards of thrombosis and haemorrhage.

The clotting mechanism. Clotting, or coagulation, is the conversion of the plasma fibrinogen into a solid mass of fibrin. The mechanism is described in Chapter 51. At this stage it is sufficient to note that the clotting is initiated by thromboplastin derived from either the blood (intrinsic) or the tissues (extrinsic). The intrinsic system is activated by a lipid factor liberated by platelets which adhere to a surface, and by a clotting factor in the plasma (Factor XII) which is activated by an abnormal surface also.

Platelets. Platelets are 2–4 μm in diameter. They have no nucleus, and their cytoplasm has many azur granules which in blood films tend to be concentrated in the centre. On electron microscopy platelets are seen to be bounded by a plasma membrane, and in their cytoplasm there are prominent dense granules which correspond to the azurophil ones seen on light microscopy. These contain hydrolytic enzymes, and also lipoprotein which is important in blood clotting. They are probably the main site at which 5-HT is bound. They also bind histamine and adrenaline. Platelets contain a few mitochondria and some vesicular elements which may be derived from the endoplasmic reticulum or the Golgi apparatus of the megakaryocyte from which they originated. Further details of platelet development and disorder are discussed in Chapter 51.

The deposition of platelets on to the intimal surface of a blood vessel is the first step in the formation of a thrombus, and it is important to understand the mechanisms whereby platelets adhere to surfaces (*adhesiveness*) and stick to each other (*aggregation*).[1]

Platelet aggregation. Platelets aggregate immediately in the presence of *adenosine diphosphate* (*ADP*). This may be demonstrated *in vitro* by the addition of ADP to a platelet-rich preparation of plasma which is kept agitated. The aggregation can be detected by measuring the ensuing decrease in optical density.[2] Adrenaline, noradrenaline, and 5-HT have a similar effect. *Thrombin* leads to aggregation, but only after a delay of 5–10 seconds. It probably acts by converting adenosine triphosphate (ATP) in the platelets to ADP.

Platelet adhesiveness.[1] Platelets adhere to a variety of foreign surfaces, and the drop in platelet count when blood is passed through a column of glass beads has been used as an *in-vitro* method of measuring platelet adhesiveness. Platelets will also adhere to vascular endothelium if it is damaged mechanically, and to *collagen*,[3] but not to pure fibrin.

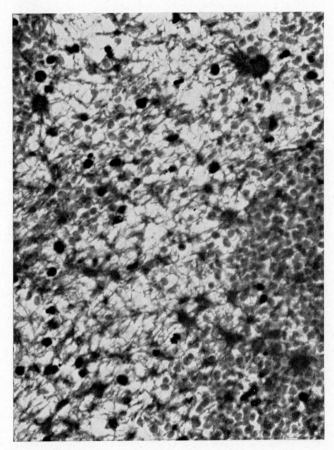

Figure 35.1
Portion of a thrombus. Strands of fibrin are seen radiating from clumps of platelets. Intermingled amongst these there are red cells and a few white cells. $\times$ 390.

The adherent platelets swell and release a variety of chemicals, including phospholipid (platelet factor 3), heparin neutralising substance (platelet factor 4), 5-HT, and ADP. The last causes platelet aggregation, and a small platelet thrombus is built up. This is unstable, and *in vivo* the platelets may break off and be released into the circulation as small emboli. Though clotting is not involved in the mechanism of platelet adhesiveness, the clotting system is soon activated by factor 3 released from the platelets and by the activation of Factor XII. Fibrin is formed, and this is thought to stabilise the platelet thrombus. In addition, the thrombin-coated fibrin leads to the further deposition of platelets.

Platelet adhesion is stimulated by ADP and inhibited by ATP. Both aggregation and adhesion take place only in the presence of ionic calcium, but whereas aggregation does not occur at low temperatures, adhesion can still take place. It is noteworthy that aspirin affects the function of platelets by preventing the release of ADP from them.[4, 5]

The healing of vascular damage. Minor degrees of injury are being constantly sustained by blood vessels, and a layer of platelets is soon laid down to retain the integrity of the wall and prevent haemorrhage. A small amount of fibrin is also formed. The process has been studied in detail under the electron microscope.[6] At first the platelets adhere in loose masses to the area of damage, and then these become compact. At first there is little morphological change in the platelets, and there is no tendency to fusion, for the plasma membrane remains intact. Later the platelets tend to apply themselves to the neighbouring cells, and close packing and distortion of shape become evident.[7] These morphological changes are most prominent at the edges of the aggregations, where the platelets lose their dense granules, adhere to leucocytes, and become entangled in meshes of fibrin. Then the internal structure of the platelet disintegrates, probably due to the release of autolytic enzymes, but the plasma membrane remains intact for a long time. Ultimately the platelets are found widely spread amid much fibrin. The close aggregation of platelets is traditionally called *viscous metamorphosis* as seen under the light microscope, but the illusion of fusion of platelets to form an amorphous mass is refuted electron-microscopically.

This deposit of platelets and fibrin is rapidly covered by endothelial cells, so that the smooth lining of the vessel is restored and further deposition ceases. The platelet deposit is removed by phagocytosis as well as by autolysis, and the fibrin is dissolved by fibrinolysins. The factors that limit the clotting tendency of circulating blood, confronted so frequently with vascular damage, are (a) naturally occurring anticoagulant substances, like heparin, (b) the fibrinolytic mechanism, which removes fibrin by the enzyme plasmin (see p. 616), and (c) the rapid endothelialisation of damaged areas, which limits the amount of clotting factors liberated into the circulation whether from aggregated platelets or damaged tissue.

THROMBOSIS[8]

Thrombosis is the formation of a solid mass in the circulation from the constituents of the streaming blood. The mass itself is called a *thrombus*, and as can be seen from the above description, consists of aggregated platelets and fibrin in which the red and white cells are trapped.

The initial stage of thrombosis is the deposition of platelets on a vascular surface. This occurs under three circumstances: (a) When the endothelial lining is damaged or removed. Exposure of collagen in the vessel wall may be of importance. (b) When there is vascular stasis; the platelets fall out of the axial stream and impinge on the wall, (c) When the streamline of the blood is disrupted and eddy currents are produced; these deflect the platelets on to the wall of the vessel. It will be recalled that ADP causes aggregation of platelets *in vitro* only if the mixture is agitated. Eddy currents probably act in this way. If a number of platelets adhere to a damaged surface they release ADP, and a thrombus is steadily built up as more platelets impinge on the surface.

The resulting thrombus is called a *pale*, or *platelet*, *thrombus*. It is, as already described, composed of a small amount of fibrin as well as the platelets, but if it is not speedily endothelialised, or if there is stasis, the fibrin increases in amount and in its meshes there are trapped red cells and leucocytes. Furthermore, the fibrin surface encourages more platelet deposition, and so the thrombus increases markedly in size. At this stage it is the blood clot which is the major component, and the mass is called a *red*, or *coagulation*, *thrombus*. Most thrombi have both pale platelet and red clot components, and are then called *mixed thrombi*.

Since the process starts with platelet deposition on a vascular surface, it can occur only in a flowing stream and is therefore encountered spontaneously only in a living animal. The clotting is a secondary phenomenon, and can occur in any column of static blood whether in the living animal or in a test-tube. Therefore a clot is not the same as a thrombus; the important feature of the latter is the platelet scaffold which is lacking in a clot.

Normally thrombosis is obviated by the smooth endothelial lining of the vessels and the streamline of blood in the complex circulatory pathways, which results in the formed elements being restricted to the central axial stream. This streamline of blood can be disturbed by obstruction of the vascular lumen through *rigid valves*, *spasm*, *intrinsic disease of the wall*, and *adjacent cicatrisation. Diffuse dilatation*, e.g. in an aneurysm, also disturbs the flow.[8] All these lesions lead to statis as well as to eddy currents, and the deposition of platelets performs a remedial function in that it smooths out the contour of the wall and restores the streamline of blood in the vessel (Fig. 35.2). The small amount of thromboplastin that is generated is dissipated in the flowing blood. It is when this dissipation is retarded that the thrombus increases in size.

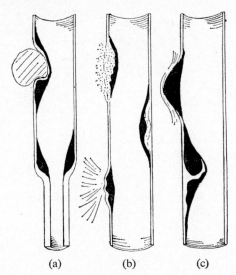

(a)   (b)   (c)

Figure 35.2
This diagram shows seven different causes of a disruption of the
normal streamlining of the blood flow, and the manner whereby
platelets (shown in black) are laid down to restore the architecture.
(*a*) Bulging due to external pressure and spasm.
(*b*) Endothelial swelling and damage due to inflammation, a
   plaque of intimal thickening, e.g. atheroma, and corrugation
   due to adjacent cicatrisation.
(*c*) Aneurysm and a sclerotic, rigid valve.
(*From Hadfield, G.* (1950), Ann. roy. Coll. Surg. Engl., **6**, 219)

Causes of Thrombosis

There are three factors concerned in the causation of
thrombosis:
   1. **The vessel wall,** especially its endothelial lining.
   2. **The flow of blood.**
   3. **The constituents of the blood,** notably the platelets
and clotting factors.
Derangements of these constitute *Virchow's triad* of
factors which determine the occurrence of thrombosis.
Changes in the vessel wall. These various anatomical
changes have already been considered. In general, they are
especially important in the pathogenesis of arterial and
cardiac thrombosis. In the veins and atria of the heart these
factors are less important, with the exception of thrombophlebitis where the inflamed vein wall is the cause of the
thrombosis.
Changes in the blood flow. The most important is
stasis, which is the usual cause of venous and atrial thrombosis. It also plays a part in the thrombus occurring in
aneurysmal sacs. Where the viscosity of the blood is increased, whether locally in acute inflammation or systemically in polycythaemia vera and dehydration, there is a
tendency to thrombosis. Thrombi in which stasis plays a
prominent part are red or mixed.
   The other alteration in blood flow is *eddy current* formation, which is important in fast-flowing streams in the arteries
and heart. The thrombus is mixed with a predominant pale
component.

Changes in the composition of the blood. *Platelets.*
Conditions associated with an increased platelet count
(thrombocytosis) are not infrequently complicated by
thrombosis. This increased count may be transient, as after
parturition, trauma, and severe haemorrhage, or it may be
persistent as in polycythaemia vera. Splenectomy is followed
by a considerable thrombocytosis which may last some time.
   The tendency to thrombosis is also related to platelet
adhesiveness. There is evidence that during the early postoperative period the platelets are more adhesive, and aggregate
more strongly in the presence of ADP and noradrenaline.[1]
Increased aggregation has also been noted in patients with
brain tumours and multiple sclerosis, conditions in which
thrombosis is not unusually frequent.[9] Hyperlipidaemia
increases platelet adhesiveness and aggregation both in man
and animals. The effect of ADP on platelets is inhibited by
adenosine and especially 2-chloroadenosine. Heparin in
large doses has a similar effect. The increased adhesiveness
in hyperlipidaemic rats is not inhibited by either adenosine
or heparin, but both together have an inhibitory effect.[10, 11]
Heparin is of little use clinically in diminishing platelet
adhesiveness.
   Clotting factors.[12] The clotting time is shortened after
severe haemorrhage, and to a lesser extent after trauma and
during the course of severe infections, e.g. typhoid fever.
Glucocorticosteroids[13, 14] and oestrogen also cause a decreased clotting time. Thrombosis sometimes complicates
these conditions or follows the administration of these drugs.
The oral contraceptive may lead to venous and cerebral
thrombosis, and it is probable that its oestrogen component
is responsible.[15, 16] Hyperlipidaemia both shortens the
clotting time and inhibits fibrinolysis. Heparin, in addition
to being an anticoagulant, clears the chylomicrons which
appear in the blood after a fatty meal.

VENOUS THROMBOSIS

Though the veins are apparently less commonly subject to
disease than the arteries, thrombosis is commoner in them
than in arteries. The venous system is capacious, and of low
pressure and velocity; it is therefore particularly liable to
bear the brunt of stasis. There are two types of venous
thrombosis: *phlebothrombosis*, which is due to stasis of blood
in uninflamed veins, usually in the calves of the legs, and
thrombophlebitis, in which the vein wall is inflamed. Though
some types of thrombosis are difficult to classify, the distinction is useful both theoretically and clinically.

PHLEBOTHROMBOSIS

This condition is the most important of all the complications that follow major surgery. Modern methods of detection have revealed that deep vein thrombosis of the leg occurs
in about 35 per cent of patients after major surgery, and it is
even more frequent in cases of recent myocardial infarction.[17]

It is a particularly common postoperative hazard of splenectomy, surgery on the hip joint, and retropubic prostatectomy.[18] The incidence is greatest in the older age group, but young people who are immobilised for any length of time are also prone to this non-infective thrombosis of the leg veins.

The Pathogenesis of Phlebothrombosis[8]

Five stages can be recognised (Fig. 35.3 and Fig. 35.6).

Primary platelet thrombus. Due perhaps to some trivial intimal damage platelets adhere to the vein wall and aggregate to form a pale thrombus as has already been

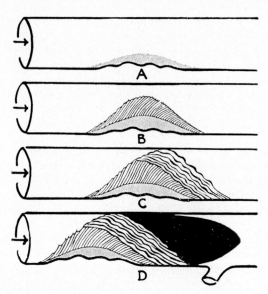

Figure 35.3
The pathogenesis of phlebothrombosis.
 A. Primary platelet thrombus.
 B. Coralline thrombus.
 C. Occluding thrombus.
 D. Consecutive clot to the next venous tributary.
(From Hadfield, G. (1950), Ann. roy. Coll. Surg. Engl., 6, 219)

described. The process has been likened to the formation of a snowdrift during a snowstorm. This would not proceed further were it not for the stasis which allows clotting factors to accumulate in the area. These promote an increase in the fibrin element which stabilises the mass of platelets and leads to the next stage.

The coralline thrombus. The fibrin deposition on the primary platelet thrombus encourages further platelet accumulations, which take the form of upstanding laminae growing across the stream. They are bent in the direction of the blood flow by the force of the stream. These laminae anastomose to form an intricate structure which resembles coral (Fig. 35.4). Between the laminae there is complete stasis, and fibrin is deposited; in it there are trapped numerous red and white blood cells. This is an example of a mixed thrombus, as it is composed of both platelet masses and blood clot.

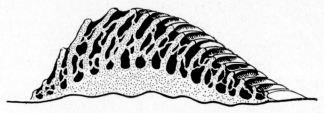

Figure 35.4.
Diagram showing the structure of the coralline thrombus and the underlying platelet thrombus.
(From Hadfield, G. (1950), Ann. roy. Coll. Surg. Engl., 6. 219)

On section it is seen to consist of alternate layers of fused platelets and fibrin with entrapped blood cells (Fig. 35.5). The retraction of the fibrin layers leads to the characteristically ribbed ("ripple") appearance seen when the surface of the thrombus is examined. The elevated platelet ridges are called the *lines of Zahn*, and they are best seen with the aid of a hand-lens. They are often conspicuous in thrombi

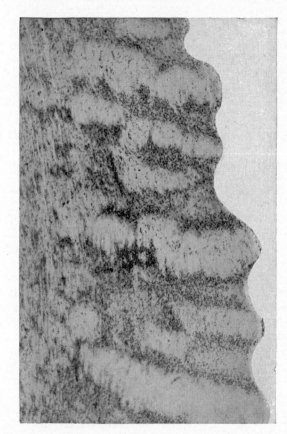

Figure 35.5
Coralline thrombus. Photomicrograph of vertical section including free surface of a coralline thrombus adherent to the wall of a large artery. Pale platelet laminae are seen projecting from the surface. Coagulated plasma containing leucocytes lies between them. Many leucocytes are adherent to the platelet laminae.
(From Hadfield, G. (1950), Ann. roy Coll. Surg. Engl., 6, 219)

formed in a fairly rapid stream of blood, e.g. in the aorta (Fig. 36.1, p. 466). Up to this stage it is possible for the process to cease, and for endothelialisation of the thrombus to occur.

Occluding thrombus. The growth of the coralline thrombus progressively occludes the lumen of the vein, and the ensuing stasis rapidly leads to the formation of more thrombus which completely occludes the lumen and trails away from the coralline thrombus in the direction of the blood flow. In this way there is formed an occluding thrombus which is composed of blood clot with a smaller platelet element. It is therefore red.

Consecutive clot. Once the vein is occluded, blood flow stops; with it stops thrombosis, which by definition can occur only in streaming blood. The stationary column of blood beyond the occluding thrombus undergoes coagulation, forming a *consecutive clot*, which extends up to the entrance of the next venous tributary. At this point the edge of the clot may become endothelialised, in which case spread, or *propagation*, is halted, but otherwise there is the development of more thrombus or clot.

Propagated clot. Propagation can occur by two methods (Fig. 35.6):

(*a*) The clot which reaches to the entrance of the venous tributary may lead to the formation of another platelet and coralline thrombus, so that there is occlusion of the ostium

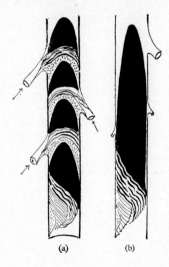

Figure 35.6
Methods of propagation in phlebothrombosis.
(*a*) With thrombus formation at each entering tributary.
(*b*) Clotting *en masse* in an extensive length of vein.
(*From Hadfield, G. (1950), Ann. roy. Coll. Surg. Engl., **6**, 219)*

of the tributary (Fig. 35.6(*a*)). Consecutive clot will then form up to the ostium of the next venous tributary. Eventually a long piece of propagated clot may be produced, which is well anchored at each successive ostium.

(*b*) Sometimes the column of blood above the consecutive clot is so stagnant, due to stasis of the venous circulation of the whole limb, that it clots *en masse*, forming one long cord of clotted blood, anchored only at the original site of thrombus formation. This length of clot retracts, and lies loose in the vein except at its one point of anchorage. It is easy to imagine how it might break off, and be carried to the heart as a massive pulmonary embolus. It is this type of propagation which is particularly dangerous to life (Fig. 35.6 (b)).

This account of propagation is necessarily simplified, and in practice it is probably a complex process in which both mechanisms described above play their part. It is quite likely that part of the propagated clot may be well attached to the points of entry of venous ostia, and that higher up it may be unattached. A great deal depends on the vigour of the circulation. A complicating factor is that the propagated clot retracts so that the circulation becomes re-established. This may lead to the deposition of a coating of thrombus over the original clot.

CAUSES OF PHLEBOTHROMBOSIS

Changes in the Vessel Wall

Frequently there is no evidence of damage at all, but a possible factor is pressure on the veins exerted by the heavy calf tissues themselves when the patient is immobilised in bed. This may be aggravated by the effect of local hypoxia due to pressure on the arteries. Sometimes of course, there are more obvious precipitating factors, e.g. direct trauma by fracture edges, and the effects of ill-applied tourniquets and plasters.

Changes in the Blood Flow

Stasis is without doubt the most important factor. It is most likely to occur in the leg veins; whenever the cardiac output is reduced, it is here that the effects of stasis are most marked, and thrombosis is most likely to occur. In addition, local factors may be responsible for regional venous stasis, and again it is the leg veins that are most vulnerable. The causes of venous stasis may be classified under the following headings:

I. GENERAL CONDITIONS
Reduced cardiac output, due to
    (i) Heart failure.
    (ii) Shock following haemorrhage, trauma, burns, and dehydration.
    (iii) Low metabolic rate, e.g. during rest in bed.
Impaired venous return due to shallow respiration.

II. LOCAL CAUSES
Lack of Muscular Activity. The venous return from the legs is greatly facilitated by the squeezing action of the surrounding muscles. This important mechanism is in abeyance in the bedridden patient. The arms are less likely to be affected, being in constant use in all conscious patients.
Incompetent Valves. The effect is somewhat debatable.

Pressure from outside, e.g. tumours, ascites, plasters, and bandages. A particularly good example of this was seen in England during the war in 1940. Many people retired to their air-raid shelters to spend the night in a deck-chair. While sheltering from the bombs, they exposed their popliteal veins to the pressure of the wooden bar, with the result that phlebothrombosis developed. The pressure of the calves on the mattress may be a factor in the bedridden and after an operation.

Changes in the Composition of the Blood

The decreased clotting time, increased platelet count, and the tendency to increased platelet adhesiveness and aggregation are important contributory factors in postoperative and post-traumatic phlebothrombosis.[1]

It is evident that although venous stasis is the most important aetiological factor in phlebothrombosis, there are also many subsidiary causes.

Merely confining a patient to bed is liable to jeopardise the venous flow in his legs both by reducing the cardiac output and inhibiting muscular activity. If in addition to this there is cardiac failure or shock, conditions are ideal for the occurrence of thrombosis. The dangers of the postoperative period are obvious, especially when respiration is painful as after chest and upper abdominal surgery. In recent years the incidence of clinically significant phlebothrombosis has diminished due to the practice of early ambulation and teaching the patient to exercise his legs in bed. But there is abundant evidence that venous thrombosis often starts during the course of the operation, especially if it is of long duration. Indeed, studies of the incidence of thrombosis using more refined modern methods of detection indicate that most of it starts very early in the postoperative period, and the use of electrical stimulation of the leg muscles during the course of the operation has been found to decrease the incidence of the condition considerably. Heparin may also be of value.[19]

Sites Affected and Naked-Eye Appearances

Phlebothrombosis commonly starts in the deep veins of the calf, and then spreads to the posterior tibial vein (Fig. 35.7). From here it may extend to involve the popliteal, femoral, and iliac veins, and even the inferior vena cava. Careful dissections have, however, shown that thrombosis sometimes starts at points higher up, e.g. at the beginning of the femoral vein or even in the external iliac vein just above the inguinal ligament. Indeed, it is not rare for thrombus to arise independently at several sites in the venous system of the lower limb.[20, 21] The pressure of the right common iliac artery on the left common iliac vein probably explains why iliac thrombosis is more common on the left side.

The most obvious feature of the affected veins is the long propagated clot, or *tail*, which may extend up to 45 cm (18 in.) This is deep red in colour, but following retraction some

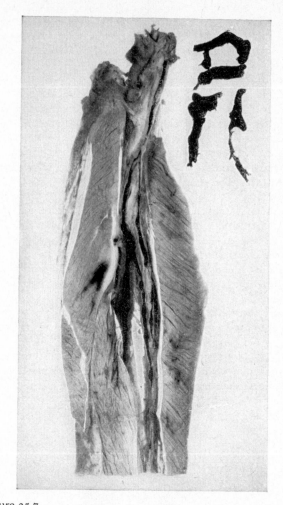

Figure 35.7
Phlebothrombosis. The muscles of the calf have been dissected to show extensive thrombosis of the main veins and their muscular branches. Several thrombi removed from the pulmonary artery are also displayed. Their calibre and branching reveal their origin from the leg. (C 40.3, *Reproduced by permission of the President and Council of the R.C.S. Eng.*)

blood may pass around it giving it a thin pale covering of platelets. The *head* (platelet and coralline thrombus) is small and firmly attached to the vein wall. By contrast, the tail is loosely attached.

Clinical Features

Clinically phlebothrombosis is remarkably silent. There is little spasm of the vessel walls and little pain. Direct pressure produced by squeezing the calf muscles may elicit tenderness, while forced passive dorsiflexion of the foot may produce pain by stretching the veins (*Homans's sign*). Oedema may develop distal to the obstructed veins, but this is neither invariable nor marked. Indeed, careful measurement may be needed to detect it. Frequently the first indication of phlebothrombosis is the occurrence of pulmonary embolism.

Specialised diagnostic procedures.[22-25] As already noted, modern methods of detection have indicated that deep vein thrombosis of the legs is much more common than is clinically evident. Furthermore, some cases in which there are signs suggestive of thrombosis prove negative to specialised tests. The most important diagnostic procedures are:

(a) *Phlebography*, in which a contrast medium is injected into a foot vein, and the venous circulation of the leg and thigh studied.

(b) *Radio-active iodine-labelled fibrinogen test*. In this test ^{125}I-labelled human fibrinogen is administered intravenously (after giving suitable doses of potassium iodide to block uptake of the radio-active iodine by the thyroid gland). The labelled fibrinogen in incorporated into forming thrombi, and the concentration of the isotope in the local area is detected and assessed by an external counter.

(c) *Ultrasound*, using a special apparatus that detects a flow of blood by the production of ultrasound that is heard from a loudspeaker. If there is thrombosis there is complete silence.

Complications

(a) Massive pulmonary embolism.

(b) Smaller pulmonary emboli, with or without pulmonary infarction.

(c) Repeated episodes of silent embolisation leading to a syndrome of progressive pulmonary hypertension.[26] This is occasionally seen as a complication of pregnancy.

THROMBOPHLEBITIS

Inflammation of a vein wall causes damage to the endothelial lining, and on this platelets are deposited. The blood flow is either normal or accelerated because of the inflammation, so that if thrombosis proceeds to complete obstruction, there is much less tendency for propagation to occur; if it

"sclerosing solutions". Strong dextrose solutions given intravenously rapidly induce thrombosis. They are therefore delivered directly into the superior vena cava through a long piece of plastic tube introduced into a forearm vein. They do not cause thrombosis of the vena cava as they are immediately diluted with a large volume of blood. It has been found that when rubber tubing is used in intravenous transfusion sets, the incidence of thrombosis is greater than when plastic tubing is used.[27]

Bacterial inflammation. Veins in the region of an infected area may become inflamed and undergo thrombosis. In pyogenic infections the organisms may invade the thrombus, soften it, and cause its disintegration. This suppurative thrombophlebitis results in the release into the circulation of numerous infected emboli, i.e. *pyaemia*. It is occasionally seen in the appendicular veins in acute appendicitis, and can complicate infected haemorrhoids; *portal pyaemia* results, and this may be accompanied by suppurative thrombophlebitis of the portal vein itself (*pylephlebitis suppurativa*). Suppurative mastoiditis similarly leads to thrombophlebitis of the lateral sinus. It must be noted that the emboli of pyaemia are tiny as compared with the massive ones frequently seen in phlebothrombosis.

Clinical Aspects of Thrombophlebitis

Spasm of the affected vein occurs, and pain is a marked feature. There are signs of acute inflammation if the vein is superficial. The condition is therefore clinically obvious. Embolism is rare when the thrombus is sterile.

Complications

(a) Pyaemic embolisation in infective cases.

(b) Venous engorgement. This is liable to occur when a large extent of venous drainage has been obliterated. It leads to residual oedema, and in very severe cases to infarction (see p. 480). After iliofemoral thrombophlebitis the superficial leg

TABLE 35.1 Comparison between phlebothrombosis and thrombophlebitis

	Phlebothrombosis	*Thrombophlebitis*
Major Cause	Stasis.	Inflammation of vein wall.
Size of Primary Thrombus	Small.	Larger—depending upon the extent of the phlebitis.
Size of Propagated Clot	Long and often poorly anchored.	Usually none; if present, short and well anchored.
Emboli	Common and massive. Sterile.	Rare except in infective cases. Pyaemic.
Site	Usually calf veins.	Anywhere.
Clinical Picture	Silent—few signs or symptoms.	Obvious—pain and signs of acute inflammation.

does, the clot is well anchored to the vein wall. The thrombus is so firmly adherent to the wall that the danger of embolism is negligible, except when the inflammation is due to pyogenic bacteria.

Sterile inflammation may be produced by direct trauma, ionising radiations, and chemicals. It is induced deliberately in varicose veins and haemorrhoids by the injection of

veins become varicose, and it is important to test the patency of the deep veins before varicose veins are ligated.

Other Types of Venous Thrombosis

There are some examples of venous thrombosis which cannot readily be classified as either phlebothrombosis or thrombophlebitis, and these are best considered separately.

Iliofemoral thrombosis[28] occurs from time to time in debilitated, bedridden patients. It was a well-recognised late complication of typhoid fever in days gone by. Two important variants are

(*a*) *Phlegmasia alba dolens*, which is the "white leg" of late pregnancy and the puerperium. Its cause is unknown. In addition to the venous involvement, there is apparently some arterial spasm causing the pallor.[29] It is possible that there is also lymphangitis. The condition is very painful. Massive pulmonary embolism sometimes occurs, but it probably arises from an unsuspected phlebothrombosis in the other leg in some cases. On the other hand, residual oedema and varicose leg veins are common sequelae.

(*b*) *Phlegmasia caerulea dolens* (see p. 480).

Thrombophlebitis migrans.[30] In this condition there are recurrent thrombotic episodes in the superficial and deep veins, especially of the extremities. Many cases are idiopathic, or form a part of Buerger's disease, and these show a diffuse inflammatory reaction. The condition is also a well-known complication of deep-seated cancer—this was first noted by Trousseau in 1865.[31] The usual sites of the primary tumour are the pancreas (tail and body), lung, stomach, and female genital tract.[32, 33] The cause of the phlebitis is unknown, and there is often little inflammatory reaction in the vein wall.

Primary mesenteric vein thrombosis is an important cause of infarction of the bowel; its aetiology is unknown.

The inferior and superior venae cavae may undergo thrombosis in the course of disease involving the retroperitoneal and mediastinal regions. The symptoms are those of venous obstruction (see Chapter 39); embolism does not occur.

THROMBOSIS IN THE ATRIA OF THE HEART

Atrial thrombosis is generally due to stasis, the condition being analogous to phlebothombosis. The atrial appendages are usually involved, because it is here that stasis is most marked. Mitral stenosis is a common cause of thrombosis in the left atrium, especially when complicated by fibrillation. It may occur in either atrium in heart failure. With valvular regurgitation there are also eddy currents.

The thrombi may become detached and lead to embolism. Precautions must be taken to prevent this when operating on the heart, e.g. when performing a mitral valvotomy. Rarely the thrombus remains in the atrium after becoming detached: this leads to the classical *ball-thrombus* that is occasionally encountered in the enormously dilated left atrium of long-standing mitral disease with combined regurgitation and stenosis. It remains free in the chamber, increases in size, and may finally block the atrioventricular orifice and cause sudden death.

Thrombi on the valves (vegetations) and in the ventricles are considered in the next chapter, because they are not associated with stasis.

GENERAL READING

HUDSON, R. E. B. (1965). *Cardiovascular Pathology*. London: Arnold. This book now in three volumes is useful for reference.

REFERENCES

1. Leading Article (1968). *Lancet*, i, 285.
2. BORN, G. V. R. (1962). *Nature, London*, **194,** 927.
3. SPAET, T. H. and ZUCKER, M. B. (1964). *American Journal of Physiology*, **206,** 1267.
4. O'BRIEN, J. R. (1968). *Lancet*, i, 789 and 894.
5. Leading Article (1969). *British Medical Journal*, iii, 371.
6. FRENCH, J. E. (1967). In *Modern Trends in Pathology*, Volume 2, p. 208. Edited by T. Crawford. London: Butterworths.
7. STEHBENS, W. E. and BISCOE, T. J. (1967). *American Journal of Pathology*, **50,** 219.
8. HADFIELD, G. (1950). *Annals of the Royal College of Surgeons of England*, **6,** 219.
9. Annotation (1968). *Lancet* i, 134.
10. BORN, G. V. R. and PHILP, R. B. (1965). *British Journal of Experimental Pathology*, **46,** 569.
11. BORN, G. V. R. (1965). *Annals of the Royal College of Surgeons. England*, **36,** 200.
12. INNES, D. and SEVITT, S. (1964). *Journal of Clinical Pathology*, **17,** 1.
13. COSGRIFF, S. W., DIEFENBACH, A. F. and VOGT, W. (1950). *American Journal of Medicine*, **9,** 752.
14. MENCZEL, J. and DREYFUSS, F. (1960). *Journal of Laboratory and Clinical Medicine*, **56,** 14.
15. INMAN, W. H. W. and VESSEY, M. P. (1968). *British Medical Journal*, ii, 193.
16. VESSEY, M. P. and DOLL, R. (1968). *British Medical Journal*, ii, 199.
17. Leading Article (1971). *British Medical Journal*, i, 305
18. KEMBLE, J. V. H. (1971). *British Journal of Hospital Medicine*, **6,** 721.
19. Leading Article (1971). *Lancet*, ii, 693.
20. GIBBS, N. M. (1957). *British Journal of Surgery*, **45,** 209.
21. SEVITT, S. (1960). *Lancet*, i, 384.
22. EVANS, D. S. and COCKETT, F. B. (1969). *British Medical Journal*, ii, 802.
23. O'BRIEN, J. R. (1970). *Lancet*, ii, 396.
24. EVANS, D. S. and NEGUS, D. (1971). *British Journal of Hospital Medicine*, **6,** 729.
25. THOMAS, M. L. (1971). *British Journal of Hospital Medicine*, **6,** 735.
26. GOODWIN, J. F., HARRISON, C. V. and WILCKEN, D. E. L. (1963). *British Medical Journal*, i, 701 and 777.

27. MOLLISON, P. L. (1972). *Blood Transfusion in Clinical Medicine*, 5th edn, p. 592. Oxford: Blackwell.
28. McLACHLIN, J. and PATERSON, J. C. (1951). *Surgery, Gynecology and Obstetrics*, **93,** 1.
29. OCHSNER, A. (1947). *Surgery, Gynecology and Obstetrics*, **84,** 659.
30. LYNN, R. B. (1953). *Angiology*, **4,** 374.
31. SPROUL, E. E. (1938). *American Journal of Cancer*, **34,** 566.
32. LIEBERMAN, J. S. *et al.* (1961). *Journal of the American Medical Association*, **177,** 542.
33. AZZOPARDI, J. G. (1966). In *Recent Advances in Pathology*, 8th edn, p. 115. Edited by C. V. Harrison. London: Churchill.

SOME COMMON ARTERIAL DISEASES

In the previous chapter the general features of thrombus formation have been described. In the high-velocity arterial system the most important cause of thrombosis is disease of the arterial wall itself. This acts in three ways:

1. Eddy-current formation leads to the deposition of platelet aggregation and deposition.

2. Ulceration of the endothelial lining contributes to platelet aggregation.

3. Disease of the arterial wall may so weaken it that aneurysmal dilatation occurs; this leads to stasis which favours thrombosis and clotting.

The causes of arterial thrombosis are those of arterial damage. Spasm, which may also initiate thrombosis, is considered in Chapter 38.

CAUSES OF ARTERIAL DAMAGE

Inflammation

1. **Trauma.** The arterial wall may be damaged by sharp spicules of bone in fractures, by adjacent missiles, or by operative procedures. The continual rubbing of the subclavian artery over a cervical rib may lead to thrombosis.[1, 2] In arterial injuries there is an important additional factor of vascular spasm.

2. **Infective and chemical lesions.** Arterial damage may occur in any acute inflammatory lesion, e.g. a carbuncle, but it is of much less importance and frequency than similar damage to veins. It is of much greater importance in chronic infective diseases, where it leads to *endarteritis obliterans*. This may be complicated by thrombosis, e.g. the cerebral vessels in syphilis and the arteries in the wall of a tuberculous cavity in a lung. It is of great importance in preventing massive haemorrhage, e.g. in peptic ulcers.

3. **Idiopathic inflammatory conditions.** *Thrombo-angiitis obliterans* (*Buerger's disease*). The disease, originally described by Buerger in 1908, is characterised by a diffuse inflammation involving segments of arteries, veins, and surrounding connective tissue. It was originally described in Jews, but there is in fact no definite racial incidence. It affects males almost exclusively. The highest incidence is during the third and fourth decades. A virus infection and hypersensitivity to tobacco have both been incriminated as aetiological agents.

Arterial thrombosis occurs in the course of the disease, and it is the medium-sized arteries (with their venae comitantes) of the leg which are most frequently affected. Intermittent claudication and gangrene are the usual clinical manifestations. The visceral vessels are seldom involved.

There is considerable controversy as to whether Buerger's disease is a distinct entity or merely the end-result of atheroma occurring in young men. Most pathologists believe that it is a specific disease of blood vessels, and its distinguishing features are the age and sex of its victims, its relationship to smoking (though atheroma is also aggravated by smoking[3]), and the tendency to attacks of superficial thrombophlebitis migrans. Histologically the diffuse inflammation, the highly cellular thrombus, and the absence of lipid material in the wall do not suggest atheroma.[4, 5, 6]

Polyarteritis nodosa. This disease is described in Chapter 16. There is an acute necrotising inflammation of a segment of the wall of an artery. Thrombosis is a common sequel. Thrombosis occasionally occurs in the related "collagen diseases", systemic lupus erythematosus and the arteritis associated with rheumatic fever and rheumatoid arthritis.

Giant-cell arteritis.[7] This disease occurs in elderly subjects, and affects the arteries of the scalp, eyes, and brain predominantly, but on occasion it involves the aorta and its branches also. There is an inflammatory reaction involving the intima and the inner part of the media. The internal elastic lamina is fragmented, and there is a conspicuous giant-cell reaction around it. Thrombosis is a common sequel, and in the ophthalmic artery it leads to retinal infarction and blindness.[8] The nature of the disease is unknown.

Neoplastic Infiltration

Tumours which invade arteries (and veins) are soon covered by thrombus. This is quite often seen in cancer of the lung, which is a notorious invader of blood vessels.

Arteriosclerosis

This term is used loosely to describe any condition in which the arterial wall is thickened and hardened. It includes atheroma as well as a number of conditions associated with hypertension and the ageing process. Inflammatory disease, e.g. polyarteritis, and that of known aetiology, e.g. syphilitic arteritis, are by convention excluded.

Arteriosclerosis obliterans.[9] Progressive thickening of the intima by fibrous tissue appears to be a feature of the ageing process in many vessels. It is found frequently in the leg arteries of patients with peripheral vascular disease. It is often accompanied by atheroma, but whereas the atheromatous element is well marked in the proximal arteries (femoral and iliac), the more distal ones show fibrosis and hyalinisation of the intima. It is not known whether this is related to atheroma, or indeed whether arteriosclerosis obliterans represents a distinct entity. Probably some of the lesions described under this heading are organised thrombi or thrombo-emboli.

Mönckeberg's medial sclerosis. This affects the large arteries of the lower limbs predominantly, and it consists of isolated rings of calcification in the media. The intima is normal. It is considered in relation to calcification in Chapter 47. It produces dramatic radiological appearances, but it does not cause ill-effects. Although commoner in elderly people, it is sometimes discovered accidentally in comparatively young adults who are otherwise healthy.

Diffuse hyperplastic sclerosis. This occurs in the small, muscular arteries, e.g. in the kidney and spleen, and in its fully-developed form it is typical of benign systemic hypertension. There is muscular hypertrophy of the media, thickening of the intima due to fibrous and elastic overgrowth, and reduplication of the internal elastic lamina.

In malignant hypertension there is intimal thickening with cellular fibrous tissue which produces an onion-skin appearance. Frequently there is an excess of acid mucopolysaccharide, so that the intima has a distinctly mucoid appearance. Similar changes are found in arterioles, particularly of the kidney. Similar changes occur in scleroderma (see p. 214).

Arteriolosclerosis

It is convenient at this point to consider also the arteriolar changes which lead to ischaemia.

Hyaline arteriosclerosis. In this condition the wall is thickened, and converted into a uniform hyaline ring. Hyalinisation of some arterioles, e.g. of the white pulp of the spleen and the ovary, is part of the normal ageing process, but when it affects the *afferent renal arterioles*, it is pathognomonic of benign systemic hypertension whether essential or secondary.

Diabetic angiopathy.[10] The arteriolar lesion of diabetes mellitus is very similar to that described as hyaline arteriolosclerosis. However, the hyaline intimal material has a high glycoprotein content, and therefore stains strongly with the PAS method.

Arteriolar necrosis. This is a fibrinoid necrosis of part or the whole of an arteriolar wall, and it leads to diffuse haemorrhage in the vicinity. It is seen in malignant hypertension of whatever cause, and it can affect many viscera, being especially prominent in the kidney. The necrosis is apparently due to the tension of an extremely raised blood pressure on the arteriolar wall. A similar lesion has been noted in the mesenteric arterioles after the successful surgical repair of a coarctation of the aorta. In this instance the previous hypo-tension of the lower part of the body has been suddenly replaced by a normal blood pressure, which is too high for the unprepared arterioles of the gut.[11] Extensive arteriolar necrosis may also lead to thrombosis and infarction; the condition resembles polyarteritis in its effects, and indeed arteriolar necrosis is a feature of some types of arteritis.

Atheroma

Without doubt this is the commonest cause of arterial thrombosis. It is the commonest killing disease in Britain (next in frequency come cancer and chronic respiratory disease), and is present to some degree in almost all adult members of the community. Indeed, its early lesions are said to commence at birth. Although of such importance and frequency, exact definition of the disease presents extreme difficulty, the reasons for which will shortly become apparent.

The disease characteristically affects the large systemic arteries like the aorta and its main branches. Of the medium-sized vessels the coronary and cerebral vessels are the most commonly involved. This is extremely unfortunate in view of the vital nature of the organs they supply, and it accounts for the lethal effects of atheroma. Atheroma may be considered as consisting of two types of condition:[12]

TYPE 1. **Yellow plaques in the tunica intima (fatty streaking).** Foam cells accumulate in the subendothelial layer, and later break down to release their fatty contents into the intima. In this way there are produced the yellow plaques or streaks which are a common *post-mortem* finding in the aorta at all ages. Although they may also be found in smaller arteries, they do not produce narrowing of the lumen. When the vessels are examined in their contracted state at necropsy, the plaques appear to be elevated. However, if the arteries are distended with fixative, the plaques more closely resemble their form in the living state: they become flattened, and far from causing narrowing of the lumen, the wall may be sufficiently weakened to allow a degree of dilatation to take place. There is some indirect evidence to suggest that the yellow plaques can be removed.

TYPE 2. **The accumulation of fatty material in the intima with additional fibrosis.** This is the common type of lesion seen in middle and old age. It is sometimes referred to as *atherosclerosis*, and may cause varying degrees of stenosis when smaller vessels are affected. Characteristic lesions are seen in the aorta.

The plaques consist of masses of foamy macrophages with much fibrous reaction around them. Later in the course of its evolution, the lesion is composed of a central mass of fatty, yellow, porridge-like material (*athere* is Greek for porridge), which consists predominantly of cholesterol and its esters, and is surrounded by dense fibrous tissue which gives the plaque a white pearly appearance. In advanced lesions ulceration with superadded thrombosis is common (Fig. 36.1). The fatty material frequently undergoes dystrophic calcification.

Figure 36.1
Thrombosis of aorta. This specimen was removed from
an aged woman who died of hypostatic pneumonia. The
aorta shows advanced atheroma, on the basis of which
there are two areas of thrombosis. These thrombi probably
formed shortly before death, when the circulation was
unduly sluggish. The lines of Zahn on the surfaces of the
thrombi are unusually well-marked.

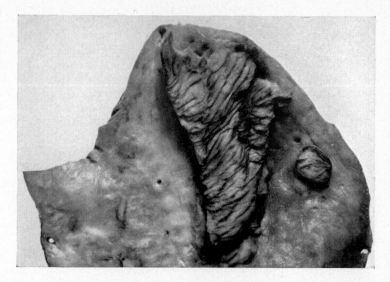

Atheroma of this type often has a capricious distribution.
Sometimes the coronary vessels are severely affected, while
the cerebral ones show minimal change. The thoracic aorta
is less severely affected than the abdominal part. It always
tends to be particularly severe in areas of vascular stress, e.g.
over syphilitic aortitis. It is more marked in hypertensive
than normotensive subjects of the same age, and it tends to
occur in the pulmonary arteries when there is pulmonary
hypertension.

Aetiology

It is evident that the two types of atheroma described
above are distinct. It is not known for certain whether the
first leads on to the second, or even whether the causative
factors are the same.

There are two classical theories regarding the aetiology of
atheroma:

The imbibition theory proposes that atheroma is due to
accumulation of fats in the intima which are derived from the
circulating lipoproteins. The evidence for this is threefold.

(*a*) Anitschkow and Chalatow as long ago as 1913 found
that rabbits fed on excessive amounts of cholesterol developed yellow atheromatous plaques.[13] This observation
has been repeatedly confirmed, but it must be remembered
that the rabbit is an herbiverous animal, and normally has a
low blood cholesterol. In carniverous animals like rats
atheroma is much more difficult to produce by cholesterol
feeding. Presumably the same would apply to man. Histologically these lesions consist of accumulations of foamy
macrophages surrounded by cellular fibrous tissue.[14] This
fibrous component is less marked than in human atheroma,
and there is no vascular occlusion, but nevertheless the lesion
is not mere fatty streaking. Rabbits fed on a diet rich in fat,
e.g. with 10–40 per cent beef fat or corn oil, get a much more
fibrous type of lesion than they do with cholesterol.[15]
Various mammals, and especially birds, have been found to

develop atheroma spontaneously; sometimes it is fatty and
sometimes more fibrous.[16]

(*b*) In man atheroma is common in a few conditions accompanied by hypercholesterolaemia. It is the cause of the
juvenile coronary thrombosis seen in patients with hyperlipoproteinaemia (p. 554), and it is unusually marked in
myxoedematous subjects. Atheroma occurs at an earlier
age and is more severe in diabetics than in the general
population.[10] This might be the result of a raised level of
blood lipids, but in well-controlled patients these are usually
normal.

(*c*) Human cases of atheroma may have an abnormal lipid
pattern in their blood.[14] The subject is complex and controversial, but most authorities recognise that the β-lipoproteins
(which include cholesterol) are elevated. Since the diet
influences the blood lipids, much work has been done on this
subject. It has been found that unsaturated fats of vegetable
origin lower the blood cholesterol level. This may be due to
the fats themselves or to the steroid content, for it is known
that some steroids, e.g. oestrogens, lower the blood cholesterol level. Choline has the same effect.

While it may be accepted that diet influences the blood
lipid level, it should not be forgotten that the body manufactures about 2 g of cholesterol daily, whereas only about
400 mg is derived from the diet. The blood cholesterol level
in fact appears to be dependent more upon the total quantity
and type of fats ingested than upon their actual cholesterol
content.

If atheroma is to be explained on a lipid basis, it must be
assumed that the β-lipoproteins are absorbed into the
arterial intima through the endothelium, which is known to
contain fat droplets when overlying a plaque. How the fat
traverses the endothelial cells is not clear: lipid–containing
macrophages can be seen to pass through the endothelium on
electron microscopy, but in which direction they are travelling is not known.[17] It is understandable that areas of damaged

endothelium should be particularly permeable to lipid. Once the β-lipoprotein is in the intima, it splits up into cholesterol and its esters which are retained, and the other lipid components, e.g. phospholipids, which are easily removed. Normally the cholesterol is kept in solution by phospholipids. The cholesterol has to diffuse outwards as far as the middle of the media before it reaches any lymphatic system which can remove it. The cholesterol in the intima could then stimulate a fibrous tissue reaction, for it is found experimentally that cholesterol injected into the tissues causes an acute inflammatory reaction, which is much less severe if phospholipid is injected at the same time.[18]

The thrombosis (incrustation) theory. Rokitansky in 1842 regarded atheroma as an incrustation of fibrin, which had become organised on the vessel walls. Virchow, however, disagreed, and the theory remained unpopular till 1946 when it was revived by Duguid.[19, 20] He noted that an artery, which in one place contained a recanalised thrombus, showed typical "atheroma" in an immediately adjacent area.

Thrombosis can be induced in an artery by transfixing its lumen with a piece of silk; the thrombus so produced undergoes organisation and then resembles atheroma. The fatty material is presumably derived from broken-down red cells entrapped in the thrombus.

The thrombotic theory has much to recommend it.[21, 22] The obstructive nature of the lesions is easily understood. Thrombosis causing complete obstruction would then no longer be considered a complication of atheroma, but merely a continuation of the same process which produced the plaque. A powerful objection to the theory is that, since thrombosis is more common in veins, atheroma ought also to be found in these vessels. A possible explanation of this paradox may lie in the disposition of the vasa vasorum in the two types of vessel. In veins these small vessels, which supply the wall itself, penetrate its whole thickness. A thrombus can therefore be easily invaded by capillaries from the media as well as the surface endothelium. In the larger arteries the vasa vasorum from the adventitia penetrate only as far as the outer half of the media. A thrombus can therefore be organised only from the surface endothelium. Presumably this process is slow, with the result that the deeper parts of the thrombus tend to break down. The production of the avascular fatty material characteristic of atheroma is the result.[23]

A considerable amount of fibrin can be demonstrated immunologically even in a small fatty plaque.[24] It is possible that it is derived from fibrinogen that leaks through the endothelium. In the fully developed lesion platelet debris can also be shown immunologically.[24]

The current trend is to combine the imbibition and incrustation theories. Simple fatty plaques do occur in man; they do not cause obstruction, and may well be produced by lipid imbibition. As was noted on p. 457, hyperlipidaemia (as after a fatty meal) shortens the clotting time[25, 26] and inhibits fibrinolysis[27] as well as rendering platelets more adhesive. Thus thrombosis is likely to occur over areas of slight

intimal irregularity engendered by the fatty plaques. Whatever may be the aetiology of the early plaque, there is little doubt that the atheromatous lesion grows by thrombotic incrustation.[24]

At present there is no satisfactory explanation for the peculiar localisation of the lesions. It is evident that there are many gaps in our knowledge of atheroma regarding both its cause and the structure of the lesions. There is no definite proof that the fatty lesions are related to the sclerotic ones, nor indeed that coronary, cerebral, and aortic atheroma are identical. Perhaps "atheroma" includes a number of different disorders which have no common cause.

Be this as it may, for the present we can only define atheroma or atherosclerosis as "a common disease of arteries manifested as a patchy thickening of the intima and an accumulation of lipid".

Effects of atheroma. *Gradual obstruction*: this is most frequent in the coronary and cerebral vessels.

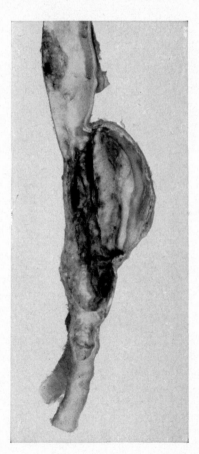

Figure 36.2
Atheromatous aneurysm of abdominal aorta. The abdominal aorta is the seat of advanced atheromatous ulceration, and just above its bifurcation there is a saccular aneurysm. It is almost completely occluded with alternate layers of white and red thrombus; this is laminated thrombus. (C 31b.7, *Reproduced by permission of the President and Council of the R.C.S. Eng.*)

Sudden complete obstruction: this may be due either to *thrombosis* or to *haemorrhage into a plaque*. Rupture of the vasa vasorum in the degenerate central region of the plaque will lead to haematoma formation. This may completely block the vessel, and is thought by some authorities to be an important factor in acute coronary occlusion. The bleeding vessels may be the high pressure capillaries coming straight off the lumen.[28]

Dilatation and aneurysm formation. Though atheroma is regarded as the prime cause of obstruction in the arterial circulation, it is very common, especially in elderly women, to find coronary arteries diffusely affected and yet widely dilated. Indeed, this type of lesion may be related to the longevity of the patient. It has been suggested that atheroma

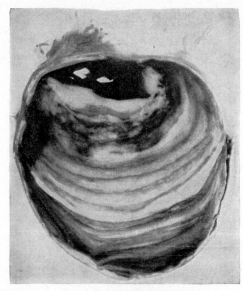

Figure 36.3
Laminated thrombus in an aneurysmal sac. This is a cross-section of an atheromatous aneurysm of the abdominal aorta, and it is almost completely filled with laminated thrombus. This specimen was removed *post-mortem* from an old man who died of an inter-current disease. (C 31b.4, *Reproduced by permission of the President and Council of the R.C.S. Eng.)*

uncomplicated by thrombotic episodes is prone to cause dilatation,[29, 30] and this again indicates the multiformity of the factors in the causation of the condition. In the abdominal aorta there is such severe weakening of the tunica media that the dilatation often progresses to aneurysm formation (Fig. 36.2 and Fig. 36.3).

Embolism. Atheromatous and thrombotic material from the aorta and its major branches sometimes becomes detached and embolises distally. The effects of this are considered on page 478.

ANEURYSMS

An aneurysm is a local dilatation of an artery or a chamber of the heart due to a weakening of its wall. It may be localised and saccular or diffuse and fusiform. The commonest site is the aorta, and then follow the arteries of the leg (especially the popliteals), the carotids, the subclavians, and the innominate.

Causes of Aneurysm Formation

Trauma, especially of the leg arteries. Subclavian aneurysm may be related to a cervical rib.

Inflammation. Syphilitic aortitis (see p. 255) was the commonest cause, but is now very rare. Polyarteritis nodosa and mycotic arteritis, i.e. following the invasion of the vessel wall by pyogenic organisms usually during pyaemia, are other examples.*

Atheroma. This is the commonest cause of aortic aneurysms, and is discussed above.

Congenital defects in the wall. The most important example is the berry aneurysm of the circle of Willis. Aneurysm of the aorta may occur proximal to a coarctation, and Marfan's syndrome may lead to dissecting aneurysm of the aorta.

Two different lesions, misleadingly called aneurysms, should be noted: (a) *arteriovenous aneurysm*, a sac of connective tissue surrounding an arteriovenous fistula, and (b) *cirsoid aneurysm*, a leash of dilated intercommunicating arteries and veins, usually on the scalp; it is congenital and a type of vascular hamartoma.

Effects. Aneurysms cause harm in the following ways:

Pressure. A good example is pressure of an aortic aneurysm on the oesophagus and the recurrent laryngeal nerve causing dysphagia and aphonia. Likewise pressure atrophy of the spinal column or sternum may occur.

Thrombosis. The main factors involved are eddy currents following the disruption of the streamline of blood entering a dilated sac, irregularity of the diseased wall, and stasis in the sac which favours clotting. Eventually a classical *laminated thrombus* develops, consisting of alternate layers of pale platelet thrombus and red blood clot. The parallel laminae result from the expansile force of the arterial pulse compressing the layers against the vessel wall (Fig. 36.3). The process is slow, but eventually the sac becomes filled with thrombus.

Haemorrhage. Unfortunately repair of an aneurysm is not effective because of the avascularity of the vessel wall. Rupture frequently follows, not so much at the apex of the aneurysm which is full of thrombus as at the sides. External haemorrhage may be impeded by the thrombus, and it is not uncommon for some small leaks to precede the final fatal gush. A good example is the recurrent haemoptysis produced by a syphilitic aortic aneurysm eroding the trachea. A ruptured aortic aneurysm is now a common cause of death.

Ischaemia. This is produced by pressure of the aneurysm on nearby branches and by the contained thrombus occluding the ostia of emerging vessels.

* The origin of the term mycotic is obscure. It is not used in the sense that fungi are involved. Perhaps it indicates that the aneurysmal bulges are mushroom shaped. It is used in this context in mycosis fungoides.

Dissecting Aneurysms of the Aorta[31]

This is the second most frequent type of aortic aneurysm, and is due to haemorrhage occurring in the media which is thereby split, or dissected, for a variable distance. The basic cause is generally medionecrosis, a condition first described histologically by Erdheim. Pools of mucopolysaccharide accumulate in the media, and there is associated fragmentation and loss of elastica.

The initial bleeding is thought to be due to a rupture of one of the vasa vasorum in the media. A small dissection results, and this eventually leads to a rupture of the intima through into the lumen, generally 2–3 cm above the aortic valve. The aneurysmal sac is then subjected to the full force of the arterial blood pressure. Rapid dissection occurs in all directions between the inner two-thirds and the outer third of the media. It extends down the aorta and into the origins of its large branches. Sometimes there is a rupture back into the lumen, and in this way a double-barrelled aorta results. However, it is much more usual for the aneurysmal sac to rupture externally—often into the pericardial sac causing acute cardiac tamponade. Clinically the disease starts as a sudden rending pain in the chest, followed by shock and the effects of obstruction of the various branches of the aorta. The blood pressure is often unequal in the two arms, as are the pulses. Ischaemia in the distribution of any branch may produce a characteristic syndrome. Involvement of the spinal arteries can cause necrosis of the spinal cord and paraplegia, involvement of the coronary arteries angina and myocardial infarction, and involvement of the renal arteries renal failure.

THROMBOSIS IN THE HEART

Thrombosis in the Atrium

This has already been described (see p. 462).

Thrombosis in the Ventricles

Thrombosis occuring on the ventricular wall is generally associated with some underlying damage to the myocardium, e.g. myocardial infarction, especially if this has progressed to aneurysm formation. It is the left ventricle which is almost always affected. Myocarditis is occasionally complicated by thrombosis. In the right ventricle a thrombus composed largely of clot is sometimes found loosely adherent to the wall. It is formed as a terminal event, presumably as the result of slowing of the blood stream, and is called an *agonal thrombus*.

At other times the blood in the right ventricle clots to form a *post-mortem clot*. In conditions accompanied by a high ESR its upper part may consist largely of plasma, when it is called "chicken-fat clot". The post-mortem clot and the agonal thrombus are of no functional significance, and should not be confused with a massive pulmonary embolus (see p. 474).

Thrombosis on the Valves

This occurs only when their endothelial covering is damaged, usually as the result of inflammation. The resulting thrombi are by tradition called *vegetations*.

Acute rheumatic fever (see Chapter 16). This affects the heart as a whole, and the oedematous endocardium is liable to be damaged along the line of contact of the valve cusps. The mitral valve is most often affected. The vegetations are of pin's-head size, and are pinkish-grey in colour. They are firmly attached to the endocardium, and never undergo embolisation. Microscopically they consist of aggregations of platelets with an admixture of fibrin, and they are invariably sterile (Fig. 36.4).

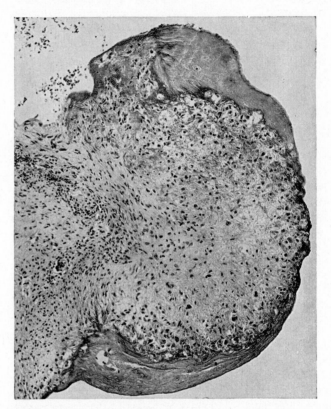

Figure 36.4
Organising rheumatic vegetation. The mass is surmounted by a layer of fibrin, in which no doubt there are aggregated platelets. The base of the thrombus consists of granulation tissue, which is invading the thrombus from below. ×110.

There is often some mitral regurgitation in the acute stage, and the jet of regurgitated blood may damage the endocardium lining the posterior wall of the left atrium, which is already the seat of severe rheumatic inflammation. This area, 1–2 cm above the mitral ring, is called *MacCallum's patch*, and is a common site of thrombus formation.[32] It is particularly liable to be implicated in subacute infective endocarditis.

The vegetations are eventually organised (Fig. 36.4), and the valve may be rendered stenotic or incompetent.

Non-bacterial thrombotic endocarditis.[33, 34] Small warty or friable vegetations along the line of closure of the mitral or aortic valves are not uncommon as a *post-mortem* finding. The vegetations are sterile, and the valves may be normal or deformed by disease, generally rheumatic. The condition is also termed *terminal, marantic,* or *cachectic* endocarditis, and has been described in association with cancer, particularly of the stomach, pancreas, and lung. It is probable that the vegetations are more common than is generally assumed, and are only regarded as terminal because they happen to be found at necropsy. Occasionally the vegetations become detached: cerebral embolism may result. Organisation can lead to the formation of a papillary tumour-like nodule called a *Lambl's excrescence.*[35, 36] The vegetations may form the site of infection for infective endocarditis.[34] Usually, however, the vegetations of non-bacterial thrombotic endocarditis are of no significance and are removed, probably by lysis.

Subacute infective (bacterial) endocarditis (and endarteritis). The adjective "subacute", hallowed by tradition, is meaningless; the course of the disease is chronic. It is much more helpful to describe the condition in terms of the causative organism than its course.[37] The usual organism is *Strept. viridans,* but sometimes other bacteria, e.g. *Staph. albus, Strept. faecalis,* anaerobic streptococci, *H. influenzae,* and coliform organisms, are responsible. The organism involved is one of relatively low virulence. The adjective infective is more appropriate than bacterial, since fungous cases are now recognised, and a special rickettsial endocarditis may occur in Q-fever and also in psittacosis.[38]

The disease occurs typically on vascular endothelium which has been previously abnormal, usually as the result of rheumatic fever. Sometimes a congenital lesion, e.g. a bicuspid aortic valve, coarctation of the aorta, or patent ductus arteriosus, is the seat of trouble, indicating that the condition need not always be an endocarditis. The disease is being encountered more frequently in the elderly than it was previously, and usually there is no obvious preceding valvular disease to account for its localisation.[39, 40] Perhaps minor degenerative lesions are present in the affected valve.

The organisms reach the heart by the blood stream. *Strept. viridans* is a commensal organism in the mouth. A transient bacteraemia is frequent after dental extraction, and it is possible that it occurs after vigorous mastication in those who have infective oral disease. However, *Strept. viridans* endocarditis has been reported on a number of occasions in edentulous people as well as in those without dental disease, and it seems probable that in these cases the source of the organism has been the nose, throat, or gastrointestinal tract. It is not understood why the other members of the copious bacterial flora of these areas do not colonise the heart valves.[41, 42]

At any rate, this bacteraemia is of no consequence in a healthy person, but in a patient with organic valvular disease there is a distinct danger of the organism colonising the valve and setting up endocarditis. The mechanism whereby this happens is not known, but the coincidental presence of non-bacterial thrombotic endocarditis is a possibility.[34] As a prophylactic measure any patient known to have a valvular lesion should be given antibiotic cover before being subjected to dental extraction or other manipulation of a potentially infected area, e.g. the urinary tract. It should be given immediately before the operation—if given too early, there will be a chance of more resistant organisms replacing those eliminated.[43] A recurrence of the endocarditis can occur in edentulous patients, and the wholesale extraction of sound teeth is not recommended for the prophylaxis of this disease.[44, 45]

Valve lesions. The vegetations are much larger and redder than those of acute rheumatic fever. They are friable and are liable to break off and embolise. Histologically they consist of thrombus containing numerous bacterial colonies which are well protected from the blood stream. The vegetations are attached to the valve by means of granulation tissue, but this is neither profuse nor does it penetrate far into the vegetation. The organisms are once more beyond the reach of the blood. The poor vascularity of the valve cusps is the explanation of this inadequate organisation. It is a good example of frustrated repair, and as such is typical chronic inflammation. The vegetations spread on to the mural endocardium, and are often found on MacCallum's patch.

Features of the condition. The disease pursues a chronic course in which a persistent low-grade pyrexia is typical. Multiple embolic phenomena are characteristic. Large emboli may cause infarction of the brain, intestine, kidney, or spleen; smaller ones are presumed to be responsible for the splinter haemorrhages of the nails, the Osler nodes, and the haematuria. *It is important to note that the emboli behave as if they were sterile.* The organisms which they contain are exposed to the bactericidal action of the blood when once they break off from the valves. It is known that the patient's blood contains a high content of antibodies against the causative organisms. As a result of the bacteraemia there is considerable reticuloendothelial hyperplasia which is reflected in the splenomegaly usually present.

One of the curious features of this disease is that organisms of relatively low virulence are able to survive in the presence of a high degree of immunity. Their inaccessibility in the thrombus appears to be the explanation.

Final diagnosis is dependent upon a positive blood culture. Frequent episodes of bacteraemia occur, but the organism is often difficult to isolate, and grows slowly (see Appendix II).

Prior to the days of antibiotics the disease was invariably fatal. With modern treatment cure is possible, but the healed valves are often grossly distorted and show calcification. The usual cause of death is heart failure[46] due not only to progressive valvular destruction, but also to a concomitant myocarditis. Other modes of death are embolism causing

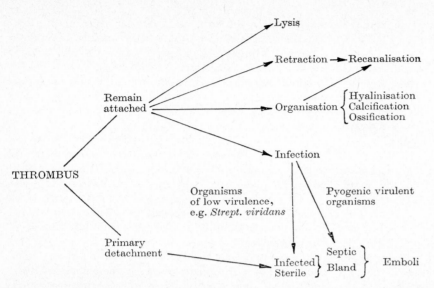

Figure 36.5

THROMBUS
- Remain attached
  - Lysis
  - Retraction → Recanalisation
  - Organisation → Recanalisation
    - Organisation {Hyalinisation, Calcification, Ossification}
  - Infection
    - Organisms of low virulence, e.g. *Strept. viridans*
    - Pyogenic virulent organisms
- Primary detachment
  - Infected / Sterile
  - Septic / Bland } Emboli

infarction of vital organs, and uraemia due to progressive glomerulonephritis in which there is a characteristic focal necrosis of the glomerular tufts. This "flea-bitten" kidney is believed to be of immune-complex origin.[47]

Acute bacterial endocarditis. In this variety of bacterial endocarditis the organism is virulent, and it usually colonises the valve during a septicaemia.

The vegetations are large and friable, and embolism is invariable. Often the disease is masked by the accompanying septicaemia and is discovered *post mortem*. The infected emboli become impacted in arteries where they lead to acute arteritis with weakening of the wall and the formation of mycotic aneurysms. Rupture may follow. The organs show septic infarcts and pyaemic abscesses. There is great destruction of the affected valve which may undergo rapid perforation. Thus the diagnosis may be suggested by changing heart murmurs in a desperately ill patient.

Chronic verrucous endocarditis. This is the Libman-Sacks lesion of systemic lupus erythematosus (see Chapter 16).

Thrombi in the Coronary Arteries

These almost invariably occur on the basis of pre-existing atheromatous plaques, although rarely other arterial diseases, like polyarteritis nodosa, are responsible. Ischaemic heart disease is less common in women before the menopause than amongst men of comparable age—an effect generally attributed to the protective action of oestrogens.[48]

FATE OF THROMBI

Figure 36.5 summarises the possible fate of thrombi.

(*a*) Some thrombi undoubtedly undergo lysis and leave no trace of their previous existence; plasmin may be of importance in this process, and it is of interest that there is a fibrinolytic enzyme, an activator of plasminogen, in the

intima of large veins. With venous stasis there is an increase in blood fibrinolytic activity, probably because of a release of this enzyme. In the superficial veins the fibrinolytic

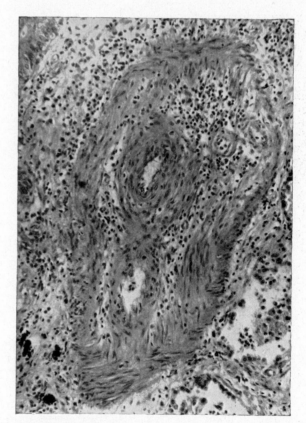

Figure 36.6
Recanalisation of a small thrombosed artery. Note the muscular arteriole in the centre of the old vessel. The diffuse cellular infiltration is due to surrounding infection. The section was taken from a bronchiectatic lung. × 130.

activity is confined to the vasa vasorum, and it is higher in the arms than in the legs both in normal subjects and in those with venous thrombosis.[49–51]

(*b*) If an occluding thrombus in an artery or vein contains much clot, it may retract sufficiently for blood to pass by, forming a new channel. Endothelium quickly lines the passage; this is one way in which recanalisation can occur.

(*c*) In arteries the thrombus may become converted into an atheromatous plaque (see incrustation theory of atheroma, p. 467).

(*d*) A thrombus which is not removed becomes organised. In veins the granulation tissue invades it from the mural aspect, and endothelium grows over the thrombus from the adjacent uncovered intima.

It has been suggested that arterial thrombi are not vascularised from the vasa vasorum, as these extend only as far as the tunica media and do not penetrate the internal elastic lamina. Instead there may be retraction of the clot with the formation of channels, which become lined by endothelium derived either from the adjacent vessel wall or else deposited from the circulation, in which endothelial cells may normally be present. Whatever their origin, these endothelial cells also contribute to the vascularisation of the thrombus. The granulation tissue is at first vascular, but later becomes dense and avascular. The blood vessels link up longitudinally, and by opening on to the luminal surface constitute another method of recanalisation (Fig. 36.6).[52] There is no significant circulation of blood through these newly-formed channels.

(*e*) The fibrosed thrombus may undergo hyalinisation and calcification. This occurs in the pelvic veins, where the calcified thrombi are known as *phleboliths*. They may be seen during radiological examinations of the pelvic area.

(*f*) Thrombi may become detached to form emboli. This depends on their anchorage, which is poor in phlebothrombosis and atrial thrombosis. The emboli produced are *bland*, or *non-infective*.

Embolisation may also follow invasion of a thrombus by bacteria. These are usually pyogenic, the emboli are *septic*, and the condition is one of pyaemia. If the organisms are of low virulence, the emboli are "bland" in behaviour (as in *Strept. viridans* endocarditis).

GENERAL READING

HUDSON, R. E. B. (1965). *Cardiovascular Pathology*, 3 vols. London: Arnold.

REFERENCES

1. SHUCKSMITH, H. S. (1963). *British Medical Journal*, ii, 835.
2. Annotation (1963). *Lancet*, ii, 1263.
3. Leading Article (1969). *British Medical Journal*, i, 460.
4. McKUSICK, V. A. *et al.* (1962). *Journal of the American Medical Association*, **181**, 5.
5. McPHERSON, J. R., JUERGENS, J. L. and GIFFORD, R. W. (1963). *Annals of Internal Medicine*, **59**, 288.
6. SZILAGYI, D. E., DeRUSSO, F. J. and ELLIOTT, J. P. (1964). *Archives of Surgery*, **88**, 824.
7. HORTON, B. T., MAGATH, T. B. & BROWN, G. E. (1934). *Archives of Internal Medicine*, **53**, 400.
8. RUSSELL, R. W. R. (1959). *Quarterly Journal of Medicine*, **28**, 471.
9. ALLEN, E. V., BARKER, N. W. and HINES, E. A. (1962). *Peripheral Vascular Diseases*, 3rd edn, p. 293. Philadelphia: Saunders.
10. Leading Article (1965). *British Medical Journal*, ii, 603.
11. TRUMMER, M. J. and MANNIX, E. P. (1963). *Journal of Thoracic and Cardiovascular Surgery*, **45**, 198.
12. SCHWARTZ, C. J. and MITCHELL, J. R. A. (1962). *Postgraduate Medical Journal*, **38**, 25.
13. ANITSCHKOW, N. and CHALATOW, S. (1913). *Zentralblatt für allgemaine Pathologie und pathologische Anatomie*, **24**, 1.
14. FRENCH, J. E. (1970). In *General Pathology*, 4th edn, p. 573. Edited by H. W. Florey. London: Lloyd-Luke.
15. GRESHAM, G. A. and HOWARD, A. N. (1962). *Archives of Pathology*, **74**, 1.
16. FINLAYSON, R., SYMONS, C. and T-W-FIENNES, R. N. (1962). *British Medical Journal*, i, 501.
17. Leading Article (1967). *Lancet*, ii, 1239.
18. ADAMS, C. W. M. *et al.* (1963). *Journal of Pathology and Bacteriology*, **86**, 431.
19. DUGUID, J. B. (1946). *Journal of Pathology and Bacteriology*, **58**, 207.
20. DUGUID, J. B. (1948). *Journal of Pathology and Bacteriology*, **60**, 57.
21. DIBLE, J. H. (1958). *Lancet*, i, 1031.
22. PICKERING, G. (1964). *British Medical Journal*, i, 517.
23. CRAWFORD, T. and LEVENE, C. I. (1952). *Journal of Pathology and Bacteriology*, **64**, 523.
24. CRAWFORD, T. (1967). In *Modern Trends in Pathology*, 2, p. 238. Edited by T. Crawford. London: Butterworths.
25. FULLERTON, H. W., DAVIE, W. J. A. and ANASTASOPOULOS, G. (1953). *British Medical Journal*, ii, 250.
26. POOLE, J. C. F. (1958). *Britsh Medical Bulletin*, **14**, 253.
27. HOWELL, M. (1964). *British Medical Bulletin*, **20**, 200.
28. GEIRINGER, E. (1951). *Journal of Pathology and Bacteriology*, **66**, 201.
29. DUGUID, J. B. and ROBERTSON, W. B. (1955). *Lancet*, i, 525.
30. DUGUID, J. B. and ROBERTSON, W. B. (1957). *Lancet*, i, 1205.
31. HIRST, A. E., JOHNS, V. J. and KIME, S. W. (1958). *Medicine (Baltimore)*, **37**, 217.
32. MacCALLUM, W. G. (1924). *Bulletin of the Johns Hopkins Hospital*, **35**, 329.
33. MacDONALD, R. A. and ROBBINS, S. L. (1957). *Annals of Internal Medicine*, **46**, 255.
34. Leading Article (1967). *British Medical Journal*, iii, 812.

35. MAGAREY, F. R. (1949). *Journal of Pathology and Bacteriology*, **61**, 203.
36. POMERANCE, A. (1961). *Journal of Pathology and Bacteriology*, **81**, 135.
37. VOGLER, W. R., DORNEY, E. R. and BRIDGES, H. A. (1962). *American Journal of Medicine*, **32**, 910.
38. LEVISON, D. A. *et al.* (1971). *Lancet*, ii, 844.
39. WALLACH, J. B. *et al.* (1955). *Annals of Internal Medicine*, **42**, 1206.
40. ANDERSON, H. J. and STAFFURTH, J. S. (1955). *Lancet*, ii, 1055.
41. Leading Article (1971). *Lancet*, ii, 589.
42. HILSON, G. R. F. (1970). *Proceedings of the Royal Society of Medicine*, **63**, 267.
43. GARROD, L. P. and WATERWORTH, P. M. (1962). *British Heart Journal*, **24**, 39.
44. CROXSON, M. S., ALTMAN, M. M. and O'BRIEN, K. P. (1971). *Lancet*, i, 1205.
45. SIMON, D. S. and GOODWIN, J. F. (1971). *Lancet*, i, 1207.
46. ROBINSON, M. J. and RUEDY, J. (1962). *American Journal of Medicine*, **32**, 922.
47. GUTMAN, R. A. *et al.* (1972). *Medicine (Baltimore)*, **51**, 1.
48. Annotation (1963). *British Medical Journal*, ii, 1487.
49. ASTRUP, T. (1966). *Federation Proceedings*, **25**, 42.
50. FEARNLEY, G. R. (1965). *Fibrinolysis*, p. 56. London: Arnold.
51. PANDOLFI, M. *et al.* (1967). *Lancet*, ii, 127.
52. DIBLE, J. H. (1958). *Journal of Pathology and Bacteriology*, **75**, 1.

Chapter 37. Embolism

An *embolus* is an abnormal mass of undissolved material which is transported from one part of the circulation to another. The most satisfactory classification is based upon its composition.

Types. Five categories may be recognised.

1. THROMBI AND CLOT. This may be bland or infected ("septic").
2. GAS: Air and nitrogen.
3. FAT.
4. TUMOUR.
5. MISCELLANEOUS.

1. Emboli Composed of Thrombus or Clot

Pulmonary embolism. Thrombi most frequently become detached in the veins, and are then carried to the pulmonary circulation. The effects are largely related to the size of the embolus: the long, loosely-attached, propagated clot of phlebothrombosis frequently becomes detached and produces the syndrome of *massive pulmonary embolism*.[1,2]

In this condition a clot 20–45 cm. long is detached from the femoral or popliteal vein, and is carried to the heart where it reaches the right ventricle. There is often sudden death, and the embolus may then be found coiled in the right ventricle with part of its length projecting into the main pulmonary artery. The embolus may be found straddled across the bifurcation of the pulmonary trunk, or forced into one of its two branches. It is important to distinguish between such an embolus and an *agonal thrombus* or *post-mortem clot*. In the latter conditions the clot is moist, shiny, and gelatinous. It is loosely inserted into the pulmonary trunk, and its shape conforms to that of the situation where it is found. The clot may extend into the pulmonary vessels, and on withdrawal a cast of the pulmonary tree is obtained. Massive embolic clot, on the other hand, is dry, friable, and granular, as it has already retracted in the leg veins; ripples of platelets may be visible on its surface. The shape of the embolus does not conform to that of its surroundings, and it is so tightly inserted into the pulmonary tree that removal is difficult. The coiled mass is usually bound together by recent thrombus (Fig. 37.1).

The *cause of death* in massive pulmonary embolism is obvious enough when the main trunk is obstructed. Not infrequently, however, only one of its branches is blocked, and death under these circumstances is more difficult to explain, because it is known that a pulmonary artery can be occluded suddenly without apparent untoward effects, e.g. during pneumonectomy. Some form of reflex "shock" or pulmonary vasoconstriction has been suggested, but never substantiated. The symptoms (dyspnoea, substernal pain, and cough) may be due to underventilation of the under-perfused lung (see also p. 485).

Experimentally, death from pulmonary embolism occurs only when there is *extensive mechanical obstruction*, caused

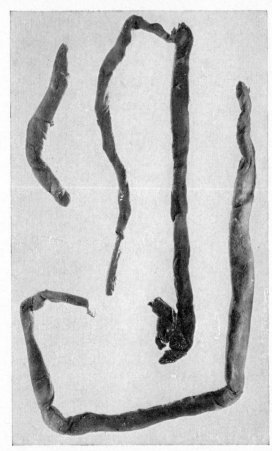

Figure 37.1
Massive pulmonary embolism. These thrombi were removed as one large coiled mass from the pulmonary arteries of a man who died a week after operation. There was extensive phlebothrombosis in both calves. It is apparent that the calibre of the unfolded thrombi corresponds with the lumina of the leg veins. (C 40.5, *Reproduced by permission of the President and Council of the R.C.S. Eng.*)

either by the emboli themselves or by superadded thrombosis. It is possible that in man the final lethal embolus may merely be one of many which have produced increasing arterial obstruction. Even in a patient who has died from a massive embolus, smaller pieces of clot may be found in branches of the pulmonary tree.

An alternative to this theory of mechanical blockage is the suggestion that the embolus, or associated thrombus, liberates 5-hydroxytryptamine, which causes *spasm* of the remainder of the pulmonary tree.[3, 4] It must be admitted that the cause of death in many cases of this important condition is not understood.

It should be noted that pulmonary embolism does not always produce the clinical picture regarded as characteristic of the condition. Emboli, frequently unsuspected during life, were found in one series of cases in about 25 per cent of elderly folk dying of various causes.[5] Such "quiet" pulmonary embolism is easily mistaken for bronchopneumonia, heart failure, etc., especially in elderly, obese, bedridden patients in whom clinical and x-ray examination is difficult.

Smaller pulmonary emboli[6] also arise from the calf veins and the right atrial appendage, and these may lead to pulmonary infarction, as is described in the next chapter. Recurrent episodes of minor pulmonary embolism may so damage the lungs as to lead to progressive pulmonary hypertension.[7, 8] Persistent hypertension is rare after a single episode of pulmonary embolism.[9]

Small septic pulmonary emboli may arise in the course of suppurative thrombophlebitis.

There is a tradition that in severe pulmonary hypertension emboli in the right side of the heart may traverse a patent foramen ovale to enter the systemic circulation. Such an event is called "paradoxical embolism". It is extremely rare, though apparently a few authentic cases have been reported.[10, 11] Usually, however, the thrombosis has in fact occurred either in the left atrium or else in the pulmonary veins. It is possible that pulmonary embolism may cause sufficient stasis in the pulmonary veins to produce thrombosis. Detachment of these thrombi would result in systemic embolism. Since pulmonary embolism also produces pulmonary hypertension, the conditions are ideal for the syndrome of "paradoxical embolism".

Fate of pulmonary emboli.[9] In those who survive, the thrombus is either lysed or organised. Bands or webs may be the only residua of previous occlusive emboli, and as with thrombi in systemic arteries, their organisation and incorporation into the vessel wall can produce plaques of atheroma.

Systemic embolism. Emboli arising in the heart are generally systemic. They may arise in the left atrium, e.g. in mitral stenosis, on the mitral or aortic valves, e.g. in infective endocarditis, or in the left ventricle, e.g. following infarction. The possibility of pulmonary-vein thrombosis has already been mentioned.

Emboli arise from the larger arteries from time to time.

The importance of thrombotic embolism from atheromatous plaques is described later in this chapter. More occasionally, atheromatous material from the aorta and its major branches becomes detached and embolises distally. The kidney, pancreas, intestine, spleen, heart, brain, and limbs are all sites where this has been described.[12, 13]

Effects of systemic emboli. The effects of impaction of any embolus are those of obstruction. It may be broken up by the pounding of the arterial pressure, and in this way move on to more distant branches; thrombosis or clotting beyond the block usually occurs.

In the peripheral vasculature severe local pain may occur, and is generally attributed to spasm of the vessel wall. Pain, however, is not a feature of embolisation in internal organs, e.g. kidney and brain. The effects of ischaemia on various tissues are considered in Chapter 38.

Bland emboli produce no other effects, whereas *septic emboli* set up secondary foci of suppuration. According to local anatomical circumstances, pyaemic abscesses, septic infarcts, or mycotic aneurysms are produced.

2. Gaseous Emboli

Air.[14] Air may be introduced into a systemic vein under the following conditions:

Operations on the head and neck. The accidental opening of a large vein, like the jugular, may allow air to be sucked in.

A mismanaged blood transfusion. This is likely to be of serious consequence only when positive pressure is being employed with old-fashioned equipment.

During haemodialysis for renal failure.[15]

Insufflation of the fallopian tubes.

Interference with the placental site during criminal abortion.

During the procedure of artificial pneumoperitoneum.

The air enters the right side of the heart, and is churned up into a froth. During systole the heart merely compresses this froth, but scarcely any blood actually enters the pulmonary artery. The effects are therefore very similar to massive pulmonary embolism. The characteristic churning noise, which may be heard without the aid of a stethoscope, serves to distinguish the two conditions clinically. It will be readily appreciated that in order to produce this effect, large quantities of air must be introduced suddenly. In dogs about 9 ml per kg is regarded as a lethal amount.[16] In man it is probably considerably less (see p. 634). Small quantities are unimportant, because they pass through the heart and become impacted in a branch of the pulmonary artery. Air, however, is readily absorbed, and the effects of the block are not usually long-lasting enough to be serious.

Air may be introduced into a pulmonary vein during the induction of a pneumothorax. This may block the ostium of a vital coronary or cerebral artery, so that only a few ml are necessary to cause serious, even fatal, effects.[16, 17] This is one of the causes of the clinician's "pleural shock". Air may also reach the systemic circulation from the venous side in the air embolism that complicates haemodialysis.[15]

Nitrogen. The important example is *decompression sickness*, also called *caisson disease*.[18] This occurs in people who have been exposed to a high pressure, e.g. divers, tunnellers, and those encased in a caisson (diving-bell), and then return to a normal atmospheric pressure too rapidly, or in those exposed to a low pressure after having been at a normal atmospheric pressure, e.g. airmen. As the pressure is reduced, bubbles of air come out of solution from the blood and interstitial fluid; whereas oxygen and CO_2 are readily absorbed and removed, the inert nitrogen remains in the tissues for some time and causes damage. As it is fairly soluble in fat, much is present in the subcutaneous tissues and the central nervous system. When it comes out of solution, it leads to tissue disruption, particularly in areas of poor blood supply where absorption is delayed. This effect is most important in the lower dorsal region of the spinal cord and the peripheral nerves. Considerable damage may be done, causing severe pain (the "bends") and sometimes permanent paraplegia or death. Damage is marked around the ends of long bones; aseptic necrosis occurs, and this leads to severe osteo-arthritis.

Several cases of decompression sickness have been reported in which there were large air cysts in the lungs. It has been suggested that these cysts discharge bubbles of air into the pulmonary veins during decompression, and so aggravate the condition.[19] Caisson disease can be averted by slow decompression or by using a helium and oxygen mixture instead of air.

In fact, the pathogenesis of decompression sickness is by no means clear. In a recent review of the subatmospheric variety of decompression sickness,[41] gaseous emboli were not found with certainty in the tissues in fatal cases. The noteworthy feature of fatal cases was severe shock, and at necropsy there were effusions into the serous cavities, pulmonary oedema, and fatty change of the liver. Fat emboli were found in small numbers in the lungs in many cases; they were less common in the systemic vascular beds—it is possible that they arose from the liver, but in any case they were too sparse to have contributed significantly to death. Evidence of cerebral ischaemia varied and was frequently absent, while spinal-cord involvement was exceptional.

3. Fat Emboli[20]

Globules of fat may enter small veins after a fracture, and in the case of multiple injuries this embolisation may be quite extensive. Actual fragments of bone marrow may be found in the pulmonary arterioles. This is commonly seen in patients who have sustained multiple fractures of the ribs as a result of vigorous external cardiac massage. A similar event has been reported in sickle-cell disease as a rare complication of the patchy infarction of the bone marrow which is seen quite often in this condition (Fig. 37.2).[21] The clinical features vary according to whether or not the emboli pass through the lung barrier. Cerebral fat and silicone

emboli are commonly found in patients who have recently undergone unsuccessful cardio-bypass operations.

Pulmonary fat embolism. The presence of fat globules in the capillaries of the lung is a frequent *post-mortem* finding in fracture patients, but the tremendous vascular bed of the lung is not likely to be appreciably obstructed by these small droplets of fat. Occasionally, however, pulmonary fat

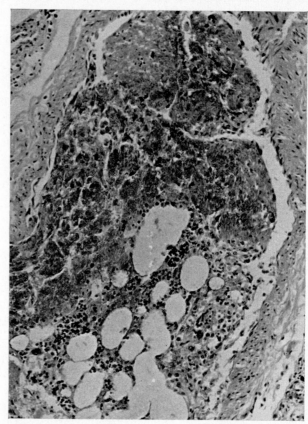

Figure 37.2
Bone-marrow embolism. This small pulmonary artery contains a fragment of fatty bone marrow. Around the fat spaces haemato-poietic tissue is recognisable. The remainder of the lumen is occluded by blood clot. The patient was a Jamaican Negress who had sickle-cell disease. She died suddenly in a state simulating massive pulmonary embolism, and at necropsy many of the pulmonary arterioles were found to contain fat and bone-marrow emboli. The latter occluded so much of the pulmonary vascular bed that death ensued. There were no systemic emboli, such as are encountered in post-traumatic fat embolism. × 130.

embolism may be extensive enough to be the immediate cause of death.[42] In the investigation of accidents like air crashes the presence of fat emboli provides evidence of survival after the injury.

Systemic fat embolism. Sometimes the emboli pass through the pulmonary bed, and become lodged in the capillaries of the brain, kidney, skin, and other organs.

In severe cases the patient becomes comatose within a few

hours of injury, and dies within 1–2 days. More usually symptoms occur 24–48 hours after injury: these include fever, restlessness, respiratory distress, and cerebral symptoms. If the brain damage is severe, coma results and death follows. A petechial skin eruption is helpful diagnostically, but is not usually manifest until the second or third day.[22] There may be subconjunctival and retinal haemorrhages also.

The important effect of systemic fat embolism is cerebral damage; this dominates the clinical picture, and is the cause of death. It is blamed also for the respiratory symptoms,[23] which may be severe and associated with multiple areas of pulmonary haemorrhage and oedema. At necropsy the brain shows striking changes: numerous petechial haemorrhages are present in the white matter (the grey matter is also severely affected by the fat emboli, but perhaps because of better anastomosis does not show many petechiae).[24] Fat emboli are found in the glomeruli and in the skin petechiae. Pulmonary involvement is always marked.

During life fat may be found in the sputum, but its presence only indicates pulmonary involvement. Examination of the urine may reveal fat, but the test is unreliable. Renal involvement has also been detected by needle biopsy.

The mechanism of fat embolism is imperfectly understood. While there can be little doubt that mechanical entry of fatty tissue into the veins is of great importance, it sometimes seems inadequate to explain the extent of the lesion in comparison with the mildness of the trauma. It has been suggested that there is also an alteration in the emulsion stability of the circulating blood lipids, so that the chylomicrons aggregate and form composite globules of fat emboli.[25, 26] This theory, which has some experimental substantiation,[27] would explain the increase in size of the globules after passing through the lungs prior to being trapped in the systemic capillaries. It has been suggested that the effects of fat embolism are due not so much to ischaemia as to the toxic action on the vascular endothelium of the fatty acids which are derived from the broken-down fat.[25] Such a mechanism would explain the delay in onset of symptoms.

Soft tissue injuries unassociated with fractures are said to cause fat embolism occasionally, but it may be that a fracture was missed in these cases. If, however, a fatty liver is injured, fat embolism may certainly ensue;[23] indeed, it has occurred spontaneously in cases of fatty liver.[28–30]

4. Tumour Emboli

It is probable that all malignant tumours invade the local blood vessels at an early stage of the disease, and that isolated malignant cells are of frequent occurrence in the circulation. The tumour cells are covered by thrombus, and the majority of these emboli are destroyed, leaving only a small percentage to develop into metastatic deposits. Multiple small tumour emboli, by leading to fibrin deposition, may initiate a consumptive coagulopathy (see p. 623).

Some tumours, notably hypernephroma and carcinoma of the lung, tend to invade larger blood vessels, and occasionally a mass of tumour becomes detached to produce a large embolus (see p. 370).

5. Miscellaneous Emboli

Foreign bodies. Bullets,[31] silk, talc, etc., are all reported to have been carried from one part of the body to another by the blood stream. Drug addicts who inject themselves intravenously with impure material containing talc can develop extensive non-caseating granulomata in the lungs.

Polythene tubing may embolise during intravenous therapy and cardiac catheterisation.[32, 33] There is a great danger of it acting as a nidus for infection and thrombosis.

Parasites. Various parasites and their ova are carried by the blood stream. Schistosomes and their ova may lodge in the branches of the portal vein in the liver, and induce a fibrosis of "pipe-stem" type (Fig. 37.3). They may pass on to the lung and produce an inflammatory reaction around the

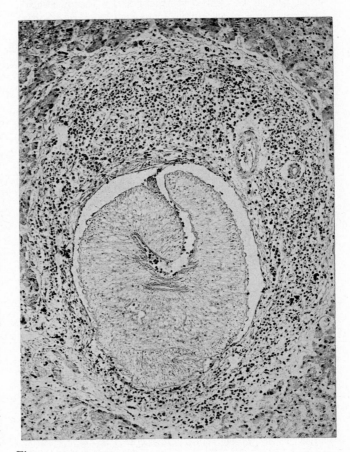

Figure 37 3
Parasitic embolus. This is a cross-section of a portal vein in which there is the parasitic trematode *Schistosoma haematobium*. Surrounding the vein there is a wide zone of small round cells, and at the periphery liver tissue is recognisable. The perivascular infiltration is the precursor of the later "pipe-stem" fibrosis. × 110.

pulmonary arterioles, which may lead to pulmonary hypertension.[34, 35]

Red-cell aggregates. Blockage of small vessels by aggregates of red cells is commonly seen in infections and following trauma. The condition is generally called *sludging*, and is considered in detail on pp. 427–428.

Red-cell aggregations also occur in the exposed limbs when cold autohaemagglutinins are present. This is the cause of the Raynaud-like phenomenon seen in patients with acquired haemolytic anaemia of the cold antibody type.

Microemboli.[36] White bodies can sometimes be seen in the retinal vessels, and by plugging them produce microinfarcts. Some of these bodies appear to consist of atheromatous material probably derived from plaques in the carotid arteries. Others are platelet aggregates or fibrin derived perhaps from the heart in cases of rheumatic heart disease. During open-heart surgery emboli may consist of calcium (from calcified valves), silicone, or fat.[37] The role of these emboli in disease is conjectural. In the *eye* they have been blamed for transient attacks of unilateral blindness (amaurosis fugax), but it appears more likely that the sudden onset of blindness is due to a reduced perfusion and flow in the retinal vessels from other causes and that platelet aggregation is a secondary phenomenon.[38] Platelet emboli have also been blamed for *transient strokes*,[39] and progressive obliteration of the microcirculation of the lower limbs is probably an important contibutory factor in the pathogenesis of peripheral vascular disease. It is difficult to prove this because examination of the vasculature of the legs is tedious and time consuming. However, it is quite common to find small arterioles in the kidney obstructed by atheromatous material. Often there is a foreign-body, giant-cell reaction to this cholesterol containing material, and since the vessels are small it is reasonable to assume that the atheromatous material is embolic, for atheroma does not affect such small vessels.

Amniotic fluid.[40] Amniotic fluid containing meconium and squamous cells may enter the uterine veins and travel to the lungs. The condition usually occurs during labour and concealed accidental haemorrhage, and is characterised by shock and a generalised bleeding tendency. The plasmin system is activated, and since this enzyme digests fibrinogen as well as fibrin, acute afibrinogenaemia occurs. It is possible that the symptoms are due to a type of anaphylactic shock rather than a direct effect of the amniotic emboli themselves.

REFERENCES

1. BAUER, G. (1946). *Lancet*, i, 447.
2. BYRNE, J. J. (1955). *New England Journal of Medicine*, **253**, 579.
3. SMITH, G. and SMITH, A. N. (1955). *Surgery, Gynecology and Obstetrics*, **101**, 691.
4. THOMAS, D. P. *et al.* (1965). In *Pulmonary Embolic Disease*, p. 59. Edited by A. A. Sasahara and M. Stein. New York: Grune and Stratton.
5. TOWBIN, A. (1954). *Journal of the American Medical Association*, **156**, 209.
6. Annotation (1964). *Lancet*, i, 91.
7. GOODWIN, J. F., HARRISON, C. V. and WILCKEN, D. E. L. (1963). *British Medical Journal*, i, 701 and 777.
8. FLEISCHNER, F. G. (1967). *New England Journal of Medicine*, **276**, 1213.
9. Annotation (1967). *Lancet*, ii, 1291.
10. JOHNSON, B. I. (1951). *Journal of Clinical Pathology*, **4**, 316.
11. HORLICK, L. (1961). *Canadian Medical Association Journal*, **85**, 889.
12. GORE, I. and COLLINS, D. P. (1960). *American Journal of Clinical Pathology*, **33**, 416.
13. KAPLAN, K., MILLAR, J. D. and CANCILLA, P. A. (1962). *Archives of Internal Medicine*, **110**, 218.
14. Annotation (1963). *Lancet*, i, 96.
15. WARD, M. K. *et al.* (1971). *British Medical Journal*, iii, 74.
16. KENT, E. M. and BLADES, B. (1942). *Journal of Thoracic Surgery*, **11**, 434.
17. VAN ALLEN, C. M., HRDINA, L. S. and CLARK, J. (1929). *Archives of Surgery*, **19**, 567.
18. DEWEY, A. W. (1962). *New England Journal of Medicine*, **267**, 759 and 812.
19. COLLINS, J. J. (1962). *New England Journal of Medicine*, **266**, 595.
20. LOVE J. and STRYKER, W. S. (1957). *Annals of Internal Medicine*, **46**, 342.
21. SHELLEY, W. M. and CURTIS, E. M. (1958). *Bulletin of the Johns Hopkins Hospital*, **103**, 8.
22. STEPHENS, J. H. and FRED, H. L. (1962). *Archives of Dermatology*, **86**, 515.
23. SEVITT, S. (1962). *Fat Embolism*, pp. 181 and 29. London: Butterworths.
24. SEVITT, S. (1972). *Lancet*, i, 848.
25. NEWMAN, P. H. (1962). *Journal of Bone and Joint Surgery*, **44B**, 761.
26. EVARTS, C. M. (1965). *Journal of the American Medical Association*, **194**, 899.
27. ADKINS, R. B. and FOSTER, J. H. (1962). *Annals of Surgery*, **156**, 515.
28. HARTROFT, W. S. and RIDOUT, J. H. (1951). *American Journal of Pathology*, **27**, 951.
29. KENT, S. P. (1955). *American Journal of Pathology*, **31**, 399.
30. LYNCH, M. J. G., RAPHAEL, S. S. and DIXON, T. P. (1959). *Archives of Pathology*, **67**, 68.
31. KINMONTH, J. B. *et al.* (1961). *British Medical Journal*, ii, 1666.
32. UDWADIA, T. E. and EDWARDS, A. E. (1963). *British Medical Journal*, ii, 1251.
33. BENNETT, P. J. (1963). *British Medical Journal*, ii, 1252.
34. CORTES, F. M. and WINTERS, W. L. (1961). *American Journal of Medicine*, **31**, 808.
35. SPENCER, H. (1968). *Pathology of the Lung*, 2nd edn, p. 345. Oxford: Pergamon Press.

36. Leading Article (1970). *Lancet*, ii, 350.
37. WILLIAMS, I. M. (1971). *Lancet*, ii, 688.
38. Leading Article (1972). *British Medical Journal*, iii, 67.
39. Leading Article (1971). *British Medical Journal*, iii, 723.
40. AGUILLON, A. *et al.* (1962). *Obstetrical and Gynecological Survey*, **17**, 619.
41. FRYER, D. I. (1969). *Subatmospheric Decompression Sickness in Man*, 343 pp. Slough: Technovision Services.
42. Leading Article (1972). *Lancet*, i, 672.

Chapter 38. Ischaemia and Infarction

Ischaemia is defined as a condition of inadequate blood supply to an area of tissue. It produces harmful effects in three ways:

1. Hypoxia

Oxygen deprivation is by far the most important factor producing damage in ischaemic tissue. It is especially so when considering the effect on very active cells, e.g. muscle. On the other hand, it plays no part in the lesions produced by pulmonary arterial obstruction, because the alveolar walls derive their oxygen supply directly from the air.

2. Malnutrition

This is probably of little importance, because the blood contains much more glucose and amino acids than could be metabolised by the amount of oxygen which it contains.[1]

3. Failure to Remove Waste Products

The accumulation of metabolites is the most probable explanation of pain in muscle ischaemia. The presence of waste products or the failure to maintain important electrolyte (or other) balances is the probable cause of necrosis in pulmonary infarction.

Hypoxia is a state of impaired oxygenation. Four types are described:

Hypoxic, due to a low oxygen tension in the arterial blood, as in lung disease and cyanotic congenital heart disease with a right-to-left shunt.

Anaemic, due to a low level of haemoglobin, which carries the oxygen in the blood.

Stagnant or *ischaemic*, due to an inadequate blood supply to the tissues. This, as will be seen, is due either to heart failure or some local vascular obstruction.

Histotoxic, due to cellular intoxication, which prevents the uptake of oxygen, e.g. cyanide poisoning.

The subject of hypoxia is dealt with in standard physiology textbooks, and will not be considered further.

CAUSES OF ISCHAEMIA

General

Ischaemia may be caused by an inadequate cardiac output; not all tissues are equally affected because of the redistribution of the available blood. Symmetrical gangrene of the extremities is an occasional manifestation of myocardial infarction (see p. 505).[2,3]

In the *Stokes-Adams syndrome* of complete heart block, and during ventricular arrest or fibrillation the blood supply to the whole body is stopped. The manifestations are confined to a single organ, the brain, which is particularly sensitive to hypoxia. If the arrest continues for 15 seconds consciousness is lost, and if the condition lasts more than about 4 minutes irreparable damage is done.[4] The neurones degenerate and replacement gliosis occurs, which is exactly similar to that produced by the acute hypoxic hypoxia that may occur as the result of a poorly administered anaesthetic. If cardiac arrest lasts for more than 8 minutes death is inevitable.

Local Causes of Ischaemia

By far the most important cause of ischaemia is obstruction to the arterial flow. It should not, however, be forgotten that extensive venous and capillary damage can also produce ischaemia.

Arterial obstruction. Most of the causes of obstruction have already been described in Chapter 36. They will therefore only be summarised:

Thrombosis.

Embolism. The effects of the embolus are potentiated by the reflex spasm of the arterial wall, and completed by the rapid development of thrombus over the embolus.

Spasm. This includes not only local spastic conditions, but also states of generalised vasoconstriction that follow haemorrhage and dehydration.

Atheroma produces partial obstruction in medium-sized vessels, e.g. cerebral, coronary, and renal.

Occlusive pressure from without, e.g. tourniquets and tightly-fitting plasters.

Venous disease. Extensive venous obstruction leads to engorgement of the areas drained by the affected veins. This may reach such an intensity that blood flow is impeded and ischaemia results. There are many good examples of this:

Mesenteric venous thrombosis, leading to intestinal infarction.

Strangulation of a hernia. The venous obstruction at its neck leads to damage long before the arterial blood flow is implicated. The same applies to volvulus and intussusception (see p. 492).

Phlegmasia caerulea dolens. This is a rare variant of iliofemoral thrombosis, in which there is sudden intense venous engorgement followed by gangrene of the limb. It has been proved by subsequent dissection that the main arteries are not affected, but that there is almost complete venous obstruction by thrombosis.[5–7]

Cavernous-sinus thrombosis leads to retinal-vein thrombosis and retinal changes resulting in blindness.

Varicose veins of the leg. Venous stasis secondary to varicose veins of the leg leads to ischaemic changes of the skin (stasis dermatitis). Ultimately indolent ulcers develop, often being precipitated by local trauma.

Capillary damage. In considerations of vascular disease the capillaries are usually forgotten. There are nevertheless many conditions in which so many capillaries and small vessels in an area are occluded that ischaemia results. An additional effect is bleeding; haemorrhage is a common feature of capillary damage even when the extent of the vascular occlusion is not enough to lead to local ischaemia.

Frost-bite. The harmful effect of cold on exposed parts is due in large measure to damage to the small blood vessels. There is initial arteriolar spasm, and the ischaemia is aggravated by stasis of blood in the damaged capillaries. In the most severe cases extensive intracapillary blockage causes infarction of the area. Even if necrosis does not occur, the capillary damage leads to the development of large bullae when the circulation is restored after the part is warmed. Pain may be severe. Severe freezing injury promotes ice-crystal formation in the cells, and this causes further damage.[8–11]

Occlusion of capillaries by red cells, e.g. in sickle-cell disease, cerebral malaria, and conditions associated with severe autoagglutination, e.g. acquired haemolytic anaemia due to cold antibodies. Sludging of the blood may also cause capillary obstruction (p. 427).

Occlusion by fibrin. This occurs in the defibrination syndrome, see p. 623.

Occlusion by antigen-antibody interaction. In immune-complex reactions the vessel walls are damaged, and the accumulation of polymorphs and the depostion of thrombus occlude the small vessels. This is a feature of the Arthus reaction (p. 180), and is also the probable explanation of the petechial haemorrhages and renal lesions of subacute infective endocarditis.

Occlusion by precipitated cryoglobulins. (See p. 551.)

Occlusion of capillaries by white cells. Clumping of the abnormal white cells in chronic myeloid leukaemia may be responsible for the infarcts that occur in this condition, e.g. of spleen.

Fat embolism.

Decompression sickness.

External pressure, e.g. bedsores.

The Effects of Arterial and Capillary Obstruction

The effects depend largely upon the degree of ischaemia produced, and may range from sudden death to virtually no damage at all. The following are the possibilities:

1. There may be *no effects* on the tissue supplied by the vessel, if ischaemia is obviated by collateral channels.

2. There may be *functional disturbances*. The collaterals supply sufficient blood during inactivity, but cannot sustain normal exercise, e.g. angina pectoris and intermittent claudication. In sudden coronary arterial occlusion there may be ventricular fibrillation; this can follow quite small occlusions, and if death is averted by defibrillation, the resulting infarct may not be large.

3. There may be *cellular degeneration* affecting the parenchyma, e.g. cloudy swelling and fatty change which may terminate in necrosis. This is a patchy affair, and leads to atrophy. It is accompanied by *replacment fibrosis* or, in the central nervous system, *gliosis*. This is seen under a variety of conditions: sudden complete arterial obstruction of short duration, e.g. of brain, and partial arterial obstruction of gradual onset, e.g. atheroma affecting the cerebral vessels.

Pressure atrophy is an example of this type of lesion; it is due to gradual ischaemia at capillary level in which there is time for atrophy to occur. The affected cells not only become smaller, but also ultimately undergo necrosis. The connective tissue framework is left behind, e.g. in the capsule of a benign tumour, because it is more resistant to the effects of ischaemia. This is not replacement fibrosis, because the expanding lesion that has caused the pressure atrophy provides the extra tissue.

It is doubtful whether ischaemia of the heart ever leads to atrophy; if ischaemic myocardium is examined microscopically it is seen to consist of foci of avascular fibrous tissue, interspersed amongst which there are surviving muscle cells. These, on the whole, are hypertrophied, no doubt a compensatory phenomenon.

4. Both arterial and venous obstruction may lead to a circumscribed necrosis of tissue; this is called *infarction*, and will be described in detail later. Complete occlusion of the capillary bed either by frost-bite or pressure produces a similar result. The latter is well illustrated by the formation of bedsores.[12]

Factors Determining the Extent of Ischaemia in Arterial Obstruction

There are three crucial factors:

1. Speed of Onset

If the obstruction is sudden the effects are more severe than if it is gradual, because there is less time for an effective collateral circulation to develop.

2. The Extent of Obstruction

A complete obstruction is obviously much more serious than a partial one. This is well illustrated in the heart: partial coronary occlusion due to atheroma may be well tolerated, while complete obstruction usually causes infarction and sometimes death.

3. The Anatomy of the Collateral Circulation

Some arteries have no anastomotic channels. These are called *end arteries*; the central artery of the retina is a classical example, as are also the smaller vessels of the cerebral cortex. Others, like the larger cerebral vessels, the coronary arteries, the interlobular arteries of the kidney, and the splenic arteries, have so inadequate an anastomosis that, should they be blocked, some degree of infarction would be inevitable. They are indeed functional end arteries. The branches of the superior mesenteric artery have an extensive arcade of vessels emerging from them, but even here the anastomosis between each branch is poor. The inferior mesenteric artery is much more effectively arrayed with anastomotic branches, and infarction is less common in the distal colon than in the small intestine and proximal colon. The stomach has the benefit of three separate arterial supplies all derived from the coeliac axis, and it is not surprising that it is the least frequently infarcted part of the gastro-intestinal tract.

The lungs and liver are peculiar in having a double blood supply, and this modifies the effect of occlusion of one set of vessels to these organs.

Four other subsidiary factors modify the effects of arterial blockage:

(*a*) **The pathology of the collateral circulation.** A collateral circulation severely affected with spasm, atheroma, or other condition is of little value in maintaining a good alternative blood supply.

(*b*) **The state of oxygenation of the blood,** in respect of arterial Po_2 and haemoglobin level.

(*c*) **The efficiency of the heart.**

(*d*) **The nature of the affected tissue.** Brain and heart are more vulnerable to ischaemia than are any other organs. Connective tissue survives much better than does the parenchyma of an organ.

THE PROCESS OF INFARCTION

Infarction usually leads to a circumscribed area of coagulative necrosis, which is subsequently organised into scar tissue. The process is as follows:

(*a*) There is death of the cells in the area deprived of its blood supply. Blood usually continues to seep into the devitalised area for a short time due to three possible processes:

(i) An opening-up of peripheral anastomotic channels. This is particularly well marked in the lung because of its double blood supply.

(ii) Blood may continue to trickle in through the occluded artery (which is atonic distally), because the obstruction is not complete initially.[1] The aperture between the obstruction and the vessel wall is, however, soon occluded by thrombus.

(iii) There may be venous reflux.

At all events most infarcts contain a great deal of blood in the early stages, and are swollen and red in colour. The red cells entering the affected area escape through the damaged capillaries, and lie free in the dead tissue. There is also a great deal of fibrin derived from the blood (*infarcire* = to stuff). Infarcts of lax structures, e.g. lung and intestine, are much more engorged than those of compact organs, e.g. kidney and heart.

(*b*) The dead tissue undergoes necrosis; in solid organs the associated swelling of the cells may squeeze the blood out of the infarct. In this way it becomes paler. It is very important to note that until necrosis is visible, the ischaemic area cannot be called an infarct. Histochemical or electron-microscopic changes may be detected very shortly after cardiac muscle has been rendered ischaemic, but in human material *post-mortem* changes are superimposed on these. In practice it takes from 12 to 24 hours for a myocardial infarct to become macroscopically recognisable, while the first microscopical changes of necrosis can be seen only from 6 to 12 hours after the ischaemic episode.

(*c*) There is progressive autolysis of necrotic tissue and haemolysis of the red cells.

(*d*) At the same time the surrounding tissue undergoes an acute inflammatory reaction, stimulated presumably by products of autolysis. The initial polymorph response, which is quite marked (Fig. 38.1), is followed after a few days by a macrophage infiltration.

(*e*) There is an outward diffusion of tissue breakdown products and free haemoglobin, which are ingested by macrophages. Bilirubin and haemosiderin are produced locally. By this stage, approximately a week after occlusion, the infarct is firm and dull yellow in colour, and is surrounded by a red zone of inflammation.

(*f*) This phase of demolition is followed by a shrinkage of the infarct, which becomes white in colour. In some organs, notably the kidney, the necrotic tissue is so well preserved that its outlines are recognisable as ghosts without nuclei for many months. There is a slow but progressive ingrowth of granulation tissue from the periphery, and eventually the infarct is organised into a fibrous scar which later undergoes hyaline change. Dystrophic calcification may occur in the midst of the infarct, and also in the area of scarring. Around many infarcts there is a residual zone of pigmentation. This consists mostly of haemosiderin, but there may also be lipofuscin derived from broken-down parenchymatous cells, especially heart muscle.

The process is somewhat different in infarcts of the central nervous system:

(*a*) The necrotic tissue undergoes rapid colliquative necrosis.

(*b*) There is an infiltration of macrophages, derived from the monocytes and the microglia, which demolish the debris and ingest the disintegrated myelin. These swell up, and in their cytoplasm there is lipid material and some pigment which consists of variable amounts of haemosiderin derived

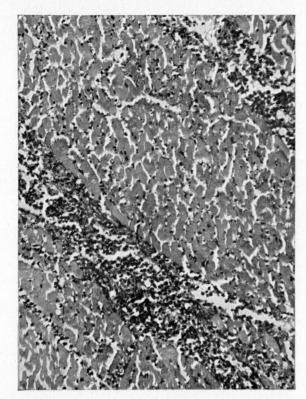

Figure 38.1
Myocardial infarction. The muscle fibres are necrotic, but their structure is easily recognisable. There is a profuse cellular infiltration, including many polymorphs, around the necrotic tissue. ×150.

from the small amount of blood in the infarct and lipofuscin from the disintegrated neurones. These macrophages are called *compound granular corpuscles* (Fig. 30.2, p. 399). Polymorphs are absent unless the meninges are involved.

(c) Repair by gliosis ensues, but sometimes a cyst surrounded by a layer of glial tissue remains.

The Morbid Anatomy of Infarcts

Infarcts of solid organs are usually wedge-shaped, with the apex directed internally in relation to the occluded artery and the base on the surface of the organ. Cerebral infarcts are ill-defined, soft, and pulpy; this is called *cerebral softening*.

Infarcts have been classified according to their colour, but this is of limited value. It is apparent that most start by being red, and become white as blood is squeezed out and as the free haemoglobin is later removed. Cerebral infarcts are usually initially white because there is virtually no anastomosis, and the vessels occluded are often so small that obstruction is usually complete right from the beginning. On the other hand, pulmonary infarcts seldom become white because of the enormous amount of blood trapped in the necrotic alveolar sacs. They are organised in the red stage.

Infarcts may be classified as *bland* and *septic* (or *infected*), according to whether they are sterile or contain organisms. As explained in Chapter 36, the infarcts of *Strept. viridans* endocarditis behave in a bland way, because the organisms in the emboli are rapidly destroyed at the site of impaction. In septic infarction there is a rapid transition from the stage of necrosis to one of suppuration, and the result is a large ragged abscess. Septic emboli which become impacted in vessels supplying tissue which does not normally show infarction, lead to a local acute inflammatory reaction terminating in suppuration. In this way multiple pyaemic abscesses are formed in the liver (portal pyaemia) and lung.

General Effects of Infarction

It should finally be noted that infarction of any significant extent is accompanied by constitutional effects. There is fever, a neutrophil leucocytosis, and a raised ESR. These effects are presumably caused by products of autolysis (see p. 55). In addition the necrotic tissue may release its enzymes into the circulation, and these may be of diagnostic help. In myocardial infarction the serum glutamate-oxaloacetate transaminase (aspartate aminotransferase) rises from a normal level of 5–35 units to over 200 units per 100 ml (see p. 541). This is useful diagnostically in the first few days, but then the level drops.

Other enzymes that are liberated include creatine phosphokinase (CPK) and lactate dehydrogenase (LDH). The creatine phosphokinase, like the SGOT, rises early and returns to normal within three days. The LDH, on the other hand, begins to rise by 12 hours, reaches a maximum at 48 hours, and returns to normal by the eleventh day. There are five isoenzyme bands of LDH as revealed by electrophoresis. The fast-moving components LDH_1 and LDH_2 are found in heart, kidney, and red cells. A rise in LDH_1 is a useful indicator of myocardial infarction. The slow-moving band LDH_5 is present in liver and muscle, and its level is a useful gauge of the extent of liver necrosis. $LDH_{2, 3, and 4}$ are present in lung and, together with LDH_1 from broken-down red cells, are found in increased quantities in pulmonary infarction. α-Hydroxybutyrate dehydrogenase (HBD) measures the same enzymatic activity as does LDH_1, and its serum level has the same significance as that of LDH_1.[13]

THE EFFECTS OF ISCHAEMIA ON VARIOUS ORGANS

It is instructive to conclude by considering the effects of ischaemia on a few tissues.

Heart

Myocardial ischaemia and infarction can occur in hearts with normal coronary arteries when the coronary perfusion is impaired by extreme tachycardia, shock, or severe aortic stenosis. Nevertheless, in most cases there is an organic stenosis of the vessels. Syphilitic occlusion of the ostia, coronary embolism, and dissecting aneurysm of the aorta are occasional causes, but atheroma and the intimal thickening that is part of the ageing process are by far the most common and important. Gradual occlusion of a coronary artery may be symptomless for a long time, and is accompanied by the development of considerable anastomotic channels between branches of the coronary system. Eventually the occlusion may become severe enough to lead to functional insufficiency during exercise and cause angina pectoris. If the patient dies at this stage the heart will show appreciable areas of fibrous replacement of myocardium. In addition microscopic areas of myocardial necrosis may be present; and it is noteworthy that these do not show the acute inflammatory reaction which is so marked in large infarcts. The anginal pain has not been adequately explained. A "factor P" produced by ischaemic muscle was suggested by Lewis, but it has never been isolated. Pain-producing substances are produced by ischaemic muscle, e.g. K^+ ions leaking out of cells, lactic acid, and phosphates, and perhaps these are responsible.[14] It is possible that vasodilator metabolites released from ischaemic muscle open up anastomotic channels, but hypoxia is more important.

Two patterns of myocardial infarction are seen:

Regional infarction. This is the usual finding in patients who die of acute heart attacks after surviving for more than twelve hours. If the anterior descending branch of the left coronary artery is occluded the anterior wall and septum of the left ventricle are affected, while blockage of the circumflex branch involves the posterior wall. Occlusion of the right artery also implicates the postero-inferior and posteroseptal wall of the left ventricle, and may spread to the posterior wall of the right ventricle. Regional infarction is often accompanied by thrombosis of the associated artery, and it is generally assumed to be secondary to the occlusion. However, this is by no means proven. In one series it was found that patients who survived an acute attack of myocardial ischaemia showed a thrombosis in 16 per cent of cases if they lived for one hour, in 37 per cent if they lived for one to twenty-four hours, and in 54 per cent if they lived for over 24 hours.[15] Such a finding leads to the unorthodox view that myocardial ischaemia and infarction occur first, and that the thrombosis is secondary. A possible explanation is that showers of small platelet thrombi are shed into the coronary circulation. They might have been formed on atheromatous plaques and released into the fast coronary flow before fibrin formation stabilised them (p. 456). Experimentally, infusion of ADP into the coronary artery of a pig leads to the formation of small platelet thrombi and the subsequent development of myocardial infarction.[16] Whatever the mechanism, there seems little doubt that infarction can occur in man without large occlusive arterial thrombi.[17, 18] Indeed, angina and myocardial infarction have been described in a nineteen-year-old-man with no coronary occlusion or other apparent cause.[19]

Subendocardial infarction. This is less common than regional infarction: a wide zone of subendocardial muscle shows infarction. This generally occurs when all the major coronary arteries are severely stenosed, but not completely obstructed by thrombosis.

Myocardial infarcts are coagulative in type and heal to form a fibrous scar. Pericarditis, either localised to the infarcted area or else generalised, is common, and so also is endocardial involvement leading to mural thrombosis and embolism. If the scar is extensive and thin, as occurs after infarction of the whole thickness of the wall, the lesion may proceed to aneurysmal dilatation of the ventricle. The wall becomes heavily calcified and the sac filled with laminated thrombus. Rupture of the aneurysm is uncommon. Recent infarcts sometimes rupture, and the process is usually called colliquative necrosis (*myomalacia cordis*). In fact, the muscle is friable rather than liquefied. It is occasionally seen in elderly people, usually women, and may be virtually symptomless until sudden rupture leads to a fatal haemopericardium.

Sudden death is common in occlusive coronary disease and is most common during the first twenty-four hours after the onset of the pain; sometimes a thrombus is found but often there is only generalised stenosis. The muscle may show little abnormality, and death is attributed to ventricular fibrillation. Patients who experience an episode of ventricular fibrillation and are successfully resuscitated have as good a prognosis as those who do not.[20]

NERVOUS TISSUE

The nervous tissue has a high rate of metabolism and cannot tolerate oxygen lack for long. With complete ischaemia, functional changes occur within seconds and cell death within a few minutes. The peripheral nerves and the nerve tracts within the central nervous system survive ischaemia for a very much longer period than does the neurone itself. Thus a lesion of the cervical cord may cause permanent lower-motor-neurone paralysis of the arms while sparing the long tracts to the legs.

Cerebral infarction. The two important causes of cerebral infarction are cerebral thrombosis and embolism from the heart. Thrombosis of the cerebral arteries most often occurs as a complication of atheroma, and is particularly common in hypertensive subjects. As already noted, there is colliquative necrosis, which may in the most severe cases implicate much of a hemisphere. The infarct usually remains pale, but with cerebral embolism it sometimes becomes haemorrhagic. This is ascribed to the restoration of some blood flow when the embolus breaks up or is pushed further down the vascular tree.

Generalised cerebral ischaemia follows cardiac arrest and severe haemorrhage; in fatal cases there is no obvious infarction, but the neurones may show early degenerative changes. Some cases of infarction do not show particularly severe cerebral arterial disease, and in these the ischaemia is often produced by marked extracerebral arterial atheroma.[21] In addition, there may be hypotension and sludging. The possible importance of thrombotic embolism from atheromatous plaques in causing transient ischaemic attacks ("encephalopathies") has been noted on p. 478.

Haemorrhagic infarction of the brain follows extensive venous-sinus thrombosis. A good example is the superior-sagittal-sinus thrombosis (marantic thrombosis) that occasionally occurs in weakly newborn infants. At necropsy much of the cerebral cortex is found to be infarcted.

Kidney

Renal infarction is also due either to local renal arterial disease, or more commonly, to embolism. Renal arterial atheroma is an important cause of progressive hypertension in young adults, and this is not due to ischaemia but to a fall in renal arterial pulse pressure.[22] Renal infarcts are wedge-shaped areas of coagulative necrosis, and heal to form depressed scars.

Renal ischaemia of a more generalised type occurs after the arterial vasoconstriction which complicates states of shock, haemorrhage, incompatible blood transfusion, and concealed accidental haemorrhage.[23] This last condition occasionally proceeds to bilateral symmetrical cortical necrosis, a fatal condition in which the outer two-thirds of the cortex of both kidneys is infarcted (see Fig. 32.4, p. 424). A similar effect is seen in the experimentally-produced generalised Sanarelli (Shwartzman) phenomenon. The mechanism of this appears to be generalised renal arterial vasoconstriction involving especially the outer part of the cortex.

In the *crush syndrome* tubular necrosis is probably caused by ischaemia. The condition arises when a casualty has sustained a continuous compression to one or more limbs. On being released, there is a temporary improvement in the clinical state, but this is followed by progressive renal impairment which culminates in acute renal failure and death.[24, 25] It resembles tourniquet shock (see p. 425).

Selective spasm, of the renal vessels has also been suggested as the explanation of "reflex anuria" in the following conditions: hysteria; passage of a ureteric stone; handling of the ureters during operation; following catheterisation.

Spleen

Infarction of the spleen is usually postembolic, but any enlarged spleen is liable to undergo infarction, possibly because its blood supply becomes inadequate. Localised infarcts are especially common in the enormous spleen of chronic myeloid leukaemia.

Splenic infarction is coagulative, and the base of the infarct often impinges on the peritoneal surface (Fig. 38.2). The focal perisplenitis so caused leads to severe pain in the left hypochondrium. Sometimes the infarct undergoes later softening. Healing is accompanied by fibrosis and shrinkage.

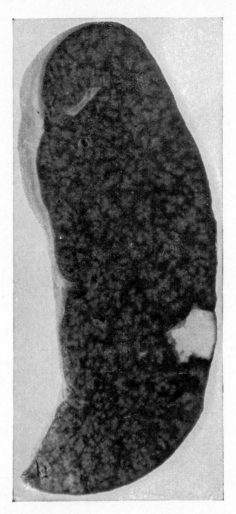

Figure 38.2
Infarct of spleen. This specimen was removed during the necropsy on a patient who died of subacute infective endocarditis. A section through the spleen shows a pale, circumscribed, wedge-shaped infarct under the capsule. The lymphoid follicles are unduly prominent. *(H 26.1, Reproduced by permission of the President and Council of the R.C.S. Eng.)*

Lung

Effects of pulmonary-artery obstruction.[26, 27]   The syndrome of massive pulmonary embolism due to clot has been described on p. 474. Surprisingly enough, occlusion of the right or left pulmonary artery in an unanaesthetised man (by inflating a balloon at the tip of a cardiac catheter) produces neither pain nor discomfort.[28, 29] An immediate increase in airways resistance occurs, and this results in a decrease in ventilation of the affected lung.[30, 31] The underventilation of the underperfused lung is partly mediated by the alterations in gas tensions. Thus it can be prevented by supplying 5 per cent CO_2 in air to the lung through the bronchospirometry tube. The local release of 5-hydroxytryptamine may also be a factor in causing collapse, for

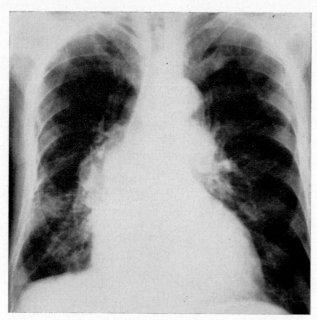

Figure 38.3
Pulmonary embolism. This is a straight chest radiograph in a patient whose right pulmonary artery has been occluded. Note the relatively normal appearance of the right lung field.

this agent produces bronchospasm which impedes ventilation by increasing airways resistance. The administration of heparin reduces bronchospasm, presumably by preventing further platelet deposition.

Figure 38.4
Pulmonary embolism. This is a lung scan (on the same patient as Fig. 38.3) using macro-aggregated radioactive-iodine labelled human albumin. Note the ischaemic right lung field.

Figures 38.3 and 38.4 are from photographs provided by Dr. H. P. Demshar, Department of Nuclear Medicine, Toronto General Hospital.

Poor ventilation of the affected lung accounts for the elevated diaphragm seen radiographically, and it sometimes leads to collapse. Nevertheless, collapse is neither invariable nor complete, and it follows that a lung scan using macro-aggregated ^{131}I-labelled human albumin shows an ischaemic lung field whereas a ^{133}Xe-ventilatory lung scan reveals a relatively normal field.[32] (Fig. 38.3 and 38.4.)

In the experimental animal occlusion of one branch of the pulmonary artery is followed by collapse of that lung. Recovery commences within a week or two, but the lung always remains smaller than normal and shows some scarring.[33] It has been suggested that the collapse is due to a deficiency of surfactant.[33] Furthermore, a reduction in the amount of this layer, or the presence of an inhibitor, may also be a factor in causing the collapse which follows open-heart surgery, when the lungs are not perfused for an hour or more.[34]

Pulmonary infarction.[27] Infarction does not occur in healthy people even if a main pulmonary artery is occluded. This is because of the additional bronchial arterial supply, which provides well-aerated blood. It is in heart failure, and especially mitral stenosis, that pulmonary infarction occurs, for there is an inadequate cardiac output due to left ventricular failure or inadequate filling of the left ventricle in mitral stenosis. The bronchial arterial supply is thus reduced, and blockage of a pulmonary artery may lead to infarction of the lung.

The usual cause of pulmonary infarction is an embolus arising from the leg veins in phlebothrombosis. About 90

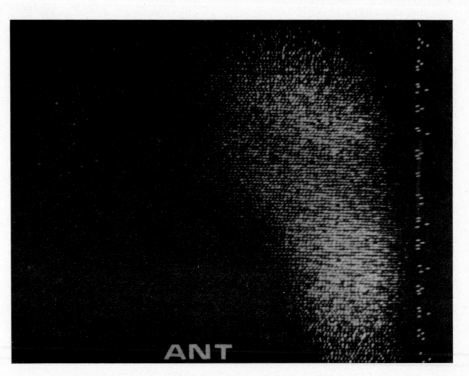

per cent of pulmonary emboli arise in this way, and the other 10 per cent come from the right atrial appendage in the course of heart disease, especially mitral stenosis. Pulmonary infarction may also follow a primary thrombosis of the pulmonary arteries, which occasionally occurs in severe pulmonary hypertension.

Pulmonary infarcts are generally described as being conical in shape and deep red in colour (Fig. 38.5). The

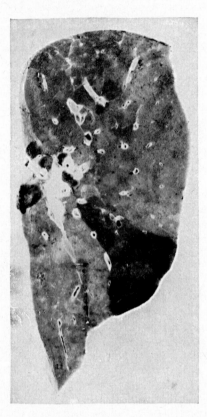

Figure 38.5
Pulmonary infarct. This vertical section through the left upper lobe shows a typical dark, wedge-shaped infarct. (R 27.3, *Reproduced by permission of the President and Council of the R.C.S. Eng.)*

broad base is certainly on the pleural surface, but the apex of the lesion is often not infarcted so that the infarct has the shape of a truncated cone;[35] pleural effusions of a haemorrhagic character sometimes complicate pulmonary infarction. The engorgement of pulmonary infarcts is due to the pre-existing chronic venous congestion of the lungs which is the result of heart failure. Blood pours into the alveoli through the damaged walls, and some of it is expectorated from the bronchioles; haemoptysis is a frequent accompaniment of pulmonary infarction. Organisation proceeds rapidly because of the comparatively good vascularity of the surrounding lung. The infarct is eventually converted into an insignificant pigmented scar, concealed by surrounding

lung tissue which shows compensatory overdistension. Large infarcts can become pale with the passage of time, and the centre occasionally breaks down to form a cavity.

It is not uncommon for a patient to develop the symptoms of pulmonary infarction together with an X-ray shadow that lasts for a few days and then disappears. Pathologically this consists of oedema and bleeding into the alveoli, as in an early infarct, but there is no progression to necrosis of the alveolar walls. Resolution can therefore be rapid. Technically this lesion cannot be called an infarct since there is no necrosis.[35]

The lung is the first site for pyaemic abscesses resulting from suppurative thrombophlebitis of the systemic veins. They usually cause empyema because of their close proximity to the pleural surface.

Liver

Hepatic infarction is very uncommon, presumably because spontaneous occlusion of the hepatic artery is rare. Nevertheless, it has been proved both experimentally and clinically (following the accidental ligation of the vessel during cholecystectomy) that occlusion of the hepatic artery can lead to extensive white infarction of the liver.[36, 37] Likewise, patchy infarction can occur if the branches of the hepatic artery are involved in polyarteritis nodosa. It would therefore appear that the portal vein contributes blood of so low an oxygen tension as to be inadequate for the survival of the parenchyma.

It is not surprising that thrombosis of the portal vein, while having serious effects on the abdominal viscera, does not lead to hepatic infarction. Pyaemic abscesses occur in the liver secondary to suppurative thrombophlebitis of the portal vein (portal pyaemia).

Focal acute congestion and haemorrhagic infarction is seen after thrombosis of the hepatic vein, which is a rare complication of polycythaemia vera and tumour invasion. It should be noted that the so-called *infarcts of Zahn* are not infarcts but focal, well-delineated areas of congestion. They are usually multiple and their pathogenesis is obscure.

Intestine

The usual cause of intestinal ischaemia is an obvious mechanical obstruction to the blood supply in such regional conditions as hernial strangulation, volvulus, and intussusception, and the changes in an affected loop of bowel are considered on page 492. Sometimes the primary lesion is vascular. Early mesenteric arterial occlusion may cause a malabsorption syndrome and severe abdominal pain shortly after meals (*intestinal angina*), and this may later progress to infarction. In some cases the ischaemia leads merely to mucosal destruction which heals by fibrosis to produce strictures. This is seen most often in the splenic flexure and descending colon, and the condition is called *ischaemic colitis*.[38, 39] It can be mistaken for ulcerative colitis, but may be distinguished when there is a wide submucosal layer containing many haemosiderin-filled macrophages. Mucosal fibrosis is another characteristic feature.[39] It is clearly a healed infarct of part of the bowel wall.

Mesenteric venous thrombosis is another important cause of ischaemia. The process starts distally in the small venous radicles and spreads proximally to implicate the main mesenteric veins. The bowel is engorged, and fresh blood may be passed *per rectum* or vomited, and the condition may simulate acute ulcerative colitis or peptic ulceration. As in all bowel infarction there is early intestinal obstruction due to paralysis of the affected portion.

Once the whole wall is infarcted the bowel becomes stiff, plum-red in colour, and covered with a fibrinous peritoneal exudate. It is rapidly colonised by saprophytes from the faeces, and gangrene ensues. Death soon follows due to the following three factors:

(*a*) *Acute intestinal obstruction.*
(*b*) *Haemorrhage into the bowel wall and lumen.*
(*c*) *Perforation and generalised peritonitis.*

Immediate resection alone can save the patient's life.

Skeletal Muscle[40, 41]

Ischaemia of skeletal muscle results in necrosis. When this is due to arterial obstruction, the resulting fibrous replacement is not marked. When the ischaemia is produced by or accompanied by venous obstruction, the necrotic muscle is haemorrhagic and a brisk fibrosis results in contracture. This is the basis of *Volkmann's ischaemic contracture*, which generally affects the forearm but it is described also in the legs. The basic lesion is arterial occlusion, either due to pressure from fracture edges (e.g. a supracondylar fracture of the humerus), ill-applied plasters, or a haematoma, or to spasm complicating such arterial damage or pressure. The importance of venous obstruction is noted above. The result of the ischaemia is infarction of the muscles of the forearm.

In the mildest cases there is slight residual fibrosis with an attempt at regeneration of partly destroyed muscle fibres at the edge. In the worst cases, however, the muscle is replaced by dense fibrous tissue, and the patient develops a severe contracture. Sometimes there is an area of calcareous, putty-like debris in the midst. The nerves and tendons are often also involved, but the skin is left intact, and there is no gangrene.[41]

The blood supply to skeletal muscle varies considerably from one muscle to another.[40] Thus there may be only one nutrient artery, and if it is obstructed severe damage results, e.g. in gastrocnemius and biceps brachii. Some muscles have multiple nutrient arteries—either from one source (tibialis anterior from the anterior tibial artery) or from several sources (extensor digitorum longus from anterior tibial and the perforating vessels). It is obvious that muscles with the latter type of blood supply are the least likely to be rendered ischaemic following injuries.

Extremities

Infarction of the limbs, most commonly the legs, is often due to a combination of disorders which are grouped together as *peripheral vascular disease*. Atherosclerosis of the large arteries is often a major component, and it may also lead to atheromatous or thrombotic material embolising to small peripheral vessels. Alternatively the main artery may be blocked by thrombus or by a large embolus. Medium-sized arteries may show arteriosclerosis obliterans, while peripheral arterioles may be occluded by the arteriolosclerosis associated with hypertension and especially diabetes mellitus. Other causes of ischaemia are Raynaud's phenomenon, trauma with spasm, ergotism, cold autohaemagglutinins blocking capillaries, frost-bite (trench-foot), iliofemoral thrombosis, and Buerger's disease. Heart failure following coronary-artery disease often aggravates the ischaemia.

There may be no effect of vascular occlusion for a long time if the collateral circulation is adequate. Eventually the blood supply becomes inadequate to sustain muscular exercise, in which case intermittent claudication occurs. At this stage the skin of the feet begins to show trophic changes: glossiness, loss of hair, and a tendency towards ulceration with colonisation by extraneous organisms which would normally be eradicated by the decontaminating mechanisms of the area. Any ulcers that form tend to persist and spread, as ischaemia weakens the tissue's response to infection (see Chapter 8).

In due course ischaemia may become severe enough to lead to infarction. This is usually precipitated by thrombosis (or else embolism from the heart). The infarcted area becomes dry, shrivelled, and black (due to an alteration in the haemoglobin consequent on desiccation and perhaps putrefaction). A red *line of demarcation*, the equivalent of the inflammatory zone of an internal infarct, develops around the area of union of dead and living. The dead area undergoes mummification (loosely called "dry gangrene"), and is amputated spontaneously at the line of demarcation if it is not resected surgically beforehand.

In many cases, however, the dead tissue is colonised by saprophytes, and putrefaction occurs; this is "wet gangrene". There is concomitant infection by organisms of low virulence around the line of demarcation, and the stump is implicated. The progressive infection of the stump accentuates the effects of ischaemia, and is itself augmented by the ischaemia; thus the necrosis and gangrene spread rapidly. It is for this reason that amputation should be carried out as soon as possible in the presence of gangrene. The question of "wet" and "dry" gangrene is considered in Chapter 4.

There is a marked contrast between the natural history of an infarct of an internal organ and one of an extremity. In one there is organisation to form a scar, and the free haemoglobin is metabolised in the RE cells to haemosiderin and bilirubin. In an extremity the infarcted area is spontaneously amputated, and there is no attempt at replacement. The haemoglobin remains *in situ*, and undergoes changes due to desiccation or putrefaction.

VASCULAR SPASM

Although vascular occlusion is generally caused by an organic lesion, there are a number of conditions in which spasm of the vessel wall plays a most important part. Spasm may occur in both veins and arteries, but it is debatable whether the capillaries are capable of independent contraction.

Venous Spasm

Trauma applied directly to the vessel wall can cause marked spasm; this may be a source of great difficulty during an inexpert venepuncture, e.g. for transfusion purposes.

Generalised venospasm has been postulated as occurring during heart failure, and is a feature of hypovolaemic shock.

Arterial Spasm

The thick wall of the muscular arteries and arterioles is admirably designed for reducing the size of the lumen of these vessels. This property is of immense value in the regulation of blood flow to the various organs. In this way, blood is diverted to the muscles and heart during exercise, to the skin when heat has to be lost, and to glands when secretion is required. Following haemorrhage, arterial spasm is an important factor in maintaining the blood pressure.

Local trauma to arteries frequently causes local spasm, a function which may be of life-saving importance. Cases of avulsion of a limb are on record in which, due to spasm of the main artery, the patient did not die of massive haemorrhage. The contraction of the vessel may in part be mediated by 5-hydroxytryptamine liberated from platelets (see p. 613).

The ability of arteries to contract can be utilised by the surgeon who is inadvertently faced with a large haemorrhage during the course of an operation. It is a wise policy to pack the wound and await the onset of spasm, rather than make heroic though blind efforts with a pair of haemostats.[42]

Certain syndromes or diseases are recognised as being due to arterial spasm:

Raynaud's phenomenon.[43] The digital arteries appear to be unduly sensitive to cold. Measurements of blood flow show that it is decreased: dry gangrene may develop.

Ergot poisoning. Arterial spasm may lead to gangrene of the extremities.

Traumatic damage. Not only may spasm occur when an artery is severed, but also when it is subjected to relatively trivial injury. Thus, a missile or a fractured bone end may cause sufficient damage to an artery to be a precipitating factor. Even pressure from a plaster or a tourniquet can cause spasm which may last for many hours. Clinical and experimental work has indicated that this spasm is produced by a nervous reflex, and that it can spread to vessels not directly damaged.

In the rabbit the application of a tourniquet to a leg can cause spasm not only at the site of application, but also of the arteries distally and proximally.[44] It may extend to the aorta and even to the opposite limb. Similar extensive arterial spasm can be produced by electrical stimulation of the proximal end of the divided sciatic nerve or the distal end of the severed splanchnic nerve. This spasm also affects the kidney, and in the rabbit the outer two-thirds of the cortex becomes pale.

In man there seems little doubt that arterial spasm can occur in response to trauma, and that it can spread to involve vessels not primarily damaged.

Generalised arteriolar spasm has been suggested as the primary factor in the causation of essential hypertension, but as yet the pathogenesis of this common condition is not known.

REFERENCES

1. WRIGHT, G. P. (1958). *An Introduction to Pathology*, 3rd edn, pp. 427 and 353. London: Longmans.
2. COTTON, R. T. and BEDFORD, D. R. (1956). *American Journal of Medicine*, **20**, 301.
3. COHEN, H. (1961). *British Medical Journal*, ii, 1615.
4. DICKINSON, C. J. and PENTECOST, B. L. (1968). In *Clinical Physiology*, 3rd edn, p. 64. Edited by E. J. M. Campbell, C. J. Dickinson and J. D. H. Slater. Oxford: Blackwell.
5. BOYD, D. P. and CLARKE, F. M. (1962). *Surgery*, **51**, 19.
6. GILLENWATER, J. Y., BRESLOW, I. H. and LISKER, S. (1962). *Circulation*, **25**, 39.
7. FOGARTY, T. J. *et al.* (1963). *Archives of Surgery*, **86**, 256.
8. MERYMAN, H. T. (1957). *Physiological Reviews*, **37**, 233.
9. WASHBURN, B. (1962). *New England Journal of Medicine*, **266**, 974.
10. BIGELOW, D. R. and RITCHIE, G. W. (1963). *Journal of Bone and Joint Surgery*, **45B**, 122.
11. GOLDING, M. R. *et al.* (1963). *Surgery*, **53**, 303.
12. HUSAIN, T. (1953). *Journal of Pathology and Bacteriology*, **66**, 347.
13. Various Authors (1970). *Journal of Clinical Pathology*, **24**, suppl. (Association of Clinical Pathology), **4**, 1 *et seq.* Enzyme Assays in Medicine.
14. KEELE, C. A. and ARMSTRONG, D. (1964). *Substances Producing Pain and Itch*, p. 326. London: Arnold.
15. SPAIN, D. M. and BRADESS, V. A. (1960). *American Journal of Medical Science*, **240**, 701.
16. JØRGENSEN, L. *et al.* (1967). *Laboratory Investigations*, **17**, 616.
17. EHRLICH, J. C. and SHINOHARA, Y. (1964). *Archives of Pathology*, **78**, 432.

18. MORE, R. H. and HAUST, M. D. (1961). In *International Symposium*: Anticoagulants and Fibrinolysins, p. 143. Edited by R. L. MacMillan and J. F. Mustard. Philadelphia: Lea and Febiger.
19. SIDD, J. J., KEMP, H. G. and GORLIN, R. (1970). *New England Journal of Medicine*, **282**, 1306.
20. LAWRIE, D. M. (1969). *Lancet*, ii, 1085.
21. Leading Article (1971). *British Medical Journal*, iii, 723.
22. DE WARDENER, H. E. (1967). *The Kidney*, 3rd edn, pp. 111 and 100. London: Churchill.
23. SHEEHAN, H. L. and MOORE, H. C. (1952). *Renal Cortical Necrosis*. Oxford: Blackwell.
24. OLIVER, J., MacDOWELL, M. and TRACY, A. (1951). *Journal of Clinical Investigation*, **30**, 1305.
25. SEVITT, S. (1959). *Lancet*, ii, 135.
26. COMROE, J. H. (1962). In *Pulmonary Structure and Function*, a Ciba Foundation Symposium, p. 176. Edited by A. V. S. de Reuck and M. O'Connor. London: Churchill.
27. SASAHARA, A. A. and STEIN, M. (1965). Editors. *Pulmonary Embolic Disease*, 312 p. New York and London: Grune and Stratton.
28. CARLENS, E., HANSON, H. E. and NORDENSTRÖM, B. (1951). *Journal of Thoracic Surgery*, **22**, 527.
29. HANSON, H. E. (1954). *Acta Chirurgica Scandinavica, Supplement*, **187**.
30. SEVERINGHAUS, J. W. *et al.* (1961). *Journal of Applied Physiology*, **16**, 53.
31. SWENSON, E. W., FINLEY, T. N. and GUZMAN, S. V. (1961). *Journal of Clinical Investigation*, **40**, 828.
32. DeNARDO, G. L. *et al.* (1970). *New England Journal of Medicine*, **282**, 1334.
33. FINLEY, T. N. *et al.* (1960). *Physiologist*, **3**, 56.
34. TOOLEY, W. H., FINLEY, T. N. and GARDNER, R. (1961). *Physiologist*, **4**, 124.
35. HAMPTON, A. O. and CASTLEMAN, B. (1940). *American Journal of Roentgenology*, **43**, 305.
36. PARKER, R. G. F. (1955). *Journal of Pathology and Bacteriology*, **70**, 521.
37. CARROLL, R. (1963). *Journal of Clinical Pathology*, **16**, 133 and *Journal of Pathology and Bacteriology*, **85**, 349.
38. MARSTON, A. *et al.* (1966). *Gut*, **7**, 1.
39. McDONALD, G. S. A. and HOURIHANE, D. O'B. (1972). *Journal of Clinical Pathology*, **25**, 99.
40. ADAMS, R. D., DENNY-BROWN, D. and PEARSON, C. M. (1962). *Diseases of Muscle*, 2nd edn, pp. 522 and 85. London: Kimpton.
41. SEDDON, H. (1964). *British Medical Journal*, i, 1587.
42. WATSON-JONES, R. (1952). In *Fractures and Joint Injuries*, 4th edn, Volume 1, p. 105. Edinburgh: Livingstone.
43. Leading Article (1972). *British Medical Journal*, iii, 782.
44. TRUETA, J. *et al.* (1947). *Studies of the Renal Circulation*. Oxford: Blackwell.

Chapter 39. Oedema

Oedema may be defined as an excessive extravascular accumulation of fluid. In its usual context it is applied to the morbid accumulation of fluid in the interstitial tissues. It is particularly liable to occur in the various preformed serous sacs, giving rise to ascites, hydrothorax, and hydropericardium, as effusions into the peritoneal, pleural, and pericardial cavities are specifically called. When generalised it is called *anasarca*. It is, of course, also possible to have intracellular oedema, as in hydropic degeneration (see Chapter 4), but for the remainder of the discussion only the interstitial type will be considered. It is necessary first to understand the normal mechanisms which regulate the distribution of fluid in the body.

MECHANISMS OF NORMAL CONTROL IN THE SYSTEMIC CIRCULATION

Local

Starling postulated that the movement of fluid between the vessels and the extravascular spaces was determined by the balance of the hydrostatic and osmotic forces acting upon it.[1, 2]

THE FORCES TENDING TO DRIVE FLUID OUT OF THE BLOOD VESSELS ARE:

The hydrostatic pressure in the vessel. This is generally accepted as 32 mm Hg at the arterial end of the capillary and 12 mm Hg at the venous end, in the skin of man at heart level.

The colloid osmotic pressure of the interstitial fluid. Since the vascular wall is completely permeable to water and crystalloids, the only effective osmotic forces are those due to the colloids (mainly proteins). The interstitial fluids normally have a low protein content, and this is therefore not an important factor in the formation of the extravascular fluids under normal conditions. Furthermore, those proteins which do escape into the tissue spaces are normally removed by the lymphatics.

THE FORCES DRAWING FLUID INTO THE BLOOD VESSELS ARE:

The tissue tension. This is low (3–4 mm Hg). It is of importance in relation to the distribution of the oedema. For instance, lax areas, like the eyelids, ankles, scrotum, and over the sacrum, tend to accumulate fluid, while tense areas, like the palms and soles, are never the site of marked oedema. A rise in tissue tension is probably an important factor in limiting interstitial-tissue fluid formation in the legs under normal conditions, and also in acutely inflamed parts.

The osmotic pressure of the plasma proteins. The osmotic pressure of a substance in solution is determined by the number of molecules present. Albumin, with its higher concentration and lower molecular weight (65 000), therefore exerts a much greater osmotic force than do the other plasma proteins, e.g. globulins with molecular weight 90 000–10⁶. The plasma proteins exert a force of 25 mm Hg. The crystalloids of the plasma exert a much larger osmotic pressure, but as they pass freely into the interstitial fluid, this force is neutralised by the osmotic pressure of the interstitial fluid crystalloids. The importance of the normal vascular permeability in regulating the distribution of fluid between the intravascular and extravascular compartments cannot be over-emphasised. In the event of increased permeability there is the formation of an exudate rich in protein, e.g. in acute inflammation.

Oedema can indeed be placed in one of two categories:

Exudates, which are morbid accumulations of fluid due to an increased vascular permeability, and *transudates*, which are morbid accumulations of fluid due to a hydrostatic imbalance between the intravascular and extravascular compartments, despite normal vascular permeability.

The basis of an exudate is the free passage of plasma proteins to the extravascular compartment, so that there is a balance between the osmotic pressures of the plasma and the interstitial fluid. There is virtually nothing, except the mounting tissue tension, to hinder the outward flow of plasma.

Table 39.1 indicates the main differences between exudates and transudates.

The mode of passage of crystalloids and water through the wall of a capillary is discussed in Chapter 6.

The importance of the lymphatics should not be forgotten. They form an elaborate network in most tissues, and their function is to drain away fluid and protein. The fluid in the lymphatics has a considerably higher protein content than that of the interstitial fluid itself.

The various factors involved in Starling's hypothesis are depicted in Fig. 6.4 (p. 73). It must be realised, however, that this merely represents an average state of affairs found in many capillaries at the level of the heart. Pressures in individual vessels show considerable variation.

TABLE 39.1

	Exudate	Transudate
Total Protein Content.	High as in plasma.	Less than 1 g per 100 ml.
Distribution of Proteins.	As in plasma.	Nearly all albumin (smallest molecule).
Fibrinogen	Present. It clots spontaneously.	Not present. No tendency to coagulation.
Specific Gravity.*	High.	Low.
Cells.	Plentiful; those of inflammation, e.g. polymorphs or lymphocytes depending on the cause.	Few present; nearly all mesothelial cells.

* The specific gravity of plasma is normally about 1·027, and it is related to its protein content. A protein-free filtrate of plasma has a SG of 1·010, and this is also the SG of the urine secreted by a failing kidney which has lost its power of concentration (see Chapter 42). A transudate with its low content of protein will have a SG of about 1·012, whereas an exudate will have a SG of over 1·018.

Over-all Fluid Balance

The total amount of fluid in the body is governed by a balance between the amount ingested and produced by metabolic activity on the one hand, and that lost in the urine, sweat, etc. on the other. The regulating mechanisms involve the sensation of thirst, the secretion of antidiuretic hormone from the posterior pituitary, and the secretion of aldosterone from the adrenal cortex (see Chapter 34).

In the causation of any type of oedema there are usually a combination of factors. Starling himself recognised that dropsy was probably never due to the derangement of a single mechanism only.

TYPES OF OEDEMA

Oedema may be local or generalised (widespread). The local oedemas are simpler to understand, because there are usually fewer factors involved.

Local Oedema

Acute inflammatory oedema. The formation of an exudate due to an increased vascular permeability to proteins is basic to the inflammatory response. The causes have been fully considered in Chapter 6, and will merely be summarised at this point:

(a) Increased vascular permeability.
(b) Increased osmotic pressure of interstitial fluid due to the protein of the exudate, and its breakdown into osmotically-active smaller molecules.
(c) Increased hydrostatic pressure in the capillaries.
(d) Increased fluidity of ground substance.
The extent of the oedema is related to the tissue tension.

Hypersensitivity (allergic oedema). Oedema is present in all lesions of immediate-type hypersensitivity, and is due to an increase in vascular permeability. It is a true exudate. The oedema of anaphylaxis is widespread.

Oedema is also seen in the acute inflammatory response of delayed-type hypersensitivity reactions.

Oedema of venous obstruction. A rise in venous pressure leads to an increase in the capillary pressure. The result is the formation of a transudate. This is seen even in normal people whose work entails long periods of standing, and is particularly evident after thrombophlebitis, e.g. pregnancy "white leg", when there is often much residual oedema.

Oedema of a limb may be produced experimentally by applying a cuff or tourniquet; under these circumstances there is an additional factor of lymphatic obstruction. If the venous pressure is maintained at 40 mm Hg or more, the vascular permeability alters, allowing protein to leak through.[3] Hypoxia has a similar effect.[4]

By enclosing a limb, or part of a limb, in a plethysmograph the rate of accumulation of transudate in response to a given increase in venous pressure can be measured. A coefficient of vascular permeability can be expressed in ml increase in volume/min/mm Hg increase in pressure/100 ml of tissue. Such measurements have shown an increased value in patients with rheumatoid arthritis, especially those who develop oedema of the legs. In many cases the fluid has a low protein content, and presumably the oedema is produced by an increase in filtration rate rather than an increase in vascular permeability.[5] It is apparent therefore that the oedema following venous obstruction depends on a number of factors: the venous pressure, the presence of hypoxia, and the degree of lymphatic obstruction.

This is illustrated by the changes in a loop of bowel which is undergoing volvulus or strangulation. The first effect is venous obstruction causing congestion of the gut wall, and there is considerable haemorrhage into the lumen. The turgid tissue increases the pressure around the constricted neck and so progressively aggravates the venous obstruction. The oedema first has the character of a transudate, but its protein content soon rises as the pressure increases. Lymphatic obstruction, increased venous pressure, hypoxia, infection, and inflammation all contribute to its formation. Finally venous thrombosis may occur. In due course the arterial supply is occluded either by direct pressure or thrombosis. Infarction results, and the necrotic bowel is at once colonised by putrefactive saprophytes native to the faeces; gangrene follows, and the bowel ruptures.

Lymphatic oedema. Extensive lymphatic obstruction

can produce an oedema of rather high protein content (though not as high as that of an exudate). If it persists it stimulates an overgrowth of fibrous tissue, and therefore has a brawny consistency and does not pit easily on pressure. In due course the fibrous-tissue and epithelial overgrowth may become so pronounced that *elephantiasis* results. A good example of this is the tropical disease filariasis due to the nematode *Wuchereria bancrofti*, which in its adult stage lives in the lymphatics of the groin. While alive the worm causes little disability to its host, but when it dies it stimulates an inflammatory reaction. The lymphangitis leads to lymphatic obstruction, and elephantiasis of the legs and external genitalia is a common result. A similar effect is produced by recurrent bacterial lymphangitis, and in lymphogranuloma venereum there is vulval elephantiasis.

The lymphatic oedema of the arm and the *peau d'orange* appearance of the breast are the results of obstruction to the axillary and mammary lymphatics through premeation by a breast carcinoma. The arm oedema is often aggravated by postoperative radiotherapy.

Oedema is sometimes seen in patients with hemiplegia. It usually affects the arm rather than the leg, and it may be confined to a hand. The fluid has a high protein content, and it may be that the oedema is due to impaired lymphatic drainage resulting from reduced muscular activity. It is interesting that in heart failure, oedema is sometimes especially marked and persistent in a paralysed limb. Patients with acute nephritis have more peri-orbital oedema on awaking in the morning than they do later in the day; the oedema is dispersed by constant blinking.

Primary lymphoedema[6] is a special variety of lymphatic oedema due to a malformation of the lymphatics of the lower limbs—hypoplasia, varicose dilatation, and obstruction have all been reported.[7] If the condition is hereditary and congenital it is called *Milroy's disease*[8]; this is inherited as an autosomal dominant of variable penetrance. Usually the oedema is not hereditary and appears in childhood. It may be unilateral, but frequently it affects both legs, which become greatly disfigured. The condition persists throughout life.

There is an association between primary lymphoedema, recurrent pleural effusions (due to lymphatic oedema), and yellow finger and toe nails. The explanation of this last feature is not understood, but it is probably due to poor lymphatic drainage.[9]

Generalised Oedema

Cardiac oedema. Although the oedema of congestive cardiac failure is familiar enough, the mechanisms involved are by no means simple or clearly understood. In right-sided and congestive cardiac failure the oedema is accompanied by a general retention of fluid, as is shown by an increase in body weight. Its distribution is influenced by gravity: when the patient is ambulant, the legs are first involved, and swelling of the ankles is often the first symptom. When he is recum-

bent, the oedema appears in the sacral and genital areas. Oedema may occasionally also develop in the upper limbs and jaw. The oedema pits readily on pressure.

The mechanism of cardiac failure is described in Chapter 40. If the back-pressure hypothesis is accepted, it would seem that the main factor leading to oedema is a *rise in the central venous pressure*, which is transmitted backwards to the venous end of the capillaries. This would have the effect of causing a transudation, as already described. Generalised oedema of any type should lead to a decrease in blood volume because of the diversion of a large amount of fluid to the extravascular compartment. This in turn stimulates anti-diuretic hormone and aldosterone secretion (see Chapter 34), and there is water and salt retention. In this way the oliguria and salt retention of heart failure could be explained, as well as the increase in body weight. Unfortunately, the facts do not fit the case. There is an increased blood volume in heart failure,[10] and it may occur before there is any rise in central venous pressure. Furthermore, oedema itself may occur before there is any rise in venous pressure, and it is manifested by an increase in body weight. In addition, the amount of oedema is not proportional to the height of the venous pressure;[11] some cases of superior mediastinal obstruction have a venous pressure much higher than that encountered in heart failure,[12] and yet there is no peripheral oedema. Oedema of the legs is not produced after the ligation of the inferior vena cava below the renal veins.[12, 13] It seems that the increased venous pressure acting together with gravity determines the situation rather than the formation of cardiac oedema.

If the theory of forward-failure is accepted, it would appear that the vascular endothelium suffers from *stagnant hypoxia*. This leads to an increased permeability. If this were the case, the oedema would have the protein content of an exudate. In fact it is a typical transudate, though it is worth qualifying this objection by remembering the lymphatics could be responsible for removing some of the protein that might be present. In heart failure there is mild proteinuria, which is presumably due to a slight increase in permeability of the glomerular capillaries.

It is obvious that neither of these two theories can explain all the features of cardiac oedema satisfactorily.

Hypoproteinaemia is not a factor, because the plasma proteins are well maintained and do not fall to that level (about 5 g per cent) at which oedema might be expected.

It has been suggested that there is an element of *lymphatic obstruction*, because dyes injected into the subcutaneous tissue of oedematous legs do not stream up the lymphatics as they do normally.[14] In fact, lymphatic drainage is dependent on muscular activity, which is poor in such patients, and also on the venous pressure, in that all lymphatics finally drain into the veins. The low protein content of cardiac oedema does not point to any important degree of lymphatic obstruction.

Finally, the question of *altered tissue tension* has to be considered. One of the limiting factors in oedema formation is the rise in tissue tension. In a cardiac patient, once oedema has developed and stretched the tissues sufficiently, there is an increased tendency for the oedema to recur.

As none of the local conditions explains the oedema satisfactorily, much attention has been focused on the renal changes of heart failure: *oliguria* and *salt retention*. If salt is withheld, cardiac oedema lessens; it recurs when salt is administered. The daily glomerular filtrate amounts to nearly 180 litres, which contains about 1 200 g of salt. Ninety-nine per cent of this is reabsorbed by the tubules, and even a slight upset in this absorption mechanism could cause a marked change in salt balance.

In congestive cardiac failure there is renal vasoconstriction due to sympathetic overactivity. In addition, the renal vasoconstriction diverts the blood away from the superficial part of the cortex, and the juxtamedullary glomeruli filter most of the urine. There is evidence to suggest that there is more complete reabsorption of sodium in these nephrons than in those whose glomeruli lie in the superficial cortex.[17] The renal blood flow may be reduced to about a half of normal,[15] and the glomerular filtration rate from 120 to about 70 ml per minute. Normally about 80 per cent of the sodium in the glomerular filtrate is reabsorbed by the proximal tubule, but if the filtration rate is reduced a larger amount could be reabsorbed. The smaller amount thus passed on could then be more completely reabsorbed by the distal tubule. Therefore some of the sodium retention could be explained in terms of a reduced glomerular filtration rate.[16] Furthermore, the vasoconstriction mobilises the renin-angiotensin system, and this leads to the secretion of aldosterone, the urinary excretion of which is raised in most patients with right-sided heart failure, but not usually in those with left-sided failure. The plasma level of aldosterone is often somewhat raised in heart failure, but not to the heights found in the nephrotic syndrome or hepatic cirrhosis. Normally the continuous administration of mineralocorticosteroids leads to only a transient retention of sodium and water, and after a few days there is an escape from the control of the hormones. The nature of this escape is unknown, and it appears to be in abeyance in cases of heart failure. Perhaps it is related to the shift in action to the juxtamedullary glomeruli.[17] It is possible that sodium reabsorption from the proximal tubule is also under the control of a hormone, but it is as yet undefined.[18–19]

The factors concerned in cardiac oedema are obscure, but a possible mechanism is as follows: the reduction in cardiac output leads to renal vasoconstriction which in turn facilitates the reabsorption of sodium both by nephrons served by juxtamedullary glomeruli and by increasing the secretion of aldosterone.[17] The resulting salt and water retention produces an expansion of the extracellular fluid compartment. Conditions are therefore propitious for the development of oedema, and local factors act to precipitate its actual occurrence, e.g. raised venous pressure and local tissue overstretching.

Renal oedema. *Acute glomerulonephritis.* Oedema is often the first symptom of the disease. It affects the face and eyelids predominantly; the ankles and genitalia are also often affected, but the oedema is seldom severe. There is no entirely satisfactory explanation for the facial distribution of the oedema; it can hardly be postural, since it is often first noticed when the patient is still ambulant. Its cause is equally obscure. At one time an allergic effect on the capillaries was blamed, but the protein content of the fluid is low (about 0·4 g per 100 ml) and not in keeping with vascular damage. It is not due to hypoproteinaemia, because it occurs at a time when the plasma proteins are not appreciably reduced. An important factor is probably heart failure produced by the sudden systemic hypertension, and aggravated by a raised blood volume due to fluid retention. This is a result of oliguria, which may be quite severe, and is due to glomerular damage. It is noteworthy that the anuria caused by tubular necrosis is not usually accompanied by peripheral oedema.

Nephrotic syndrome. The outstanding feature here is a heavy proteinuria. This results in a low plasma protein level affecting especially the albumin fraction. On Starling's hypothesis the diminished osmotic pressure of the plasma proteins can easily explain the generalised oedema, and this is undoubtedly an important factor. However, once again there are other considerations. A salt-free diet reduces the oedema, especially if combined with diuretics. In the nephrotic syndrome there is a reduced blood volume.[20] This in turn stimulates the secretion of aldosterone (which is found in considerable amounts in the urine) and ADH. There is ensuing water retention, as already described, and oliguria is present as the oedema accumulates. If the plasma volume is expanded with albumin or dextran, the oedema is checked and a considerable diuresis occurs. There may also be spontaneous diureses during the course of the disease, in which the oedema is cleared though the level of plasma proteins remains unaltered. The syndrome is described on pp. 528–529.

Chronic glomerulonephritis. This is almost invariably associated with hypertension. The oedema is due to heart failure. The pulmonary oedema of uraemia is considered on page 527.

Famine oedema (nutritional oedema).[21, 22] The oedema that is seen after prolonged starvation is usually confined to the legs, but sometimes it is more generalised. At first sight it would appear to be explicable in terms of hypoproteinaemia, but in fact there is no close correlation between the level of plasma proteins and the presence of oedema; it is sometimes extensive when the plasma proteins are normal. The true explanation of famine oedema is unknown. An important factor appears to be a loss of compact tissue (mostly fat) and its replacement by a loose connective tissue which can accumulate fluid without a rise in tissue tension. When the patient is confined to bed, there is a diuresis and the oedema decreases rapidly, even if the diet is unaltered. This is merely an accentuation of the normal diuretic effect of recumbency (see page 443), and testifies to the considerable degree of fluid retention in famine oedema. It is interesting that cachectic patients with cancer do not generally exhibit oedema, therefore a mere loss of tissue mass cannot be the whole answer. In some of the victims of starvation there is heart failure due to thiamine deficiency (beri-beri), and perhaps this is an additional factor in some cases of famine oedema.

An interesting condition of malnutrition accompanied by marked oedema is *kwashiorkor*.[*][21, 23] It occurs in infants at the time of weaning, and is prevalent in Africa, Asia, and Latin America. There is also a failure of growth, normocytic anaemia, reduced plasma albumin, and an enlarged fatty liver which may be the precursor of a later cirrhosis. The cause of the condition is a dietary deficiency of protein. It can be cured by a high-protein diet in assimilable form, e.g. milk. There is often pronounced skin involvement with muco-cutaneous ulceration, depigmentation of the hair (which may have a reddish hue), and pellagroid eruptions. Though the oedema is presumably related to the protein lack, there are multiple dietary deficiencies in many cases.

Protein-losing enteropathy. Oedema is a prominent feature of this rare condition (see p. 550).

Hepatic oedema (see Chapter 43). Its main manifestation is ascites, and in a way it falls midway between the local and generalised oedemas. However, there may sometimes be a more widespread oedema affecting the legs also. The factors involved are lymphatic obstruction, a fall in the level of plasma proteins, an increase in the regional venous pressure due to portal hypertension, and a failure in the hepatic inactivation of aldosterone.

Oedema due to adrenal hormones. Salt retention occurs during the therapeutic administration of cortisone and ACTH. There is an increase in weight, and oedema may develop. Hypertension is another common effect. These manifestations are also seen in Cushing's syndrome. The cause of the oedema is complex, being due to several mechanisms.

(*a*) There may be an increased blood volume due to sodium retention. As mentioned in Chapter 34, cortisol has a mild mineralocorticoid action.

(*b*) There may be a change in the ground substance of the connective tissue, rendering it more water-soluble. The typical "moon face" might well be due to a local oedema of this type.

(*c*) There may sometimes be heart failure secondary to hypertension.

* The word comes from a Ghanaian dialect. It means "first-second", i.e. the first child is deposed from the breast by the next child. Kwashiorkor is a disease the child gets when the next baby is born.

Primary hyperaldosteronism (Conn's syndrome) does not cause oedema despite considerable sodium retention. It seems that aldosterone secretion aggravates the tendency to oedema rather than producing it initially.[24]

Pregnancy. Retention of fluid over and above that required for the uterine contents is normal in pregnancy, and in some women is manifest as oedema of the ankles and occasionally of a more generalised distribution.[25, 26] Oedema is also a feature of pre-eclampsia, and is accompanied by hypertension and proteinuria.

Unexplained oedema. Generalised oedema sometimes occurs in the absence of any known cause, and although such cases are uncommon, they indicate that factors other than those already discussed may operate even in the common types of oedema.

A well-recognised condition is *cyclical*, or *periodic*, *oedema*,[*] in which there are recurrent attacks of oedema involving skin, mucous membranes, joints, or even internal organs, e.g. the brain. In some cases the oedema is widespread and the attacks so severe that the loss of fluid and plasma proteins from the circulation can lead to hypovolaemic shock and death.[30] Usually, however, the area involved is more localised. Thus, one patient is recorded as having pain and swelling of the left hand on alternate Wednesdays, lasting one week, for 18 years.[31] The immediate cause of the oedema appears to be an increase in vascular permeability, and both hereditary factors and allergy[32] have been blamed. Cyclical oedema is more common in women and is often related to the menstrual cycle; attacks may cease after the menopause.[33]

In the familial variety of *angio-oedema* the C1 esterase inhibitor is either absent[34] or present in an abnormal and inert form.[35] The inhibitor is present in normal people, and is presumably important in preventing the unwanted activation of the complement system with the production of permeability factors (p. 81). Another consideration is that the C1 esterase inhibitor also inhibits the capacity of activated Hageman factor to convert kallikreinogen to kallikrein and plasminogen proactivator to activator. It also directly inhibits kallikrein, plasmin, and plasma thromboplastin antecedent (factor XI). The acute attacks are probably related to activation of Hageman factor but the precipitating cause remains obscure.[36]

It is normal for there to be some salt and water retention during the premenstrual phase, but this is not associated with a change in vascular permeability.[37] It is also found that psychological factors may influence electrolyte and water balance both in the normal individual[38] and in those with congestive heart failure.[39] Hypnosis has been used to treat "allergic" diseases, like asthma, and has also been shown to influence the exudative component of the Mantoux test and the P-K reaction.[40] It is evident that the complex relation-

* Other periodic syndromes are also described, e.g. fever, arthrosis, neutropenia, paralysis (familial periodic paralysis), purpura, peritonitis, vomiting, and headaches.[27-29]

TABLE 39.2

	Increased venous pressure	Low plasma proteins	Lymphatic obstruction	Sodium and water retention
Cardiac Oedema	+ +	—	±	+ + + +
Acute Nephritis	+	±	—	+ + +
Nephrotic Syndrome	—	+ + + +	—	+ + + +
Hepatic Oedema (Ascites)	+ (portal hypertension)	+ +	+ + +	+ + + +
Famine Oedema	—	+ +	—	+ +
Adrenal Steroids	±	—	—	+ + +

ships between allergy, vascular permeability, and the nervous system are poorly understood at the present time.

Table 39.2 summarises the main factors in the causation of generalised oedema.

PULMONARY OEDEMA

The hydrostatic balance of the lung capillaries is somewhat different from that of the systemic circulation.

The blood pressure in the pulmonary circuit is about 15–25 mm Hg systolic and 6–12 mm Hg diastolic. The capillary pressure varies from 3–13 mm Hg, being highest at the base and lowest at the apex.

The interstitial fluid pressure is negative due to the elastic recoil of the lungs. The negative intrathoracic pressure is about —10 mm Hg in forced inspiration, and about —5 mm Hg in expiration. Both these forces tend to drive fluid out of the capillaries into the interstitial tissue, from where it escapes with ease into the alveoli.

The plasma and interstitial fluid osmotic pressures are like those elsewhere in the body. It therefore follows that the plasma is kept in the capillaries by the osmotic pressure exerted by the plasma proteins, which is normally more than adequate to cope with the situation. The lungs are "dry"; saline introduced into them is soon absorbed, though serum is removed more slowly.[41]

The capillaries derive their oxygen supply from the alveolar air, and if the alveoli are full of fluid the cells become hypoxic. The vascular permeability increases, and a protein-rich fluid accumulates and spreads to adjacent alveoli both through the pores of Kohn and *via* the alveolar ducts. In this way pulmonary oedema, once formed, spreads rapidly and asphyxiates the patient. Furthermore, the protein-containing fluid favours bacterial proliferation.

Acute fulminating pulmonary oedema is quite common, and whatever the cause, increased vascular permeability increases its extent. The following are important conditions leading to its production:

Heart failure. In left ventricular failure there is a rise in pulmonary venous pressure which presumably leads to the formation of a transudate. Acute pulmonary oedema is a frequent complication of left ventricular failure, and is also common in mitral stenosis. It may occur prior to the fluid retention which is so important in peripheral cardiac oedema. This suggests that a local redistribution of fluid is the basis of acute pulmonary oedema. The back-pressure theory, while intellectually satisfying, is not the whole explanation.

It is probable that peripheral vasoconstriction also plays an important role in precipitating the pulmonary oedema of heart disease.[42] In mitral stenosis and the "low output" failures there is widespread vasoconstriction (see p. 499). It is to be expected that this will lead to the displacement of blood from the systemic to the pulmonary circulations. Support for this contention is provided by the finding that adrenaline has a considerable effect on the pulmonary circulation: there is a moderate rise in pulmonary arterial pressure, and the pulmonary blood flow is greatly increased.[42] Acute pulmonary oedema is a well-known hazard of adrenaline administration, and it is relieved by the ganglion-blocking drugs which cause systemic vasodilatation.[43]

In the dramatic paroxysmal dyspnoea, which is described on page 503, there is a rise in blood pressure and systemic vasoconstriction. It may well be that the attack is precipitated by a raised pulmonary venous pressure accentuated during recumbency (the pulmonary blood flow is greater in the horizontal than in the upright position), and that it is continued by the adrenaline secreted as the result of fear and anxiety. This would explain the ameliorative effects of cerebral depressants like morphine and anaesthetics, and the lethal effect of adrenaline. Once the acute stage is survived, the oedema is rapidly removed *via* the pulmonary lymphatics which are very extensive. There are none in the alveolar walls, but they commence in the ducts and form large channels in the peri-bronchial tissue. In due course the situation is further remedied by constriction of the pulmonary arterioles, which limits the pulmonary blood flow, and by a thickening of the connective tissue around the alveolar capillaries, which impedes the outward flow of plasma to the alveoli.

The oedema of the lungs that follows overloading of the circulation with intravenous saline solutions is no doubt attributable to left ventricular failure. Clinically the danger of blood transfusions and other intravenous therapy in patients with heart failure is well known.

Withdrawal of effusions. Pulmonary oedema may follow the aspiration of fluid or air from a pleural cavity. This hazard is most likely to follow the rapid removal of a large amount of fluid or air that has been present for at least a few days. The oedema is often confined to the lobe rendered airless by the compression of the fluid, and it usually resolves quite rapidly. Less often it becomes widespread and may cause death. The mechanism of this pulmonary oedema is obscure. It may be that the prolonged collapse and airlessness leads to a deficiency of surfactant, and when there is a sudden increase in negative intrathoracic pressure following the aspiration, the lungs re-expand less easily. The trauma incurred may engender leakage of fluid from the pulmonary capillaries into the connective tissue and the alveolar spaces. A similar effect may follow the removal of a massive ascites. Clearly all large effusions should be drained slowly, especially if they are chronic.[44]

Cerebral damage. It is apparent from the above discussion that neurogenic factors play an important part in pulmonary oedema. A fulminating oedema, rich in protein, occurs in rats and rabbits when a fibrin-forming mixture is injected into the basal cisternae. If the animal is vagotomised beforehand no pulmonary oedema forms, and it appears that the permeability of the lung capillaries is affected by an outflow of stimuli from the brain stem *via* the vagus nerves.[45] The nature of the reflex is obscure.

Pulmonary oedema is seen occasionally in patients with head injuries and lesions involving the hind-brain. It is also a dangerous complication of neurosurgery. These conditions are attended by peripheral vasoconstriction (the animals mentioned above also have systemic hypertension and a raised right atrial pressure), and it is probable that sympathetic overaction is an important factor.[46, 47] As already described, it leads to pulmonary displacement of blood. Local alterations in the pulmonary blood vessels are apparently also important, for the oedema is sometimes sharply confined to one lung or even one lobe.[48]

Experimentally pulmonary oedema can be produced by the administration of large doses of adrenaline, the induction of prolonged hypoglycaemia (which probably acts by adrenaline release), and the infliction of cerebral trauma of various kinds. Cerebral depressant drugs and sympathetic inhibitors ameliorate the effects of these experiments. Even in phosgene poisoning, where there is a primary action on the vascular endothelium of the lung, these drugs are helpful; this suggests an additional neurogenic factor in phosgene poisoning.

Acute inflammation. Acute pulmonary oedema was a notorious feature of the 1918 influenza pandemic, during which over 15 million people died of this dread complication. It is also encountered from time to time in fulminating bronchopneumonia due to *Strept. pyogenes*, *B. anthracis*, and *Y. (Past.) pestis*.

Irritant gases, e.g. nitrous fumes, chlorine, and phosgene, produce a similar fulminating oedema. Some chemicals after absorption, e.g. thiourea derivatives, like α-naphthyl thiourea used as a rat-poison, also produce pulmonary oedema.[49] It may follow radiotherapy to the chest.

Other conditions. Pulmonary oedema is also seen in uraemia, where it has a peculiarly fibrinous consistency, and in many terminal conditions, where it is probably due to heart failure. High concentrations of oxygen, when breathed for long periods especially if under high pressure, may also precipitate it. Even at a partial pressure of one atmosphere, an exposure to pure oxygen for 6–30 hours can produce toxic effects in some individuals. The lungs become inelastic, congested, oedematous, and haemorrhagic, and show hyaline-membrane formation. These changes are not specific and are similar to those produced by other factors, e.g. heart failure and shock. Nevertheless, an increased partial pressure of oxygen appears to be toxic to the lung, and can add to the respiratory difficulties of a critically ill patient, especially if on a respirator.[50, 51]

Acute pulmonary oedema is an occasional complication of "mountain fever", and is seen in mountaineers, often the young and healthy members of a party, who climb too high too fast.[52] It occurs between 12 and 72 hours after going above 9 000 feet. The pathogenesis is uncertain. Hypoxia is certainly involved, and it may cause capillary damage in the lungs directly. It also leads to a lowering of the arterial PCO_2, which induces peripheral vasoconstriction causing deviation of blood from the peripheral circularion to the pulmonary bed. Exposure to cold has a similar effect. High-altitude pulmonary oedema is becoming more common in these days of rapid, cheap air travel, and is seen in tourists as well as soldiers engaged in manoeuvres in mountainous areas.

Conclusions

In pulmonary oedema there is always an accumulation of a fluid of high protein content, indicating a change in vascular permeability. Although the explanation of the oedema may sometimes appear obvious, as in phosgene poisoning, in many instances the mechanism is obscure. A nervous reflex causing peripheral vasoconstriction may well be of great importance. When once oedema has commenced, the resulting deprivation of oxygen supply explains its rapid spread and high protein content.

REFERENCES

1. STARLING, E. H. (1896). *Journal of Physiology (London)*, **19**, 312.
2. LANDIS, E. M. (1927). *American Journal of Physiology*, **82**, 217.
3. LANDIS, E. M. *et al.* (1932). *Journal of Clinical Investigation*, **11**, 717.
4. LANDIS, E. M. (1928). *American Journal of Physiology*, **83**, 528.
5. JAYSON, M. I. V. and BARKS, J. S. (1971). *British Medical Journal*, ii, 555.

6. Leading Article (1963). *British Medical Journal*, ii, 1483.
7. KINMONTH, J. B. *et al.* (1957). *British Journal of Surgery*, **45,** 1.
8. MILROY, W. F. (1892). *New York Medical Journal*, **56,** 505.
9. Leading Article (1972). *British Medical Journal*, iv, 130.
10. SCHREIBER, S. S. *et al.* (1954). *Journal of Clinical Investigation*, **33,** 578.
11. ALTSCHULE, M. D. (1938). *Medicine (Baltimore)*, **17,** 75.
12. WOOD, P. (1968). *Diseases of the Heart and Circulation*, 3rd edn, p. 319. London: Eyre and Spottiswoode.
13. RAY, C. T. and BURCH, G. (1947). *Archives of Internal Medicine*, **80,** 587.
14. McMASTER, P. D. (1937). *Journal of Experimental Medicine*, **65,** 373.
15. MAXWELL, M. H., BREED, E. S. and SCHWARTZ, I. L. (1950). *Journal of Clinical Investigation*, **29,** 342.
16. THOMPSON, D. D. and PITTS, R. F. (1952). *American Journal of Physiology*, **168,** 490.
17. BROD, J. (1972). *British Medical Journal*, i, 222.
18. DE WARDENER, H. E. *et al.* (1961). *Clinical Science*, **21,** 249.
19. MILLS, I. H. *et al.* (1961). *Clinical Science*, **21,** 259.
20. GARNETT, E. S. and WEBBER, C. E. (1967). *Lancet*, ii, 798.
21. PASSMORE, R. and DRAPER, M. H. (1964). In *Biochemical Disorders in Human Disease*, 2nd edn, pp. 24 and 34. Edited by R. H. S. Thompson and E. J. King. London: Churchill.
22. EALES, L. (1961). In *Recent Advances in Human Nutrition*, p. 198. Edited by J. F. Brock. London: Churchill.
23. HANSEN, J. D. L. (1961). In *Recent Advances in Human Nutrition*, p. 267, *loc. cit.*
24. LUETSCHER, J. A. (1967). In *The Adrenal Cortex*, p. 646–650. Edited by A. B. Eisenstein. London: Churchill.
25. Leading Article (1967). *British Medical Journal*, iii, 3.
26. Leading Article (1967). *Lancet*, ii, 197.
27. Leading Article (1963). *Lancet*, ii, 563.
28. CULLEN, K. J. and MACDONALD, W. B. (1963). *Medical Journal of Australia*, **2,** 167
29. REIMANN, H. A. (1962). *American Journal of Medical Science*, **243,** 727.
30. CLARKSON, B. *et al.* (1960). *American Journal of Medicine*, **29,** 193.
31. ABBOTT, W. D. (1933). *Journal of the American Medical Association*, **100,** 1328.
32. WEINBREN, I. (1963). *Lancet*, ii, 544.
33. THORN, G. W. (1957). *American Journal of Medicine*, **23,** 507.
34. DONALDSON, V. H. and EVANS, R. R. (1963). *American Journal of Medicine*, **35,** 37.
35. ROSEN, F. S. *et al.* (1965). *Science*, **148,** 957.
36. ROSEN, F. S. and AUSTEN, K. F. (1969). *New England Journal of Medicine*, **280,** 1356.
37. ROGERS, J. (1958). *New England Journal of Medicine*, **259,** 676.
38. SCHOTTSTAEDT, W. W. *et al.* (1958). *American Journal of Medicine*, **25,** 248.
39. BARNES, R. and SCHOTTSTAEDT, W. W. (1960). *American Journal of Medicine*, **29,** 217.
40. Annotation (1963). *British Medical Journal*, i, 968.
41. COURTICE, F. C. and PHIPPS, P. J. (1946). *Journal of Physiology (London)*, **105,** 186.
42. HARRIS, P. and HEATH, D. (1962). *The Human Pulmonary Circulation*, pp. 235 and 116. Edinburgh: Livingstone.
43. SARNOFF, S. J., GOODALE, W. T. and SARNOFF, L. C. (1952). *Circulation*, **6,** 63.
44. TRAPNELL, D. H. and THURSTON, J. G. B. (1970). *Lancet*, i, 1367.
45. CAMERON, G. R. and DE, S. N. (1949). *Journal of Pathology and Bacteriology*, **61,** 375.
46. SARNOFF, S. J. and SARNOFF, L. C. (1952). *Circulation*, **6,** 51.
47. SARNOFF, S. J., BERGLUND, E. and SARNOFF, L. C. (1953). *Journal of Applied Physiology*, **5,** 367.
48. RICHARDS, P. (1963). *Brtish Medical Journal*, ii, 83.
49. ROBERTS, K. B. (1970). In *General Pathology*, 4th edn, p. 391. Edited by H. W. Florey. London: Lloyd-Luke.
50. NASH, G., BLENNERHASSETT, J. B. and PONTOPPIDAN, H. (1967). *New England Journal of Medicine*, **276,** 368.
51. HEDLEY-WHYTE, J. (1970). *New England Journal of Medicine*, **283,** 1518.
52. Leading Article (1972). *British Medical Journal*, iii, 65.

Chapter 40. Heart Failure

Heart failure may be defined as a condition where the output of the heart is insufficient to meet the demands of the tissues, despite satisfactory venous filling.[1] This definition serves to eliminate extracardiac circulatory failure due to haemorrhage and vasovagal syncope. It also excludes constrictive pericarditis and cardiac tamponade, conditions in which the failure in the circulation is due to impaired atrial filling as the result of external compression.

The normal cardiac output at rest is 4·5–5 litres per minute. Since the heart can normally expel all the venous blood reaching it, it follows that the cardiac output is determined by the venous return. This is the volume of blood draining all the tissues and organs of the body, and is itself directly related to their arterial blood supply. The blood supply of a tissue is determined mainly by the local autoregulatory mechanisms.[2] The cardiac output is therefore governed by extracardiac factors, namely the metabolic requirements of the body as a whole. Thus the cardiac output can be increased four-fold during strenuous exercise. Indeed, a young man can increase his cardiac output to about 25 litres per minute in steady, severe exertion.

The range of the normal systemic blood pressure at rest is $\frac{120–150 \text{ mm Hg systolic}}{60–90 \text{ mm Hg diastolic}}$, and a reading above 150/90 is suggestive of systemic hypertension, especially in a young person. The range of "normal" blood pressures is, however, wide, and a figure above 180/110 would be considered more indicative of systemic hypertension in an elderly subject.

By the time the blood reaches the capillaries the pressure has dropped to 32 mm Hg, and on the venous side it is about 12 mm Hg (these figures refer to a capillary at heart level). There is a steady drop in the venous circulation. Measurements of blood pressure in the chambers of the right side of the heart and the pulmonary circulation are obtained during cardiac catheterisation.[3] Cardiologists measure these pressures at a point somewhere near the centre of the heart, e.g. 5 cm below the sternal angle with the patient lying recumbent. Under these conditions the right atrial pressure averages 4 mm Hg, and the right ventricular pressure 24/4 mm Hg. The pulmonary arterial pressure averages 24/10 mm Hg, and a figure over 30/15 mm Hg indicates pulmonary hypertension. The left atrial pressure averages 7 mm Hg, which is about 10 mm Hg lower than the pulmonary arterial pressure.

The normal heart rate is about 70 beats per minute, and the normal stroke volume about 70 ml per beat. The ventricles do not empty completely with each beat, and there is a residual volume of about 50 ml; the ventricular end-diastolic volume is therefore about 120 ml.[4]

THE MECHANISM OF HEART FAILURE[1]

There are two classical approaches to heart failure:

The back-pressure theory of James Hope (1832), which attributes failure to an inadequate discharge of blood from the ventricles. The accumulation of blood behind them leads to atrial and venous engorgement.

The forward-failure theory of James Mackenzie (1913), which states that the heart fails as a whole, so that there is insufficient propulsion of blood from behind.

In fact there is a great deal of truth in both these concepts, which can usefully be combined. Most of the pathological effects of heart failure are due to forward failure, which is the basis of *stagnant hypoxia*, i.e. hypoxia due to an inadequate blood supply consequent on a poor cardiac output, while most of the signs and symptoms of heart failure, e.g. engorged jugular veins, hepatomegaly, and peripheral oedema, are due in no small measure to the effects of venous back-pressure.

THE CAUSES OF HEART FAILURE

An inadequate cardiac output occurs under the following three circumstances:

Overburdening due to a sustained increase in ventricular pressure. This occurs in systemic (and pulmonary) hypertension and valvular stenosis and regurgitation. In such conditions the heart has progressively greater difficulty in maintaining a normal output, and eventually a state of *low output failure* results.[5] In order to conserve the blood as efficiently as possible, there is peripheral vasoconstriction with a small thready pulse.

Overburdening due to a sustained increase in cardiac output. There is a group of widely diverse conditions which have one feature in common: the necessity for an increased cardiac output to supply the demands of the tissues. The cardiac output may rise to 10 litres per minute at rest, and eventually the heart fails under the strain. Such conditions are:

Anaemia, where under the stress of anaemic hypoxia the tissues need more blood.

Thyrotoxicosis, where the metabolic needs of the tissues are increased.

Arteriovenous fistulae, which shunt so much blood that only a greater cardiac output can meet the demands of the deprived area of tissue.

Chronic pulmonary heart disease ("cor pulmonale") where there is hypoxic hypoxia, and also possibly a pulmonary-bronchial arterial anastomosis that acts as a shunt.

Extensive Paget's disease of bone, where there are innumerable arteriovenous shunts in the affected bones, which are extremely vascular.[6]

Generalised erythrodermas, e.g. exfoliative dermatitis and erythrodermic psoriasis.[7, 8]

Advanced liver disease. Anastomoses between the portal and pulmonary veins *via* the azygos and bronchial veins have been demonstrated. The failure of detoxification of a vaso-depressor substance has also been suggested.[9]

Beri-beri. The cause is not known.

All these conditions are associated with a hyperkinetic circulatory state: the hands are warm, the pulses throbbing, and the forearm veins distended. This is *high output failure*.[5] Though the cardiac output is raised relative to the normal, it is still insufficient to meet the demands of the body.

Although it is often easy enough to explain the vasodilatation on a teleological basis, i.e. in terms of an increased demand for blood due to hypoxia or greater tissue metabolism, it must be admitted that there is considerable ignorance about the actual reflexes brought into action to produce it. Furthermore, while it is understandable that there should be local vasodilatation in a limb with a large arteriovenous fistula, so that as much blood as possible may pass the shunt and reach the tissues peripheral to it, it is less understandable why there should also be generalised vasodilatation.

Myocardial disease. This may be *hypoxic*, as in anaemia and ischaemia due to coronary-artery disease, or hypotension occurring in shock, *metabolic*, as in amyloidosis, myxoedema, and glycogen-storage disease, *toxic*, as in diphtheria, or due to a *specific myocardial lesion*, e.g. acute rheumatic fever, virus myocarditis, systemic lupus erythematosus, and tumours of the heart. Into this last group fall the *cardiomyopathies*,[10] in which there is cardiac enlargement and eventual failure in the absence of obvious valvular, coronary, or specific myocardial disease. In some cases there is subvalvular stenosis, usually aortic, and in these as well as in some without outflow obstruction there is a familial tendency. Endomyocardial fibrosis is common in East Africa, but its cause is unknown. Cardiomyopathy occurs in chronic alcoholics;[11] its pathogenesis may be related to the cardiac effects of beri-beri. Some cases have been attributed to cobalt poisoning following the addition of cobalt salts to beer during its manufacture.[12] But there is, in addition, both clinical and experimental evidence that alcohol has a directly damaging effect on the myocardium. Most of these cases are well nourished, and respond to bed rest with abstinence from alcohol.[13]

Myocardial disease is by far the most important cause of heart failure. It often acts with the other two factors, e.g. in syphilitic aortic regurgitation there may be myocardial ischaemia due to occlusion of the coronary ostia, and in hypertensive heart disease there is often ischaemia due to coronary-artery disease.

The contributory factors to a state of heart failure include *anxiety*, which raises the heart rate and blood pressure, *exertion* and *infection*, which increase the cardiac output, and *pregnancy*, which increases the strain on the heart as the result of an increased blood volume. *Arrhythmias* are also important. Those that cause tachycardia interfere with diastolic filling and the coronary blood flow, while those that cause marked bradycardia decrease the cardiac output directly.

Sometimes the brunt falls on the left side of the heart, e.g. in systemic hypertension and aortic-valve disease, and then the condition is called *left ventricular failure*. Less often the right side is first affected, e.g. in pulmonary stenosis and pulmonary hypertension, and this is called *right ventricular failure*. Most commonly the heart fails as a whole (this occurs in myocardial disease), and *congestive cardiac failure* ensues. Left ventricular failure eventually progresses to congestive cardiac failure if the patient survives long enough.

THE EFFECTS OF HEART FAILURE[1]

The effect of forward-failure, i.e. an inadequate cardiac output, is that some organs obtain an insufficient blood supply. The arteriovenous oxygen difference (normally 50 ml per litre) is increased, as more oxygen is extracted by the tissues in order to obtain their necessary supply. This leads to a reduction of the tissue oxygen tension, and the resulting hypoxia is called "stagnant hypoxia". If the blood supply is further diminished, the actual amount of oxygen available to the tissues becomes so inadequate that its quantity as well as its tension is reduced. Degenerative changes culminating in necrosis then occur.

Not all organs suffer equally.

The cerebral circulation is maintained at a volume near normal. Terminally it may decrease enough to cause symptoms.

The coronary blood flow is also well maintained until terminally. Severe arrhythmias, e.g. paroxysmal atrial or ventricular tachycardia, endanger this circulation. Severe systemic hypotension has the same effect.

The renal blood flow can drop from 1·1 litre to about 0·5 litre per minute, and the glomerular filtration rate from 120 ml to 70 ml per minute. These effects are the result of arteriolar vasoconstriction. Diuresis is preceded by an increase in the renal flow, which may be independent of any change in cardiac output.

The hepatic blood flow is normally about 1·5 litre per minute, and is reduced in proportion to the reduction of cardiac output. The stagnant hypoxia is most severe in the peripheral areas of the acini of the liver, and it is here that the most marked changes occur (see p. 505).

Blood flow to the extremities. Peripheral vasoconstriction causes a reduction in blood flow; the skin then becomes pale and cold. In vascular areas like the lips and face the effect of stagnant hypoxia on the dammed-up venous blood often produces visible cyanosis (of the peripheral type).

As has already been noted, these changes are seen in the low output type of heart failure but not in the high output type. Here there is generalised vasodilatation, which is still insufficient to meet the tissues' demands.

The effects of back-pressure. The rise in ventricular diastolic pressure causes a corresponding rise in the left atrial and pulmonary venous pressures in left ventricular failure. Similarly the rise in right ventricular pressure raises the systemic venous pressure, and leads to liver engorgement.

The pulmonary symptoms of left ventricular failure are due largely to venous engorgement, and the peripheral oedema of congestive cardiac failure owes its situation to the effects of an increased venous pressure.

A very important factor in heart failure is the early rise in blood volume discussed in Chapter 39. It is related to increased salt and water retention by the kidneys.

THE CARDIAC RESERVES[1]

Despite an organic lesion of the heart, the individual may not only have a normal cardiac output at rest, but also be able to undertake moderate exercise with ease. This is the state of *compensation*, when with the aid of the cardiac reserves, a damaged heart can supply an output of blood which is sufficient to meet the tissues' needs even during exercise. In due course the reserves may fail and exercise tolerance becomes poorer and poorer. Eventually with all the reserves utilised the cardiac output is only just adequate at rest. This is the state of total *decompensation*, and the patient is in the terminal stages of heart failure.

There are four cardiac reserves:

The strength of the cardiac contraction. Despite the *all-or-none law* of cardiac contraction, the heart as a whole can nevertheless beat more vigorously to meet an extra load. The intrinsic state of the muscle may change from beat to beat, e.g. increased sympathetic tone strengthens the cardiac contraction and increased vagal tone weakens it. This adrenergic activity is the first reserve, and it comes into play at once during exercise to increase the ventricular emptying. The effect of digitalis on the heart muscle is still not understood, but it presumably increases the strength of contraction.[14]

Cardiac hypertrophy. This is a long-term method of increasing the strength of contraction. The muscle fibres increase in size, but not in number. Unfortunately, there is no increase in the number of capillaries supplying each muscle fibre, and the enlarged heart eventually suffers from ischaemia.[15]

Increased heart rate. The cardiac output rises with an increase in rate until a critical speed is reached (180 beats per minute). As most of the ventricular filling occurs in early diastole, a moderate tachycardia does not interfere much with the stroke volume.[16] At great rates, however, the shortness of diastole does interfere with ventricular filling, and furthermore, the coronary blood flow, which is mostly diastolic, is impaired. Finally, the mechanical efficiency of the heart itself declines. Acting together with increased adrenergic activity, which strengthens the cardiac contraction, an increased heart rate is the main mechanism whereby the cardiac output is increased in exercise. It also comes into play in most cardiac conditions.

Increased filling pressure and cardiac dilatation. According to *Starling's "Law of the Heart"*, the energy of contraction is proportional to the initial length of the cardiac muscle fibres.[17] This means that the increase in stroke volume that follows an increased filling pressure depends on the degree to which the ventricular muscle is stretched at the end of diastole. There is a critical point beyond which any further dilatation of the ventricles results in a fall of output. In a classical graph (Starling) the resting cardiac output is plotted against the central venous filling pressure (this is the right atrial pressure minus the negative intrathoracic pressure). Ascent represents compensation, and descent decompensation (Fig. 40.1).

Starling's Law has been accepted as a significant factor in the normal heart.[18] Refined radiographic techniques have demonstrated an increase in the end-diastolic volume of the exercising heart. In exercise the stroke volume can double itself—this is due both to the increased end-diastolic volume and to a reduction of the residual volume.[18] The effects of exercise are an increased heart rate (to about $2\frac{1}{2}$ times the normal) and a 5-fold rise in cardiac output.[4, 18]

But it is in heart failure that Starling's Law is especially important. The failing heart resembles a heart-lung preparation more closely inasmuch as the reserves of rate and autonomic stimulation are already in operation and are proving inadequate. It is at this point that an increased central venous pressure becomes vitally important (see Fig. 40.2).[19]

The central venous pressure may rise under the following conditions:

(*a*) When there is an increased back-pressure behind a raised ventricular diastolic pressure, as previously described. The obstruction behind a stenosed mitral valve has a similar effect.

(*b*) When the blood volume is increased. This occurs in heart failure.

(*c*) A primary reflex venoconstriction stimulated as a compensatory mechanism has been suggested, but as yet there is no direct evidence to support it.[20, 21]

Beyond a critical point, the ventricle cannot respond to an increase in filling pressure by an increase in output; distension

Figure 40.1
Relationship of cardiac output to
venous filling pressure (Starling's
curve). *(From Paul Wood (1956),
Diseases of the Heart and Circulation,
2nd ed. London : Eyre and Spottiswoode)*

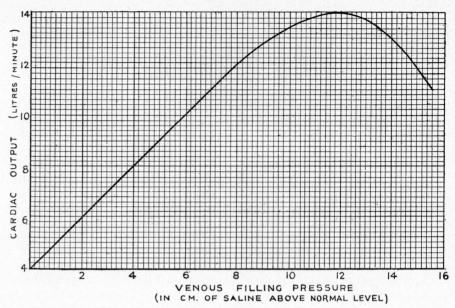

Figure 40.1
Relationship of cardiac output to
venous filling pressure (Starling's
curve). *(From Paul Wood (1956),
Diseases of the Heart and Circulation,
2nd ed. London : Eyre and Spottiswoode)*

actually decreases the cardiac output. The diastolic volume
and pressure rise, and the venous pressure increases. This is
decompensation, and it may be precipitated by sodium and
water retention. It is easy to understand how a therapeutic
venesection could relieve congestive failure at this stage.

To summarise, the main reserve of a failing heart is a
raised central venous filling pressure acting to increase the
stroke volume. Autonomic influences on the strength of
contraction and tachycardia are important at first, but as
these mechanisms fail to be effective, they later play only a
subsidiary part. Hypertrophy is a long-term matter. It is
worth noting that an increased central venous pressure leads
to tachycardia due to the atrial reflex of Bainbridge. Fig.

40.2, summarises the cardiac reserves during exercise and in
states of high and low output.

LEFT VENTRICULAR FAILURE

The most important causes are:

Systemic hypertension.
Aortic stenosis or regurgitation.
Mitral regurgitation.
Myocardial ischaemia (including infarction, which nearly
always involves the left ventricle).
Coarctation of the aorta.
Finally, it occurs as a part of *congestive cardiac failure.*

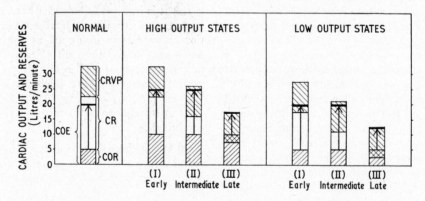

Figure 40.2
In the normal individual the resting cardiac output (COR) is shown as 5 litres/min. Severe exercise, depicted by the arrow, increases
this to 20 litres/min. (COE) by utilising especially those cardiac reserves not involving an increase in venous pressure (CR). The reserve of increased venous pressure (CRVP) is not greatly used under physiological conditions.

In a high output state, the cardiac output at rest is shown as 10 litres/min., and on severe exercise the reserve of increased venous
pressure must be utilised (I); this causes symptoms. The other cardiac reserves fail, and symptoms occur on even modest exercise (II).
Finally, the venous pressure is raised even at rest and severe exercise is no longer possible (III).

In low output states the reduction in those cardiac reserves not involving a venous pressure rise (e.g. due to myocardial damage)
necessitates the increase in venous pressure to attain a satisfactory cardiac output. At first this occurs only on severe exercise (I), but
later as the reserves fail, symptoms occur on modest exercise (II), and finally at rest (III)

Morbid Physiology

When the left ventricle fails to discharge its contents adequately, the cardiac output tends to fall. The diastolic pressure rises, and this is followed by an increase of pressure in the left atrium and pulmonary veins. A similar rise in pressure occurs in mitral stenosis, where the cause is an obstruction at the entrance of the left ventricle, and not a failure of the ventricle itself. The rise in pulmonary venous pressure is extremely serious because of the imminent danger of acute pulmonary oedema (see Chapter 39): a pressure above 35 mm Hg is dangerous to life. It is not uncommon for patients with mitral stenosis to experience attacks of pulmonary oedema quite early in the course of the malady. These are usually precipitated by exertion and emotion, and may be fatal. Later on, both in left ventricular failure and mitral stenosis the pulmonary circulation is made more capable of accommodating the dammed-up blood. This appears to be brought about by a redistribution of the total blood volume, more of which is held in the lungs, and less in the systemic circulation than before.[22] In left ventricular failure the increased diastolic stretch engendered by the raised pulmonary venous and ventricular diastolic pressures may increase the left ventricular output for a time, and so balance the ouputs of the two ventricles. This balance is always precarious, and as the left ventricle fails, the danger of pulmonary oedema increases.

In due course more far-reaching mechanisms come into play, whereby the amount of blood entering the lung is reduced:

(*a*) There is a rise in pulmonary arterial pressure due to active arteriolar vasoconstriction. In this way the amount of blood entering the lungs is decreased, the venous pressure tends to fall, and the risk of oedema is obviated.

(*b*) There may be a shift of the interventricular septum, so that the right ventricle is somewhat occluded. In this way less blood enters it. This is called the *Bernheim effect*,[23] and although it is sometimes a prominent *post-mortem* finding, opinions vary as to its importance in reducing the pulmonary blood flow.

The first mechanism leads to secondary pulmonary hypertension; in mitral stenosis high pressures are common. Although this succeeds in protecting the patient from the immediate danger of pulmonary oedema, it soon leads to right ventricular failure. Systemic venous congestion ensues. But it is worth noting that the increased central venous filling pressure acts to increase the cardiac output to near normal levels.[24]

Clinical Features of Left Ventricular Failure

Undue breathlessness of effort. This is due to the pulmonary venous congestion decreasing the compliance of the lungs. Breathing is therefore rendered more arduous. It is not due to carbon dioxide retention or arterial hypoxia.

Orthopnoea. The patient breathes most comfortably in the upright position. When he is recumbent, the vital capacity is reduced due to the elevation of the diaphragm. Furthermore, the right atrial pressure is increased by the inflow of blood from the lower parts of the body, because the effect of gravity is minimised in the recumbent posture. There is a corresponding increase in the output of the right ventricle, and more blood reaches the left atrium. The left atrial pressure rises accordingly. The inadequate left ventricle does not respond properly by increasing its output. Pulmonary engorgement and dyspnoea, which are already present, are further aggravated.

Paroxysmal (nocturnal) dyspnoea. The patient wakes up breathless in the early hours of the morning with a sense of oppression in the chest. He sits up, but the dyspnoea increases. Increasing restlessness drives him out of bed to seek the fresh air at the window. The sense of suffocation becomes intense and with it there is profound distress. The skin has an ashen cyanosis; sweat breaks out and is profuse. The patient may cough up blood-stained sputum, and in severe cases profuse pulmonary oedema develops with dramatic suddenness. The blood pressure is raised at first, but as pulmonary oedema develops both the breathing and the pulse weaken, and death finally ensues.

The complete explanation of this paroxysmal dyspnoea is not known. During the attack the jugular venous pressure, the systemic blood pressure, and the cardiac output are all raised. One possible explanation is that the ambulant cardiac patient already has oedema of the legs. When he retires to bed, the fluid is absorbed. The pulmonary oedema might therefore be due to a sudden increase in blood volume, similar to that seen after the administration of excessive saline infusions. Dependent oedema is not, however, a feature of left ventricular failure. Another explanation is sudden imbalance between the outputs of the two ventricles. This is rather begging the question, since the cause of the hypothetical imbalance is unknown.

It is very probable that a neurogenic factor is involved, because there is usually dramatic relief after the administration of morphine, which is the specific treatment of this emergency (see p. 496).

Finally, bronchospasm is often a marked feature of left ventricular failure, and when this element of spasm is prominent, the condition is called *cardiac asthma*. It is important to distinguish it clinically from bronchial asthma, because morphine is detrimental in the bronchial type, while adrenaline is often fatal in the cardiac type.

X-ray signs. The hilar fan-shaped shadow of pulmonary congestion and oedema is characteristic. Bilateral hydrothorax is common, and usually more marked on the left side.

Other signs. There is a prolongation of the pulmonary circulation time. The arm-tongue time (normally 9–18 seconds) is increased to about 30 seconds in left heart failure. This test is performed by injecting saccharin into an arm vein, and noting the time taken before the substance is tasted in the tongue.

The other manifestations of left ventricular failure, e.g.

Cheyne-Stokes respiration, gallop rhythm, and pulsus alternans, are dealt with in physiology text-books. Indeed, there is no satisfactory explanation of the various types of gallop rhythm.

RIGHT VENTRICULAR FAILURE

There is a rise of pressure in the right atrium and the venae cavae. This is manifested by general venous engorgement and an enlarged, tender liver.

Sometimes the failure is primarily right-sided as in pulmonary hypertension secondary to *lung disease*, e.g. pulmonary fibrosis due to tuberculosis, pneumoconiosis, or bronchopneumonia, and also chronic bronchitis and emphysema; *massive pulmonary embolism*; *multiple emboli* composed of blood clot, tumour, or schistosomal parasites; *post-pneumonectomy*; and finally as an idiopathic condition called *primary pulmonary hypertension*.

It may also be due to certain congenital heart lesions, notably pulmonary stenosis and atrial septal defect.

The commonest cause, however, is as a secondary event in left ventricular failure and mitral stenosis.

In conditions in which the heart fails as a whole, e.g. high output failure and myocarditis, there is a prominent right-sided element.

Where there is a combined left- and right-sided failure, the condition is called *congestive cardiac failure*. In fact, pure right-sided failure is uncommon; in most chronic lung diseases there is high output failure as well as pulmonary hypertension.

Features

Elevated venous pressure is a most important sign. The pressure may be normal at rest, but with exercise it rises. Normally the jugular venous pressure falls on exertion, because there is a lowered mean intrathoracic pressure due to the increased ventilation.

Enlargement and tenderness of the liver. This is due to chronic venous congestion. Liver function tests show no abnormality other than a slight rise in serum bilirubin.[25] The spleen is slightly enlarged in congestive cardiac failure, but it is rarely clinically palpable. Jaundice occasionally occurs in heart failure complicated by extensive pulmonary infarction, when there is a vigorous breakdown of haemolysed red cells in the lung.

Oedema. The extent of cardiac oedema is very variable. As noted in Chapter 39, the important factor in its production is fluid retention, and its site is related to the raised venous pressure acting with gravity. Hydrothorax, often right-sided, is a frequent accompaniment; ascites is rare except in tricuspid valve lesions and constrictive pericarditis.

Other Features include:

Cerebral effects, e.g. fatigue, confusion, and impaired ability to concentrate. These are terminal features due to an impaired cerebral blood flow.

Renal effects. There is moderate oliguria. The urine is of high specific gravity, for the concentrating ability of the kidney is good. The blood urea is seldom raised except terminally. There is often slight proteinuria.

Venous thrombosis is a common complication of heart failure (see Chapter 35). Pulmonary infarction is the result of subsequent embolism.

Haematological effects. There is a depression of the ESR, the cause of which is unknown. This occurs even during the course of an inflammatory condition, e.g. acute rheumatic fever.[26] The peripheral blood sometimes contains nucleated red cells, perhaps due to the effect of hypoxia on the bone marrow.

Metabolic effects. The BMR is raised by about 20 per cent; the cause of this is unknown. Some patients with long-standing cardiac disease develop "cardiac cachexia". This may be due to the combined effects of a raised BMR and a poor dietary intake due to anorexia.

MORBID ANATOMY OF HEART FAILURE

Acute Left Ventricular Failure

The lungs are deeply congested and the alveoli contain a variable amount of serous fluid. Sometimes this oedema is so marked that the lungs have a solid consistency resembling the consolidation of pneumonia, but usually they are bulky and crepitant, and on pressure exude an abundant blood-stained, frothy fluid. The basal parts of the lung show the severest change. Bronchopneumonia may be superadded at a later stage (see p. 226). The mechanism of pulmonary oedema is considered in Chapter 39.

Chronic Venous Congestion of Lung

This occurs in chronic left ventricular failure and especially in mitral stenosis.[27] The lungs are tougher in consistency than normal, and have a brownish colour. The condition is known as *brown induration of the lungs*. Histologically there are three features:

(1) The alveolar septa are widened as the result of distension of the capillaries with blood.

(2) The septa show a mild increase in connective tissue which contributes to the thickening, and is the cause of the toughness of the lung. It is possible that this fibrous thickening may prevent fluid entering the alveoli, and so diminish the tendency to oedema.[28]

(3) Small haemorrhages are present within the alveoli. Clinically these can be correlated with the frequently occurring haemoptyses that are a feature of the condition. The lungs also show abundant evidence of previous haemorrhage. The alveoli are filled with macrophages containing haemosiderin; it is these "heart-failure cells" which give the lung its brown colour.

It must not be thought that the presence of heart-failure cells is pathognomonic of cardiac disease. They are found wherever haemorrhage has occurred, e.g. around infarcts and tumours. In mitral stenosis the haemosiderosis is sometimes especially well marked, and its focal distribution in groups of alveoli gives a characteristic mottled appearance radiologically.[29]

Finally, the frequent occurrence of pulmonary infarcts in heart failure (especially in mitral stenosis) must be borne in mind.

Congestive Cardiac Failure

The clinical onset of congestive heart failure is a serious event: about 50 per cent of patients will have died within five years.[30] The changes seen in the various organs in congestive cardiac failure are classically described as those of *chronic venous congestion.* However, the decreased blood supply to many of the tissues is of even greater importance than the congestion.

Skin and extremities. The vasoconstriction of low output failure may rarely produce sufficient ischaemia to cause necrosis. "Dry gangrene" may then affect the nose and ears.

This complication is occasionally seen in severe myocardial infarction.

Liver. The *acinus of the liver*, as described by Rappaport,[31] has an arteriole in its centre, and it is the *peripheral zone* which is most hypoxic and shows the most severe damage. The cells undergo degenerative changes and finally die, so that the area is composed of capacious, blood-filled, vascular channels, among which there is often brown pigment derived from the liver cells. An element of venous back-pressure contributes to the congestion. The central area of the acinus is less affected, and merely shows the yellow coloration of

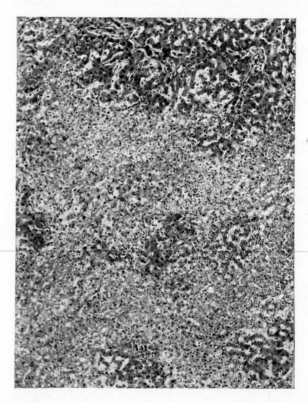

Figure 40.4
Nutmeg liver. In this section many liver cells have disappeared, and are replaced by dilated sinusoids filled with blood. The periportal liver cells show marked degenerative changes. × 90.

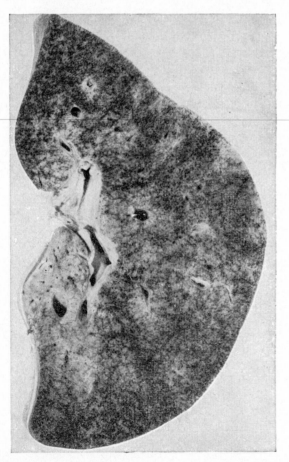

Figure 40.3
Nutmeg liver. The alternating pattern of dark congestion and pale fatty change is apparent. (A 95.2, *Reproduced by permission of the President and Council of the R.C.S. Eng.)*

fatty change. This red and yellow mottling produces the characteristic *nutmeg liver* (Figs. 40.3 and 40.4). It is often debated whether it is the venous back-pressure or the hypoxia which is responsible for the changes of "chronic venous congestion" in the liver. Probably both play a part, for a similar picture can be produced by venous obstruction, e.g. following hepatic-vein thrombosis. The term chronic is not always appropriate, for the appearances of a nutmeg liver can be produced in a few days, e.g. when a patient dies shortly after a myocardial infarct. It should be noted that if the liver is pictured in terms of the classical *lobule*, it is the *central zone* which shows the congestion. However, the concept of the acinus is more helpful in understanding the features of nutmeg liver.

With long-standing disease the liver may show fine fibrosis and even some evidence of regeneration (cardiac cirrhosis),[32] but this is of no great functional significance.

The spleen is slightly enlarged, deeply congested, and resilient (*cyanotic induration of the spleen*). The sinuses are dilated, and their walls somewhat thickened. The congestion is greater, and the fibrosis less, than in the congestive splenomegaly of hepatic cirrhosis.

Kidney. Although changes in renal function appear to play an important part in the causation of cardiac oedema, there is remarkably little to be seen in the way of structural damage. The organ is congested (cyanotic induration), and the tubules may show degenerative changes like cloudy swelling and fatty change. The glomeruli may show mesangial proliferation.

William Harvey, in his grandiloquent dedication of "De Motu Cordis" to King Charles I, describes the heart of animals as "the foundation of their life, the sovereign of everything within them, the sun of their microcosm, that upon which all growth depends, from which all power proceeds" (translated by Robert Willis in 1847).

The pathologist is certainly humiliated when called upon to explain the manifold clinical features of heart failure in terms of the meagre findings noted at necropsy. In few other conditions is the inadequacy of current pathological techniques so apparent. The mysterious feature of heart failure is the progressive nature of the process. There is no satisfactory explanation of why an overburdened heart fails.[33] Until more accurate methods are at hand to investigate cellular dysfunction at a biochemical level, the nature of heart failure will elude exact explanation.

REFERENCES

1. WOOD P. (1968). *Diseases of the Heart and Circulation*, 3rd edn, p. 291. London: Eyre & Spottiswoode.
2. GUYTON, A. C. (1967). *New England Journal of Medicine*, **277**, 805.
3. HARRIS, P. and HEATH, D. (1962). *The Human Pulmonary Circulation*, p. 39. Edinburgh: Livingstone.
4. DICKINSON, C. J. and PENTECOST, B. L. (1968). In *Clinical Physiology*, 3rd edn, p. 40. Edited by E. J. M. Campbell, C. J. Dickinson and J. D. H. Slater. Oxford: Blackwell.
5. McMICHAEL, J. (1947). *Advances in Internal Medicine*, **2**, 64.
6. EDHOLM, O. G., HOWARTH, S. and McMICHAEL, J. (1945). *Clinical Science*, **5**, 249.
7. SHUSTER, S. (1963). *Lancet*, i, 1338.
8. FOX, R. H. *et al.* (1965). *British Medical Journal*, i, 619.
9. HUDSON, R. E. B. (1965). *Cardiovascular Pathology*, p. 262. London: Arnold.
10. Ciba Foundation Symposium on Cardiomyopathies (1964). Edited by G. E. W. Wolstenholme and M. O'Connor, London: Churchill.
11. Leading Article (1967). *Lancet*, ii, 457.
12. HALL, J. L. and SMITH, E. B. (1968). *Archives of Pathology*, **86**, 403.
13. Leading Article (1972). *British Medical Journal*, ii, 247.
14. KOCH-WESER, J. (1967). *New England Journal of Medicine*, **277**, 417, and 469.
15. KATZ, L. N. (1954). *Circulation*, **10**, 663.
16. RUSHMER, R. F. and CRYSTAL, D. K. (1951). *Circulation*, **4**, 211.
17. STARLING, E. H. (1918). *The Law of the Heart Beat* (*Linacre Lecture*). London: Longmans.
18. LINDEN, R. J. (1963). In *Recent Advances in Physiology*, 8th edn, p. 330. Edited by R. Crese. London: Churchill.
19. McMICHAEL, J. (1952). *British Medical Journal*, ii, 525.
20. SHARPEY-SCHAFER, E. P. (1944). *Clinical Science*, **5**, 125.
21. McMICHAEL, J. (1949). *American Journal of Medicine*, **6**, 651.
22. WOOD, P. (1954). *British Medical Journal*, i, 1051 and 1113.
23. BERNHEIM (1910). *Revue de Médecine (Paris)*, **30**, 785.
24. McMICHAEL, J. and SHARPEY-SCHAFER, E. P. (1944). *British Heart Journal*, **6**, 33.
25. SHERLOCK, S. (1951). *British Heart Journal*, **13**, 273.
26. WOOD, P. (1936). *Quarterly Journal of Medicine*, **5**, 1.
27. ARNOTT, W. M. (1963). *British Medical Journal*, ii, 765 and 823.
28. HAYWARD, G. W. (1955). *British Medical Journal*, i, 1361.
29. LENDRUM, A. C. (1950). *Journal of Pathology and Bacteriology*, **62**, 555.
30. McKEE, P. A. *et al.* (1971). *New England Journal of Medicine*, **285**, 1441.
31. RAPPAPORT, A. M. *et al.* (1954). *Anatomical Record*, **119**, 11.
32. KOTIN, P. and HALL, E. M. (1951). *American Journal of Pathology*, **27**, 561.
33. BRAUNWALD, E., ROSS, J. and SONNENBLICK, E. H. (1967). *New England Journal of Medicine*, **277**, 794, 853, 910, 962 and 1012.

Chapter 41. Respiratory Failure

The cells of the higher animals show considerable diversity in their specialisation, but insofar as energy production is concerned each cell is self-sufficient. Energy is produced by the oxidation of substances derived from the food and brought to the cell by the blood stream. Although the oxidative process, centred around the Krebs cycle, is referred to as intracellular respiration, respiration in its broadest context involves four other processes. Gases are *transported* to and from the tissues by the blood stream, while in the capillaries actual *exchange* occurs between blood and cells. In the lungs the gases exchange with the alveolar air by *diffusion* across the alveolar walls. The final act of respiration is the exchange between alveolar air and the atmosphere mediated by the *ventilation* produced by the lungs. Respiration in its clinical sense is restricted to those aspects which directly concern the lungs, and *respiratory failure* is defined as a condition in which there is a fall in arterial blood Po_2*(below 60 mm Hg) or a rise in arterial blood Pco_2* (over 49 mm Hg) due to dysfunction of the lungs.[1] The causes are nearly always to be found in the lungs themselves, and it is therefore necessary to consider their normal structure and function.

STRUCTURE OF THE LUNG AND AIR PASSAGES

The trachea is lined by a pseudostratified columnar ciliated epithelium containing in addition numerous goblet cells. How the secretion of these cells is regulated is not known, but local "irritation", e.g. trauma and chemicals, leads to an increased discharge of mucus. Opening on to the surface are the ducts of compound mucous and seromucous glands. Vagal stimulation produces secretions from these glands, an action blocked by atropine. The wall of the trachea contains hoops of cartilage, incomplete posteriorly; this allows considerable change in size of the lumen. Thus, on inspiration there is an increase, and on expiration a decrease in size. During coughing the trachea can be occluded almost completely, and foreign bodies and accumulations of mucus can be speedily ejected. Muscle and elastic fibres complete the wall, together with a small amount of collagenous connective tissue.

The bronchi, as they enter the substance of the lung, divide

* The following abbreviations are used in this chapter:

Po_2—partial pressure of oxygen; Pco_2—partial pressure of carbon dioxide. In each case the site will be designated, e.g. in arterial or venous blood or in alveolar gas.

into smaller branches and ultimately into bronchioles. The structure of the bronchial wall is very similar to that of the trachea except that the cartilage rings are replaced by irregular plates that completely surround the bronchus. These prevent collapse of the bronchi, but nevertheless, as in the trachea, some alteration in size does occur with respiration. It follows therefore that a mass nearly occluding a bronchus will not prevent air entering the affected lung, but will effectively block its escape on expiration. The lung, therefore, becomes overdistended. Contraction of the bronchial muscle on expiration helps to reduce the anatomical dead-space to a minimum (see p. 510).

As the bronchi decrease in size their walls become thinner, and at about 1 mm in diameter the bronchioles lose their cartilage. At this point the glands also disappear. The smallest bronchiole that is found without alveoli budding from its wall is called the *terminal bronchiole*. It is the last part of the bronchial tree to receive an oxygenated bronchial arterial supply, and also the last part to act purely in a conducting capacity.

That part of the lung distal to the terminal bronchiole is called the *acinus*, or the *unit of the lung*. Several units are together grouped to form the lobules which can be seen on the lung surface, when outlined by carbon deposits. Each terminal bronchiole divides into a number of *respiratory bronchioles*, of which there are usually three generations. They are about 0·5 mm in diameter, and are lined at their commencement by ciliated columnar epithelium devoid of goblet cells. Lower down the cilia disappear, and the epithelium becomes low cuboidal. In the wall there is muscle, collagen, and elastic fibres. A few alveoli bud off directly from the respiratory bronchiole (hence its name). The respiratory bronchioles themselves branch into 2–11 *alveolar ducts* which follow a long, tortuous course, and finally divide into *air sacs*. The alveolar ducts and sacs have no mucosal lining, and their walls consist of the orifices of the numerous alveoli which open into them. Elastic fibres are disposed in the walls at the entrances of the alveoli.

The alveoli are polygonal in shape, like soap bubbles packed closely together, and it is in their walls that gaseous exchanges take place between blood and air. Electron microscopy reveals that they are lined by a complete layer of flattened cells which is separated from the capillary endothelial cells by a thin space containing basement membrane, reticulin, and an occasional elastic fibre (Fig. 41.1).[2] The alveolar surface is covered by a layer of lipoprotein, rich in

Figure 41.1
Blood-air pathway of the normal human lung. The
alveolar air space (Alv) is separated from the basement membrane (Bm) by an alveolar epithelial
cell (Ep). On the other side of the basement
membrane there are two endothelial cells (End),
the cell membranes of which overlap (Cm). The
space internal to the endothelial cells is the pulmonary capillary (Cap). ×42 000. *(From Schulz,
H. (1962), In "Pulmonary Structure and Function",
a Ciba Foundation Symposium, Fig. 2(a), p. 205.
London : Churchill)*

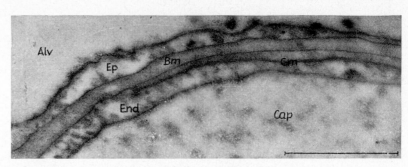

dipalmitoyl lecithin,[3] which has important surface-active
("surfactant") properties.[4, 5] Two types of epithelial cell are
described (Fig. 41.2). Type I pneumocytes are more abundant, and the lateral extensions of their cytoplasm form the
major part of the continuous epithelial lining. Type II
pneumocytes usually occur singly, are larger, and on electron

described by Lambert,[7] connecting bronchioles directly
with alveoli. It therefore follows that the only complete
separation of lung tissue occurs at the anatomically distinct
septa, and it is for this reason that collapse due to bronchial
obstruction is frequently lobar in distribution. Blockage of
smaller bronchi does not always produce collapse.

Figure 41.2
Electron micrograph of normal mouse lung. The red
cell lies in a capillary (Cap), which is bounded on
each side by an alveolus. A type II pneumocyte lines
part of one alveolus. The cytoplasm contains several
mitochondria (m) and osmophilic inclusions (Inc),
and the free border of the cell has numerous microvilli
(mv) extending into the alveolar space. The remainder
of the alveolar surface is covered by the thin lateral
extensions of Type I cells. One such extension partially covers the Type II cell, and forms a junctional
complex (jc) at the luminal surface. Uranyl acetate
and lead hydroxide stain. ×13 000. *(From Curry,
R. H. (1968), "A Morphologic Study of Mouse Lung,
the Adenomatous Tumours of Mice", M.Sc. Thesis,
University of Toronto. Reproduced by permission of
the Director, School of Graduate Studies)*

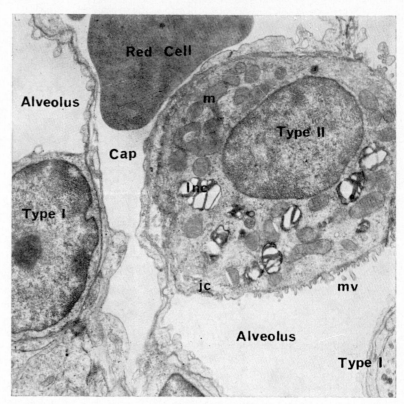

microscopy are seen to contain characteristic osmophilic
granules, or inclusions. These cells are thought to secrete
surfactant, since fetal lung shows a simultaneous appearance
of surfactant and inclusions. Furthermore, animals exposed
to a high concentration of oxygen or subjected to bilateral
vagotomy show a loss of both surfactant and inclusions.[3]

Although each respiratory unit has a separate anatomical
integrity, defects of the walls between adjacent alveoli
(forming the pores of Kohn[6]) result in an air communication
with neighbouring units. Furthermore, there are channels,

In the alveoli there are free macrophages. In tissue cultures
of lung inconspicuous cells in the septa (*septal cells*) assume
a typical macrophage appearance and function, and these
probably are a reservoir of macrophages (see Fig. 7.2, p. 89).

THE CONTROL OF BREATHING[8]

Breathing is accomplished by the contraction of the
respiratory muscles, which causes expansion of the thorax
and overcomes the elastic resistance (elastance) of the lungs

and also the resistance of the airways to the flow of air through them. The rate, depth, and rhythm of breathing are determined by nerve cells in the reticular system. There is no anatomically localised respiratory centre, but rather a diffuse system of neurones in the brain-stem. It appears to have an intrinsic rhythmicity of its own, but is influenced by a variety of extramedullary functions:

The cortex. Impulses from the higher centres are probably an important factor in the causation of the increased ventilation of voluntary exercise.

Proprioceptive impulses from the muscles of respiration.[9] The tension developed in the inspiratory muscles is integrated with the movement produced. Any decrease in the volume of inspired air produced by an additional load, e.g. airways obstruction, therefore produces an abnormal sensation. This stimulates an increase in inspiratory effort to overcome the obstruction.

Blood Pco_2 and pH. The volume of respiration is finely regulated by arterial Pco_2, an increase stimulating and a decrease depressing it. A fall in blood pH also stimulates ventilation.

Blood Po_2. Hypoxia stimulates breathing, not through a direct effect on the chemoreceptors of the reticular formation, but indirectly *via* the aortic and carotid-body receptors. If pure oxygen is given to a normal subject, ventilation is depressed, indicating that the control of breathing is influenced by the Po_2 level. However, this response is less sensitive than that to changes in Pco_2. At high altitudes the hypoxia stimulates breathing so much that the Pco_2 of the blood is permanently lowered and the central chemoreceptors have their sensitivity adjusted to a lower level. In chronic lung disease the hypoxia acts as a spur to respiration, and if it is relieved by oxygen administration, the drop in ventilation may cause so great a rise in arterial Pco_2 that coma ensues (CO_2 narcosis).

Factors Governing Respiratory Gas Exchange in the Lungs

The primary function of the lung is to arterialise the mixed venous blood. This involves the controlled elimination of CO_2 and absorption of O_2 such that the blood-gas tensions are maintained at their correct levels. The exchange of gas depends upon three factors:

Ventilation. This includes both the *volume* and the *distribution* of the inspired air which ventilates the alveoli.

Diffusion. The passages of gases between the alveoli and blood in the alveolar capillaries.

Pulmonary capillary blood flow (perfusion). This involves the total *volume* of blood and its *distribution* to all the ventilated alveoli.

Control of the Volume of Ventilation[8]

Ventilation involves two phases: inspiration and expiration.

Inspiration is carried out by the contraction of the diaphragm and intercostal muscles, assisted if necessary by the accessory muscles of inspiration. The result is an increase in the negative intrathoracic pressure,* which is about -5 cm H_2O (about -4 mm Hg) when the muscles are inactive and there is no airflow. The inspiratory muscles are opposed by two forces:

The elastic force, which has two approximately equal components.

(*a*) The elastic properties of the lung substance.
(*b*) The surface tension of the fluids lining the airways (see below).

The non-elastic or resistive load. This is chiefly due to the frictional resistance of the respiratory passages to airflow.

The elastic load is commonly measured as the *compliance of the lung*, i.e. the increase in lung volume per unit increase in distending pressure, and is measured by dividing the volume of air inspired by the change in negative intrathoracic pressure. It is normally 0·12–0·25 litres per cm H_2O.

Expiration[10] is achieved by the elastic recoil of the lungs, during which the inspiratory muscles relax. During forced expiration there is contraction of the accesssory muscles of expiration, e.g. those of the abdominal wall.

The elastic properties of the lung are obviously of great moment in allowing the lung both to be inflated and emptied. It was noticed nearly 40 years ago that for a given distending pressure, a cat's lung would inflate to twice the volume when filled with water as opposed to air. This is due to the water abolishing the surface-tension effect of the fluid-gas interface that normally exists in the lungs, and which provides half the elastic resistance to inflation.[11]

The surface-tension resistance of the lung is less than would be expected were the alveoli lined by either saline or plasma. The surface tension of the film lining the alveoli is lowered by the lipoprotein surfactant agent. Its presence thus decreases the work needed to expand the lungs in each inspiration, and its absence leads to stiffness and loss of compliance.

In addition this lipoprotein lowers the surface tension of a saline film, *especially when the film is compressed*. During expiration the lining of the alveoli is compressed and its surface tension is rapidly lowered. It is thus of importance in preventing the collapse of alveoli following their emptying during expiration. A loss of this surfactant property of the lung lining is recognised in the respiratory distress syndrome of the newborn (hyaline-membrane disease) and in the "post-perfusion lung" syndrome that follows open-heart surgery (see p. 486), but it is not certain whether it causes or merely follows these conditions.[8]

The *tidal volume* (the volume of air which enters and

* This is the pressure outside the lung but inside the thoracic cage, and is measured intrapleurally or intra-oesophageally. It must be distinguished from the alveolar pressure, which is equal to the mouth pressure when there is no airflow.

leaves the lungs during normal quiet breathing) is normally 500 ml, and at a rate of 15 respirations per minute, 7·5 litres are inspired and expired each minute. The *amount* of air that is inspired depends on the compliance of the lungs. The *rate* of airflow is related to the calibre of the airways. This forms the principal part of the non-elastic resistance to ventilation, the other factor being the displacement of tissues and blood in the lungs themselves. The last 100–170 ml of each breath (500 ml) is expended in filling the conducting airways, and does not reach the alveoli—it is called the *anatomical dead-space.*

It is obvious that the compliance and the non-elastic resistance are important factors in influencing the depth and rate of respiration. With a low compliance or a high non-elastic resistance a greater pressure difference or a longer time is required for proportional ventilation as compared with a high compliance or a low non-elastic resistance. When compliance is low, the work of breathing is increased, and it is most advantageous to take frequent shallow respirations. The rate and depth of respiration are optimally adjusted in relation to dead-space volume, compliance, and non-elastic resistance. Exactly how this is brought about is not known, but it appears to be a function of the reticular centres.

Distribution of Ventilation in Relation to Perfusion[8]

From the point of view of maintaining the normal gaseous composition of the arterial blood, the distribution of ventilation relative to pulmonary capillary blood flow (*perfusion*) is

Figure 41.3
Diagrammatic representation of the lung showing two alveoli with ideal $\frac{\text{ventilation}}{\text{blood flow}}$ relationships. The oxygen tensions are in mm Hg, and the figures in brackets are the percentage oxygen saturation of the blood. (*After Comroe, J. H. et al.* (1963), *"The Lung: Clinical Physiology and Pulmonary Function Tests", 2nd ed., Fig. 26, p. 88. Chicago: Year Book Medical Publishers*)

very important. Considering the lung as a whole, under normal conditions the ratio

$$\frac{\text{Alveolar ventilation}}{\text{Perfusion of capillaries}} \text{ * is approximately unity.}$$

The situation in an ideal lung is shown in Fig. 41.3. Although in the normal lung the alveolar ventilation and perfusion are closely coordinated, there are areas where ventilation exceeds perfusion. Thus, in the erect position the apices of the upper lobes receive relatively little blood in comparison with the volume of air ventilating them.

Some effects of badly correlated ventilation and perfusion are shown in Fig. 41.4. The following points are noteworthy:

1. There is a rise in the P_{O_2} of the blood leaving alveolus A, but because of the nature of the oxygen dissociation curve (Fig. 41.5) this does not appreciably raise the oxygen saturation. Hence it does not compensate for the desaturated blood leaving alveolus B. The excess ventilation of alveolus A is therefore wasted, and when added to the anatomical dead-space constitutes the *physiological dead-space.* This in itself leads to an increase in ventilation.

2. The mixed venous blood reaching alveolus B is not as fully arterialised as in the "ideal lung". This wasted blood produces the same effect as a direct *right-to-left shunt.*

* Generally written $\dfrac{\dot{V}_A}{\dot{Q}_C}$ the dot indicating that the volumes are in unit time. Thus, in a normal subject at rest

$$\frac{\dot{V}_A}{\dot{Q}_C} = \frac{4 \text{ litres per min}}{5 \text{ litres per min}} = 0.8.$$

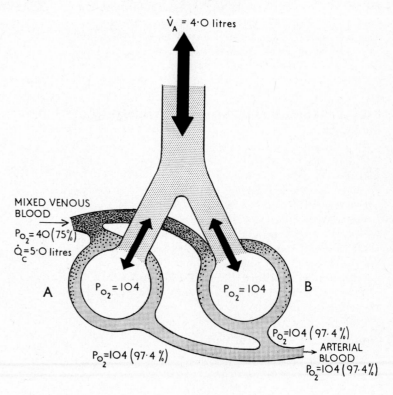

$\dot{V}_A = 4.0$ litres

MIXED VENOUS BLOOD →
$P_{O_2} = 40 (75\%)$
$\dot{Q}_C = 5.0$ litres

A $P_{O_2} = 104$ $P_{O_2} = 104$ B

$P_{O_2} = 104 (97.4\%)$

$P_{O_2} = 104 (97.4\%)$
ARTERIAL BLOOD →
$P_{O_2} = 104 (97.4\%)$

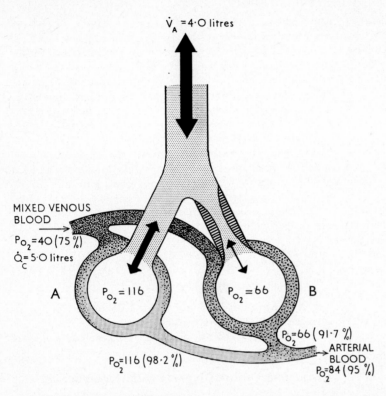

$\dot{V}_A = 4 \cdot 0$ litres

MIXED VENOUS
BLOOD

$P_{O_2} = 40\,(75\,\%)$

$\dot{Q}_C = 5 \cdot 0$ litres

A $P_{O_2} = 116$ $P_{O_2} = 66$ B

$P_{O_2} = 66\,(91 \cdot 7\,\%)$
ARTERIAL
BLOOD
$P_{O_2} = 116\,(98 \cdot 2\,\%)$ $P_{O_2} = 84\,(95\,\%)$

Figure 41.4
Diagrammatic representation of the lung showing two alveoli which are unevenly ventilated but uniformly perfused. Note how the over-ventilation of one alveolus does not compensate for the underventilation of the other, with the result that some arterial desaturation occurs and the P_{O_2} is considerably reduced. *(After Comroe, J. H. et al.* (1963), "The Lung: Clinical Physiology and Pulmonary Function Tests", *2nd ed., Fig. 28, p. 94. Chicago: Year Book Medical Publishers)*

3. The increased ventilation of alveolus A has the effect of washing out an excessive quantity of CO_2 from the blood perfusing it. This tends to compensate for the raised P_{CO_2} of the blood leaving the under-ventilated alveolus B.

4. The mixed arterial blood is desaturated (P_{O_2} 84 mm Hg), while the P_{O_2} of the mixed alveolar gas is raised (106 mm Hg). This difference therefore appears as a *diffusion defect*.

5. The desaturated mixed arterial blood causes an increase in the total ventilation as a compensatory mechanism. This reduces the P_{CO_2} to near normal levels, and also increases the arterial saturation because alveolus B is better ventilated. However, the alveolar P_{O_2} is also raised, and the alveolar-arterial P_{O_2} difference remains.

A similar situation arises if the ventilation of alveoli is uniform but the perfusion is non-uniform. In the alveolus receiving little blood there is wasted ventilation, but the blood leaving it is fully oxygenated. In the alveolus receiving the excess blood there is not enough ventilation to oxygenate the blood fully or to reduce the P_{CO_2} to normal. Arterial desaturation and an increase in the physiological dead-space bring about similar compensatory changes to those described above.

Imbalance between distribution of perfusion and ventilation thus introduces great inefficiency in the act of respiration, and it is not surprising that there are mechanisms for co-ordinating these two parameters. These mechanisms are not well understood. If one lung is ventilated with gas of a low P_{O_2} or a high P_{CO_2}, or if there is bronchial obstruction, the

blood flow through that lung is dramatically reduced. The gas tensions therefore regulate blood flow. Furthermore, a reduced blood flow, e.g. due to arterial obstruction, is followed by reduced ventilation, probably as a result of increased airways resistance and reduced compliance.

Diffusion[8, 12]

In the normal lung the barrier between the alveolar gas and the blood consists of the alveolar cell, the endothelial cell and the thin layer of intervening connective tissue. In addition to this membrane barrier there is also the red-cell envelope, which constitutes a further barrier. Diffusion depends on the difference between the partial pressures of the gas in the alveolar air and the interior of the red cell, the solubility and molecular weight of the gas, the thickness of the barriers mentioned above, and the speed of the physico-chemical processes in the red cell. Apart from these conditions, diffusion also depends upon the area over which the blood gases and alveolar gas can interchange. This is related to the total volume of functioning lung and the balance between perfusion and ventilation.

CO_2 is much more soluble than O_2, and diffuses 20 times as readily through the pulmonary membranes. The arterial P_{CO_2} is therefore the same as that of the alveolar gas, both in health and when there are defects of diffusion. The arterial P_{O_2}, on the other hand, is slightly lower than the alveolar gas P_{O_2} even in the normal individual, due to the fact that his lungs are not "ideal". Arterial desaturation is characteristic of diffusion defects.

The pulmonary diffusing capacity can be estimated clinically, being measured in ml of oxygen or carbon-monoxide transfer each minute for each mm Hg pressure difference of oxygen or carbon monoxide across the lung. The diffusing capacity is impaired under the following circumstances:

1. When there is a decrease in the anatomical area available for diffusion, e.g. following lung destruction or resection.

2. When there is a decrease in the *functional* alveolar-capillary surface due to *impaired distribution*. It therefore follows that *distribution and diffusion defects produce the same functional end-results, and respiratory failure due to these causes may be considered together.*

It was formerly believed that the diffusing capacity could be decreased when there was an increase in the distance between the alveolar gas and the red cell. This was called the "alveolar-capillary block syndrome", and was described in many fibrotic conditions of the lung (see p. 513). It is now believed that the diffusion defect in these conditions is due either to destruction of lung tissue or an impaired ventilation-perfusion ratio.

Blood-gas Transport[8]

The relation between the P_{O_2} of the arterial blood and the volume of O_2 carried in the blood is demonstrated by the classical S-shaped dissociation curve (Fig. 41.5). The normal arterial P_{O_2} is 80–110 mm Hg, and the arterial saturation 93–98 per cent. A considerable reduction of arterial P_{O_2} causes no significant change in the oxygenation of the

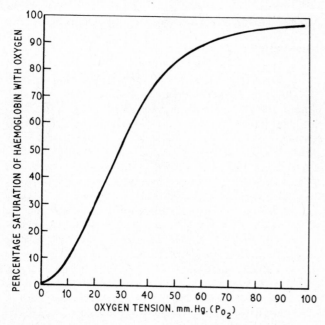

Figure 41.5
Oxygen dissociation curve of blood. *(After Starling and Lovatt Evans (1962), "Principles of Human Physiology", 13th ed., p. 79. Edrs. Davson, H. and Eggleton. M. G. London : Churchill)*

arterial blood, e.g. an arterial saturation reduction below 90 per cent does not occur until the P_{O_2} is less than 60 mm Hg.

It is evident that a fall of ventilation by almost half causes little decrease in the arterial saturation, but below 60 mm Hg a further drop produces disproportionate desaturation. Overventilation of parts of the lung to compensate for the underventilation elsewhere cannot alter the arterial saturation much, for a raised P_{O_2} above normal leads to only a negligible increase in arterial O_2 saturation.

The CO_2 dissociation curve in the physiological range is much steeper, and greater changes in saturation occur for a change in partial pressure that would have little effect on O_2 saturation (Fig. 41.6).

Therefore overventilation of the lungs can remove CO_2 not properly eliminated by areas of underventilated alveoli.

TYPES OF RESPIRATORY FAILURE[1]

Two main types are recognised:

1. Ventilatory failure due to an inadequate volume of inspired air available for exchange.

2. Impaired alveolar-arterial gas exchange due to failure of distribution or diffusion.

Ventilatory Failure (Hypoxia with Hypercapnia)[1]

This is caused by (*a*) *airways obstruction** due usually to chronic bronchitis, emphysema, and asthma, which are considered on p. 515, (*b*) *restriction of thoracic movement*, e.g. in severe kyphoscoliosis, scleroderma, pneumothorax, pleural effusion, ascites, and pregnancy, (*c*) *neuromuscular impairment*, e.g. in poliomyelitis, polyneuritis, or curare poisoning, and (*d*) *disturbances of the reticular centres*, e.g. due to organic disease or depressant drugs such as an overdosage of barbiturates.

Effects. Since arterial $P_{CO_2} \propto \dfrac{CO_2 \text{ production}}{\text{alveolar ventilation}}$ and at rest the CO_2 production is constant, it follows that when alveolar ventilation is reduced, the arterial P_{CO_2} is increased, and there is an arithmetically equivalent fall in P_{O_2}. Thus, if the P_{CO_2} rises from 40 to 60 mm Hg, then the P_{O_2} falls from 100 to 80 mm Hg. As already explained above, a drop of P_{O_2} of this order does not greatly affect the oxygen saturation of the arterial blood; desaturation, with cyanosis, is a late event in ventilatory failure.

The main effect is a raised arterial P_{CO_2} (*hypercapnia*), and the symptoms are referable to this.[14] The pulse is rapid and bounding, the hands moist and warm, pupils small, and the blood pressure raised. If there is severe CO_2 retention, confusion, drowsiness, coarse tremors, and coma may ensue. The reflexes are depressed, and the plantar response is extensor. Papilloedema is an uncommon though well recog-

*This is defined as persistent widespread narrowing of intrapulmonary airways, at least on expiration, causing increased resistance to airflow[13].

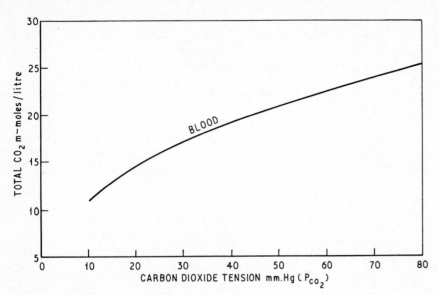

Figure 41.6
Carbon-dioxide dissociation curve of blood. *(After Starling and Lovatt Evans* (1962), "Principles of Human Physiology", 13*th ed., p.* 89. *Edrs. Davson, H. and Eggleton, M. G. London : Churchill)*

nised effect of prolonged, very severe hypercapnia, and it is a manifestation of the cerebral vasodilatation caused by CO_2 excess.[15] Dyspnoea is often absent.

The plasma bicarbonate level is high. There is a raised arterial P_{CO_2}, and a respiratory acidosis ensues. As the difference between arterial and venous P_{CO_2} at rest is slight (6 mm Hg in a normal person), the mixed venous P_{CO_2} is often measured. The *rebreathing method* is very easy:[16, 17] the patient rebreathes from a bag containing a CO_2 mixture. The contents of the bag and lungs mix, and the CO_2 mixture equilibrates with the pulmonary blood. This equilibrium persists until the blood recirculates around the body and returns to the lungs with an increased CO_2 tension, and therefore after 20 seconds the CO_2 content in the bag is ascertained and the CO_2 tension calculated.

Impaired Alveolar-Arterial Gas Exchange (Hypoxia without Hypercapnia)[1]

In this type of failure there is a reduction of alveolar-capillary surface available for gas exchange. This may occur as a result of either lung destruction or resection or of an imbalance between the distribution of perfusion and ventilation. Frequently these factors are combined, and of the two maldistribution is much more important and becomes prominent in all progressive lung disease. It is indeed the usual cause of cyanosis in lung disease.

Impaired alveolar-arterial gas exchange occurs in emphysema and severe chronic bronchitis, especially postoperatively (see p. 514). It is a feature of pulmonary embolism and chronic obstructive pulmonary vascular disease. It is also seen in such diffuse fibrotic lung conditions as asbestosis, berylliosis, rheumatoid arthritis, scleroderma, radiation damage to the lung, and allergic reactions in the alveoli following the inhalation of organic dusts—a good example is farmer's lung due to actinomycetes in mouldy hay. If the

fibrosis is idiopathic the condition is called *diffuse fibrosing alveolitis,*[18, 19] or the *Hamman-Rich syndrome.* In a number of cases of idiopathic fibrosing alveolitis there is also a tendency to polyarthritis, active chronic hepatitis, Sjögren's syndrome, and thyroid disease, conditions with a background of immunological abnormality. Non-organ-specific antibodies are sometimes present, and sometimes deposits of immune complexes have been found in alveolar walls. But other cases have no immunological basis, and may be related to infection or extrinsic inhaled agents.[20]

Effects. There is an interference with O_2 uptake, and, as on exercise the venous blood becomes more desaturated, increasing arterial desaturation also occurs. A useful clinical sign of this is *central cyanosis.* Cyanosis is taken to indicate the presence of more than 5 g of reduced Hb per 100 ml blood in the capillaries. It is best detected in the mucosa of the mouth, where the blood flow is always good; in this situation *peripheral cyanosis* (due to stasis) does not occur. When destructive lung disease is a major factor there is little unsaturation at rest, but a dramatic fall in saturation accompanies exercise, and cyanosis rapidly develops.[8] Severe hypoxia leads to neurological disturbances ranging from impairment of intellectual function to convulsions and coma.

Although in impaired alveolar-arterial gas exchange there is a severe interference with O_2 uptake, CO_2 elimination, on the other hand, is little impaired. In the distribution-failure group some alveoli are underventilated relative to alveolar perfusion. This is remedied by overventilation of the remainder of the lung. This serves to eliminate more CO_2 from the blood, but it cannot compensate for an unequal O_2 uptake, for, as has been shown, overventilation does not produce an appreciable increase in the amount of O_2 taken up by the blood above the normal level.

In some cases of distribution failure where some alveoli are poorly ventilated, an increased respiratory effort may so improve the ventilation of the affected areas that oxygenation of the blood is corrected. The P_{CO_2} is, however, lowered. The administration of 30 per cent O_2 produces the same effect, and this may be used as a diagnostic measure.

Other Manifestations of Lung Disease

Tachypnoea,[8] an increased rate of respiration, is seen when pain restricts respiratory movements, as in pleurisy and Bornholm disease, and when the lung compliance is decreased; rapid shallow respiration results. It is also seen when there is an increased need for ventilation, due to exercise or to chemical changes in the blood, e.g. hypercapnia, hypoxia (hypoxic or anaemic), and metabolic acidosis. High external temperatures may have a similar effect. Usually it is accompanied by an increase in depth of breathing, and the term *hyperpnoea* embraces both conditions. *Hyperventilation* means breathing in excess of the metabolic need, and is seen occasionally in hysterical people.

Dyspnoea is best restricted to a condition in which the act of breathing causes distress. It occurs under two main conditions:

1. When tachypnoea or hypernoea are of marked degree.
2. When the ventilatory effect produced on inspiration is small in comparison with the muscular effort needed to produce that effect. This occurs in any disease interfering with the respiratory excursions of the lung. It is seen when there is decreased compliance due to fibrosis, pneumonia, or venous congestion. Airways obstruction, whether due to pulmonary disease like chronic bronchitis or to strangulation, has a similar effect and produces severe dyspnoea. However, this is not invariable, for sometimes airways obstruction does not produce severe dyspnoea; instead the changes in blood-gas tensions are tolerated, and polycythaemia develops (see "blue bloaters", p. 515).

Although dyspnoea is a common symptom, there is little precise information about the mechanisms involved in its production. Conditions which apparently cause severe dyspnoea in one patient may be found in another who suffers little discomfort. Psychological factors certainly play a part. Thus, the sudden blockage of a tube through which a person is breathing occasions intense dyspnoea. However, if the subject is asked to block the tube himself, the manoeuvre causes no immediate discomfort.

Right-sided heart failure. This is due to a variety of causes of which pulmonary hypertension is the most obvious, and probably the most important. Pulmonary hypertension is due in part to the destruction of the pulmonary capillary bed (as in emphysema), and also, it is believed, to functional vasoconstriction secondary to abnormalities in alveolar gaseous tensions. The increased tension in the right ventricular myocardium which develops during systole has the effect of reducing the coronary blood flow. Myocardial ischaemia therefore contributes to the right ventricular failure.

An aggravating factor is the secondary polycythaemia which not only increases the load on the heart, but also predisposes to pulmonary arterial and systemic venous thrombosis (with subsequent embolism).

The respiratory acidosis leads to an increased reabsorption of sodium and bicarbonate ions from the glomerular filtrate. This sodium retention increases the blood volume, thus causing an additional strain on the heart. Peripheral oedema is not uncommon in chronic lung disease and may in part be due to right-sided heart failure. Patients with chronic obstructive airways disease have an impaired ability to excrete water in response to a standard water load (20 ml/kg body weight).[21]

RESPIRATORY EFFECTS OF VARIOUS CONDITIONS

General Surgical Procedures[22]

The use of general anaesthesia produces important changes in carbon dioxide excretion. During the operation the P_{CO_2} of the blood rises due to the depressant effect of the anaesthetic agent on the brain. If respiration is actively assisted by the anaesthetist, the P_{CO_2} may actually be lower than normal. In either event the arterial P_{CO_2} remains above normal after the operation for a few hours as a result of the continued action of the anaesthetic agent. This is particularly important in curarised patients whose breathing is completely controlled by the anaesthetist; if the curare-effect is not promptly counteracted after the operation, there may be a dangerous rise of the blood P_{CO_2}.

There is also a danger of hypoxia. This is not usually due in any great measure to poor ventilation except in unusual circumstances, but rather to an error of distribution. This is not important in healthy people, but is of great moment in patients predisposed to airways obstruction through chronic bronchitis. The cause is probably partial collapse of some air-spaces, resulting in a reduced ventilation-perfusion ratio. There is a danger of massive segmental collapse ensuing. The predisposing factors are the increased amount of sputum (which is said to be very viscous after operations[23]), impaired cough reflex and ciliary action due to the anaesthetic, the aspiration of vomitus and blood during the induction of anaesthesia, and later a decreased power of coughing after thoracic and abdominal surgery. It is advisable to administer oxygen for some time after an operation on chronic bronchitic subjects.[24]

Conditions associated with Abnormal Blood-Gas Transport

In *anaemia* (and also methaemoglobinaemia and sulphaemoglobinaemia) the volume of O_2 taken up is reduced, but the arterial P_{O_2} and P_{CO_2} are normal. If the anaemic hypoxia is severe, it stimulates breathing *via* the aortic and carotid chemoreceptors, and the P_{CO_2} falls below the normal. The hyperpnoea does not usually cause much distress.

In *metabolic acidosis* the increased hydrogen-ion concentration of the blood stimulates breathing and reduces the blood Pco_2. *Metabolic alkalosis* has the opposite effect—in fact, the depression of respiration is usually not very marked[8] (see p. 451).

Left-Sided Heart Failure and Mitral Stenosis

Pulmonary venous engorgement decreases the compliance of the lungs; it leads to brown induration which aggravates this effect. Engorgement of the bronchi causes a ventilatory impairment comparable with that of chronic bronchitis; indeed, recurrent "chronic bronchitis" is a frequent complaint of victims of mitral stenosis. The tendency to pulmonary oedema interferes with the distribution of the gases. Finally, the increased pulmonary arterial pressure leads to vascular changes which interfere with the perfusion of the lungs. It is the lungs that bear the brunt of left-sided heart disease, and their dysfunction is an important cause of death.

CHRONIC NON-SPECIFIC LUNG DISEASE[25, 26]

This collective title includes chronic bronchitis, emphysema, and asthma, so frequently diagnosed together though often in fact found separately. Their aetiology is unknown, and it is advisable to consider each as a separate condition.

Chronic Bronchitis

This is defined as a condition in which there is a chronic or recurrent increase in the volume of mucoid bronchial secretion, sufficient to cause expectoration, and which is not due to localised broncho-pulmonary disease.[26, 27] At first the expectoration is intermittent, and worse on rising in the morning, but eventually it becomes continuous. It is much commoner in tobacco-smokers than in non-smokers, but chronic bronchitis may occur in those who do not smoke at all. Atmospheric pollution is another contributory factor, but much less important than tobacco smoking.[28] Morphologically the bronchial mucosa is thickened due to hyperplasia of the mucous glands,[29, 30] and there is an increase in the number of goblet cells in the lining epithelium. Chronic inflammation is not a constant feature, and Laennec's term "bronchial catarrh" is peculiarly apt.[31] At this stage there is little interference with respiratory function and the condition is called *simple chronic bronchitis*.[32]

Recurrent inflammation is a common complication, especially in urban areas. It is due to infection with respiratory-tract viruses, pneumococci, and *H. influenzae*, and is aggravated by chemical irritants—smog is particularly dangerous. The clear mucoid sputum with its predominance of macrophages becomes purulent. In the acute stage of infection there may be constitutional symptoms, but these wane as chronicity follows.

The main effect of progressive chronic bronchitis is obstruction of the airways due to such factors as mucous-gland hyperplasia, mucosal oedema, and fibrosis following localised bronchopneumonia. The excess mucus in the lumen also plays a part, and together with bronchospasm produces acute episodes which can be reversed by treatment. The airways obstruction leads to progressive ventilatory failure, and the condition is called *chronic obstructive bronchitis*.[32]

In some patients with chronic bronchitis there is, despite the airways obstruction, little dyspnoea; in fact there is hypoventilation with progressive hypercapnia. There is also arterial desaturation due to poor distribution of ventilation. It is not known why these patients tolerate the changes in blood-gas tensions with so little discomfort. However, there is cyanosis, and later the low Po_2 leads to secondary polycythaemia. There is sodium retention and right-sided heart failure. These cyanosed, oedematous people have been called "blue bloaters".* A similar picture is found in some patients with brain damage who do not breathe normally (*primary alveolar hypoventilation*).[1]

If the hypoxia is relieved by oxygen administration, the ventilation can sometimes become so depressed that CO_2 retention occurs,[14] leading to the effects described on p. 512. On the other hand, the vasodilator effect of CO_2 excess ensures that the brain receives an adequate blood supply,[33, 34] and vigorous artificial ventilation of the lungs to relieve the hypercapnia may produce such a fall in the blood Pco_2 that generalised vasoconstriction results.[35] This leads to cerebral ischaemia, and serious sequelae may occur.[34, 36] In the treatment of respiratory failure it is the hypoxia and acidosis rather than the hypercapnia which demand the most attention.

Emphysema

The word, introduced by Laennec, is derived from the Greek, meaning an inflation. It is defined as a condition in which there is an increase beyond the normal in size of the acini, due either to dilatation or destruction of the walls.[26] Such emphysema used to be called "vesicular" in contrast to the interstitial variety in which air was present in the connective tissues of the lung, but nowadays this adjective is regarded as redundant. Though emphysema is suspected clinically by signs of hyperinflation and decreased vascularity of the lung, the final diagnosis is made by the pathologist on the properly-fixed, inflated lung. This is prepared by distending the organ by controlled intrabronchial infusion of fixative prior to sectioning.[37]

Dilatatory emphysema.[26] Emphysema due to dilatation of the air passages occurs as a compensatory phenomenon following removal or collapse of adjacent lung. It also follows a partial bronchial block. If the dilatation affects mainly the larger respiratory bronchioles the emphysema is

* The concept of pink puffers and blue bloaters has apparently been derived from the teaching of Professor A. C. Dornhorst, who pointed out the distinction between those patients with chronic respiratory difficulty that were "pink and puffing" and those that were "blue and bloated".[31]

centrilobular (or *centriacinar*), while if third-generation respiratory bronchioles and alveolar ducts are also involved, the whole acinus is affected and the emphysema is called *panacinar*. Centrilobular emphysema is also described in coal-miner's lung, in which it appears to be related to the deposits of carbon around the respiratory bronchioles, and is called "focal dust emphysema".[38] Neither type is of any great importance as a cause of respiratory failure.

Destructive emphysema.[26] This is of great moment, so much so that the WHO Committee on Chronic Cor Pulmonale has defined emphysema simply as an increase in the size of the air spaces distal to the terminal bronchioles with destruction of their walls.[27]

There are two main varieties of destructive emphysema:

(*a*) *Panacinar*, in which there is a uniform enlargement of air spaces throughout the acini comprising the lobules—it is the alveolar ducts which are principally enlarged due to destruction of the alveoli comprising their walls; (*b*) *centrilobular* (or *centriacinar*), in which there is a large air space in the centre of each lobule—this is the enlarged respiratory bronchiole. The terminal bronchioles may show chronic inflammatory changes, and some authorities have maintained that bronchiolitis and adjacent bronchopneumonia are major aetiological factors in centrilobular emphysema. This, however, is debatable, and the true cause is unknown. Both types of destructive emphysema may be *localised* to a few lobules, or else be *widespread* (a better term than generalised, which could be confused with panacinar).

There is probably a spectrum of clinical types with pure chronic bronchitis at one end and pure emphysema at the other, while most patients have a mixture of both conditions. Emphysema, particularly the centrilobular type, may be accompanied by airways obstruction, but this is probably the result rather than the cause of the condition.[39] The obstruction is probably brought about by a collapse of the bronchioles deprived of their support by the destruction of the walls of the surrounding air spaces. The absence of emphysema in asthma of long duration is further evidence that obstruction is not a factor in its pathogenesis. An inherited factor in the aetiology of emphysema is likely. Homozygous subjects with α_1-antitrypsin deficiency tend to develop emphysema, and so, but to a lesser extent, may the heterozygotes with a low enzyme level. The precise relationship between enzyme deficiency and emphysema has yet to be clarified.[46*]

The effects of emphysema vary. A widespread panacinar type is quite common in the aged, and it produces little functional impairment.[40] Likewise there may be widespread centrilobular emphysema in symptomless people.[40] On the other hand, there can be a variety of functional effects. Airways obstruction has already been referred to, and in addition there may be impaired alveolar-arterial gas exchange

---

* α_1-antitrypsin deficiency is also associated with neonatal hepatitis which progresses to cirrhosis,[47] and with cirrhosis of the liver in adults.[48] In both age-groups the liver cells contain PAS-positive globules which are characteristic.

due to diffusion failure following the loss of capillary surface. Another important factor is an increase in the physiological dead-space due to the ventilation of large avascular bullae.

All these effects cause dyspnoea, which is often severe. As ventilation is maintained, the Pco_2 is normal or even rather below normal, and these patients remain pink in spite of the difficulty they have in maintaining this ventilation. They are called "pink puffers" (see footnote, p. 515). The blood-gas tensions are kept normal, and there is no right-sided heart failure until terminally. Despite their bright appearance these patients are the victims of a relentlessly progressive disease, and little can be done to help them. On the other hand, the "blue bloater", despite his alarming appearance, can usually be tided over his attack of acute infection with antibiotics. "Pink puffers" can be given oxygen without the danger of CO_2 retention.[41, 42]

Chronic bronchitis is said to be more common in Britain—the "English disease"—than in the USA, where emphysema is said to predominate, but the difference may lie more in terminology than in incidence.[43]

Asthma[44]

This is a condition of widespread narrowing of the bronchial airways, which changes its severity over short periods of time either spontaneously or under treatment, and is not due to cardiovascular disease.[26] It is characterised clinically by paroxysms of wheezing dyspnoea, relieved by bronchodilator drugs. The airways obstruction is caused partly by contraction of the bronchial muscle which is hypertrophied, and partly by plugging with thick viscid mucus.

A considerable amount of asthma is *extrinsic* and associated with hypersensitivity reactions to inhaled agents. This usually starts in childhood and is often associated with atopic eczema and hay-fever. It is due to IgE antibodies against such antigens as pollen and animal danders. The reaction is immediate and transient, and eosinophilia is prominent.

Extrinsic asthma should not be confused with *external allergic alveolitis*, which is an immune-complex reaction mediated by sensitising IgG and is not characterised by asthmatic symptoms (see p. 183).

Asthma with pulmonary infiltrates and esosinophilia and *broncho-pulmonary aspergillosis* are described on page 183. Asthmatic attacks are also characteristic of *progressive allergic granulomatosis* (p. 213). An *intrinsic* asthma often complicates chronic bronchitis in later life, but sometimes it arises *de novo*. It may sometimes also have an allergic basis, e.g. to an infecting organism. The pathogenesis of asthma is complicated by strong hereditary and psychological factors.

The disease can terminate fatally in status asthmaticus, and it is interesting that the lungs seldom show emphysema even if the condition has persisted for many years.[45] Indeed, if status asthmaticus can be prevented, the ultimate prognosis is much better than in chronic bronchitis and emphysema.

ASSESSMENT OF RESPIRATORY FUNCTION[8]

Respiratory function may be assessed under the following headings:

Clinical examination in respect of symptoms, e.g. cough, dyspnoea, expectoration, and cyanosis, and physical examination of the chest.

Radiographic appearances of the lungs. The diagnosis of chronic bronchitis and emphysema is notoriously difficult.

Blood-gas analysis is desirable, since respiratory failure is defined in terms of arterial P_{O_2} and P_{CO_2}.

Tests of ventilation, distribution, and gas diffusion.[8] Many of these are highly complicated, and involve knowledge and apparatus which are available only at certain specialised centres. Detailed monographs should be consulted.

Three simple tests will be described here:

Vital capacity. This is the volume of air expelled by a maximum voluntary expiration after a maximum voluntary inspiration (normally 4·5–5 litres in a man). The amount of air left is called the *residual volume* (normally 1 200 ml.). As maximum inspiration depends on the chest volume, the bony cage, the muscles of respiration, and the compliance of the lung, and maximum expiration on the patency of the airways, it is evident that the vital capacity is reduced in nearly all the conditions mentioned in this chapter. Its main use is a measure of progress in any condition.

Forced expiratory volume and time. Normally over 80 per cent of the vital capacity can be expelled in one second, and the other 20 per cent in another 2–3 seconds. In airways obstruction less than 40 per cent is expelled in the first second, and the remainder takes much longer, in fact it may be incompletely removed before the next inspiration is made. A spirometer or a kymograph is used to measure the amount of expired air. This is a diagnostic test for obstructive respiratory disease.

The ratio: $\dfrac{\text{forced expiratory volume in one second}}{\text{vital capacity}}$ or $\dfrac{FEV_1}{VC}$, is a useful measurement of the degree of airways obstruction. Normally it exceeds 70 per cent. In restrictive lung disease the vital capacity is low because of the limited chest expansion. The FEV_1 is much less affected, and therefor the ratio $\dfrac{FEV_1}{VC}$ is either normal or high.

A useful clinical test on the same lines is the "match test". The patient is asked to blow out a lighted match after taking a deep breath. Normally this can be done at a distance of 3–4 inches, but with obstructive disease the distance is much less.

Maximum Breathing Capacity. The patient breathes as rapidly and deeply as possible for about 15 seconds. The volume is measured in a bag or recorded on a spirogram in litres per minute.

Results of all these tests are abnormal in airways obstruction; in ventilatory failure due to restriction, e.g. kyphoscoliosis, the match test is relatively normal; the forced expiratory volume in one second is reduced, but it remains normal in proportion to the vital capacity, i.e. over 75 per cent.

CONCLUSIONS

The advances in respiratory physiology over the last 20 years have been most impressive and have revolutionised our understanding of the clinical and functional aspects of lung disease. There has also been a mounting knowledge of the morbid anatomy of common pulmonary disease, such as chronic bronchitis, emphysema, and asthma.[40] The mortality figures for chronic respiratory disease are nevertheless still extremely high. In 1969 over 34 000 people in England and Wales died of this group of diseases, and 1 327 of them succumbed to asthma.

GENERAL READING

COMROE, J. H., FORSTER, R. E., DUBOIS, A. B., BRISCOE, W. A. and CARLSEN, E. (1962). *The Lung: Clinical Physiology and Pulmonary Function Tests*, 2nd edn, 390 pp. Chicago: Year Book Medical Publishers, Inc.

REFERENCES

1. CAMPBELL, E. J. M. (1965). *British Medical Journal*, i, 1451.
2. LOW, F. N. (1953). *Anatomical Record*, **117**, 241.
3. ASKIN, F. B. and KUHN, C. (1971). *Laboratory Investigation*, **25**, 260.
4. SCARPELLI, E. M. (1968). *The Surfactant System of the Lung*, 269 pp. Philadelphia: Lea and Febiger.
5. MORGAN, T. E. (1971). *New England Journal of Medicine*, **284**, 1185.
6. LOOSLI, C. G. (1937). *Archives of Pathology*, **24**, 743.
7. LAMBERT, M. W. (1955). *Journal of Pathology and Bacteriology*, **70**, 311.
8. CAMPBELL, E. J. M. (1968). In *Clinical Physiology*, 3rd edn, p. 93. Edited by E. J. M. Campbell, C. J. Dickinson and J. D. H. Slater. Oxford: Blackwell.
9. CAMPBELL, E. J. M. and HOWELL, J. B. L. (1962). In *Ciba Foundation Symposium on Pulmonary Structure and Function*, p. 29. Edited by A. V. S. de Reuck and M. O'Connor. London: Churchill.
10. MEAD, J. (1961). *Physiological Review*, **41**, 281.
11. COMROE, J. H. (1962). In *Ciba Foundation Syposium on Pulmonary Structure and Function*, p. 180, *loc. cit.*
12. FORSTER, R. E. (1957). *Physiological Review*, **37**, 391.
13. Medical Research Council Committee on Aetiology of Chronic Bronchitis (1965). *Lancet*, i, 775.

14. WESTLAKE, E. K., SIMPSON, T. and KAYE, M. (1955). Quarterly Journal of Medicine, **24**, 155.
15. Annotation (1963). *British Medical Journal*, ii, 1486.
16. CAMPBELL, E. J. M. and HOWELL, J. B. L. (1960). *British Medical Journal*, i, 458.
17. CAMPBELL, E. J. M. and HOWELL, J. B. L. (1962). *British Medical Journal*, ii, 630.
18. SCADDING, J. G. (1964). *British Medical Journal*, ii, 686 and 941.
19. SCADDING, J. G. and HINSON, K. F. W. (1967). *Thorax*, **22**, 291.
20. WARWICK, M. T. (1972). *British Journal of Hospital Medicine*, **7**, 697.
21. WHITE, R. J. and WOODINGS, D. F. (1971). *British Medical Journal*, ii, 561.
22. HOBSLEY, M. (1963). *Annals of the Royal College of Surgeons of England*, **33**, 105.
23. BLANSHARD, G. (1960). *Diseases of the Chest*, **37**, 75.
24. NUNN, J. F. and PAYNE, J. P. (1962). *Lancet*, ii, 631.
25. SCADDING, J. G. (1959). *Lancet*, i, 323.
26. Report of a Ciba Guest Symposium (1959). *Thorax*, **14**, 286.
27. Report of an Expert Committee (1961). *World Health Organisation Technical Report Series*, **213**, 15.
28. LOWE, C. R. (1969). *British Medical Journal*, i, 463.
29. REID, L. (1954). *Lancet*, i, 275, and (1960). *Thorax*, **15**, 132.
30. RESTREPO, G. L. and HEARD, B. E. (1963). *Thorax*, **18**, 334 and *Journal of Pathology and Bacteriology*, **85**, 305.
31. SCADDING, J. G. (1963). *British Medical Journal*, ii, 1425.
32. STRUART-HARRIS, C. (1972). *British Journal of Hospital Medicine*, **7**, 719.
33. KETY, S. S. and SCHMIDT, C. F. (1948). *Journal of Clinical Investigation*, **27**, 484.
34. Leading Article (1965). *Lancet*, i, 94.
35. SCHMIDT, C. F. and PIERSON, J. C. (1934). *American Journal of Physiology*, **108**, 241.
36. HAMILTON, J. D. and GROSS, N. J. (1963). *British Medical Journal*, ii, 1092 and 1096.
37. HEARD, B. E. (1958). *Thorax*, **13**, 136.
38. HEPPLESTON, A. G. (1947). *Journal of Pathology and Bacteriology*, **59**, 453 and (1953). *Ibid.*, **66**, 235.
39. GOUGH, J. (1960). In *Recent Advances in Pathology*, 7th edn, p. 69. Edited by C. V. Harrison. London: Churchill.
40. REID, L. (1967). *The Pathology of Chronic Bronchitis*, 372 pp. London: Lloyd-Luke.
41. BURROWS, B. *et al.* (1964). *American Review of Respiratory Diseases*, **90**, 14.
42. MITCHELL, R. S. *et al.* (1966). *American Review of Respiratory Diseases*, **93**, 720.
43. Leading Article (1967). *British Medical Journal*, iv, 436.
44. PEPYS, J. (1972). *British Journal of Hospital Medicine*, **7**, 709.
45. GOUGH, J. (1955). *Lancet*, i, 161.
46. Leading Article (1973). *British Medical Journal*, i, 1.
47. PORTER, C. A. *et al.* (1972). *British Medical Journal*, iii, 435.
48. BERG, N. O. and ERIKSSON, S. (1972). *New England Journal of Medicine*, **287**, 1264.

Chapter 42. Renal Failure

Renal failure is a state in which the body's metabolism is deranged as a consequence of dysfunction of the kidneys. There are numerous manifestations of metabolic disturbance. Most of these are attributable to an imbalance between the rates of production of various chemical substances by the body and their rates of excretion by the kidney. The kidney is the most important regulator of the extracellular fluid; it controls the concentration of its various electrolytes, it is essential for acid-base balance, and it is responsible for the excretion of nitrogenous waste products. In addition the kidney may play a part in the maintenance of the blood pressure, and it is concerned in erythropoiesis.

From a clinical point of view renal failure is a common and very serious condition, in which the retention of nitrogenous substances like urea and creatinine is the most conspicuous biochemical finding. This condition is called *uraemia*, though few of its clinical manifestations can be directly attributed to urea retention. The failure in acid-base regulation and the disordered handling of electrolytes are of much greater importance. A true conception of renal failure demands a much broader scope than this, for there are many renal lesions which produce metabolic disturbances in which neither nitrogenous retention nor uraemic symptoms are present. Examples of such conditions are the nephrotic syndrome, in which the kidney excretes large amounts of plasma proteins, and certain tubular defects, in which there is a selective loss of amino acids and various electrolytes.[1] In order to comprehend the diverse manifestations of renal failure, it is important first to consider certain aspects of urine formation.

PHYSIOLOGICAL ASPECTS OF URINE FORMATION

The secretion of urine by the kidney entails two distinct processes: (*a*) the passive filtration of plasma through the glomeruli with the formation of a fluid identical with plasma except that it contains only a trace of protein, and (*b*) the passage of this glomerular filtrate through a complex system of tubules in which much of the water and many of its solutes are absorbed back into the blood stream, while some substances are secreted directly into the tubules from the blood. The resulting urine differs very considerably from the glomerular filtrate from which it was derived, not only in the concentration of its solutes but also in its hydrogen-ion concentration.

Glomerular Filtration

The glomerular capillary wall consists of an endothelial cell layer, an epithelial cell layer, and a basement membrane, 50–100 nm, lying between them. The epithelial cells are called *podocytes*, for they are suspended in the fluid of Bowman's capsule and make contact with the basement membrane only by innumerable terminal foot processes, or *pedicels*.

The hydrostatic pressure of the blood forces a "protein-free" filtrate from the plasma through the walls of the glomerular capillaries, which act as if they were ultrafilters perforated by pores 7·5–10 nm in diameter. In fact, such pores have never been demonstrated by electron microscopy. The structural basis of the impermeability to colloids may bear a relation to the "slit pores" lying between the pedicels of the epithelial cells, but the essential factor is the basement membrane which allows small molecules in the aqueous phase to pass through, but restricts larger proteins[2] (see Fig. 42.1).

The rate of glomerular filtration is about 120 ml per minute, and it is intimately influenced by the renal blood flow. The concept of *clearance* is used in assessing the glomerular filtration rate, for it measures the volume of plasma "cleared" of any substance by the kidney in a given time. It is calculated by the formula $\frac{UV}{P}$, where U and P are the concentrations in mg per 100 ml of the substance in the urine and plasma respectively, and V is the volume of urine in ml per minute. In man inulin is neither absorbed nor secreted by the tubules, therefore its clearance provides a good estimate of the glomerular filtration rate. In the dog the creatinine and inulin clearances are identical, indicating that both substances are treated similarly by the kidney. However, in man there is also some tubular secretion of creatinine, so that its clearance value is somewhat higher than that of inulin. The inulin clearance test is technically difficult and time consuming and the creatinine clearance is often used clinically as a measure of glomerular filtration rate. The normal range is 90–130 ml per minute. In a diseased kidney, however, the creatinine clearance sometimes greatly overestimates the glomerular filtration rate, so that a single normal value does not necessarily indicate normal renal function.[3]

In practice, urea is more often used, because it is more easily measured. In the urea clearance test the patient is

Figure 42.1
Electron-micrograph of a glomerular
capillary loop of the rat. In the centre there
is the capillary lumen, which is bounded by
flattened endothelial cells supported on a
dense, amorphous basement membrane.
On the other side of this basement membrane there are the epithelial cells, or
podocytes. They are suspended in the
fluid of Bowman's capsule, and make
contact with the basement membrane by
numerous terminal foot processes, or
pedicels. The spaces between the pedicels
are called slit pores. ×20 000. *(From
Farquhar, M. G., Wissig, S. L. and Palade,
G. E. (1961), J. exp. Med.,* **113,** 47*)*

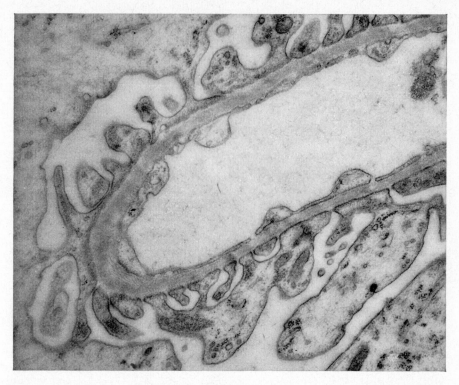

often given a dose of 15 g of urea, though this may be simplified (and improved) by omitting the urea, and merely
measuring the excretion of endogenous urea. In this case
there is no alteration in the plasma urea. The clearance of urea
is less than that of inulin, because some of it is reabsorbed by
the tubules. If the urine flow is greater than 2 ml per minute,
the urea clearance is five-eighths of the normal glomerular
filtration rate, i.e. 75 ml per minute (range 60–100 ml per
minute). This is called the "maximal urea clearance". If the
urine flow is less than 2 ml per minute, the factor of tubular
reabsorption becomes even more important, as more urea is
absorbed at a slower rate of flow. An estimation called "standard urea clearance" is often calculated, using a revised
formula $\dfrac{U\sqrt{V}}{P}$, but the adequacy of this is open to doubt. It
is better not to employ the test if the volume passed is less
than 2 ml per minute, but rather to administer sufficient
water so that the volume is subsequently adequate for the
proper calculation.

The simplest, though crudest and most imprecise, method
of assessing glomerular filtration is by estimating the plasma
concentrations of urea (normally 15–35 mg per 100 ml, or
10–20 mg per ml if expressed as blood urea nitrogen, BUN)
and creatinine (normally 0·15–1·2 mg per 100 ml). These
concentrations depend on two factors: the rate of production
in the body and the rate of excretion through the glomeruli.
A drop in filtration to half the normal rate will lead to a corresponding rise in the plasma levels of these substances, e.g.
the plasma urea will rise from 20 to 40 mg per 100 ml, which

is just outside the "normal" range. With greater drops in rate
the rise in level becomes much more obvious, e.g. a four-fold
drop in rate results in a plasma urea of 80 mg per 100 ml.
When filtration drops to 10–15 per cent of normal, uraemic
manifestations are imminent.

It is important to understand that, though an estimation of
the blood urea is the first step to be taken in assessing renal
efficiency, a normal value is compatible with a considerably
decreased filtration rate. Even a small rise in the level of the
blood urea is evidence of a serious decrease in glomerular
filtration. Furthermore, the concentration of urea is related
to the diet. It is low in patients on a low protein diet. On the
other hand, it is raised after gastro-intestinal haemorrhage.
This is in part due to the digestion of free blood in the bowel,
but there is also often acute renal failure.

In the event of a normal blood urea, clearance studies are
necessary to reveal lesser degrees of renal dysfunction. These
tests need not be performed if the blood urea is raised.

Tubular Function

Tubular reabsorption starts in the proximal convoluted
tubule where about 80 per cent of the water of the glomerular
filtrate is returned to the blood stream. In particular, glucose,
amino acids, and the trace of protein that passed the glomerular filter are completely reabsorbed. Sodium reabsorption
is incomplete, and urea passes through almost without
hindrance. The absorption of electrolytes is such that the
luminal fluid is isotonic with the plasma, a process called
isosmotic absorption.

In the ascending limb of the loop of Henle there is a considerable transfer of sodium chloride from the lumen to the interstitial fluid of the medulla. As this part of the loop of Henle is impermeable to water, it follows that the filtrate within it becomes progressively more hypotonic as compared with the plasma, whilst the interstitial fluid becomes hypertonic.

In the distal tubule the pH of the filtrate and its electrolyte composition are finally adjusted, and in the collecting tubule a certain amount of its water and urea is absorbed from the lumen to the medullary interstitial fluid. At this stage the glomerular filtrate has the full composition of urine.

Water excretion. When the hypotonic filtrate leaves the loop of Henle and enters the distal tubule, it becomes isotonic with plasma once more, as this part of the nephron is fully permeable to water. In its course through the collecting tubules the filtrate, being surrounded by the hypertonic interstitial fluid of the medulla, tends to attain osmotic equilibrium by transferring some of its water to the interstitial tissue. In this way the filtrate attains the final hypertonicity characteristic of urine as compared with plasma. The permeability of the distal and collecting tubules is related to the circulating level of ADH, which renders these tubules permeable to the passage of water from the lumen to the interstitial fluid. An excess of the hormone is therefore productive of a highly concentrated urine, whereas its deficiency leads to a hypotonic polyuria. This passive absorption of water is said to be accompanied by a similar passage of urea to the interstitial fluid of the medulla.

This rather detailed discussion of water excretion is relevant, because one of the most widely employed tests of renal function, the tubular ability to concentrate urine (the *water concentration test*), is based on an application of its mechanism. It is well known that when a patient is deprived of fluid for about 24 hours, or alternatively if he is given ADH in the form of an injection of vasopressin tannate in oil, he passes a highly concentrated urine. The degree of concentration of the urine reflects its osmolality (i.e. its concentration of particles in solution), and can to some extent be correlated with its specific gravity. The specific gravity of the urine is, however, related also to the weight of the dissolved particles. In the absence of abnormal solutes like albumin or glucose, the specific gravity of the urine is determined by its urea concentration. After water deprivation or vasopressin administration it should exceed 1·025 on at least one occasion, and should certainly be higher than 1·020.

The ability to concentrate depends upon three factors:

(*a*) *The secretion of ADH* (see p. 444). This is reduced in diabetes insipidus, which may complicate hypothalamic and pituitary lesions.

(*b*) *The capacity of the tubules to respond to the hormone*, which is defective in congenital nephrogenic diabetes insipidus. A similar defect may occur in acquired renal disorders like those associated with hypercalcaemia and hypokalaemia.

(*c*) *The solute load*. If there is an increased amount of solute to be removed by the kidneys, an increased amount of water is excreted in order to contain it. This is called *osmotic diuresis*, and it occurs even in the presence of ADH. An osmotic diuresis is induced by glycosuria, and this accounts for the polyuria so typical of diabetes mellitus. It is noteworthy that the specific gravity of the urine in this condition is high, because the abnormal solute glucose is a heavy molecule. An osmotic diuresis following the administration of urea will be attended by the production of a urine of much lower specific gravity, because urea has a much lower molecular weight.

If three-quarters of the functioning renal tissue of an animal is removed, the remaining quarter has to cope with the entire endogenous solute load, i.e. the nitrogenous products, which are mostly urea, produced in the course of the body's metabolism. This renal tissue, even if functionally normal, cannot produce a concentrated urine because of the large solute load relative to the amount of renal tissue. The blood urea rises four-fold, because the glomerular filtration rate is reduced to a quarter. An osmotic diuresis in the remaining tubules is essential to remove all the normal waste products of the body: it is the increased urea in the glomerular filtrate that stimulates the diuresis. In due course there is an enlargement of the remaining nephrons due to a proliferation of the cells of the glomeruli and tubules, and the blood urea level drops.

A similar sequence is seen in all morbid conditions in which there is a great destruction of nephrons. Eventually so few survive that renal failure is inevitable. In clinical practice a failure of urine concentration is more often due to extensive renal destruction than to tubular dysfunction.

Another test often used, the *water dilution test*, measures the kidney's ability to produce a dilute urine after the patient has been loaded with water. Three-quarters of such a load should be excreted within 4 hours, and the specific gravity of the urine should fall below 1·004. This test is unpredictable, because the water diuresis is sometimes unaccountably delayed or else precipitously accelerated by nervous factors. There is an inability to secrete a water load properly in both renal failure and Addison's disease.

The cause of this failure in Addison's disease is unknown; it is reversed with cortisol. In renal failure it is possibly related to the destruction of nephrons and a consequent water retention. The inability to produce a urine of very low specific gravity is in part explicable in terms of the poor water diuresis, but the most important factor is the persistent osmotic diuresis. Just as the presence of much urea prevents the formation of a urine of high specific gravity by its diuretic effect, so its continual presence during the water dilution test serves to prevent the production of a very hypotonic urine. It is this osmotic diuretic effect of urea that causes the fixity of the urine's specific gravity in progressive renal disease.

A state of affairs eventually comes about in which the

kidneys can produce neither a hypertonic nor a hypotonic urine. Usually the failure of a concentration precedes that of dilution. A stage is finally reached in which the kidney produces a urine of fixed specific gravity (about 1·010), a condition called *isosthenuria*. At this stage the osmolality of the urine is similar to that of plasma.

It is also well known that there is a normal diurnal rhythm of urine formation. During the night there is a diminished excretion of water and electrolytes, and pH falls, and the concentration rises. The nature of this phasic pattern of urine formation is ill understood. An abolition of the diurnal rhythm is an early manifestation of renal failure, but it also occurs in many other conditions, especially those associated with the production of generalised oedema, e.g. cardiac failure, cirrhosis of the liver, malnutrition, and the nephrotic syndrome.

Control of acid-base equilibrium. The kidney plays a vital part in the control of the acid-base balance of the body by varying the rate of secretion of hydrogen ions.

Secretion of hydrogen ions occurs throughout the whole tubular system including the collecting ducts, but is greatest in the distal convoluted tubules. As the hydrogen ions enter the lumen, there is a return into the blood of bicarbonate ions (see p. 449). The hydrogen ions in the filtrate also combine with buffer base radicals, particularly phosphate, and with ammonia to form ammonium ions. These are then excreted in the urine. Ammonia formation follows the enzymatic breakdown of glutamine by glutaminase and α-amino acids by α-amino oxidases, all of which are present in the cells of the distal tubules.

In acidosis, whether metabolic or respiratory, there is an increased excretion of hydrogen ions into the tubular fluid and an increased reabsorption of bicarbonate ions into the plasma. There is a concomitant formation of large amounts of ammonia to combine with the hydrogen ions.

The handling of electrolytes. *Sodium.* About 80 per cent of the sodium contained in the glomerular filtrate is reabsorbed together with chloride and bicarbonate ions in the proximal tubules. A variable amount of the remaining sodium is reabsorbed in the distal and collecting tubules, where the process appears to be a selective one, as compared with the isosmotic absorption of electrolytes that takes place in the proximal tubule. Chloride ions follow the actively absorbed sodium ions, while hydrogen and potassium ions travel in the opposite direction into the filtrate. The absorption of sodium ions in the distal tubules is influenced by aldosterone (see p. 443).

Potassium. Some of the potassium in the glomerular filtrate is reabsorbed in the proximal tubule, but there is an active secretion from the distal tubule which, as noted above, follows the reabsorption of sodium into the cells of the distal tubule. Aldosterone increases potassium excretion, apparently secondarily to its effect on sodium absorption. Potassium ions compete with hydrogen ions for the available transport systems in the distal tubule; it follows that an

alteration in the secretion of one of them affects that of the other also.

Calcium. There is reabsorption of calcium from the proximal tubules, and if an excessive amount is present, from the distal and collecting tubules also. Parathormone actually increases calcium absorption, but as it also mobilises calcium from the bones, the total effect is one of increased calcium excretion in the urine (*hypercalcuria*). Hypercalcaemia damages the tubular cells (see p. 569).

Phosphate. The excretion of phosphate, like that of urea, is closely related to the glomerular filtration rate. Parathormone increases phosphate excretion in the urine, probably by depressing its reabsorption in the proximal tubules. Whenever there is nitrogenous retention due to renal disease, there is always an associated rise in the blood phosphate level. This in turn induces a fall in the blood calcium level which stimulates parathormone secretion. Nevertheless, although there may be a considerable hyperplasia of the parathyroid glands, the parathormone secreted cannot lower the phosphate to a normal level.

SYNDROMES OF RENAL INSUFFICIENCY

The two most characteristic syndromes of renal insufficiency, *acute renal failure* and *chronic renal failure*, are both associated with a retention of nitrogenous waste products in the blood. In both of them clinical uraemia is encountered. Though many of the manifestations of uraemia are still unexplained, it is possible to correlate some of its symptoms with known disturbances in renal function. Both the mechanisms and the manifestations of acute and chronic renal failure are so distinct that it is better to consider them separately, while always remembering that many cases of chronic failure are complicated by acute exacerbations during their course.

ACUTE RENAL FAILURE[4]

In this condition there is a sudden drop in the urinary output of the kidneys to below 400 ml per day. It must be clearly distinguished from urinary retention in the bladder secondary to prostatic enlargement or urethral obstruction.

Causes of Acute Renal Failure

Renal vasoconstriction. Sudden vasoconstriction of the renal arteries is by far the most important cause of acute renal failure. The normal renal blood flow is about 1 200 ml per minute, and *if the flow is impaired*, there is a decrease in the glomerular filtration rate.

A fall in the arterial pressure will also decrease the glomerular filtration rate, and with a systolic pressure below 60 mm Hg glomerular filtration stops. In emergency, e.g. after haemorrhage or fluid loss, there is an additional vasoconstriction mediated by the renal nerves, which are solely vasoconstrictor in function; this is important in conserving blood for the heart and brain. It is probable that humoral agents liberated into the blood stream after injury accentuate the vasoconstriction. This vasoconstriction is seen in the following conditions:

(i) *Following a sudden decrease in blood volume* due to haemorrhage, or severe plasma loss as in burns, or a great decrease in extracellular fluid due to prolonged vomiting, diarrhoea, or even profuse diuresis as in diabetic coma. These conditions all fall into the category of "shock".

(ii) *Cardiac failure* is attended by a fall in renal blood flow sometimes to less than 500 ml per minute. Renal effects are seldom marked except occasionally in myocardial infarction, where there may be sudden severe vasoconstriction with anuria.

(iii) *The presence of free haemoglobin and myoglobin in the circulation*, especially when they are suddenly released in large quantities, leads to a degree of vasoconstriction. If it is associated with antibodies against red cells, e.g. in incompatible blood transfusions and blackwater fever, the effect of haemoglobinaemia is more severe.

The renal failure of the *crush syndrome*, in which there is extensive contusion of the muscles of the leg, is due to free myoglobin in the circulation and also to fluid loss into the damaged muscles causing a decrease in blood volume.

(iv) *Certain complications of pregnancy*, notably eclampsia, concealed accidental haemorrhage (abruptio placentae), and abortion may be accompanied by severe renal vasoconstriction. An extreme example of this is the rare, fatal, bilateral symmetrical cortical necrosis which occasionally complicates concealed accidental haemorrhage. The renal vasoconstriction may be entirely attributable to sudden, severe blood loss, but some authorities believe that in addition an acute rise in intra-uterine pressure reflexly decreases the renal blood flow.

(v) *Acute renal failure is sometimes seen postoperatively*, and is particularly common in patients who are jaundiced. The explanation is not known, but it is claimed that the administration of mannitol helps to prevent this complication.[5]

These common conditions are all responsible for what is often called "extrarenal uraemia". This is an unfortunate term, for though the kidney itself is not primarily at fault, the subsequent effects are all due to renal dysfunction, and the patient is liable to succumb to renal failure. In the early stages there is no structural damage; complete recovery follows removal of the predisposing factors, but if these are not speedily remedied, the condition progresses to acute tubular necrosis.

Acute bilateral renal artery obstruction. The commonest cause of this is dissecting aneurysm of the aorta.

Acute tubular necrosis. This may be toxic or ischaemic. Nephrotoxic agents include the heavy metals, carbon tetrachloride, and sulphonamides; they lead characteristically to necrosis of the proximal part of the tubules. The damage is widespread, but the basement membrane is not destroyed.

The effects of ischaemia depend on its severity and duration—if transient or mild there are no obvious microscopic changes in the tubules. More severe ischaemia leads to patchy tubular necrosis, affecting particularly the terminal portions of the proximal convoluted tubules and the distal convoluted tubules, and characteristically the basement membrane is disrupted.[6] There is oedema of the interstitial tissue and sometimes an inflammatory infiltrate. The oedema is a useful histological sign of tubular necrosis, for the separation of tubules which it causes helps to distinguish tubular necrosis from *post-mortem* autolysis. Functionally the interstitial oedema probably aggravates the anuria by occluding nephrons. Severe ischaemia leads to massive cortical necrosis.

Acute renal diseases, e.g. polyarteritis nodosa, acute glomerulonephritis, and pyelonephritis with papillary necrosis, may occasionally be so fulminating that they lead to complete anuria. The prognosis is extremely grave in such cases. Certain infections, e.g. Weil's disease, yellow fever, and epidemic haemorrhagic fever, are characterised by renal damage which may progress rapidly to cause death from renal failure.

Acute urinary-tract obstruction. This may be due to a stone in the pelvis or ureter, and sometimes a calculus in one ureter causes a reflex "calculous anuria" on the other side; the cause of this is unknown, but it might be vascular in origin. Sometimes the obstructing agents are intrarenal, e.g. sulphonamide crystals in the tubules or uric-acid obstruction in leukaemia or polycythaemia vera, especially after cytotoxic drugs have been given. It has been suggested that the anuria of acute renal failure is in part due to tubular blockage by casts composed of a urinary mucoprotein,[7] which is probably derived from the tubular epithelium.[8]

Acute renal failure may be superimposed on chronic renal failure following the uraemic manifestations of profuse vomiting and diarrhoea.

Effects of Acute Renal Failure

The most important type of acute renal failure is that following tubular necrosis. The functional effects are divided into an oliguric phase which corresponds to the period of necrosis, and a diuretic phase (provided the patient survives) in which there is epithelial regeneration.

The oliguric phase is associated with the necrosis already mentioned. Histologically the glomeruli appear normal, and it is possible that the filtrate is entirely reabsorbed through the damaged tubules. The effective glomerular filtration may be zero. A very common finding is the presence of blood-stained casts in the tubules. These are called *pigment casts* and contain haemoglobin; they were originally thought to be peculiar to cases of incompatible blood transfusion, but are in fact encountered in ischaemic tubular necrosis from whatever cause. They are more likely to be the result of the tubular damage than the cause of the anuria, though, as mentioned above, casts of mucoprotein may aggravate the anuria by obstructing the tubules.

The functional changes are:

(i) *The passage of small amounts of dark urine* containing protein, blood products, and cell debris. Its specific gravity is about 1·010.

(ii) *The extreme retention of nitrogenous substances* (like urea and creatinine), potassium, magnesium, phosphate, and other anions in the blood. There is also a mounting metabolic acidosis. The main source of these substances is from the endogenous breakdown of muscle protein. The rise in blood potassium is particularly serious, and is accentuated by the retention of hydrogen ions which tend to be deviated intracellularly, while the potassium ions are released into the extracellular fluid. The blood calcium is somewhat lowered secondarily to the raised blood phosphate. These changes are aggravated by the administration of protein to the patient.

(iii) *A considerable increase in extracellular water* with a decrease in the serum concentrations of sodium and chloride. The most probable explanation of these lowered levels despite the retention of sodium and chloride is an intracellular deviation, while potassium and various anions are released into the extracellular fluid. The effect is aggravated by injudicious water administration.

(iv) *A rapidly developing anaemia.* This may be accentuated by the diluting effect of an increased blood volume secondary to water retention, but there is a severe haemolytic process in uraemia. There is also a neutrophil leucocytosis.

The usual modes of death in this phase are (i) potassium intoxication causing cardiac arrest. Its effect is potentiated by the lowered level of serum calcium; (ii) overhydration leading either to water intoxication or else to an overexpansion of the extracellular compartment with congestive cardiac failure; (iii) concomitant infection, much of which is due to hospital cross-infection; (iv) a gradual clouding of consciousness which terminates in coma. It seems that waste-products of unidentified nature are responsible. There is often a dramatic relief of symptoms following dialysis even if the dialysing fluid has the same urea and electrolyte concentrations as the patient's plasma; (v) haemorrhagic manifestations.

Hypertension is not usual in acute anuria.

This phase of oliguria may last for many days, and is accompanied by persistent renal ischaemia,[9] the cause of which is unknown; it might be due to vasoconstrictor substances liberated from the damaged tubular cells.

The diuretic phase is the functional counterpart of the epithelial regeneration. This is particularly satisfactory in toxic necrosis, because the basement membrane remains intact and complete recovery can be expected. In ischaemic necrosis there is some destruction of the basement membrane with a tendency to the ingrowth of granulation tissue, so that a complete restoration of all the tubules may be impossible. However, the lesions are usually patchy, and a considerable degree of recovery can be expected. The regenerating cells are flattened and atypical, and lack a brush border; the

tubule is merely a channel for the filtrate. Soon, however, the cells differentiate, and normal function is acquired.

The diuretic phase occurs quite dramatically. The urinary output rises rapidly and soon exceeds a litre a day. The urine at first is little more than a protein-free plasma filtrate, for its other constituents are present in concentrations similar to those found in plasma. The regenerating tubules soon start to conserve sodium and to concentrate urea, yet the urine remains isotonic with the plasma for quite a long time. There is a similar delay in the recovery of the acidifying function of the tubule.

It is interesting that, despite dramatic clinical improvement the blood urea often shows no fall whatsoever for at least a week after the commencement of the diuresis. This demonstrates the minor role played by urea retention in the production of uraemic symptoms.

The diuresis is principally attributable to the excretion of accumulated fluid and waste products by the newly-functioning nephrons. It is accentuated by the osmotic effect of a high blood urea and the poor concentrating capacity of the nephrons. The patient's life is now in jeopardy because of dehydration, which is apt to be complicated by acute sodium and potassium loss.

In due course renal function tends to be restored to a satisfactory extent, but perfect recovery is unusual.

CHRONIC RENAL FAILURE[10]

The causes of chronic renal failure are extremely numerous:

Chronic destructive renal disease. This is the most important group, and it includes such conditions as chronic pyelonephritis (which is the commonest cause of chronic renal failure), chronic glomerulonephritis, systemic lupus erythematosus, polyarteritis nodosa, scleroderma, bilateral renal tuberculosis, and radiation nephritis.

Chronic renal vascular disease. Malignant hypertension, renal-vein thrombosis, and bilateral occlusion of the renal arteries with infarction of the kidneys are all associated with progressive renal failure. Non-malignant ("benign") hypertension causes only minor impairment of renal function; death is due either to heart failure or to cerebral haemorrhage.

Obstruction to the outflow of urine. This is manifested by bilateral hydronephrosis, and occurs secondarily to urethral obstruction following a stricture, prostatic enlargement, or carcinoma of the cervix (often complicated by radiation fibrosis), which may also occlude both ureters.

Congenital lesions like polycystic disease and certain tubular defects may eventually lead to severe renal failure.

Metabolic conditions, e.g. hypercalcaemia, multiple myeloma, hypokalaemia, amyloidosis, gout, and diabetic nephropathy, may all lead to serious renal dysfunction, especially if they are of long duration.

Effects of Chronic Renal Failure[11]

The metabolic disturbances that may occur in chronic renal failure are diverse and very complex. They result from a primary inadequacy of the kidney to regulate the internal environment of the body. It is not surprising that there may be rapid fluctuations from dangerous excesses to severe depletions of water and various electrolytes consequent on dietary indiscretions or gastrointestinal disturbances, which may be either primary, or else secondary to the renal condition itself.

Disturbances in water metabolism. The inability of the failing kidney to concentrate urine adequately or to cope with an increased load of water has already been discussed. Nocturia and moderate polyuria are early symptoms of renal failure. The polyuria is due to the effect of osmotic diuresis, and it is not severe because of the decreased number of functioning renal elements. It is especially marked in chronic pyelonephritis, as the concentrating part of the medulla is affected early. There is usually a mild degree of dehydration which is manifested by thirst. As soon as the patient ceases to maintain an adequate fluid intake, or if there is persistent "uraemic" diarrhoea and vomiting, dehydration becomes severe. This in its turn by decreasing the blood volume causes renal vasoconstriction and leads to acute renal failure.

On the other hand, injudicious administration of fluids, especially those given intravenously, may precipitate the very serious syndrome of water intoxication (see p. 446).

Disturbances in sodium balance. An adequate excretion of sodium is compatible with even a severely decreased glomerular filtration rate, and sodium retention is not a feature of chronic renal failure. On the other hand, there is a persistent tendency towards sodium depletion, due primarily to the inevitable loss of sodium that attends the osmotic diuresis already mentioned. There is a compensatory secretion of aldosterone in order to retain sodium, but eventually the distal tubules may become less responsive to this hormone. There is a rare condition of *salt-losing nephritis*, almost always a late result of chronic pyelonephritis, in which the tubules are completely unresponsive to aldosterone. The clinical picture is very similar to Addison's disease, but in salt-losing nephritis there is a functional hyperplasia of the adrenals with an increased aldosterone production, whereas in Addison's disease there is adrenal destruction or atrophy with a diminished production of aldosterone.[1] Obviously any gastrointestinal upset leads to further sodium depletion.

Disturbances in potassium balance. The loss of potassium is not altogether dependent on the glomerular filtration rate, for some that passes into the filtrate is reabsorbed by the proximal tubules. The excretion of potassium by the distal tubules is an active process, and is accompanied by an active reabsorption of sodium ions into the cells. In chronic renal failure there is commonly a mild retention of potassium which may become severe terminally.

Potassium depletion is very unusual in chronic renal failure. A primary *potassium-losing nephritis* is almost invariably associated with a failure of the tubules to acidify the urine due to their inability to secrete hydrogen ions.[1] As a consequence the tubules secrete more potassium ions in place of hydrogen ions, in order to counterbalance the opposing movement of sodium ions into the tubular cells. The loss of potassium during the diuretic phase of acute tubular necrosis is explained by the inability of the newly-regenerated cells to acidify the urine in this way.

Any tendency to potassium retention is aggravated by the administration of potassium citrate, while diarrhoea and vomiting lead to potassium depletion.

Disturbances in acid-base balance. Progressive renal failure is attended by a metabolic acidosis due to a relative failure of acidification of the urine. There is predominantly an impairment in ammonia production; the ability to secrete hydrogen ions is less severely impaired. Dietary or therapeutic indiscretions, like the administration of ammonium chloride, aggravate the acidosis, as also does diarrhoea with its inevitable faecal loss of hydroxyl ions in excess of hydrogen ions.

Alkalosis is very rare in uncomplicated renal failure. Potassium depletion leads to alkalosis, because there is an intracellular deviation of hydrogen ions to replace the lost potassium ions. It therefore comes about that renal failure secondary to potassium depletion in Conn's syndrome is accompanied by an alkalosis (see p. 447).

Disturbances in calcium and phosphorus metabolism.[12] In chronic renal disease where there is a persistent retention of phosphate, there is sometimes a considerable secondary parathyroid hyperplasia. The parathormone mobilises calcium and phosphate from the bones, and may give rise to a picture reminiscent of osteitis fibrosa cystica. Another feature of some cases of chronic renal disease is an impaired absorption of calcium from the bowel. This is relatively resistant to vitamin D. Both osteomalacia (renal rickets) and the lesions of hyperparathyroidism can therefore occur in chronic renal disease, and the serum alkaline phosphatase may be moderately increased.

Light has recently been shed on the vitamin-D resistant rickets that may occur in chronic renal failure. Normally vitamin D is converted in the liver into 25-hydroxycholecalciferol (25-HCC), which is believed to be the main form of the vitamin in the blood in man. But the kidney can hydroxylate 25-HCC to 1,25-dihydroxycholecalciferol (1,25-DHCC), which is the most powerfully active form of vitamin D. When the diet is low in calcium, more 1,25-DHCC is formed by the kidney, and *vice versa*. It has also been found that parathormone suppresses the conversion of 25-HCC to 1,25-DHCC, and increases the production of a much weaker form, 21,25-DHCC. This is apparently due to a direct effect by parathyroid hormone on the kidney. It would seem probable that the rickets of renal failure is at least in part attributable to the high level of circulating parathormone interfering with the metabolism of vitamin D.[13, 14]

The serum calcium is somewhat reduced, apparently as an inverse response to the raised serum phosphate and also perhaps due to impaired intestinal absorption. The bone lesions cannot be directly correlated with the levels of serum phosphate and calcium. They are commoner in children than adults. Despite the normal or low level of serum calcium (which is important in distinguishing primary renal disease with skeletal changes from primary hyperparathyroidism with secondary renal failure due to hypercalcuria) there is sometimes widespread metastatic calcification and patchy osteosclerosis. The occurrence of metastatic calcification despite a rather low serum calcium level is apparently due to the very high serum phosphate level. It is usually a terminal manifestation.

The parathyroid hyperplasia is not always relieved by successful renal transplantation. Symptoms of hyperparathyroidism may persist, necessitating a parathyroidectomy, when adenomatous change may be found.[12] This "tertiary hyperparathyroidism" indicates an autonomous change in the hyperplastic parathyroids, and demonstrates how a hyperplasia can develop neoplastic potentialities. Sometimes there is only a generalised hyperplasia similar to that found in some cases of primary hyperparathyroidism.[15]

Disturbance of carbohydrate metabolism. Impaired glucose tolerance is common and may lead to diagnostic confusion with diabetes mellitus. It rarely causes clinical symptoms and its pathogenesis is not understood.

Retention of waste products. These include urea, uric acid, creatinine, phenol derivatives, various ill-defined anions ("the anuric anions"), and urochromogen.

Hypertension.[16] Many chronic renal diseases are complicated by hypertension which may progress to a malignant phase, i.e. one in which there is frank necrosis of arterioles. Examples of such diseases are chronic pyelonephritis, chronic glomerulonephritis, polyarteritis nodosa, polycystic disease, and diabetic nephropathy. Stenosis of the renal arteries is particularly liable to be complicated by severe, rapidly progressive hypertension. Furthermore, unilateral renal disease, e.g. hydronephrosis or the stenosis of one renal artery, also tends to produce hypertension, which may be reversed if the kidney (or the arterial obstruction) is removed in time. Renal compression by a haematoma is another cause of reversible hypertension.

When the renal artery of a dog is partially occluded, hypertension develops, and will persist if the other kidney is removed; in some other animals the mere constriction of one renal artery leads to permanent hypertension. The kidney liberates a proteolytic enzyme called *renin*. This acts on an α_2-globulin called *angiotensinogen*, which is present in the plasma and acts as a substrate. The product *angiotensin I* is a decapeptide with feeble pressor activity, but it is converted into *angiotensin II*, a powerfully pressor octapeptide, by another plasma enzyme. Angiotensin is degraded by *angiotensinase*, which is present in many tissues, including the kidney. There is histochemical evidence that renin is formed in the juxta-glomerular complex, possibly in the cells of the afferent arterioles. The two important stimuli leading to the release of renin are a reduction in afferent arteriolar pressure and sodium depletion.

Angiotensin in man is not only a powerful vasoconstrictor but it also stimulates aldosterone secretion from the adrenal. This leads to sodium retention by the tubules, an effect potentiated by angiotensin which has a direct action on the tubules as well.[16] It is noteworthy that the hypertension of Conn's syndrome is relieved by spironolactones, thus proving that the changes in sodium metabolism brought about by aldosterone can be important in causing hypertension. It might be expected that the plasma renin level would be raised in renal hypertension, but in fact there is a remarkably wide scatter in renin values in even such a condition as renal artery stenosis, which mimics the experimental renal arterial occlusion in animals. The level of plasma renin is closely related to the level of plasma sodium, the highest renin levels being found where the sodium is lowest. There may well be a relation between the extracellular fluid volume, angiotensin, and the presence of hypertension, but at present no definite statement can be made.[16]

In animals two types of renal hypertension have been described: (a) *vicious-circle renal hypertension*, in which a sustained hypertension is produced even when the original occlusion to the renal artery is removed. This depends on hypertensive changes that have developed in the other kidney, for if it is now removed, the blood pressure returns to normal, and (b) *renoprival hypertension*, which follows bilateral nephrectomy.

Earlier experiments suggested that even if the animals were maintained in good condition by dialysis they still developed hypertension, but more recent work in totally nephrectomised human subjects indicates that the blood pressure does not rise if the sodium and water balance is kept perfect by dialysis. Apparently the increased sodium and water load in undialysed patients is important in the initiation of hypertension, but it is not known why such patients are so susceptible to alterations in sodium and water balance. It is probable that the normal kidney inactivates some extrarenal pressor agent; certainly the hypertension is reversed as soon as a fresh kidney is transplanted. In some species bilateral adrenalectomy prevents the hypertension following renal artery occlusion, but in man adrenalectomy is disappointing in the treatment of renal hypertension.[16] There is no evidence that essential hypertension has a renal basis.

Haematological effects. A severe normocytic, normochromic *anaemia* is common in the later stages of renal failure. It may be related to an impaired production of erythropoietin, which is normally formed in the kidney (see p. 587), or more probably the erythropoietin may not act properly (see p. 596).

Another frequent feature of renal failure is *purpura*, which is probably due to a qualitative deficiency in the platelets (see p. 620).

URAEMIA[11]

Uraemia is a clinical syndrome which is associated with a retention of nitrogenous waste products in the blood. Its manifestations are protean, and most of them cannot be explained in terms of recognisable renal dysfunction. It is instructive to consider those features which may be related to known biochemical abnormalities:

Symptoms related to disturbances of sodium and water metabolism. There may be dehydration or water intoxication. These are discussed in detail in Chapter 34. Water intoxication (cellular overhydration) may be responsible for the nausea, vomiting, headache, convulsions, and stupor seen in terminal uraemia especially in acute renal failure. If the extracellular compartment is overhydrated, symptoms of pulmonary oedema and heart failure may develop.

Symptoms related to disturbances of potassium metabolism. In acute renal failure there may be hypotension and paraesthesiae due to hyperkalaemia, and death from cardiac arrest and ventricular fibrillation may ensue.

Symptoms related to disturbances in acid-base balance. The deep, sighing respiration so typical of uraemia can be attributed to metabolic acidosis. It may also account for the clouding of consciousness, coma, and the cardiovascular complications which may cause sudden death.

Disturbances in calcium metabolism. The hypocalcaemia is seldom severe enough to cause tetany especially while there is an acidosis, which maintains the ionised fraction of the blood calcium near normal levels. If the acidosis is suddenly corrected, attacks of tetany may ensue. Likewise any tendency towards alkalosis leads to severe tetany by diminishing the blood level of the ionised fraction of calcium. It is possible that the irregular muscle twitchings seen in uraemic coma may be indirectly related to a lowered level of blood calcium, for intravenous calcium salts often abolish them.

The retention of waste products. It has been suggested that the raised blood urea plays a part in producing the severe gastritis and colitis sometimes seen in uraemia.[17] The urea diffuses into the gastric and colonic secretions where it is converted into ammonia by the resident organisms of the bowel, and also by the enzyme urease which is present in the gastric mucosa. The ammonia so produced is absorbed and used in the synthesis of amino acids in the liver.[18] An excess might irritate the mucosa, and lead to persistent vomiting and diarrhoea. Rarely the urea excretion in the sweat may be so great that it crystallises out as "urea frost". The excretion of urea in the saliva and its breakdown into ammonia gives rise to an unpleasant taste in the mouth and an ammoniacal odour in the breath.

Some of the other retained waste products, e.g. the phenol derivatives and the "anuric anions", are possibly responsible for the deepening coma of uraemia, but there is no certain evidence of this.

A retention of the normal pigment of the urine, urochromogen, may explain the pale colour of the urine, and this has even been postulated as the cause of the earthy pigmentation of the skin so characteristic of chronic renal disease.

There are many features of uraemia which elude explanation. These include hiccup, pruritus, and a terminal sterile fibrinous pericarditis which is often clinically silent. It is possible that these manifestations are due to toxic waste products circulating in the blood stream and damaging nerve endings and endothelial surfaces, but at present no such substances have been isolated. Of the various substances implicated, certain derivatives of the guanidines appear to be most liable to reproduce some of the symptoms of uraemia, e.g. nerve damage, convulsions, red-cell destruction, and gastric ulceration.[11] The pruritus is sometimes related to hyperparathyroidism, for it may be dramatically relieved by parathyroidectomy.[19]

The associated hypertension may lead to heart failure. An interesting condition occasionally seen in uraemic, hypertensive patients is *uraemic lung*.[20, 21] There are dense radiological opacities extending from the hila of the lungs out to the midzones. Although the condition is usually seen in association with left ventricular failure, the diagnosis is made on radiological, not clinical, grounds. Histologically there is much fibrinous exudate (unassociated with infection) as well as oedema fluid in the affected alveoli. It has been suggested that there is a failure of the normal fibrinolytic mechanism in uraemic lungs.[22]

Acute exacerbations of hypertension may be yet another factor in the causation of the cerebral manifestations of uraemia. The so-called hypertensive encephalopathy may lead to epileptiform convulsions. The retinal changes typical of renal disease are all due to the associated hypertension.

Many patients with chronic renal disease ultimately succumbing to uraemia remain normotensive throughout the course of their illness. Indeed, the presence of mounting hypertension is of particularly bad omen.

THE PROTEIN-LOSING KIDNEY[1, 23]

Normally only a trace of protein passes through the glomerular filter, and all this should be reabsorbed by the proximal tubule. The urine may in fact contain a minute amount of protein, which is undetectable by the routine clinical tests. In nearly all renal disease of clinical significance there is some degree of proteinuria due to an increased permeability of the glomerular filter and perhaps accentuated by tubular dysfunction.[24] The degree of proteinuria is no indication of the severity of the disease, because in progressive renal failure the glomerular filtration rate may fall so much that with the onset of uraemia the urine may contain only a trace of protein.

There is, however, a syndrome in which massive proteinuria is the main feature. This is the *nephrotic syndrome*. It sometimes arises idiopathically, and several types are described.

In *idiopathic membranous glomerulonephritis* the glomeruli show, on light microscopy, a thickening of the basement membrane—a change described as "membranous". Electron microscopy reveals that this membranous change is due to the deposition of material on one or other side of the lamina densa of the true basement membrane (p. 64). In the adult type of idiopathic membranous glomerulonephritis the deposits are on the epithelial side of the basement membrane, while in the childhood type they are on the endothelial side. In additions there are striking changes in the foot processes of the podocytes, described as "fusion of the foot processes", because the basement membrane is covered by a continuous layer of epithelial-cell cytoplasm. Some authorities maintain that this appearance is not due to actual fusion of the processes but rather to the retraction of some of them and the spreading-out of the others.[25]

In *lipoid nephrosis*, which generally occurs in childhood, the glomeruli appear normal on light microscopy. Electron microscopy reveals some thickening of the basement membrane and fusion of the foot processes as described above (Fig. 42.2). The latter change is in fact a concomitant of marked proteinuria irrespective of cause, and opinions are divided as to whether it is the cause or the effect of the proteinuria. It is probably the effect of protein leakage, and the fundamental cause of proteinuria is a defect in the basement membrane.

The nephrotic syndrome may also appear during the course of other renal disease, e.g. chronic glomerulonephritis particularly of the lobular type (p. 204), systemic lupus erythematosus, diabetic glomerulosclerosis, amyloidosis, and as an occasional complication of benign quartan (*P. malariae*) malaria and a rare one of secondary syphilis; in these last two conditions it appears to be related to the deposition of immune complexes in the glomeruli.[26, 27] It is a common feature of renal-vein thrombosis, which occasionally complicates renal tumours and amyloidosis.[28]

Finally, it can also be produced by drugs, e.g. troxidone and mercury. Mercurial preparations used as teething powders or diuretics are dangerous, and the nephrotic

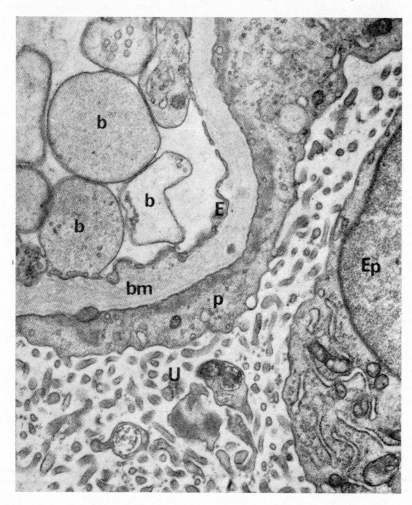

Figure 42.2
Lipoid nephrosis in a 6-year-old child. The basement membrane (bm) is thickened, and its structure is fibrillar in places. The endothelium (E) is fenestrated, but it is swollen in some regions and forms balloons (b) of variable density. The foot processes (p) are completely spread out. The podocyte (Ep) is swollen. In the urinary space (U) there are numerous cytoplasmic fragments which somewhat resemble foot processes. ×19 800, *(From Simon, G. T. and Chatelanat, F. (1969), In "The Kidney", p. 304, vol. 1, edrs. Rouiller, C. and Muller, A. F. New York and London: Academic Press)*

syndrome has also been reported as an occupational hazard in those using mercury.[29]

Effects of the Protein-Losing Kidney

Gross proteinuria. The loss is usually 10–15 g a day, but it may be much greater than this. Albumin, the smallest of the protein molecules, is lost in greatest bulk, but the globulins are also excreted; a_2-globulin is retained because of its greater molecular size. The cells of the proximal tubules often contain large "hyaline droplets" composed of protein material absorbed from the glomerular filtrate (see p. 52).

Hypoproteinaemia. There is an enormous fall in the total protein content of the plasma, and the albumin level commonly drops below 1 g per 100 ml. There is a fall in the globulin fractions also, except for a_2-globulin, the level of which rises considerably.

Oedema (see Chapter 39). The lowered plasma protein level causing a decrease in the plasma osmotic pressure is partly responsible for the anasarca so typical of nephrosis, and the fluid retention is aggravated by an increased secretion of aldosterone.

Increased blood lipids. This is constantly present, and the blood cholesterol may sometimes exceed 1 000 mg per 100 ml. The cause of this hyperlipoproteinaemia is unknown.

Increased susceptibility to infection. Death from pneumonia, peritonitis, and other pyogenic infections is very common, and is probably related to the low level of immunoglobulin in the serum, which results from its loss in the urine.

Renal function is usually very good, and often the glomerular filtration rate is raised in the early stages. The blood urea may be abnormally low, due to the combined effects of a raised filtration rate and a negative nitrogen balance. Sometimes there is a degree of potassium depletion as a result of endogenous aldosterone secretion, exogenous cortisone administration, and the use of diuretics.

In due course nitrogen retention usually supervenes. The glomerular filtration rate falls, and the protein content of the urine may drop quite considerably. Death from uraemia is the usual outcome, though in the idiopathic group spontaneous remissions and even permanent cure may sometimes occur.

The blood pressure is normal, but it may rise as renal function fails. In amyloid disease a normal blood pressure usually persists to the end.

DEFECTS OF TUBULAR FUNCTION

There is an uncommon, though very interesting, group of renal conditions in which the defect is primarily one of tubular dysfunction. This may be either an inability to reabsorb certain constituents of the glomerular filtrate, or more rarely, an excessive reabsorption of such constituents. Most of these conditions are congenital, but occasionally they may be acquired in later life.

Impaired water reabsorption—nephrogenic diabetes insipidus.[30] It is an example of a disease often inherited as a sex-linked recessive characteristic.* It manifests itself in infancy with symptoms of pyrexia, dehydration, vomiting, and collapse. There is severe polyuria, as the kidney does not respond to antidiuretic hormone.

Impaired glucose reabsorption—renal glycosuria.

Impaired phosphate reabsorption—familial hypophosphataemia, or vitamin-D resistant rickets. This condition is interesting in being inherited as a sex-linked dominant characteristic. There is an increased renal excretion of phosphate and also an impaired absorption of calcium from the bowel. The serum calcium is usually normal, but the serum phosphate is very low, and osteomalacia ensues.

An adult type of hypophosphataemia is also described: it affects both sexes equally, and there is also muscle weakness which is not found in the familial type of hypophosphataemia.[32]

Impaired amino-acid reabsorption[33]—cystinuria. There are small amounts of certain amino acids like glycine, taurine, and alanine normally present in the urine, but in some conditions there are much larger amounts of other amino acids in addition. In cystinuria there is much cystine in the urine, while small amounts of arginine, lysine, and ornithine are also present. The danger is the formation of cystine calculi, which are very insoluble in acid solution. The condition is inherited as an autosomal recessive character. About a third of heterozygotes excrete small quantities of cystine and lysine in their urine (the excretion of arginine and ornithine is usually normal), while the other two-thirds have a normal urinary amino-acid excretion.[34]

Impaired xanthine reabsorption—xanthinuria. There is a defect in the conversion of xanthine to uric acid due to the absence of xanthine oxidase in the liver. The xanthine is excreted by the kidney, and is not absorbed owing to a tubular defect. In this condition there are apparently two congenital defects which are quite distinct. Xanthine calculi may be formed. The blood uric acid is very low in xanthinuria.

Impaired reabsorption of amino acids, glucose, and phosphate. This is usually called the *Fanconi syndrome*. When congenital, it appears to be inherited as an autosomal recessive characteristic. Such cases have widespread deposits of cystine crystals in their tissues, hence the alternative names "cystinosis" and "cystine-storage disease" that are sometimes used. The amino-aciduria is more extensive in variety, but much less copious than in cystinuria, and only small amounts of cystine are present in the urine. The condition is frequently attended by other renal defects as well: (*a*) proteinuria; (*b*) an inability to secrete hydrogen

*It is of interest that the "water drinker's curse" which affects certain families in the Maritime provinces of Canada and in New England was known in the folklore to affect males but be passed on by the females for more than a hundred years before Mendel proposed his laws of heredity.[31]

ions, so that the urine is imperfectly acidified. This in turn is accompanied by excessive potassium excretion and symptoms of hypokalaemia; (c) impaired glomerular filtration leading to renal failure, which is the usual cause of death.

There is in addition osteomalacia with a low serum phosphate and a normal serum calcium as described in hypophosphataemia.

Inability to secrete hydrogen ions—renal tubular acidosis.[30] In this condition the distal tubules cannot transfer hydrogen ions to the filtrate. Whereas the normal kidney can acidify the urine to a pH of 4·4, in renal tubular acidosis the pH remains at a higher level (over 6) despite a severe metabolic acidosis. The serum bicarbonate concentration is low, while the serum chloride is raised. Hyperchloraemic acidosis is produced (see p. 451). As in the Fanconi syndrome there is an associated hypokalaemia.

In addition, calcium is lost in the urine; this has been ascribed to the chronic acidosis bringing calcium and phosphate out of the bones. The loss is increased as the result of inadequate tubular reabsorption. Nephrocalcinosis and stone formation frequently ensue; perhaps the relative alkalinity of the urine facilitates the precipitation of the calcium and phosphate. Osteomalacia and calcium deficiency are common findings.

There is no abnormality in the absorption of amino acids,

glucose, or phosphate as seen in the Fanconi syndrome. The disease is most common in early childhood, but an adult type is also described. Its aetiology is uncertain; it is familial in some cases.

Excessive reabsorption of phosphate—pseudohypoparathyroidism. In this very rare condition the renal tubules are congenitally unresponsive to parathormone. The serum phosphate is raised and the serum calcium is low. The patient suffers from severe tetany which does not respond to parathormone. Other features of this condition are a flat round face, stumpy hands, and mental retardation.

The above conditions are all congenital, but similar defects of tubular reabsorption may occur during the course of other diseases. Galactosaemia and Wilson's disease, for example, damage the tubules and lead to amino-aciduria, while chronic pyelonephritis may be associated with defective hydrogen-ion production by the distal tubule.[30] An acquired Fanconi syndrome may follow the toxic action on the tubules of heavy metals like mercury and lead, and may complicate the copper intoxication of Wilson's disease. The acquired syndrome is not accompanied by cystinosis.

These tubular defects are of the greatest theoretical interest, because they throw fresh light on the more obscure aspects of renal function.

GENERAL READING

BLACK, D. A. K. (1967). *Renal Disease*, 2nd edn, 798 pp. Oxford: Blackwell.
DE WARDENER, H. E. (1967). *The Kidney*, 3rd edn, 408 pp. London: Churchill.
PITTS, R. F. (1968). *Physiology of the Kidney and Body Fluids*, 2nd edn, 266 pp. Chicago: Year Book Medical Publishers.

REFERENCES

1. PLATT, R. (1959). *Lancet*, i, 159.
2. FARQUHAR, M. G., WISSIG, S. L. and PALADE, G. E. (1961). *Journal of Experimental Medicine*, **113,** 47.
3. KIM, K. E. *et al.* (1969). *British Medical Journal*, iv, 11.
4. SCHREINER, G. E. (1967). In *Renal Disease*, p. 309, *loc. cit.*
5. Leading Article (1968). *Lancet*, i, 1183.
6. OLIVER, J., MacDOWELL, M. and TRACY, A. (1951). *Journal of Clinical Investigation*, **30,** 1305.
7. PATEL, R., McKENZIE, J. K. and McQUEEN, E. G. (1964). *Lancet*, i, 457.
8. GRANT, G. H. (1959). *Journal of Clinical Pathology*, **12,** 510.
9. BRUN, C. *et al.* (1955). *Proceedings of the Society of Experimental Biology and Medicine*, **89,** 687.
10. ROSENHEIM, M. L. and ROSS, E. J. (1967). In *Renal Disease*, p. 327, *loc. cit.*
11. MERRILL, J. P. and HAMPERS, C. L. (1970). *New England Journal of Medicine*, **282,** 953 and 1014.
12. STANBURY, S. W. (1967). In *Renal Disease*, p. 665, *loc. cit.*
13. Leading Article (1972). *Lancet*, i, 1000.
14. GALANTE, L. *et al.* (1972). *Lancet*, i, 985.
15. ANDERSON, T. J. and BOYLE, I. T. (1971). *Journal of Pathology*, **105,** 211.
16. PEART, W. S. (1967). In *Renal Disease*, p. 665, *loc. cit.*
17. MASON, E. E. (1952). *Annals of Internal Medicine*, **37,** 96.
18. Leading Article (1971). *Lancet*, ii, 1407.
19. HAMPERS, C. L. *et al.* (1968). *New England Journal of Medicine*, **279,** 695.
20. DONIACH, I. (1947). *American Journal of Roentgenology*, **58,** 620.
21. DONIACH, I. (1949). *Lancet*, ii, 911.
22. MacLEOD, M., STALKER, A. L. and OGSTON, D. (1962). *Lancet*, i, 191.
23. ROBSON, J. S. (1967). In *Renal Disease*, p. 275, *loc. cit.*
24. CHINARD, F. P. *et al.* (1954). *Journal of Clinical Investigation*, **33,** 621.
25. SIMON, G. T. and CHATELANAT, F. (1969). In *The Kidney*, p. 261, Vol. 1. Edited by C. Rouiller and A. F. Muller. New York and London: Academic Press.
26. Memorandum on Immunology of Nephritis in Africa (1972). *Bulletin of the World Health Organisation*, **46,** 387.

27. BRAUNSTEIN, G. D. *et al.* (1970). *American Journal of Medicine*, **48,** 643.
28. BARCLAY, G. P. T., CAMERON, H. M. and LOUGHRIDGE, L. W. (1960). *Quarterly Journal of Medicine*, **29,** 137.
29. KAZANTZIS, G. *et al.* (1962). *Quarterly Journal of Medicine*, **31,** 403.
30. MUDGE, G. H. (1958). *American Journal of Medicine*, **24,** 785.
31. BODE, H. H. and CRAWFORD, J. D. (1969). *New England Journal of Medicine*, **280,** 750.
32. Leading Article (1971). *Lancet*, i, 1343.
33. MILNE, M. D. (1964). *British Medical Journal*, i, 327.
34. WOOLF, L. I. (1961). *British Medical Bulletin*, **17,** 224.

Chapter 43. *Hepatic Failure and Jaundice*

Hepatic failure is a condition in which there is a disturbance of the body's metabolism due to a derangement in the function of the liver. The functions of the liver are manifold: amongst those that immediately come to mind are bile excretion, protein, carbohydrate, and fat metabolism, vitamin storage, and detoxification. In its widest application the concept of hepatic failure includes conditions in which any of these functions is impaired.[1]

In its clinical connotation, however, liver failure is a very serious condition indeed. It is the result of severe structural damage to the liver, and is attended by such characteristic manifestations as jaundice, ascites, bleeding tendencies, and neuro-psychiatric distrubances. The syndrome is sometimes called *cholaemia*, and it is often fatal. Much of the ensuing account will be devoted to an analysis of the principal manifestations of cholaemia, and an attempt will be made to assess which of them is attributable directly to hepatocellular failure, and which to extraneous factors like biliary obstruction and portal venous hypertension.

CAUSES OF LIVER FAILURE

The functional reserve capacity of the liver is remarkable. In man it is a commonly observed finding that, though the liver may be extensively infiltrated with metastatic cancer, there is seldom any obvious failure of its function. Likewise, large amoebic abscesses and hydatid cysts are not attended by symptoms of liver dysfunction, and jaundice is seldom encountered during their course. The remarkable regenerative capacity of the hepatocytes is an additional safeguard against hepatic failure secondary to such relatively localised lesions. The presence of very extensive lesions is an exception. Thus the rare alveolar type of hydatid disease, in which the entire liver is permeated by cystic spaces, kills as a result of liver failure.

Liver failure is the result of *hepatocellular necrosis* causing widespread destruction of parenchymatous tissue or of *cirrhosis*.

Necrosis. The question of hepatic *necrosis* and its relationship to cirrhosis have already been discussed in Chapter 10. Focal necrosis need not be attended by any evidence of liver dysfunction, although the widespread lesions of virus hepatitis do cause biochemical changes. Zonal necrosis also causes dysfunction, and massive necrosis is a very important antecedent of cholaemia.

Cirrhosis. Hepatic failure is an important complication of cirrhosis, whether macronodular or micronodular. It may be precipitated by bleeding from oesophageal varices or episodes of hepatocellular necrosis. Cardiac cirrhosis causes no disturbance other than a mild hyperbilirubinaemia. Biliary cirrhosis is attended by the symptoms of obstructive jaundice; liver failure occurs only terminally.

Vascular lesions. Infarction of the liver is uncommon and is considered on p. 487. If extensive it leads to rapidly developing liver failure. A slow idiopathic occlusion of the hepatic veins leads to the *Budd-Chiari syndrome*, in which there is marked hepatic congestion, ascites, and progressive liver failure. A rather similar effect is seen in *veno-occlusive disease*, in which the small radicles of the hepatic vein undergo progressive intimal fibrosis. The result is a reverse-type cirrhosis similar to that of cardiac disease, but unlike cardiac cirrhosis it leads to liver failure. The condition is especially common in Jamaica, and is said to be due to the ingestion of "bush-teas" which are toxic to the liver.

ACCOMPANIMENTS OF LIVER DISEASE

JAUNDICE (ICTERUS)

Of all the symptoms of liver disease icterus is the most immediately apparent. It is due to an excessive amount of bilirubin in the plasma, the normal range being 0·1–0·8 mg per 100 ml. When the level reaches about 3 mg per 100 ml, jaundice becomes clinically obvious, and is especially noticeable in the sclerae, skin, and palatal mucosa.

Bilirubin is demonstrated qualitatively and estimated quantitatively by means of the *diazo reagent*. This is diazotised sulphanilic acid (sulphanilic acid treated with a mixture of sodium nitrite and hydrochloric acid), and in the presence of bilirubin a red compound, azobilirubin, is formed. It has been known for some time that bilirubin which has passed through the liver cells gives an immediate reaction with the diazo reagent, and this is called a *direct van den Bergh reaction*. On the other hand, there is no reaction between the diazo reagent and bilirubin which has not passed through the liver, until alcohol has been added to the mixture, when an immediate red colour appears. This is called an *indirect van den Bergh reaction*. In order to understand the different types of jaundice, it is necessary to consider the metabolism of the bile pigments.

Bilirubin Metabolism[2, 57]

By far the largest amount of the body's bilirubin is derived from the porphyrin moiety of the haemoglobin of effete red cells which are broken down in the RE system. It is known that bilirubin is not the only breakdown product of haem, but the alternative metabolic pathway is unknown.[3] The fact that such an alternative pathway exists, however, helps explain why the blood bilirubin level becomes stable even when excretion by the liver is completely stopped. In animal studies in which ^{15}N-labelled glycine has been administered, it has been shown that of the labelled bilirubin, about 85 per cent is excreted at about 120 days. Glycine is utilised in the synthesis of haemoglobin, and this excretion is as a result of the red-cell destruction. From 15–20 per cent of the labelled bilirubin is excreted within ten days of the administered glycine. Some of this is derived from the bone marrow during the formation of haemoglobin (*ineffective erythropoiesis*). Although the amount of bilirubin formed in this way is small under normal circumstances, it may be increased in some diseases, e.g. thalassaemia and pernicious anaemia,[4] and contribute to the jaundice. It has been described as a primary cause of jaundice in one family.[5] The early labelled bilirubin which is not derived from haemoglobin synthesis is produced during the metabolism of enzymes, such as the cytochromes, and possibly myoglobin.

Bilirubin is soluble in lipids but insoluble in water. It is kept in solution in the plasma by being tightly bound to albumin. It is removed from the circulation in the liver, where at the surface of the liver cells it is detached from the albumin. It is then bound by proteins in the liver. Two have been identified and designated Y and Z. Y protein is the principal binding protein, and it is quantitatively deficient in the newborn guinea-pig. The administration of phenobarbitone increases the amount of this protein. Z protein is less important, and is competitively inhibited by flavaspidic acid, the active agent in male fern used in the treatment of tape worm. Its administration can cause jaundice.[6] In the liver cell the bilirubin is conjugated into a water-soluble pigment, *bilirubin diglucuronide*, by a specific enzyme called bilirubin-UDP-glucuronyl transferase, which is located in the smooth endoplasmic reticulum. The amount of this enzyme can be increased by the administration of phenobarbitone or dicophane by a process of *enzyme induction*.[7] For this reason, and for the effect on protein Y, these drugs are useful in the treatment of enzyme-deficient jaundice (p. 535).

Some of the bilirubin diglucuronide in the liver cells is reconverted into bilirubin and excreted.[8] This has been demonstrated in the Gunn strain of rat. This animal lacks the necessary conjugating enzyme in the liver. If bilirubin is injected intravenously, none of the pigment appears in the bile. If bilirubin glucuronide is injected, both free and conjugated bilirubin appear in the bile.

The conjugated bilirubin is excreted *via* the bile-ducts into the intestine. It is excreted as a micellar complex with cholesterol, phospholipids, and bile salts. The large molecule of bilirubin diglucuronide is not absorbed in the gallbladder or small bowel, but in the colon it is hydrolysed to the unconjugated form by bacterial glucuronidases, and is then reduced to *stercobilinogen*, nearly all of which is excreted

The structural formula of haem. Note the protoporphyrin ring structure which is composed of four pyrrole rings joined by methene (= CH—) bridges.

in the faeces. This pigment is well absorbed from the small bowel but minimally from the colon. That which is absorbed into the portal circulation is carried to the liver and re-excreted into the bile, apparently as bilirubin, for stercobilinogen has not been identified in the bile. There is therefore a considerable enterohepatic recirculation of bile pigments. The normal liver removes most of the stercobilinogen from the portal blood, and the little that escapes it is excreted in the urine as *urobilinogen*. A damaged liver may fail to perform this function adequately, and an excess of urobilinogen appears in the urine. The normal daily excretion of stercobilinogen in the faeces is 40–280 mg.

The differences between conjugated and unconjugated bilirubin. It is apparent that conjugated bilirubin gives a direct reaction with the diazo reagent because it is water soluble. Unconjugated bilirubin cannot react until it is brought into aqueous solution by the presence of alcohol. The basis of its indirect reaction depends entirely on its insolubility in water.

Furthermore, conjugated bilirubin enters the glomerular filtrate with ease, and is excreted in the urine. Unconjugated bilirubin, being insoluble in water, cannot escape into the glomerular filtrate on its own; it remains bound to the plasma albumin. This explains why haemolytic jaundice is "acholuric", i.e. without bilirubin in the urine.

On the other hand, the lipid-solubility of unconjugated bilirubin has distinct dangers: when in high concentration it exhausts the binding capacity of the albumin, and it is then absorbed by lipid-rich areas in the brain. At a serum concentration of about 20 mg per 100 ml the basal ganglia may become deeply bile-stained, and there is irreparable damage to the neurones. The condition is called *kernicterus*. Bilirubin is indeed to be regarded as a toxic substance, and its conjugation is a part of the detoxifying function of the liver. Even

BILIRUBIN

The iron has been split off, and the porphyrin ring has been opened. The pyrrole rings are now disposed in a straight line.

UROBILIN

A reduction product of bilirubin.

the most severe obstructive jaundice is never complicated by kernicterus, because conjugated bilirubin is not soluble in lipids.

It is noteworthy that certain drugs, notably sulphonamides and salicylates, compete with bilirubin for albumin.[9] The free, unbound, unconjugated bilirubin becomes redistributed in the tissues, and by traversing the blood-brain barrier can lead to kernicterus. The danger of giving such drugs in the early neonatal period is obvious. In this circumstance a serum bilirubin level considerably below 20 mg per 100 ml can be dangerous.

It is also interesting that the blood-brain barrier against unconjugated bilirubin is poorly developed at birth, but that it increases considerably in childhood. In the Crigler-Najjar syndrome, which is mentioned later, if the infant is protected against kernicterus by early exchange transfusions, it may survive and develop normally. Despite high levels of serum bilirubin, it does not develop subsequent kernicterus in later childhood. It therefore does not require repeated exchange transfusions.

Unconjugated bilirubin is very susceptible to photo-oxidation by white light. The end-products are water soluble and not toxic, and this property has been utilised in the treatment of neonatal jaundice. Exposure of the infant's body to bright light lowers the blood level of bilirubin, and it appears to be quite harmless provided overheating is avoided.[10]

Types of Jaundice

Jaundice can conveniently be divided into three types: haemolytic, obstructive, and hepatocellular. The first two are relatively clear-cut, though there is invariably some hepatic dysfunction associated with them. Hepatocellular jaundice, on the other hand, can seldom be explained entirely in terms of a single mechanism.

Haemolytic jaundice. This is due to an increased bilirubin load consequent on an excessive breakdown of red cells. The conditions that cause it are those associated with haemolytic anaemia, as described in Chapter 49. Though the cause of the jaundice is an excess of unconjugated bilirubin, there is an additional factor of hepatic dysfunction due to anaemia. The main biochemical features of a haemolytic jaundice are:

(i) An increased amount of indirectly-reacting bilirubin in the serum.

(ii) An increased amount of stercobilinogen in the faeces.

(iii) An increased amount of urobilinogen in the urine. This is the result of the absorption of so much stercobilinogen from the bowel that some escapes hepatic metabolism.

(iv) An absence of bilirubin in the urine.

The jaundice is not often severe; the serum bilirubin seldom rises above 5–10 mg per 100 ml, except in the neonatal haemolytic anaemia called erythroblastosis fetalis, in which intense jaundice and kernicterus are frequently encountered.

Obstructive jaundice. This occurs when there is an obstruction to the passage of conjugated bilirubin from the liver cells to the intestine. The condition is called *cholestasis*, and the obstruction may be intrahepatic or extrahepatic.

Extrahepatic cholestasis is very well recognised, because it comes into the category of "surgical jaundice". The best known examples of this are: (*a*) blockage of the common bile-duct by gall-stones; (*b*) occlusion of the duct by a carcinoma of the head of the pancreas; (*c*) pressure from without by enlarged lymph nodes in the porta hepatis; and (*d*) a carcinoma of the duct itself, either at the ampulla of Vater or else higher up. Another example is *primary biliary cirrhosis*,[11] which occurs chiefly in middle-aged women. There is a progressive obstructive jaundice which usually kills in about five years. The main bile-ducts are normal, but there is a destruction of the cholangioles, which are surrounded by a chronic inflammatory reaction. Later on severe periportal fibrosis develops. The nature of the disease is obscure, but an autoimmune aetiology is suggested (see p. 205).

Intrahepatic cholestasis may occur from time to time in the absence of obstruction to the bile ducts; it is a rare complication in the last trimester of pregnancy, and is probably due to the effects of oestrogen.[12] Some women who take the oral contraceptive have likewise exhibited cholestatic jaundice due to its oestrogen content. Infants may develop jaundice when breast fed: the factor in milk appears to be an unusual steroid 3α, 2β pregnanediol, which inhibits glucuronyl transferase. Another rare cause of neonatal jaundice is the familial *Lucey-Drescoll syndrome*; a factor present in the mother's serum is believed to be responsible but it has not been identified.

Intrahepatic cholestasis is produced by drugs, and is called *cholestatic drug jaundice*.[13] There are two types: (*a*) that associated with chlorpromazine and other phenothiazine derivatives, and more rarely arsphenamine, para-amino-salicylic acid, and thiouracil. About 1 per cent of patients on chlorpromazine develop icterus after a month's therapy, irrespective of dosage. It is probable that drug allergy is responsible, for there is a heavy cellular infiltration containing many eosinophils in the portal tracts. *Halothane* occasionally causes hepatic damage, and in fatal cases there is massive necrosis similar to that seen in virus hepatitis. Leucocytosis and eosinophilia occur, and hypersensitivity to the drug appears to be the explanation. (*b*) that associated with those steroids which have in common the substitution of an alkyl group in the C17 position; the most important is methyl-testosterone (testosterone propionate has no effect). Steroid icterus affects all patients given a large enough dose, and does not produce portal-tract infiltrations.

In these conditions the liver cells are either normal or else show only minor degenerative changes. In all types of intrahepatic cholestasis abnormalities have been described, at electron-microscopic level, in the microvilli lining the bile canaliculi.[14, 15]

The main biochemical manifestations of an obstructive jaundice are:

(i) An increased amount of directly-reacting bilirubin in the serum.

(ii) A decreased amount of stercobilinogen in the faeces, which are pale in colour. Not only is bilirubin excluded from the bowel, but so also are the bile salts which are important in aiding the absorption of fat. The stool is therefore bulky and frothy, and in long-continued cases the patient may suffer from a malabsorption syndrome. In particular there is an impairment of absorption of vitamin K, and the consequent deficiency of prothrombin may lead to a bleeding tendency. This can be remedied by the parenteral administration of vitamin K.

(iii) A complete absence of urobilinogen in the urine.

(iv) The presence of bilirubin and bile salts in the urine.

(v) A raised serum alkaline phosphatase (see p. 541).

Patients with obstructive jaundice are often subject to severe pruritus, and this is usually attributed to the bile salts in the circulation, but apparently there is no direct correlation between the two.[1]

There is generally also hypercholesterolaemia, which is due to an overproduction by the liver itself rather than retention in the bile. The serum lipids are combined with peptides to form lipoprotein fractions, one of which migrates electro-

phoretically with the α_2-globulin portion of the serum proteins.[16] It is for this reason that there is an increase in α_2-globulin in obstructive jaundice.

In prolonged obstruction there is also hepatocellular damage due to the back-pressure of dammed-up bile.

Hepatocellular jaundice. In this type of jaundice the van den Bergh reaction usually shows both a directly and an indirectly-reacting type of bilirubin, and it is often called *biphasic*. This points both to a failure in the conjugating mechanism within the liver cells, and to an obstruction to the escape of conjugated bilirubin either from the cells into the canaliculi, or from the canaliculi themselves (which constitutes intrahepatic cholestasis). It is also well established that the time of red-cell survival is reduced in conditions of liver failure,[17, 18] so that there is the additional factor of an increased bilirubin load. Despite the complex nature of hepatocellular jaundice, it is helpful to note a few conditions in which the mechanism seems fairly definite.

Enzyme deficiency. During the first few days of life there is a deficiency of glucuronyl transferase necessary for the conjugation of bilirubin. This is the primary cause of *icterus neonatorum*. In addition there is an increased bilirubin load because of haemolysis of some of the fetal red cells; the newborn infant produces bilirubin at a rate of about three times that of the adult.[19] All these effects are aggravated in premature infants. It is hardly to be wondered at that a baby with erythroblastosis fetalis runs a great risk of kernicterus. Severe bacterial infections in the newborn also cause jaundice that is predominantly haemolytic.[20] It is occasionally severe enough to produce kernicterus.

A deficiency of the transferase enzyme is seen in the rare *Crigler-Najjar type of congenital jaundice*,[21] which leads to severe jaundice and kernicterus. A similar condition is seen in the Gunn strain of rat. In some types of Crigler-Najjar jaundice there is a complete absence of the enzyme, but in others the defect is partial and they respond to the enzyme-inducing effect of phenobarbitone (p. 533).

A less severe variant is *Gilbert's disease*, which is the commonest form of unconjugated familial hyperbili-rubinaemia.[22, 23] It is probably inherited as a dominant characteristic, and is manifest as episodes of benign, intermittent jaundice starting from childhood. Needle biopsies have shown a considerable reduction of the conjugating enzyme; in addition there is probably also a defect in uptake of bilirubin into the cell and a mild degree of haemolysis associated with a slightly decreased red-cell survival time. Phenobarbitone induces the enzyme and relieves the jaundice; this also occurs in neonatal jaundice.

The Dubin-Johnson type of jaundice.[24] This is a chronic, intermittent jaundice seen in young people. It is a benign condition and is often familial. The icterus is due to conjugated bilirubin (which escapes into the urine). An interesting though obscure feature is the presence of much brown pigment in the liver cells; it is a lipofuscin. Macroscopically the liver has a greenish-black colour. The defect appears to be one of failure of transport of conjugated bilirubin from the cells into the canaliculi. The picture is one of an obstructive jaundice in the presence of normal canaliculi and bile ducts.

A similar type of jaundice is seen in the *Rotor syndrome*,[25] but here the liver cells do not show pigmentation. The Dubin-Johnson and Rotor syndromes are closely related and may occur in various members of a single family.[26, 27] Sometimes features of Gilbert's disease are mixed with those of the Dubin-Johnson and Rotor syndromes.[28]

Intrahepatic cholestasis complicating liver-cell damage. In some liver diseases, in addition to hepatocellular damage, there is also intrahepatic cholestasis. This may be due to defective transport of conjugated bilirubin into the canaliculi, as described in the Dubin-Johnson syndrome. Acute cholestasis may complicate virus hepatitis to such an extent that a laparotomy may be necessary to rule out the possibility of an organic obstruction to the bile-ducts. The "acute fatty liver" of the alcoholic may lead to obstructive jaundice, due perhaps to pressure on the canaliculi by the distended liver cells. An obstructive element may occur in the course of severe neonatal jaundice, and be due either to inspissated bile in the canaliculi or to frank hepatocellular damage leading to defective transport of conjugated bilirubin to the canaliculi.

It is obvious that in a common condition like virus hepatitis there may be several patterns of jaundice. In the early stage the obstructive element usually predominates. Later on it subsides, and the urine contains an excess of urobilinogen. In the absence of a haemolytic anaemia this is always a valuable sign of liver disease; it indicates that the liver is unable to cope with the absorbed stercobilinogen, which is passed straight on to the systemic circulation.

Cirrhosis is seldom associated with marked jaundice except during phases of acute exacerbation and terminally; indeed its presence is of evil omen. There is, however, a constant excess of urobilinogen in the urine.

Post-operative jaundice is not uncommon, but does not represent a separate entity since many factors can be involved. Amongst these are hepatic necrosis following a period of shock, hepatitis due to drugs or halothane, red-cell destruction in areas of bleeding, and haemolysis of transfused red cells.

THE PORTAL CIRCULATION IN LIVER DISEASE

The normal portal blood-flow is from 1 000 to 1 200 ml per minute. The pressure, normally 3–13 mm Hg, may be measured directly by the insertion of a catheter either through a patent umbilical vein[29] or directly into the vessel at operation. Two other methods are available:

The wedged hepatic venous pressure. Under fluoroscopic control a catheter is passed through an antecubital vein, past the heart, and into a radicle of the hepatic vein into which it is wedged. This gives a measure of the pressure at the venous end of the hepatic sinusoids (*postsinusoidal pressure*).

The intrasplenic pressure. A thin needle is introduced through the skin into the splenic pulp. The pressure recorded is approximately the same as that in the portal vein, and is therefore a measure of the *presinusoidal pressure*. Splenic puncture may usefully be followed by the injection of diodone, which rapidly enters the portal vein and can be seen by radiography.

Portal Venous Occlusion

Mechanical obstruction of the portal blood-flow results in a rise in pressure (*portal hypertension*). The obstruction can occur in the portal vein itself, within the liver, or in the hepatic veins. However, from a functional point of view it is more useful to consider two types:

Postsinusoidal obstruction. This is seen in the Budd-Chiari syndrome, which may be either idiopathic or a result of hepatic-vein thrombosis related to trauma, polycythaemia, tumour invasion, or contraceptive pills.[30] Obstruction is also a feature of veno-occlusive disease.

Presinusoidal obstruction. This may be extrahepatic due to portal-vein thrombosis, or intrahepatic in conditions where there is fibrosis around the portal triads, as for instance in schistosomiasis.

In the common types of hepatic cirrhosis the obstruction is predominantly of the postsinusoidal type. In addition anastomoses develop between the small branches of the hepatic artery and the portal vein. This shunt contributes to the portal hypertension, as may be demonstrated by temporarily occluding the hepatic artery at operation and observing the fall in portal venous pressure.

Effects of Portal Hypertension

The abdominal viscera are engorged with blood, the portal vein and its tributaries are distended, and anastomoses develop between them and the systemic venous circulation.

Portal-systemic anastomoses. The most important site for these portal-systemic anastomoses is the lower end of the oesophagus, where the resulting varices may bleed and cause haematemesis. Not only is there an immediate danger of death from exsanguination, but it may also precipitate cholaemia either by causing shock and hepato-renal necrosis, or by adding to the alimentary protein load (p. 539). Anastomoses between the superior and inferior haemorrhoidal veins may result in the development of haemorrhoids. In practice this is not a common complaint in cirrhosis. A rare but classical sign is the *caput medusae* at the umbilicus, where veins of the abdominal wall drain blood from the umbilical vein, or if this is not patent, from the plexus which surrounds it. Other sites of anastomosis are lieno-phrenic, lieno-colic, lieno-renal, and in the retroperitoneal tissues around the duodenum. These may pose technical problems during surgery on patients with cirrhosis.

In advanced cirrhosis, most of the portal blood by-passes

the liver and enters the systemic circulation, mostly *via* the azygos veins which in life are often demonstrably enlarged on a radiograph. The liver in these cases relies upon hepatic-artery blood, and is usually small.

Portal-pulmonary anastomoses. In addition to the portal-systemic anastomoses, branches of the left gastric vein may form portal-pulmonary communications. This shunt can result in some degree of arterial desaturation as well as contributing to the high cardiac output.

Congestive splenomegaly. An enlarged spleen is the single most important diagnostic sign of portal hypertension. The sinuses are dilated, and their walls show prominent lining cells and some increase in reticulin fibres. Hyper-splenism may result in depression of any or all of the circulating cells of the peripheral blood. It was indeed this aspect of cirrhosis that led to the original description of Banti's syndrome as a separate entity.

Atheromatous change in the portal vein with terminal thrombosis. This leads to rapid deterioration and intractably severe ascites.

Portal-systemic shunting of blood. The by-passing of the liver by the portal blood is an important feature of chronic liver disease:

1. Toxic substances from the intestine pass into the systemic circulation and contribute to the *neuro-psychiatric manifestations* described on p. 539.

2. *An oral glucose tolerance test is abnormal*, since the absorbed glucose passes directly into the systemic circulation.

3. *The ammonia tolerance is impaired*. If ammonium salts are administered by mouth, the liver normally converts the ammonia to urea, and the blood level of ammonia scarcely rises. Except as a terminal event liver disease is never severe enough to upset this mechanism. Hence any rise in blood ammonia in the test is due to portal-systemic shunting of blood rather than to hepatocellular damage.

4. Organisms from the gut can gain access to the general circulation and cause septicaemia. *Gram-negative endotoxic shock* is sometimes seen as a terminal manifestation.

5. *Peptic ulcer*. This is due apparently to the release of a gastric secretogogue from the bowel and its by-passing the liver which would normally degrade it.

6. *Liver-cell failure* due to decreased hepatic blood flow. Hepatocellular necrosis is not uncommon as a terminal event in cirrhosis.

Hepatocellular Dysfunction

The main manifestations of dysfunction in hepatic disease are related to the processes of protein and carbohydrate metabolism and detoxification.

Disturbances of protein metabolism. The liver is responsible for the synthesis of most of the plasma proteins, the most notable exception being the immunoglobulins. It therefore follows that in progressive liver disease there is a fall in plasma albumin and sometimes in α and β-globulins

also. The hypoalbuminaemia leads to a fall in the osmotic pressure of the plasma and is a considerable factor in producing the ascites of liver failure. Most liver disease is accompanied by a rise in the level of γ-globulins, which is reflected by the empirical flocculation tests that are used clinically, e.g. zinc sulphate turbidity, thymol turbidity, and cephalin cholesterol flocculation tests.

The cause of this hypergammaglobulinaemia is not entirely understood. Possible factors involved include antibodies against a causative organism or against necrotic liver cells (autoantibodies). It has also been found that patients with liver disease have high titres of antibodies against organisms that are normally resident in the bowel. It may be that antigens from these organisms pass directly into the systemic circulation *via* a portal-systemic shunt and stimulate antibody formation; normally such antigenic products would be removed by the Kupffer cells in the liver. Thus either a failure of Kupffer cells or a by-passing of them might lead to antibody formation and a consequent hypergammaglobulinaemia.[31]

The most marked hypergammaglobulinaemia occurs in *active chronic hepatitis** seen mostly in young people. In this condition there are usually antinuclear antibodies and antibodies against smooth muscle, and the LE-cell phenomenon is sometimes positive. The condition has therefore been called "lupoid hepatitis", but it is in fact unrelated to SLE. It develops as a relentlessly progressive destruction of liver cells (piecemeal necrosis) and their replacement by fibrous tissue heavily infiltrated by lymphocytes and plasma cells. Thus there is a severe cirrhosis. It appears to be autoimmune in aetiology, and is sometimes accompanied by Sjögren's syndrome, renal tubular acidosis, fibrosing alveolitis, thyroiditis, ulcerative colitis, and arthritis.[32]

The liver is also responsible for the synthesis of most of the clotting factors, many of which are β-globulins. It is hardly surprising that liver disease is often accompanied by a haemorrhagic diathesis (see Chapter 51).

The liver is the principal seat of deamination of amino acids,[33] and it is probably the only organ which can convert the ammonia so produced into urea. In severe liver failure there may be an "overflow" type of amino-aciduria as the

---

* The terminology of chronic hepatitis is confusing.[40] The essential histological feature is a chronic inflammatory reaction with fibrosis in the portal triads. The term *chronic persistent hepatitis* is used to describe the condition when there is good preservation of lobular structure and little or no hepatic-cell necrosis. If groups of cells adjacent to the triads show necrosis (*piecemeal necrosis*), there is usually a heavier inflammatory infiltrate, often with plasma cells, and the liver shows progressive loss of lobular structure with fibrosis. This type of hepatitis is termed *chronic aggressive hepatitis*: it terminates in cirrhosis and death. No doubt other patterns of reaction can be recognised,[41] but as yet the histological pattern cannot be correlated with the aetiology. Alcohol, drugs, hypersensitivity, autoimmunity, and virus infection may all be involved. Whether active chronic hepatitis, which often shows chronic aggressive hepatitis histologically, is a distinct entity is not known.

result of increased blood levels of amino acids. This is to be contrasted with the renal type of amino-aciduria due to tubular defects (see Chapter 42).

Ammonia is also manufactured in the intestine by the bacterial decomposition of protein material. If the ammonia cannot be converted adequately into urea, the level of ammonia in the blood rises and it may interfere with cerebral metabolism. Ammonia intoxication is a possible cause of the neuro-psychiatric symptoms of cholaemia.[34, 35]

Disturbances of carbohydrate metablism[36] Following total hepatectomy in an experimental animal death is due to hypoglycaemia. Such is the hepatic reserve that hypoglycaemia is rarely a feature of human liver disease. It is occasionally seen in acute hepatic necrosis and following an acute episode of alcoholic debauchery. Impaired gluconeogenesis is the mechanism.

The impaired glucose tolerance in liver disease is due to portal-systemic shunting, and if hypoglycaemia occurs, the development of a hepatoma should be suspected, for this tumour is sometimes associated with hypoglycaemia. The mechanism is not clear, but it is usually assumed that the tumour metabolises glucose at a high rate. There is, however, some evidence that the tumour forms an insulin-like substance.

Failure of Detoxification. The usual method of detoxification is by conjugation, either with an organic or mineral acid, e.g. glucuronic acid or sulphuric acid, or with amino acids, e.g. glycine and glutamic acid. These conjugated products are then excreted in the bile or the urine. The conjugation of bilirubin is a classical example of this type. Bromsulphalein is conjugated with glycine, glutamic acid, and as a mercaptide, and though it can be excreted in the bile without conjugation, its clearance from the plasma is an excellent test of liver function.

Morphine is conjugated as a glucuronide in the liver, and intolerance to this drug is an important feature of hepatocellular disease. A small dose may precipitate hepatic coma.[37]

The steroid hormones are conjugated in the liver prior to being excreted in the urine.[1] On the whole, their metabolism is not seriously impaired even in severe liver failure, but a few abnormalities are worth noting: (a) a reduced urinary output of 17-oxosteroids and 17-hydroxycorticoids; (b) an increased urinary output of aldosterone,[38] apparently the liver cannot convert it into biologically inert substances; (c) a tendency towards oestrogen retention.[39]

OTHER MANIFESTATIONS OF HEPATIC DYSFUNCTION

Although the liver plays an important role in *fat metabolism*, there does not seem to be much significant disturbance in liver failure. There is evidence, however, that ketogenesis in response to starvation is reduced in patients with liver disease. The liver manufactures cholesterol, and low serum levels are found in advanced liver failure.[1]

Damaged liver cells release many of their chemical contents into the circulation. This accounts for the raised serum levels of *enzymes*,[42] e.g. transaminases, dehydrogenases, glucose 6-phosphatase, aldolase, and glutathione reductase, *iron*[43, 44], and *vitamin B_{12}*[45] encountered in hepatocellular disease.

Ascites[2]

Ascites is a common manifestation of hepatic cirrhosis and its pathogenesis is complex. There is considerable controversy concerning the relative importance of the many factors involved. In the experimental animal ascites can be produced easily by obstructing the hepatic veins but not by ligating the portal vein. The blood in the hepatic sinusoids normally communicates with fluid in the space of Disse through pores between the endothelial cells. From here the fluid, virtually of the same composition as plasma, is drained by the hepatic lymphatics and reaches the thoracic duct. In cirrhosis the major vascular obstruction is postsinusoidal, and the *flow of lymph is considerably augmented*. The lymphatic vessels, including the thoracic duct, are dilated, but they nevertheless appear inadequate to deal with the increased volume of lymph. Fluid oozes from the liver surface, and while the patient suffers the liver weeps. It has been observed that if the thoracic duct is drained the ascites rapidly diminishes. Since external loss of protein-rich lymph is undesirable, the creation of a lymphatic-venous fistula is one approach to the treatment of ascites.

Other factors in the pathogenesis of ascites are *hypoalbuminaemia*, for if this is combined experimentally with portal-vein obstruction ascites develops, and *salt retention* due to hyperaldosteronism (this is more important in relation to the later generalised oedema). Finally there is the increased capillary pressure secondary to *portal obstruction*, but this appears to be of minor importance. It has been found that there is a rapid turnover of ascitic fluid, about 50 per cent being replaced every hour. Its protein content varies from 1 to 3 g per cent, and it must be concluded that ascites is a type of lymphoedema, with salt and water retention and hydrostatic forces acting as contributory factors.

The Systemic Circulation in Liver Disease

In hepatic failure the plasma volume is increased, but due to the pooling in the splanchnic area the effective volume is decreased. As described in Chapter 39 this causes water and salt retention. The latter may be aggravated by poor inactivation of aldosterone by the damaged liver. Salt retention is often marked in liver failure, and although it may be a factor in the production of ascites, it is probably of greater importance in causing the generalised oedema that occurs in the later stages of liver disease.

The cardiac output is increased in some cases of cirrhosis and there is a hyperkinetic circulation. The hands are warm, the forearm veins dilated, and the pulses full. Congestive cardiac failure of high output type may rarely supervene. The pathogenesis of these effects is complex and uncertain. The arteriovenous shunting in the liver and the portal-pulmonary anastomoses have already been described. The opening-up of many normally inactive arteriovenous anastomoses by a vasodepressor material (VDM) released from the damaged liver has been suggested (this agent is reduced ferritin).[46]

In progressive liver disease there sometimes develop numerous *vascular spiders* on the skin of the face, chest, and upper limbs. These consist of a central dilated arteriole from which emerges a leash of small vessels, and pressure on the central area causes blanching of the whole lesion.[47] Another finding is *palmar erythema* (liver palms); both it and the vascular spiders are also seen in some cases of rheumatoid arthritis and occasionally during pregnancy. The cause is unknown.

Neuro-psychiatric manifestations (portasystemic encephalopathy).[48] These include abnormalities of behaviour, nocturnal ramblings, and attacks of screaming. Convulsions and coma may ensue. Ataxia and a characteristic "flapping" tremor of the outstretched hands are also noteworthy accompaniments. The electroencephalograph shows changes typical of a metabolic disturbance of cerebral function. Sometimes the syndrome is acute, as in the course of massive necrosis or in advanced cirrhosis complicated by a precipitating factor like morphine intoxication, gastro-intestinal haemorrhage, or even a heavy protein meal. On other occasions it is chronic, and may last intermittently for many years. It is this group of patients which is the most pathetic, for they exhibit personality changes, mental deterioration, and other neurological symptoms. It is one of the complications of portacaval shunt operations.

Animals with a portacaval (Eck) fistula become comatose and die if given a meat meal ("meat intoxication"). It is believed that these manifestations are caused by nitrogenous substances which are formed in the bowel, perhaps as a result of bacterial action. They escape detoxification because of the portal-systemic shunt, and thereby reach the brain where they cause this *portasystemic encephalopathy*. A similar chain of events occurs in man either spontaneously in liver disease or else following portacaval anastomosis.

As already mentioned, ammonia is the product chiefly incriminated. The liability to coma after gastro-intestinal haemorrhage is explained by the large amount of extra protein in the bowel. The administration of broad-spectrum antibiotics, e.g. neomycin, reduces the severity of portasystemic encephalopathy by diminishing the bacterial activity in the intestine. It is in fact doubtful whether hepatic coma is attributable to any one single substance absorbed from the bowel.

It seems that the brain is peculiarly vulnerable to toxic and metabolic insults during the course of liver failure, and that such diverse factors as morphine, ammonia excess, electrolyte imbalance, infection, and hypoxia can all produce the non-specific picture of hepatic coma in susceptible subjects.

Foetor hepaticus.[49] The offensive faecal odour of the breath of patients with liver disease is probably due to the passage of foul-smelling products from the gut into the systemic circulation, either through anastomotic channels or through a poorly-functioning liver. The nature of the offensive substances is unknown.

Endocrine changes. The gynaecomastia, testicular atrophy, and loss of body hair sometimes seen in male patients with cirrhosis have been attributed by oestrogen excess due to inadequate inactivation. On the other hand, women may exhibit breast atrophy and amenorrhoea. It is evident that the causation of these effects is complex.

Fever. A low-grade pyrexia, uninfluenced by antibiotics or diet, is not uncommon during the course of progressive cirrhosis. Its cause is unknown; suggested factors are pyrogens liberated from necrotic cells and the failure of the liver to inactivate pyrogenic steroids, e.g. aetiocholanolone.[50]

Anaemia. Patients with advanced liver disease are sometimes anaemic, and this is due to iron deficiency consequent on recurrent gastro-intestinal haemorrhage, hypersplenism, and a diminished rate of red-cell survival. Red-cell fragility is decreased and target cells may be present. A folic-acid deficiency megaloblastic anaemia is rarely present.

Bleeding tendencies.[2] These are due to a failure of synthesis of such clotting factors as fibrinogen, prothrombin, Factor V, and Factor VII. Indeed, the only factor that does not appear to be made in the liver is Factor VIII (antihaemophilic globulin factor). Vitamin K given parenterally does not help, as it cannot be utilised. Other causes of a bleeding tendency are a *defibrination syndrome* sometimes encountered in liver failure, and *thrombocytopenia* secondary to hypersplenism.

Terminal manifestations of hepatic failure. As the patient's condition deteriorates, certain ill-understood biochemical disturbances may supervene. These consist of hyponatraemia and nitrogen retention. A fall in plasma sodium is common to many terminal states, but in liver failure it is particularly severe. Unlike the low-sodium state that follows salt depletion, symptoms are not alleviated by the intravenous administration of saline solutions. On the contrary such treatment may hasten death. The hyponatraemia is not due to sodium loss, nor is there evidence that it is a dilution effect secondary to water retention. Perhaps it is due to intracellular deviation of sodium.[51]

Terminal nitrogen retention, manifest by a rising blood-urea level, is not uncommon, and the combination of renal failure with severe hepatic failure is known as the *hepato-renal syndrome*.[52] Its existence as an entity is denied by some workers, but the frequency with which the combination occurs warrants its recognition. Nevertheless, the pathogenesis varies from case to case, and there is no constant finding to explain the renal failure. The following mechanisms may be postulated:

1. The agent causing the liver damage may also affect the

kidneys, e.g. leptospirosis, carbon tetrachloride poisoning, and tetracycline overdosage.

2. Chronic liver disease may be accompanied by a chronic nephritis in which there is mesangial proliferation and eventual glomerular destruction.[53] The pathogenesis is not known.

3. The renal blood flow is reduced in cirrhosis of the liver and this is usually associated with a redistribution of blood within the kidney, such that the flow through the outer cortex is reduced while that through the juxta-medullary cortex and medulla is maintained.[54] This may explain why patients with cirrhosis rapidly develop oliguric renal failure in response to a relatively minor reduction in blood volume.

4. Renal shut-down, terminating in renal tubular necrosis if the patient lives long enough, can complicate shock. This may be precipitated by haemorrhage, hypovolaemia secondary to rapid accumulation of ascitic fluid following paracentesis, septicaemia, or endotoxaemia. Renal shut-down is particularly common in jaundiced patients, and is a danger when operating on them. It is also common after cholecystectomy, and the infusion of mannitol to maintain renal perfusion is claimed to be of prophylactic value.

Another finding that usually heralds imminent death is the presence of large amounts of various amino acids in the urine. A rise in the level of plasma amino acids and their overflow into the urine is a sign of very severe hepatic dysfunction.

The patient gradually sinks into cholaemic coma in which deepening jaundice, haemorrhagic manifestations, ascites, remittent pyrexia, and circulatory collapse are the main features. A final haematemesis often precedes death.

TESTS OF LIVER FUNCTION

In the light of what has been discussed it is possible to adopt a rational approach to the testing of hepatic function.

It is still as true as ever that most of the tests at our disposal assess only gross dysfunction. The following tests should be performed as a routine:

Estimation of the serum bilirubin, together with an assessment of the bilirubin and urobilinogen contents of the urine, and an inspection of the faeces for stercobilinogen. By this procedure pure haemolytic jaundice can easily be distinguished from pure obstructive jaundice, as has already been described. It is seldom possible to distinguish between hepatocellular and obstructive jaundice on the basis of tests of pigment metabolism. As diagnostic aids in liver disease they are of limited value.

Estimation of serum proteins. The changes in serum albumin and globulin in progressive liver disease have been fully described. No change is found in haemolytic jaundice, while in obstructive jaundice there may be an increase in α_2-globulin. In addition to a total estimation of serum albumin and globulin, electrophoretic examination of the various globulin fractions should be performed. The non-specific serum flocculation tests already mentioned are other useful indications of the presence of an increased γ-globulin fraction, which is seen typically in hepatocellular disease.

Bromsulphalein (BSP) clearance. In the absence of jaundice this is the best available test of liver function. A 5 per cent solution of BSP is injected slowly intravenously; the dose is 5 mg per kg body weight. Its concentration in the plasma is measured colorimetrically, and after 45 minutes there should be less than 3 per cent retention. In the presence of jaundice this test is rendered unreliable from a colorimetric point of view. In any case it is then unnecessary, for there is obvious retention in the plasma of another substance, bilirubin, normally conjugated in the liver and excreted into the bile. There is an increased BSP retention in nearly all cases of cirrhosis, except the most compensated. In heart failure, BSP excretion is generally within normal limits.

TABLE 43.1   Liver function tests in the various types of jaundice

	Haemolytic jaundice	Hepatocellular jaundice	Obstructive jaundice
(a) Pigment Metabolism			
Serum Bilirubin	Indirectly-reacting.	Usually biphasic.	Directly-reacting.
Faeces	Darkly coloured.	Usually normal.	Pale.
Urine	No bilirubin.	Variable bilirubin.	Bilirubin ++.
	Urobilinogen ++.	Urobilinogen ++.	No urobilinogen.
(b) Serum Alkaline Phosphatase (in King-Armstrong units)	3–13.	15–30.	>30.
(c) Serum Proteins	Normal.	Increased γ-globulin. Positive flocculation tests. In progressive cases diminished serum albumin, α_2- and β-globulin.	Increased α_2-globulin. Negative flocculation tests.
(d) Serum Transaminase	Normal.	Great increase in acute necrosis. Moderate increase in cirrhosis.	Mild increase.

SERUM ENZYMES IN LIVER DISEASE[55, 56]

Alkaline phosphatase. Various alkaline phosphatase isoenzymes may be found in the serum, and they differ in their source, electophoretic mobility, and stability to heating and urea. Five sources may be described:

1. *Bone.* This alkaline phosphatase is the least heat-stable, and is considered on page 573.

2. *Liver.* This isoenzyme is usually the major component of serum and is of intermediate stability.

3. *Intestine.* The amount of this stable enzyme depends on the diet. The highest quantity is found in people who are of blood groups B and O and who are also secretors and Le+.

4. *Placental.* This is the most heat-stable, and is present during the third trimester.

5. *Tumour.* This type of alkaline phosphatase is indistinguishable from the placental type, and is most frequently found in patients with cancer of the lung.

The normal level of alkaline phosphatase in the serum is 3–13 King-Armstrong units per ml.

In obstructive liver disease, the liver's content of alkaline phosphatase is increased due to overproduction. The enzyme regurgitates into the blood, and in obstructive jaundice values of over 30 units per 100 ml are the rule. In hepatocellular disease the level varies from 15–30 units, while normal values occur in haemolytic jaundice.

In bile-duct obstruction the alkaline phosphatase that is reabsorbed is in a macromolecular form and is not readily excreted. The conjugated bilirubin which is reabsorbed at the same time is easily excreted by the kidney. It follows therefore that if some of the bile ducts are obstructed, the blood level of bilirubin can be normal while that of the alkaline phosphatase is raised. Any infiltrating lesion of the liver can produce this picture of a raised alkaline phosphatase level in the face of normal values for other tests of liver function. A common cause in practice is a tumour, either primary or secondary.

Serum transaminase activity. The liver is the second richest source of glutamate-oxaloacetate transaminase (GOT), and the richest of glutamate-pyruvate transaminase (GPT). It is not surprising that any marked necrosis of liver cells leads to an escape of these enzymes into the blood. In acute hepatitis both these enzymes are increased, sometimes ten or even a hundred fold. The increase affects the serum GPT (normally 5–25 units per ml) even more than the serum GOT (normally 5–35 units per ml), and these changes may precede the onset of clinical jaundice. In cirrhosis and to a lesser extent obstructive jaundice there is also an increase in these transaminases. The rise is less pronounced than in acute necrosis, and the serum GOT is somewhat higher than the serum GPT. The terminology of these transaminases has recently been amended. Glutamate-oxaloacetate is now called aspartate aminotransferase (As-At) and glutamate-pyruvate is alanine aminotransferase (Al-At).

Other enzymes. Other enzymes released from necrotic liver cells are 5'-nucleotidase, leucine aminopeptidase, and D-glutamyltransferase. More important is one of the isoenzymes of *lactate dehydrogenase*. LDH_5 is found in large amounts in the liver, and the level in the blood is raised in destructive liver disease (see also p. 483). Of all the enzymes liberated from disintegrating liver cells, these two—alanine aminotransferase and lactate dehydrogenase—are the most important diagnostically, as they occur predominantly in hepatic tissue.

In hepatocellular disease there is a fall in the *pseudocholinesterase activity of the serum*. This is in contrast to the other enzymes, the blood levels of which rise after liver damage. Pseudocholinesterase is a mucoprotein, an α-globulin, synthesised by the liver. Its level drops also in malnutrition.

GENERAL READING

Sherlock, S. (1968). *Diseases of the Liver and Biliary System*, 4th edn, 809 pp. Oxford Blackwell.
Schiff, L. (1972). Editor. *Diseases of the Liver*, 3rd edn, 1102 pp. Philadelphia and Toronto: Lippincott.

REFERENCES

1. Sherlock, S. (1961). In *The Scientific Basis of Medicine Annual Reviews*, p. 216. London: Athlone Press.
2. Sherlock, S. (1971). *British Journal of Hospital Medicine*, **6,** 785.
3. Ostrow, J. D., Jandl, J. H. and Schmid, R. (1962). *Journal of Clinical Investigation*, **41,** 1628.
4. Klatskin, G. (1961). *Annals of Reviews in Medicine*, **12,** 211.
5. Israels, L. G. and Zipursky, A. (1962). *Nature (London)*. **192,** 73.
6. Levi, A. J., Gatmaitan, Z. and Arias, I. M. (1969). *Journal of Clinical Investigation*, **48,** 2156 and (1969). *Lancet*, ii, 139.
7. Leading Article (1969), *Lancet*, ii, 144.
8. Okolicsanyi, L., Magnenat, P. and Frei, J. (1968). *Lancet*, i, 1173.
9. Odell, G. B. (1959). *Journal of Clinical Investigation*, **38,** 823.
10. Lucey, J. F. (1969). *Pediatrics*, **44,** 155.
11. Sherlock, S. (1968). *British Medical Journal*, iii, 515.
12. Leading Article (1967). *British Medical Journal*, iv, 499.
13. Sherlock, S. (1968). *British Medical Journal*, i, 227.
14. Eliakim, M. et al. (1966). *Archives of Internal Medicine*, **117,** 696.
15. Phillips, M. J. (1967). *Postgraduate Medicine*, **41,** 3.
16. Hobbs, J. R. (1967). *Proceedings of the Royal Society of Medicine*, **60,** 1250.

17. CHAPLIN, H. and MOLLISON, P. L. (1953). *Clinical Science*, **12**, 351.
18. PITCHER, C. S. and WILLIAMS, R. (1963). *Clinical Science*, **24**, 239.
19. MOLLISON, P. L. (1948). *Lancet*, i, 513.
20. HAMILTON, J. R. and SASS-KORTSAK, A. (1963). *Journal of Pediatrics*, **63**, 121.
21. CRIGLER, J. F. and NAJJAR, V. A. (1952). *Pediatrics*, **10**, 169.
22. POWELL, L. W. *et al.* (1967). *New England Journal of Medicine*, **277**, 1108.
23. BLACK, M. and BILLING, B. H. (1968). *New England Journal of Medicine*, **280**, 1266.
24. DUBIN, I. N. and JOHNSON, V. B. (1954). *Medicine (Baltimore)*, **33**, 155.
25. ROTOR, A. B., MANAHAN, L. and FLORENTIN, A. (1948). *Acta Medica Philippina*, **5**, 37.
26. SAGILD, U., DALGAARD, O. Z. and TYGSTRUP, N. (1962). *Annals of Internal Medicine*, **56**, 308.
27. ARIAS, I. M. (1961). *American Journal of Medicine*, **31**, 510.
28. WOLF, R. L. *et al.* (1960). *American Journal of Medicine*, **28**, 32.
29. MALT, R. A., CORRY, R. J. and CHÁVEZ-PEÓN, F. (1968). *New England Journal of Medicine*, **279**, 930.
30. CHAMBERLAIN, D. W. and WALTER, J. B. (1969). *Canadian Medical Association Journal*, **101**, 618.
31. Leading Article (1972). *Lancet*, i, 80.
32. Leading Article (1971). *British Medical Journal*, iv, 126.
33. WU, C., BOLLMAN, J. L. and BUTT, H. R. (1955). *Journal of Clinical Investigation*, **34**, 845.
34. SHERLOCK, S. *et al.* (1954). *Lancet*, ii, 453.
35. SHERLOCK, S. (1960). *Annals of Reviews of Medicine*, **11**, 47.
36. Leading Article (1971). *British Medical Journal*, ii, 416.
37. LAIDLAW, J., READ, A. E. and SHERLOCK, S. (1961). *Gastroenterology*, **40**, 389.
38. YATES, F. E., URQUART, J. and HERBST, A. L. (1958). *American Journal of Physiology*, **194**, 65.
39. TAGNON, H. J. *et al.* (1952). *Journal of Clinical Investigation*, **31**, 346.
40. SCHEUER, P. J. (1968). *Liver Biopsy Interpretation*, 138 pp. London: Baillière, Tindall and Cassell.
41. BAGGENSTOSS, A. H. *et al.* (1972). *Human Pathology*, **3**, 183.
42. WILKINSON, J. H. (1961). In *The Scientific Basis of Medicine Annual Reviews*, p. 108. London: Athlone Press.
43. CHRISTIAN, E. R. (1954). *Archives of Internal Medicine*, **94**, 22.
44. SCHAMROTH, L. *et al.* (1956). *British Medical Journal*, i, 960.
45. COWLING, D. C. and MACKAY, I. R. (1959). *Medical Journal of Australia*, **2**, 558.
46. SHORR, E. (1954–55). *Harvey Lectures*, **50**, 112. New York: Academic Press Inc.
47. BEAN, W. B. (1953). *Circulation*, **8**, 117.
48. SHERLOCK, S. (1967). In *The Liver*, p. 241. Edited by A. E. Read. London: Butterworths.
49. CHALLENGER, F. and WALSHE, J. M. (1955). *Lancet*, i, 1239.
50. TISDALE, W. A. and KLATSKIN, G. (1960). *Yale Journal of Biology and Medicine*, **33**, 94.
51. TALSO, P. J., STRUB, I. H. and KIRSNER, J. B. (1956). *Journal of Laboratory and Clinical Medicine*, **47**, 210.
52. Leading Article (1969). *British Medical Journal*, ii, 201.
53. BLOODWORTH, J. M. B. and SOMMERS, S. C. (1959). *Laboratory Investigation*, **8**, 962.
54. KEW, M. C. *et al.* (1971). *Lancet*, ii, 504.
55. KAPLAN, M. M. (1972). *New England Journal of Medicine*, **286**, 200.
56. WIEME, R. J. and DEMEULENAERE, L. (1970). *Journal of Clinical Pathology*, **24**, Supplement (Association of Clinical Pathologists), **4**, 51.
57. SCHMID, R. (1972). *New England Journal of Medicine*, **287**, 703.

Chapter 44. Amyloid Disease

Amyloid disease was first described by Rokitansky in 1842. Virchow, who gave amyloid its name, found that, like the corpora amylacea of the brain, it stained violet with iodine and sulphuric acid, and he attributed this to its cellulose or starch-like nature. The salient feature of amyloid disease is the extracellular deposition of an eosinophilic hyaline material. Occasionally this occurs in an isolated area, but in most instances the deposits are widely distributed, though usually some organs, for example the liver, spleen, and kidneys, are more severely affected than others. The deposits tend to be adjacent to or within the walls of small blood vessels. Amyloid is a relatively inert substance, for its deposition excites little tissue response; rarely there is a foreign-body giant-cell reaction to it.[1] The parenchyma of the affected organ shows atrophy due perhaps to pressure, but more probably to interference with its blood supply.

CLASSIFICATION OF AMYLOIDOSIS[2]

The nature of amyloidosis is not understood, and there is no acceptable classification which embodies all the known facts. As with tumours it is convenient to use several classifications, each based on a different facet of the disease.

Classification According to Staining Properties

Three empirical staining methods are in common use:

Iodine staining. This may be used either on the specimen itself or on a histological section. Amyloid is coloured mahogany brown, and if sulphuric acid is added may turn violet.

Methyl violet. This is a metachromatic histological stain because, whereas all other tissues become violet, amyloid appears rose pink.

Congo red. This dye is soluble in amyloid and can therefore be used to stain sections: the amyloid stains an orange colour, and when the stained slide is viewed in a polarising microscope a characteristic green birefringence is imparted. Apart from electron microscopy this is the most reliable method available for identifying amyloid.[2]

Various other dyes have been used, but each lacks specificity. The fluorochrome *thioflavine-T* reacts strongly with amyloid, but it has been found to be more useful in demonstrating the juxtaglomerular apparatus of the kidney which also takes up the dye.[3]

Amyloid which reacts characteristically with these stains is called *typical*, while if the stains are negative it is called

atypical, or sometimes *paramyloid*. This classification is unsatisfactory, since the staining is dependent upon the way the sections are prepared and the precise technique used. Both methyl violet and congo red stains work better on cryostat sections than on the usual paraffin ones.

Classification According to Organs or Tissues Involved

Typical generalised amyloid. The common type of severe generalised amyloid affects the *liver, spleen, kidneys*, and sometimes *intestine, adrenal, lung, lymph nodes*, and other sites to a lesser extent. This distribution is described as typical, the amyloid usually stains typically, and it is deposited external to the endothelial cells of the sinusoids and small blood vessels.[4]

Atypical generalised amyloid.[4] A less common severe generalised amyloidosis affects the collagenous connective tissue of heart, blood vessels, tongue, and gastro-intestinal tract. The amyloid often shows atypical staining with methyl violet and iodine.

Localised amyloid deposits, or "tumours". Localised deposits of amyloid, either single or multiple, may occasionally be found in various sites—urethra, bladder, eye, lung, bronchi, larynx, and skin.

Classification According to Fibres Associated with Amyloid[5]

It has been postulated that amyloid is deposited in tissue in relationship to pre-existing fibres. On this basis two types are described:

1. Perireticular, as when amyloid is deposited in spleen, liver, and kidney.

2. Pericollagenous, as in amyloid deposited in the adventitia of the blood vessels, heart, etc.

This classification has little to recommend it, since electron microscopy has shown amyloid deposition to be unrelated to collagenous fibrils. Furthermore, the two types described are in fact a reiteration of the classification proposed previously. Perireticular deposition corresponds to the type of amyloid described as of typical distribution, whilst the pericollagenous type corresponds to the localised tumours and amyloid of generalised atypical distribution.

Classification According to Associated Conditions

This is the most useful classification because the amyloidoses are grouped on a clinical basis.

Senile amyloid. In elderly people it is common to find amyloid in the brain as senile plaques, in the walls of arterioles of the heart, and in the islets of Langerhans.[6] Amyloid may in fact be a substance which is laid down as part of the aging process. In the heart the deposits may lead to heart failure.[7]

Primary amyloid.[8] Deposition of amyloid may occur in association with no known factors. Two types are described:

(i) Localised deposits forming tumour-like masses as described previously.

(ii) Generalised amyloidosis. Usually the distribution is atypical: involvement of the heart is sometimes a salient feature. Nevertheless, the typical distribution is not uncommon. In some cases of "primary" amyloidosis Bence-Jones proteinuria may be found, and it is possible that these are atypical or occult cases of multiple myeloma.[9] A diagnosis of primary amyloidosis should be made only after excluding myeloma, other gammopathies, and the causes of secondary amyloidosis.

Hereditary and familial amyloid.[2] Several syndromes are described:

Familial amyloid polyneuropathy.[10] In the Portuguese type, inherited as an autosomal dominant trait, the amyloid is deposited in the blood-vessel walls of many tissues. The peripheral nerves, especially those of the legs, are affected most severely. Other types have been described, and in these the eye, liver, and spleen may also be involved.

Amyloid nephropathy in familial Mediterranean fever.[11, 12] This is inherited as an autosomal recessive trait, and is found in people of Mediterranean stock, especially Jews and Armenians. Periodic attacks of fever and polyserositis are associated with the development of generalised blood-vessel amyloid deposits. Renal involvement is marked and often leads to death. Curiously enough, the liver is spared.

Familial amyloid heart disease.[13] One family in Denmark has been described.

Urticaria-deafness-nephropathy syndrome.[14] This curious combination was first described in a family in Derbyshire. An urticarial rash and fever in adolescents is followed by deafness, glaucoma, and subsequent death in uraemia.

Familial cutaneous amyloid.[15] Localised deposits of amyloid in the skin have been described in several families.

These various syndromes are rare; indeed, some have been described only in a few patients. Nevertheless, it is obvious that special attention should be paid to genetic factors whenever cases of primary amyloid are encountered.

Amyloid in medullary carcinoma of the thyroid.[16] This tumour, described on p. 336, often has extensive deposits of amyloid in its stroma. The tumour may show a familial pattern and be associated with phaeochromocytoma. Amyloid is sometimes found in the stroma of other tumours; it is not uncommon in basal-cell carcinoma of the skin.

Secondary amyloidosis. This is the common type of amyloid disease. At one time it was a not infrequent sequel to tertiary syphilis, chronic pulmonary tuberculosis, and chronic suppurative disease such as osteomyelitis and bronchiectasis. These conditions are now rarities, and amyloidosis is more commonly seen as a complication of *leprosy,*[17] *rheumatoid arthritis,*[18] *decubitus ulceration* and *suppurative pyelonephritis* in paraplegia,[19] and *malignant disease,*[20] in particular Hodgkin's disease.[21] The amyloid disease which occurs in these conditions is usually generalised and of typical distribution and staining. An exception to this is the amyloid disease which may complicate *multiple myeloma.*[2] In this the amyloid is often of atypical distribution.

Specific Organ Involvement in Amyloid Disease[2]

Spleen. The organ is enlarged and firm. The common type shows a focal distribution. Amyloid is laid down in the walls of the arterioles of the white pulp, and it subsequently replaces the malpighian bodies (Fig. 44.1). The cut surface of the spleen then presents the characteristic appearance of numerous translucent nodules scattered throughout the red pulp (*sago spleen*). A diffuse type of amyloid spleen is also recognised, in which the amyloid is laid down in the walls of the sinuses, and tends to spare the follicles.

Liver. The organ is enlarged, heavy, pale, and firm. Amyloid is deposited in the walls of the sinuses in the space

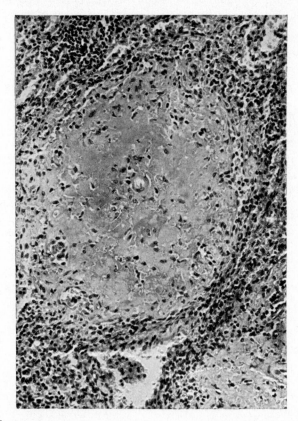

Figure 44.1
Amyloidosis of spleen. This is part of a "sago spleen", for the amyloid infiltration is confined to the malpighian bodies. × 160.

of Disse between the endothelium and the liver cells, at first in the midzone, and later extending to the remainder of the lobule. The liver cells undergo atrophy (Fig. 44.2). The clinical effects of amyloidosis of the liver are often remarkably

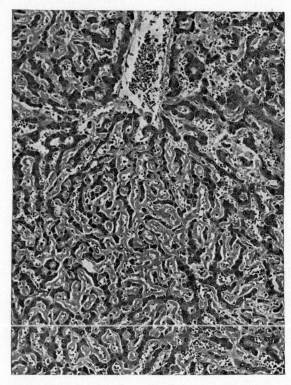

Figure 44.2
Amyloidosis of liver. There is an extensive deposition of amyloid in the space of Disse surrounding the sinusoids throughout the liver lobule. The adjacent liver cells are compressed and atrophied. × 120.

slight even in the presence of marked involvement. Signs of liver failure with an increased blood bilirubin level may rarely occur; likewise portal hypertension with oesophageal varices has been described.

Kidney. Amyloid is deposited in the glomeruli, in the arterioles, and in the interstitial tissue between the tubules. The organ is usually enlarged and pale, but in long-standing disease secondary ischaemic changes may result in a small scarred kidney. Renal involvement in amyloidosis is common and is the most serious manifestation, since its effects are often the presenting feature as well as the major cause of death. The common result of renal amyloidosis is a *nephrotic syndrome. Renal-vein thrombosis* is an occasional terminal manifestation.[22] Persistent haematuria is sometimes seen, and occasionally the involvement of the medulla is sufficient to prevent water reabsorption; a clinical picture of nephrogenic diabetes insipidus has been reported.[23]

Heart. Cardiac involvement is the major manifestation of primary amyloidosis and that which occurs in multiple myeloma. It usually occurs in elderly people. The heart is enlarged and its muscle is extremely rigid and firm. Histologically there is widespread deposition of amyloid in the interstitial tissue surrounding and replacing muscle fibres as well as in the walls of small blood vessels. Clinically there is cardiomegaly with intractable heart failure. The rigidity of the muscle may lead to the condition mimicking constrictive pericarditis. Heart block and arrhythmias are common, and the patients are particularly susceptible to the effect of digitalis.

Gastro-intestinal amyloidosis. Involvement of the gastro-intestinal tract is common and may affect any part. Enlargement and rigidity of the tongue may cause dysphagia as may also involvement of the oesophagus. Plaque-like lesions of the bowel wall may occur at any level. The effects of gastro-intestinal involvement include obstruction, ulceration, malabsorption, haemorrhage, protein loss, and diarrhoea.

Respiratory tract. Amyloidosis of the upper respiratory tract, although not common, may lead to the production of nodules which cause severe effects and even death when they occur in crucial anatomical locations. Amyloidosis of the lungs may produce localised nodules or diffuse involvement of lung parenchyma and tracheobronchial tree. Haemoptysis and respiratory failure may result.

It is evident that the deposition of amyloid in any tissue can produce a variety of effects. The organ may become rigid, and this is particularly important if it has a mechanical function to perform, as for example the tongue or the heart. There is atrophy of the parenchyma of the tissue, and whilst in an organ like the liver which has an abundant reserve this is unimportant, in peripheral nerve the effects are severe. Affected vessels tend to bleed easily and therefore repeated haemorrhages are to be expected; thus in amyloid of the skin purpuric spots appear, whilst epistaxis, haemoptysis, haematemesis, melaena, and haematuria are not uncommonly seen when the respective systems are involved. Since almost any tissue can be involved in amyloidosis the clinical picture may be extremely varied, and the diagnosis should always be kept in mind when one is presented with an unusual case.

Diagnosis of Amyloid Disease in Life[2]

Congo red test. A known quantity of Congo red is injected intravenously, and its concentration in the plasma measured at 4 minutes and again 60 minutes later. If over 80 per cent of the circulating Congo red has been removed from the plasma, amyloid disease may be diagnosed with confidence. Values between 60 and 80 per cent indicate that amyloid is probably present; below 40 per cent the test is negative. As with any test this investigation is not infallible. Furthermore, fatal anaphylactic reactions to Congo red have been reported, and the test is not popular.

Biopsy. Amyloid may be demonstrated in biopsy material

obtained from bone marrow, spleen, liver, kidney, and intestine. The gastro-intestinal tract is frequently involved in most types of amyloidosis. Biopsy of the gingiva or rectal mucosa is a useful procedure, and has advantages over other sites in that, should haemorrhage occur, it can readily be treated. As noted previously, tissue involved with amyloid disease has a tendency to bleed when subjected to trauma.

PATHOGENESIS OF AMYLOID[2, 24, 25]

The composition of amyloid has been the subject of much investigation and speculation. The early view that it was composed of carbohydrate, such as chondroitin sulphate, has been disproved, and the current concept is that amyloid, or at least some types of amyloid, is a protein consisting of a fragment of the light chains of an immunoglobulin molecule. Considerable evidence has been amassed to show that amyloid is produced as a result of a long-continued immune response or of abnormal immunoglobulin production. This evidence may be summarised as follows:

1. Secondary amyloid is commonly seen as a complication of chronic infection and rheumatoid arthritis.

2. It occurs as a complication in about 10 per cent of cases of multiple myeloma, a disease in which an abnormal immunoglobulin is produced.

3. Amyloidosis is found in horses used for the production of diphtheria antitoxin and in mice given injections of sodium caseinate.[26]

4. Fluorescent-tracer techniques have shown that amyloid contains γ-globulin.[27, 28] This has been confirmed using classical immuno-chemical methods.[29]

The immunoglobulin origin of amyloid does not explain the pathogenesis of primary amyloidosis, and the theory has not gone unchallenged. Some investigators have failed to demonstrate immunoglobulin determinants in amyloid;[30] others have identified fibrinogen, complement, and lipoprotein in it, thereby suggesting that all these substances and others also, such as immunoglobulin, could be deposited as a secondary phenomenon but need not themselves be part of the amyloid molecule itself. Amyloidosis has been reported in patients with agammaglobulinaemia,[31, 32] and it will develop in some mice given sodium caseinate even though the animals are rendered tolerant to this antigen.[33, 34]

High-resolution electron microscopy has revealed that amyloid consists of *fibrils* (Fig. 44.3), and that these are made up of 1–4 laterally aligned *filaments* each 7·5 nm in diameter (Fig. 44.4).[2, 35] These filaments are themselves made up of 5 protofibres, each 2·5–3·5 nm in diameter (Fig. 44.5).[35] This filamentous structure is comparable to that of other proteins, for example keratin, and is not like that of antigen-antibody precipitates. Other structural arrangements for amyloid have been proposed. Thus one group of workers have identified amyloid as rod-shaped structures, 10 nm in diameter, and made up of pentagonal subunits piled one on top of another to give the fibre a 4 nm periodicity.[36] It is

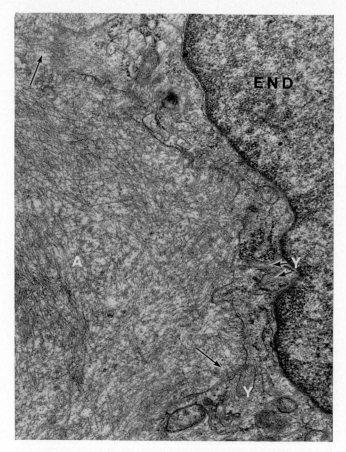

Figure 44.3
Amyloid-laden rabbit spleen. The amyloid fibrils (A) fill most of the space near the endothelial cell (END), whose plasma membrane bears an intricate relationship to the fibrils, especially in the areas marked by arrows. In several areas (Y) fibrils appear to be intracellular. Osmium-fixed, Epon-embedded tissue, stained with lead citrate. ×24 000. *(From Cohen, A. S.* (1965), in "International Review of Experimental Pathology" vol. 4, p. 159, eds. Richter, G. W. and Epstein, M. A. New York and London: Academic Press)

doubtful whether these filaments are in fact composed of amyloid.

The difficulties which research workers have encountered in identifying the chemical nature of amyloid have been due to the difficulties inherent in analysing insoluble substances —and amyloid fibrils are very insoluble. It has recently been found that they can be dissolved in 6 M guanidine hydrochloride solution, and amino-acid-sequence analysis has indicated that the solubilised fibrils contain the same amino-acid sequence as is found in the amino-terminal variable segment of the light chains of immunoglobulin, usually of the λ type.[25] Further evidence of the close relationship between light chains and amyloid has come from a study of patients with multiple myeloma. Bence-Jones protein from some patients has been digested *in vitro*, and the fraction

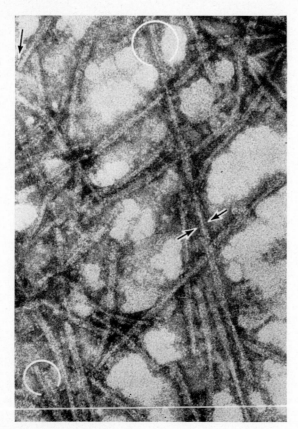

Figure 44.4
Amyloid filaments stained negatively with phosphotungstate. In some portions fine linear structures, protofibrils, can be seen either beside the filaments (arrows) or on the filaments (circle) × 200 000. *(From Shirahama, T. and Cohen, A. S. (1967), J. Cell Biol., 33, 679)*

containing the variable portion of the molecule forms fibrils which have the same properties as amyloid.[37] In summary, this work shows that amyloid is a fibrillar protein with an x-ray diffraction pattern indicating a β-pleated structure; it has a molecular weight of 5 000–18 000, and is composed of a fraction of the light chain of the immuno-globulin molecule. It has been postulated that certain light-chain variable regions possess an "amyloidogenic" structure, while others do not. Furthermore, other fractions of the immunoglobulin molecule could also form the same β-pleated sheet and be deposited as amyloid. Indeed, there is as yet no proof that all varieties of amyloid have a similar type of chemical structure, and one example of amyloid has been reported in which the amino-acid sequence does not correspond to any known protein sequence.[25] Amyloid as recognised histologically may therefore be less homogeneous than has been believed, and this may account for the widely differing views which have been put forward concerning its composition and pathogenesis.

Although the composition of amyloid and its relationship to immunoglobulin have been clarified by recent work, the mechanism of amyloid deposition remains obscure. It is possible that antigen-antibody complexes are phagocytosed by macrophages and broken down to produce amyloid which is deposited locally. Certainly it is often found in organs with a high content of reticulo-endothelial cells, for instance the spleen and liver. Alternatively, a soluble amyloid or a precursor could be present in the circulating blood and be deposited extracellularly; amyloid is frequently found around blood vessels and in the glomeruli. Soluble sub-stances with antigenic similarity to amyloid have been found in the plasma of amyloid-affected subjects. However, if amyloid is derived from immunoglobulin this is not alto-

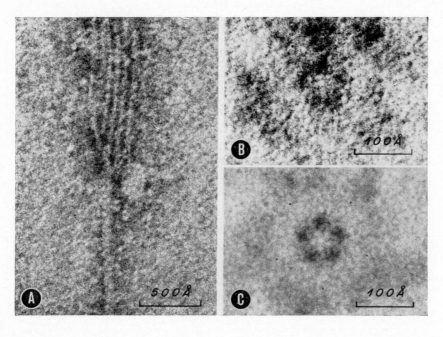

Figure 44.5
(A) An amyloid filament about 7·5 nm wide (bottom half of the photomicrograph) has been dispersed into several (probably five) protofibrils (upper half of the picture) by treatment with urea. Negatively stained with phosphotungstate. × 320 000.
(B) A cross-section of an amyloid filament in a positively stained section. It measures 8–9 nm in diameter, and consists of five subunits of about 3 nm diameter, which are pentagonally arranged around an electron-lucent core of about 2 nm diameter. × 1 470 000.
(C) Same as (B), but five separate exposures have been given and superimposed on one another. Between each, the negative has been rotated through 72° around an axis in the centre of the filament. This confirms that the filaments contain five peripheral, evenly-spaced subunits. *(From Shirahama, T. and Cohen, A. S. (1967), J. Cell Biol., 33, 679)*

gether surprising, and the observation is of dubious significance.

Amyloid may even be a normal component of the body, and an excessive accumulation might arise by augmented production or reduced metabolism, perhaps as a result of some enzyme defect or impaired immune response. The stimulus for this is not known, but the list of known predisposing factors includes inherited abnormality, senility, and a variety of infections, chemical agents, and tumours. It must be concluded that it is still a mystery why amyloid is formed or deposited at certain sites under particular conditions.

REFERENCES

1. WEISS, L. (1960). *American Journal of Clinical Pathology*, **33**, 318.
2. COHEN, A. S. (1967). *New England Journal of Medicine*, **277**, 522, 574, and 628.
3. LEHNER, T. (1965). *Nature (London)*, **206**, 738.
4. KING, L. S. (1948). *American Journal of Pathology*, **24**, 1095.
5. HELLER, H. *et al.* (1964). *Journal of Pathology and Bacteriology*, **88**, 15.
6. SCHWARTZ, P. (1965). *Transactions of the New York Academy of Sciences*, **27**, 393.
7. POMERANCE, A. (1965). *British Heart Journal*, **27**, 711.
8. SYMMERS, W. St. C. (1956). *Journal of Clinical Pathology*, **9**, 187.
9. BARTH, W. F. *et al.* (1969). *American Journal of Medicine*, **47**, 259.
10. HORTA, J. DA S., FILIPE, I. and DUARTE, S. (1964). *Pathology and Microbiology*, **27**, 809.
11. HELLER, H. *et al.* (1961). *Archives of Internal Medicine*, **107**, 539.
12. GAFNI, J., SOHAR, E. and HELLER, H. (1964). *Lancet*, i, 71.
13. FREDERIKSEN, T. *et al.* (1962). *American Journal of Medicine*, **33**, 328.
14. MUCKLE, T. J. and WELLS, M. (1962). *Quarterly Journal of Medicine*, **31**, 235.
15. SAGHER, F. and SHANON, J. (1963). *Archives of Dermatology*, **87**, 171.
16. SCHIMKE, R. N. and HARTMANN, W. H. (1965). *Annals of Internal Medicine*, **63**, 1027.
17. SHUTTLEWORTH, J. S. and ROSS, H. (1956). *Annals of Internal Medicine*, **45**, 23.
18. MISSEN, G. A. K. and TAYLOR, J. D. (1956). *Journal of Pathology and Bacteriology*, **71**, 179.
19. TRIBE, C. R. and SILVER, J. R. (1969). *Renal Failure in Paraplegia*, p. 54. London: Pitman Medical.
20. KIMBALL, K. G. (1961). *Annals of Internal Medicine*, **55**, 958.
21. AZZOPARDI, J. G. and LEHNER, T. (1966). *Journal of Clinical Pathology*, **19**, 539.
22. FRASER, J. G. and KAYE, M. (1961). *Canadian Medical Association Journal*, **85**, 967.
23. CARONE, F. A. and EPSTEIN, F. H. (1960). *American Journal of Medicine*, **29**, 539.
24. COHEN, A. S. (1965). In *International Review of Experimental Pathology*, Volume 4, p. 159. Edited by G. W. Richter and M. A. Epstein. New York: Academic Press.
25. GLENNER, G. G., EIN, D. and TERRY, W. D. (1972). *American Journal of Medicine*, **52**, 141.
26. COHEN, A. S., CALKINS, E. and LEVENE, C. I. (1959). *American Journal of Pathology*, **35**, 971.
27. MELLORS, R. C. and ORTEGA, L. G. (1956). *American Journal of Pathology*, **32**, 455.
28. VAZQUEZ, J. J. and DIXON, F. J. (1956). *Journal of Experimental Medicine*, **104**, 727
29. SCHULTZ, R. T. *et al.* (1966). *American Journal of Pathology*, **48**, 1.
30. CATHCART, E. S. and COHEN, A. S. (1966). *Journal of Immunology*, **96**, 239.
31. TEILUM, G. (1964). *Journal of Pathology and Bacteriology*, **88**, 317.
32. MURRAY, W. D. and COOK, I. A. (1968). *Journal of Clinical Pathology*, **21**, 32.
33. CLERICI, E., PIERPAOLI, W. and ROMUSSI, M. (1965). *Pathologie et Microbiologie*, **28**, 806.
34. DRUET, R. L. and JANIGAN, D. T. (1966). *American Journal of Pathology*, **49**, 1103.
35. SHIRAHAMA, T. and COHEN, A. S. (1967). *Journal of Cell Biology*, **33**, 679.
36. BLADEN, H. A., NYLEN, M. U. and GLENNER, G. G. (1966). *Journal of Ultrastructure Research*, **14**, 449.
37. GLENNER, G. G. *et al.* (1971). *Science*, **174**, 712.

Chapter 45. The Plasma Proteins

The only proteins of the body which are readily available for study in man are those of the plasma. Although these, of course, represent but a small fraction of the total protein content of the body, they form an important group for both the pathologist and the clinician.

The plasma proteins have been classified in various ways. One approach has been to describe each protein in terms of its physico-chemical structure insofar as this is known. Alternatively, a plasma protein can be described in terms of its known function. Ideally a combination of both methods is used, but in practice this is not always possible.

Separation of Plasma Proteins on the Basis of Physico-Chemical Properties

The name attached to a plasma protein is often a reflection of the method used in its separation and identification. It is instructive therefore to outline how the present rather complex system has been evolved. *Fibrinogen* presents no great problem; it is a protein which during coagulation forms an insoluble fibrin clot. The remaining serum was thought, until the middle of the nineteenth century, to contain a single protein called "albumin". It was then shown that by half-saturation with ammonium sulphate, part of this could be precipitated (now called *globulin*) leaving the remainder in solution (the *albumin*). The normal levels are:

Albumin	4·0–5·7 g/100 ml.
Globulin	1·5–3·0 g/100 ml.
Fibrinogen	0·1–0·5 g/100 ml.
Total	6·2–8·2 g/100 ml.

A simple method of subdividing the globulin fraction depends upon *solubility in distilled water*. The *pseudoglobulins* are soluble, but the *euglobulins* are insoluble. This method of fractionation is not much used. A more complex separation was devised by Cohn. It involves the precipitation of many fractions by alteration of temperature and pH, and with differing ethanol concentrations. The method is used commercially for the preparation of plasma components.

For clinical practice a more useful separation is obtained by *electrophoresis*: many different components can be separated, but for most purposes recognition of albumin and the α_1, α_2, β, and γ-globulin fractions is sufficient (Fig. 45.1). Many more components can be detected by the technique of immuno-electrophoresis (see Fig. 1.4, p. 6).

Molecular size has also been investigated. Fibrinogen has a molecular weight of 400 000, albumin 65 000, and the globulins range from 45 000 to several million. A further separation can be made by means of the *ultracentrifuge*. When human serum is centrifuged, three main components can be sedimented:

THE 4S FRACTION. This consists of albumin, the β-globulins, and some of the α-globulins.

THE 7S FRACTION. Composed of γ-globulins.

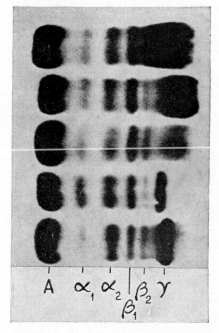

Figure 45.1
Paper electrophoresis in various disease. In hepatic cirrhosis and systemic lupus erythematosus there is a diffuse increase in the γ-globulins. This contrasts with the narrow band seen in myeloma and macroglobulinaemia. *(From Waldenström, J. (1958), Triangle, the Sandoz Journal of Medical Science, 3, 262)*

THE 19S FRACTION. Composed of α-globulins and γ-globulins.

The rapidly sedimenting material in the 19S fraction consists of large molecules, which are therefore called the *macroglobulins*.

Some proteins precipitate out of solution in the cold. These are called *cryoglobulins*.[1] Finally, some proteins may contain lipid or carbohydrate. The former are called *lipoproteins*, and the latter *glycoproteins*. These may also be divided electrophoretically into the conventional globulin fractions.

Separation of Plasma Proteins on the Basis of their Function[1]

Many proteins, or groups of proteins, can be recognised by virtue of their function:

Immunoglobulins. These proteins have antibody activity and have been described in Chapter 12. Most of them are γ-globulins, but some fall within the α and β range on electrophoresis. They may be further characterised by precipitin and other reactions as well as by the composition of their polypeptide chains.

The Proteins Concerned with Clotting.
The Proteins Concerned with Fibrinolysis.
The Components of Complement.
Hormones, e.g. of the anterior lobe of the pituitary.
Enzymes, e.g. alkaline phosphatase.
Carrier Proteins, e.g. caeruloplasmin (copper), transferrin (iron), haptoglobins (haemoglobin), haemopexin (haematin), thyroxine-binding globulin, and corticosteroid-binding globulin.[2] Albumin itself has an important carrier role, e.g. bilirubin, free fatty acid, and sulphonamides. The water-insoluble lipids, e.g. cholesterol and phospholipids, are combined with globulins to form the lipoproteins (see later).

It is evident from the above account that an individual protein may be described and named in various ways: a single substance can be labelled a macroglobulin, immunoglobulin, glycoprotein, β_2-globulin, or 19S-globulin.

Source of the Plasma Proteins[1]

The principal plasma proteins are all made in the liver, with the notable exception of the immunoglobulins, the protein hormones, and some enzymes. This has been elegantly demonstrated by experiments which showed that an isolated perfused rat's liver incorporated radioactive-labelled lysine into plasma albumin, α-globulin, β-globulin, and fibrinogen.[3] In the eviscerated rat, however, labelled lysine was incorporated into the γ-globulins, and to a lesser extent into the β-globulins, but not into the albumin.[4]

The serum immunoglobulins of the normal newborn child are of maternal origin, and their level diminishes after birth. Production of antibodies does not normally commence for some weeks (pp. 141 and 164).

Fate of the Plasma Proteins

There is a regular turnover of the plasma proteins but the sites of catabolism are poorly defined. The liver and probably other organs are concerned with the breakdown of γ-globulin,[5] and there is good evidence that albumin is secreted into the gastrointestinal tract where it is broken down and its constituent amino acids reabsorbed.

Abnormalities of Plasma Proteins

There are three types of abnormality of any protein group. The level may either be raised or lowered, or else an abnormal form of the protein may be present. The term *dysprotein-*

aemia indicates that there is an imbalance between the proportions of the various plasma proteins. It is generally used to describe the conditions where the changes are marked, as when an M protein is present, or where a major component is absent (see dysgammaglobulinaemia, p. 172).

ALBUMIN

Hypoalbuminaemia

During *starvation* the protein reserves are metabolised, and the plasma protein level falls. This principally affects the albumin, the globulins remaining little altered. During *acute infections* and following *trauma* or *surgery* the albumin level drops due to its increased catabolism. This is accompanied by a rise in the α-globulins (especially the α_2-globulin), and the appearance of C-reactive protein (see p. 553). This *acute reaction to stress* is non-specific, and is probably mediated by the release of adrenal hormones.[6] In *chronic liver disease* like cirrhosis, the plasma albumin falls due to a failure in its manufacture.

A low blood albumin is also found whenever there is an excessive loss, e.g. the *nephrotic syndrome*, with rapidly accumulating exudates, and following haemorrhage, burns, and severe injury.

An uncommon cause of hypoproteinaemia is the syndrome of *protein-losing gastroenteropathy.*[7-10] Clinically this is characterised by oedema and a low plasma albumin level, but with no obvious source of protein loss. The syndrome is associated with a variety of local gastrointestinal lesions, e.g. gastric cancer, hypertrophic gastritis, Whipple's disease, Crohn's disease, steatorrhoea, ulcerative colitis, and intolerance to milk,[11] and their cure may lead to its correction. Sometimes no such lesion is found, but instead the jejunum shows uniform thickening due to oedema. The lymphatics are dilated, and the gut wall is brown due to the presence of pigment within the muscle fibres and the phagocytes between the fibres (see p. 564). Tracer techniques using [131]I- and ^{51}Cr-labelled albumin demonstrate the gastrointestinal loss, but the relationship between this and the organic lesions listed above is not clear.

The preponderance of albumin together with its low molecular weight make this protein an important factor in the maintenance of the non-crystalloid osmotic pressure in plasma. A low plasma albumin level therefore contributes to oedema formation (see Chapter 39).

Analbuminaemia has been described as a rare genetic metabolic error. Curiously enough, symptoms (e.g. oedema) are remarkably slight.[1,13]

Hyperalbuminaemia is seen in haemoconcentration.

Bisalbuminaemia.[14] In this rare condition, of which there are several variants, the serum shows two closely adjacent peaks of albumin on electrophoresis instead of the usual one.

THE GLOBULINS

The globulins include a wide array of plasma proteins. The immunoglobulins form a major component, being present in the γ fraction and to a lesser extent the α and β. The normal level appears to be maintained by contact with micro-organisms. Thus in germ-free rats the γ-globulin level is reduced to about one-fifth. The α_2 and β fractions are also lowered. When the intestinal flora of such animals is restored, the plasma proteins return to normal.[15] It is probable that even non-living antigens in the diet can stimulate antibody production.

Agammaglobulinaemia and **hypogammaglobulin-aemia** are described in Chapter 13, since they are associated with various immunologically deficient states.

Hypergammaglobulinaemia

The immunoglobulins form the major component of the plasma globulin, and it follows that hyperglobulinaemia is invariably due to an increase in this fraction. Two main patterns are described.

Polyclonal gammopathy. This occurs whenever there is a prolonged and marked immune response, and is therefore common in chronic infections, e.g. tuberculosis, chronic osteomyelitis, leprosy, and kala-azar. It is also a feature of certain diseases which have an autoimmune component, such as systemic lupus erythematosus and rheumatoid arthritis. Whether this is the explanation of the hyperglobulinaemia of hepatic cirrhosis, active chronic hepatitis, and sarcoidosis is not known. Hypergammaglobulinaemia occasionally develops in the absence of detectable disease and is then labelled idiopathic.

The electrophoretic pattern in these conditions is that of a broad-based elevation of the γ globulins as well as some increase in the β and even the α fractions. There is an increase in many classes of immunoglobulin, and it is assumed that many clones of antibody-forming cells are involved, hence the term polyclonal gammopathy. A rise in the globulin level is sometimes seen when there is a marked hypoalbuminaemia, as in analbuminaemia and the nephrotic syndrome. In the latter there is sometimes a marked increase in the α_2 fraction, and this may simulate an M protein.[16]

Monoclonal gammopathy.[17] In some cases of hyperglobulinaemia there is a marked increase in the level of one type of globulin, which appears as a heavy, narrow band on electrophoresis, or as a spike when the result is expressed graphically. The protein is homogeneous, and contains one type of heavy chain and one type of light chain. It is therefore postulated that only one clone of cells is involved in its production. The condition occurs commonly in *m*ultiple *m*yeloma, Waldenström's *m*acroglobulinaemia, as well as in a few cases of *m*alignant lymphoma. The term *M protein** is aptly applied, but some writers use the term *paraprotein*, on the assumption that the protein is an abnormal one. In fact

* It is not to be confused with the M protein of *Stept. pyogenes.*

it is not known whether the appearance of an M protein is due to the production of an abnormal protein, or to the overproduction of one present normally but in low concentration.

Characteristics of the M proteins. An M protein belongs to one of the five classes of immunoglobulin, and is homogeneous in that it contains only one type of light chain. In the latter respect it differs from normal immunoglobulins, which occur as mixtures of K and L types. Rarely an M band consists only of light or heavy chains.

Effects of hypergammaglobulinaemia. Hypergammaglobulinaemia generally presents itself as a biochemical abnormality which requires further investigation. The patient's symptoms are those of the primary disease—commonly a lymphoma when an M protein is present. Sometimes, however, the plasma-protein abnormality may directly lead to secondary effects:

Hyperviscosity syndrome. The presence of a high concentration of protein, especially a macroglobulin, increases the viscosity of the blood and impedes the peripheral circulation. In the eye the retinal veins are dilated, and characteristically there are localised narrowings which give a "link sausage" appearance. Haemorrhage is common. Sudden paresis may occur, and can progress to coma and death when the cerebral vessels are involved. The heart, kidney, and digits may also suffer, and prompt and repeated plasmapheresis is indicated.

Cryoglobulinaemia.[18, 19] The presence of proteins which precipitate when the serum is cooled may lead to Raynaud's syndrome through vascular blockage in the extremities. When the skin is involved, purpuric lesions appear. Cryoglobulinaemia has been described in macroglobulinaemia, multiple myeloma, kala-azar, malaria, systemic lupus erythematosus, and other connective-tissue diseases, all of which are associated with hypergammaglobulinaemia. It may also occur as an isolated idiopathic condition.

Haemolytic anaemia. Cold agglutinins directed against the I red-cell antigen are not uncommon in mycoplasmal and other infections, but they rarely lead to trouble. In macroglobulinaemia and lymphocytic lymphoma the antibody activity can be sufficiently marked to produce a severe haemolytic anaemia.

Bence-Jones proteinuria. The massive Bence-Jones proteinuria of multiple myeloma may so overload the resorptive capacity of the renal tubles that these structures are damaged. Protein casts form in the tubules, obstruct the lumen, and provoke a foreign-body reaction. The renal damage of multiple myeloma is due partly to this lesion, but to it may be added the effects of ischaemia caused by the hyperviscosity of the blood, amyloidosis, hypercalcaemia, and pyelonephritis.

Protein interactions. Abnormal proteins may interact and bind to other plasma components, such as calcium, platelets, and the proteins of the clotting system. A bleeding tendency may ensue.

Susceptibility to infection. Although M proteins belong to the immunoglobulins chemically, they have little if any antibody activity. Indeed, the production of antibody immunoglobulin is often inhibited, and this leads to an increased tendency to infection. Multiple myeloma often terminates in this manner.

Conditions under which M proteins are found. M proteins are found most commonly in *multiple myeloma* and *Waldenström's macroglobulinaemia.* In these two diseases there is an abnormal proliferation of cells of the plasma-cell series. Recently a third member has been added—*Franklin's disease.* These are described below. In addition, M proteins may occur in other lymphoreticular proliferative disorders, most commonly lymphatic leukaemia. Occasional cases are encountered in which two or more M proteins are present in the same patient. These biclonal or triclonal gammopathies usually progress to a monoclonal state. Presumably one type of neoplastic cell replaces the others.

The routine screening of large numbers of sera has revealed subjects who have none of the diseases mentioned, but in whom an M protein is present.[20, 21] Some have other diseases, e.g. carcinoma, hepatic cirrhosis, or a collagen disease, while others appear healthy. In this latter group a number of cases subsequently develop multiple myeloma or macroglobulinaemia, but the residue remain healthy and have been called "essential monoclonal benign hyper-gammaglobulinaemia". Some cases appear to be familial. The level of M protein is generally low, and neither albumin nor normal γ-globulin is greatly reduced. Bence-Jones protein is not present in the urine. These features help to distinguish the benign condition from the malignant varieties, but a careful follow-up is essential.

Multiple Myeloma[22]

Multiple myeloma is characterised by a neoplastic proliferation of the plasma-cell series. These cells produce an M protein which is usually of the IgG type (55 per cent of cases) or IgA (23 per cent). IgD type protein occurs in about 1 per cent of cases, while IgE myeloma is extremely rare, and in about 20 per cent of cases there are only light chains without a complete M protein in the plasma. By investigating myeloma proteins the classes of immunoglobulin have been delineated. IgD was discovered thus.

About 50 per cent of the patients excrete Bence-Jones protein in the urine. This substance has a molecular weight of about 22 000, and consists of light chains which are of the same type as those present in the M protein. It is recognised by its property of precipitating in urine heated to a temperature of 60–80°C, and then redissolving at higher temperatures. When cooled, it precipitates through the same temperature range, and then redissolves. Bence-Jones protein is produced by the myeloma cells, and since in any one patient it is homogeneous, the urine of patients with this disease is an invaluable source of light-chain polypeptide for chemical analysis.

Macroglobulinaemia of Waldenström[22]

This condition is characterised by anaemia, a high ESR, lymphocytosis, and a tendency to haemorrhages from mucous membranes, especially the gums, either spontaneously or after dental extraction. Retinal haemorrhages also occur. Generalised lymphadenopathy, hepatomegaly, and splenomegaly are common. The disease runs a prolonged course and does not terminate in frank leukaemia. The serum has remarkable features: it is viscous, the globulin level is very high, and the albumin low. When a drop is allowed to sink in a cylinder of water, a heavy precipitate of euglobulin is formed (Fig. 45.2). This simple water dilution test is not

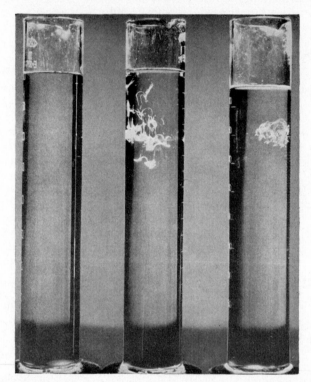

Figure 45.2
The water-dilution test. Left: normal serum; centre: macro-globulinaemic serum; right: kala-azar serum. Note the precipitation of euglobulin. *(From Waldenström, J.* (1958), *Triangle,* Sandoz Journal of Medical Science, **3**, 262)

specific, for it is also positive in some other hyperglobulinaemias, e.g. kala-azar. It is also called the *Sia test.* The ultracentrifuge shows a high level of macroglobulin due to the presence of an M protein of the IgM class. Monomer 7S IgM may also be found in the plasma both in this disease and in other examples of malignant monoclonal macroglobulinaemia.[23] Microscopically, the lymph nodes and bone marrow are crowded with lymphocytes or atypical plasma cells.

Franklin's Disease (Heavy-Chain Disease)[22, 24, 25]

This uncommon disease is characterised by painful enlargement of the lymph nodes with fever, splenomegaly, and recurrent bacterial infections. An odd feature is transient, though sometimes severe, oedema and erythema of the palate, similar to that seen in infectious mononucleosis. In this condition, unlike multiple myeloma, skeletal lesions are not found, but the bone marrow and lymph nodes are crowded with atypical plasma cells. Both the blood and urine contain an abnormal peak on electrophoresis, which is in the fast γ or slow β region. It consists of a fragment of the γ chain resembling the Fc fragment (p. 143). α and μ heavy-chain disease have been described in patients with intestinal lymphoma and chronic lymphatic leukaemia respectively.

C-reactive protein[26, 27] is so named because it reacts as a precipitin with the C-polysaccharide of the pneumococcus. Described originally as occurring in human serum in cases of pneumonia, it is found also in infections due to other organisms, in rheumatoid arthritis, and following trauma. The significance of this is not known. Its appearance is closely related to a rise in the ESR.

Genetic Variation in the Plasma Proteins[13, 14]

The formation of the plasma proteins, like that of other proteins, is determined by genetic factors, and it is therefore not surprising that sometimes the structure of a protein of one person differs slightly from that of another. This variation, or polymorphism, may be detected by electrophoresis or immunoelectrophoresis, and although the various types of a particular protein do not seem to differ functionally, their detection is of considerable interest in anthropological studies. Some examples have already been described. Thus with the immunoglobulins, variations occur in both light and heavy chains, and are determined by alleles at each of the independent loci *Gm* and *Inv* (p. 144). Bisalbuminaemia is noted on p. 550. Other examples are known in the group-specific component, haptoglobin, and transferrin (see below).

The group-specific component.[14, 28] The α_2-globulin band contains several fractions whose function is unknown. Amongst these is a protein which shows polymorphism. This is the group specific component, and its variants are directed by the genes *Gc*[1] and *Gc*[2] to give the three common phenotypes Gc 1-1 (fast), Gc 2-2 (slow), and Gc 2-1 (in which both fast and slow components are present).

Haptoglobin.[14] Three main types are known, Hp 1-1, Hp 2-1, and Hp 2-2, and are determined by the two alleles *Hp*[1] and *Hp*[2]. Haptoglobin has the property of binding any free haemoglobin which is released in the circulation, and is further described on p. 588.

Transferrin.[14] The iron in serum is bound to a β-globulin called transferrin, or siderophilin: each molecule binds two atoms of ferric iron. No less than seventeen variants are known and can be distinguished by their mobilities in starch-gel electrophoresis.

GLYCOPROTEINS[29, 30]

The glycoproteins are proteins other than nucleoproteins, which contain more than 1 per cent of sugar. Certain well-

known proteins, e.g. prothrombin, caeruloplasmin, haptoglobins, and the 19S macroglobulins, are included in this group, as are also some hormones—gonadotrophin, thyroid-stimulating hormone, and thyroglobulin. In general the carbohydrate is firmly bound to the protein, in contrast to the acid mucopolysaccharide-protein complex of connective tissue mucoproteins, which are only loosely bound. The plasma level of glycoproteins is raised in many conditions, including cancer, rheumatoid arthritis, acute rheumatic fever, and tuberculosis; the reason for this is unknown.

Glycoproteins are important components of the ground substance. They are not sulphated nor do they contain uronic acid, and have on this account been called neutral mucoproteins. However, this is a misnomer, because they contain the nine-carbon amino sugar sialic acid, which gives them acidic properties. Epithelial mucins and the blood-group substances belong to this general group.

LIPOPROTEINS[14, 31]

The lipids of the blood form a heterogeneous group which includes phospholipids (such as lecithin), cholesterol and its esters, neutral fat (glyceryl triesters), free fatty acids, carotenoids, vitamin A, and vitamin E. They are carried in the blood as complexes with each other and with certain plasma proteins. Four proteins are involved:

Albumin, which is the carrier of free fatty acids.

Three globulins, named apoprotein A, B, and C, which are manufactured in the liver and exist only in the plasma in combination with lipid. Apoproteins A and B combine with lipid to form the α- and β-lipoproteins respectively. In combination, the three apoproteins form the protein moiety of the chylomicrons and the pre-β-lipoproteins (see below).

The lipoproteins have been separated and characterised by three important techniques:

Chemical Analysis.

Density, as quantitated in the ultracentrifuge and measured in Svedberg units of flotation (Sf).

Electrophoresis.

Lipoproteins Found in the Blood

Free fatty acid is mostly combined with the albumin. This fraction is derived from the adipose tissues, and is the form in which lipid is transported from the fat depots to the tissues.

Chylomicrons. These are particles, over 0·1 μm in diameter, which on electrophoresis do not migrate from the point of application. They have a high neutral fat (triglyceride) content, and are formed in the intestine following the absorption of dietary fat.

Low density lipoproteins (density 1·006–1·063, Sf 0–20). These are β-lipoproteins and contain much cholesterol.

Very low density lipoproteins (density less than 1·006, Sf 20 to 400+). This fraction appears on paper electrophoresis between the α and the β bands. It is called the *pre-β-lipo-*

protein fraction and contains much triglyceride of endogenous origin. It is made in the liver from carbohydrate or lipid sources, and is the form in which triglyceride is transported in the fasting individual.

High density lipoproteins (density 1·063–1·21). These are the *α-lipoproteins* and contain much phospholipid and fatty acid.

Abnormalities of the Plasma Lipoproteins

Hyperlipoproteinaemia is a common finding and indicates an increase in the level of one or more of the lipoprotein fractions described above. In *hypercholesterolaemia* there is an increase in the cholesterol content, due to a raised level of β-lipoproteins or the "broad beta" lipoprotein (see below).

Two major groups of hyperlipoproteinaemia are recognised:

Primary, or familial, hyperlipoproteinaemia.

Secondary hyperlipoproteinaemia, in which the lipid abnormality is associated with some disease which is presumed to be its cause.

The first satisfactory subdivision of each group was that proposed by Fredrickson.[31] Five types or patterns were recognised, based on the lipoprotein fraction which was elevated. This classification has subsequently been modified by a committee of the WHO, which subdivided the original Type II into two subgroups depending on whether the elevated level of low-density lipoprotein occurred alone or was accompanied by an additional elevation of very low-density lipoprotein.[32-34] The memorandum also drew attention to a previously poorly-defined lipoprotein—the *sinking pre-β-lipoprotein.* This has pre-β mobility on electrophoresis, but unlike normal pre-β-lipoprotein, it has a density of 1·050–1·080 and is therefore relatively heavy. Its presence is unrelated to any hyperlipoproteinaemia and is found in about 11 per cent of subjects. It must be taken into account when interpreting the results of lipoprotein analyses. The current classification, which like its predecessor is to be regarded as provisional, is as follows:

Type I. Elevated chylomicron level.
Type II. (a) Elevated β-lipoproteins.
        (b) Elevated β-lipoprotein and pre-β-lipoprotein.
Type III. Presence of an abnormal lipoprotein which appears as a broad band in the β region ("broad beta"). It is rich in both cholesterol and triglyceride, and is therefore of lower density than normal β-lipoprotein. It is also called "floating beta" for this reason.
Type IV. Elevated pre-β-lipoproteins.
Type V. Elevated chylomicrons and pre-β-lipoproteins.

So far as the **primary group** is concerned, the five types have been recognised. Thus *type I*, or *familial fat-induced hyperlipaemia*, is characterised by a raised triglyceride level, and there is a creamy, lipaemic plasma. It is a disease of infancy, and recurrent abdominal pain and pancreatitis are common. *Type II*, or *familial hyper-β-lipoproteinaemia*, is the most common variety, and has a high plasma cholesterol. In this type, and also in types III and IV, there is a tendency for the patients to develop atherosclerosis at an early age.[35] They should therefore be remembered when a young person develops occlusive arterial disease or myocardial ischaemia. In all varieties of familial hyperlipoproteinaemia there is a tendency for focal collections of foam cells to occur in the skin or tendons. *Xanthomata* are therefore common particularly in type III. Eruptive xanthomata of the skin are invariably associated with a raised blood triglyceride level, and are therefore seen in types I and V.

It must be stressed that the lipoprotein pattern of an individual depends, to a considerable extent, on the diet immediately preceding the test. Abnormal patterns may be produced by an abnormal diet even in the absence of genetic error or associated disease. Before testing the lipoproteins therefore, a patient must be on a standard, reasonable diet and have the blood drawn after a sixteen-hour fast.[35] Types III, IV, and V have been called carbohydrate induced, because the abnormal lipid pattern is related to carbohydrate in the diet. An abnormal glucose tolerance is present, and there is often a family history of diabetes mellitus.

In **secondary hyperlipoproteinaemia**, apart from type III, the same spectrum of lipoprotein patterns is found. Thus, in obstructive jaundice there is an increase in plasma cholesterol and β-lipoproteins, while in diabetes mellitus it is the chylomicrons and pre-β-lipoproteins which are elevated. Other diseases characterised by hyperlipoproteinaemia are acute alcoholism, pancreatitis, hypothyroidism, and the nephrotic syndrome. As with the primary group the lipid pattern is influenced by diet, and there may be a change from one type to another.

Apart from correlating the various types of hyperlipoproteinaemia with the presence of arterial disease and various types of xanthomata, the classification is useful because it indicates a line of treatment.[33] Thus, if there is an increase in the level of chylomicrons, containing triglyceride of exogenous origin, as in types I and V, limitation of dietary fat is indicated. If the pre-β-lipoprotein is elevated, as in type IV, carbohydrate restriction is likely to be effective. In hypercholesterolaemia (Types II) treatment with drugs is often necessary. In mixed types, IIb, III, and V, a combination of methods is required.

Hypolipoproteinaemia

Tangier disease, or *familial alpha-lipoprotein deficiency*. In this rare disease, named after Tangier Island (in Chesapeake Bay), which was the home of the first recognised case, there is an absence of the high-density, α-lipoprotein fraction. Cholesterol esters are stored in the RE system, and this storage is responsible for the remarkable enlargement of the tonsils which have a characteristic orange colour—a unique and virtually diagnostic sign.

Abeta-lipoproteinaemia.[36] This syndrome is characterised by steatorrhoea, crenation of the red cells, retinitis pigmentosa, and cerebellar ataxia.

THE ERYTHROCYTE SEDIMENTATION RATE (ESR)[37]

When a column of blood mixed with anticoagulant is allowed to stand vertically, the red cells steadily gravitate downwards because their density is greater than that of plasma. The speed at which this sedimentation occurs is dependent upon many complex factors, chief of which are the degree of rouleaux formation and the extent of sludging. Both these phenomena are related to the composition of the plasma rather than to any change in the red cells themselves. Any increase in the plasma content of high-molecular-weight substances is found to increase the ESR. Thus an increase in fibrinogen or globulin (especially α and β fractions) has this effect; the 7S γ-globulins are the least effective, while excess albumin delays red-cell sedimentation. For this reason a raised ESR is particularly characteristic of macroglobulinaemia and myeloma, and also follows the infusion of high-molecular-weight dextrans.[38] It is also raised in conditions of hypoalbuminaemia, e.g. nephrosis.[39]

The ESR is higher in normal women than in men, and it shows a significant rise with age. The upper limits of normal by the Westergren method may be taken as 15 mm for men and 20 mm for women under the age of 50 years and 20 mm and 30 mm respectively for those over that age.[40, 41] It is usually raised during infection and following tissue necrosis, e.g. myocardial infarction. Presumably an alteration in the balance between the plasma components is responsible, but the factors concerned are ill-defined. A raised ESR is usually accompanied by the appearance of C-reactive protein. The non-specific nature of the ESR limits its value in diagnosis, but nevertheless it is a useful investigation.

The presence of a raised ESR must always be taken to indicate disease, if anaemia and pregnancy are excluded—oral contraceptives are reported to raise it slightly.[42] However, a normal ESR does not rule out organic lesions. It is of value in following the course of a known disease, e.g. tuberculosis and rheumatoid arthritis.

It should be noted that the Westergren method is generally regarded as more meaningful than the Wintrobe method. For an account of various technical difficulties which attend the performance of the ESR a text-book of haematology should be consulted.

GENERAL READING

PUTNAM, F. W. (1965). In *The Proteins*, 2nd edn, vol. III, pp. 153–267. Edited by H. Neurath. New York and London: Academic Press.

REFERENCES

1. HAUROWITZ, F. (1961). In *Functions of the Blood*, p. 527. Edited by R. G. Macfarlane and A. H. T. Robb-Smith. Oxford: Blackwell.
2. Leading Article (1963). *British Medical Journal*, ii, 696.
3. MILLER, L. L. and BALE, W. F. (1954). *Journal of Experimental Medicine*, **99**, 125.
4. MILLER, L. L., BLY, C. G. and BALE, W. F. (1954). *Journal of Experimental Medicine*, **99**, 133.
5. COHEN, S., GORDON, A. H. and MATTHEWS, C. (1962). *Biochemical Journal*, **82**, 197.
6. PETERMANN, M. L. (1961). *Annals of the New York Academy of Sciences*, **94**, 144.
7. JARNUM, S. (1963). *Protein-losing Gastroenteropathy*. Oxford: Blackwell.
8. DAWSON, A. M. (1965). In *Recent Advances in Gastroenterology*, p. 126. Edited by J. Badenoch and B. N. Brooke. London: Churchill.
9. Leading Article (1967). *British Medical Journal*, iii, 510.
10. WALDMANN, T. A. (1969). *New England Journal of Medicine*, **281**, 1170.
11. Leading Article (1967). *Lancet*, ii, 347.
12. BENNHOLD, H., KLAUS, D. and SCHEURLEN, G. P. (1960). *Lancet*, ii, 1169.
13. HARRIS, H. (1961). *British Medical Bulletin*, **17**, 217.
14. STANBURY, J. B., WYNGAARDEN, J. B. and FREDRICKSON, D. S. (1972). Editors. *The Metabolic Basis of Inherited Disease*, 3rd edn, p. 1778. New York: McGraw-Hill.
15. WAGNER, M. and WOSTMANN, B. S. (1961). *Annals of the New York Academy of Science*, 94, 210.
16. SUNDERMAN, F. W. (1964). In *Serum Proteins and the Dysproteinaemias*, p. 324. Edited by F. W. Sunderman and F. W. Sunderman, Jr. Philadelphia: Lippincott.
17. Leading Article (1968). *British Medical Journal*, i, 460.
18. KORNGOLD, L. (1961). *Annals of the New York Academy of Sciences*, **94**, 110.
19. MELTZER, M. and FRANKLIN, E. C. (1966). *American Journal of Medicine*, **40**, 828.
20. HÄLLÉN, J. (1966). *Acta medica scandinavica*, supplement, **462.**
21. HOBBS, J. R. (1967). *British Medical Journal*, iii, 699.
22. HUMPHREY, J. H. and WHITE, R. G. (1970). *Immunology for Students of Medicine*, 3rd edn, pp. 337–347. Oxford: Blackwell.
23. CARTER, P. M. and HOBBS, J. R. (1971). *British Medical Journal*, ii, 260.
24. FRANKLIN, E. C. et al. (1964). *American Journal of Medicine*, **37**, 332.
25. FRANKLIN, E. C. (1970). *New England Journal of Medicine*, **282**, 1098.
26. Leading Article (1954). *Lancet*, i, 350.
27. Leading Article (1956). *British Medical Journal*, ii, 145.
28. CLEVE, H. and BEARN, A. G. (1961). *Annals of the New York Academy of Sciences*, **94**, 218.
29. SHETLAR, M. R. (1961). *Annals of the New York Academy of Sciences*, **94**, 44.

30. HEISKELL, C. L. *et al.* (1961). *Annals of the New York Academy of Science*, **94**, 183.
31. FREDRICKSON, D. S., LEVY, R. I. and LEES, R. S. (1967). *New England Journal of Medicine*, **276**, 34, 94, 148, 215 and 273.
32. Memorandum (1970). *Bulletin of the World Health Organisation*, **43**, 891.
33. LEHMANN, H. and LINES, J. G. (1972). *Lancet*, i, 557.
34. Leading Article (1971). *Lancet*, ii, 806.
35. Leading Article (1971). *Lancet*, i, 117.
36. Editorial (1971). *New England Journal of Medicine*, **284**, 848.
37. Leading Article (1960). *British Medical Journal*, i, 1717.
38. SALSBURY, A. J. (1967). *British Medical Journal*, iv, 88.
39. ARNEIL, G. C. (1961). *Lancet*, ii, 1103.
40. BÖTTIGER, L. E. and SVEDBERG, C. A. (1967). *British Medical Journal*, ii, 85.
41. BOYD, R. V. and HOFFBRAND, B. I. (1966). *British Medical Journal*, i, 901.
42. BURTON, J. L. (1967). *British Medical Journal*, iii, 214.

The pigments of biological origin are frequently striking and of brilliant colour. Less marked in man than in many animals, they nevertheless exhibit obvious abnormalities in disease processes.[1-3]

The common pigments in the human body, e.g. melanin and haemoglobin, are manufactured by specialised cells: they are therefore termed *endogenous*, in contrast to other pigments, e.g. carbon and β-carotene, which are absorbed entire and are called *exogenous*.

Superficially satisfying, this classification is somewhat arbitrary, because exogenous pigments undergo some modification in the tissues. A good example of this is mercurial pigmentation, which is generally classified as exogenous. It is, in fact, produced after the absorbed mercury has been converted into mercuric sulphide.

In this chapter only the more important pigments will be considered in detail. Three main groups are found: the melanins, pigments derived from haemoglobin, and those associated with fat.

THE MELANINS[4-6]

Melanin constitutes the colouring matter of hair,[7] skin, and the eye. It is also present in the leptomeninges, adrenal medulla, and certain nerve cells, e.g. those of the substantia nigra and the locus caeruleus. Limited pigmentation may also occur in the juxtacutaneous mucous membranes, e.g. mouth and vagina.

The pigment usually colours the tissue yellow-brown or, when in large quantities, black. It appears microscopically as brown intracellular granules. Under certain conditions its dispersion and situation may be such that it appears blue or even green.[1] This occurs in the iris of fair-haired individuals, in the sexual skin of certain baboons, and most strikingly of all in many fish.* Melanin reduces an ammoniacal silver-nitrate solution to metallic silver, and is stained black in a section. It is bleached by oxidising agents, such as hydrogen peroxide and potassium permanganate.

The function of melanin in nature appears to be largely protective. This is well exemplified by the "ink" of the cuttle-fish and the changing colour of the chameleon.[2] In man the melanin of skin appears to protect against sunlight.

---

* Fish have additional reflecting cells, or iridocytes. These contain guanin instead of melanin, and are responsible for the beautiful iridescent metallic sheen of many fish.[1]

Thus the effects of sunburn are less severe in dark-skinned individuals, and in the tropics cancer of the exposed parts is more common in the white races.

Site of melanin formation. In skin, melanin is formed in *melanocytes* or their precursors, the *melanoblasts*. They are generally believed to be derived from the neural crest and to migrate during development to their definitive position. In H. and E. sections of skin they appear as large clear cells in the basal layer of the epidermis, but special staining techniques reveal that they possess dendritic processes with which they appear to make contact both with other melanocytes and the epithelial cells. It is through these processes that melanin is donated to the basal cells of the epidermis, which are thereby pigmented.[8] The dermis of normal skin may also contain pigmented macrophages, or *melanophores*, which contain melanin but cannot produce it.

Melanocytes contain enzymes capable of bringing about the production of melanin from tyrosine (see Fig. 46.1). The most defined of these is tyrosinase, a copper-containing enzyme which slowly oxidises tyrosine to dihydroxyphenylalanine (DOPA), which is then more rapidly oxidised to a quinone. After several further stages a closed-ring indol quinone is produced, which polymerises to melanin. This then combines with various proteins to form a melanoprotein (Fig. 46.1). The pigment therefore probably has a variable composition.[4, 5] It is probable that the synthesis of tyrosinase takes place in relationship to the rough endoplasmic reticulum. It is transferred to the Golgi apparatus, and finally enclosed in a membrane-bound organelle called a *melanosome*. This develops an internal structure, and in it melanin is produced and stored.

Although melanocytes have tyrosinase, they do not always contain melanin. The presence of the enzyme can, however, be detected by incubating a section of tissue in a solution of either tyrosine or DOPA. The enzyme, if present, leads to a darkening of the cells due to the production of melanin. This *DOPA reaction* is occasionally of value in distinguishing an amelanotic melanoma from other anaplastic tumours. The reaction with tyrosine is more specific but slower than that with DOPA.

The distribution and extent of skin pigmentation are governed by many factors.

The *number of melanocytes* present varies from one site to another. Thus there are fewer in the palmar epidermis than in that of the dorsum of the hand.

The formation of tyrosinase in melanocytes appears to be

controlled by *genetic factors*. In albinism the cells are present, but are DOPA-negative, and lack the ability to form melanin. The common freckles are also genetically determined. The degree of pigmentation is, of course, also racially determined; the increased pigmentation in dark-skinned races is due to the increased activity of the melanocytes rather than an increase in their number.

In view of the neural origin of melanoblasts and the similarity between the formulae of adrenaline and melanin and its precursors, it is not surprising that pigmentary and

in Addison's disease, presumably because, with the absence of adrenal secretions, the normal feed-back mechanism is interrupted and the pituitary manifests hyperactivity. The administration of cortisone diminishes pigmentation. Pallor is a feature of hypopituitarism: ACTH has slight melanocyte-stimulating activity because it has an amino-acid sequence in common with MSH.[2] The administration of ACTH therefore causes hyperpigmentation.

The sex hormones also play a part in the control of melanin pigmentation.[9] *Progesterone* causes darkening of frogs' skin,

Figure 46.1
Stages in the formation of melanoprotein from tyrosine. The formulae of adrenaline and noradrenaline are shown for comparison with tyrosine. (*After Lerner, A. B.* (1955), Amer. J. Med., **19**, 902)

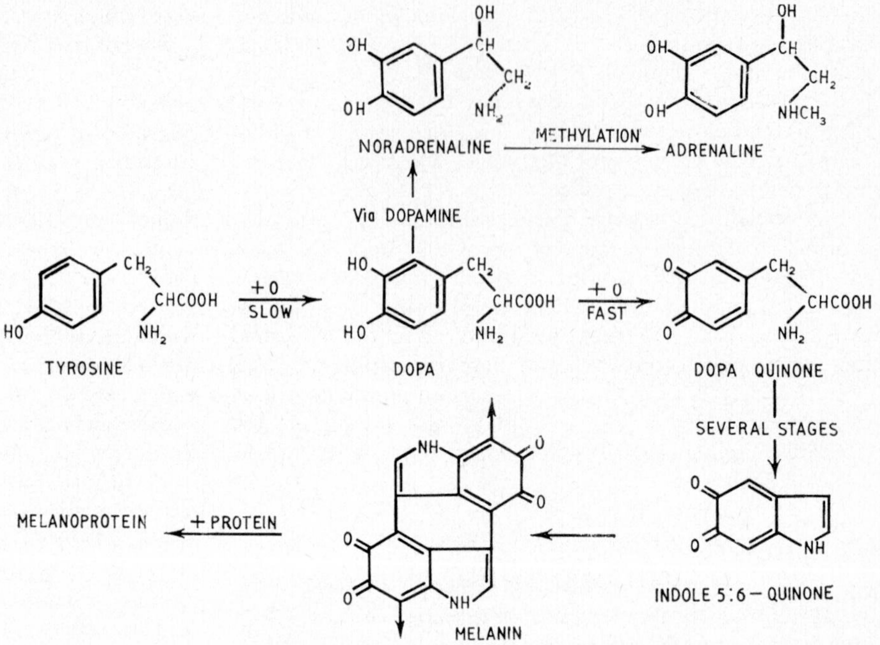

nervous abnormalities may coexist. The best example of this is neurofibromatosis, in which there is an increased incidence of phaeochromocytoma as well as a tendency to focal pigmentation.

The depth of colouring of the skin depends not only upon the number of melanocytes, but also upon the amount of melanin present and its distribution within these cells. This is related to certain *hormones* of the pituitary,[9] and to a lesser extent of the gonads.

The pituitary (pars intermedia) of amphibians secretes a *melanocyte-stimulating hormone* (MSH), which is a polypeptide, and is capable of causing darkening of small, isolated pieces of frogs' skin. This it does by causing the melanin in melanocytes to become dispersed throughout the cytoplasm. This hormone probably regulates the rapid colour changes seen in reptiles: blanching is due to pigment concentrating around the nucleus. Adrenaline inhibits the action of MSH, and the pigmentation of Addison's disease may in part be related to this.[6]

In man MSH is formed in the anterior lobe of the pituitary, and can be detected in urine. Increased amounts are excreted

but its role in man is not known. *Oestrogen* also increases pigmentation if given systemically, as is seen in men treated with large doses for prostatic cancer. This might also explain the hyperpigmentation which sometimes occurs in chronic liver disease and pregnancy, and in women taking contraceptive pills. The action of oestrogen appears to be a direct one, for local application to a guinea-pig's nipples causes pigmentation.

In the male *androgens* are important for normal pigmentation. It is found that eunuchs are burnt by sunlight, but do not tan.

The most potent agent known to lighten the colour of frogs' skin is *melatonin*,[6, 10] which like 5-HT, is found in the pineal gland, and has been identified as N-acetyl-5-methoxytryptamine. It acts by causing the melanin granules to aggregate around the nucleus. Whether it plays any part in the regulation of skin pigmentation in man is not known.

Development of pigmentation. In the white races very little pigment is present in the skin at birth, and the hair is often fair. With increasing age progressive darkening occurs, usually reaching its maximum at puberty.

ABNORMALITIES IN PIGMENTATION[5]

Excessive Pigmentation

Generalised hyperpigmentation. A generalised increase in pigmentation is seen in a variety of conditions. In *Addison's disease* it is most marked in exposed parts and those areas normally pigmented. It is also conspicuous in areas of skin subject to repeated trauma, and is typically noted in the buccal mucosa. The hyperpigmentation seen in *acromegaly* and after *prolonged ACTH administration* is less severe, but is also attributable to the effect of excessive pituitary hormones.

Production of excessive pigmentation by oestrogens has already been mentioned. In pregnancy there is increased pigmentation of the nipples and genitalia, and sometimes a blotchy appearance of the face producing the "pregnancy mask". The term *chloasma* is applied to this condition, which is not uncommon in dark-complexioned women. In *chronic arsenical poisoning* a characteristic pigmentation with raindrop markings may occur, the mechanism of which is unknown. A generalised increase in skin pigmentation is quite often seen in *haemochromatosis*, and also in occasional cases of *chronic malnutrition, cachexia, rheumatoid arthritis* (especially in *Felty's syndrome*), *thyrotoxicosis*, and *pellagra*.

A curious melanosis may follow prolonged treatment with *chlorpromazine*.[11] It affects the eye (lens, cornea, conjunctiva, and retina) and also those areas of skin exposed to sunlight, which become violaceous or even slate-grey in colour. The substances deposited are melanin and a drug metabolite, and on occasions internal organs are also affected. It is possible that chlorpromazine melanosis is endocrine in origin, perhaps due to an increased secretion of MSH or an inhibition of pineal melatonin production.

Focal hyperpigmentation. Scattered areas of pigmentation are common on the skin of normal people and are called freckles, or *ephelides*. There is an increased amount of pigment in the basal layer of the epidermis but the number of melanocytes is not increased.

Café-au-lait spots are large pigmented macules which resemble freckles microscopically apart from a mild increase in the number of melanocytes. They are encountered in two uncommon systemic disorders, (*a*) *neurofibromatosis* (see p. 360), and (*b*) *Albright's syndrome*,[12, 13] a non-hereditary condition which comprises a triad of polyostotic fibrous dysplasia, pigmentation, and precocity (sexual and skeletal).

Another rare condition associated with focal pigmentation is the *Peutz-Jeghers syndrome (familial gastrointestinal polyposis)*,[14–16] inherited as an autosomal dominant characteristic and comprising multiple polyposis of the stomach and bowel, leading to transient, recurrent intussusception, and a brownish pigmentation peppered around the mouth and lips (Fig. 46.2), and sometimes in the skin elsewhere. The intestinal lesions do not become cancerous and are probably hamartomatous in nature. The condition is to be contrasted with polyposis coli, in which the polyps are confined to the colon, cancer invariably ensues, and there is no pigmentation.

Another focal pigmented lesion is the *lentigo*, which differs from the above in showing a great increase in the number of melanocytes in the basal layer of the epidermis. *Lentigo senilis* is a common condition in the elderly, in which there are multiple, smooth "liver spots" on the dorsa of the hands, the face, neck, and arms. *Lentigo maligna* also affects

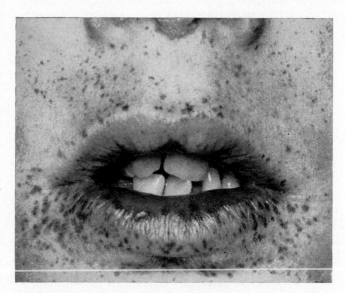

Figure 46.2
Peutz-Jeghers syndrome. Linear streaks and brown spots of circumoral pigmentation. *(Sheward, J. D.* (1962), Brit. med. J., **1**, 921)

the elderly, but is usually solitary and on the face. There are many atypical melanocytes in the basal layer, and the condition is to be regarded as premalignant; about 25 per cent of cases develop invasive melanoma after some years (see p. 358). These tumours are less malignant than melanomata arising from junctional naevi or normal skin,[17] but this is disputed.[18] The good prognosis may be merely an expression of the difficulty in distinguishing between lentigo maligna with marked cellular anaplasia and a malignant melanoma.

Finally, hyperpigmentation of a focal type follows exposure of the skin to ionising radiations, ultraviolet light (sun-tan), and heat. The last is called *erythema ab igne*, and is seen on the legs of people who habitually sit close to an open fire. Pigmentation also follows chronic irritation, and is therefore a feature of pruritic skin diseases. Skin nodules commonly pigmented are naevocellular naevi, malignant melanomata, seborrhoeic keratoses, and basal-cell carcinomata.

Lack of Pigmentation[5]

Generalised hypopigmentation. The most extreme example is *albinism*. In this defect characteristic dendritic melanocytes are present, but tyrosinase activity is defective, and little or no melanin is produced. Electron microscopy has confirmed the presence of these cells with their characteristic granules but lacking in pigment. In *universal albinism* the body contains no pigment-producing melanocytes, the skin is milk-white, the hair pale, the irides transparent, and the pupils pink. The condition occurs in animals, but no proven human case is known. In *generalised albinism* some melanin is produced in the iris and occasionally elsewhere; it is usually inherited as an autosomal recessive characteristic. The patient suffers from nystagmus and photophobia. In adult albinos the presence on the exposed parts of solar keratoses, and squamous-cell and basal-cell carcinomata emphasises the importance of melanin as a protective agent.

Generalised pallor is a feature of panhypopituitarism, male eunuchoidism, and phenylketonuria. In the last condition the great excess of phenylalanine which accumulates probably competes for tyrosinase, and inhibits melanin formation. Thus pigment production in hair can be promoted

either by increasing the intake of tyrosine[19] or by lowering that of phenylalanine.[20]

Focal hypopigmentation. A striking example is *cutaneous partial albinism*, variously called *congenital leucoderma* and *piebaldness*. It produces white patches on the skin which may be quite extensive (Fig. 46.3). It is usually inherited as an autosomal dominant character. Another type of localised albinism is *ocular albinism*, in which the eye alone is affected. It is inherited as a sex-linked recessive trait.

Acquired focal depigmentation is common in leprosy and following the healing of wounds—especially chemical burns. However, by far the most common cause of focal depigmentation is *vitiligo*, a disease which is said to affect about 1 per cent of the population: there are sharply defined areas of depigmentation on the skin, especially that of the exposed parts. In the affected areas melanocytes are absent, and little or no melanin is present. The cause and pathogenesis are unknown, but in some cases a familial tendency is evident.

Pigments Related to Melanin

Ochronosis,[21] first described by Virchow, is a condition in which a melanin-like pigment is present in the cartilages of the ear, larynx, trachea, and joints, in the tendons of the hand, and in ligaments and fibrous tissue generally. In the sclera it occurs midway between the cornea and the canthi.

Ochronosis generally occurs in alcaptonuria, and the pigment is presumably formed from homogentisic acid. A similar pigmentation also occurred in chronic phenol poisoning, in the days when this disinfectant was often applied to wounds.

Melanosis coli. Macrophages laden with brown pigment are found in the mucosa of the large gut in this condition. It is usually associated with chronic constipation, and the pigment is probably a derivative of emodin, an anthraquinone compound found in cascara.[22]

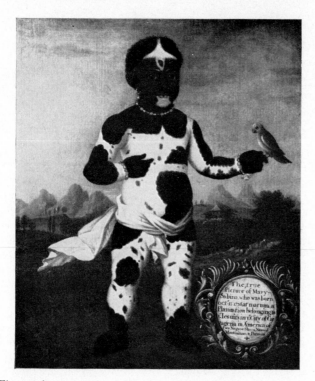

Figure 46.3
Cutaneous partial albinism. This reproduction of a painting in the Royal College of Surgeons of England shows a Negro child. Note the segmental distribution of the areas of depigmentation, and the symmetry of the lesions on the forehead. The caption reads "The true picture of Mary-Sabina, who was born on Oct. 12, 1736, at Matuna, a plantation belonging to ye Jesuits in ye city of Cartagena in America of two Negro slaves, named Martiniano and Patrona". This rare type of cutaneous partial albinism should not be confused with the common vitiligo which usually first appears in early adult life.

PIGMENTS DERIVED FROM HAEMOGLOBIN

Haemoglobin may form a variety of pigments:

1. Methaemoglobin and sulphaemoglobin are considered in Chapter 49. Carboxyhaemoglobin is a bright pink pigment produced from the combination of carbon monoxide and haemoglobin. These three pigments are all intracorpuscular.

2. The porphyrin moiety following haemoglobin breakdown is converted into bilirubin* (see jaundice, p. 533).

3. The porphyrins* in porphyria are described below.

4. The iron released following haemoglobin breakdown is stored in the body as either ferritin or haemosiderin (see p. 562).

* Like haemoglobin, the porphyrins are composed of four substituted pyrrole nuclei joined to form a ring. In the bile pigments like bilirubin, the nuclei are joined to form a chain (see pp. 533 and 534).

Pigmentation due to porphyrins—the porphyrias[23-25]

In the *porphyrinurias* there is an increased excretion of coproporphyrin in the urine secondary to haemolytic anaemia or lead poisoning. The latter may simulate acute intermittent porphyria but the increased porphyrin metabolism is not thought to be related to the symptoms.

The *porphyrias* are an uncommon group of diseases in which there is an abnormality in porphyrin metabolism. The metabolic pathways involved in porphyrin synthesis are outlined in Fig. 46.4. It should be noted that the porphyrins

should be noted that delta–aminolaevulinic acid (ALA), porphobilinogen (PBG), and uroporphyrin are excreted mainly in the urine, coproporphyrin is excreted preferentially in the bile but may overflow into the urine in liver disease, while protoporphyrin is excreted entirely in the bile.

Erythropoietic porphyrias. *Congenital erythropoietic porphyria.* This is a rare inborn error of metabolism, probably inherited as an autosomal recessive trait, which first manifests itself in infancy. The urine is Burgundy-red in

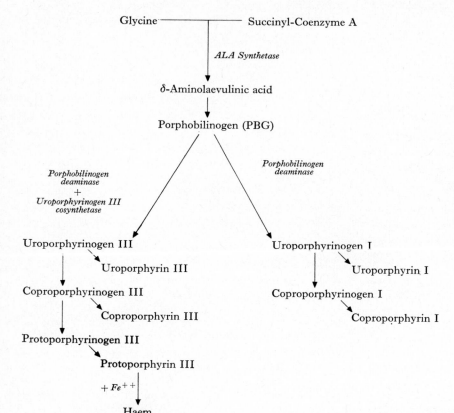

Figure 46.4
Diagram to illustrate the metabolic pathways involved in the synthesis of haem. The condensation of glycine and succinyl coenzyme A in the presence of ALA synthetase results in the formation of δ-aminolaevulinic acid (ALA). Two molecules of this condense to form porphobilinogen (PBG). Normally about 99 per cent of this is converted into uroporphyrinogen III by the combined activity of two enzymes porphobilinogen deaminase and uroporphyrinogen III cosynthetase (also called porphobilinogen-isomerase). Porphobilinogen deaminase acting alone leads to the production of series-I products. These together with uroporphyrin III and coproporphyrin III cannot be used in the synthesis of haem, and are excreted.

of series I are by-products, and are not utilised. Series III, on the other hand, are intermediates in the production of haem in the red-cell precursors, and in other cells (predominantly in the liver) for the synthesis of enzymes such as catalase, cytochromes, and peroxidase. Abnormalities in porphyrin metabolism may therefore be divided into two main groups: (*a*) *erythropoietic porphyria*, in which the abnormality is in the red-cell precursors of the bone marrow, and (*b*) *hepatic porphyria*, in which the erythroid cells are normal, but the liver contains and produces excess quantities of porphyrins.

A remarkable feature of some of the porphyrins is that their presence in the skin causes a sensitivity to light and trauma. This is most marked with uroporphyrin, less so with coproporphyrin, and least with protoporphyrin. Finally it

colour and contains an excess of uroporphyrin I and coproporphyrin I. There appears to be a defect in uroporphyrinogen III cosynthetase activity, so that an excessive amount of PBG is converted into the photosensitising uroporphyrin I. The skin in fact exhibits marked photosensitivity: bullae followed by infection and scarring occur both after trauma and exposure to light (*hydroa aestivale*). Deposits of porphyrin impart a red-brown discoloration to the bones and teeth. A haemolytic anaemia is sometimes present.

Erythropoietic protoporphyria. The red cells and faeces contain a great excess of protoporphyrin, but there is no excess of porphyrin in the urine. Urticaria and chronic eczema develop in areas of skin exposed to light, but the bullae and sensitivity to trauma so characteristic of congenital erythropoietic porphyria are not present.

Erythropoietic coproporphyria has also been described, and is associated with light sensitivity.

Hepatic porphyria. *Acute intermittent porphyria.* This disease is the most common of the porphyrias and is inherited as an autosomal dominant. It is associated with increased delta-aminolaevulinic acid synthetase activity, which results in an overproduction of ALA in the liver. Excess ALA and porphobilinogen are present in the urine. The disease is characterised by acute episodes which may be of three patterns, either singly or in combination:

1. Abdominal—the symptoms closely resemble those of an "acute abdomen".

2. Neurological—a polyneuritis, predominantly paralytic in effect.

3. Psychotic—acute delirium.

Photosensitisation of the skin does not occur. The disease may be latent, and acute attacks can be precipitated by various factors, e.g. pregnancy, infection, and drugs—especially the barbiturates.

Variegate porphyria (porphyria cutanea tarda hereditaria). Many cases of this disease have been reported from South Africa, and most of them can be traced to a Dutch couple who married at the Cape of Good Hope in 1688. As in acute intermittent prophyria, there are acute abdominal and nervous manifestations which may be precipitated by drugs. There is a persistent elevation of the amount of protoporphyrin and coproporphyrin in the faeces, and during the attacks there is in addition an excess excretion of porphobilinogen in the urine. Photosensitivity of the skin occurs, and the disease is usually first noted during the third decade.

This mixed, or variegate, porphyria is of historical interest, for many members of the Royal Houses of Hanover, Prussia, and Stuart are thought by some authorities to have been its victims.[26] Frederick the Great's hemiplegia at the age of 35 years, George III's periods of madness, and Mary Queen of Scot's attacks of colic and fits which earned her the unenviable title of one of the great invalids of history, may all have been manifestations of this unusual disease.

Hereditary coproporphyria is very rare, and is characterised by an increased excretion of coproporphyrin in the urine. Clinically the disease resembles variegate porphyria.

Porphyria cutanea tarda symptomatica. During attacks of this type, the urine contains an excess of uroporphyrin and appears red. Photosensitisation is present and is the presenting symptom. The repeated formation of subepidermal bullae leads ultimately to considerable scarring of the sun-exposed parts. Hyperpigmentation is common, and so also is an increased growth of hair (hypertrichosis)—an unexplained feature which is also found in other types of porphyria. The patients usually have obvious liver disease, and many of them are alcoholics.

Although the metabolism of the porphyrins is well understood, the precise defect in the various types of porphyria is not known. There appears to be an overproduction of porphyrins, either in the bone marrow or in the liver. Photosensitivity can usually be explained by the presence of porphyrins in the skin, but the pathogenesis of the abdominal and nervous manifestations is not known. In some types there is a genetic basis, but even in these the disease may be precipitated by other factors like liver disease or the administration of drugs; sometimes indeed a toxic substance appears to be the major factor. This is well illustrated by the outbreak of porphyria that occurred in Turkey in 1956 due to the accidental ingestion of hexachlorbenzene used as a fungicide in wheat. The present classification of the porphyrias must therefore be regarded as tentative and subject to future change.

IRON-CONTAINING PIGMENTS[27, 28]

Iron occurs in many forms in the body: it is present in such enzymes as the cytochromes and peroxidases, but the largest quantities are present in the red cells as haemoglobin, in muscle as myoglobin, and in the RE system stores as ferritin. The total body content of iron is about 4 g.

In order to remain in balance the normal adult absorbs about 0·6 mg of iron daily, while the menstruating female requires about 1·2 mg. Since the diet contains about 15 mg, it is evident that the intestine plays a crucial part in preventing iron overloading. The mechanism is described on p. 587.

Iron is normally stored in the ferric state and combined with a β-globulin (*apoferritin*) as *ferritin*,[29] a compound containing about 23 per cent ferric iron. It does not give a Prussian-blue reaction, and cannot be seen under the light microscope in routine paraffin sections. On electron microscopy, however, molecules of ferritin are readily visible as groups of four electron-dense particles.

When abnormally large quantities of iron have to be stored, ferritin can take up a greater amount of iron to produce *haemosiderin*. This contains about 36 per cent of iron, and appears as brown insoluble granules which give a Prussian-blue reaction. Haemosiderin is found in any situation where excessive quantities of iron are being stored. This may occur as a local phenomenon or may be generalised.

Localised Haemosiderin Deposits

Whenever there is a haemorrhage, the iron from the broken-down red cells is found in the nearby macrophages in the form of haemosiderin. This is seen around organising haematomata, haemorrhagic infarcts, fractures, etc. A yellow discoloration around a brain cyst is therefore good evidence of its origin from an infarct. One other instance of localised haemosiderin deposition is important: the *sclerosing haemangioma* (p. 352), which is often deeply pigmented and can be mistaken both clinically and pathologically for a malignant melanoma unless special stains are used.

The cells of the renal tubules can also convert haemoglobin

to haemosiderin. This pigment is therefore seen in the renal tubular cells after haemoglobinuria.

Pulmonary Haemosiderosis

The small haemorrhages which occur in the lungs in mitral stenosis and left ventricular failure are responsible for the formation of "heart failure cells". These are alveolar macrophages containing haemosiderin. A mild diffuse fibrosis may occur in long-standing cases to produce *brown induration*. In children and sometimes young adults pulmonary haemosiderosis may arise without obvious cause. This idiopathic haemosiderosis[30, 31] is manifested clinically by a progressive anaemia accompanied by miliary x-ray shadows in the lungs. One variety is accompanied by acute glomerulonephritis; it is called *Goodpasture's syndrome* and has an immunological aetiology (see p. 204).

Generalised Haemosiderosis

If the body is overloaded with iron, haemosiderin is formed in excessive amounts. Two patterns are seen.[28]

Parenchymatous deposition. When the overloading is due to excessive absorption from the intestine, the haemosiderin is deposited in the parenchymatous cells of the liver, pancreas, kidney, and heart, and considerable damage may be inflicted on these organs. This type of deposition is seen (a) when the normal regulating mechanism for iron absorption is impaired, as in haemochromatosis, (b) when there is increased erythropoietic activity, as in chronic haemolytic anaemia (especially thalassaemia), and (c) when there is a great increase in the iron content of the diet.[28, 32]

Generalised haemosiderosis in refractory anaemias with a hyperplastic bone marrow is attributable to an increased rate of iron absorption from the bowel. The haemosiderosis is most severe in those conditions where few viable red cells are delivered to the circulation.

A similar type of haemosiderosis is met with in the South African Bantu, whose diet has a high iron content. Over 100 mg a day may be ingested, much being derived from the iron containers used in the preparation of alcoholic drinks.[28] In these conditions the haemosiderin distribution resembles that of haemochromatosis, but, for an unknown reason, causes less severe parenchymatous damage. Sometimes, however, cirrhosis and diabetes mellitus develop.[28]

RE Deposition. This is seen following parental iron administration or repeated blood transfusions. Haemosiderosis following transfusion affects the RE system primarily. However, the iron content of the body may exceed that attributable to the transfusion, in which case it is evident that there has been an excessive intestinal absorption.[33]

Haemochromatosis.[28, 34, 35] Also known as "bronzed diabetes", this disease is usually considered to be an inborn error of metabolism, and inherited as an autosomal dominant character. It is postulated that there is some abnormality of the mechanism regulating the absorption of iron. This results in excessive absorption of iron (2–3 mg daily), and

over a period of years the body builds up a large store of haemosiderin. The finding that many of the relatives of patients with haemochromatosis have an increased absorption of iron supports this genetic concept. Furthermore, it has been claimed that patients with haemochromatosis lack an iron-binding protein called gastroferrin which is said to be present in the gastric juice.[36, 37] The concentration of this protein is also low in iron-deficiency anaemia, and its secretion may form part of the mechanism which regulates iron absorption from the gut.[38]

Haemochromatosis most commonly affects men, women presumably being protected by their menstrual loss. The pigment is found in the liver cells, pancreas, heart, and other organs. The liver may contain over 50 g of iron. The pigment seems to cause damage, and in the fully-developed disease this results in cirrhosis, diabetes mellitus, and heart failure. A progressive polyarthritis occurs in about half the patients, and it usually starts in the small joints of the hand.[39–41] Other joints, e.g. the wrists, elbows, hips, knees, and ankles may become involved, the pattern somewhat resembling that of rheumatoid arthritis. In about half the cases there are x-ray changes of chondrocalcinosis (p. 569), and attacks of acute synovitis occur.

The plasma iron level is raised and the transferrin is almost completely saturated (see p. 587). The diagnosis is confirmed by liver biopsy or skin biopsy—the pigment is present in the cells of the sweat glands. It is interesting that these patients also show increased melanin pigmentation, and sometimes a lipofuscin pigmentation as well. The reason for this is unknown.

Not all workers accept the genetic basis of haemochromatosis.[42] The repeated failure to produce the disease in the experimental animal by iron overloading alone has led to the view that haemochromatosis is not a distinct entity, but merely represents cirrhosis of the liver in an iron-overloaded patient. Certainly alcoholism is common in haemochromatosis, and some beverages, for example wine, are rich in iron.

Haematin Pigmentation

When the ferrous iron of haem is oxidised to the ferric form, a bluish-black pigment, *haematin*, or *methaem*, is produced. As an intracorpuscular pigmentation, methaemoglobinaemia is described on p. 597. Sometimes, however, particles of black pigment are found in macrophages and lying free in the connective tissue in chronic malaria and schistosomiasis, both infections in which the parasites live in the blood stream, and presumably utilise the red cells during their own metabolism (see Fig. 30.1, p. 398). This pigment is believed to be haematin—it does not give the Prussian-blue reaction, is bleached by formic acid, and is insoluble in strong acids, but is extracted by alkalies. It accounts for the blackish colour of malarial organs.[43, 44]

Formalin pigment, which is produced when tissue containing much blood is subjected to prolonged formalin fixation, is also believed to be haematin. The pigment is birefringent with polarised light; this provides a rapid method of distinguishing it from haemosiderin.

PIGMENTS ASSOCIATED WITH FAT

The term *lipopigment* is best applied to any pigment which is related to fat: it includes two main groups, the lipochromes and the lipofuscins.*[1]

The lipochromes, or carotenoids are yellow pigments, soluble in fat and entirely exogenous, being derived from ingested vegetables. They are hydrocarbons, and constitute the colouring matter of beetroot,[45] carrots, tomatoes, etc. There are two groups: the *carotenes*, the best known of which are β-carotene and its isomer lycopene, and the *xanthophylls*, or *oxycarotenoids*.[46]

These pigments are found dissolved in the fat of the body, and are responsible for the yellow colour of atheromatous plaques, the adrenal cortex, and corpora lutea, as well as that of the fat depots. The actual quantity and proportion of each carotenoid in the tissues depends upon the diet, and occasionally if excessive quantities of coloured vegetables are ingested, there is sufficient coloration of the plasma and skin to simulate jaundice.[47] This is said to occur also in diabetes mellitus, but in all probability it is due to a high dietary intake and not primarily to the disease itself.

Lipofuscins.[1] The brown pigments which are included under the name lipofuscins form an ill-defined group. Other names, like ceroid and haemofuscin, have been applied to some of them. They are all thought to be derived from lipids by oxidation, and are thus endogenous in origin. They are present in residual bodies (p. 24). They usually stain with the Sudan fat stains, and also retain basic fuchsin, i.e. they are acid fast.

The pigments tend to occur in old age and in atrophic conditions—whence the alternative name of "wear and tear" pigment. One of the best examples is encountered in brown atrophy of the heart, which is seen in senility and severe wasting. The small muscle fibres contain caps of brown pigment in the cytoplasm at each pole of their centrally-placed nuclei. Although a small amount of pigment is normally found in this position, it is greatly increased in brown atrophy. Lipofuscins are found in the seminal vesicles and nerve cells in old age, and similar pigments are also found in the liver. "Ceroid"[48] is a pigment found in the liver cells of animals on deficient diets, and a similar pigment is often seen in cirrhosis. "Haemofuscin" is found in haemochromatosis. Both are included in this rather vague group of pigments derived from fat. An extreme instance of fuscous pigmentation of the liver cells occurs in Dubin-Johnson jaundice.

In some cases of protein-losing gastro-enteropathy the small intestine is pigmented due to the presence of lipo-

* The suffix "fuscin" is derived from the Latin *fuscus* meaning dark or sombre. It must not be confused with the fuchsin dyes, which are red in colour.

fuscin in the muscle fibres and in the many phagocytes found between the fibres (see p. 550). The liver and skeletal muscles are also pigmented. Lipofuscin deposition can be produced in animals by a diet deficient in vitamin E.[22] This vitamin is said to be an antioxidant, and since lipofuscinosis of the bowel can also occur in the malabsoprtion syndrome due to many causes—coeliac disease, chronic pancreatitis, Whipple's disease, etc.—it is possible that vitamin-E deficiency is also important in man.

MISCELLANEOUS PIGMENTS

Pigments Containing Copper[49, 50]

The curious association between hepatic cirrhosis and degeneration of the basal ganglia found in Wilson's disease has stimulated research into copper metabolism. This metal, when given by mouth, is absorbed into the blood stream where it first becomes attached to albumin. Within 24 hours it is found more firmly bound to a specific copper-containing α_2-globulin fraction of the plasma proteins, which, because of its blue colour, is called *caeruloplasmin*.

In *Wilson's disease* copper absorption from the gut and its excretion in the urine are both increased. The serum caeruloplasmin level is low, and the copper remains attached to albumin. Presumably this loosely-bound copper is more easily deposited in the basal ganglia and liver. There is no doubt that high levels of copper are found in these sites, and most likely account for the degeneration. Another metal, manganese, is also known to produce a similar type of brain and liver damage. Deposition of copper in the cornea produces the golden-brown *Kayser-Fleischer ring*, pathognomonic of the condition. The disease shows an autosomal recessive inheritance pattern and is to be regarded as an inborn error of metabolism. The basic defect appears to be an impaired production of the copper-binding globulin fraction of the plasma proteins.

Myoglobin[51, 52]

Occasionally this pigment is released from the muscles, and is excreted in the urine. The mechanism is obscure. It may occur as the result of severe injury to muscle, following strenuous exercise in healthy people, after ingestion of poisonous substances ("Haff disease"), and finally as an acute idiopathic condition. The urine is a dark portwine colour, and gives the usual chemical tests for haemoglobin. The condition may be associated with acute renal failure secondary to vasoconstriction and tubular necrosis.

Pigmentation Due to Absorption of Heavy Metals

Silver and gold become deposited in the skin and produce permanent grey pigmentation. The silver pigmentation is called *argyria*,[53] and was quite frequent in the days when silver nitrate was used as a disinfectant and in nasal drops.

Lead reacts with sulphides produced by bacteria around

the gingival margin to form lead sulphide. This substance causes the characteristic "blue line". Mercury salts similarly produce a green gingival discoloration. It should be noted that the skin pigmentation of arsenical poisoning is due to melanin; it has a characteristic rain-drop appearance with most of the melanin disposed peripherally.

Pigmentation of the Lungs by Inhaled Particles

The lungs of most people, especially town-dwellers, show black discoloration due to the accumulation of carbon. This is especially marked in coal-miners, and is called anthracosis. The brilliant brick-red discoloration of haematite-miner's lung also comes into this category. Haematite is an iron oxide ore (iron sesquioxide, Fe_2O_3).

Pigmentation of Skin by Topically Applied or Injected Dyes

Carbon and cinnabar are deliberately introduced into the dermis in the process of tattooing to produce blue and red colouring respectively. This is a true exogenous pigmentation, and it may occur accidentally when dirt is driven into wounds. The prolonged use of ointments containing mercury can lead to a slate-grey discoloration of the skin at the site of application.

REFERENCES

1. Fox, D. L. (1953). *Animal Biochromes and Structural Colours.* Cambridge University Press.
2. Knowles, F. (1963). *Triangle,* **6,** 2.
3. Wolman, M. (1969). Editor. *Pigments in Pathology,* 551 pp. New York and London: Academic Press.
4. Lerner, A. B. and Fitzpatrick, T. B. (1950). *Physiological Reviews,* **30,** 91.
5. Lerner, A. B. (1955). *American Journal of Medicine,* **19,** 902.
6. Lerner, A. B. (1961). *Scientific American,* **205,** No. 1, 99.
7. Gjesdal, F. (1959). *Acta pathologica et microbiologica scandinavica,* **47,** Supplement 133, 1.
8. Woodruff, M. F. A. (1960). In *The Transplantation of Tissues and Organs,* p. 33. Springfield, Illinois: Thomas.
9. Annotation (1961). *British Medical Journal,* ii, 634.
10. Annotation (1963). *British Medical Journal,* i, 139.
11. Leading Article (1967). *British Medical Journal,* iii, 630.
12. Albright, F. *et al.* (1937). *New England Journal of Medicine,* **216,** 727.
13. Albright, F. (1947). *Journal of Clinical Endocrinology,* **7,** 307.
14. Dormandy, T. L. (1957). *New England Journal of Medicine,* **256,** 1093, 1141 and 1186.
15. Sheward, J. D. (1962). *British Medical Journal,* i, 921.
16. Burdick, D., Prior, J. T. and Scanlon, G. T. (1963). *Cancer (Philadelphia),* **16,** 854.
17. Mishima, Y. (1967). *Cancer (Philadelphia),* **20,** 632.
18. Jackson, R., Williamson, G. S. and Beattie, W. G. (1966). *Canadian Medical Association Journal,* **95,** 846.
19. Snyderman, S. E., Norton, P. and Holt, L. E. (1955). *Federal Proceedings,* **14,** 450.
20. Armstrong, M. D. and Tyler, F. H. (1955). *Journal of Clinical Investigation,* **34,** 565.
21. O'Brien, W. M., La Du, B. N. and Bunim, J. J. (1963). *American Journal of Medicine,* **34,** 813.
22. Leading Article (1968). *British Medical Journal,* ii, 574.
23. Wintrobe, M. M. (1967). In *Clinical Hematology,* 6th edn, p. 187. Philadelphia: Lea & Febiger.
24. Gray, C. H. (1970). In *Biochemical Disorders in Human Disease,* 3rd edn, p. 215. Edited by R. H. S. Thompson and I. D. P. Wootton. London: Churchill.
25. Marver, H. S and Schmid, R. (1972). In *The Metabolic Basis of Inherited Disease.* Edited by J. B. Stanbury, J. B. Wyngaarden and D. S. Fredrickson. 3rd edn, p. 1087. New York: McGraw-Hill.
26. MacAlpine, I., Hunter, R. and Rimington, C. (1968). *British Medical Journal,* i, 7.
27. Chanarin, I. (1970). In *Biochemical Disorders in Human Disease,* p. 161, *loc cit.*
28. Charlton, R. W. and Bothwell, T. H. (1970). In *Biochemical Disorders in Human Disease,* p. 201, *loc cit.*
29. Crichton, R. R. (1971). *New England Journal of Medicine,* **284,** 1413.
30. Leading Article (1963). *Lancet,* i, 979.
31. Ognibene, A. J. and Johnson, D. E. (1963). *Archives of Internal Medicine,* **111,** 503.
32. Wallerstein, R. O. and Robbins, S. L. (1953). *American Journal of Medicine,* **14,** 256.
33. Cappell, D. F., Hutchison, H. E. and Jowett, M. (1957). *Journal of Pathology and Bacteriology,* **74,** 245.
34. Pollycove, M. (1966). In *The Metabolic Basis of Inherited Disease,* p. 780, *loc. cit.*
35. Leading Article (1967). *British Medical Journal,* i, 446.
36. Davis, P. S., Luke, C. G. and Deller, D. J. (1966). *Lancet,* ii, 1431.
37. Morgan, O. S. *et al.* (1969). *Lancet,* i, 861.
38. Luke, C. G., Davis, P. S. and Deller, D. J. (1967). *Lancet,* i, 926.
39. Annotation (1968). *Lancet,* i, 1186.
40. Leading Article (1969). *British Medical Journal,* iii, 191.
41. Leading Article (1971). *British Medical Journal,* ii, 182.
42. MacDonald, R. A. (1964). *Haemochromatosis and Hemosiderosis,* 374 pp. Springfield, Illinois: Thomas.
43. Johnson, F. B., Hamilton, P. K. and Gridley, M. F. (1954). *Journal of Histochemistry and Cytochemistry,* **2.** 481.
44. Pearse, A. G. E. (1972). In *Histochemistry, Theoretical and Applied,* 3rd edn, Volume 2, p. 1075. London: Churchill.
45. Annotation (1963). *British Medical Journal,* ii, 948.
46. Goodwin, T. W. (1954). In *Biochemical Society Symposia,* No. 12, p. 71. Cambridge University Press.
47. Reich, P., Shwachman, H. and Craig, J. M. (1960). *New England Journal of Medicine,* **262,** 263.

48. PAPPENHEIMER, A. M. and VICTOR, J. (1946). *American Journal of Pathology*, **22**, 395.
49. BEARN, A. G. (1972). In *The Metabolic Basis of Inherited Disease*, p. 1033, *loc. cit.*
50. THOMPSON, R. H. S. and CUMINGS, J. N. (1970). In *Biochemical Disorders in Human Disease*, p. 476, *loc. cit.*
51. ZIERLER, K. L. (1970). In *Biochemical Disorders in Human Disease*, p. 510, *loc. cit.*
52. Leading Article (1961). *Lancet*, i, 704.
53. OLCOTT, C. T. (1948). *American Journal of Pathology*, **24**, 813.

Chapter 47. Heterotopic Calcification

The deposition of calcium salts in tissues other than osteoid and enamel is called *heterotopic calcification*. Because these salts are radio-opaque, their deposition is conspicuous on x-ray examination, and calcification has therefore come to assume an importance in diagnostic radiology which far outweighs its pathological significance (Fig. 47.1).

Two quite distinct types are recognised:

Dystrophic calcification, the deposition of calcium salts in dead or degenerate tissue. The blood levels of calcium and

silver-impregnation method of von Kóssa in fact stains phosphate and carbonate. Nevertheless, these ions are almost always associated with calcium when in particulate, insoluable form.

The amount of calcium revealed by staining methods does not correlate well with the amount present as estimated chemically.[1, 2] Electron-probe analysis promises to be more useful. In this a beam of electrons is focused on a small spot of tissue in a vacuum, and the emitted x-rays are analysed by

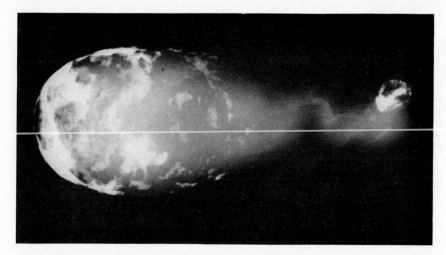

Figure 47.1
Calcified gall-bladder. The patient had had a history of gall-bladder dyspepsia for many years. There was a palpable tumour in the right hypochondrium, and x-rays showed a calcified gall-bladder with a calculus impacted in the neck. The specimen was x-rayed after excision, and the patchy calcification of the walls of the fundus is well shown. *(EA 117.2, Reproduced by permission of the President and Council of the R.C.S. Eng.)*

phosphorus are usually normal, and local conditions are presumably of overriding importance. The calcium deposits are localised.

Metastatic calcification, the precipitation of calcium salts in apparently normal tissues as the result of a generalised upset in calcium-phosphorus metabolism. There is usually hypercalcaemia.

The deposition of calcium salts in calculi is a special example of pathological calcification and is considered in the next chapter.

Appearance of heterotopic calcification. Microscopically calcium salts appear as granular deposits which stain a very deep blue colour with haematoxylin. They simulate bacterial colonies, which are also deeply basophilic, but lack the uniformity in size and shape exhibited by micro-organisms. Calcium deposits typically form an incrustation on such surfaces as the elastic fibres of the lung and arteries, and on ova. Calcium deposits can be identified by their red staining with alizarin red S. The more commonly used

a spectroscope. The presence of a given element is recognised by its characteristic spectrum, and its concentration is determined by the intensity of the emission.[3]

DYSTROPHIC CALCIFICATION

The cause of dystrophic calcification can be considered under two headings: (*a*) calcification in dead tissue, and (*b*) calcification in degenerate tissue. Though the distinction between the two may be somewhat arbitrary, this forms a convenient division.

Calcification in Dead Tissue

Caseous material. Calcification is of frequent occurrence in caseous material, and remains as a permanent landmark of previous tuberculous infection. It is seen in healed Ghon foci and the associated nodes, and also in the mesenteric nodes of "primary" intestinal infection. Calcification is not confined to childhood infection, nor indeed need the lesion be healed, for it is also seen in chronic adult tuberculosis, e.g. in the wall of a psoas abscess. It should furthermore not be forgotten that well-calcified tuberculous lesions sometimes contain living bacilli, which may cause future disease. Calcification is also seen in the healed lesions of histoplasmosis and coccidioidomycosis.

Dead parasites. Many parasites undergo calcification, but this occurs only after their death (Fig. 47.2). *Trichinella spiralis*, hydatid cysts, schistosome ova, and the lesions of

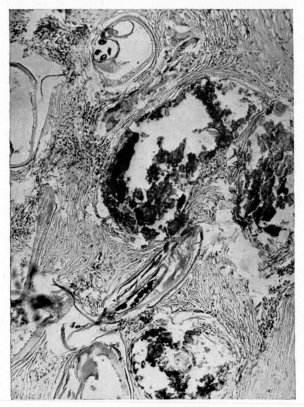

Figure 47.2
Dystrophic calcification. This is a section through a subcutaneous nodule produced by the filarial worm *Onchocerca volvulus*. There are segments of necrotic worm, some of which are heavily incrusted with darkly-staining calcium salts. Note also the chronic inflammatory reaction in the surrounding connective tissue, and the foreign-body giant cells at the side of one of the calcified segments. × 40.

cysticercosis are common examples. The dead fetus may also be included under this heading. In the rare occurrence of ruptured tubal pregnancy in which the fetus survives for a while, its subsequent calcification converts it into a *lithopoedion*.

Fat necrosis. This is seen after acute pancreatitis as well as in traumatic lesions of the breast (see p. 54).

Infarcts. Some infarcts have a peculiar liability to undergo calcification. Experimentally, infarcts in the rat kidney invariably calcify.

Thrombi. Thrombi in veins may calcify to produce *phleboliths*; these are quite commonly seen radiologically in the pelvic veins. Arterial thrombi are less liable to calcification, unless, of course, atheroma is included under this heading (see p. 467).

Haematomata. Although collections of blood in any situation may undergo calcification, this is particulary common when the haematoma is in close association with bone. It is seen in the traumatic subdural haematoma. In traumatic myositis ossificans there is calcification and subsequent ossification of the haematoma in a muscle. The bone-forming cells have presumably been derived from the periosteum.

Calcification in Degenerate Tissue

Scars. The fibrous tissue of scars may undergo hyaline degeneration and subsequent calcification. Some individuals show a definite predisposition to this.

Chronic inflammatory granulation tissue. Dystrophic calcification is quite common in the degenerate tissue of chronic inflammatory lesions. It is seen in the walls of chronic abscesses. It is important in constrictive pericarditis, and is prominent in the scarred valves of rheumatic heart disease and healed infective endocarditis.

Atheroma. Calcification in the degenerate tissue of atheroma is of very frequent occurrence in the aorta and coronary vessels. This intimal calcification must be clearly distinguished from the medial lesions of Mönckeberg's sclerosis.

Mönckeberg's sclerosis. The hyalinised tunica media in this condition regularly becomes calcified, thereby converting the artery into a rigid tube. The calcified tissue is disposed in the form of rings, as it has the same distribution as the muscle coat which it replaces.

Senile degenerate tissue. Calcification is not uncommon in the pineal gland after middle age, and forms a useful landmark in x-ray examinations of the brain. The dura mater may calcify in old age. Degeneration and calcification in the supraspinatus tendon is possibly a senile change, but previous traumatic vascular damage probably also plays a part. The lone calcareous aortic stenosis seen in the middle-aged and elderly is the end-result of a congenital valvular malformation.[4]

Degenerate colloid goitres and so-called adenomata of the thyroid. Flecks of calcification are present in many nodular goitres; this may be of value in the detection of retrosternal goitres.

Cysts. Many cysts of long standing show calcification of their walls. Good examples are afforded by epidermoid and pilar cysts of the skin.

Degenerate tumours. Large uterine fibroids often undergo extensive calcification, usually after the muscle element has undergone necrosis and become replaced by hyaline fibrous tissue. Some tumours show circumscribed spherules of calcification; the psammoma bodies of meningiomata are outstanding examples, and similar structures are seen in some papillary cystadenocarcinomata, especially of the ovary. Many tumours show foci of calcification which may well have followed necrosis; this has been put to practical use in the diagnosis of breast cancer[5,6] (Figs. 47.3 and 47.4)

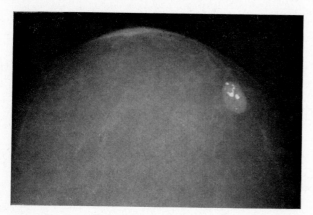

Figure 47.3
Typical radiographic appearance of a benign lesion in a breast. This patient, a 66-year-old woman, had a very hard mass which was discovered on routine examination. It proved to be a fibro-adenoma. *(From Egan, R. L. (1964), "Mammography", Springfield, Ill. : Thomas)*

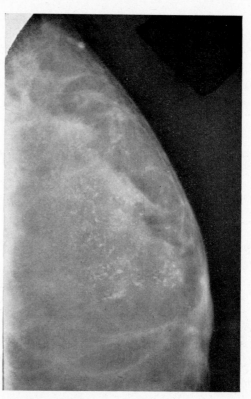

Figure 47.4
This patient presented with a vague nodularity of the breast. Mammograms revealed no mass, but showed a fine stippled calcification which is characteristic of many intraduct carcinomata. The lesion was removed, and study revealed a 2·5 cm adeno-carcinoma of the breast with no axillary lymph-node metastases. *(From Egan, R. L. (1964), "Mammography", Springfield, Ill.: Thomas)*

Sundry lesions. Pulmonary alveolar microlithiasis[7] is a remarkable condition in which calcified laminated structures are found in the alveoli. Presumably they are formed by the calcification of successive accumulations of secretion, so as to produce the typical laminated structures reminiscent of starch granules. A similar condition occurs in the prostate (corpora amylacea), and again calcification may occur.

Calcinosis.[8,9] In this rare condition abnormal deposits of calcium salts are laid down in skin, subcutaneous tissues, muscles, and tendons. The cause is unknown, and the condition should not be confused with fibrodysplasia ossificans progressiva (see p. 308). Calcinosis of the finger pulps is a common feature of scleroderma.

Chondrocalcinosis.[10] This is characterised by the deposition of calcium pyrophosphate crystals in cartilage. Fibrocartilage is most commonly involved, particularly the menisci of the knee and the triangular cartilage of the wrist, but articular hyaline cartilage may also calcify. A chronic arthritis results, and its course is sometimes aggravated by attacks of acute synovitis during which crystals of calcium pyrophosphate are present in the joint fluid. The condition is also called *pseudogout*, and as in gout, the crystals in the joint fluid are phagocytosed by polymorphs. A release of damaging lysosomal enzymes is the probable pathogenesis of the synovitis in both conditions. Chondrocalcinosis may occur as a complication of other diseases, e.g. ochronosis, haemochromatosis, hyperparathyroidism, and gout, or it may appear as an idiopathic isolated condition.

Heterotopic bone formation may occur at any site of dystrophic calcification, and is considered in Chapter 24.

METASTATIC CALCIFICATION[11]

This name should, strictly speaking, be applied only to those conditions in which calcium salts are removed from the bones and deposited in the tissues. It is caused by a disordered metabolism of calcium and phosphate, and although in the common type (hyperparathyroidism) the calcium salts are truly metastatic, there are other conditions in which the excess calcium is derived from the gut. Nevertheless, it is convenient in practice to use the term "metastatic calcification" to cover both these varieties, and it will be used in this context in the account that follows.

Generalised metastatic calcification is usually due to hypercalcaemia, but occasionally, as in renal osteodystrophy, a high blood phosphate appears to be the precipitating factor. The bone salts are deposited in certain sites of election:

Kidney. This is the most frequent and important site. Deposition occurs especially around the tubules, where severe damage is produced. The condition is called *nephro-calcinosis*, and it may lead to renal failure (see Chapter 42). In addition calculi often form in the pelvis and ureter, where they may predispose to infection and cause further renal damage. *Renal failure is therefore a prominent feature of generalised metastatic calcification whatever may be the primary cause* (Fig. 47.5).

An important factor in the causation of nephrocalcinosis is hypercalcuria. While this is usually caused by hypercalcae-mia, e.g. in primary hyperparathyroidism, it may on

cation, it is important to consider briefly some general aspects of calcium metabolism.

Calcium Metabolism[12–14]

Calcium exists in the plasma in three forms:

1. Ionised calcium, which is diffusible and which constitutes about 65 per cent of the total plasma calcium. This is the most important fraction, and its level is regulated by the secretions of the parathyroid glands and the C cells

Figure 47.5
Diagrammatic representation of the important effects of disturbed calcium metabolism. The effects of parathormone and dietary calcium intake on vitamin D are not shown (see pp. 525 and 571).

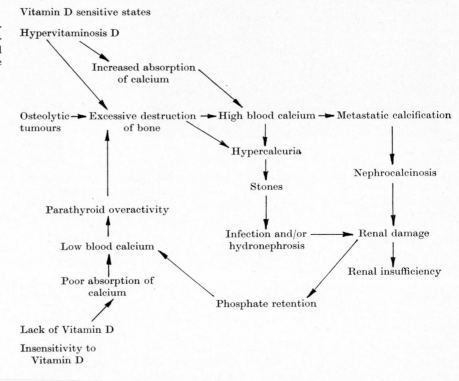

occasion be found with low blood levels, e.g. in renal tubular acidosis, see p. 530. Nephrocalcinosis may therefore occur as an isolated event.

Lung. Calcium is deposited in the alveolar walls, where it forms an incrustation on the elastic fibres. These are thereby prominently outlined in blue on routine H. and E. staining.

Stomach. Calcification occurs around the fundal glands. It has been suggested that as these glands secrete hydrochloric acid, the tissues are left relatively alkaline, and that this favours calcification.

Blood vessels. The coronary vessels (and even the heart) may be affected. Sometimes the internal elastic lamina is incrusted as has already been described with regard to the lungs.

Cornea. A site frequently affected is the cornea of the eye, and the condition can be discovered by slit-lamp examination during life.

Before describing in detail the causes of metastatic calcifi-

found predominantly in the thyroid gland. The intake of vitamin D also plays a minor role.

2. Protein-bound calcium. This is nearly all attached to albumin, and it is therefore non-diffusible.

3. Non-ionised, diffusible calcium, which exists for the most part as citrate, and constitutes the smallest fraction.

It is the total plasma calcium that is usually measured in clinical practice, and in the absence of a marked alteration in the level of plasma proteins it is a good guide to the level of the ionised fraction. The normal concentration is between 9·2 and 10·4 mg per 100 ml, and is remarkably constant in health due to the efficiency of the regulating mechanisms. Even drastic attempts to alter the plasma calcium level fail.[15] Presumably the vast area (estimated at about 100 acres) of bone salt is in equilibrium with the tissue-fluid calcium and therefore the plasma calcium.

Parathormone.[13] The concept of parathormone's main action on calcium metabolism being mediated by its increasing the excretion of phosphate is no longer accepted even by Albright, who himself originally suggested it. Although it does increase the kidney's output of phosphate, the main action of parathormone appears to be its ability to mobilise calcium from the bones. Experimentally, parathyroid tissue transplanted heterotopically into bone causes localised osteoclastic activity and bone destruction, evidently due to a direct action of the secreted hormone. These two actions of parathormone are probably independent of each other. Parathormone secretion is thought to be regulated by the level of ionised plasma calcium. Parathormone has another important effect on calcium metabolism: it depresses the synthesis of 1,25-dihydroxycholecalciferol (see below).

The view that calcium can be directly removed from bone by a process of diffusion, or *halisteresis*, is not generally accepted. It is thought that osteoclastic activity is always necessary before calcium can be removed. The two views are not in fact irreconcilable: if bone salts are removed by diffusion, the exposed osteoid may be removed by osteoclastic activity.

Calcitonin.[16-18] Calcitonin is a polypeptide hormone secreted by cells of ultimobranchial origin. These cells in some species form a separate body, but in mammals are incorporated into the thyroid gland. In man they exist as the parafollicular, or C, cells which lie on the basement membrane of the thyroid acini and are separated from the colloid by the follicular cells. They contain characteristic granules on electron microscopy. Man, unlike the lower mammals, also has calcitonin-secreting cells in the parathyroids and thymus.[19, 20]

The existence of calcitonin was indicated by experiments in which the perfusion of the thyroid-parathyroid region with a high-calcium-containing fluid produced a more rapid reduction of serum calcium than did total parathyroidectomy. Hence the effect could not have been due to a reduction of parathormone secretion, but could be attributed to a new calcium-lowering hormone.

The action of calcitonin is primarily on the bone: it causes a reduction of bone resorption by inhibiting osteoclastic activity. A fall in plasma calcium level follows. The precise role of calcitonin in calcium homeostasis has not yet been delineated, but it could clearly complement parathormone, since the stimulus for its secretion is hypercalcaemia. Calcitonin has been used with some success in the treatment of Paget's disease of bone and hypercalcaemia.[51]

Medullary carcinoma of the thyroid has now been recognised as a tumour of the C cells. It contains large quantities of calcitonin, but there is no outstanding change in serum calcium levels.[21]

Vitamin D. Various forms of vitamin D exist.[52] The first apparently pure compound was called D_1, but in fact was a mixture. The irradiation of ergosterol produces an active substance called vitamin D_2, or ergocalciferol, and this is present in a diet containing fortified foods. Natural vitamin D is produced in the skin by the irradiation of 7-dehydro-

cholesterol, and is called D_3, or cholecalciferol. Both vitamins D_2 and D_3 are hydroxylated in the liver to 25-hydroxy compounds (25-hydroxycholecalciferol, 25-HCC in the case of vitamin D_3) and this is the form in which they circulate in the blood and are carried by specific binding protein. 25-HCC is further hydroxylated to 1,25-dihydroxycholecalciferol (1,25-DHCC) in the kidney, and this is currently believed to be the final active metabolite. This final hydroxylation is promoted by a low blood calcium level. In the presence of a high blood level of parathormone 21,25-DHCC is formed, and this is much less active (see p. 525).[53]

Vitamin D appears to aid the absorption of calcium from the gut, and it also has a parathormone-like action. In excessive doses it leads to a rise in blood and urinary calcium levels. Deficiency results in hypocalcaemia and a diminution or complete abolition of calcification. In the growing child provisional calcification of dead cartilage does not occur at the growing ends of the bones. This uncalcified material is inadequately removed, and as cartilaginous growth continues, the epiphyses show considerable enlargement. The result is *rickets*.[22] In the normal adult, bone is continually being removed by osteoclastic activity and replaced by osteoid, which promptly calcifies to form bone. If this calcification fails, the bones gradually become replaced by osteoid, and the result is *osteomalacia*. The causes of rickets and osteomalacia are:[14, 23]

1. Dietary lack of vitamin D combined with lack of sunshine. A diet rich in phytate can prevent the absorption of calcium and have the same end-result as vitamin D deficiency.[24]

2. The malabsorption syndrome,[14] e.g. coeliac disease and steatorrhoea.

3. Chronic renal failure (p. 525).

4. Hypophosphatasia (see p. 574).

5. Familial hypophosphataemia — vitamin D-resistant rickets[25] (see p. 529).

6. Fanconi syndrome (see p. 529).

7. Renal tubular acidosis (see p. 530).

CAUSES OF METASTATIC CALCIFICATION

It must be acknowledged that the actual basis of metastatic calcification is not understood. Although it is usually associated with hypercalcaemia, a normal or low blood calcium level may be found in certain syndromes. In these the site of calcification may be atypical, e.g. the basal ganglia in hypoparathyroidism, or confined to the kidney in renal tubular acidosis. In renal osteodystrophy calcification occurs in the subcutaneous tissues as well as in the arteries, kidneys, and other more usual sites.

The following causes of metastatic calcification can be recognised:

Hyperparathyroidism—Hyperplasia—primary or secondary.
Neoplasia.

Excessive absorption of calcium from the bowel
>   Hypervitaminosis D.
>   Vitamin-D sensitive states, e.g.
>   idiopathic hypercalcaemia of
>   infants and sarcoidosis.
>   Compulsive milk drinking.

Hypophosphatasia
Destructive bone lesions
Hypoparathyroidism
Renal tubular acidosis

Hyperparathyroidism[26-29]

Excessive secretion of the parathyroid glands may occur as a primary or a secondary condition.

Primary hyperparathyroidism. The first account of this disease was published in 1743 by a Welshman Sylvanus Bevan. It is generally due to an idiopathic hyperplasia of the parathyroids, but sometimes a simple adenoma is responsible; rarely the tumour is malignant.[30]

Primary hyperparathyroidism can present in a variety of ways. The best known is classical *osteitis fibrosa cystica*, or *von Recklinghausen's disease of bone*, in which intense osteoclastic resorption leads to porosis and cystic changes involving many bones. Pathological fractures are common, and sometimes tumour-like masses ("brown tumours") may simulate giant-cell tumours (see p. 323).

More commonly the osteoporosis is generalised, and the bone disorder is inconspicuous. In these cases the hypercalcaemia causes characteristic symptoms, e.g. tiredness, weakness, muscular asthenia, and mental disturbances, and the ensuing hypercalcuria leads rapidly to renal failure. Polyuria and thirst are pronounced, for as mentioned on p. 521, calcium intoxication causes the renal tubules to become unresponsive to ADH.[31]

Another well-known presentation of hyperparathyroidism is recurrent renal-calculus formation. These cases are usually of long standing, bone lesions may be absent, and the systemic effects of hypercalcaemia are often mild. The incidence of peptic ulcer is increased in cases of primary hyperparathyroidism; presumably this is due to an effect of parathormone on gastric acid secretion.

The biochemical changes of hyperparathyroidism are a raised level of plasma calcium (it may rise to 22 mg per 100 ml),* a lowered level of plasma phosphate, and an increased urinary output of calcium. As the disease progresses the plasma phosphate level may rise owing to secondary renal failure, and the urinary calcium may fall as the result of the reduced glomerular filtration rate (in addition parathormone aids calcium reabsorption—see p. 522).[33, 34] Metastatic calcification in the usual sites is common, and is aggravated when renal failure develops.

Secondary hyperparathyroidism.[14] Hyperplasia of the parathyroids occurs in many types of osteomalacia and rick-

---

* Normocalcaemia occasionally occurs in hyperparathyroidism, especially in cases that show themselves with renal calculi.[32]

---

ets; probably there is an associated increased parathormone secretion, but this is difficult to prove as there is no simple assay method available. It is the hypocalcaemia that stimulates the glands into activity. In some cases this is sufficiently marked to initiate osteoclastic activity in the bones, and therefore in addition to the changes of rickets or osteomalacia there develop those of osteitis fibrosa cystica. This type of response occurs only occasionally, and renal disease is the usual antecedent.

Renal osteodystrophy (renal rickets).[14] Chronic renal disease, especially in young people, is sometimes attended by skeletal lesions which comprise a mixture of calcification defects—osteomalacia (or rickets according to age) and osteitis fibrosa cystica. Metastatic calcification affecting principally the kidneys, arteries, and subcutaneous tissues sometimes occurs,[12] and may be worsened by dialysis unless hyperphosphataemia is controlled. Corneal and conjunctival deposits can be detected by slit-lamp examination in patients with conjunctivitis.[35] In addition, there may also be osteosclerosis, which in the vertebral bodies tends to occur in the areas adjacent to the intervertebral discs. The central parts of the bodies are osteoporotic, and therefore a radiograph of the spine presents a banded appearance—the so-called rugger-jersey spine. The pathogenesis of the condition is discussed on page 525.

Tertiary hyperparathyroidism.[36, 37] It is now recognised that some cases of long-standing parathyroid hyperplasia secondary to malabsorption or chronic renal failure may undergo adenomatous change. Hypercalcaemia then develops (see p. 526).

Excessive Absorption of Calcium from the Bowel

Hypervitaminosis D. Excessive administration of this vitamin leads to hypercalcaemia and generalised metastatic calcification. The parathormone-like activity of vitamin D is responsible for the hypercalcaemia. The vitamin helps regulate the equilibrium between bone and blood calcium.

Vitamin-D sensitive states. There are several conditions which resemble hypervitaminosis D, but in which there is no evidence of excessive dietary intake. An increased susceptibility to the actions of the vitamin is postulated,[25] but this theory cannot be regarded as proven. Two conditions are worth noting:

Sarcoidosis. The hypercalcaemia which is occasionally seen in this condition is due to increased calcium absorption rather than bone destruction.[38] Exposure to sunlight appears to increase the hypercalcaemia.[39, 40]

Infantile hypercalcaemia.[13, 41, 42] This condition, first described in 1952,[43] is seen in infants between the ages of 6 weeks and 8 months. Two types are recognised:

A BENIGN FORM is characterised by anorexia, vomiting, constipation, and marked hypotonia of the limbs. The serum level of calcium is over 12 mg per 100 ml and the blood urea is raised. After some months of illness recovery generally ensues.

THE MALIGNANT FORM[44] of the disease is accompanied by marked physical and mental retardation. The face shows a characteristic "elfin" appearance. Severe nephrocalcinosis is reflected in nitrogen retention. Hypertension may be present. The bones may show sclerosis of an intensity reminiscent of Albers-Schönberg disease. Extensive metastatic calcification occurs. There is probably no absolutely distinct line between the two forms of the disease, and intermediate types are described.

Although the condition closely resembles hypervitaminosis D, the evidence for excessive intake is not conclusive. Some cases were receiving 1 000–3 000 units daily, a dose not generally regarded as toxic. However, the disease has been prominent in Great Britain, where milk and foods are artificially fortified, whereas it is unknown in North America. Furthermore, it has not been reported in breast-fed babies; cows' milk contains four times as much calcium as does human milk. An alternative suggestion that the disease is due to an abnormal sensitivity to vitamin D has not been convincingly substantiated. The high blood cholesterol level often present has led to the suggestion that faulty steroid metabolism may be a factor.

Compulsive milk drinking.[13] Subjects with this neurosis absorb excess calcium from the bowel, and the consequent hypercalcaemia leads to nephrocalcinosis. The most severe examples are met with in patients suffering from peptic ulceration, in whom the situation is aggravated by concomitant alkali administration (*milk-alkali syndrome*). The ensuing alkalosis aggravates the nephrocalcinosis, and severe renal failure may result.

Hypophosphatasia

Hypercalcaemia and hypercalcuria may lead to nephrocalcinosis (see p. 574).

Destructive Bone Lesions

Extensive involvement of the skeleton in secondary carcinoma, multiple myeloma, and Hodgkin's disease may result in metastatic calcification. Hypercalcuria, usually without hypercalcaemia, is seen in cases of osteoporosis due to prolonged immobilisation, and may lead to nephrolithiasis (see p. 304).

Hypoparathyroidism[13]

It is paradoxical that bilateral symmetrical calcification occurs in the basal ganglia of the brain in hypoparathyroidism. This may be seen in the idiopathic cases, following surgery,[45] and in pseudohypoparathyroidism, a curious condition in which the glands are normal and the hypocalcaemia does not respond to parathormone (see pp. 308 and 530).

Renal Tubular Acidosis

There is hypercalcuria and nephrocalcinosis in this condition (see p. 530).

MECHANISM OF CALCIFICATION

The composition of the calcium salts laid down in heterotopic calcification is the same as that of normal bone. It may be inferred that the process of calcification is similar in both cases. However, the mechanism of normal calcification is not understood. The exact composition of bone salt is not known, but it is generally considered to have a hydroxyapatite structure. In addition to calcium and phosphate there are also present the anions chloride, fluoride, and citrate. There are in addition sodium, magnesium, and potassium, and rare trace elements. In bone the salts occur as very small crystals 20–45 nm long and 1·5–2 nm wide, and are probably situated within the collagen fibrils. The theories concerning the mechanism of calcification are centred around the formation of these crystals. It is assumed that they are formed when the product (*concentration of calcium*) × (*concentration of phosphate*) reaches the level at which precipitation occurs. Of the four main theories three attempt to explain the occurrence of a local rise in the ionic concentration of calcium or phosphate, while the fourth concerns the "seeds", or centres, around which the crystals may grow.

The calcium soap theory. The original observations on dystrophic calcification stressed its occurrence in fatty tissue, e.g. atheroma, caseous material, and fat necrosis. It was suggested that the following reactions took place:

$$\text{Fatty acid} + \text{Calcium ion} \rightarrow \text{Calcium soap.}$$
$$\text{Calcium soap} + \text{Phosphate} \rightarrow \text{Calcium phosphate.}$$

There is, however, little evidence that this soap hypothesis is true. In the first place, the calcium soaps have never been isolated in the lesions. It could be argued, of course, that they are formed, but that this intermediate stage proceeds too fast for the soaps to be detectable.

Secondly, it is found that if calcium soaps are injected into an animal, they are absorbed, and calcification does not occur. It seems unlikely that the soap theory can provide an answer to the puzzle of calcification.

The phosphatase theory.[46, 47] High alkaline-phosphatase activity is found in growing bone, and has been claimed at sites of dystrophic calcification. It is present in high concentrations in osteoblasts, and the blood level rises during active bone formation. The enzyme breaks down hexosemonophosphate at pH 9, and by liberating free phosphate ions could theoretically so raise the local concentration that precipitation of calcium phosphate would ensue. However, alkaline phosphatase is also found in granulation tissue, liver, kidney, and intestinal mucosa (see p. 541), and in these situations calcification does not normally occur. Although the exact function of alkaline phosphatase in normal calcification is not known, it probably plays an important part in the process, if not in the actual calcification then in the formation of the organic matrix of bone. In the rare condition of *congenital hypophosphatasia*,[14, 48] which is inherited as an autosomal recessive trait, the blood and tissues have a low level of alkaline phosphatase. Bone formation is abnormal, and a condition resembling rickets develops. An excess of phosphorylethanolamine is found in the plasma and urine, which suggests that this is (or is derived from) the normal substrate of the enzyme.

The binding property of the matrix. *For phosphate.* It has been suggested that the chemical nature of the matrix is important. Cartilage contains glycogen before calcification, and this disappears as calcification proceeds. Possibly, glycogen binds phosphate as follows:

$$\text{Glycogen} + \text{Inorganic Phosphate} \xrightarrow{\text{Phosphorylase}} \text{Glucose 1-Phosphate}$$

This might therefore form a storage mechanism for phosphate.

For calcium. The sulphate and glucuronic-acid groups of ground substance can bind calcium. In this way both calcium and phosphate might be concentrated locally, if the ground substance were of suitable composition.

Target or epitactic theory. It has been supposed that the structure of bone matrix plays an important part in initiating crystal formation by a process of seeding, or *epitaxy*.[49, 50] The collagen or its associated acid mucopolysaccharides might provide centres, or targets, from which the bone crystals could grow, even in the presence of a subsaturated solution of salts.

This theory fails to explain why calcification does not normally occur in tendon, fascia, and other collagenous material, nor can it explain how calcification occurs in non-collagenous tissue like enamel, caseous material, etc.

The following table summarises the main changes in the blood levels of calcium, inorganic phosphate, and alkaline phosphatase found in some of the conditions mentioned in this chapter.

TABLE 47.1

	Calcium	Phosphate	Alkaline Phosphatase
Normal	9·2–10·4 mg %	2·4–4·5 mg %	3–13 units %
Osteoporosis	Normal	Normal	Normal
Primary hyperparathyroidism	Raised (greatly)	Lowered, except with renal failure	Raised (moderately)
Hypoparathyroidism	Lowered (greatly)	Raised (greatly)	Normal
Osteomalacia, dietary and malabsorption	Normal or lowered	Lowered	Raised (moderately)
Renal tubular acidosis	Normal or lowered	Lowered	Normal or raised
Hypophosphataemia	Normal	Lowered	Normal or raised
Renal rickets (uraemia)	Lowered	Raised (greatly)	Normal or raised
Hypophosphatasia	Normal or raised	Normal	Lowered
Paget's disease of bone	Normal	Normal	Raised (greatly)
Osteolytic metastases	Normal or raised	Normal	Normal
Osteosclerotic metastases	Normal	Normal	Normal or raised

REFERENCES

1. BLUMENTHAL, H. T., LANSING, A. I. and GRAY, S. H. (1950). *American Journal of Pathology*, **26,** 989.
2. ANDERSON, M. *et al.* (1959). *Archives of Pathology*, **68,** 380.
3. ROBERTSON, A. J. *et al.* (1961). *Lancet*, i, 1089 and Leading Article (1966). i, 696.
4. CAMPBELL, M. (1968). *British Heart Journal*, **30,** 514 and 606.
5. EGAN, R. L. (1963). *American Journal of Surgery*, **106,** 421.
6. KOEHL, R. H. *et al.* (1970). *American Journal of Clinical Pathology*, **53,** 3.
7. SPENCER, H. (1968). In *Pathology of the Lung*, 2nd edn, p. 695. Oxford: Pergamon Press.
8. BELL, E. T. (1956). In *A Text Book of Pathology*, 8th edn, p. 125. London: Kimpton.
9. ROBBINS, S. L. (1967). In *Textbook of Pathology*, 3rd edn, p. 407. Philadelphia: Saunders.
10. RUSSELL, R. G. G. *et al.* (1970). *Lancet*, ii, 899.
11. MULLIGAN, R. M. (1947). *Archives of Pathology*, **43,** 177.
12. FOURMAN, P. (1963). In *Bone Metabolism in Relation to Clinical Medicine*, p. 12. Edited by H. A. Sissons. London: Pitman.
13. FOURMAN, P. and ROYER, P. (1968). *Calcium Metabolism and the Bone*, 2nd edn, 656 pp. Oxford: Blackwell.
14. BALL, J. (1960). In *Recent Advances in Pathology*, 7th edn, p. 293. Edited by C. V. Harrison. London: Churchill.
15. HASTINGS, A. B. and HUGGINS, C. B. (1933). *Proceedings of the Society of Experimental Biology and Medicine*, **30,** 458.
16. Proceedings of the Symposium on Thyrocalcitonin and the C Cells (1968). Edited by S. Taylor, 402 pp. London: Heinemann.
17. Leading Article (1968). *British Medical Journal*, iv, 67.
18. FOSTER, G. V. (1968). *New England Medical Journal*, **279,** 349.
19. GALANTE, L. *et al.* (1968). *Lancet*, ii, 537.
20. Leading Article (1968). *Lancet*, ii, 1379.
21. TUBIANA, M. *et al.* (1968). *British Medical Journal*, iv, 87.
22. Leading Article (1962). *Lancet*, i, 1168.

23. DENT, C. E. (1963). In *Bone Metabolism*, p. 79, *loc. cit.*
24. WILLS, M. R. *et al.* (1972). *Lancet*, i, 771.
25. FANCONI, G. (1956). In *Bone Structure and Metabolism*, a CIBA Foundation Symposium, p. 187. Edited by G. E. W. Wolstenholme and C. M. O'Connor. London: Churchill.
26. Leading Article (1961). *Lancet*, ii, 641.
27. DENT, C. E. (1962). *British Medical Journal*, ii, 1419 and 1495.
28. ROTH, S. I. (1962). *Archives of Pathology*, **73**, 495.
29. PYRAH, L. N., HODGKINSON, A. and ANDERSON, C. J. (1966). *British Journal of Surgery*, **53**, 245.
30. DONIACH, I. (1960). In *Recent Advances in Pathology*, 7th edn, p. 258, *loc. cit.*
31. BECK, D., LEVITIN, H. and EPSTEIN, F. H. (1959). *American Journal of Physiology*, **197**, 1118.
32. WILLS, M. R. (1971). *Lancet*, i, 849.
33. KYLE, L. H., BEISEL, W. R. and CANARY, J. J. (1962). *Annals of Internal Medicine*, **57**, 957.
34. Leading Article (1965). *Lancet*, i, 361.
35. Leading Article (1972). *British Medical Journal*, i, 762.
36. DAVIES, D. R., DENT, C. E. and WATSON, L. (1968). *British Medical Journal*, iii, 395.
37. Leading Article (1968). *British Medical Journal*, iii, 389.
38. ANDERSON, J. *et al.* (1954). *Lancet*, ii, 720.
39. Annotation, (1963). *British Medical Journal*, i, 1629.
40. TAYLOR, R. L., LYNCH, H. J. and WYSOR, W. G. (1963). *American Journal of Medicine*, **34**, 221.
41. Leading Article (1956). *British Medical Journal*, i, 159.
42. Leading Article (1956). *Lancet*, i, 1052.
43. LIGHTWOOD, R. (1952). *Proceedings of the Royal Society of Medicine*, **45**, 401.
44. SCHLESINGER, B. E., BUTLER, N. R. and BLACK, J. A. (1956). *British Medical Journal*, i, 127.
45. Leading Article (1961). *Lancet*, ii, 1441.
46. BOURNE, G. H. (1956). Editor. *The Biochemistry and Physiology of Bone*, p. 251. New York: Academic Press.
47. KING, E. J. and MOSS, D. W. (1963). In *Bone Metabolism*, p. 42, *loc. cit.*
48. ENGFELDT, B. and ZETTERSTRÖM, R. (1956). In *Bone Structure and Metabolism*, p. 258, *loc. cit.*
49. FROST, H. M. (1963). In *Bone Remodelling Dynamics*, p. 48. Springfield, Illinois: Thomas.
50. NEUMAN, W. F. and NEUMAN, M. W. (1958). *Chemical Dynamics of Bone Mineral*, p. 169. Chicago: University of Chicago Press.
51. Leading Article (1973). *British Medical Journal*, i, 371.
52. RAISZ, L. G. (1972). *New England Journal of Medicine*, **287**, 926.
53. Leading Article (1972). *Lancet*, i, 1000.

Chapter 48.   Calculi

A calculus is a mass of precipitated material derived from a secretion and deposited in an excretory duct. The mode of calculus formation is obscure. It is usually assumed that in any secretion the crystalloids are held in solution by adsorption on to colloidal particles,* and that when the concentration of crystalloids increases or the colloid content decreases, the crystalloids will precipitate out. The colloidal matrix in which the crystalloids of low molecular weight deposit varies according to the secretion; in urinary calculi it consists mostly of mucoprotein and muco-polysaccharide with smaller amounts of plasma proteins.

The important calculi are *urinary, biliary, salivary, pancreatic,* and *prostatic.* It is the calcium (and magnesium) content of a calculus that renders it radio-opaque; it follows that stones composed of the phosphate, carbonate, oxalate, or bilirubinate of calcium are revealed by straight x-rays. Calculi composed of uric acid and xanthine can be detected only by the appearance of a filling defect during pyelography, and pure cholesterol stones are demonstrated similarly during cholecystography. Cystine stones usually contain a sufficient amount of calcium to be faintly radio-opaque.

Causes of Calculus Formation

An increase in the crystalloid content of the secretion. The effect is a precipitation of some of the crystalloid, and the resulting calculus is called *primary,* or *metabolic,* i.e. it is formed without prior inflammation.

The presence of a solid mass acting as a nidus around which the crystalloids precipitate. Such a nidus may be formed by a foreign body, fibrin, necrotic epithelial cells, clumps of organisms, or a primary metabolic stone. This type of calculus is sometimes called *secondary.* It may also be called a *concretion.* Chemically it consists predominantly of calcium phosphate and calcium carbonate.

CALCULI OF THE URINARY TRACT

These are usually found in the renal pelves, but may also occur in the ureters and bladder. The common primary calculi are:

* A colloid is a state of matter intermediate between a true solution and a suspension or emulsion. A colloidal solution (or sol) is one in which the dispersed particles have a diameter between 1 and 100 nm. The colloid is the discontinuous phase, and the medium the continuous phase (as distinct from solute and solvent). In a medium it is possible to separate crystalloid from colloid by means of a membrane, e.g. parchment or collodion, which is permeable to crystalloids only. This process is called *dialysis.*

Urate stones, composed of uric acid with sodium and ammonium urate. These are brown in colour, smooth and hard, and on section show concentric lamination (Fig. 48.1).

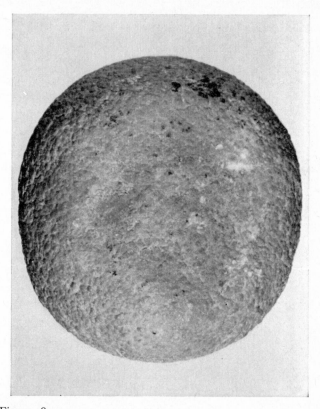

Figure 48.1
Uric acid calculus. The surface of this stone, which measured 7 cm in diameter, is light brown in colour and has an evenly granular ("tuberculated") contour. *(Reproduced by permission of the President and Council of the R.C.S. Eng.)*

Calcium oxalate stones, which are dark brown, and have characteristically spiky surfaces, which cause much mucosal trauma and bleeding. They are very hard, and are also laminated (Figs. 48.2 and 48.3).

Cystine stones, which are pale yellow or white.

Xanthine stones, which are brownish-red.
These last two varieties of calculus are rare.

Silica stones are very rare, or at least have rarely been reported. They follow the long-continued ingestion of magnesium trisilicate for indigestion.[28]

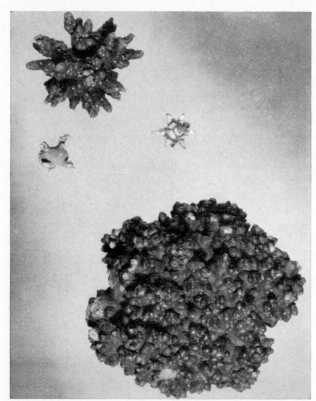

Figure 48.2
Calcium oxalate calculi. These stones of varying size all show the salient features of dark coloration and spiky irregularity of surface. *(Reproduced by permission of the President and Council of the R.C.S. Eng.)*

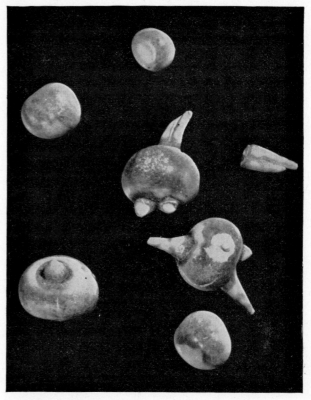

Figure 48.3
Small calcium oxalate calculi. The little spiky oxalate stones used to be called jackstones. Jackstones (also called checkstones, or dibstones) is a centuries-old children's game in which small round pebbles (or sheep's knuckle-bones) are tossed up in a small basket and caught again as they fall. These small calculi were presumably alleged to resemble the pebbles or knuckle-bones used in the game.

Some of the stones photographed are finely polished, and have a smooth contour. This is not unusual when the stones have been present for a long time. *(Reproduced by permission of the President and Council of the R.C.S. Eng.)*

Secondary calculi may arise *de novo* following infection of the urinary tract or the introduction of a foreign body into the bladder. In the course of time they also form around primary calculi, and the result is a *mixed stone*. They are composed of **calcium phosphate** and **magnesium ammonium phosphate** together with a variable amount of **calcium carbonate.** In appearance they are white and smooth, and have a soft, friable consistency (see Fig. 48.6).

Calculi composed of calcium salts, usually a mixture of oxalate and phosphate, are by far the most common in the urinary tract, and many are not due to infection. In conditions of hypercalcuria mentioned below it is this type of calculus that is formed. About 90 per cent of urinary calculi are composed of calcium salts, and 4–10 per cent of uric acid.

Aetiology of Primary Urinary Calculi[1]

The majority of primary urinary stones arise in an unknown way, but a few factors are worthy of consideration:

Increased content of crystalloids (or abnormal crystalloids) in urine. In the rare metabolic disorders of *xanthinuria* and *cystinuria* it is understandable that poorly soluble substances like cystine and xanthine should precipitate out of solution.

Another uncommon metabolic disease, *oxalosis*, is associated with the precipitation of calcium-oxalate crystals in many tissues.[2] There is hyperoxaluria with a tendency to oxalate-calculus formation. Nevertheless, in most patients with oxalate calculi there does not appear to be any error in oxalate metabolism.

Uric-acid stones are not uncommon in patients with *chronic gout*, and are related in part to the increased excretion of uric acid often found, but in addition gouty patients tend to secrete an unusually acid urine (see p. 578).

An increased calcium excretion in the urine may also lead to calculus formation, e.g. in *hyperparathyroidism, sarcoidosis*, and in *patients immobilised in bed for a long time*, when the skeleton undergoes progressive demineralisation as the result of disuse atrophy. Such stones are composed of variable amounts of calcium phosphate and oxalate. About 20 per cent of cases of hyperparathyroidism, however, do not form calculi despite marked hypercalcuria.[3] Conversely, many patients who form calculi repeatedly do not excrete calcium in excessive amounts.[1] There is also a syndrome of idiopathic hypercalcuria and renal lithiasis despite a normal serum calcium level; sometimes the serum phosphate level is reduced.[4, 5] It is possible that the cause of the hypercalcuria is an increased absorption of calcium from the bowel.[6] Another hypercalcuric syndrome associated with stones is renal tubular acidosis (see p. 530). An acquired type due to chronic pyelonephritis may manifest itself with renal calculus.[7]

The mechanism of formation of calcium-containing calculi in those many instances in which there is no obvious abnormality in calcium metabolism is not known. It has been found that the concentration of calcium in the renal papilla is normally considerably greater than in the other parts of the kidney; in fact it is unknown how this high concentration of calcium is kept in solution. Hypercalcuria should be most dangerous in a hyperosmolal urine,[8] and indeed people who live in hot desert areas may develop renal stones. Likewise stones are quite common in some tropical areas, but not in all of them. It has been found that the incidence of stone in the South African Bantu is much less than that in South Africans of European stock. It has also been noted that the Bantu excretes much more sodium ions in his urine than does his fair-skinned neighbour, who excretes only a little more calcium than does the Bantu.[8] It would seem that hypercalcuria is dangerous in urine with a low sodium concentration, whereas an increase in the amount of both ions is relatively harmless. In fact, hypercalcuria is most dangerous in a hypo-osmolal urine. Thus the traditionally held deleterious effect of *dehydration* on stone formation needs reconsidering. While it probably is of importance, it is evident that the osmolality of the urine must also be considered when large amounts of water are prescribed as a prophylactic measure in those prone to calculus formation; this osmolality is mostly a function of sodium ions.[8] Whether other substances that hold calcium in solution are also present normally but deficient in those who form stones is not known —amongst such agents have been postulated citrate, amino acids, ascorbic acid, and pyrophosphate, but none has been substantiated.[1, 5]

Foci of calcification in the kidney (nephrocalcinosis) acting as a nidus for calculus formation. *Randall's plaques.*[9, 10] Randall described foci of dystrophic calcification in the renal papillae arising secondarily to injury; these ulcerated through the pelvic mucosa, and acted as a nidus for calculus formation. Such plaques are fairly common, but are usually not associated with stone formation. Conversely, stones may occur in kidneys without Randall's plaques. It is probable that these lesions are a result of the high calcium content of the papillary area of the kidney already noted.[8]

Renal microliths. Small flecks of calcium salts are present in the interstitial tissue of all kidneys, and are probably situated in the renal lymphatics.[11] It has been suggested that if the lymphatic system is blocked or overloaded, these microliths might coalesce to form calculi.[12] They might then ulcerate into the pelvis, and form the nidus of an even larger calculus. Though interesting, this hypothesis lacks proof.

Stasis plays no part in the formation of primary stones with the probable exception of those calculi that develop in immobilised patients, in whom it is possible that the calcium salts may separate out in the calyces by a gravitational effect. In this example the stasis merely determines the site of stone formation. Obstruction leads to secondary calculus formation because it predisposes to infection.

Urinary pH. Uric-acid stones form in an acid urine, and patients who develop these calculi are often unable to secrete an adequate amount of ammonia in their distal renal tubules.[13] Oxalate and cystine stones also precipitate in an acid urine.

On the other hand, the phosphates of calcium and magnesium ammonium deposit in an alkaline urine. The presence of urea-splitting organisms, notably *Proteus* species, in the urine leads to ammonia formation and alkalinity. It is not surprising that phosphate stones occur in severe urinary-tract infection. It is, however, interesting how seldom calculi are found in the very common condition of chronic pyelonephritis.

Vitamin-A deficiency may lead to renal stones in rats,[14] but there is no evidence that it plays any part in human calculus formation.[15]

Ureteric calculi are usually renal in origin, as are also many *vesical calculi*. Stones may also be produced in the bladder as the result of severe, persistent cystitis secondary to obstruction to the outflow of urine, or in narrow-necked diverticula. They also form around foreign bodies introduced from the outside, e.g. pieces of catheter and safety-pins. Such calculi are composed of calcium and magnesium ammonium phosphate.

BILIARY CALCULI

Gall-stones are described classically as being either *primary* or *secondary*.[16] There are three primary, or metabolic, types:

Cholesterol stones are characteristically solitary. They are pale yellow in colour, ovoid, and have a smooth surface. The cut surface shows a radiating, glistening, crystalline pattern. *Strawberry gall-bladder*, or *cholesterolosis of the gall-bladder*, in which the mucosa is thrown up into yellow plaques containing accumulations of fat-filled macrophages, is not usually accompanied by stones.

Calcium bilirubinate stones (pigment stones). These are multiple, jet-black in colour, irregular in shape, and rather friable in consistency.

Calcium carbonate stones are rare, and are chalky in appearance.

In fact, pure stones are not found, and the above classification is not regarded with favour by research workers, although it is of some clinical value. All stones contain variable amounts of bile pigments, cholesterol, calcium carbonate, and apatite, and their core usually consists of bile pigments or mucoprotein, which is secreted by the gall-bladder epithelium.[17–19] The gall-bladder is usually normal structurally.

Aetiology of Gall-stones[20]

Cholesterol stones.[20] The basis of the common cholesterol stone appears to be a precipitation of cholesterol which is not kept adequately in solution. Cholesterol, which is insoluble in water, is carried in solution in the bile in a mixed micelle consisting of bile salts, phospholipid, and the cholesterol itself. The micelle is a polymolecular aggregate comparable, in this instance, with a detergent molecule, and it is the bile salts, and to a lesser extent the phospholipid, that bring the cholesterol into solution. Patients with cholesterol stones sometimes secrete a bile that is saturated or supersaturated with cholesterol.

The bile secreted in the liver is abnormal in patients with cholesterol stones. They have a reduced bile-salt pool, and it seems that the defect is a lack of bile salts rather than an excess of cholesterol. Gall-stones are a common accompaniment of cirrhosis, where there is often a reduction in the bile-salt pool and a decrease in the bile-salt content of the bile. The nature of the hepatic defect is unknown, but it may be related to the lipoprotein plasma membrane of the bile canaliculi.

The gall-bladder plays a secondary part in allowing the cholesterol crystals to precipitate and form a stone. It may also provide a nidus for seeding in the form of mucous secretion, and stasis enhances the growth of the stone. This probably accounts for the increased incidence of gall-stones in women, for there is stasis during pregnancy, especially in the last trimester. Stones can form in the bile ducts of those who have undergone a cholecystectomy, thus proving that the gall-bladder is not essential for stone production.

Attempts are being made to expand the bile-salt pool and thereby increase the bile-salt content of the bile. *Chenodeoxycholic acid*[21] expands the pool and alters the bile composition towards favouring cholesterol solubility (cholic acid has no effect on the composition of the bile). It may be a means of dissolving cholesterol stones, thereby treating the condition medically. It will not dissolve calcareous material, and therefore an accurate assessment of the nature of the stone is important before the agent is given.

There is a dietary and perhaps also a genetic factor in cholesterol stone formation, for this type of calculus is far commoner in Europeans than in the Oriental groups.[22]

Pigment stones are an important complication of some congenital haemolytic anaemias (see p. 595), but not of the acquired ones. They are much commoner in African and Asian people than in Europeans.[22] Apparently another factor, in addition to hyperbilirubinaemia, is operative in their production. Since most of the bile pigments are excreted as the soluble diglucuronide, increased activity of the enzyme β-glucuronidase may be a factor in promoting the release of bilirubin, which is subsequently precipitated as the calcium salt. An inhibitor of β-glucuronidase, identified as glucaro-1, 4-lactone, is present in the normal bile. Its activity may be overcome by the β-glucuronidase activity of *Esch. coli*, thereby providing another link between infection and calculus formation.[23]

Secondary biliary calculi are produced as the result of cholecystitis, which often occurs in a gall-bladder that already harbours stones. Secondary infective stones are more obviously "mixed" than the "primary" cholesterol type; they consist of variable quantities of cholesterol, calcium bilirubinate, and calcium carbonate, which produce a predominantly brown colouring. Mixed stones are characteristically multiple, no doubt forming around organisms and necrotic inflammatory debris. It usually happens that a family of stones form at the same time, and as they grow at a regular rate, they tend to press on each other. This leads to the typically faceted surfaces of mixed stones (Fig. 48.4).

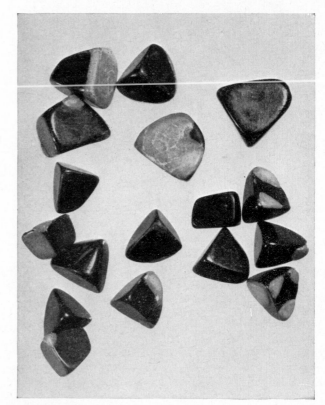

Figure 48.4
A family of "mixed" gall-stones. They are all of approximately the same size, and their surfaces are smoothly faceted. Their predominantly dark colour testifies to the large amount of bile pigment present in them, while the pale areas are due to cholesterol. *(Reproduced by permission of the President and Council of the R.C.S. Eng.)*

On section the stones present a characteristic concentric laminated appearance, and it is of interest that the laminae are parallel to the surface even of the faceted stones. Their shape is therefore determined during growth, and is not produced by mechanical erosion of one stone against another.

A second type of mixed stone is the *mulberry stone*. Occasionally it is solitary, but more usually there are multiple stones of one or more generations.

Another type of secondary calculus is one that develops around a primary cholesterol stone. It enlarges progressively

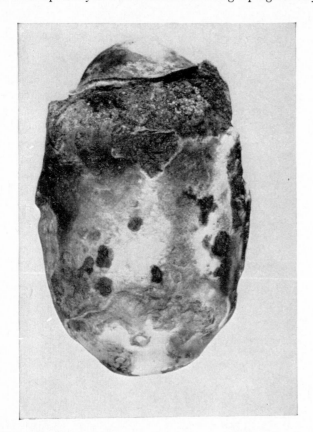

Figure 48.5
Barrel stone. This large calculus forms a complete cast of an enlarged gall-bladder. *(Reproduced by permission of the President and Council of the R.C.S. Eng.)*

by the concentric precipitation of calcium salts, bile pigments, and cholesterol. It is called a *combination stone*, and may be accompanied by other stones of mixed type. Sometimes a combination stone remains solitary, and by its steady growth eventually fills and distends the gall-bladder. This is called a *barrel stone* (Fig. 48.5).

A final type of mixed stone is earthy, soft, and laminated. It is formed in the bile ducts, and is smooth and egg-shaped or sausage-shaped. The formation of this type of stone is generally attributed to *stasis*.

SALIVARY CALCULI[24]

Found most commonly in the submandibular duct, these consist of calcium phosphate and carbonate, i.e. they are of the secondary type. Their mode of formation is obscure, but it is probable that they form around a central nidus composed of desquamated epithelial cells and masses of organisms, e.g. actinomyces. Infection leads to calculus formation, and calculi predispose to infection. In this vicious circle it is impossible to decide which comes first.

PANCREATIC CALCULI[25, 26]

These are uncommon. They consist of calcium phosphate and carbonate. They are found in association with chronic pancreatitis, which is itself an obscure condition. The stones

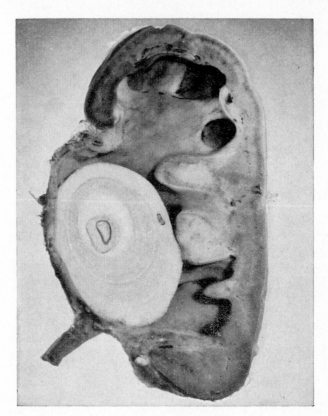

Figure 48.6
Renal calculus. This is a hydronephrotic kidney, in the pelvis of which there is a large, round phosphatic calculus. It has been sectioned to show its laminated construction. It has been built up by the layering of successive deposits of phosphates on the original central phosphate piece. *(U 25.3, Reproduced by permission of the President and Council of the R.C.S. Eng.)*

are found in the larger ducts, the epithelium of which shows squamous metaplasia. The mode of production of these stones is unknown.

PROSTATIC CALCULI[27]

These are found not infrequently in the hyperplastic prostates of elderly men, and occur in the smaller ducts. They consist of calcium phosphate and carbonate. They are typically small and multiple. The secretions of the acini often become inspissated in the ducts to form *corpora amylacea*, and these are probably the nuclei around which the calcium salts precipitate. Sometimes necrotic inflammatory debris and blood clot also act as a central nidus.

EFFECTS OF CALCULI

Calculi are often silent, and are discovered accidentally during radiological or *post-mortem* examinations. They may, however produce definite pathological effects:

Pain. The sudden distension or spasm of a hollow muscular viscus produced by a stone leads to pain. Spasm itself causes a typical colic. Urinary calculi, by abrading the mucosa, also cause **haemorrhage.**

Obstruction. A ureteric or renal calculus may obstruct the outflow of urine completely or partially. If obstruction is sudden and complete, the kidney stops secreting urine, and undergoes slow disuse atrophy. If obstruction is partial or intermittent, there is a dilatation of the ureter and pelvis proximal to the stone, so that a considerable hydronephrosis may eventually develop (Fig. 48.6).

Likewise an intermittent obstruction of the cystic duct leads to a mucocele of the gall-bladder. A blockage of the common bile duct results in obstructive jaundice, which is characteristically intermittent and fluctuant in intensity. A barrel stone may rarely ulcerate through the wall of the gall-bladder into the duodenum. In its subsequent passage down the bowel it may impact in the lumen, and lead to intestinal obstruction.

A salivary calculus leads to a painful distension of the associated salivary gland, especially during mastication.

Infection. Where there is any element of stasis in an out-flowing secretion, infection is bound to be superadded in due course. The organisms may come from the exterior, as in the salivary duct, or be derived from the excretion of the viscus itself, as in the kidney and liver. A pyonephrosis eventually complicates a hydronephrosis, and acute "ascending" cholangitis stones in the common bile duct. An empyema of the gall-bladder is a well-known sequel to a stone in the cystic duct. Suppurative sialadenitis is a frequent accompaniment of salivary calculi. The presence of infection leads to secondary calculus formation, and sets up a vicious circle.

Malignancy. Carcinoma of the gall-bladder is very frequently superimposed on a chronically-inflamed organ that contains stones. On the other hand, it is an uncommon form of cancer, and there may well be little causal relationship between the stones and the subsequent malignancy (see Chapter 29).

Pancreatic and prostatic calculi seldom produce definite symptoms, and are usually discovered incidentally.

REFERENCES

1. McGeown, M. G. and Bull, G. M. (1957). *British Medical Bulletin*, **13,** 53.
2. Archer, H. E. *et al.* (1957). *Lancet*, ii, 320.
3. Hellström, J. (1955). *British Journal of Urology*, **27,** 387.
4. Albright, F. *et al.* (1953). *Proceedings of the Royal Society of Medicine*, **46,** 1077.
5. Leading Article (1963). *Lancet*, i, 34.
6. Peacock, M., Knowles, F. and Nordin, B. E. C. (1968). *British Medical Journal*, ii, 729.
7. Cochran, M. *et al.* (1968). *British Medical Journal*, ii, 721.
8. Leading Article (1972). *Lancet*, i, 825.
9. Randall, A. (1937). *Annals of Surgery*, **105,** 1009.
10. Rosenow, E. C. (1940). *Journal of Urology*, **44,** 19.
11. Anderson, L. and McDonald, J. R. (1946). *Surgery, Gynecology and Obstetrics*, **82,** 275.
12. Carr, R. J. (1954). *British Journal of Urology*, **26,** 105.
13. Henneman, P. H., Wallach, S. and Dempsey, E. F. (1958). *Journal of Clinical Investigation*, **37,** 901.
14. Higgins, C. C. (1935). *Journal of the American Medical Association*, **104,** 1296.
15. Council on Pharmacy and Chemistry (1935). *Journal of the American Medical Association*, **105,** 1983.
16. Aschoff, L. (1924). In *Lectures on Pathology*, p. 208. New York: Hoeber.
17. Annotation (1968). *Lancet*, i, 1416.
18. Russell, I. S., Wheeler, M. B. and Freake, R. (1968). *British Journal of Surgery*, **55,** 161.
19. Bouchier, I. A. D. and Freston, J. W. (1968). *Lancet*, i, 340.
20. Bouchier, I. A. D. (1971). *Lancet*, i, 711.
21. Leading Article (1972). *Lancet*, i, 360.
22. Maki, T. (1961). *Archives of Surgery*, **82,** 599.
23. Small, D. M. (1968). *New England Journal of Medicine*, **279,** 588.
24. Husted, E. (1953). *Acta chirurgica scandinavica*, **105,** 161.
25. Haggard, W. D. and Kirtley, J. A. (1939). *Annals of Surgery*, **109,** 809.
26. Edmondson, H. A., Bullock, W. K. and Mehl, J. W. (1950). *American Journal of Pathology*, **26,** 37.
27. Gentile, A. (1947). *Journal of Urology*, **57,** 746.
28. Joekes, A. M., Rose, G. A. and Sutor, J. (1973). *British Medical Journal*, i, 146.

Chapter 49. Some Disorders of the Blood

I—THE RED CELL

The science of haematology is now so complicated that many haematologists confine themselves to a single facet of the speciality, e.g. the haemolytic anaemias, the leukaemias, or the disorders of clotting, and relegate other aspects of blood disease to colleagues more expert than themselves. Despite this disheartening prospect it is still possible for the interested observer to learn a great deal about the common blood disorders through a grasp of elementary pathological principles. Once this has been achieved, the standard text-books are at his disposal for further enlightenment.

THE NORMAL LIFE CYCLE OF THE RED CELL

Development

The original haematopoietic cell in the fetus is believed to be a migrating multipotential *stem cell* that arises in the yolk-sac and migrates to the liver, spleen, bone marrow, lymph nodes, and thymus.[1] In all these organs there is a period of haematopoiesis during fetal life, but at birth all blood formation is confined to the bone marrow, apart from small foci of haematopoiesis in the liver that disappear after a few days. The postnatal stem cell resides in the bone marrow and travels to distant sites from there. Whether this is the same stem cell that gives rise to RE cells, fibroblasts, and other cells mentioned in Chapter 30 is not certain; perhaps the original stem cell first differentiates into the haematopoietic stem cell, which in this case would be identical with the *haemocytoblast* described in text-books as the most primitive recognisable blood cell, which can form red cells, white cells, and platelets. At any rate it is impossible to distinguish categorically between the stem cell and the haemocytoblast in terms of morphology. If the haemocytoblast is "committed" to red-cell development, it passes through the following four stages:

Pronormoblast. A large cell with deeply basophilic cytoplasm and a large nucleus containing fine clumps of chromatin and several nucleoli.

Basophilic (early) normoblast. A slightly smaller cell with deeply basophilic cytoplasm. There are no nucleoli in its nucleus. Some authorities do not separate it from the pronormoblast.

Polychromatic (intermediate) normoblast. The cell is somewhat smaller, and the cytoplasm has a greenish tint due to the first appearance of haemoglobin. The nucleus is smaller and its chromatin is condensed into thick clumps (Fig. 49.1).

Pyknotic (late) normoblast. The cell is much smaller, and contains a dense pyknotic nucleus which is later extruded.

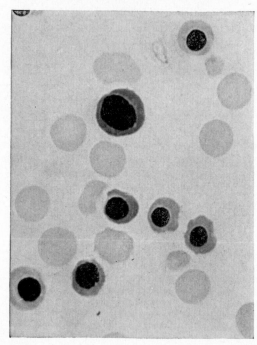

Figure 49.1
Normoblasts in peripheral blood. The patient was a newborn infant with erythroblastosis fetalis due to Rh-haemolytic disease. One intermediate normoblast and six late normoblasts are shown. × 960.

The cytoplasm is usually reddish (orthochromatic) due to an abundance of haemoglobin.

It should be noted that the word "erythroblast" refers to any nucleated red cell, both the normal normoblast series described above, and the megaloblast series typical of pernicious anaemia. A table illustrating the cellular components of the bone marrow and indicating their derivation is given in the next chapter (p. 599).

THE NORMAL RED CELL[2]

The mature red corpuscle appears greenish-yellow in unstained preparations, and is roughly circular in shape.

Seen on edge it is a biconcave disc. It is brightly eosinophilic in blood films, using the usual Romanowsky techniques,* because of its content of haemoglobin. This is distributed uniformly throughout the cell, but the centre is somewhat paler than the periphery due to the biconcavity.

A young erythrocyte often contains remnants of the basophilic ribonucleic acid (RNA), which is very conspicuous in the cytoplasm of the early normoblasts. Such a red cell may stain a bluish or greyish colour with Romanowsky dyes, and this is called *polychromasia* (or diffuse basophilia). Sometimes the RNA is aggregated in discrete granules, so producing *punctate basophilia* (or basophilic stippling). The most important appearance of this RNA, however, is as filamentous skeins that cannot be demonstrated by Romanowsky methods, which need preliminary fixation with methyl alcohol. If blood is stained supravitally with brilliant cresyl blue, these basophilic threads are outlined; they are the "reticulum" of the *reticulocyte*. Polychromasia, punctate basophilia, and reticulocytosis are all manifestations of residual RNA in newly-formed red cells; the difference lies in the form that the RNA assumes and in the presence or absence of prior fixation. Electron microscopy shows it in the form of ribosomal aggregates.

In practice a *reticulocyte count* is the most accurate method of assessing an increase in the number of these young red cells; they should not exceed 2 per cent of the total. A rise in the reticulocyte percentage indicates an accelerated rate of red-cell formation. This may be secondary to red-cell depletion, as after haemorrhage or haemolysis, or it may follow the successful treatment of a chronic anaemia like pernicious anaemia or iron-deficiency anaemia. In this case the reticulocytosis is temporary, and heralds a progressive increase in the red-cell count. Reticulocytes are larger than older red cells, therefore any condition accompanied by a reticulocytosis has a mildly macrocytic blood picture. In very severe haemolytic anaemias there may also be nucleated red cells in the peripheral blood, a feature especially typical of Rh-haemolytic disease.

EXAMINATION OF THE RED CELL

The most useful method of examining red cells is to inspect them in a well-made, well-stained blood film. By this means an experienced haematologist can diagnose many common blood disorders. Quantitative indices are of value, but they merely state in figures what a trained eye can relate

---

* The Romanowsky dyes (which include such well-known stains as Leishman, Jenner, May-Grünwald, and Giemsa) consist of a carefully blended mixture of methylene blue and eosin. Derivatives of the mixture stain the blood cells admirably. Acidic groupings in the nucleic acids of the nuclei and primitive cytoplasm take up variable amounts of basic methylene blue, while basic groupings on the haemoglobin molecule have an affinity for acidic eosin. An important derivative, *methylene blue azure*, stains the "azurophil" granules of monocytes and promyelocytes, as well as the nuclei of malarial and other parasites, a reddish-purple colour.

---

in form. A *haemoglobin estimation* is certainly essential in order to assess the presence and degree of anaemia. It is a simple and easily reproducible procedure. A *packed cell volume* is also useful and reliable, but it necessitates a venepuncture, whereas a blood film and haemoglobin estimation can be performed on capillary blood. A *red-cell count* has so great a margin of error that it cannot be recommended as a routine investigation, unless the laboratory is equipped with an electronic cell counter. There are three *absolute values*, which are of use provided accurate measurements are made.

Mean corpuscular volume (MCV), which is obtained thus:

$$\frac{\text{Percentage packed cell volume}}{\text{Red cell count in millions per } \mu l} \times 10 \text{ (expressed in nl)}$$

Mean corpuscular haemoglobin (MCH), obtained thus:

$$\frac{\text{Haemoglobin in g per 100 ml}}{\text{Red cell count in millions per } \mu l} \times 10 \text{ (expressed in pg)}$$

Mean corpuscular haemoglobin concentration (MCHC), obtained thus:

$$\frac{\text{Haemoglobin in g per 100 ml}}{\text{Percentage packed cell volume}} \times 100 \text{ (expressed as a percentage)}$$

This index, unlike the MCH, assesses the degree of haemoglobinisation of the red cells irrespective of their size. Red cells cannot be over-haemoglobinised, but they can be deficient in haemoglobin, and the MCHC is particularly useful in assessing the extent of under-haemoglobinisation, thus confirming the appearance in a well-stained film.

Another investigation that is occasionally performed is a measurement of *mean corpuscular diameter* (MCD) using an eyepiece micrometer. It is a simple procedure but little more informative than a well-made blood film. The following table summarises the range of red-cell values in a normal man:

TOTAL RED-CELL COUNT	4·6–6·2 million per μl (mm³)
HAEMOGLOBIN	14–18 g per 100 ml
PACKED CELL VOLUME	40–54 per cent
MEAN CORPUSCULAR VOLUME (MCV)	80–92 nl (μm^3)
MEAN CORPUSCULAR HAEMOGLOBIN (MCH)	27–31 pg
MEAN CORPUSCULAR HAEMOGLOBIN CONCENTRATION (MCHC)	32–36 per cent
MEAN CORPUSCULAR DIAMETER (MCD)	6·7–7·7 μm*

There are some physiological variations in the levels of haemoglobin, total red cells, and packed cell volume. Thus,

---

* This is the average red-cell diameter in a film. In an isotonic medium, the average red cell is 8·4 μm in diameter.[2]

the newborn infant has a high level of circulating red cells, but there is such a precipitous drop within the first month of life that the subsequent level is distinctly below the adult standard. After the fifth year there is a steady rise to the adult level, which is finally attained at puberty. The red-cell count in women is about half a million cells per c.mm less than in men, and the haemoglobin level is about 2 g per 100 ml lower. Another important factor influencing the red-cell count is the barometric pressure. People who live at high altitudes have a moderate polycythaemia to compensate for the low oxygen tension of the surrounding air.

The normal red cell is described as *normocytic* and *normochromic*, i.e. it is normal in size and haemoglobin concentration as defined by the above table. If it is larger in volume than normal it is called a *macrocyte*, and if smaller, a *microcyte*. Marked variation in size of a population of red cells is called *anisocytosis*, and a marked variation in shape, *poikilocytosis*. Cells with a reduced concentration of haemoglobin are described as *hypochromic*, and in a stained film they are easily recognisable by their colourless centres, which may be so extensive that only a narrow rim of haemoglobin is left around the periphery ("pessary forms"). In addition, the cells may contain a small central aggregation of haemoglobin surrounded by the extensive colourless zone; these are called *target cells*. The term *leptocyte* is used to include all such abnormally thin, under-haemoglobinised red cells.

Although macrocytes often appear extremely well-coloured, they do not contain a greater concentration of haemoglobin than normal. The appearance is due to the increased cell thickness which obliterates the mild central pallor normally present. There is therefore no such condition as hyperchromia.

Another pathological type of red cell is the *spherocyte*, a small, darkly-staining cell which is almost perfectly spherical in shape. Although it appears small, its volume is normal because of an increased thickness. This accounts for its deep staining despite a normal concentration of haemoglobin.

"Burr" cells, or acanthocytes,[3] are mature red cells which possess one or several spiky projections on their periphery. They are characteristic of those haemolytic anaemias in which mechanical trauma is believed to damage the red cells, e.g. microangiopathic haemolytic anaemia. They are also found in uraemia and abeta-lipoproteinaemia (p. 554).

HAEMOGLOBIN

Haemoglobin is a conjugated protein. The molecule consists of four haem groups attached to the protein globin, which in turn is composed of two pairs of polypeptide chains, designated α and β respectively. A haem group is attached to each polypeptide chain (Fig. 49.2).

Haem is a metal complex. It consists of an iron (Fe^{++}) atom in the centre of a porphyrin structure, which is in fact a protoporphyrin. Porphyrins are tetrapyrroles. The four pyrrole rings are united by four methene bridges to produce the porphin nucleus. The structural formula of haem is shown on p. 533.

The biosynthesis of porphyrins starting with a simple, acetate salt has been elucidated. It is a very complex process, and it is found that, in addition to the protoporphyrin bound in the haem group, there are two other by-products

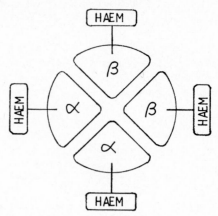

Figure 49.2
Diagrammatic representation of haemoglobin. The four polypeptide chains of globin are labelled α and β. *(After Wintrobe, M. M. (1967), Clinical Hematology, 6th ed., Fig. 3–7, p. 139. Philadelphia: Lea & Febiger)*

formed (see Fig. 46.4, p. 561). These are called *coproporphyrin* and *uroporphyrin*, because they were first discovered in the faeces and urine respectively. Coproporphyrin is excreted in small amounts both in the faeces and the urine. The amount is raised whenever there is increased erythropoiesis, and it is also high in chronic lead poisoning. Liver disease is associated with an increased urinary excretion and a diminished faecal excretion of coproporphyrin. Despite its name, uroporphyrin is present in the urine in an even smaller amount than coproporphyrin.* In the *porphyrias* there is a defect in pyrrole metabolism, which is either inherited or due to liver disease (see p. 561).

From a haematological point of view the *globin* moiety of haemoglobin is even more interesting than its haem group. An important group of blood dyscrasias is now known to be due to *abnormal haemoglobins* and the abnormality of these haemoglobins resides in their globin portion. The study of the *haemoglobinopathies*[4] is so specialised that it now forms a separate branch of haematology. Chemical analysis of the globin moiety has revealed that it consists of two pairs of polypeptide chains of which five types are known—α, β, γ, δ, and ε. Four normal types of haemoglobin have been recognised:

Haemoglobin A. This is the major component of normal adult human haemoglobin. Its globin consists of two α

* About 250 mg of prophyrin are made each day during haem synthesis. Nearly all of this is protoporphyrin. Less than 1 mg is excreted as coproporphyrin (about 300 μg in the faeces and 200 μg in the urine) and uroporphyrin (about 10 μg in the urine).

chains and two β chains, and the haemoglobin is therefore designated $\alpha_2\beta_2$.

Haemoglobin A$_2$. About 2 per cent of normal haemoglobin is designated Hb-A$_2$, and the β chains are replaced by δ. It is therefore $\alpha_2\delta_2$.

Fetal haemoglobin. Hb-F is the normal haemoglobin found in the fetus and during early infancy. Its formation may continue abnormally in infancy as a result of any type of anaemia causing marrow overactivity. Hb-F is designated $\alpha_2\gamma_2$.

Embryonic haemoglobin. This is found only in the very early embryo and is depicted as $\alpha_2\varepsilon_2$; an ε_4 has also been described.

There are two types of inherited disorders of haemoglobin synthesis. There may be a structural abnormality in one of the polypeptide chains, usually the α or β chains of Hb-A. Thus Hb-S has a replacement of glutamic acid in the sixth position of the β chain by valine. In the second type of abnormality, the thalassaemia syndromes, there is a gross reduction in the rate of synthesis of one of the globin sub-units and overproduction of another. Thus in the common type of thalassaemia there is deficient β chain production, and an excess of Hb-F and Hb-A$_2$ is produced (p. 592). The actual structure of the haemoglobins is normal.

The various haemoglobins differ from the normal Hb-A in such physico-chemical attributes as electrophoretic mobility, resistance to alkali denaturation, solubility, and antigenicity. New variants were allotted a new letter, but this method of nomenclature soon proved inadequate (see later). The clinical effects of abnormal haemoglobins vary; some, such as Hb-G, Hb-J, and Hb-K are apparently symptomless. Others, by adding a new property, may have serious effects: the insolubility of Hb-S leads to the vascular occlusive effects of sickle-cell disease, while Hb-M leads to the formation of an abnormal methaemoglobin and so impairs the oxygen-carrying capacity of the red cells. The most important effect of abnormal haemoglobins is haemolytic anaemia (see p. 592).

The electrophoretic mobility of most abnormal haemoglobins is slower than that of normal adult haemoglobin, though a few rare ones are somewhat faster.

Normal adult haemoglobin (Hb-A) is rapidly denatured by an alkali, like potassium hydroxide, so that it cannot combine with oxygen any longer. Fetal haemoglobin (Hb-F) is much more resistant to alkali denaturation, and is easily distinguished from adult haemoglobin by this means. Hb-F is often present among the abnormal haemoglobins of different haemoglobinopathies, and is particularly conspicuous in β-thalassaemia major.

Haemoglobin-S, the abnormal haemoglobin of sickle-cell disease, is much more insoluble in its reduced state than as the oxy-compound. It is this property that enables sickling to be so easily demonstrated when the haemoglobin is reduced.

The abnormal haemoglobins are genetically determined; for instance large populations in Africa are heterozygous for Hb-S and often for Hb-C as well, whereas many South-East Asians are heterozygous for Hb-E. It has been well established that the Hb-S trait is associated with a relative immunity to *P. falciparum* malaria. The geneticist and the anthropologist are as interested in abnormal haemoglobins as is the haematologist.

The nomenclature of the haemoglobins is complicated.[5] For a while capital letters were used according to the haemoglobin's electrophoretic mobility. If several haemoglobins occupied the same position on the strip, the geographical area where the abnormal haemoglobin was first found was appended, e.g. Hb-G(Baltimore), Hb-G(Honolulu), Hb-G(Norfolk), and Hb-G(Philadelphia).

It was finally decided to discontinue designating new variants by letter. New variants are named by the area or hospital where the haemoglobin was discovered, e.g. Hb-Dakar. The most logical nomenclature is to record the haemoglobin in terms of its structure; thus Hb-S is $\alpha_2\beta_2^s$ or better still, since the exact abnormality is known in this case, $\alpha_2\beta_2^{\,6\,\text{glu}\,\rightarrow\,\text{val}}$.

HAEMOGLOBIN AND OXYGEN CARRIAGE

Haemoglobin must be maintained in a reduced state to function as an oxygen carrier. However, in the presence of a high concentration of oxygen it is readily oxidised to methaemoglobin. This is useless for oxygen transport, but it can be reduced to haemoglobin by NADH$_2$. The energy to do this and to extrude sodium and thereby maintain a high level of intracellular potassium is derived from the glycolytic pathway (p. 46). Glycolysis results in the phosphorylation of ADP to ATP and in the reduction of NAD to NADH$_2$. An additional pathway of glucose metabolism is the oxidative hexosemonophosphate shunt (p. 23). In this NADP is reduced to NADPH, a co-enzyme necessary for the conversion of oxidised glutathione (GSSH) to the reduced state (GSH) through the glutathione reductase reaction. This GSH is a vital component of the red cell, for it helps to maintain the readily oxidisable SH groups of haemoglobin and red-cell enzymes. In the process GSH becomes oxidised to GSSH. NADPH$_2$ cannot act as a hydrogen donor and reduce methaemoglobin to haemoglobin except in the presence of methylene blue (p. 597).

The important function of oxygen carriage by the haemoglobin of red cells has recently been found to be regulated by the concentration of 2:3-diphosphoglycerate (DPG) in the cells.[52] This substance complexes with reduced haemoglobin and inhibits its oxygen binding capacity; this facilitates the unloading of oxygen to the tissues. Variation in the DPG content of red cells is an important regulating mechanism, the details of which are not yet clear. Thus ascent to a high altitude causes a substantial increase in the DPG level, and oxygen is therefore made more readily available to the tissues. A similar increase occurs in other conditions of hypoxia such as in heart failure, chronic lung disease, and anaemia. The importance of DPG as a regulator is illustrated by comparing the well-tolerated anaemia of pyruvate-kinase deficiency, which has a high red-cell DPG level, with the poorly tolerated anaemia of hexokinase deficiency, in which DPG is deficient (see p. 593).

REQUIREMENTS FOR RED-CELL PRODUCTION

Protein, including the essential amino acids.

Vitamin B. The essential factors are *folic acid (pteroyl-glutamic acid)* and *vitamin B_{12} (cyano-cobalamin)*.[6] In the absence of either (or both) the red-cell precursors undergo a characteristic perversion of development called *megaloblastic erythropoiesis*. A *megaloblast* is a nucleated red cell which is larger than a normoblast in the corresponding stage of development. It has a large nucleus containing chromatin arranged in a delicate, stippled pattern instead of the coarse clumps characteristic of a normoblast (Fig. 49.3). When the

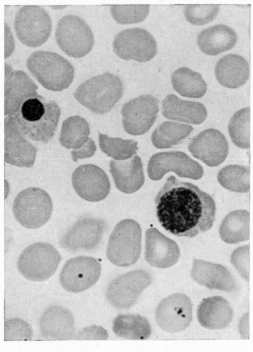

Figure 49.3
A megaloblast. Note the large size of the cell and its stippled nuclear chromatin as compared with the much smaller normoblast and its pyknotic nucleus. The smear was from the marrow of a patient with pernicious anemia. × 960.

nucleus is finally extruded a macrocyte is produced. Pathological megaloblasts are very similar in appearance to the nucleated red cells seen in normal fetal marrow.

Folic acid is water-soluble and easily absorbed from the bowel. Vitamin B_{12} cannot be so absorbed, unless given in massive doses, except in the presence of *intrinsic factor*, a mucoprotein which is normally secreted by the epithelium of the stomach. Vitamin B_{12} is the *extrinsic factor*. Both vitamin B_{12} and folic acid are stored in the liver. The metabolic functions of these two substances are very complex; both are essential for the biosynthesis of purines, pyrimidines, and consequently nucleic acids. Nevertheless, a folic-acid deficiency anaemia often does not respond well to vitamin B_{12}, and *vice versa*. Apparently each plays a part at a different point in nucleic-acid synthesis.[6]

The normal level of vitamin B_{12} in the serum ranges from 200 to 900 pg per ml. In pernicious anaemia it is usually below 100 pg per ml. It is particularly low in subacute combined degeneration of the cord, which sometimes manifests itself before there is any anaemia. Folic acid produces a considerable haematological response in pernicious anaemia, but it is powerless against the neurological effects, and is therefore contra-indicated in the therapy of the disease.

The *Schilling test* is used to assess the absorption of vitamin B_{12} from the bowel. A test dose of the vitamin labelled with radioactive cobalt is given *orally*, and the patient is loaded with unlabelled vitamin *intramuscularly* to block the body's stores, so that the labelled vitamin is flushed out. The urine is collected for 24 hours, and the excretion of labelled vitamin measured. Normally more than 15 per cent is excreted. If the excretion is less than 5 per cent the test is repeated, this time mixing intrinsic factor with the labelled vitamin. If this restores excretion to normal, the defect is gastric (e.g. pernicious anaemia), but if it has no effect, there is an intestinal lesion. It is important first to exclude renal disease as a cause of poor excretion.

The normal serum folate level is 5 to 21 ng per ml, and the red-cell folate is 160 to 640 ng per ml of packed cells. A serum folate below 4 ng per ml and a red-cell folate below 140 ng per ml indicates folic-acid deficiency. Another useful test of folic-acid deficiency is the formiminoglutamic acid (Figlu) test. Histidine is degraded into Figlu when it is metabolised, and this in turn is acted on by folic acid. In cases of deficiency there is an accumulation of Figlu in the urine after an oral dose of histidine.

Pyridoxine (vitamin B_6) is also important in red-cell production. The cofactor pyridoxyl phosphate is essential for an early stage of porphyrin synthesis. Deficiency in animals leads to a hypochromic, microcytic anaemia despite great sideraemia and siderosis. In man there is seldom any anaemia until the deficiency is very severe. Isoniazid therapy tends to interfere with the activity of pyridoxine, and may lead to symptoms of its deficiency.[7]

Ascorbic acid. The part that vitamin C plays in erythropoiesis is still uncertain. Scurvy is usually attended by multiple deficiencies which complicate the blood picture. Ascorbic acid is necessary for the conversion of folic acid to folinic acid (citrovorum factor), which is also essential for nucleic-acid synthesis. Ascorbic acid deficiency may occasionally be associated with megaloblastic erythropoiesis especially in infancy, and cases are on record in which pernicious anaemia remained unresponsive to vitamin B_{12}

until ascorbic acid was also administered. There may be a haemolytic element in the anaemia of scurvy.[8]

Minerals

Iron.[9, 10] This is obviously an essential mineral, as it forms an integral part of the haem group. Most iron is absorbed from the bowel in the ionic form, ferrous ions being more easily absorbed than ferric ions. The solubility of iron is decreased by phytates (present in cereals), phosphates, and an alkaline medium. It is for this reason that hydrochloric acid aids iron absorption, most of which occurs in the duodenum and upper portion of the small intestine, and little in the colon. Ascorbic acid also assists iron absorption, presumably because it reduces ferric iron to the ferrous state. In practice, however, neither hydrochloric acid nor ascorbic acid is necessary unless there is a considerable deficiency of iron in the diet.

Iron can also be absorbed directly from haem without prior digestion to an ionised form. This is derived from haemoglobin and myoglobin in the diet, and is important in Western diets. The haem appears to be absorbed into the mucosal cell as an intact porphyrin complex, and its absorption is not affected by gastric acidity, ascorbic acid, or phytate.

The absorption of iron by the mucosal cells of the small intestine depends on the ferritin mechanism which traps the iron and prevents its further absorption into the body, and a second mechanism responsible for its bodily absorption. It is believed that the amount of iron absorbed is determined by the ferritin content of the epithelial cells. This itself is determined by the body's requirements at the time of the cell's formation in the crypts of Lieberkühn: this ferritin remains as the cells migrate towards the tips of the villi. Thus, in iron-deficiency states the epithelial cells contain little ferritin, which would arrest the absorbed iron, and therefore iron absorption can take place from the gut lumen. With iron overload the epithelial cells contain much ferritin, and absorption does not take place. The explanation of increased iron absorption in iron-loaded states with augmented erythropoiesis is that, since iron is utilised by the marrow, it is not available to the gut epithelial cells. The nature of the transport of the ferrous iron across the mucosal cell is not known.

Iron is carried in the blood in the ferric state bound to a globulin called *iron-binding protein, transferrin,* or *siderophilin*. The total iron-binding capacity of the plasma (i.e. the plasma transferrin level) is 300–360 μg per 100 ml, and it is normally a third saturated with iron. The iron-binding capacity is increased in the latter part of pregnancy and in iron-deficiency anaemia, but it is reduced in chronic infection, rheumatoid arthritis, cancer, cirrhosis of the liver, and the nephrotic syndrome. The normal level of iron in the plasma is 60–200 μg per 100 ml, and it is much reduced in iron-deficiency anaemia (*sideropenia*), while in most other types of anaemia it is moderately or greatly raised (*sideraemia*). The plasma iron is also raised in liver necrosis (see p. 538), and especially in transfusional siderosis and haemochromatosis, in which two conditions the iron-binding capacity of the plasma is saturated.

Iron is stored as ferritin and haemosiderin in the RE cells of the liver, spleen, and bone marrow, and small amounts are also present in the parenchymal cells. It would appear that the function of transferrin is to transport iron from the RE cells to the red-cell precursors. In cases of absence of transferrin there is severe iron-deficiency anaemia and heavy siderosis.[11] Apparently transferrin is not essential for the transport of iron from the bowel.

The iron is incorporated by the normoblasts into haemoglobin, but in from 20 to 60 per cent of normoblasts small granules of haemosiderin can be demonstrated by Prussian blue staining. This number is decreased in sideropenic anaemias and increased in sideraemic ones. Siderotic normoblasts are called *sideroblasts*. Occasionally siderotic granules are found in mature red cells, which are then called *siderocytes*. These are seen especially after splenectomy (see p. 610).

Iron excretion is small in men, in whom minute losses occur from the faeces, urine, hair, and nails. In women greater losses occur during menstruation and pregnancy.

Copper. There is some experimental evidence that copper facilitates iron metabolism, but in clinical practice there is no convincing evidence that pure copper deficiency leads to anaemia.

Cobalt. Deficiency in animals leads to a severe anaemia, and excess cobalt may induce a polycythaemia. Its role in human nutrition is unknown. It is a constituent of vitamin B_{12}.

Hormonal Factors

Erythropoietin.[12] This is a plasma factor, a glycoprotein, which has a stimulating effect on erythropoiesis. The production of the factor is governed by a balance between the supply of oxygen to the tissues and their demand. Raised levels of erythropoietin have been reported in many different types of anaemia, but there is no correlation between the severity and duration of the anaemia and the plasma level of the factor. Its site of production is the kidney, probably in the juxtaglomerular cells, but it is possible that there are extrarenal sources also. Whether the renal erythropoietic factor is identical with the plasma factor, or is a precursor that is activated by normal serum is not known. It appears to act on the stem cell, which once directed to erythroblastic differentiation, does not require any further erythropoietin stimulation. Erythropoietic depression occurs when there is a reduced demand for oxygen, e.g. after hypophysectomy and starvation.

Thyroxine. Lack of thyroxine decreases the rate of production of red cells, and there is a decreased use of iron for the synthesis of haemoglobin. Myxoedema sometimes causes a moderate normochromic, macrocytic anaemia with a hypocellular bone marrow. It is slowly reversed with thyroxine.

Androgen. This stimulates erythropoiesis, probably by potentiating the action of erythropoietin. It is useful in some types of aplastic anaemia, e.g. in myxoedema and hypopituitarism.

Adrenocorticosteroids. These too stimulate erythropoiesis, but the mode of action is unknown. Polycythaemia may occur in Cushing's syndrome, and marrow aplasia in hypopituitarism. Addison's disease is associated with a normocytic, normochromic anaemia which is masked by the concomitant haemoconcentration.

The Disposal of the Red Cell

Two methods used to study the life-span of the red cell are *differential agglutination* using transfused compatible, though immunologically different, red cells, and *isotopic labelling* with radioactive elements, notably ^{51}Cr, which are incorporated metabolically into the patient's red cells. The cells are labelled with the chromate *in vitro*, and are then re-injected into the individual. Both these procedures indicate that the normal life-span of a red cell is about 120 days.

The manner in which the effete red cell is destroyed is still uncertain. The process of ageing precedes and is responsible for eventual destruction, and it is possible that the cell undergoes fragmentation in the circulation prior to its ultimate removal by the RE cells of the liver, bone marrow, and spleen.

Inside the RE cell the haemoglobin is broken down. The globin portion is released, degraded, and returned to the body's pool of amino acids. The porphyrin part of the haem molecule is converted into bilirubin (see Chapter 43), while the iron combines with apoferritin to form ferritin, and is then transported with transferrin to be used again.

Any free haemoglobin reaching the plasma is bound to an α_2-globulin called *haptoglobin*. There are three main types of haptoglobins, and these are genetically distinct. Like the blood-group antigens and the abnormal haemoglobins, the haptoglobins are of anthropological and genetic interest. The haptoglobin concentration (normally 100–150 mg per 100 ml) rises in inflammatory conditions similarly to the ESR.

If haemoglobin in excess of the haptoglobin binding capacity of the plasma is released, the excess haemoglobin breaks down into a ferric protoporphyrin complex, haematin, which is immediately bound by two proteins, a β_1-globulin called *haemopexin* and albumin. Of the two haemopexin has the greater affinity, but any excess haematin combines with albumin to form a brown pigment called *methaemalbumin*. The haptoglobin, haemopexin, and albumin combinations are all metabolised in the body, and none escapes into the urine. The presence of methaemalbumin in the plasma is a reliable indication of an abnormal amount of intravascular haemolysis; normally only traces of haemoglobin can be detected in the plasma.

Thus, after severe intravascular haemolysis haptoglobin is first lost from the cirulation; then haemopexin disappears as the level of methaemalbumin increases. In acute haemorrhagic pancreatitis, extravasated haemoglobin is converted into haematin which is absorbed into the circulation and forms complexes with haemopexin and albumin. The result is methaemalbuminaemia, a low haemopexin, and a *normal level of haptoglobin*; this finding has been described as a useful diagnostic test for the haemorrhagic variety of pancreatitis.[13]

Persistent haemoglobinaemia and haemoglobinuria occur only when all these binding proteins have been saturated. The tubular epithelium of the kidneys produces haemosiderin from the free haemoglobin. *Haemosiderinuria* is therefore seen whenever there is persistent haemoglobinaemia. It is a common finding in patients with a heart-valve prosthesis.

THE ANAEMIAS

Anaemia may be defined as a condition in which there is a fall in the quantity of red cells or haemoglobin in a unit volume of blood in the presence of a low or normal total blood volume. In anaemia the total blood volume may be reduced due to a decrease in the number of red cells, but often, as in pernicious anaemia, this is offset by an absolute increase in the plasma volume. On the whole, the reduction in blood volume in anaemia is very small.

The question of blood volume and anaemia is important in relation to pregnancy.[14] A moderate fall in the levels of red cells and haemoglobin is common during the latter part, and is followed by a slow recovery in the puerperium. There is a raised blood volume (due to a considerable increase in plasma volume) in pregnancy, and it is probable that much of the "physiological anaemia" is due to simple haemodilution. However, there is often an additional element of iron deficiency.

There is no completely satisfactory classification of the anaemias. A *morphological classification* is extremely useful, but there is great overlapping, e.g. macrocytic anaemia is seen both in vitamin-B_{12} deficiency and in many haemolytic anaemias. Classifications based on *aetiology* or *pathogenesis* are also very helpful, but in some anaemias there are several mechanisms at work, e.g. pernicious anaemia has a haemolytic element as well as a maturation defect. Furthermore, some anaemias have no certain aetiology. The anaemia of chronic renal failure is described as "toxic", but is probably secondary to deficient erythropoietin activity. The following classification is of practical value:

ACUTE POSTHAEMORRHAGIC ANAEMIA	Typically normochromic and normocytic. It is diagnosed clinically, and has been described on p. 421.
IRON-DEFICIENCY ANAEMIA	Typically hypochromic and microcytic.

MEGALOBLASTIC ANAEMIA	Typically normochromic and macrocytic. The marrow contains megaloblasts.
HAEMOLYTIC ANAEMIA	Excessive red-cell destruction with subsequent regeneration (reticulocytosis) is the predominant feature.
ANAEMIA OF BONE-MARROW INADEQUACY	This is usually normocytic and normochromic, and there is little evidence of effective regeneration.

Anaemia results from the failure of the bone marrow to meet the demands of the body. This may be due to a massive haemorrhage depleting the blood mass too rapidly for it to be compensated, or to an absence of essential haematopoietic agents like iron, folic acid, or vitamin B_{12}, or else to excessive red-cell breakdown incompletely compensated by regeneration. In the anaemia of bone-marrow inadequacy there is reduced output, which can be assessed by studies of plasma and erythrocytic iron metabolism (ferrokinetics). The term *dyshaemopoietic anaemia* is not used, as it includes the iron-deficiency and megaloblastic group as well as some bone-marrow inadequacy states.

The pathological effects of anaemia are due to hypoxia. The cardiac output is increased in order to meet the oxygen demands of the tissues, but eventually heart failure of the high output type occurs.

The basal metabolic rate is raised, and in severe degrees of anaemia pyrexia is quite common. The cause of this is unknown.

The morbid anatomy of chronic anaemia is that of pallor and severe fatty change of the viscera. In days gone by, untreated pernicious anaemia was a frequent object of *post-mortem* study, and profound fatty change was described in the liver, kidneys, and even the heart. The "thrush-breast", or "tabby-cat", yellowish streaking of the papillary muscles, due to fatty change of the myocardium, was a classical finding. Nowadays death from chronic anaemia is very uncommon. Patients with incurable blood disorders, like aplastic anaemia and leukaemia, are kept at adequate haemoglobin levels by repeated red-cell transfusions until the final fatal episode.

IRON-DEFICIENCY ANAEMIA[15]

Causes

Chronic blood loss, e.g. from a bleeding peptic ulcer, gatro-intestinal cancer, haemorrhoids, or menorrhagia. This is the most important cause in clinical practice.

Nutritional deficiency. Iron-deficiency anaemia is not uncommon in *infants*. If was quite frequent in adolescent girls about 50 years ago, and was called *chlorosis* because of a alleged greenish tinge of the skin. It was probably related to the onset of menstruation and poor diet, and is no longer common. Iron-deficiency anaemia is very common in *pregnant women*, in whom there is an increased demand by the growing fetus, especially if there is dietary deficiency. In women between the ages of 30 and 50 years an *idiopathic hypochromic anaemia* is well recognised. There is typically achlorhydria, and sometimes a family history both of this condition and of pernicious anaemia. It is doubtful whether it is a distinct entity, for in most cases there is dietary deficiency and also often menorrhagia. It is very uncommon in men.

Inadequate absorption. Iron-deficiency anaemia is a usual complication of *gastrectomy* because of the intestinal hurry that follows the removal of the gastric reservoir. From it chyme is normally expelled slowly enough to come into optimal contact with the intestinal mucosa. The lack of hydrochloric acid is a secondary factor. *Intestinal lesions* causing malabsorption also lead to iron deficiency.

Ankylostomiasis.[16] While blood loss caused by the hookworms accounts for some of the iron deficiency, most cases occur in underprivileged communities in whom there are multiple dietary deficiencies.

Haematological Findings

There is a moderate fall in red-cell count with a greater reduction in the haemoglobin level. The MCV, MCH, and MCHC are all reduced. Of these the MCHC is the most reliable, and is usually 25–30 per cent. The red cells are microcytic and hypochromic, with a moderate degree of anisocytosis and poikilocytosis. Target cells are quite common (see Fig. 49.4). The reticulocyte count is normal or depressed except after a recent haemorrhage, when there is a temporary reticulocytosis.

The white cells and platelets are usually normal.

The bone marrow shows normoblastic hyperplasia. The number of sideroblasts is greatly reduced.

Biochemical Findings

A reduced plasma iron, usually below 30 μg per 100 ml. The iron-binding capacity of the plasma is increased.

The serum bilirubin is normal or low, for there is no increased haemolysis. There may be *achlorhydria* in some cases, especially in the idiopathic anaemia of the middle-aged.

Pathological Findings

Oral manifestations occur in about 40 per cent of cases. The commonest is a degree of atrophy of the filiform papillae of the tongue, and there may also be angular stomatitis. Dysphagia may also be present, and then the condition is called the *Plummer-Vinson syndrome* (see p. 382). There has been doubt cast on the relationship between the dysphagia and iron deficiency, but the consensus of opinion strongly associates the two.

Atrophic gastritis is a common accompaniment of chronic iron deficiency, which both causes the stomach lesion and is aggravated by it. This leads to marked hypochlorhydria.

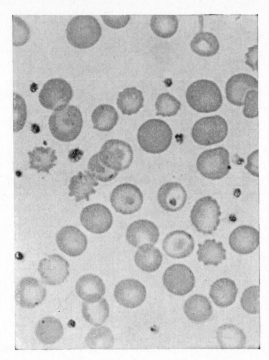

Figure 49.4
Iron-deficiency anemia. This film of peripheral blood contains red cells that are hypochromic. Quite a number show a target-like distribution of their haemoglobin. There are numerous platelets present. ×960.

Koilonychia—spoon-shaped, brittle, lustreless finger-nails—occurs in about a third of cases of chronic iron-deficiency anaemia.

An extension of red marrow into the shafts of the long bones.
Splenomegaly. This is sometimes seen in the "idiopathic" type of anaemia; its cause is unknown.

MEGALOBLASTIC ANAEMIA[17, 18]

This is due to a deficiency of vitamin B_{12} or folic acid either alone or else in combination.

Causes

Nutritional defects. A nutritional megaloblastic anaemia is seen quite often in India, especially in pregnant women. It has been called "tropical macrocytic anaemia", though it occurs in temperate climates also. It is due to folic-acid deficiency. Occasionally there is also a degree of vitamin-B_{12} deficiency.

A true vitamin-B_{12}-deficiency anaemia has rarely been reported in vegans, strict vegetarians who do not eat any animal products. It is interesting that few vegans become anaemic despite the low level of vitamin B_{12}.

Pregnancy. A nutritional megaloblastic anaemia is not uncommon in pregnant women living in temperate areas like Britain and the USA. It is due to folic-acid deficiency

following poor intake and the demands of the fetus. Megaloblastic anaemia has been noted in infants, and is once more due to a deficiency of folic acid.

Gastric defects. Since intrinsic factor is secreted by the gastric mucosa, it is to be expected that total gastrectomy would lead to megaloblastic anaemia. So great are the stores of vitamin B_{12} in the liver that it takes about 4 years for anaemia to develop. Partial gastrectomy may also lead to vitamin-B_{12} deficiency.[19, 20] The intestinal malabsorption due to intestinal hurry (see p. 589) acts together with the reduction in the amount of available intrinsic factor.

By far the most important gastric cause of megaloblastic anaemia is the mucosal atrophy that affects the upper two-thirds of the stomach in *pernicious anaemia*. This disease occurs most often in Northern Europeans, and shows a familial tendency. It is commonest in subjects of blood group A. It is probable that the tendency to mucosal atrophy is inborn, and that achylia gastrica (the absence of pepsin and hydrochloric acid in the gastric juice) is established before megaloblastic anaemia develops. In exceptional cases free hydrochloric acid is present in the gastric juice.

It is found that 90 per cent of patients have antibodies against parietal cells and 57 per cent have antibodies against intrinsic factor in their serum. The presence of auto-antibodies against intrinsic factor appears to be specific for pernicious anaemia, apart from rare cases of thyroid disease and atrophic gastritis. It has been suggested that pernicious anaemia is an autoimmune disease in which patients react abnormally to the frequent episodes of trauma to which the stomach is prone. The antibodies cause mucosal atrophy with an ensuing lack of secretion. On the other hand, it is possible that the autoantibodies are merely an indication of gastric disease. At any rate, an assessment of intrinsic factor antibodies is a useful diagnostic aid in some cases of pernicious anaemia. There is an increased incidence of disorders of a possibly "autoimmune" type, e.g. thyroid disease, Addison's disease, vitiligo, and hypoparathyroidism, in near relatives, and some patients with pernicious anaemia have myxoedema or Graves's disease.

Cases of juvenile pernicious anaemia have been known in which there was no mucosal disease or autoantibodies.[21] It is postulated that there is a genetic failure of the mucosal cells to produce intrinsic factor in these children.

Intestinal malabsorption. This, whether due to intrinsic mucosal disease such as idiopathic steatorrhoea or sprue, or to strictures, anastomoses, or fistulae which alter the bacterial flora of the bowel, is often associated with megaloblastic anaemia. In the first group there is a primary failure to absorb, whereas in the other "surgical" conditions it appears that the bacteria that flourish behind strictures or in blind loops between anastomoses, or are introduced through fistulae either compete with the mucosa for the folic acid or vitamin B_{12} or else prevent its absorption by causing chronic enteritis. On the whole it is folic-acid deficiency that predominates in most of these conditions. The absorption of vitamin B_{12} is confined to the terminal ileum, and so it is most likely to be seriously impaired in regional lesions such as Crohn's disease. In malabsorption secondary to bacterial contamination of the bowel oral tetracyclines sometimes have a good effect on the anaemia.

Fish-tapeworm infestation. This parasite, *Diphyllobothrium latum,* competes with its host for vitamin B_{12}. The megaloblastic anaemia is found only in Finland despite the wide distribution of the worm elsewhere in the world.

Chronic liver disease. Megaloblastic anaemia due to folic-acid deficiency is occasionally noted in alcoholic cirrhosis. This effect is due to alcoholism. Vitamin-B_{12} deficiency is not a significant factor.

Drugs. A folic-acid deficiency megaloblastic anaemia may follow the administration of such anticonvulsants as primidone and phenytoin sodium.[22] The antimetabolites used as cytotoxic agents also produce a megaloblastic anaemia; indeed, some are folic-acid antagonists. Vitamin B_{12} may also have some ameliorative effect. It is not known how anticonvulsants cause the anaemia; it is in any case a rare side-effect.

Haematological Findings

There is a considerable fall in red-cell count with a smaller reduction in the haemoglobin level. The MCV and MCH are greatly raised, but the MCHC is normal. The red cells are macrocytic and normochromic. Both anisocytosis and poikilocytosis are very marked (Fig. 49.5). Polychromasia

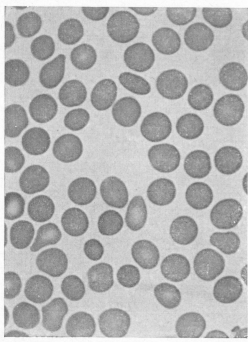

Figure 49.5
Megaloblastic anemia. This film of peripheral blood contains well-haemoglobinized red cells which show considerable variation in size and shape. Large forms (macrocytes) predominate. ×800.

and sometimes punctate basophilia may be noted, but the reticulocyte count is usually within normal limits. The peripheral blood often contains a few nucleated red cells. In the malabsorption syndrome there may be concomitant iron deficiency producing a "dimorphic" blood picture.

There is a marked neutropenia, and some of the neutrophils are large and have multi-segmented nuclei (*macropolycytes*). A few myelocytes are often present in the peripheral blood.

The platelet count is reduced. Both the leucocyte and platelet abnormalities are more marked in pernicious anaemia than in the other magaloblastic anaemias.

The bone marrow shows megaloblastic hyperplasia, though normoblasts are also present in varying numbers. There is considerable myeloid hyperplasia also, and giant myelocytes are of diagnostic importance. Megakaryocytes may be reduced in number. It is evident that the dyshaematopoiesis of the megaloblastic anaemias is by no means confined to the red cells.

Biochemical Findings

There is a mild haemolytic process, which is most marked in classical pernicious anaemia. This is manifested by a slightly raised serum bilirubin (1–3 mg per 100 ml), an increased excretion of urobilinogen in the faeces, and moderate urobilinuria. The red-cell survival rate is considerably reduced, and in addition, the ineffective erythropoiesis adds to the bilirubin load. Patients given labelled glycine show an increased excretion of early labelled bilirubin (p. 533).

The plasma iron level is raised.

Achlorhydria is almost invariable in pernicious anaemia, but is inconstant in the other megaloblastic anaemias.

Pathological Findings

Severe fatty change of the liver, kidneys, and heart.

Marked haemosiderosis of the liver, bone marrow, kidneys, and spleen. This is due to a continued absorption of iron which is not adequately used for erythropoiesis.

The changes of subacute combined degeneration of the spinal cord: demyelination of the lateral and posterior columns without any gliosis. There may also be degenerative changes in the peripheral nerves and in the brain. These neurological manifestations are peculiar to vitamin-B_{12} deficiency, and are not seen in folic-acid deficiency.

Atrophy of the mucosa of the tongue with disappearance of the filiform papillae. This is typical of pernicious anaemia, and produces the characteristic raw, beefy tongue. Glossitis is also seen in sprue, but is not constant in the other megaloblastic anaemias.

Atrophy of the gastric mucosa in pernicious anaemia has already been mentioned. It is the pathognomonic change of this disease.

Evidence of increased haematopoiesis: the marrow is deep red in colour, and extends into the shafts of the long bones where it replaces the fatty marrow. There may be extramedullary haematopoiesis in the spleen and liver. Moderate splenomegaly is typical of pernicious anaemia. In the malabsorption syndrome, on the other hand, splenic atrophy sometimes occurs.

There is evidence that a generalised cellular dystrophy attends folic-acid and vitamin-B_{12} deficiency: many of the body's cells are larger than normal, and have a delicate chromatin network in their nuclei. This is seen not only in the cells of the bone marrow but also in the epithelial cells of the mouth and stomach (see p. 309).

THE HAEMOLYTIC ANAEMIAS[23, 24]

Though there is a haemolytic element in many types of anaemia, in the true haemolytic anaemias the factor of increased red-cell destruction is paramount. This destructibility is due either to some intrinsic defect in the red cells, or to some extracorpuscular factor acting on the red cells from without. If the defect is primarily corpuscular, the red cells of the patient will not survive long when transfused into a healthy recipient, whereas the patient's plasma will not destroy normal red cells. On the other hand, if the cause of the haemolysis is extra-corpuscular, normal red cells will be eliminated in the same way as those of the patient, while the patient's red cells will survive well in a normal recipient. The diagnostic feature of a haemolytic anaemia is a persistent reticulocytosis in the absence of haemorrhage or bone-marrow replacement.

CORPUSCULAR DEFECTS

The most important of these are:

Hereditary spherocytosis (congenital acholuric jaundice). There is a spherocytic malformation of the red cell. The condition is inherited as an autosomal dominant characteristic. The abnormality lies in the cell membrane, but its underlying nature is obscure. Secondary effects on the membrane include a loss of phospholipid leading to spherocytosis, an abnormal permeability to sodium ions, and the change in shape predisposing to sequestration of the red cells in the spleen, where they are avidly phagocytosed and destroyed. Of all the haemolytic anaemias this one responds best to splenectomy. It is interesting that despite a dramatic amelioration of the anaemia and a greatly increased red-cell survival, the spherocytic malformation persists.[25]

Hereditary elliptocytosis. This is another malformation inherited as an autosomal dominant characteristic. The red cells are oval in shape, and occasionally there is a moderate haemolytic anaemia. Splenectomy is of some value.

The haemoglobinopathies. The conditions associated with abnormal haemoglobins have been discussed on p. 585 and their ethnic significance stressed. If a patient inherits the gene from one parent only, i.e. if he is heterozygous, he shows minimal signs of the disease, but if he is homozygous, a haemolytic anaemia may result. The following haemoglobinopathies are of special importance:

Sickle-cell disease. This is the haemoglobinopathy *par excellence* of Negroes. In a stained film sickled red cells are not conspicuous, but when a drop of blood is sealed under a cover-slip on a slide, and especially if a reducing agent like sodium dithionite is added, bizarre sickling of the cells soon becomes apparent. As already explained, this is due to the insolubility of reduced Hb-S.

Haemoglobin-C disease. This is encountered especially in West-African Negroes. In a stained film target cells are frequent. The condition is less severe than sickle-cell disease.

The thalassaemia syndromes.[26] Two types of thalassaemia are recognised according to whether the α or β chain synthesis is defective.

β-thalassaemia. This is the best known type, and is the common haemoglobinopathy of the Mediterranean races. In *homozygous β-thalassaemia, Cooley's anaemia,* or *thalassaemia major,* there is a considerable increase in the amount of Hb-F, and the main effects are anaemia, splenomegaly, hepatomegaly, leg ulcers, fever, and skeletal changes (which are seen also in other hereditary haemoglobinopathies) characterised by widening of the marrow space and the formation of subperiosteal bone, which in the skull gives a "hair-on-end", or "brush", appearance. The poor synthesis of haemoglobin causes the red cells to be very hypochromic, and extreme leptocytosis is characteristic. The blood film resembles that of a severe iron-deficient anaemia. In *β-thalassaemia minor,* which is the heterozygous state, there is a mild anaemia and a tendency to develop gall-stones. The level of Hb-A_2 is increased as also may be that of Hb-F.

α-Thalassaemia. In the homozygous state there is a complete inability to produce α chains, and the major component is Hb-Bart's (γ_4). The condition of *α-thalassaemia major* is incompatible with life. *α-thalassaemia minor,* found in individuals who are heterozygotes for the α-thalassaemia gene, is symptomless and difficult to detect. There is, however another gene which alone is silent, but which when combined with one α-thalassaemia gene, leads to a mild anaemia. This is *Hb-H disease,* and the red cells contain Hb-H (β_4) together with some Hb-Bart's (γ_4).

Combinations of these haemoglobinopathies are quite common. The most important are sickle cell-Hb-C disease, sickle cell-thalassaemia, and Hb-C-thalassaemia. None of these conditions is as severe as sickle-cell disease or thalassaemia major.

The mechanism of haemolysis is largely mechanical in sickle-cell disease; the sickled cells are fragile and are destroyed in the circulation. The same explanation is probably true for the leptocytes of thalassaemia. In *hereditary Heinz-body anaemia* (see p. 594) there is an unstable haemoglobin unduly liable to be converted to methaemoglobin, and here too haemolysis is increased.[27] In *haemoglobin-Zurich disease,* severe crises of haemolysis are precipitated by the administration of sulphonamides and primaquine. Once again this haemoglobin is unstable, this time in the presence of oxidant drugs.[28]

Paroxysmal nocturnal haemoglobinuria.[29] In this disease, which is not familial and is acquired in adult life, there is an episodic haemolytic anaemia manifested by attacks of haemoglobinuria usually occurring at night. The defect resides in the red cells, especially the reticulocytes, which are easily haemolysed by complement present in the plasma (p. 163). Such cells are very susceptible to haemolysis in acid solutions at pH 6·8, or when mixed with 20 per cent sucrose solution. It has been suggested that the nocturnal haemolysis is due to the rise in Pco_2 which occurs during sleep, but the evidence is unconvincing, and treatment with alkalis is ineffective. The nature of the defect remains to be elucidated; it is probably an abnormality of the cell membrane.

Enzyme-deficient red cells.[30–32] It was the finding that American Negroes were much more susceptible to haemolytic anaemia after the administration of the antimalarial drugs pamaquin and primaquine than were white-skinned Americans that led to the discovery that many drug-induced anaemias were due to hereditary enzyme defects. The most important is a deficiency of *glucose 6-phosphate dehydrogenase (G6PD)*[33] in the red cells, which impedes the hexose monophosphate shunt (p. 23 and p. 585).[33] One type of G6PD deficiency is seen in Caucasians living in the Mediterranean area, while another type occurs in Negroes of West-African stock. They are inherited as incomplete dominant sex-linked characteristics. In both types the subjects are especially liable to haemolysis after exposure to oxidant drugs like those mentioned above, and also sulphones, sulphonamides, probenecid, phenacetin, acetanilid, aspirin, and para-aminosalicylic acid. The acute haemolytic anaemia *favism* that occurs occasionally after contact with or ingestion of fava beans (*Vicia faba*) is seen only in the Mediterranean type of G6PD deficiency, and is perhaps due also to an additional genetic effect.* Rare cases of chronic haemolytic anaemia associated with G6PD deficiency have been described.

Pyruvate kinase deficiency haemolytic anaemia. This disease is inherited as an autosomal recessive trait, and is characterised by a non-spherocytic haemolytic anaemia, often presenting in early childhood. It is the commonest type of enzyme-deficient haemolytic anaemia in people of North-European stock.

Non-spherocytic haemolytic anaemia can be caused by other enzyme deficiencies, but they are rare: included are a deficiency of glutathione, glutathione reductase, hexokinase, and triosephosphate isomerase.

EXTRACORPUSCULAR FACTORS

The following conditions are important:

Autoantibodies[34] (see also Chapter 16). Autoantibodies against red cells usually arise idiopathically, but from time to time they occur during the course of another disease such as

---

* Pythagoras counselled his followers never to walk in bean fields, and is reputed to have suffered from favism.[33]

Hodgkin's disease or systemic lupus erythematosus, when they may lead to a secondary haemolytic anaemia. Some infective diseases, notably mycoplasmal pneumonia and syphilis, are occasionally attended by characteristic autoantibodies against the patient's red cells.

Most autoantibodies against red cells are agglutinins. Some of these agglutinate red cells in saline suspension, and are called *complete antibodies*; they are IgM. Others are *incomplete*, for although they coat the red cells and lead to their destruction in the body, they are incapable of agglutinating red cells *in vitro*. However, these coated red cells can be agglutinated *in vitro* by an antihuman-globulin serum. This is the basis of the *Coombs*, or *antiglobulin*, *test* which is described in detail on p. 629. These antibodies are IgG.

The complete antibodies are amboceptors, and lead to *in-vitro* haemolysis in the presence of complement. There is indeed one antibody which acts primarily as a haemolysin, the *Donath-Landsteiner antibody*. By contrast, the incomplete antibodies are feebly haemolytic *in vitro*.

Some of these antibodies are most active at 37°C, and are called *warm antibodies*. Nearly all are incomplete IgG antibodies directed against Rh antigens. Clinically they are responsible for the most severe cases of autoimmune haemolytic anaemia. The autoantibodies that occasionally occur in systemic lupus erythematosus and lymphomata come into this category.

Cold antibodies are virtually inactive at 37°C, but become increasingly powerful *in vitro* as the temperature drops to 0°C. Such antibodies are complete IgM and usually anti-I. One type of chronic haemolytic anaemia caused by complete cold antibodies ("cold agglutinins") occurs predominantly in elderly subjects. The main features of this *cold-haemagglutinin syndrome* are a moderate anaemia, haemoglobinuria, and a Raynaud-like phenomenon. This follows blockage of the vessels of the extremities by red cells, which are agglutinated at the low surface temperature. A similar, though more acute, condition occasionally complicates mycoplasmal pneumonia, in which a raised titre of cold agglutinins is characteristic, and has been known to lead to an acute haemolytic anaemia with renal failure.[35]

In paroxysmal cold haemoglobinuria, a rare disease which is usually a complication of tertiary syphilis, there are dramatic episodes of severe haemolysis occurring shortly after exposure to the cold. This is due to the Donath-Landsteiner cold haemolysin. It sensitises the red cells at a low temperature, but only when the temperature rises once more does gross haemolysis occur. The phenomenon is easily reproducible *in vitro*.

Clinically all these autoantibodies lead to rapid red-cell destruction. The level of complement in the serum is lowered, since haemolysis involves its activation and consumption. These anaemias are sometimes accompanied by falsely positive serological reactions for syphilis, due presumably to autoantibodies formed against normal lipid constituents of the body.

The mode of red-cell destruction is largely due to complement activation in the intravascular types of haemolysis associated with cold-antibody haemoglobinuria. In the warm-antibody conditions red-cell destruction is extravascular, and it is the RE cells that remove the sensitised red cells rapidly from the circulation. Extravascular destruction may also be the major event in some cases of the cold-haemagglutinin syndrome; in these complement is fixed to the red cells, but for reasons which are not clear it fails to produce lysis. The spleen acts as the most sensitive filter, but the liver plays the dominant role in red-cell destruction when haemolysis is massive or when the spleen is overloaded or removed. The bone marrow is also active, accepting the overflow from liver and spleen. In the cold-antibody anaemias there is also prominent erythrophagocytosis in the RE cells, expecially those of the liver.

Alloantibodies. These are discussed in Chapter 52. The common alloantibody anaemia is erythroblastosis fetalis, in which the red cells of a Rhesus-positive infant are destroyed by antibodies from its Rhesus-negative mother, who has been sensitised beforehand either by a transfusion of Rh-positive blood or by a previously-born Rh-positive child. It is well established that fetal red cells commonly enter the maternal circulation during pregnancy. These can be demonstrated by the property of fetal haemoglobin to resist acid elution—fetal cells retain their haemoglobin in strong acid solution, whereas adult cells are decolorised.[36] The most dangerous period is during parturition, especially if the labour is complicated. With a subsequent pregnancy, Rhesus antibodies (of a "warm" incomplete type) cross the placenta. The infant's red cells, which give a positive Coombs test, are rapidly haemolysed. A group-A fetus may likewise be the victim of anti-A antibodies from his group-O mother.

An advance of great importance is the discovery that the administration of a γ-globulin containing incomplete anti-Rh of high activity can prevent the sensitisation of Rh-negative mothers by Rh-positive fetal cells provided it is given within two days of delivery. The anti-D antibody probably reacts with and neutralises the incompatible cells, which are then disposed of by the RE cells.[37–39]

Infective agents. These may produce haemolysis by the production of powerful exotoxins, e.g. *Cl. welchii*, or endotoxins, e.g. streptococci causing septicaemia. Some organisms produce haemolysis secondarily to parasitisation of red cells, e.g. the parasites of malaria and Oroya fever. Blackwater fever is a fulminating intravascular haemolysis which occurs in chronically malarial subjects who have taken quinine fitfully; its mode of production is unknown.

Drugs. As has already been mentioned, the idiosyncratic haemolytic anaemias following many drugs are associated with a congenital enzyme deficiency in the red cells or an abnormal haemoglobin. There are, however, some agents which will produce haemolysis in any subject if given in a large enough dose, e.g. phenylhydrazine, methyl chloride,

arsine, lead, and nitrobenzene. In drug-induced haemolytic anaemias, whether idiosyncratic or not, the red cells often contain fragments of denatured haemoglobin, which are called *Heinz bodies* and are useful evidence of exogenous intoxication. A hereditary Heinz-body anaemia due to an abnormal haemoglobin has already been mentioned.

Drugs may also cause haemolytic anaemia by immunological mechanisms.[40] Three such mechanisms are recognised: (a) the drug, acting as a hapten, combines with red-cell proteins, and the antibodies formed lyse the cells by activating complement. High-dose penicillin therapy may act thus when the binding power of the plasma proteins is exhausted. (b) The red cell may be an "innocent bystander" and be bound adventitiously by circulating antibodies to such drugs as stibophen, quinine, or phenacetin. These too act as haptens, but they combine with some body protein other than that of the red cell. When the red cell-antibody complex next meets antigen, complement is activated and lysis occurs. (c) Alpha-methyldopa is peculiar in stimulating antibodies that act specifically against red-cell antigens determined by the *Rh* locus. There is no drug binding as with penicillin. It would appear that the antibody produced by α-methyldopa is accidentally reactive to some of the host's antigens.

Extensive burns. The effect is a simple thermal damage to the red cells, which are then destroyed locally or else removed rapidly from the circulation by the spleen.

Other diseases. The list of diseases that may be complicated by haemolytic anaemia is quite impressive. Some, like Hodgkin's disease, chronic lymphatic leukaemia, and systemic lupus erythematosus, are usually associated with autoantibodies. Other conditions that may be complicated by haemolytic anaemia are carcinomatosis, ovarian tumours especially teratomata, thrombotic thrombocytopenic purpura, uraemia, liver failure, eclampsia, and sarcoidosis, and in these the cause of haemolysis varies.

One important mechanism is red-cell trauma following direct contact of the cells with diseased fibrin-coated blood vessels[41] in such conditions as thrombotic thrombocytopenic purpura and malignant hypertension, where diffuse vascular damage is present. This is called *microangiopathic haemolytic anaemia*, and its basic cause is usually the defibrination syndrome described on p. 622. In one type there is severe renal damage due to blockage of the glomeruli (haemolytic uraemic syndrome). This acute disease, which usually affects children or pregnant women with eclampsia, exhibits an acute haemolytic anaemia, thrombocytopenia, and acute renal failure due to a severe glomerulitis with necrosis and thrombosis in glomeruli and vessels. Several entities may be included in the haemolytic-uraemia syndrome and some may be viral or rickettsial.[42]

That physical trauma can cause red-cell destruction is demonstrated by the haemolytic anaemia that occasionally occurs in calcareous aortic stenosis as well as following the introduction of prostheses for the surgical treatment of aortic-valve disease.[43, 44] The increased cardiac turbulence leads to mechanical damage of the cells.

Another important factor leading to haemolysis is hypersplenism where there is splenomegaly, e.g. sarcoidosis, myelosclerosis, etc. (see p. 609).

Haematological Findings

There is a variable fall in red-cell count with a proportional drop in haemoglobin level. The red cells are typically normocytic and normochromic but the numerous young forms tend to produce a somewhat macrocytic picture. Anisocytosis and poikilocytosis are present in variable degree. In the congenital corpuscular defects there are characteristic malformations, e.g. spherocytes, leptocytes, and sickled forms. In the acquired anaemias due to autoimmune and alloimmune mechanisms there is also spherocytosis (Rh-haemolytic disease is an exception). Poikilocytosis is prominent in anaemias due to mechanical trauma to red cells as in the microangiopathic syndromes—some of the cells are fragmented, some bear spicules, and some have a burr or helmet outline, or are even triangular.

Polychromasia is conspicuous, and a reticulocytosis is invariable: it may exceed 30 per cent. Punctate basophilia is noteworthy in lead poisoning. Nucleated red cells may be present, especially in thalassaemia and Rh-haemolytic disease (erythroblastosis fetalis—Fig. 49.1, p. 582).

The red-cell osmotic-fragility test is an important investigation in cases of haemolytic anaemia. Normally the red cell start to haemolyse in a 0·5 per cent saline solution, and nearly all are haemolysed in a 0·35 per cent solution. The fragility is much increased when there is spherocytosis, and is decreased in the leptocytosis of thalassaemia.

There is a marked neutrophil leucocytosis during phases of acute haemolysis, and myelocytes and metamyelocytes may be present in the peripheral blood. In chronic anaemias the white-cell count is usually normal. The platelet count is normal or increased.

The bone marrow shows intense normoblastic hyperplasia.

"*Crises.*" During the course of hereditary spherocytosis and sickle-cell disease episodes of acute exacerbation of symptoms with a rapidly increasing anaemia are common. These may be due to increased haemolysis, but most crises are due to temporary aplasia of the marrow. Marrow aplasia is quite common in paroxysmal nocturnal haemoglobinuria.[29]

Biochemical Findings

There is a moderate or severe haemolytic jaundice with a raised serum bilirubin, increased excretion of urobilinogen in the faeces, and a considerable urobilinuria (see Chapter 43). In most haemolytic anaemias there is methaemalbuminaemia even when there is no obvious evidence of intravascular haemolysis, and the level of haptoglobin is reduced, as the haemoglobin-haptoglobin complex is removed more rapidly than new haptoglobin can be synthesised. This is particularly well marked in sickle-cell disease and thalassaemia.

Acute intravascular haemolysis is on occasions accompanied by dramatic symptoms, and fatal anuria may ensue. There is experimental evidence that large quantities of free haemoglobin in the circulation may lead to a decrease in the renal blood flow,[45] but acting on its own it is probably insufficient to produce serious damage.[46] Thus, patients with paroxysmal nocturnal haemoglobinuria pass large amounts of haemoglobin in their urine, and yet usually have no specific renal symptoms; their complaints are those of severe anaemia. It will be recalled that in this condition there is destruction of abnormal red cells by the normal haemolytic mechanisms of the plasma.

When there is intravascular haemolysis as the result of antibodies acting on normal cells, the symptoms are more severe. There is pain in the back and calves, often accompanied by abdominal colic, headache, fever, and rigors. This is seen in paroxysmal cold haemoglobinuria. In conditions of very severe haemolysis, e.g. blackwater fever and incompatible blood transfusions, there is also marked renal vasoconstriction, and acute renal failure may ensue. It seems probable that an antigen-antibody reaction on the red cells is accompanied by the release of powerful vasoconstrictor substances that are responsible for the pain and renal effects.[46] The matter is considered in greater detail with respect to blood-transfusion reactions in Chapter 52. Following massive intravascular haemolysis the binding power of plasma, due to haptoglobin, haemopexin, and albumin, is exhausted, and the plasma and urine are flooded with haemoglobin. This haemoglobinaemia and haemoglobinuria are accompanied by methaemalbuminaemia; jaundice and urobilinuria soon follow. In chronic cases there is haemosiderinuria as the result of the breakdown of haemoglobin by the proximal convoluted tubules.

Pathological Findings

Evidence of increased haematopoiesis. In adults the red marrow extends into the shafts of the long bones. In children these are already filled with red marrow, hence there is a tendency towards widening of the medullary cavity and absorption of the cortex of the bone. Extramedullary haematopoiesis may also be prominent.

Splenomegaly. This is common, but the histological findings are seldom remarkable. There may be erythrophagocytosis in the autoimmune types of anaemia, and the pulp is often crowded with red cells. Splenic infarction and subsequent *atrophy* is usual in sickle-cell anaemia, so that splenomegaly is not a feature of this haemoglobinopathy except in the early stages.

Haemosiderosis of liver, spleen, kidneys, and marrow. In paroxysmal nocturnal haemoglobinuria it is virtually confined to the kidneys, which are brown in colour.

Chronic leg ulcers are common in hereditary spherocytosis and sickle-cell disease, and may occur also in thalassaemia. Their cause is unknown.

Gall-stones of calcium bilirubinate (*pigment stones*) are an important complication of hereditary spherocytosis and sickle-cell disease, and sometimes also of thalassaemia. They are not unusually frequent in acquired haemolytic anaemias.

Vascular occlusion. Vascular complications are especially frequent in sickle-cell disease, where accumulations of sickled red cells, by occluding capillaries and venules, lead to infarction, especially of the bones (see p. 476), spleen, and central nervous system. Vascular occlusion is also seen in cold-antibody anaemia, and may lead to gangrene of the extremities. In paroxysmal nocturnal haemoglobinuria venous thrombosis is a common complication; perhaps the haemolysed red cells liberate clotting factors.

ANAEMIAS OF BONE MARROW INSUFFICIENCY

This group includes those anaemias which are usually normocytic and normochromic and show no evidence of increased red-cell regeneration.

The anaemia of chronic disease (e.g. chronic infection, rheumatoid arthritis, leukaemia, and some cases of cancer) though usually normocytic and normochromic, may show mild microcytosis and hypochromia. The plasma iron is low, the iron-binding capacity is reduced, and the level of saturation of transferrin is low. The percentage of sideroblasts in the marrow is reduced, yet the RE cells are crowded with haemosiderin. Thus there is sideropenia in the presence of a surfeit of iron. The basic dysfunction is not clear; perhaps it lies in disordered erythropoietin function or impaired transferrin metabolism.

The anaemia of renal failure. This rather similar anaemia occurs in chronic renal failure. It is probably due to inhibited marrow action by retained toxic products. The finding of low erythropoietin levels in some cases has led to the suggestion that the anaemia is due to a lack of this factor, but dialysis ameliorates the anaemia without altering the plasma level of erythropoietin. The haemoglobin level tends to remain at about 8g per 100 ml despite all treatment.

Endocrine anaemias, especially those of hypopituitarism, myxoedema, and Addison's disease, have been noted on pp. 587–588.

The anaemia of bone-marrow replacement—leuco-erythroblastic anaemia—is described on p. 611.

The anaemia of bone-marrow aplasia—aplastic anaemia—is described on p. 607.

Sideroblastic anaemia.[47, 48] In this condition there is a hypochromic anaemia with abnormal sideroblasts in the marrow. Not only are the sideroblasts increased in number, but they also contain increased amounts of iron in the cytoplasm, characteristically in a conspicuous ring around the nucleus in association with the mitochondria. There is also increased iron in the RE cells, and the plasma iron is usually high. The level of transferrin is reduced, but it is almost fully saturated.

A hereditary sex-linked type of sideroblastic anaemia is described, but most cases are acquired. An important cause is

pyridoxine deficiency after using the antituberculous drugs isoniazid, cycloserine, and pyrazinamide. Lead poisoning and chronic alcoholism occasionally lead to a sideroblastic anaemia, which has also been described in the malabsorption syndrome (no doubt through pyridoxine lack). Some cases complicate lymphomata, leukaemia, and myelosclerosis. One type is idiopathic. The nature of the dysfunction is not known.

POLYCYTHAEMIA

Polycythaemia is a condition in which the quantity of red cells is raised in a unit volume of blood in the presence of an increased total blood volume. It must be distinguished from the haemoconcentration that follows sodium and water deficiency (see Chapter 34). In polycythaemia the total blood volume is notably raised owing to a considerable increase in the red-cell mass. The plasma volume is normal or low, therefore the viscosity of the blood is greatly increased. In polycythaemia the ESR is decreased, whereas in anaemia it is increased.

Polycythaemia secondary to other conditions is called *erythrocytosis*, when the red-cell count, haemoglobin content of the blood, and packed cell volume are all increased, but the white-cell and platelet counts are not raised. It occurs in the following conditions:

Hypoxia due to chronic pulmonary disease, cyanotic congenital heart disease, methaemoglobinaemia, and sulphaemoglobinaemia. A marked polycythaemia is found in those who live at high altitudes. An interesting recent discovery is the existence of a number of rare abnormal haemoglobins with an unusually high affinity for oxygen. The resulting tissue hypoxia evokes a polycythaemia. This polycythaemia is hereditary, and is another example of a haemoglobinopathy, e.g. Hb-Chesapeake, Hb-Capetown, and Hb-Yakima.

Miscellaneous conditions. The occasional occurrence of polycythaemia with renal lesions, mostly hypernephroma and sometimes polycystic disease and hydronephrosis, has led to the suggestion that these lesions may promote the secretion of an erythropoietin-like factor. Indeed, such a factor has been isolated from some tumours and cysts. More rarely polycythaemia may complicate cerebellar angioma, uterine myoma, hepatoma, and Wilms's tumour. Once again an erythropoiesis stimulating factor has sometimes been found in these tumours, the removal of which leads to a haematological remission.

Cushing's syndrome.

In the primary type of polycythaemia, called *polycythaemia vera* or *erythraemia*,[49] there is a neoplastic process involving the normoblastic element of the marrow. There is a great rise in the red-cell count, sometimes up to 10 million cells per μl, with a comparable or less marked rise in the level of haemoglobin. The cells are normocytic and usually normochromic (though after a therapeutic venesection there may be temporary hypochromia); a few polychromatic and nucleated red cells are also present in the blood. In most cases there is a considerable neutrophil leucocytosis with a shift to the left, and also a thrombocytosis. These changes indicate a general proliferative change in the bone marrow, but in some cases the increase is confined to the erythroblastic element, when the condition can scarcely be distinguished from an erythrocytosis.

The pathological features of polycythaemia vera are those of intense venous engorgement which is manifested in the ruddy, plethoric, cyanotic appearance of victims of the disease. There is considerable splenomegaly, and both the spleen and liver may contain foci of extramedullary haematopoiesis. There is a marked tendency for thrombotic complications to supervene, e.g. cerebral and coronary thrombosis, and mesenteric venous thrombosis, and these are probably related to the high platelet count and the increased viscosity of the blood. Surprisingly, haemorrhagic manifestations are also common, and there is no satisfactory explanation. Hypertension is not unduly prevalent in polycythaemic subjects despite the increased viscosity of the blood. Peptic ulceration is common, and has been ascribed to thrombosis of the vessels in the gastric and duodenal mucosa.

Occasionally chronic myeloid leukaemia or myelosclerosis develops. In such an instance the polycythaemia is replaced by a normocytic, normochromic anaemia.

DISORDERS OF HAEMOGLOBIN ACCOMPANIED BY CYANOSIS[50, 51]

There are two such conditions, methaemoglobinaemia and sulphaemoglobinaemia. In *methaemoglobinaemia* the ferrous iron of normal haemoglobin is converted into the ferric form, and as such it cannot combine with oxygen. There is therefore tissue hypoxia, and a secondary polycythaemia may result. The condition is usually produced by drugs e.g. nitrates, sulphonamides, phenacetin, acetanilide, aniline, and nitrobenzene. Some of these may also cause haemolytic anaemia. The condition can be reversed by administering reducing agents, like ascorbic acid and methylene blue (see p. 585). Methaemoglobinaemia may also be due to congenital defects in the red cells. An example of this is a haemoglobinopathy due to Hb-M, which is oxidised abnormally easily. In this type of methaemoglobinaemia reducing agents are powerless.

In *sulphaemoglobinaemia* an abnormal compound is formed by the reaction of haemoglobin with inorganic sulphides and hydrogen peroxide. It may be produced by acetanilide and phenacetin. It is not reversible, and time has to elapse before it is eliminated from the body. It too interferes with the oxygen-combining power of haemoglobin.

Enterogenous cyanosis refers to methaemoglobinaemia and sulphaemoglobinaemia of unknown origin. There are often associated abdominal symptoms. It may be due to the absorption of large amounts of nitrites and sulphides from the bowel. Enterogenous methaemoglobinaemia clears up in a few days, but sulphaemoglobinaemia may take several months.

The clinical manifestation of these disorders is a slate-blue cyanosis in the absence of dyspnoea. Spectroscopic examination is essential to identify these two abnormal intracorpuscular pigments and to distinguish them from reduced haemoglobin.

GENERAL READING FOR HAEMATOLOGY

DACIE, J. V. and LEWIS, S. M. (1968). *Practical Haematology*, 4th edn, 568 pp. London: Churchill.
DE GRUCHY, G. C. (1970). *Clinical Haematology in Medical Practice*, 3rd edn, 800 pp. Oxford: Blackwell.
WINTROBE, M. M. (1967). *Clinical Hematology*, 6th edn, 1287, pp. Philadelphia: Lea and Febiger.

REFERENCES

1. Leading Article (1972). *Lancet*, i, 1056.
2. BIRD, G. W. G. (1972). *British Medical Journal*, i, 293.
3. Leading Article (1971). *British Medical Journal*, i, 683.
4. STANBURY, J. B., WYNGAARDEN, J. B. and FREDRICKSON, D. S. (1972). *The Metabolic Basis of Inherited Disease*, p. 1398 et seq., 3rd edn, New York: McGraw-Hill.
5. Recommendations by the International Society of Haematology on the Nomenclature of Abnormal Haemoglobins (1965). *British Journal of Haematology*, **11**, 121.
6. SHINTON, N. K. (1972). *British Medical Journal*, i, 556.
7. WAYNE, L. et al. (1958). *Archives of Internal Medicine*, **101**, 143.
8. GOLDBERG, A. (1963). *Quarterly Journal of Medicine*, **32**, 51.
9. DAGG, J. H., CUMMING, R. L. C. and GOLDBERG, A. (1971). In *Recent Advances in Haematology*, p. 77. Edited by A. Goldberg and M. C. Brain. Edinburgh and London: Churchill Livingstone.
10. Leading Article (1971). *Lancet*, ii, 475.
11. HEILMEYER, L. (1966). *Acta haematologica*, **36**, 40.
12. Leading Article (1972). *British Medical Journal*, i, 263.
13. NORTHAM, B. E., WINSTONE, N. E. and BANWELL, J. G. (1965). In *Recent Advances in Gastroenterology*, p. 349. Edited by J. Badenoch and B. N. Brooke. London: Churchill.
14. Leading Article (1963). *Lancet*, i, 309.
15. TURNBULL, A. (1971). *British Journal of Hospital Medicine*, **6**, 573.

16. GILLES, H. M., WILLIAMS, E. J. W. and BALL, P. A. J. (1964). *Quarterly Journal of Medicine*, **33**, 1.
17. HOFFBRAND, A. V. (1971). In *Recent Advances in Haematology*, p. 1, *loc. cit.*
18. CHANARIN, I. (1971). *British Journal of Hospital Medicine*, **6**, 581.
19. DELLER, D. J. and WITTS, L. J. (1962). *Quarterly Journal of Medicine*, **31**, 71.
20. DELLER, D. J., RICHARDS, W. C. D. and WITTS, L. J. (1962). *Quarterly Journal of Medicine*, **31**, 89.
21. DIMSON, S. B. (1966). *Archives of Diseases in Childhood*, **41**, 216.
22. FLEXNER, J. M. and HARTMANN, R. C. (1960). *American Journal of Medicine*, **28**, 386.
23. DACIE, J. V. (1960), (1962) and (1967). *The Haemolytic Anaemias*, 2nd edn, Parts 1, 2, 3 and 4. London: Churchill. An exhaustive account of the subject.
24. BRAIN, M. C. (1971). In *Recent Advances in Haematology*, p. 146, *loc. cit.*
25. BAIRD, R. N., MACPHERSON, A. I. S. and RICHMOND, J. (1971). *Lancet*, ii, 1060.
26. WEATHERALL, D. J. (1971). In *Recent Advances in Haematology*, p. 194, *loc. cit.*
27. GRIMES, A. J., MEISLER, A. and DACIE, J. V. (1964). *British Journal of Haematology*, **10**, 281.
28. RIEDER, R. F., ZINKHAM, W. H. and HOLTZMAN, N. A. (1965). *American Journal of Medicine*, **39**, 4.
29. DACIE, J. V. (1963). *Proceedings of the Royal Society of Medicine*, **56**, 587.
30. DE GRUCHY, G. C. and GRIMES, A. J. (1968). In *Recent Advances in Clinical Pathology*, Series V. Edited by S. C. Dyke. p. 225. London: Churchill.
31. PRANKERD, T. A. J. (1970). *Journal of Clinical Pathology*, **24**, Supplement (Association of Clinical Pathologists), **4**, 71.
32. BEUTLER, E. (1969). *Medical Clinics of North America*, **53**, 813.
33. Leading Article (1969). *Lancet*, ii, 1177.
34. DACIE, J. V. (1970). *British Medical Journal*, ii, 381.
35. LAWSON, D. H. *et al.* (1968). *Lancet*, ii, 704.
36. WOODROW, J. C. and FINN, R. (1966). *British Journal of Haematology*, **12**, 297.
37. FINN, R. (1970). *British Medical Journal*, ii, 219.
38. A Combined Study from Centres in England and Baltimore (1971). *British Medical Journal*, ii, 607.
39. WOODROW, J. C. *et al.* (1971). *British Medical Journal*, ii, 610.
40. WINTROBE, M. M. (1969). *Journal of the Royal College of Physicians of London*, **3**, 99.
41. BULL, B. S. and BRAIN, M. C. (1968). *Proceedings of the Royal Society of Medicine*, **61**, 1134.
42. EDELMAN, C. M. (1969). *New England Journal of Medicine*, **281**, 1072.
43. BRODEUR, M. T. H. *et al.* (1965). *Circulation*, **32**, 570.
44. SEARS, D. A. and CROSBY, W. H. (1965). *American Journal of Medicine*, **39**, 341.
45. BLACKBURN, C. R. B. *et al.* (1954). *Journal of Clinical Investigation*, **33**, 825.
46. MUELLER, C. B. and MASON, A. D. (1956). *American Journal of Clinical Pathology*, **26**, 705.
47. WEATHERALL, D. J. (1969). *Journal of the Royal College of Physicians of London*, **3**, 275.
48. BATEMAN, C. J. T. and MOLLIN, D. L. (1970). *British Journal of Hospital Medicine*, **4**, 371.
49. DAMON, A. and HOLUB, D. A. (1958). *Annals of Internal Medicine*, **49**, 43.
50. BODANSKY, O. (1951). *Pharmacological Reviews*, **3**, 144.
51. FINCH, C. A. (1948). *New England Journal of Medicine*, **239**, 470.
52. BENESCH, R. (1969). *New England Journal of Medicine*, **280**, 1179.

Chapter 50.   Some Disorders of the Blood:

II. THE WHITE CELLS, BONE MARROW, AND SPLEEN

THE CONSTITUENT CELLS

A haemocytoblast which is developing into a granulocytic leucocyte passes through the following stages:

Myeloblast. This is the most primitive of the granulocytic series. It is a large cell, very similar in appearance to a pro-normoblast. It has a scanty basophilic cytoplasm and a large round nucleus containing fine strands of chromatin and several prominent nucleoli.

Promyelocyte. This cell is transitional between a myeloblast and a myelocyte. It is smaller than the myeloblast, and has few, if any, nucleoli. On the other hand, it does not contain specific cytoplasmic granules, though a few non-specific azurophil granules may be present.

Myelocyte. This is smaller, and the specific neutrophil, eosinophil, or basophil granules are present in the cytoplasm. The nucleus is smaller and may be indented.

Metamyelocyte. A somewhat smaller cell in which the specific cytoplasmic granulation is fully developed. The nucleus is kidney-shaped and its chromatin is condensed into clumps. A later *stab cell* stage is sometimes described, in which the nucleus has assumed a horse-shoe shape.

The mature granulocyte, i.e. neutrophil, eosinophil, and basophil polymorphonuclears. In these mature cells, which are

TABLE 50.1 The cellular constituents of the normal bone marrow

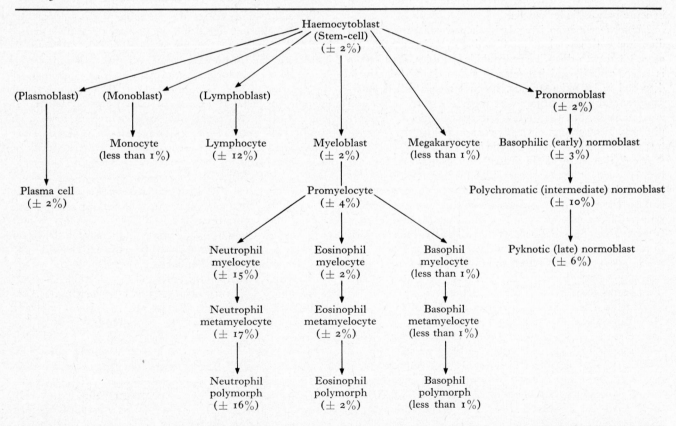

The percentages are a rough average of the normal range of the cells. Plasmoblasts, monoblasts, and lymphoblasts are not normally present.

10–15 μm in diameter, the fine lilac-coloured granules of the neutrophil, the large red granules of the eosinophil, and the very coarse purple granules which overlie the nucleus of the basophil, are the typical features, and are well shown in Romanowsky-stained films. In H. and E. sections only the eosinophil granules are clearly stained. The nuclei are separated into two or three lobes joined by fine chromatin strands. It is the peculiarly shaped nucleus that gives rise to the name "polymorph". The neutrophil leucocytes play an essential part in many acute inflammatory processes, but the function of the eosinophils and basophils is less certain (see p. 96).

The other leucocytes seen in the marrow and the peripheral blood are the lymphocyte and the monocyte. Neither contains specific granules in its cytoplasm.

The lymphocyte is a small round cell about 10 μm in diameter with a large round or indented nucleus containing dark clumps of chromatin. Its cytoplasm is scanty and basophilic. A larger form (up to 20 μm in diameter) is also seen, in which there is much more cytoplasm but a similar darkly-staining nucleus. Its precursor is the *lymphoblast*, a cell almost indistinguishable from the myeloblast, but said to have fewer nucleoli and a coarser chromatin pattern. Lymphoblasts are found in lymphoid tissue. They are not normally recognisable in a marrow film, but they predominate in acute lymphatic leukaemia.

The monocyte is an irregularly-shaped cell 12–20 μm in diameter with abundant muddy-blue cytoplasm, which is often filled with dust-like azurophilic granules. Its nucleus is large, central, and irregular in shape. Its chromatin is disposed in lace-like strands. Precursor cells called *promonocytes* and *monoblasts* are described. These are larger and have nucleoli, but they retain the typical monocytic morphology. They are not normally recognisable in the marrow, but are conspicuous in monocytic leukaemia.

A cell that is regularly present in the marrow, but not normally seen in the peripheral blood is the *plasma cell*. It is large and pear-shaped, and has deeply basophilic cytoplasm and an eccentric nucleus containing clumps of chromatin arranged like a cart wheel. The current view is that it arises from the lymphocyte. Large primitive plasma cells are seen in the marrow in multiple myeloma.

The monocytes form the second phagocytic system of the blood. The part played by these cells, the lymphocytes, and the plasma cells in the immune response is described in Chapter 12. The relationship of the lymphocyte to the "stem cell" is discussed in Chapter 30.

It will be noted that the leucoblastic elements of the marrow predominate over the erythroblastic ones in the ratio of about 4:1. This is called the *myeloid-erythroid ratio*; it is decreased and even reversed in normoblastic and megaloblastic hyperplasia of the marrow, whereas it is increased when there is leucoblastic (myeloid) proliferation, e.g. in acute pyogenic infections and leukaemia.

From the description of the development of the red and white cells it is apparent that as a blood cell matures, it undergoes the following changes:

(*a*) It becomes smaller.

(*b*) Its nucleus becomes smaller, the chromatin becomes condensed, and the nucleoli disappear.

(*c*) The cytoplasm becomes less basophilic, except with the plasma cell.

(*d*) The specific cytoplasmic constituents, e.g. haemoglobin and granules, appear.

THE NORMAL WHITE-CELL COUNT

The total white-cell count of the peripheral blood varies from 4 000 to 11 000 cells per μl. The range of the differential leucocyte count in a healthy adult is as follows:

NEUTROPHIL	
POLYMORPHONUCLEARS	40–75% (2 500–7 500 per μl)
EOSINOPHIL	
POLYMORPHONUCLEARS	1–5% (50–400 per μl)
BASOPHIL	
POLYMORPHONUCLEARS	0–1% (up to 100 per μl)
LYMPHOCYTES	20–45% (1 500–3 500 per μl)
MONOCYTES	3–7% (200–600 per μl)

The figures in brackets are the range of absolute counts, and are much more significant than a mere percentage figure. With neutropenia there is often an apparent, or "relative", increase in the lymphocyte count, when the absolute figure is normal or even lowered. Normally a small percentage of the neutrophils have unsegmented nuclei. These are called juvenile, or "stab", forms. In conditions of neutrophil leucocytosis their proportion increases, and there may be numbers of metamyelocytes and even myelocytes in the circulation. At one time a classification of the maturity of leucocytes based on their nuclear segmentation was very much in vogue. Arneth devised an exhaustive system in which the most primitive cells were tabulated on the left-hand side of a page and the most mature cells on the right-hand side. Though the Arneth count is now obsolete, the term "a shift to the left" is still useful in denoting an increase in the blood of young forms of polymorphs. The most extreme example of such a shift is the leukaemoid reaction which is occasionally encountered in severe infections and intoxications. A "shift to the right" is characteristic of pernicious anaemia with its multi-segmented macropolycyte, though there is also a tendency for a few myelocytes to enter the blood in this condition.

In the newborn infant there is a moderate neutrophil leucocytosis which usually drops to nearly normal within the first week. From then on there is a relative lymphocytosis until the fourth year, when neutrophil and lymphocyte counts are almost equal. The normal adult count is attained at puberty. Strenuous exercise, convulsions, paroxysmal tachycardia, emotional stress, and ether anaesthesia are all associated with a transient neutrophil leucocytosis. During labour this is very marked.

VARIATIONS IN THE WHITE-CELL COUNT

A total and differential white-cell count is a basic diagnostic procedure in clinical medicine. It is often an eloquent commentary on the body's reaction to infectious agents of various types, and is therefore a valuable guide in pointing to the cause of an undiagnosed pyrexial illness.

Neutrophil Leucocytosis (Neutrophilia)

The commonest alteration in the white-cell count is a leucocytosis due to an increase in the number of neutrophils. It is encountered in the following pathological conditions:

Infection (*a*) Pyogenic, both acute, e.g. staphylococcal, and chronic, e.g. actinomycotic, (*b*) other bacterial diseases, e.g. anthrax, plague, diphtheria, scarlet fever, and leptospiral jaundice (Weil's disease), and (*c*) virus disease after the prodromal period, e.g. smallpox, poliomyelitis, and zoster.

A hormone that promotes the growth of granulocytes in agar has been discovered; it is called the colony-stimulating factor, and has been isolated in human serum.[1] Whether it is important in stimulating a leucocytic response is not known.

Metabolic disorders. Uraemia, acute gout, diabetic ketosis, and eclampsia.

Intoxications. Chronic lead poisoning, mercury, digitalis, adrenaline, camphor, and arsphenamine.

Serum sickness and after *anaphylactic shock*.

After acute haemorrhage especially into a serous cavity, e.g. ruptured ectopic pregnancy.

In acute haemolytic anaemia.

In the catabolic phase of convalescence after injury.

In conditions of massive necrosis, e.g. myocardial infarction.

In rapidly-growing malignant tumours, e.g. cancer of the liver, lung, or colon, and Hodgkin's disease.

In neoplastic diseases of the bone marrow, e.g. chronic myeloid leukaemia and polycythaemia vera.

In most of these conditions, especially the acute pyogenic group, there is a variable "shift to the left". This becomes very marked in severe infections, when metamyelocytes and even myelocytes may enter the blood. *Leukaemoid blood pictures* are an extreme manifestation of this tendency. They are occasionally encountered in (*a*) severe infections, e.g. pneumonia, meningitis, plague, septicaemia, and especially miliary tuberculosis, (*b*) sudden acute haemolysis, (*c*) eclampsia, (*d*) widespread malignant disease without skeletal metastases, and (*e*) conditions associated with bone-marrow replacement (see p. 610). The peripheral blood picture may closely resemble that of myeloid leukaemia, both chronic and acute. An assessment of the *leucocyte alkaline phosphatase* level in the neutrophils may be of value in the differential diagnosis. The activity of the enzyme is moderately increased in the leucocytosis of infection and in the leukaemoid reaction, whereas it is characteristically low in chronic myeloid leukaemia.

Another test of value in assessing the origin of a neutrophil leucocytosis is the *nitroblue-tetrazolium test*,[2] which depends on the ability of neutrophils to reduce the colourless soluble dye nitroblue tetrazolium and produce a blue-black formazan precipitate. Normally less than 10 per cent of circulating neutrophils have this ability, but the percentage is much greater in systemic bacterial and fungous infections associated with a neutrophilia. There is no such increase in virus infections, allergic diseases, or surgical trauma. It would seem that the neutrophils actively concerned in phagocytosis during a natural infection are those that can reduce nitroblue tetrazolium. In children with chronic granulomatous disease (see p. 161) there is no reaction at all.

In severe infections the fine lilac granulation of the neutrophils may be replaced by irregular bluish granules, a condition called *toxic granulation*.

Leucopenia

This is invariably due to a fall in the neutrophil count, i.e. neutropenia. It is less common than a neutrophilia, and is seen in the following conditions:

Infections (*a*) Certain specific bacterial diseases, e.g. typhoid fever and brucellosis, (*b*) virus disease in the prodromal period, e.g. influenza, smallpox, measles, and infective hepatitis, (*c*) chronic protozoan disease, e.g. malaria, leishmaniasis, and trypanosomiasis, and (*d*) overwhelming bacterial infection, e.g. miliary tuberculosis, septicaemia, and pneumonia, when it is of very serious prognostic import.

Some conditions associated with splenomegaly (*hypersplenism*), e.g. Felty's syndrome, hepatic cirrhosis (Banti's syndrome), primary splenic neutropenia, and Gaucher's disease.

In pernicious anaemia, and occasionally in chronic iron-deficiency anaemia.

Systemic lupus erythematosus.

Bone-marrow aplasia (see p. 607). If the neutrophils alone are involved, the condition is called *agranulocytosis*.

Acute leukaemia. When there is a profound leucopenia the condition is often miscalled "aleukaemic leukaemia".

Anaphylactic shock and serum sickness. There is an immediate leucopenia, but a neutrophilia soon follows.

Neutropenia is almost always accompanied by a relative lymphocytosis. Occasionally the lymphocytosis may be so great that the total white-cell count is within normal limits despite the severe neutropenia.

Lymphocytosis

An absolute lymphocytosis, i.e. lymphocytic leucocytosis, is met with in a few specific conditions:

Whooping-cough. White cell counts of over 100 000 cells per μl have been reported.

Infectious mononucleosis (glandular fever). This common disease, seen most often in children and young adults, is infective in origin. The classical condition with heterophile antibodies to sheep red cells, which are discussed below, is caused by the EB virus,[3] a herpesvirus which has been noted on p. 385 with reference to Burkitt's tumour. Young adults who were initially seronegative developed infectious mononucleosis and antibodies after exposure to the virus. Many people have antibodies without having had the disease previously, an indication that subclinical infection is widespread, a situation seen also in herpes simplex. A disease clinically and haematologically indistinguishable from the EB virus infectious mononucleosis, but without heterophile antibodies, may occur in young adults with cytomegalic inclusion disease and toxoplasmosis.

The symptoms of infectious mononucleosis are protean,[4] and important features are a prolonged pyrexia, enlarged painful lymph nodes, sore throat, and an enlarged spleen. Its course is typically benign, but complications like splenic rupture, hepatic necrosis, encephalitis, and oedema of the glottis may rarely cause death.

The leucocytosis is due to the presence of variable numbers of abnormal lymphocytes in the blood. These vary in size, and have a vacuolated or foamy basophilic cytoplasm. The nucleus varies in shape, and its chromatin is disposed in coarse clumps and strands. Though the nuclear shape may resemble that of a monocyte, the chromatin lacks the lacy disposition so typical of this cell. Sometimes the white-cell count may exceed 40 000 cells per μl.

Another characteristic finding is the presence of *heterophile antibodies* in the patient's serum, which are capable of agglutinating sheep's red cells in high titre (*Paul-Bunnell test*). A rather similar antibody is found to low titre in normal people, especially after the injection of horse serum (Forssman antibody, see p. 139). It is distinctive in being absorbed by a suspension of guinea-pig kidney, which is rich in Forssman antigen, and not by ox red cells. The glandular-fever antibody, on the other hand, is absorbed by ox red cells but not by guinea-pig kidney. Differential absorption followed by a sheep red-cell agglutination test serves to distinguish between the two antibodies.

Acute infectious lymphocytosis.[5] This is an uncommon benign febrile disease of childhood in which there is a lymphocytosis of up to 100 000 cells per μl. The cells are mature, and the titre of heterophile antibodies is not increased.

Chronic infections, e.g. secondary and congenital syphilis and healing tuberculosis.

Endocrine conditions. Thyrotoxicosis may be accompanied by an inconstant lymphocytosis. The lymphocyte count is raised in adrenal insufficiency, e.g. Addison's disease.

Chronic lymphatic leukaemia.

Waldenström's macroglobulinaemia. These cells, which produce the abnormal immunoglobulin, have a copious basophilic cytoplasm rich in carbohydrate which stains with the PAS method.

Occasionally a reactive lymphocytosis may be marked enough to mimic lymphatic leukaemia. This *lymphocytic leukaemoid reaction* has been described in whooping-cough, infectious mononucleosis, infectious lymphocytosis, miliary tuberculosis, and carcinoma of the stomach.[6]

Lymphopenia

This is not common, and the fall in lymphocytes is seldom great enough to lead to a leucopenia. It is seen in the following conditions:

After whole-body irradiation (see Chapter 31).

In response to ACTH or adrenal cortical steroids.

In Hodgkin's disease. The usual white-cell picture in this condition is a moderate neutrophilia. Sometimes there may also be an absolute fall in the lymphocyte count.

Monocytosis

A rise in the monocyte count may be found in:

Infections. (*a*) Chronic bacterial diseases, e.g. tuberculosis, subacute infective endocarditis, and brucellosis. It is said to indicate activity in tuberculosis, and was regarded as an unfavourable sign in the pre-antibiotic era, (*b*) Protozoan disease, e.g. malaria, leishmaniasis, and trypanosomiasis, in which it is a characteristic finding, (*c*) In the later stages of acute pyogenic infection. It declines once resolution has occurred, but persists if chronic inflammation develops.

Tetrachlorethane poisoning.

Monocytic leukaemia.

Hodgkin's disease is sometimes accompanied by a moderate monocytosis.

Eosinophilia

T lymphocytes are necessary for the development of eosinophilia in mice and rats infected with *Trichinella spiralis*; the mechanism is not understood (see p. 96). In human pathology eosinophilia is found in:

Hypersensitivity of atopic type, e.g. bronchial asthma, hay-fever, and urticaria. Eosinophils are present in large numbers in the sputa or nasal discharges of such patients. Wherever eosinophils are being broken down Charcot–Leyden crystals are found; they are protein in nature, and are probably derived from lysosomes.[7, 8]

Interestingly, eosinophilia is not a feature of generalised anaphylaxis, though there may be some eosinophils in the exudates in the tissues. Likewise, serum sickness does not usually lead to eosinophilia except, to an extent, around the lesions in the tissues. Delayed-type hypersensitivity is not associated even with eosinophils in the local lesions, except for the rather strange retest phenomenon (see p. 187).

Certain chronic skin diseases, e.g. pemphigus vulgaris and dermatitis herpetiformis.

Infections. Eosinophilia is characteristic of all helminthic infestations which invade the tissues, e.g. schistosomiasis, trichinosis, hydatid disease, and filariasis.

Loeffler's syndrome[9] is a transient pulmonary infiltration accompanied by a marked eosinophilia. It is probably a

TABLE 50.2   The leucocytic response to some of the agents causing a prolonged pyrexia

Blood picture	Possible cause of pyrexia
NEUTROPHILIA	a. Hidden pus, e.g. subphrenic or perinephric abscess. b. Widespread malignancy including Hodgkin's disease. c. Polyarteritis nodosa (frequent).
NEUTROPENIA WITH RELATIVE LYMPHOCYTOSIS	a. Typhoid fever. b. Brucellosis. c. Systemic lupus erythematosus. d. Chronic protozoan disease.
ABSOLUTE LYMPHOCYTOSIS	a. Infectious mononucleosis—abnormal lymphocytes.
EOSINOPHILIA	a. Early helminthic infestations. b. Polyarteritis nodosa (occasional). c. Hodgkin's disease (uncommon).
MONOCYTOSIS	a. Protozoan disease. b. Subacute infective endocarditis (occasional). c. Active tuberculosis (occasional).
NORMAL	a. Subacute infective endocarditis. This is the usual white-cell count; sometimes there is a moderate leucopenia or leucocytosis. b. Tuberculosis. Usually the white-cell count is normal, though all pictures from agranulocytosis to a leukaemoid reaction are possible. c. Q-fever and mycoplasmal pneumonia. d. Widespread malignancy including Hodgkin's disease (less common than neutrophilia). e. Polyarteritis nodosa (less common than neutrophilia). f. Systemic lupus erythematosus (less common than neutropenia).

hypersensitivity reaction, and is seen most often in connexion with helminthic infestations, e.g. ankylostomiasis, ascariasis, and trichinosis. It has also been described in tuberculosis, brucellosis, and coccidioidomycosis. A related hypersensitivity of a longer duration and relapsing course has also been described. Another hypersensitivity syndrome with pulmonary infiltration, asthmatic symptoms, weight loss, and moderate splenomegaly is called *tropical eosinophilia*, because it was first described in South-East Asia. It is a reaction to various parasites, usually microfilariae[10] (see also p. 183).

Intestinal worm infestation is less commonly accompanied by eosinophilia. It is in the early stages of ascariasis and ankylostomiasis that the blood change occurs.

During most acute infections the eosinophil count drops as a result of the increased output of adrenal cortical hormones. Recovery is often heralded by an eosinophilia. *Scarlet fever* and *chorea* are sometimes associated with a marked eosinophilia.

Polyarteritis nodosa is attended by an eosinophilia in about 20 per cent of cases.

Diseases of the bone marrow. In chronic myeloid leukaemia there is an absolute eosinophilia which is overshadowed by the neutrophilia. A special "eosinophilic leukaemia" has been described. Polycythaemia vera and Hodgkin's disease are sometimes associated with a considerable eosinophilia, and so occasionally are widely metastasising tumours.

Plasma Cells and Atypical Lymphoid Cells in the Blood

Plasma cells are not commonly present in the peripheral blood. They occur typically in *rubella*, and rather less constantly in *measles* and *chickenpox*. They may occasionally be present in multiple myeloma, and are very numerous in the rare *plasma-cell leukaemia*.

Atypical lymphoid cells with very basophilic cytoplasm and resembling the immunoblasts seen in active lymph nodes are found in small numbers in the blood from time to time in *bacterial infections*, and during *immunological reactions*. The Türk cell is probably of this nature. A rare condition in which there are many abnormal lymphocytic cells in the blood is the *Sézary syndrome*.[11, 12] This is a fatal lymphomatous condition primarily of the skin and consisting of infiltrative lesions with erythroderma and intense pruritus. Similar lymphoid cells are present in the skin. The Sézary syndrome is closely related to mycosis fungoides.

Table 50. 2 relates white-cell patterns with diseases which often present themselves clinically as a prolonged *pyrexia of unknown origin*. Such pyrexia may be due to the following factors:

Infections. *Bacterial*, e.g. deep-seated suppuration, typhoid fever, subacute infective endocarditis, miliary tuberculosis, and brucellosis.

Protozoan, e.g. malaria, leishmaniasis, and trypanosomiasis.

Helminthic, e.g. trichinosis and schistosomiasis.

Due to other agents, e.g. Q-fever, mycoplasmal pneumonia, and infectious mononucleosis.

Widespread or deep-seated malignancy, e.g. hypernephroma, carcinoma of the lung and liver, and tumours of the lymphoreticular system, especially Hodgkin's disease.

Diseases in which hypersensitivity is a factor, e.g. systemic lupus erythematosus and polyarteritis nodosa.

HAEMATOLOGICAL ASPECTS OF THE LEUKAEMIAS

Leukaemia is a condition in which there is a widespread proliferation of the leucocytes and their precursors throughout the tissues of the body, with a variable circulating component. Its aetiology is unknown, and its course is nearly always fatal. As a neoplastic condition of the haematopoietic tissues it has been mentioned in Chapter 30, and it is now necessary to consider its haematological manifestations in some detail. It is worth recalling that, although the aetiology is unknown, there are a few suggestive factors:[13]

Viruses in fowl and mouse leukaemia (see Chapter 29).

Ionising radiation in human leukaemia (see Chapter 31).

Chemical agents. Myeloid leukaemia, usually acute, has been described as a complication of benzene ingestion, and acute leukaemia has occasionally been known to follow the use of phenylbutazone.[14] Nevertheless, there is little evidence that any drug predisposes to leukaemia.

Congenital chromosomal abnormalities.[13, 15] Acute leukaemia usually myeloid, is twenty times commoner in children with Down's syndrome than in normal children. There is also an increased incidence of acute leukaemia in Fanconi's hypoplastic anaemia, mentioned on p. 608, in which cultured blood cells show a high frequency of chromosomal breakage and rearrangement (see also p. 28).

Immunological deficiency syndromes are not infrequently complicated by acute leukaemia, see p. 171.

Classification

The important factors are the rapidity of the process and the type of cell involved. The more acute the process, the more primitive is the predominant cell. Nowadays acute leukaemias are often successfully checked, though in due course a relapse is to be expected. Thus a case of acute leukaemia may sometimes survive as long as some chronic leukaemias. The difference in the cell type and the clinical picture make a distinction quite easy in practice. The following classification is recommended:

CHRONIC LEUKAEMIA	(*a*) Myeloid (myelocytic)
	(*b*) Lymphatic (lymphocytic)
ACUTE LEUKAEMIA	(*a*) Myeloid (myeloblastic)
	(*b*) Lymphatic (lymphoblastic)
	(*c*) Monocytic (monoblastic)

The names in brackets allude to the predominant cell in the blood.

Chronic Myeloid Leukaemia

This disease has its maximum incidence in early and middle adult life. The organs principally involved are the bone marrow and the spleen. Lymph-node involvement occurs late in the disease, and is seldom conspicuous. The liver is frequently enlarged, and skin lesions are occasionally present.

Blood picture. *The most prominent finding is an enormous increase in the white-cell count,* a figure of 800 000 cells/μl being occasionally attained. The greatest white-cell counts are found in this disease, but sometimes the leucocytosis is smaller. The predominant cells are neutrophil polymorphs with a variable admixture of metamyelocytes and myelocytes. Myeloblasts are present only in very small numbers. There is also an increase in the number of eosinophils, basophils, and their myelocyte precursors. The blood film, on cursory inspection, resembles a normal marrow film. As the disease progresses to a fatal termination, the proportion of myelocytes and myeloblasts increases.

If the leucocytes are grown in tissue culture, some show an abnormal Ph′ chromosome (see p. 42).

The red cells may be little reduced in number in the early stages (occasionally a mild polycythaemia is encountered), but later on a severe normocytic, normochromic anaemia develops. There is some polychromasia, and a mild reticulocytosis is quite common. Nucleated red cells are present in small numbers. The cause of the anaemia is complex. There is usually a haemolytic element, and the bone marrow itself is inadequate.

The platelet count may be normal or raised in the early stages, but later on there is a moderate thrombocytopenia. These changes in the red cells and platelets are valuable in distinguishing chronic myeloid leukaemia from a leukaemoid blood picture.

The bone marrow is very hypercellular due to leucoblastic proliferation. The cells present are similar to those seen in the blood, but slightly less mature forms predominate. The normoblastic element is relatively reduced, but the megakaryocytes are often increased in number until the final stages of the disease.

Chronic Lymphatic Leukaemia

The maximum incidence of this disease is in the middle-aged and elderly. The organ principally involved is the lymph node, and generalised painless lymphadenopathy is the main clinical feature. The bone marrow and spleen are affected later in the course of the disease, and the degree of involvement is seldom as great as in the myeloid variety. The liver is often enlarged, and cutaneous lesions are commoner than in myeloid leukaemia. The tonsils, salivary glands, eyes, stomach, and gut are also sometimes affected.

Blood picture. *There is a considerable leucocytosis* varying from 20 000 to 250 000 cells/μl, a figure lower than that of the myeloid variety. The most important feature is an absolute lymphocytosis, about 90 per cent of the cells being mature, small lymphocytes. Large lymphocytes are not infrequent, but lymphoblasts are very uncommon. There is a relative reduction in the granulocytic polymorph elements.

The red cells and platelets are reduced in number as in the myeloid variety. In chronic lymphatic leukaemia there is seldom the early increase in the red-cell and platelet counts sometimes noted in the myeloid type. On the other hand, the ensuing anaemia develops rather more slowly. Acute haemolytic anaemia is common, and there may be autoantibodies in the blood.

The bone marrow may show no changes at all at first, but later on there is an absolute increase in the number of lymphocytes, which may crowd out the other cells in the terminal stages.

Course of chronic leukaemia. The average duration of life in the myeloid type from the onset of symptoms is usually about 3 years, irrespective of treatment. About 20 per cent survive for 5 years, and about 5 per cent for 10 years. Less than 1 per cent survive for 20 years. Chronic lymphatic leukaemia runs a slower course, and many cases survive for 10 years, especially elderly patients, in whom death may be due to an intercurrent disease. In myeloid leukaemia the end is usually heralded by an acute exacerbation in which the blood is flooded with myeloblasts. In the lymphatic type this is exceptional; death is usually due to progressive anaemia and secondary infection.

Acute Leukaemia

This condition can occur at any age, and it is encountered quite frequently in the first five years of life. Until puberty most acute leukaemia is lymphatic, but in the adult there is a greater incidence of the myeloid form. Monocytic leukaemia is commonest in middle life.

The onset of acute leukaemia is usually sudden and fulminating, but there is sometimes a prodromal period of malaise lasting a few months, during which there may be an obscure thrombocytopenia or anaemia.

The disease is heralded by a rapidly-developing anaemia, necrotic lesions in the mouth and throat, and generalised bleeding manifestations. A high remittent fever is so common that an infective disease is often mimicked. There is usually some enlargement of the lymph nodes, spleen, and liver, though never so marked as in chronic leukaemia. Skeletal lesions are often sufficiently severe to produce bone tenderness and joint pains.

It is impossible to distinguish between the three varieties of acute leukaemia on clinical grounds. Even the swelling and ulceration of the gums that is regarded as typical of monocytic leukaemia may be encountered in the other types also.

Blood picture. *The white-cell count* varies from a severe leucopenia of less than 1 000 cells per μl up to a leucocytosis of more than 100 000 cells per c.mm. As a rule the count is normal or low until terminally, when a great rise usually occurs. The diagnostic feature is the presence of primitive "blast" cells in the blood. Where there is a raised count these are obvious enough, but when there is a leucopenia* they may be extremely scanty. An inexperienced worker may dismiss them as lymphocytes, but a careful inspection reveals irregularities in size and nuclear pattern with nucleoli in some of the cells.

It is often extremely difficult to distinguish between myeloblasts and lymphoblasts. The best criterion is a study of the other white cells, because a "blast" cell is known by the company it keeps, e.g. the presence of myelocytes and neutrophils would suggest that the cell is a myeloblast, whereas a number of mature lymphocytes would indicate the lymphoblastic nature of an unidentified primitive cell.

There are often very few mature cells, in which case histochemistry may be useful in identifying the "blast" cells.

(*a*) *The peroxidase test*, which demonstrates the presence of peroxidase in the granules of neutrophils and monocytes (and their precursors). Lymphocytes are peroxidase-negative. In practice this method is seldom helpful, because the "blast" cells are usually too primitive to contain any granules.

(*b*) *The PAS stain*, which may show coarse masses of glycogen in cells of the lymphoid series. Myeloblasts do not contain any, but glycogen is plentiful in mature polymorphs.

(*c*) *Sudan black staining*, which shows up lipid material in myeloblasts and monoblasts. Lymphoblasts do not show sudanophilia.

Sometimes the "blast" cells have a monocytoid appearance. If there are also numerous myelocytes present, the leukaemia is to be regarded as myeloid (the Naegeli type). If only monocytes and their precursors are present, the leukaemia is truly monocytic (the Schilling type). Sometimes the predominant cell in acute leukaemia is the promyelocyte. This *promyelocytic leukaemia* resembles acute myeloblastic leukaemia except that haemorrhage due to hypofibrinogenaemia is more common and its response to treatment is less satisfactory.

A leukaemia composed of cells so immature that it cannot be classified is called a "stem-cell leukaemia".

There is a severe normochromic, normocytic anaemia. Anisocytosis and poikilocytosis are not conspicuous (this applies also to the chronic types), but there is some polychromasia and reticulocytosis. There are many nucleated red cells in the peripheral blood.

There is a profound thrombocytopenia.

---

* Acute leukaemia with a profound leucopenia is sometimes described as "aleukaemic". This name is unnecessary and confusing. Clinically it masquerades as an aplastic type of anaemia, but the bone marrow is crowded with primitive cells.

The bone marrow is always crowded out with these primitive cells, except, of course, during a remission.

Variations. Very rarely the predominant cell of a leukaemic process is of one specific type: eosinophilic, basophilic, plasma-cell, megakaryocytic, and mature neutrophilic leukaemias have all been described. Most of these run an acute course, but occasionally they are chronic.

In acute leukaemia there is usually a marked depression of the normoblastic element, but occasionally there is a considerable proliferation of erythroblasts in the marrow. Occasionally this is marked and the condition has been termed *erythroleukaemia*. In *Di Guglielmo's syndrome* the peripheral blood is flooded with erythroblasts, either early or late depending on whether it is the acute or chronic form. The marrow, liver, spleen, and other organs are infiltrated by abnormal primitive red-cell precursors. This rare syndrome may be an extreme variant of leukaemia in which the leucoblastic abnormality is overshadowed by the primitive red cells, or it may be a pure neoplastic leukaemia-like disease which affects the red cells.

Course of acute leukaemia. Untreated cases usually die within a few weeks to 6 months of the onset of symptoms. Spontaneous remissions are not uncommon, and exceptionally these have exceeded 20 years, but most soon relapse. Death is usually due to infection and massive haemorrhage, especially into the brain.

Therapy has prolonged the average survival period up to a year, and quite a number of cases have survived 5 years. A few cases have survived over 10 years, and it is probable that these are cured; a remission lasting more than 11 years is probably tantamount to a cure.[16] The lymphatic variety has a better prognosis than the myeloid and monocytic ones.

PATHOLOGICAL FEATURES OF LEUKAEMIA

The invariable feature of leukaemia is a monotonous infiltration of various organs with the primitive cells. The spleen, liver, bone marrow, and lymph nodes are particularly severely affected, but no organ is exempt. On the whole, the infiltrations of acute leukaemia are more circumscribed than those of chronic leukaemia, and there is a greater tendency for a single organ, e.g. intestine, lung, kidney, or gonad, to be massively involved.

In chronic myeloid leukaemia the *spleen* is enormously enlarged, and its architecture is submerged by an accumulation of myelocytes, whereas in chronic lymphatic leukaemia there is a diffuse infiltration of lymphocytes. In acute leukaemia there is a similar infiltration of "blast" cells.

The *lymph nodes* are affected more severely in acute leukaemia and chronic lymphatic leukaemia than in the chronic myeloid variety.

In chronic myeloid leukaemia the *liver* is diffusely infiltrated throughout its sinusoids by myelocytes (Fig. 50.1), whereas in chronic lymphatic leukaemia the lymphocytic

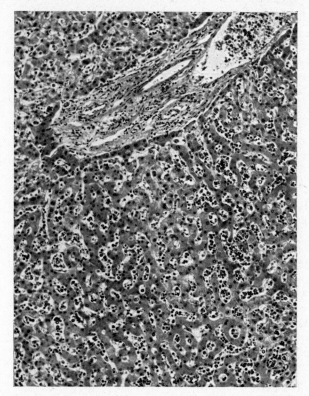

Figure 50.1
Chronic myeloid leukaemia. There is a diffuse infiltration of leukaemic cells throughout the sinusoids of the liver. × 120.

infiltration is usually more marked around the portal tracts (Fig. 50.2).

The *marrow* of the long bones is increased in amount, and is pinkish-grey in colour. Bone destruction is uncommon, but subperiosteal leukaemic infiltrations are not infrequent in acute leukaemia. A rare manifestation is *chloroma*,[17] in which there are extensive leukaemic deposits under the periosteum of the bones. The skull (especially the orbital regions) is typically the site of these tumour deposits, and exophthalmos may be a presenting symptom. The condition is peculiar to acute myeloid leukaemia. Excised chloroma tumours have a greenish tinge which fades rapidly on exposure to air. The nature of the pigmentation is unknown.

The other pathological features of the leukaemias are due to the effects of *thrombocytopenia* and *agranulocytosis*, and the *blockage of blood vessels* by leukaemic cells. Vascular occlusion produces the priapism which may be so troublesome during life, and is also the cause of the areas of infarction so typical of leukaemic spleens. Foci of necrosis and haemorrhage are common in the brain, and are often the immediate cause of death. Other frequent *post-mortem* findings are purpura and haemorrhagic extravasations into the tissues. There is almost invariably severe bacterial infection, e.g. pneumonia, tonsillitis, and enterocolitis,

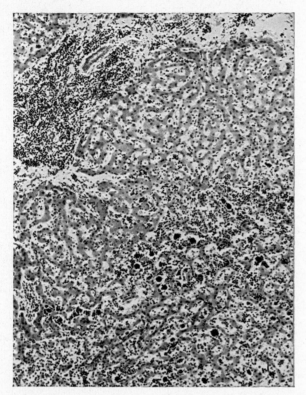

Figure 50.2
Chronic lymphatic leukaemia. The infiltration of leukaemic cells is much more dense around the portal tracts than in the sinusoids of the liver. × 100.

which is aggravated by the cytotoxic drugs used therapeutically.

MULTIPLE MYELOMA[18, 19]

Multiple myeloma is a monoclonal gammopathy, and as such is described on p. 552. There is a neoplastic proliferation of plasma cells, called *myeloma cells*, scattered throughout the skeleton. Myeloma cells are large (15–30 μm in diameter), and have a prominent eccentric nucleus with a coarse chromatin pattern which is reminiscent of that of the plasma cell. The tumours so produced are intramedullary, unlike chloroma, and they cause destruction of the surrounding cortex, seen radiologically as areas of translucency. Pathological fracture is the usual sequel.

The disease is predominantly one of the later years of life. The tumours are found usually in those bones containing red marrow, such as the vertebrae, pelvis, ribs, sternum, clavicles, skull, and the proximal portions of the humerus and femur. Multiple myeloma, unlike the leukaemias, is usually not associated with extraskeletal lesions, but occasionally the lymph nodes, liver, spleen, and other organs are involved. Solitary plasma-cell tumours have also been found in patients who appear otherwise healthy; the upper respiratory tract

and oral cavity are the usual sites of these lesions, but solitary myeloma of a bone is also encountered from time to time. These single lesions tend to terminate in multiple myeloma, and cannot be regarded as innocent.

Apart from the pain, deformity, and neurological effects of its skeletal lesions, multiple myeloma also causes profound metabolic changes. The demineralisation of the skeleton may cause *hypercalcaemia* and renal failure. The disturbances in protein metabolism, considered in detail on p. 551, also produce clinical effects. Thus the *Bence-Jones protein*, present in about half the cases, may precipitate in the tubules, blocking them, and inducing a foreign-body reaction. The tubular obliteration and fibrosis lead to progressive renal failure—the condition is called *myeloma kidney*. The *cryoglobulinaemia* sometimes present leads to vascular occlusion in cold surroundings, and the *hyperglobulinaemia* increases the viscosity of the blood and is important in causing bleeding tendencies similar to those found in macroglobulinaemia. *Amyloidosis* occurs in about 10 per cent of cases, especially those with heavy Bence-Jones proteinuria. The abnormal globulin formation also leads to an impaired production of other immunoglobulins, and *susceptibility to infection* is another complication. It is seen most often in IgG myelomata.

Blood picture. *The red cells* are moderately or severely reduced in number, and are normochromic and normocytic (or often macrocytic). There is usually little evidence of increased formation. The hyperglobulinaemia leads to marked rouleaux formation (and sludging), and is responsible for the raised ESR so characteristic of the condition.

The white-cell count shows no constant change, but there may occasionally be evidence of marrow replacement. Plasma cells may be present in small numbers in the blood, but any great invasion is rare. A few cases are associated with a high plasma-cell count, and these have been called "plasma-cell leukaemia".

The platelets are reduced in the later stages of the disease.

The usual survival period of patients with myelomatosis is from a few months to about 4 years, but occasional cases live for 10 years. The common causes of death are compression of the spinal cord often due to a pathological fracture of a vertebra, chronic renal failure, progressive anaemia, and secondary infection.

BONE-MARROW APLASIA[20]

In the conditions about to be considered there is a depression in the formation of blood cells in the marrow. This most commonly affects all three elements. *Aplasia* is a word with two different connotations in pathology (see p. 303); it is preferably applied specifically to the bone marrow, when it means a sudden cessation of division of the blood-cell precursors. These are usually destroyed by some noxious agent, but sometimes they persist and yet fail to develop into more mature forms. The mature elements in the blood are destroyed in the normal way, and are not replaced.

Pure red-cell aplasia has been described; in the better known condition of *agranulocytosis* the aplasia is confined to the granulocytic precursors. A *pure platelet aplasia* may occur in primary thrombocytopenic purpura, which is considered separately in the next chapter. A marked reduction in numbers of all three elements of the blood is called *pancytopenia*, and is met with under the following circumstances:

Leukaemias of the "aleukaemic" type. A careful inspection of the blood film reveals a few primitive cells, while the bone-marrow examination is conclusive.

Hypersplenism. This is described separately.

Aplasia due to physical and chemical agents, secondary to disease, and of familial type. This is referred to as *aplastic anaemia*.

Causes of Bone-Marrow Aplasia

Ionising radiation. Both whole-body irradiation, as in the Hiroshima victims, and continuous skeletal irradiation, as in the girls who swallowed luminous watch-paint (see Chapter 31), may be associated with bone-marrow aplasia.

Drugs.[21] Some substances lead to aplasia in all individuals, provided a large enough dose is given. Examples of these are benzene, anti-metabolites, and alkylating agents. On the other hand, a large number of drugs act unpredictably on only a few unfortunate individuals. In these cases the mysterious factor of idiosyncrasy* has to be invoked. Examples of this type of drug are chloramphenicol, arsphenamine, sulphonamides, phenylbutazone, gold salts, and mesantoin. It is not known whether these agents act directly on the stem cells or on the blood sinusoids of the marrow, thus destroying the medullary microcirculation.

Infections. Traditionally miliary tuberculosis may lead to aplastic anaemia, but this is very rare nowadays. Some virus infections are more important causes of a marrow aplasia that may last some time and is often fatal. Infective hepatitis has been complicated by aplasia on numerous occasions; it usually occurs a few months after the hepatitis.[22]

Hypopituitarism, and occasionally myxoedema.

Congenital pancytopenia. Fanconi described a familial disease in which the marrow was congenitally hypoplastic.[23] There were also multiple congenital abnormalities of the skeleton, central nervous system, and other tissues. This "Fanconi syndrome" must not be confused with the characteristic defect of the renal tubules (see Chapter 42), which he also described. It is preferable to reserve the word *hypoplasia* for conditions in which an organ or tissue does not attain full, mature size. In such a connotation Fanconi's anaemia

* A qualitatively abnormal drug reaction is termed *idiosyncrasy*, e.g. haemolytic anaemia with primaquine. It is to be distinguished from (a) *intolerance*, which is an excessive, though normal, reaction to a small dose, e.g. morphine in liver failure, and (b) *hypersensitivity*, in which an immunological reaction is involved.

is indeed "hypoplastic", as it is a true developmental defect.

Blood picture. All three elements are greatly reduced in number.

The red cells are normocytic and normochromic. There is little anisocytosis or poikilocytosis, and there is no evidence of regeneration—the reticulocyte count is very low.

The severe leucopenia is accompanied by a relative lymphocytosis, but in the worst cases there may also be a lymphopenia.

The thrombocytopenia is severe.

The bone marrow is very hypocellular, and many of the nucleated cells present may be lymphocytes. Sometimes the cellularity is normal or even increased, and it would appear that the failure of division occurs in the later stages of haematopoiesis. On the other hand, the aplasia itself may be patchy, and the marrow may have been taken fortuitously from a normal or hypercellular area; several areas of marrow should be examined. Sometimes there is a failure in maturation, or *maturation arrest*. Such hypercellularity is seen in hypersplenism.

Biochemical changes. The serum iron is raised, and the iron-binding protein may be saturated. There is an increased percentage of sideroblasts, and the RE cells also contain granules of haemosiderin. This siderosis becomes extreme in patients kept alive for long periods with transfusions.

Prognosis. This is grave. In fulminating cases death is almost invariable, but the more chronic ones may survive over four years. About 50 per cent live for 15 months, and then the chance of survival is good. Death is due to infection and haemorrhage.

A very interesting feature is the tendency for cases of chronic acquired aplastic anaemia to develop acute leukaemia or paroxysmal nocturnal haemoglobinuria later. It would appear that a clone of myeloid or erythroid cell undergoes an aberration.

Pathological features. *Haemorrhages* due to the thrombocytopenia.

Infective lesions due to the agranulocytosis.

Replacement of the red marrow by yellow fatty material, except when there is maturation arrest.

Lymphoid atrophy. The spleen may be small, and it often shows atrophy of the malpighian bodies. The liver, spleen, and lymph nodes are not usually enlarged in aplastic anaemia; an increase in size suggests that the diagnosis is wrong.

Individual Aplasias

Pure red-cell aplasia.[24] In this condition the white cells and platelets are normal. It is rare, but is well recognised as an occasional accompaniment of *thymic tumours*.[25] These are usually benign thymomata, and there may be an associated myasthenia gravis; an immunological mechanism is probably responsible. A *congenital hypoplastic anaemia* involving the red cells alone has been described by Diamond and Blackfan.[26, 27] It develops insidiously during the later neonatal period, and there is no evidence of red-cell regeneration. The bone marrow is deficient in normoblasts.

Acute red-cell aplasia may occur during the *crises* of congenital acholuric jaundice and sickle-cell disease (see p. 595).

Agranulocytosis. This is a very important condition which occurs both as a component of marrow aplasia and as a separate disease in which the defect is confined to the white cells.

The white-cell count is below 2 000 per μl and it may drop to less than 100 cells per μl. Of the cells present only 1–2 per cent are granulocytes. There is thus a relative lymphocytosis and monocytosis. In pure agranulocytosis the red-cell and platelet counts are normal. The marrow shows a great reduction of myelocytes and granulocytes, with variable numbers of myeloblasts and promyelocytes.

The agents that may lead to agranulocytosis are grouped into those that will produce it regularly if a sufficient dose is given, i.e. the agents already mentioned in relation to marrow aplasia such as ionising radiations and benzene, and those in which the condition is an occasional unpredictable occurrence (idiosyncrasy). The list of such drugs is very large: the most important are amidopyrine (the most notorious of all), thiouracil and its derivatives, phenylbutazone, chlorpromazine and other phenothiazine derivatives, sulphonamides, tridione, pyribenzamine, and dinitrophenol. The drugs that may occasionally lead to marrow aplasia can obviously be included in the list.

The mechanism of production of agranulocytosis is uncertain, and probably there is more than one process.[21] A leucocyte-agglutinating globulin has been found in the sera of patients sensitive to amidopyrine. This drug is particularly apt to lead to a rapid disappearance of granulocytes from the blood, and it may well be that they are destroyed in the capillaries after agglutination. Such leucocyte agglutinins are true autoantibodies, but the matter is not as simple as this, because similar antibodies are also found in the sera of people who have received blood transfusions. In chlorpromazine agranulocytosis no agglutinins are present; instead there is a temporary leucocytic aplasia of the marrow. The same may be seen after sulphonamides and amidopyrine. It is probable that toxic action on the proliferating cells in the marrow and a destructive action on the mature circulating granulocytes both play their part in producing agranulocytosis.

The pathological effects of agranulocytosis are those of severe infection. Necrotic lesions of the skin, mouth, throat, vagina, and gastrointestinal tract are common, and there is usually confluent bronchopneumonia. In all these lesions there is a conspicuous absence of polymorphs, only lymphocytes and plasma cells being present together with masses of bacteria. In the liver, spleen, and lymph nodes foci of necrosis are common. Perhaps they are due to the effect of infection.

Primary thrombocytopenic purpura. (See Chapter 51.)

The Prevention of Drug-Induced Marrow Aplasia

The best way to obviate the danger of aplasia is to use drugs that are relatively safe. The performance of routine blood counts may lull one into a false sense of security. When aplasia strikes, it tends to do so out of the blue. In those exposed in the course of their work to ionising radiations it is more helpful to control the doses received than to perform routine blood counts.

HYPERSPLENISM[28, 29]

The functions of the spleen.[30] These are incompletely understood. It is well known that splenectomy is followed by no obvious ill-effects, though there are minor haematological changes. The possible functions of the spleen are related to blood formation, storage, and destruction, and the body's defence against infection:

Blood formation. Except in the fetus the spleen plays no part in blood formation, though if the bone marrow is destroyed, the spleen will at once take over its role. It is this property that enables mice to survive whole-body irradiation if the spleen is shielded from the radiation (see Chapter 31).

Effect on haematopoiesis. It is possible that the spleen exerts some inhibitory effect on leucocyte and platelet production in the marrow, but the evidence for inhibition of erythropoiesis is unconvincing.

Removal of defective red cells.[31] Some newly-formed red cells contain nuclear fragments called *Howell-Jolly bodies*. Others contain granules of haemosiderin, and these cells are called *siderocytes*. Normally such cells are "scrutinised" by the spleen, and filtered off from the general circulation. The iron-containing granules of the siderocyte are removed, and the cell is then released into the circulation.

Destruction of effete red cells. As described in Chapter 49, the effete red cell is removed from the circulation by phagocytic RE cells in the liver, bone marrow, and spleen. Of these three organs the spleen plays the greatest part. The spherocytes of congenital acholuric jaundice are particularly sensitive to the destructive processes within the spleen.

The splenic reservoir. The blood reservoir of the spleen is useful in lower animals but not in man; the average adult spleen holds 20–30 ml of red cells only.[32] The sequestration of red cells is of great importance in relation to the destructive functions mentioned above.

The immune response. The lymphoid tissue of the spleen plays a prominent part in the immune response in regard to the formation of both immunoglobulins and lymphocytes (p. 150).

Defence against infection. There is clinical evidence that splenectomised children are unduly susceptible to fulminating infections like meningitis and septicaemia.[33] This may be related to the removal of a large mass of RE cells which is contained in the spleen.

Blood changes following splenectomy. As the spleen removes imperfectly-formed *red cells* from the circulation, it is not surprising that after splenectomy (or with splenic atrophy or agenesis) the blood contains numbers of nucleated red cells, most of which have Howell-Jolly bodies rather than complete nuclei. Siderocytes are also numerous. It seems that the spleen in some way ensures that red cells have a normal shape, for after splenectomy thin target cells are conspicuous. Howell-Jolly bodies, siderocytes, and target cells persist indefinitely, and afford valuable evidence of splenectomy. There is an early reticulocytosis and initially a mild anaemia, but this soon passes.

There is an immediate *neutrophil leucocytosis* greater than can be attributed merely to a surgical procedure, and this is followed by a mild increase in lymphocytes, monocytes, eosinophils, and basophils. These later changes may last for a long time.

There is also a *thrombocytosis* maximal about 3 weeks after splenectomy, and this too may persist for some time.

The relationship between the spleen and anaemia. In *hypersplenism* there is an alleged splenic over-activity which is associated with maturation arrest in the bone marrow or increased destructive changes in the peripheral blood. As has been noted, the haematological functions of the spleen are obscure, and it is not certain that any of these changes is due entirely to splenic activity. Nevertheless, it is clinically well recognised that some blood dyscrasias respond favourably to splenectomy.

Hypersplenism is suggested by the following findings taken together:

(*a*) A fall in the count of any or all of the three elements of the blood, or else a haemolytic type of anaemia.
(*b*) A normal or hypercellular marrow.
(*c*) Splenomegaly.
(*d*) Cure following splenectomy.

The paradox of an increased production of precursors and a drop in the number of mature cells in the blood is usually explained as a *maturation arrest*, i.e. there is a failure in division at the last stages of haematopoiesis, so that mature elements are not formed or released. It is equally possible that the mature cells are released into the circulation, and then rapidly destroyed by an overactive spleen.

Hypersplenism may be primary or secondary. *Primary hypersplenism* is a somewhat controversial condition. It has two possible manifestations, "primary splenic pancytopenia" and "primary splenic neutropenia".[34-36] These are chronic diseases in which there is a persistent or cyclical aplastic type of anaemia or agranulocytosis of moderate severity. There is an associated splenomegaly and a hyperplastic bone marrow. Splenectomy sometimes produces a slow improvement. The conditions are rare, and it is by no means certain that the spleen is the culprit. Primary thrombocytopenic purpura has also been classified as a primary hypersplenism affecting the megakaryocytes only.

Secondary hypersplenism is more definite, for it is well known that in the course of many diseases associated with splenomegaly there is a tendency towards pancytopenia or haemolytic anaemia. The marrow is usually hyperplastic, and splenectomy often relieves the blood manifestations even when having no effect on the primary condition.

The best-known example of this type of disease is the so-called *Banti syndrome*, in which there is a greatly enlarged spleen secondary to portal hypertension. This usually follows hepatic cirrhosis, but may also be due to a malformation of the splenic vein. A severe "splenic anaemia" follows, in which there is a normocytic, normochromic anaemia, a leucopenia, and a moderate thrombocytopenia. Recurrent haematemeses lead to an additional iron-deficiency anaemia. A splenectomy, while relieving the pancytopenia, does not diminish the portal hypertension in cases secondary to cirrhosis.

A similar type of blood picture occurs in *Felty's syndrome*, in which chronic rheumatoid arthritis is associated with splenomegaly. Here it is the red cells and leucocytes that bear the brunt of the hypersplenism. Gaucher's disease, schistosomiasis (Egyptian splenomegaly), and leishmaniasis may also produce anaemia and leucopenia.

Sometimes there is an acute haemolytic anaemia instead of an aplastic one, and this may occasionally be accompanied by autoantibodies. Acute haemolytic anaemia occurring during the course of chronic lymphatic leukaemia, Hodgkin's disease, sarcoidosis, and myelosclerosis may be due to hypersplenism, and a splenectomy may relieve this complication while having no effect on the primary condition.

INDICATIONS FOR SPLENECTOMY IN
BLOOD DISEASE

Hereditary spherocytosis, the indication *par excellence*. It is also of some value in *hereditary elliptocytosis*.

Acquired haemolytic anaemia due to autoantibodies. There is no doubt that the spleen plays a large part in removing sensitised red cells, and that a splenectomy sometimes has a temporarily beneficial effect. In due course the other organs with RE cells in them take over the splenic function.

Primary thrombocytopenic purpura.

"*Primary splenic pancytopenia*" and "*primary splenic neutropenia*".

Secondary hypersplenism associated with pancytopenia or haemolytic anaemia. In Banti's syndrome a splenectomy should not be performed unless the surgeon is prepared to undertake a venous-shunting operation at the same time.

THE SYNDROME OF
BONE-MARROW REPLACEMENT

The normal bone marrow may be replaced by fibrous tissue, bone, or some foreign element like tumour tissue. In each case a characteristic blood picture is produced, and it is called *leuco-erythroblastic anaemia* because of the presence of many primitive white and red cells in the blood.

Causes of Leuco-erythroblastic Anaemia

Tumour destruction of the bone marrow. Metastatic carcinoma from the breast, lung, and prostate is by far the commonest cause of this condition. Five per cent of cases of multiple myeloma produce it, and so occasionally does Hodgkin's disease.

Replacement of marrow by lipid-filled macrophages in Gaucher's disease and Niemann-Pick disease (see Chapter 30).

Myelofibrosis (myelosclerosis).[37] This is an interesting disease of later life in which the bone marrow is replaced by fibrous or even bony tissue. The cortex is normal, but in the medulla there is either cellular fibrous tissue or else a thickening of bone with a laying down of new trabeculae. Such changes may be recognisable radiologically, and the condition is then called osteosclerosis. Of all the bone-marrow replacement diseases this one is the most chronic, and there is widespread myeloid metaplasia of many organs, especially the spleen and liver. This has led to confusion, and a plethora of synonyms has arisen, e.g. "agnogenic myeloid metaplasia", "myeloid megakaryocytic hepato-splenomegaly", and "aleukaemic megakaryocytic myelosis".

The nature of the condition is uncertain. In many cases there is hyperplasia of the marrow early in the disease even though there is also marked extramedullary haematopoiesis. Later on the cellular elements of the marrow become sparser and fibrosis develops. Finally there is complete fibrous or bony replacement. The condition has much in common with polycythaemia vera and haemorrhagic thrombocythaemia; in all three there is a benign proliferation of red-cell, white-cell, and platelet precursors, and there are borderline cases in which all three overlap. Thus these three diseases can be grouped together as the *myeloproliferative disorders*.[38] It is better not to include chronic myeloid leukaemia among them because of the frankly malignant nature of the cellular proliferation and its much worse prognosis. Why some cases of myeloproliferative disorder should proceed to fibrosis is not clear. But it is evident that the extramedullary haematopoiesis cannot be attributed simply to the bone-marrow replacement; while this no doubt accentuates the extramedullary blood formation, it also often follows it.

Marble-bone disease of Albers-Schönberg (osteopetrosis).[39] This is a congenital disease in which there is a failure of removal of bony trabeculae and their replacement by marrow spaces. The bones are enormously thick and sclerotic, and are uniformly radio-opaque. The manifestations of this condition include spontaneous fractures, various cranial nerve palsies, hydrocephalus, and in about 25 per cent of cases, a leuco-erythroblastic anaemia.

Blood picture. *There is a variable degree of anaemia*, though in the early stages the red-cell count may be normal or even raised. The cells are normochromic and are mostly normocytic. Anisocytosis is usual and often marked, while poikilocytosis is characteristic. There are considerable numbers of nucleated red cells in the blood and often a moderate reticulocytosis.

The white-cell count varies from a moderate leucopenia to a leucocytosis of up to 50 000 cells per μl. There are numerous myelocytes in the blood and even a few myeloblasts. The picture may resemble chronic myeloid leukaemia, but the white-cell count is seldom as high as in that condition.

The platelet count is normal or reduced. Abnormally large, bizarre platelets are common, especially in myelofibrosis.

A bone-marrow examination is essential; it is the only method by which tumour cells or lipid-filled macrophages can be demonstrated. In myelofibrosis the marrow feels gritty, and hardly any can be aspirated. Sometimes, however, it may be normal or even hyperplastic. To confirm a diagnosis of myelofibrosis a surgical biopsy should be performed. Stained sections are necessary in order to study the architecture of the marrow and assess the degree of fibrosis.

In some of these conditions there may be hypersplenism producing thrombocytopenic purpura or haemolytic anaemia.

Pathology. The most profound pathological changes are encountered in myelofibrosis. There is enormous splenomegaly, and the spleen shows marked *myeloid metaplasia*, i.e. the red pulp contains all the marrow elements including many megakaryocytes. Its architecture, including the malpighian bodies, is not destroyed. In the enlarged liver the haematopoietic cells are present in the sinusoids, as is seen in chronic myeloid leukaemia and fetal haematopoiesis. The lymph nodes and connective tissue may also be sites of extramedullary haematopoiesis.

The bone marrow is replaced by fibrous tissue or bony trabeculae. Some haematopoietic tissue persists, and in it megakaryocytes are often plentiful.

In secondary carcinoma the marrow contains foci of tumour tissue surrounded by zones of active blood formation. Extramedullary haematopoiesis is seldom conspicuous, because death ensues very rapidly.

In myelosclerosis the leuco-erythroblastosis is apparently due to the spleen and other organs augmenting the marrow's function. Such organs lack the regulatory mechanism of the marrow, and are unable to prevent primitive cells from entering the blood. It is logical to regard the enlarged spleen as vital to the patient's well-being, as it is a major blood-forming organ. In practice, however, splenectomy is usually followed by no ill-effects, and the patient may actually improve if there has been an aspect of hypersplenism in his blood condition.[40] Obviously the other foci or haematopoiesis take over the spleen's function quite satisfactorily.

The mechanism of the leuco-erythroblastosis accompanying bone-marrow metastases is unknown. There is a decreased red-cell survival time in conditions of bone-marrow replacement, and it is evident that haematopoiesis does not adequately compensate for the cellular destruction.

BONE-MARROW EXAMINATION

A bone-marrow examination is useful for the following purposes:

1. To assess the over-all cellularity of the marrow as well as the development of its individual elements.

2. To determine whether erythropoiesis is normoblastic or megaloblastic.

3. To detect foreign elements in the marrow, e.g. tumour cells, myeloma cells, or lipid-filled macrophages.

4. To assess whether there is fibrous or bony replacement of functioning tissue. A surgical biopsy is necessary for this.

5. To detect (and if necessary culture) blood-borne organisms, e.g. leishmania, histoplasma, malarial plasmodia, and typhoid bacilli.

REFERENCES

1. CHAN, S. H., METCALF, D. and STANLEY, E. R. (1971). *British Journal of Haematology*, **20**, 329.
2. Leading Article (1971). *Lancet*, ii, 909.
3. Leading Article (1968). *Lancet*, ii, 1381 and (1969). *British Medical Journal*, iv, 445.
4. HOAGLAND, R. J. (1960). *American Journal of Medical Science*, **240**, 21.
5. Editorial (1968). *New England Journal of Medicine*, **279**, 432.
6. BICHEL, J. (1949). *Blood*, **4**, 759.
7. ARCHER, G. T. and HIRSCH, J. G. (1963). *Journal of Experimental Medicine*, **118**, 277.
8. ARCHER, G. T. and BLACKWOOD, A. (1965). *Journal of Experimental Medicine*, **122**, 173.
9. Leading Article (1968). *British Medical Journal*, iii, 569.
10. WEBB, J. K. G., JOB, C. K. and GAULT, E. W. (1960). *Lancet*, i, 835.
11. Leading Article (1971). *British Medical Journal*, iii, 549.
12. CROSSEN, P. *et al.* (1971). *American Journal of Medicine*, **50**, 24.
13. Leading Article (1972). *Lancet*, i, 82.
14. WOODLIFF, H. J. and DOUGAN, L. (1964). *British Medical Journal*, i, 744.
15. MILLER, R. W. (1966). *New England Journal of Medicine*, **275**, 87.
16. Leading Article (1971). *Lancet*, i, 742.
17. HUMBLE, J. G. (1946). *Quarterly Journal of Medicine*, **15**, 299.
18. OSSERMAN, E. F. (1959). *New England Journal of Medicine*, **261**, 952 and 1006.
19. OSSERMAN, E. F. (1961). *American Journal of Medicine*, **31**, 671.
20. LEWIS, S. M. (1971). *British Journal of Hospital Medicine*, **6**, 593.
21. WINTROBE, M. M. (1968). *Journal of the Royal College of Physicians of London*, **3**, 99.
22. Leading Article (1971). *Lancet*, i, 844.
23. McDONALD, R. and GOLDSCHMIDT, B. (1960). *Archives of Diseases of Childhood*, **35**, 367.
24. Leading Article (1968). *British Medical Journal*, ii, 3.
25. JAHSMAN, D. P., MONTO, R. W. and REBUCK, J. W. (1962). *American Journal of Clinical Pathology*, **38**, 152.
26. DIAMOND, L. K. and BLACKMAN, K. D. (1938). *American Journal of Diseases in Childhood*, **56**, 464.
27. KHO, L. K. *et al.* (1962). *Blood*, **19**, 168.
28. DOAN, C. A. (1949). *Bulletin of the New York Academy of Medicine*, **25**, 625.
29. DAMESHEK, W. (1955). *Bulletin of the New York Academy of Medicine*, **31**, 113.
30. PRANKERD, T. A. J. (1963). *British Medical Journal*, ii, 517.
31. NATHAN, D. G. (1969). *New England Journal of Medicine*, **281**, 558.
32. MOTULSKY, A. G. *et al.* (1958). *New England Journal of Medicine*, **259**, 1164 and 1215.
33. ERAKLIS, A. J. *et al.* (1967). *New England Journal of Medicine*, **276**, 1225.
34. REIMANN, H. A. and DE BERARDINIS, C. T. (1949). *Blood*, **4**, 1109.
35. Leading Article (1968). *Lancet*, ii, 1282.
36. KYLE, R. A. and LINMAN, J. W. (1968). *New England Journal of Medicine*, **279**, 1015.
37. PITCOCK, J. A. *et al.* (1962). *Annals of Internal Medicine*, **57**, 73.
38. WARD, H. P. and BLOCK, M. H. (1971). *Medicine (Baltimore)*, **50**, 357.
39. KELLEY, C. H. and LAWLAH, J. W. (1946). *Radiology*, **47**, 507.
40. GREEN, T. W. *et al.* (1953). *New England Journal of Medicine*, **248**, 211.

Chapter 51. Some Disorders of the Blood:

III. THE PLATELETS AND CLOTTING FACTORS

The precursor of the platelet is the *megakaryocyte*, an enormous giant cell about 100 μm in diameter with irregularly-lobed central nuclei and a light blue cytoplasm packed with azurophilic granules. Its origin is uncertain, but it is probably derived ultimately from the haemocytoblast. As a megakaryocyte develops, it becomes larger, its basophilic cytoplasm develops granules, and its nucleus undergoes many divisions without cytoplasmic fission. This is clearly an exception to the dictum that as a cell matures it becomes smaller. Megakaryocytes are found in the bone marrow, spleen, and lungs. Whether those present in the lungs represent effete cells in the process of destruction, or whether they constitute an important supply of platelets is still an unsettled problem. It is certain that the main source of platelets is the marrow.

Platelets[1] are formed by the fragmentation and detachment of delicate processes from the cytoplasm of megakaryocytes. Their morphology and function are described in Chapter 35.

The normal platelet count varies from 150 000–400 000 cells per μl. The range is wide, and no counting technique is very satisfactory. A count below 100 000 cells per μl can be taken as a definite thrombocytopenia. The newborn infant has a slightly lower count than the adult, but normal levels are attained within 3 months. The causes of a rise in the platelet count (*thrombocytosis*) have been considered on p. 457. The opposite condition of *thrombocytopenia* is associated with a bleeding tendency, and will be discussed later.

The Functions of Platelets in Haemostasis

(*a*) They seal the injured vessel by adhering to the damaged area and aggregating to form a mass known as a *haemostatic plug*. The platelet lipoprotein surface catalyses the intrinsic clotting system, and the fibrin which is formed consolidates the plug. Finally the entire aggregate contracts, probably due to the contractile protein in the platelets called thrombosthenin. Thrombin released during coagulation causes further platelet deposition as well as fibrin formation. Defects in the intrinsic system of blood clotting, such as in haemophilia, do not prevent the formation of a haemostatic plug, and therefore the bleeding time is normal (p. 616). However, the plug is not stable, and rebleeding may occur later.

(*b*) When exposed to stimuli, such as collagen, antigen-antibody complexes, and bacterial endotoxin, they release a number of chemical agents (*platelet release reaction*).[2] These include *ADP*, which causes the platelets to swell, throw out pseudopods, and adhere together, *5-HT*, which is a vasoconstrictor and important in haemostasis, and *lipoprotein*, which plays a part in clotting. Aspirin inhibits the platelet release reaction, but does not prevent ADP-induced platelet aggregation.[3]

(*c*) They are necessary for proper clot retraction.

THE CLOTTING MECHANISM

The object of the very complex clotting mechanism is the conversion of the plasma protein fibrinogen into the insoluble network of fibres which is called fibrin. In order to systematise the bewildering number of clotting factors that have been discovered, the International Committee for the Nomenclature of Blood Clotting Factors has decreed that each factor should be designated by a Roman numeral, starting with fibrinogen as Factor I.[4] It therefore comes about that the clotting process is best described by starting at the final stage, and then working backwards. As the most recently discovered factors, other than Factor XIII, are all concerned with the initial stages of the process, this is less unreasonable than would appear at first sight. The platelet lipid factors are designated by Arabic numerals; in practice the only important one is factor 3.

When plasma clots, the fluid that is subsequently expressed is called serum, and it is completely lacking in *fibrinogen* (**Factor I**). This conversion of fibrinogen to fibrin is brought about by thrombin, which is normally present as an inert precursor called prothrombin. *Thrombin*, also called *Factor IIa* to denote that it is activated Factor II, is a proteolytic enzyme that splits off two peptide fragments, fibrinopeptides A and B, from a molecule of fibrinogen; these peptides cause smooth muscle to contract. The remainder of the fibrinogen molecule is capable of spontaneous polymerisation with its fellows; in this way the fibrin monomer forms orderly molecular aggregates which reach a sufficient size to make up the network of fibres called a clot. This is easily disrupted until **Factor XIII, fibrin-stabilising factor**, creates covalent bonds between the aggregates, so turning the clot into a firm gel.[2]

Prothrombin (Factor II), like fibrinogen, is a normal plasma protein. It is a glycoprotein and migrates with the

a_2-globulins. It is converted into thrombin by **thromboplastin (Factor III)**.

This is a vague, rather unsatisfactory term, and refers to the total activity of the plasma in converting prothrombin into thrombin, but there is no one substance that can be identified as such. Thromboplastic activity can be generated in two ways. In the *intrinsic (blood) system*, contact with an abnormal surface leads to the sequential activation of Factors XII, XI, IX, VIII, and X. Activated Factor X, designated Xa, in conjunction with Factor V and platelet factor 3 results in the formation of *blood thromboplastin*, also known as *intrinsic prothrombin activator*, or *prothrombokinase*. In the *extrinsic (tissue) system*, tissue damage results in the release of a tissue factor rich in phospholipid. This in conjunction with Factor VII activates Factor X, which as in the intrinsic system interacts with Factor V and phospholipid to produce a prothrombokinase, called *tissue thromboplastin*, or *extrinsic prothrombin activator*. The tissue factor is found in large amounts in the brain, extracts of which are used as a source of it in various laboratory tests, such as the prothrombin time. The venom of the Russell viper is also rich in it.

The two pathways of blood clotting are both important, for a derangement of either leads to a serious defect in haemostasis. The intrinsic system develops much more slowly than the extrinsic one, but both are initiated by tissue damage, either by releasing tissue factor or providing an abnormal surface. In both systems there is activation of Factor X, and from then on there is a final *common pathway* involving Factor V, phospholipid, prothrombin, and fibrinogen. Some details of these systems will now be described.

In all the phases leading up to the formation of thrombin from prothrombin, **calcium ions (Factor IV)** are necessary. Calcium is not essential for the reaction between thrombin and fibrinogen, but helps to accelerate it. Its mode of action is uncertain. Clinical hypocalcaemia is never severe enough to interfere with clotting.

The two clotting systems are activated in different ways, and it is best to consider them separately. Their ultimate purpose is similar, the conversion of prothrombin to thrombin.

THE EXTRINSIC SYSTEM

As soon as there is local trauma tissue factor is produced. It leads to the formation of a prothrombin activator in the presence of the following four factors (see Fig. 51.1):

(i) Factor V, also known as **proaccelerin** and **labile factor.** This is present in normal plasma even when treated with aluminium hydroxide, but is not found in serum. A special Factor VI was also described, but has fallen out of use, as its existence is open to doubt.

(ii) Factor VII, also known as **proconvertin** and **stable factor.** This is present in normal serum, from which it is adsorbed with aluminium hydroxide. Unlike Factor V it is

resistant to heat and survives storage. The nature of Factors V and VII is obscure; both are probably globulins.

(iii) Factor X, also called the **Stuart-Prower Factor** (after the two patients in whom a deficiency was first described). It resembles Factor VII closely. Neither is consumed in the clotting process, so that both are present in serum as well as plasma. Both are adsorbed with aluminium hydroxide. Unlike Factor VII it is thermolabile.

(iv) Calcium ions.

In the extrinsic system a complex of *tissue factor*, predominantly lipid, *Factor VII*, and *calcium ions* activate Factor X. The activated product Factor Xa in turn forms a complex with Factor V, calcium ions, and platelet phospholipid factor 3. This is a thromboplastin, and leads to the conversion of prothrombin to thrombin.

THE INTRINSIC SYSTEM

In the formation of blood thromboplastin the following factors are required:

(a) Factor XII, called **Hageman factor** after the patient in whom a deficiency was first noted, is a β_2-globulin which is present both in serum and in plasma containing aluminium hydroxide. Deficiency of this factor is peculiar in having no significant clinical effect despite a greatly prolonged clotting time.

(b) Factor XI, called **plasma thromboplastin antecedent (PTA),** is also a β_2-globulin present both in serum and alumina-treated plasma. It is thermolabile, unlike Factor XII, and its activity increases when stored frozen.

(c) Factor IX, called **Christmas factor,** once again after a patient, and also **plasma thromboplastin component (PTC),** is a globulin present in serum but not in alumina-treated plasma (like Factors VII and X).

(d) Factor VIII, or **antihaemophilic factor,** or **antihaemophilic globulin (AHG),** is a globulin present in alumina-treated plasma but not in serum (like Factor V).

(e) Factor X.

(f) Factor V.

(g) Platelet factor 3. It is probable that this does not exist as a distinct entity, but is the altered lipoprotein surface of the platelets which catalyses several of the steps in clotting. Nevertheless, the term may usefully be employed to denote this activity.

(h) Calcium ions.

The activation of these various factors is believed to follow a *cascade sequence*, many of the factors being substrates that are activated by a preceding enzyme. The original theory was described independently by Macfarlane in England[5] and Davie and Ratnoff in the USA,[6] but since then a number of modifications have been discovered (Fig. 51.1).

Factor XII is first activated by the contact of blood with a foreign surface, the product being Factor XIIa. This activates Factor XI, and Factor XIa activates Factor IX

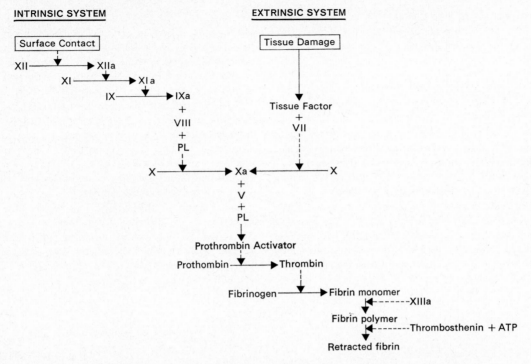

INTRINSIC SYSTEM EXTRINSIC SYSTEM

Figure 51.1
A simplified diagrammatic representation of the blood clotting mechanism. Solid arrows indicate transformation, interrupted arrows denote actions. PL denotes phospholipid which, in the formation of prothrombin activator *via* the intrinsic system, is derived from the platelets (factor 3). In the extrinsic system phospholipid is derived from the tissues. There is evidence that platelets in conjunction with Factor XII can form a platelet "tissue-factor" and thereby initiate the extrinsic system. The importance of this *in vivo* is debatable. Not shown in the diagram is the ionic calcium which is required for most of the steps shown. *(After Marcus, A. J. (1969), New Engl. J. Med., 280, 1213)*

Factor IXa forms a complex with Factor VIII, calcium ions, and phospholipid, and the complex activates Factor X. Factor Xa now forms a complex with Factor V, calcium ions, and phospholipid, and this complex activates Factor II (prothrombin) to Factor IIa (thrombin). The thrombin then converts fibrinogen to fibrin which is stabilised by Factor XIII, itself first activated by thrombin.

The earliest phase of the intrinsic system is slow. However, once thrombin is formed the process is greatly accelerated—indeed, there is a real cascade, for thrombin potentiates the activity of Factors V and VIII. It also causes platelets to aggregate and so increases the amount of phospholipid (Factor 3). This is called the *autocatalytic action of thrombin*. Interestingly, thrombin also destroys Factors V and VIII after potentiating their reactivity; in this way fibrin formation is stopped when a high concentration of thrombin has been achieved.

THE PHYSIOLOGICAL INHIBITION OF INTRAVASCULAR CLOTTING

The first natural mode of inhibition of intravascular clotting is the slowness of thrombin formation due to the exclusion of tissue thromboplastin, and the almost complete absence of blood thromboplastin, which is attributable to the stability of the various clotting factors. Once the vascular endothelium is damaged and tissue fluids enter the blood, there is a great tendency for clotting to occur intravascularly. To obviate this danger, there are several inhibitors, or anticoagulants, present in the blood:

Antithrombin. Fibrin is a natural antithrombin, in that the thrombin is removed as a result of its affinity for the fibrin surface. The fibrin threads with the adsorbed thrombin are filtered off in the capillaries and destroyed. In addition there are a number of distinct "antithrombins" which antagonise thrombin. They are probably α-globulins.

Heparin. This is a sulphated mucopolysaccharide found in most tissues of the body, and prominent in the granules of mast cells. These cells are distributed typically around small vessels and capillaries. Heparin is antithrombic because it aids the adsorption of thrombin on fibrin threads, and it inhibits the action of thrombin on fibrinogen. It is probably the cause of the increased clotting time found in anaphylactic shock in the dog (see Chapter 14). It is counteracted by protamine. Platelet factor 4 is an antiheparin agent, and like factor 3 is liberated by platelet aggregating agents.[7]

Antithromboplastin. The existence of this is debatable, but it is a fact that the titre of thromboplastin falls within a few minutes during the thromboplastin generation test.

CLOT DISSOLUTION (FIBRINOLYSIS)[8, 9]

Fibrin formed *in vitro* from normal blood usually remains intact for days or weeks provided bacterial contamination is avoided. In extravascular situations in the body large deposits may be found in the form of haematomata and inflammatory exudates, and these too are fairly stable. They are ultimately removed in the demolition phase which precedes resolution or organisation. In both instances digestion is brought about by proteolytic enzymes derived most probably from the polymorphs. There is, however, a proteolytic enzyme which is formed from the constituents of the blood, and this acts intravascularly. Although called a fibrinolysin, it can also slowly digest fibrinogen and other plasma proteins (see Fig. 51.2).

Figure 51.2
The blood fibrinolytic system.

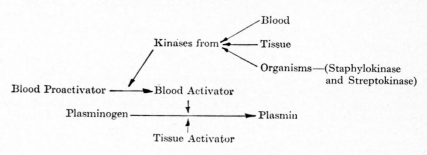

Plasminogen, a normal plasma protein, can be activated in a variety of ways to produce the active fibrinolytic enzyme **plasmin**. A proactivator exists in the blood, which by the action of enzymes (**kinases**)* is converted into an activator. These kinases are liberated from precursors in the blood or the tissues. Certain organisms, e.g. *Strept. pyogenes* and *Staph. pyogenes*, also produce kinases, of which streptokinase is the most important. *In vitro* plasminogen can be activated directly by trypsin, chloroform, the products of tissue damage, thrombin, and activated Hageman factor. The fibrinolytic system may thus be triggered off in a number of ways, but the actual mechanisms involved are not known, nor indeed are the circumstances under which it occurs. When blood clots, plasminogen is adsorbed on to the fibrin, and it is at this site that activation occurs rather than in the blood itself. Vascular endothelium contains a plasminogen activator, and this may well be an important factor in the dissolution of intravascular clot, e.g. in a thrombus, after it has become endothelialised.

Activation of the system occurs after exercise, adrenaline

* A *kinase* is a substance which activates an enzyme. It usually forms the suffix of the word indicating what is being activated, e.g. thrombokinase (now called thromboplastin) activates thrombin from prothrombin. However, in regard to fibrinolysis the word kinase is used in the context described above.

administration, injury, and stress, and has been reported in anaphylaxis. Plasmin activity probably accounts for the persistent fluidity of the blood which is so frequent a *post-mortem* finding after sudden death, haemorrhage, shock, and asphyxia. It was indeed noted by John Hunter that the blood of two deer chased to exhaustion failed to clot.

It seems apparent that the plasmin content of the blood is increased in a wide range of conditions, and is presumably a defence mechanism contrived to balance the clotting mechanism.[10] One might postulate that an imbalance between the two systems leads to intravascular clotting on the one hand and afibrinogenaemia on the other (see disseminated intravascular coagulation syndrome, p. 623).

A reduction in the quantity of tissue activator, or the presence of an inhibitor have been suggested as factors concerned in the fibrin accumulation found in the lungs in patients with uraemia[11] or subjected to thoracic radiation.[12] They may possibly play a subsidiary role in hyaline-membrane disease of the newborn.[13]

TESTS OF IMPORTANCE IN THE BLEEDING DISEASES

There is no single test which will evaluate the integrity of the complex haemostatic mechanisms of blood. Many tests are available, and an outline of the commonly used ones will be given. When evaluating the tests for clotting defects, it is convenient to consider whether the test is measuring the intrinsic system, the extrinsic system, the common pathway, or a combination of these (see Fig. 51.3). The *sensitivity* of each test must also be remembered. Thus the commonly used clotting time can be normal when one of the clotting factors involved is as low as one or two per cent of normal.

Bleeding time. This is the time taken for a small skin puncture to stop bleeding. It varies from 1–9 minutes. An increased bleeding time is due to inadequate platelet activity in sealing the puncture, or to a failure of vascular contraction; in practice both are often combined. It is invariable in thrombocytopenia and usual with defective platelet function (*thrombocytopathia*).

Capillary fragility test (Hess's test). This test assesses the degree of fragility of the capillaries to a sustained rise of blood pressure (between systolic and diastolic for 5 minutes), and a positive result is manifested by a purpuric eruption on the skin of the arm below the applied tourniquet. Presumably

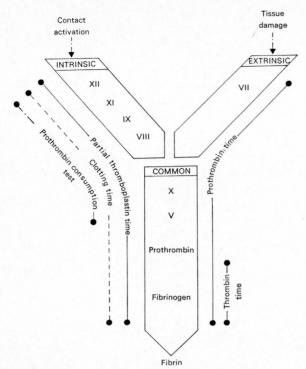

Figure 51.3
The interpretation of screening tests of blood clotting.
(From Bithell, T. C. and Wintrobe, M.M. (1970), *in* Harrison's
Principles of Internal Medicine, *6th ed., Fig.* 62.3, *p.* 323, *New
York. McGraw-Hill.)*

the capillaries are mildly damaged by the sudden rise in
pressure, and become more permeable. The platelets cover
the endothelium, and so protect it.

The test is positive in severe thrombocytopenia, but the
results correspond poorly with the platelet count. Indeed,
some normal people develop a considerable number of
petechiae when tested. This test is also positive when there is
vascular damage, e.g. scurvy, scarlet fever, and hypertension.

Platelet count has already been mentioned.

Clotting time. This is the time taken before a specimen
of whole blood clots. It is important to exclude tissue factors,
therefore the venepuncture must be "clean". The blood is
placed in an unsiliconised tube at a temperature of 37°C, and
clotting should occur within 5 to 15 minutes. If a siliconised
tube is used the clotting time is 20–60 minutes. The clotting
time is prolonged if there is a deficiency of any of the factors
concerned in the *intrinsic clotting system* or in the *common
pathway*. The test is insensitive, and a normal result can be
obtained even in the presence of very low levels of some
clotting factors. Relatively little prothrombin activator is
needed to produce a normal clotting time. The test is not
affected by the level of Factor VII (extrinsic system), but is
prolonged when a circulating anticoagulant such as heparin
is present in excess. The test is widely used to control
heparin therapy. With thrombocytopenia there is usually a

normal clotting time despite a prolonged bleeding time. This
is because clotting requires very few platelets for its initiation.
In haemophilia there is no shortage of platelets nor any
vascular abnormality. The bleeding time is therefore
normal despite a prolonged clotting time.

Prothrombin consumption test. The clotting time can
be normal even though a small amount of prothrombin
activator is produced (see above). However, much unused
prothrombin will remain and this can be measured in the
prothrombin consumption test. The test measures only
those factors concerned in the intrinsic system (XII, XI,
IX, VIII, X, and V), and is more sensitive than the clotting
time. It is also affected by platelet abnormality and thrombocytopenia.

Clot retraction. In the absence of platelets the clot is
soft and jelly-like; it lacks the firmness and adhesiveness of
a normal clot, and is less effective in producing permanent
haemostasis. Measurements of clot retraction are not done
as a routine procedure. Normal blood starts retracting
30–60 minutes after being drawn. Associated with thrombocytopenia there is a defective retraction of the clot, and this
contributes to the bleeding tendency.

Prothrombin time. In this test equal amounts of brain
extract (containing tissue factor), calcium-chloride solution,
and test plasma are incubated at 37°C, and the time taken for
clotting to occur is recorded. A control must be put up at the
same time, and this should clot in 10–16 seconds. The test is
a measure of the factors concerned in the *extrinsic system*
(Factor VII) and in the *common pathway* (Factors X, VII,
and prothrombin). The intrinsic pathway is by-passed.

This test was introduced as an indicator of prothrombin
deficiency, but it is now known that deficiencies of the three
other factors mentioned above also serve to prolong the
prothrombin time. It is nevertheless of great value in controlling anticoagulant therapy in thrombotic disorders,
because the commonly-used anticoagulants of the coumarin
and phenylindanedione types depress Factors VII and X as
well as prothrombin. Unfortunately these anticoagulants
also depress the level of Factor IX, and the test is of no value
in assessing a deficiency of this factor.

Where the prothrombin time is greatly prolonged, there
is also a prolonged clotting time. The clotting time may,
however, be normal despite a significantly increased
prothrombin time, e.g. during the administration of anticoagulants, and the patient's life is in jeopardy.

Plasma thrombin time. This is the time taken for plasma
to clot when thrombin is added. It is a measure of the
fibrinogen level, and is also affected by excess heparin and
other anticoagulants.

The Fi test. This is a rapid test for hypofibrinogenaemia.
Latex particles coated with antibody to human fibrinogen
are mixed with plasma. Normally there is aggregation, and a
failure of this to occur indicates afibrinogenaemia.

Partial thromboplastin time (PTT). This is the time
taken for plasma to clot under the following three conditions:

(*a*) The test is carried out in a glass tube—the surface causes activation of Factor XII.

(*b*) A fraction of brain extract called "cephalin" is added.* This provides excess phospholipid, and makes the test independent of the platelet count.

(*c*) Calcium chloride is added.

The PTT is a sensitive measure of the factors concerned in the *intrinsic and common pathways* (see Fig. 51.3). It is increased if any of the factors are below 15–20 per cent of normal, and is also prolonged by heparin and other inhibitors. Sometimes kaolin is added to the mixture to aid the activation of Factor XII: this is then called the *activated partial thromboplastin time*.

Thromboplastin generation test. This invaluable test assesses the factors that are of importance in *the intrinsic system*, and it depends on the fact that some of these are contained in normal plasma adsorbed with aluminium hydroxide, and others are present in normal serum. These factors produce blood thromboplastin (in the presence of ionic calcium), which at once reacts with prothrombin and leads to clotting. Normally a mixture of adsorbed plasma, serum, platelets, and calcium incubated at 37°C produces such rapid formation of thromboplastin that clotting occurs in 8–10 seconds. If clotting is delayed more than 5 seconds relative to a control mixture, the result is abnormal. The deficient factor can be determined by replacing in turn the patient's plasma, serum, and platelets with normal plasma, serum, and platelets, and repeating the test.

Table 51.1

Factor	Serum	Alumina-treated plasma
V	Absent	Present
VII	Present	Absent
VIII	Absent	Present
IX	Present	Absent
X	Present	Absent
XI	Present	Present
XII	Present	Present

Table 51.1 indicates the presence or absence of the various clotting factors in serum and alumina-treated plasma. Although Factor VII is included in the table, it plays no part in the thromboplastin generation test.

If normal adsorbed plasma induces the rapid formation of thromboplastin while normal serum has no effect, the deficiency is one of Factors V or VIII. These two can be distinguished by means of the prothrombin time which is normal in Factor-VIII deficiency and prolonged in Factor-V deficiency.

If the defect is relieved by normal serum but not by normal adsorbed plasma, there is a deficiency of Factor IX or Factor X. Factor-X deficiency leads to a prolonged proth-

* This extract is soluble in ether but not in acetone. It is not the same as the water-soluble extract used in the prothrombin time.

rombin time, which is normal in Factor-IX deficiency.

If the defect is relieved both by normal adsorbed plasma and normal serum, the deficiency is one of Factors XI or XII, and as already mentioned, Factor-XII deficiency seldom causes any clinical symptoms.

If the defect is present even when normal adsorbed plasma and normal serum are used, the fault lies in the patient's platelets, which are deficient in function (thrombocytopathia).

In practice, there are specialised laboratories which keep plasma of patients known to be deficient in these individual factors. Depending on whether or not such a plasma can be corrected by that of a fresh case, a diagnosis of specific factor deficiency can be confirmed.

The four tests which can most easily be carried out as an initial investigation of a patient with a bleeding disease are the *platelet count*, the *bleeding time*, the *partial thromboplastin time (PTT)*, and the *prothrombin time (PT)*. If both PTT and PT are normal, the defect is probably in the vessels or the platelets. If either PTT or PT is prolonged, there is probably a defect in the clotting system. If both PTT and PT are abnormal, the defect is most likely in the common pathway. If the PTT is prolonged and the PT is normal, it is the intrinsic system which is most probably at fault. A prolonged PT and a normal PTT is rare, and indicates a deficiency of Factor VII (see Fig. 51.3).

THE HAEMORRHAGIC DISEASES

A haemorrhagic tendency may be due to one or more of three factors:

(*a*) A defect in or damage to the blood vessels.

(*b*) A decreased number of platelets (or inadequately functioning platelets).

(*c*) A defect in the clotting mechanism.

In practice, (*a*) and (*b*) are often combined.

The clinical manifestation of these diseases is an increased tendency to bleed. This may occur after obvious trauma, like bruising or a surgical incision, or it may take place apparently spontaneously as petechial haemorrhages* into the skin, mucous membranes, and viscera. Such petechial haemorrhages are called *purpura*, and this type of lesion is peculiar to states of vascular damage and platelet inadequacy. It is uncommon in the disorders of clotting. Not all purpuric lesions are evidence of a generalised bleeding tendency. Quite a large number of purpuras are due to local vascular damage, and these should be separated from the generalised purpuras which are clearly important manifestations of a haemorrhagic diathesis. Localised purpuric lesions

* Haemorrhages less than 2 mm in diameter are called *petechiae*. Diffuse flat haemorrhages larger than this are *ecchymoses*, while if there is a definite swelling the lesion is called a *haematoma*. *Purpura* is defined as any condition in which there is bleeding into the skin.

include (*a*) *senile purpura*,[14] (*b*) *cachectic purpura*, in both of which the blood vessels are poorly protected against trauma in the atrophic skin and subcutaneous tissue. (*c*) *orthostatic purpura* on the legs of people who stand for long periods of time; (*d*) *mechanical purpura*, which may occur in whooping-cough, convulsions, and traumatic asphyxia, due to the rupture of many capillaries; (*e*) *purpura in women who bruise easily*, probably due to excessively fragile capillaries; (*f*) *purpura in certain rare skin diseases*, e.g. the Ehlers-Danlos syndrome,* where there is inadequate support for the capillaries,[15] (*g*) *corticosteroid purpura*, due to the mechanical rupture of poorly supported blood vessels in the atrophic skin which results from the prolonged local or systemic use of glucocorticosteroids.

The generalised purpuric diseases may be divided into those due to *platelet abnormalities*, and those due primarily to *vascular damage*.

HAEMORRHAGIC DISEASES DUE TO PLATELET ABNORMALITIES

Thrombocytopenic Purpura (Purpura Haemorrhagica)

The purpura due to a low platelet count may be primary or else secondary to drugs, other blood diseases, etc.

(i) Primary (idiopathic or essential) thrombocytopenic purpura is predominantly a disease of children and young adults. Bleeding occurs into the skin, genito-urinary and alimentary tracts, and sometimes into the central nervous system. Epistaxis, menorrhagia, and melaena are common manifestations, and excessive bleeding after operations is a serious hazard. Apart from an occasionally palpable spleen there are no other physical abnormalities. Haemarthrosis is not a feature of the disease.

The fundamental haematological change is severe thrombocytopenia. Bleeding seldom occurs until the platelet count is less than 60 000 per μl. Severe platelet depression is accompanied by (*a*) a prolonged bleeding time; (*b*) a positive capillary fragility test; (*c*) poor clot retraction. The clotting time is normal.

The red and white cells show no abnormality apart from a possible posthaemorrhagic anaemia.

The bone marrow contains an excess of megakaryocytes, but most of them are either young or else abnormal in appearance, and few appear to be giving off platelets. The main value of a marrow investigation is to exclude acute leukaemia or aplasia.

The pathogenesis of primary thrombocytopenic purpura is obscure. It is one of the blood dyscrasias that frequently responds well to splenectomy, and it has therefore been

* This consists of hyperelasticity of the skin and hyperextensibility of the joints, and is apparently due to a congenital defect of the collagen, which is sparse and thin. The skin is very fragile, and haematoma formation is a conspicuous feature.

postulated that the spleen either inhibits the formation of platelets from megakaryocytes in the marrow, or else that it is abnormally destructive to circulating platelets.

There is also evidence that some patients have platelet agglutinins in their sera, and the condition may have an immunological basis. Some of these may, however, be alloantibodies, for serologically distinct types of platelets are now identifiable, e.g. corresponding to the ABO and other blood-group systems of the red cells. There is no correlation between these antibodies and the clinical severity of the disease.[16]

In addition there is a factor of capillary defectiveness in the condition, because the bleeding is often greater than can be explained by the degree of thrombocytopenia. Splenectomy may improve the capillary fragility long before it has any effect on the platelet count.

(ii) Secondary thrombocytopenic purpura may occur in numerous conditions:

In other blood dyscrasias, e.g. acute leukaemia, marrow aplasia, and secondary hypersplenism. The thrombocytopenia of pernicious anaemia is seldom severe enough to lead to purpura, but retinal haemorrhages sometimes occur.

Following the administration of chemical and physical agents. Some will invariably produce thrombocytopenia if a sufficiently large dose is given, and a list of these has been given in connexion with marrow aplasia. Others produce a specific effect on the platelets due to idiosyncrasy, e.g. "Sedormid", organic arsenicals, quinidine, and sulphonamides. These four drugs are particularly liable to produce purpura; in addition there is an extensive list that includes all the drugs that occasionally lead to bone-marrow aplasia. "Sedormid" (allylisopropylacetyl carbamide) is peculiar in confining its attack to platelets, and there is evidence that it stimulates the formation of autoantibodies (produced against a platelet-Sedormid antigen), which agglutinate platelets and lyse them in the presence of complement.[17] The specific quinidine purpura is apparently produced in a similar way. Many drugs leading to thrombocytopenia do so by a direct action on the megakaryocytes.

Thrombocytopenic purpura may also follow physical agents like ionising radiations, burns, and heatstroke.

Thrombotic thrombocytopenic purpura (*thrombotic microangiopathy*, or *Moschcowitz's disease*)[18] is an uncommon disorder in which there is a diagnostic triad of thrombocytopenic purpura, acute haemolytic anaemia, and transient neurological signs. The terminal arterioles and capillaries of the body are occluded by fibrin in which there are entrapped platelets. It is the kidneys, brain, heart, pancreas, and adrenals that are particularly likely to suffer.

The aetiology of the disease is not understood, but the most likely pathogenesis is a primary deposition of fibrin on the blood vessels with secondary defibrination. This would account for the fluctuating neurological signs, and the fibrin-covered vessels could cause fragmentation of the red cells. But the severity of the anaemia and the cause of the defibrination remain unexplained. The course is usually acute, and only a few cases have survived.

Systemic lupus erythematosus.

Acute infections. Purpura is a frequent manifestation of severe infections, but it is seldom due to platelet deficiency. Thrombocytopenia may occasionally occur in the course of septicaemia, typhus, and smallpox. It is a well-recognised complication of infectious mononucleosis and rubella.

Extensive haemangiomata in infants are occasionally complicated by thrombocytopenia, which is relieved when the lesion is removed. Presumably the angioma sequestrates large numbers of platelets.

Following massive blood transfusions. See p. 634.

Thrombocytopathic Purpura

The term thrombocytopathia includes those conditions in which there is defective platelet function but a normal platelet count.[19] As so little is known about normal platelet function in regard to vascular integrity, it is still impossible to classify the thrombocytopathias properly, and in all probability there are a number of different platelet dysfunctions included in the term. In 1918 Glanzmann described a bleeding condition in which defective clot retraction was the only abnormal finding, and he called it *thrombasthenia*. There is now considerable doubt about the identity of the disease he described, and it has been advocated that the term thrombasthenia should be used for a defect in which there is a prolonged bleeding time, poor clot retraction, normal platelet count, and defective platelet aggregation by ADP.[20] Several such cases have been reported; they have suffered from purpura, extensive bruising, and severe post-traumatic and postoperative haemorrhage. The platelets may be abnormal in appearance.

Acquired thrombocytopathia has been described in uraemia, liver failure, and scurvy, when it may contribute to the bleeding tendencies found in these conditions. In *uraemia* platelet dysfunction is especially important, and it has been attributed to the retention of a dialysable substance that would normally be excreted by the kidney. The bleeding time is increased, platelet adhesiveness[21] and aggregation are impaired, and there is a poor release of lipid factor.[22] The bleeding noted so frequently in *macroglobulinaemia* has been attributed to a coating of abnormal protein around the platelets, thus preventing the release of lipid factor.

Thrombocythaemic Purpura[23]

In the rare disease *haemorrhagic thrombocythaemia* the platelet count may reach many millions per μl, yet there is a severe bleeding tendency marked by gastrointestinal bleeding, and occasionally haematuria, haemoptysis, menorrhagia, and postoperative haemorrhage. The platelets vary in size and show evidence of dysfunction, for example decreased adhesiveness and impaired liberation of factor 3. There is also a moderate leucocytosis and sometimes a polycythaemia, but the bleeding may lead to anaemia. The

disease bears some relationship to polycythaemia vera; there is splenomegaly, and furthermore it may be complicated by venous thrombosis despite the tendency to haemorrhagic manifestations.

HAEMORRHAGIC DISEASE DUE TO VASCULAR DAMAGE

This group comprises the non-thrombocytopenic purpuras. The haematological findings are negative. The capillary fragility test is sometimes positive.

"Anaphylactoid" ("allergic") purpura of Henoch-Schönlein. This is a disease especially of young people, which is characterised by multiform skin lesions such as urticarial weals, bullae, and purpuric spots, and also arthritic pains, severe abdominal colic, and haematuria. The abdominal symptoms are due to extravasations of blood into the bowel wall. This may simulate intussusception clinically, and also precipitate it. The joint pains are due to peri-articular lesions; haemarthrosis is not encountered.

The renal symptoms are due not merely to haemorrhages into the kidney, but are also often a manifestation of acute glomerulonephritis. This is in fact the great danger of the condition, and is the cause of death in the occasional fatal cases. The haemorrhagic manifestations do not jeopardise life on account of blood loss, and there is no tendency towards excessive bleeding after injury or operation.

The disease is an angiitis involving the arterioles and venules. There is sometimes immunofluorescence evidence of antigen-antibody complexes in the skin and kidney. Thus Henoch Schönlein purpura is an immune-complex disease related to polyarteritis nodosa.[24, 25]

Scurvy. In scurvy petechiae are first noted in the hair follicles, and this is followed by gingival bleeding in adults and extensive subperiosteal haematoma formation in infants. There is little tendency to excessive bleeding after injury, but there is a great delay in wound healing (see Chapter 9). The cause of the haemorrhagic tendency is probably poor anchorage of the blood vessels in a thin, watery intercellular substance devoid of adequate collagen fibres.

Infections. Many severe infections are accompanied by purpura, e.g. haemorrhagic smallpox, arbovirus fevers, scarlet fever, chickenpox, measles, diphtheria, and typhus. Toxic capillary damage is the probable explanation, as there is seldom a marked thrombocytopenia in these conditions. Another possibility is the defibrination syndrome, which may occur in fulminating infections, causing both infarction and diffuse haemorrhage.[26, 27] This is the most likely explanation of the *Waterhouse-Friderichsen syndrome* that characteristically complicates meningococcal septicaemia ("spotted fever") and more rarely staphylococcal, *Esch. coli*, and *H. influenzae* septicaemias. The massive adrenal haemorrhage is probably a haemorrhagic infarct.

In some infections bacterial embolism may play a part in the purpuric eruption, e.g. subacute infective endocarditis with its splinter haemorrhages into the nail-beds and typhoid fever with its rose spots on the abdomen.

Drugs and Chemical agents. These include iodides, belladonna, quinine, aspirin, phenacetin, bismuth, and mercury. Viperine snake venom produces petechial haemorrhages into many organs as the result of the diffuse vascular damage it produces.

Macroglobulinaemia. The bleeding in this condition has not been adequately explained. Vascular damage secondary to an infiltration of the wall by the abnormal protein is one possible factor. Interference by the protein with platelet function (see p. 620) and with the clotting mechanism may occur. Hyperviscosity of the plasma (p. 551) and precipitates of cryoglobulin are other mechanisms.

Hereditary Haemorrhagic Telangiectasia[28, 29]

Although this is not a purpuric condition, it merits consideration because it leads to severe haemorrhages from many areas of the body. The disease is essentially a malformation of the capillaries and venules, which has the characteristics of a generalised hamartomatous dysplasia. The telangiectases, which consist of dilated capillaries and defective venules, usually appear in adult life, though the defect is no doubt already present in childhood. There is a recurrent bleeding from the nose, mouth, and stomach, and also from damaged telangiectases in the skin. There are no conspicuous haematological findings. Capillary fragility is usually normal, though a few cases are on record in which the tourniquet test was positive. The disease is inherited as an autosomal dominant characteristic; in some individuals the manifestations are so mild that they are missed until carefully sought. Pulmonary arteriovenous fistulae and aneurysms of the splenic artery have been described in association with this condition, thereby stressing once again the generalised nature of the angiomatous malformation (see Chapter 27).

HAEMORRHAGIC DISEASE DUE TO DEFECTS IN THE CLOTTING MECHANISM

The Thromboplastin-Deficiency Syndromes

Haemophilia. This is the most classical of all conditions inherited as a sex-linked recessive characteristic; the affected males exhibit the disease while the females merely transmit it to the next generation (see Chapter 3). There is a deficiency in the production of Factor VIII (antihaemophilic globulin), which is congenital and of all grades of severity. Recently cases have been reported in which the factor has been present in normal amount but in an abnormal form devoid of activity. Similar cases of Factor IX, X, and VII defect may also occur.[42]

The bleeding of haemophilia takes place both from the natural orifices, e.g. epistaxis and melaena, and into the tissues, e.g. retroperitoneal, intrapsoas, and intracranial. It

occurs typically after injuries and incisions, e.g. dental extraction, and there is a grave danger of exsanguination. In the small vessels on the surface of a wound clotting is satisfactory because of an abundance of tissue thromboplastin, but the larger, deeper vessels are not so adequately protected. A very characteristic manifestation of haemophilia is *recurrent haemarthrosis*, which is usually preceded by a negligible injury. In due course crippling deformity ensues, and the joint cavity is obliterated by fibrous adhesions or bony ankylosis. It is interesting that although diffuse subcutaneous ecchymoses are frequent, there are seldom any petechial haemorrhages.

The blood picture is otherwise normal apart from post-haemorrhagic anaemia. The clotting time is greatly prolonged (it may be normal during periods of remission), but the bleeding time and clot retraction are normal. The prothrombin time is normal, but the thromboplastin generation test and the partial thromboplastin time reveal the abnormality. Haemophilia has occasionally been reported in the female offspring of an affected father and a mother who carried the trait. The disease is no more serious than in the male subject.

For the treatment of haemophilic bleeding a transfusion of fresh blood (if there has been much bleeding) or plasma from normal human subjects should be given. Freeze-dried plasma retains its antihaemophilic potency for years. As Factor VIII is labile, having a half-life of less than a day, repeated transfusions are necessary. Bovine and porcine plasma have a much greater antihaemophilic power, but they soon stimulate antibodies that neutralise them. Even human Factor VIII sometimes leads to the appearance of a circulating anticoagulant which is probably an antibody. The explanation of this alloimmunisation against Factor VIII is not understood, since some cases have occurred in haemophiliacs who were only partially deficient in the factor.

At present various concentrates of Factor VIII, using amino-acid precipitation or cryoprecipitation, are being used with considerable success. They are an alternative to freeze-dried plasma.

Christmas disease (Factor-IX deficiency). This too is inherited as a sex-linked recessive characteristic. It mimics haemophilia so closely that no distinction is possible without recourse to the thromboplastin generation test, or else by trying to correct the defect in the serum of a known case of Christmas disease. Christmas disease has sometimes been called *haemophilia B* in contrast with Factor-VIII deficiency, which is then called *haemophilia A*.

Factor-XI deficiency (plasma thromboplastin antecedent deficiency).[4] This is inherited as an autosomal recessive characteristic. In this condition bleeding is commonest after surgical operations, e.g. dental extractions. Spontaneous ecchymoses, purpura, and haemarthrosis are uncommon. This disease is usually much milder than haemophilia. It impairs the thromboplastin generation test, and can be diagnosed by the inability of the serum to correct the defect in the serum of a known case of the deficiency.

Factor-XII deficiency (Hageman factor deficiency).[4]
This is inherited as an autosomal recessive characteristic. It
is usually symptomless.

von Willebrand's disease.[30] This condition, first
described by von Willebrand in inhabitants of the Aland
Islands in the Baltic Sea, has aroused much interest, and the
nature of the bleeding defect is not well understood. Inherited as an autosomal dominant trait, it is characterised by
bleeding from the body orifices, haemarthrosis, and postoperative haemorrhage. The three abnormal features are a
prolonged bleeding time, reduced platelet adhesiveness, and
a deficiency of Factor VIII, resulting in a prolonged partial
thromboplastin time. Other platelet functions, e.g. count,
aggregation, and lipid factor 3, are normal as is also clot
retraction. The clotting time may be prolonged and the
thromboplastin generation test is abnormal.

There appears to be a deficiency of a factor, called the
anti-VW factor, necessary for the formation of Factor
VIII.[31] Transfusions of both normal and haemophilic
plasma raise the level of Factor VIII in the plasma of patients
with von Willebrand's disease, and allay the postoperative
bleeding tendency.[32] The factor is said to be stable and to be
present in serum as well as plasma. Why its lack should
prolong the bleeding time is obscure; perhaps it is necessary
for the adhesion of platelets prior to their aggregation into a
solid plug.[30] Nevertheless, the control of postoperative
bleeding appears to be related to the rise in Factor VIII
produced by the precursor factor, for the bleeding time often
remains prolonged.[33] Factor VIII acts more slowly and the
effect lasts longer in von Willebrand's disease than in haemophilia.[32] The plasma of a patient with von Willebrand's
disease does not alleviate haemophilia.

The Hypoprothrombinaemias[34]

At one time it was believed that hypoprothrombinaemia
was a single condition due to a deficiency of prothrombin.
However, it is now evident that this rarely occurs alone, and
that there is nearly always an associated deficiency of Factor
VII, and often of Factors X and V as well. Factors V and X
are necessary in the final common pathway of the clotting
systems, and their deficiency leads to an impaired thromboplastin generation test and partial thromboplastin time as
well as a prolonged prothrombin time. Factor VII is not
concerned in the intrinsic system, and the PTT is normal
when it is deficient; the prothrombin time alone is prolonged.
The clotting time is prolonged in severe cases of deficiency
of these factors, but, being an insensitive indicator, is often
normal when there is an increased prothrombin time. The
hypoprothrombinaemias (including Factor V, VII, and X
deficiency) may be inherited as autosomal recessive traits,[35, 36]
or they may be acquired in various conditions such as liver
failure, anticoagulant administration, and haemorrhagic
disease of the newborn.

The basic factor in most of the acquired hypoprothrombinaemias is *vitamin-K deficiency*. This fat-soluble vitamin

is imperfectly absorbed in conditions of steatorrhoea, such as
the *malabsorption syndrome* and *obstructive jaundice*, and it
cannot be used by the liver in prothrombin synthesis if there
is *hepatic failure*. When there is vitamin-K deficiency there
is a concomitant lack of Factors VII and X and occasionally
IX, but Factor V is normal in amount.

In liver disease there may also be deficiencies of Factors V
and IX; Factor VIII alone remains normal. It is obvious that
the liver plays a key role in many clotting disorders.

In the newborn there is a normal depression of the levels of
prothrombin and Factor VII (and also to some extent of
Factors IX and X, but not of Factor V, which is slightly
raised). In haemorrhagic disease of the newborn this tendency is accentuated, probably because of functional im-
maturity of the liver and poor intake of vitamin K by the
mother. Once the child develops its own intestinal bacterial
flora, it is able to synthesise its own vitamin K.

The coumarin group of anticoagulants mimic *sweet-clover
disease of cattle* (which is due to a coumarin compound), and
lead to the impaired synthesis of prothrombin, Factor VII,
and sometimes Factors IX and X as well.

The clinical manifestations of these disorders include
subcutaneous ecchymoses, epistaxis, melaena, haematuria,
and an intractable oozing type of haemorrhage after incisions.
Purpura is not a feature. Haemarthrosis has been reported
with Factor-VII deficiency.

The part played by Factor VII is intriguing, as it is not
required for blood clotting *in vitro*. It is evident that the
extrinsic system is of considerable importance in haemostasis.

The Hypofibrinogenaemias

If there is a complete absence of fibrinogen, the blood is
incoagulable. Several *congenital cases* of this type have been
recorded. Despite numerous bleeding episodes the condition
causes less inconvenience than haemophilia, and it does not
lead to haemarthrosis. In *congenital*, or *constitutional*,
hypofibrinogenaemia there is a greatly reduced plasma
fibrinogen, and also moderate thrombocytopenia. The
bleeding tendency is less severe than in congenital afibrinogenaemia. It is interesting that patients with congenital
abnormalities of fibrinogen may develop thrombotic complications as well as bleeding tendencies.

The condition of *acquired hypofibrinogenaemia* is of much
greater importance than the congenital one. As fibrinogen is
synthesised in the liver, the level may be low in hepatic
failure. The most important and dramatic types of acquired
hypofibrinogenaemia, however, are encountered in the
defibrination syndrome which may be encountered under two
circumstances:

The fibrinolytic syndrome.
Disseminated intravascular coagulation.
The fibrinolytic syndrome.[37] Activation of the plasmin
system can occur when large amounts of tissue activator are
released into the blood stream, for example during major

operations especially those involving the lungs and heart, in obstetrical accidents such as abruptio placentae, and in certain tumours, particularly carcinoma of the prostate and acute leukaemia. It also occurs in *liver disease* and congenital heart disease. The plasmin which is formed can be detected in the blood; it digests fibrinogen as well as other clotting factors, and the blood eventually becomes incoagulable. Fibrin degradation products can be detected in the blood, and are of importance because they are inhibitors of thrombin (the thrombin time is increased), they interfere with the polymerisation of fibrin, and they impair platelet aggregation. *The platelet count remains normal.* Bleeding, e.g. from an operation site, is the salient clinical feature. Treatment consists of eliminating the cause, replacing clotting factors, and administering a fibrinolytic inhibitor such as epsilon-aminocaproic acid.

Disseminated intravascular coagulation.[37] This condition, also known as *consumptive coagulopathy*, occurs under two circumstances which may occur separately or in combination:

(*a*) The release of clotting factors into the blood stream.
(*b*) Extensive endothelial damage.

The result is the formation of fibrin in the circulation and this produces vascular obstruction and micro-infarction. In addition, the extensive intravascular coagulation consumes the coagulation factors so that *afibrinoginaemia and thrombocytopenia* are characteristic features. Moreover, the formation of fibrin leads to the activation of the fibrinolytic system; whilst this removes some of the obstructing fibrin, it causes further degradation of the clotting factors and the formation of anticoagulant fibrinogen breakdown products, as noted in the fibrinolytic syndrome. Thus the two effects of consumptive coagulopathy are a severe bleeding tendency and a tendency to infarction, primarily microscopic in extent but becoming larger when fibrinolysis is inadequate. The syndrome of disseminated intravascular coagulation is seen under many circumstances:

(*a*) In abruptio placentae with amniotic-fluid embolism, when placental material enters the circulation.
(*b*) Intrauterine retention of a dead fetus.
(*c*) In incompatible blood transfusion reactions.
(*d*) After severe trauma, fat embolism, open-heart surgery with an extracorporeal circulation, and extensive lung operations.
(*e*) In the newborn after abruptio placentae, birth asphyxia, hypothermia, and Rhesus immunisation. It must be differentiated from Vitamin K deficiency by the tests mentioned below.[38]
(*f*) Severe infections. This has been discussed on p. 620; the Waterhouse-Friderichsen syndrome is probably caused in this way. So also is the generalised Shwartzman reaction described on p. 423. In both these examples there is severe infarction as well as a bleeding tendency. In the Shwartzman reaction it would seem that the first dose of endotoxin

initiates clotting, but the RE cells are able to clear the endotoxin complexes and clotting intermediates. The second dose likewise initiates clotting, but the complexes cannot be removed by a blocked RE system.

(*g*) Purpura fulminans,[39] a rare bleeding disease with extensive infarction particularly of the skin occurring usually about a week after an acute streptococcal infection. It may represent an antigen-antibody reaction in the blood. It resembles the localised Shwartzman reaction in histology and distribution.

(*h*) Metastatic cancer, usually of the prostate, and occasionally of the lung, pancreas, and stomach. This is a rare complication of disseminated cancer.

(*i*) Thrombotic thrombocytopenic purpura, see p. 619.

(*j*) Malignant hypertension.

Clinically there is postoperative bleeding, ecchymosis, and haemorrhage from the body's orifices. In addition to the severe hypofibrinogenaemia with increased fibrin breakdown products there is a fall in the level of Factors V and VIII due to the large amount of thrombin formed (see p. 615). A thrombocytopenia is also characteristic. There may also be a haemolytic anaemia (see p. 594). The condition is an emergency and is treated with transfusions of fresh blood or fibrinogen. Heparin should be administered to prevent further intravascular clotting. The fibrinolysin inhibitor ε-aminocaproic acid can be given at the same time as the heparin.

Therapeutic defibrination. From the venom of the Malayan pit viper a purified coagulant fraction called *arvin* has been prepared.[40] By converting fibrinogen into a fibrin-like substance it leads to defibrination and incoagulability of the blood. Its use as a therapeutic anticoagulant is under trial.

Factor XIII deficiency. As a congenital defect it causes ecchymoses and haematomata but apparently no bleeding from the mucosa. Defective wound healing may occur. There may be fatal umbilical haemorrhage. The condition is diagnosed by the clot solubility test, normal clot being insoluble in 30 per cent urea solution or 1 per cent monochloracetic acid. An acquired deficiency can occur in liver disease and in the hypofibrinogenaemia of abruptio placentae.

Circulating Anticoagulants[41]

Pathological circulating anticoagulants prevent the formation of blood thromboplastin, but do not usually interfere with its action on prothrombin. They may be encountered in patients with haemophilia and Christmas disease who have developed antibodies after repeated transfusions of Factors VIII and IX respectively. The condition has also been described in women who have recently passed through a pregnancy, and more rarely in elderly patients. It may complicate a number of diseases, of which systemic lupus erythematosus is the most important. The nature of the antithromboplastic substance is unknown (it often has an anti-Factor VIII action), but an immunological mechanism is probably responsible. It is reasonably attributable to autoimmunity.

The presence of a heparin-like substance in the blood of people who have been exposed to ionising radiations has been postulated to account for the delayed clotting time that occurs quite commonly, but there is little proof that this is true.

The clinical manifestation of a circulating anticoagulant is diffuse bleeding into the tissues and from the body orifices.

CONCLUSIONS

It is clear that an abnormal bleeding tendency may be due to a bewilderingly large variety of conditions. Nevertheless, certain clinical observations can assist in the elucidation of the nature of the disorder.

1. The commonest cause of regional haemorrhage is local vascular disease. Severe postoperative bleeding is much more likely to be due to badly-ligated blood vessels or secondary infection than to any of the generalised bleeding disorders. Similarly, recurrent epistaxis is usually due to a vascular abnormality in the nose, and haematuria is usually a symptom of a lesion in the urinary tract.

2. Severe postoperative bleeding may be due to a deficiency in the platelets (either quantitative or qualitative) or to an impairment of the clotting mechanism, but is rarely caused by generalised vascular damage acting on its own.

3. Petechial haemorrhages (purpura) are typical of conditions of generalised vascular damage and platelet inadequacy, but are uncommon in the clotting disorders.

4. Recurrent haemarthrosis is very suggestive of Factor VIII or IX deficiency. It is not a feature of the platelet and vascular disorders.

5. A family history should always be carefully elicited. Many of the clotting diseases and also hereditary haemorrhagic telangiectasia have a strongly familial tendency.

GENERAL READING

Biggs, R. (1972). *Human Blood Coagulation, Haemostasis and Thrombosis*, 697 pp. Oxford: Blackwell.
Biggs, R. and Macfarlane, R. G. (1966). *Treatment of Haemophilia and other Coagulation Disorders*, 391 pp. Oxford: Blackwell.
Poller, L. (1969). *Recent Advances in Blood Coagulation*, 362 pp. London: Churchill.

REFERENCES

1. Marcus, A. J. (1969). *New England Journal of Medicine*, **280**, 1213, 1278 and 1330.
2. Mustard, J. F. and Packham, M. A. (1970). *Canadian Medical Association Journal*, **103**, 859.
3. Leading Article (1969). *British Medical Journal*, iii, 371.
4. The Nomenclature of Blood Clotting Factors (1962). *Journal of the American Medical Association*, **180**, 733.
5. MacFarlane, R. G. (1964). *Nature (London)*, **202**, 498.
6. Davie, E. W. and Ratnoff, O. D. (1964). *Science*, **145**, 1310.
7. Youssef, A. and Barkhan, P. (1968). *British Medical Journal*, i, 746.
8. MacFarlane, R. G. (1961). *Functions of the Blood*, p. 335. Edited by R. G. MacFarlane and A. H. T. Robb-Smith. Oxford: Blackwell.
9. Various Authors (1964). *British Medical Bulletin*, **20**, 171–246.
10. Innes, D. and Sevitt, S. (1964). *Journal of Clinical Pathology*, **17**, 1.
11. MacLeod, M., Stalker, A. L. and Ogston, D. (1962). *Lancet*, i, 191.
12. Leading Article (1960). *Lancet*, ii, 1014.
13. Lieberman, J. and Kellogg, F. (1960). *New England Journal of Medicine*, **262**, 999.
14. Shuster, S. and Scarborough, H. (1961). *Quarterly Journal of Medicine*, **30**, 33.
15. McKusick, V. A. (1966). *Heritable Disorders of Connective Tissue*, 3rd edn, p. 179. St. Louis: Mosby.
16. Dausset, J., Colombani, J. and Colombani, M. (1961). *Blood*, **18**, 672.
17. Ackroyd, J. F. (1949). *Clinical Science*, **8**, 269.
18. Amorosi, E. L. and Ultmann, J. E. (1966). *Medicine (Baltimore)*, **45**, 139.
19. Braunsteiner, H. and Pakesch, F. (1956). *Blood*, **11**, 965.
20. Hardisty, R. M., Dormandy, K. M. and Hutton, R. A. (1964). *British Journal of Haematology*, **10**, 371.
21. Eknoyan, G. et al. (1969). *New England Journal of Medicine*, **280**, 677.
22. Leading Article (1967). *British Medical Journal*, iv, 437.
23. Fountain, J. R. and Losowsky, M. S. (1962). *Quarterly Journal of Medicine*, **31**, 207.
24. Copeman, P. W. M. and Ryan, T. J. (1970). *British Journal of Dermatology*, **82**, Supplement 5, p. 2.
25. Copeman, P. W. M. (1970). *British Journal of Dermatology*, **82**, Supplement 5, p. 51.
26. McGehee, W. G., Rapaport, S. I. and Hjort, F. P. (1967). *Annals of Internal Medicine*, **67**, 250.
27. Cronberg, S. and Nilsson, I. M. (1970). *Acta medica scandinavica*, **188**, 293.
28. Bean, W. B. (1958). *Vascular Spiders and Related Lesions of the Skin*, p. 132. Oxford: Blackwell.
29. Harrison, D. F. N. (1964). *Quarterly Journal of Medicine*, **33**, 25.
30. Dormandy, K. M. (1969). *Journal of Royal College of Physicians of London*, **3**, 211.
31. Nilsson, I. M. et al. (1957). *Acta medica scandinavica*, **159**, 179.
32. Cornu, P. et al. (1963). *British Journal of Haematology*, **9**, 189.
33. Biggs, R. and Matthews, J. M. (1963). *British Journal of Haematology*, **9**, 203.
34. Leading Article (1964). *Lancet*, ii, 1280.
35. Marder, V. J. and Shulman, N. R. (1964). *American Journal of Medicine*, **37**, 182.

36. HALL, C. A. *et al.* (1964). *American Journal of Medicine*, **37,** 172.
37. BRODSKY, I. and SIEGEL, N. H. (1970). *Medical Clinics of North America*, **54,** 555.
38. BOYD, J. F. (1967). *Archives of Diseases in Childhood*, **42,** 401.
39. ANTLEY, R. M. and McMILLAN, C. W. (1967). *New England Journal of Medicine*, **276,** 1287.
40. Leading Article (1968). *Lancet*, i, 513.
41. MARGOLIUS, A., JACKSON, D. P. and RATNOFF, O. D. (1961). *Medicine (Baltimore)*, **40,** 145.
42. Leading Article (1972). *Lancet*, i, 729.

Chapter 52. Blood Grouping and Blood Transfusion

Attempts to transfuse blood from one individual to another, both in animals and in man, were made from the fifteenth century onwards. One of the early experimenters was Dr. C. Wren, who is better known for creating the famous landmark in the City of London than for his work on blood transfusion. It was fortunate that the clotting of blood frustrated many of these early attempts.

The human red cell is a veritable mosaic of blood-group antigens. With the major exception of the ABO and Rhesus antigens these are weak, and when once methods were devised for matching individuals with respect to these groups, blood transfusion became a practical and useful procedure. Antibodies are produced against leucocytes and platelets, but these are rarely a cause of serious trouble.

Antibodies to the less well-known blood-group antigens are sometimes a cause of serious trouble, and blood transfusion can no longer be regarded as a minor procedure to be left to the most junior resident on the hospital service. While the management of transfusions should be the responsibility of well-trained specialists in the field, it is desirable that all clinicians should have a working knowledge of the red-cell antigens and the precautions necessary to prevent transfusion reactions.

It is remarkable that, although the albumin of an animal of one species acts as a potent antigen when introduced into a member of a different species, it is not antigenic to other members of the same species. Transfusions containing the various allotypes of the immunoglobulins, transferrins, β-lipoproteins, etc. may lead to the formation of alloantibodies. However, these are rarely a cause of trouble, and even following repeated transfusions anaphylactic shock is rare; transfusions are now commonplace, and are often repeated in the same patient.

The term "blood groups" is applied to the genetically determined antigens which can be detected on the red-cell surface by specific antibodies. At the present time there are twelve well-defined systems of antigens, and of these, two, the ABO and Rhesus systems, are of great clinical importance. The other ten systems are named MNSs, P, I, Lutheran, Lewis, Kell, Duffy, Kidd, Diego, and Xg. The last is the only one which is inherited as a sex-linked trait. Many other red-cell antigens are known, and more no doubt remain to be discovered. Some (*public*) are present in almost all individuals, while others are restricted to a few individuals (*private antigens*). The antigens associated with the blood groups other than the ABO and Rhesus systems are occasionally the cause of transfusion reactions; approximately 1 per cent of hospital patients possess antibodies outside the ABO and Rhesus systems.

THE ABO AND RELATED BLOOD GROUPS[1]

The ABO blood groups are determined by genes which govern the presence of antigens on the cells, in particular the red cells. In addition, similar substances may be present in the body fluids, and these are determined by the Lewis and Secretor genes. Although not strictly red-cell antigens, they are conveniently considered here.

A glycoprotein precursor substance is converted into H substance under the influence of the *H* gene. Nearly all individuals are of genotype *HH* or *Hh** and their red cells contain H substance. The *A* and *B* genes are at a different locus, and by their presence some H substance is converted into A or B substance. *O* is an amorph and leaves H unchanged. There are therefore four major blood groups, as the following table shows.

Table 52.1

Genotype	Phenotype (blood group)	Antibody normally present in serum
AA or *AO*	A	anti-B
BB or *BO*	B	anti-A
AB	AB	none
OO	O	anti-A and anti-B

The serum of each person generally contains antibodies to those antigens which he does not possess. Such antibodies are called *alloantibodies* because they are capable of agglutinating the red cells of normal people who happen to be of a different blood group, but are incapable of agglutinating the individual's own red cells. The prefix *iso-* has been used previously in connexion with these antibodies. Unfortunately *iso-* and *syn-* are now used in transplantation immunology to indicate genetic identity. Individuals of a species who differ genetically are called allogeneic, therefore antibodies formed

* *h* (like *O* and *le*) is an amorph, i.e. a gene which has no detectable product. The cells of an individual of genotype *hh* therefore contain neither H, A, nor B antigen. The serum contains anti-H, anti-A, and anti-B. This very rare condition was first described in two people in Bombay, and is therefore called the "Bombay", or O_h, phenotype.

by one individual against antigens possessed by another should be called alloantibodies, alloagglutinins, etc. This terminology has now been adopted by Mollison. Alloantibodies must be distinguished from *autoantibodies*, which are capable of agglutinating or damaging the individual's own red cells (see Chapter 49).

The anti-A and anti-B antibodies are naturally occurring. Those present in an infant at birth are passively acquired from the mother. The child begins to develop his own antibodies at the age of 3–6 months. It is unknown how such antibodies can develop in the absence of the appropriate antigenic stimulus. It may be that these agglutinins develop as a response to substances which are antigenically similar to the human blood-group substances, and which are inhaled or ingested. Such antigens are widely distributed in nature, being present in animal tissues, e.g. horse serum, and in bacteria.* It has been noted that chicks reared in a germ-free environment do not develop heteroagglutinins against human B cells, such as are found in chicks reared normally.[2] This might be related to the finding that many Gram-negative bacteria have high concentrations of blood-group specific substances.[3] If this is the correct explanation, the term "naturally-occurring antibody" is a misnomer, since the antibody is specifically stimulated. Nevertheless, the matter is by no means settled, and it is convenient to retain the term. *Naturally-occurring* antibodies to the ABO group antigens are always present, and may also be accompanied by other naturally-occurring antibodies, e.g. anti-P_1. They are predominantly IgM, and react more strongly at lower temperatures than at 37°C. The anti-A and anti-B are in fact active at 37°C, but anti-P_1 is seldom active above 25°C, and so is not a significant transfusion risk.

Naturally-occurring antibodies are generally capable of agglutinating red cells in saline suspension, and for this reason have been termed *complete*. Antibodies which are formed as a result of a definite antigenic stimulus, e.g. pregnancy, transfusion, or injection of red-cell antigens, are termed *immune antibodies*. They are generally IgG, most active at 37°C, and often fail to agglutinate red cells in saline suspension. In contrast to the naturally-occurring antibodies they are therefore called *incomplete*.

Subgroups of group A. About 80 per cent of European persons of group A or AB belong to the subgroup A_1 or A_1B, and there is a specific antibody (anti-A_1) which reacts with these cells. The remaining 20 per cent of group A and AB individuals belong to the subgroups A_2 or A_2B. The A_2 antigen appears to be a weaker form of A_1, and although A_2 and A_2B red cells are agglutinated by anti-A they are not agglutinated by anti-A_1. There is no specific anti-A_2. This nomenclature is very confusing. It is evident that "*anti-A*

* It is interesting to note also that agglutinins are found in extracts of the seeds of certain plants, e.g. Lima beans. These substances are called *lectins*. One of them is of use in being highly specific for A_1 cells.

serum" contains two *antibodies*— anti-A and anti-A_1. Anti-A antibody agglutinates all cells containing either A_1 or A_2 antigen, while the antibody anti-A_1 reacts only with cells containing A_1.

The importance of this subgrouping is that A_2 cells, and particularly A_2B cells, sometimes react weakly with an anti-A serum and are therefore mislabelled as group O or B respectively. The serum of an A_2 or an A_2B subject often contains anti-A_1. An A_1B or an A_1 individual's serum may contain anti-H, which agglutinates O and A_1 cells.

Secretor status. About 80 per cent of the population possess the secretor gene *Se* (genotype *SeSe* or *Sese*), and are able to form water-soluble glycoproteins which have the antigenic specificity of H substance (as well as that of A and B, if the *A* and *B* genes are also present). Such people are called "secretors", and have H (and A and B) antigens in their secretions such as saliva and gastric juice. "Non-secretors", who lack the *Se* gene (genotype *sese*), in fact secrete a glycoprotein, but it has no H, A, or B activity. Le^a is secreted if the Lewis gene *Le* is present (see below). The classification of secretor status ignores the presence of Lewis substances and of non-specific glycoprotein; only ABH antigens are considered.

The Lewis antigens. Two Lewis antigens are known, Le^a and Le^b, together with the corresponding antibodies anti-Le^a and anti-Le^b. The antigens are found primarily in the body fluids such as plasma and saliva, but also become attached to the red cells by adsorption. The formation of the Lewis antigens is dependent upon the presence of a single gene *Le* (genotype *LeLe* or *Le le*) acting in conjunction with the *Se* gene (see above).

The *Le* gene acting alone leads to the formation of Le^a antigen, found in the plasma, saliva, and on the red cells, which are therefore of phenotype Le(a+b−). *Such people never secrete A, B, or H substances in their saliva.* The *Le* gene acting in conjunction with the secretor gene (genotype *SeSe* or *Sese*) leads to the formation of Le^b, red-cell phenotype Le(a−b+). Such a person secretes Le^b, and also some Le^a and H substance. If the *A* and *B* genes are present there is also A and B substance in the saliva of Le(a−b+) persons. The gene *le* is an amorph, and individuals of the genotype *lele* form no Lewis antigen, and their red cells are of group Le(a−b−). They secrete H (and A and B) if the *Se* gene is present.

ABO grouping. The ABO grouping of a blood sample is performed on a tile or in tubes, preferably at room temperature. Two drops of a 2 per cent red-cell suspension in normal saline are mixed with 1 drop of potent anti-A and anti-B serum respectively, and the development of agglutination is noted. If this occurs with anti-A, the cells are group A, and with anti-B, group B. If both sera agglutinate the red cells, they are group AB, and if there is no agglutination with either, they are group O. An additional safeguard is to test the cells with a group O serum (containing anti-A and anti-B). This agglutinates all cells which are not group O, and is a safeguard against mistaking an A_2 subject for group O. Agglutination is easily recognisable with the naked eye, but should be confirmed microscopically. As a routine procedure the patient's serum is tested with group A, B, and O cells to confirm the presence of the expected alloagglutinins, anti-A and anti-B, according to the table on p. 626. This is termed "reverse grouping".

Apart from alloagglutination, the red cells may be clumped under the following conditions:

Pseudoagglutination. This is the clumping of red cells by non-immunological means, and is due to rouleaux formation such as occurs in multiple myeloma and macroglobulinaemia.

Autoagglutination due to cold agglutinins. The effect is overcome by carrying out the reverse grouping at $37°C$.

Panagglutination. This is a non-specific agglutination of *contaminated red cells*, particularly liable to occur in old blood samples. The agglutination is due to the unmasking of an antigen (T antigen) which is present in all human red cells. Such "changed" red cells are agglutinated by normal human serum which contains anti-T. The change can be brought about by bacteria *in vitro*, and it may rarely occur *in vivo*. Cells which have become panagglutinable (also called polyagglutinable) can readily be detected by the use of an anti-T lectin extracted from peanuts.

The anti-A and anti-B sera are prepared by blood transfusion centres. They are collected from blood donors, and are selected for their potency. It is most important to be sure that the anti-A serum will reliably detect the weak forms of the A antigen.

Immune anti-A and anti-B

If a patient is transfused with blood of an incompatible A or B group, he develops a high titre of *immune anti-A or anti-B*. This antibody is normally present only in traces, but its titre rises after an incompatible transfusion or after the injection of A or B substance obtained from the tissues of certain animals, e.g. pigs. Preparations of diphtheria and tetanus toxoid are particularly liable to stimulate these antibodies, apparently because the medium on which the organisms are grown contains peptone derived from hog's stomach, which is very rich in these substances. Immune anti-A and anti-B are stronger agglutinins at $37°C$ than are their naturally-occurring counterparts, and furthermore haemolyse red cells in the presence of complement. It therefore follows that grouping sera are always heated to inactivate complement before being issued by blood transfusion centres; haemolysis is less easy to interpret than agglutination, for it might also be due to badly-cleaned tubes.

Some of these immune antibodies are IgM, but others are IgG and IgA. The IgG antibodies can traverse the placenta (see p. 594) and cause a neonatal haemolytic anaemia. This usually occurs when the mother is group O and the fetus group A. Unlike Rh-haemolytic disease, it commonly affects the firstborn, some of whose group A cells have entered the mother's circulation during pregnancy and acted as a booster to the already present maternal anti-A antibody. The condition is quite common, but only occasionally is the anaemia severe enough to require treatment.

Nature of the ABO blood-group substances. Ovarian-cyst fluid has provided a rich source of human blood-group substances for chemical analysis. The *soluble* ABO group and Lewis antigens are glycoproteins which consist of a protein backbone with many short polysaccharide side-chains; the composition of the side-chains determines specificity. Each step in the sequence: precursor glycoprotein $\rightarrow$ H substance $\rightarrow$ A or B substance, involves the addition of a single sugar, e.g. *N*-acetylgalactosamine for A specificity and D-galactose for B specificity. Likewise, the production of the Lewis antigens involves the addition of a sugar unit. Since each of these steps is determined genetically, it is evident that the red-cell antigens are not the direct product of genetic activity. Each gene gives rise to a specific glycosyltransferase; these enzymes are present in the serum and secretions. The ABO specificity of *red cells* is determined by glycoproteins and by glycolipids each carrying the same immunodominant sugar. These blood-group antigens are also present on the membranes of all vascular endothelial cells and some epithelial cells. Hence the importance of ABO matching with renal and other allografts (p. 198).

Relationship between ABO groups and susceptibility to disease. There is statistical evidence that gastric cancer is unusually common in group A subjects, and duodenal ulceration in those of group O. Pernicious anaemia is also found most frequently in group A people. Secretor status has also been related to disease: non-secretors are more liable to duodenal ulceration and acute rheumatic fever than are secretors. The significance of these findings is not understood.

THE RHESUS (Rh) SYSTEM

If the red-cells of *Rhesus* monkeys are injected into other animals, an anti-Rhesus serum is produced which will agglutinate the red cells of about 85 per cent of white-skinned people.* These cells are designated Rh-positive. Subsequent investigations have shown that the gene involved in the Rhesus groups is complex and is responsible for the formation of several different antigens, one of which (D or Rh_0) is the antigen present in Rhesus-positive cells. There are two main theories concerning the nature of the Rhesus groups, and these have led to two separate systems of nomenclature.

The *linked gene theory* of Fisher and Race supposes that

---

* This discovery was made in 1940 by Landsteiner and Wiener, but the antibodies they discovered are now known to be distinct from, though closely related to, those now called Rhesus antibodies. The *LW* gene (named after the discoverers) leads to the production of the LW antigen. This reacts with true anti-Rhesus antibody—i.e. serum from a guinea-pig immunised against *Rhesus*-monkey red cells. Both LW and Rhesus antigens are probably derived from a common substrate under the influence of the *LW* and *Rh* genes.

there are three very closely linked loci occupied by the genes
C, D, and E or their alleles c, d, and e. These genes give rise
to the red-cell antigens C, D, E, c, and e. There is no d
antigen, but it is convenient to use the symbol *d* in writing
Rh genotypes. Each person inherits one trio of genes from
each parent. Thus an individual of the genotype *CDe/cdE*
inherited *CDe* from one parent and *cdE* from the other. He
has the antigens C, c, D, E, and e on his red cells. It should
be noted that the genes are very closely linked, and crossing
over almost never occurs. The Fisher–Race nomenclature
has the asset of simplicity. Cells containing D are termed
Rhesus (Rh) positive, and those which lack it Rh negative.
In practice D-negative donors are also tested with anti-C
and anti-E, and only those donors who are *cde/cde* are labelled "Rhesus negative" for transfusion purposes.

The Rhesus antigens are more complex than the above
account would suggest. There are other alleles as well, e.g.
four of C (C^w, C^v, C^u, and C^x), one of D (D^u), and two of E
(E^u and E^w), and these are associated with corresponding
antigens. Furthermore, genes in combination on one
chromosome (e.g. *Cde*) sometimes produce a compound
antigen (e.g. Ce). The antibody to this antigen (anti-Ce)
reacts with a sample of *Cde/cDE* cells but not *cde/CDE* cells.

The second theory is that of Wiener, and it supposes that
there is a single locus which can be occupied by any of a large
number of alleles. This *multiple allele theory* supposes that a
single gene can give rise to several antigens of different
specificities. In the Wiener classification the common antigens are called rh′ (C), hr′ (c), rh″ (E), hr″ (e), and Rh_o (D).
In brackets are the corresponding antigens of the Fisher–
Race nomenclature. Table 52.2 shows a comparison of Rh
gene nomenclature according to the two theories. Thus it
will be seen that the allele R^1 gives rise to the antigens Rh_o,
rh′, and hr″; these correspond to D, C, and e. The Wiener

TABLE 52.2 The common Rh genes

Wiener notation	Fisher notation
R^1	CDe
r	cde
R^2	cDE
R^0	cDe
r″	cdE
r′	Cde
R^Z	CDE
r^Y	CdE

Table showing the Rhesus genes arranged in descending order
of frequency. The first column shows the symbols for the genes
based on the notation of Wiener. The corresponding genes of the
CDE notation are shown in the second column. It should be
noted that the capital *R* always indicates the presence of the gene
responsible for the antigen D; *r* implies its absence. The most
common genotypes in a Caucasian population are *CDe/cde*,
CDe/CDe, and *cde/cde*. There is some evidence that the actual
order of the genes is *DCE* rather than *CDE*.

theory is more difficult to learn and work with, but its main
assertion, that the Rh antigens are determined by a series of
alleles at a single locus, is probably correct. Nevertheless,
the simple Fisher–Race nomenclature is commonly used
and is adequate for most purposes. It has the great advantage
of being the only notation readily useful for communicating
information between workers in blood-transfusion laboratories. For research work a numerical nomenclature has
been described.[4] Each phenotype is defined in terms of
the reaction of the red cells with specific antisera, to which
numbers have been assigned.

In practice it is the D antigen that is of crucial importance,
and most transfusion reactions due to Rh incompatibility
involve this antigen. Occasionally reactions occur as a result
of c and E incompatibilities.

The Rh antigens appear to be confined to the red cells;
evidence of their presence in white cells, platelets, and body
secretions is not convincing. The chemical nature of the Rh
antigens is not known.

Rhesus Antibodies

Naturally-occurring Rhesus antibodies are rare, though a
number of cases of anti-E and anti-C^w have been reported.
Such antibodies are usually more active at lower temperatures than at 37°C.

On the other hand, *immune Rhesus antibodies* are commonly
met with following the sensitisation of Rh-negative individuals with Rh-positive cells: (*a*) by transfusion, and (*b*) by
the transplacental passage of fetal cells.

Early in the course of Rh sensitisation complete IgM
antibodies are formed. These are not passed across the
placenta. Later on they are succeeded by IgG antibodies,
which are able to pass the placental barrier. These IgG
antibodies act best at 37°C, and are *incomplete*, that is, incapable of agglutinating red cells in saline suspension, but
capable of agglutinating them under the following three
conditions:

(*a*) If the red cells are suspended in a colloid medium
before the serum is added. A suitable medium is provided
by a concentrated protein solution such as 30 per cent
bovine albumin.

(*b*) If the red cells are first incubated at 37°C with the
serum, then washed three times to remove all traces of
serum proteins, and finally mixed with an antiglobulin serum
prepared by injecting human globulin into a rabbit. This is
called the *Coombs*, or *antiglobulin*, *test*. It detects the presence
of globulin on the surface of the red cells.

(*c*) If the red cells are treated with such enzymes as trypsin
or papain before the addition of the serum. The most sensitive procedure of all is an antiglobulin test on enzyme-treated
red cells.

Antiglobulin (Coombs) test. In the Coombs test, as
outlined above, the antibody combines with the cells *in vitro*.
This is the *indirect test*; it detects incomplete antibody in the

patient's serum, and is invaluable in cross-matching blood. In haemolytic anaemia due to antibodies, the patient's red cells have already been exposed to the incomplete antibody *in vivo*, and they will undergo agglutination *in vitro* once they have been thoroughly washed and then mixed with an antiglobulin serum. This is the *direct test*; it detects globulin already adsorbed on to the cells. In the "direct" Coombs test all that needs to be done is to treat the washed cells with the antiglobulin serum, whereas in the "indirect" test the cells have first to be incubated with the test serum.*

Red-cell agglutination. It has been found that red cells possess a surface negative charge and that they normally repel one another. This electrical property is due to the carboxyl group of sialic acid, and treatment with neura-minidase, trypsin, or papain liberates a sialomucopeptide. The result is a great reduction in their negative charge, and incomplete antibodies are helped in their agglutinating action. A colloid medium like albumin also reduces the electric repulsion between red cells and so facilitates their agglutination.

Most IgG are incomplete antibodies—those against A and B antigens are exceptions—while most IgM are complete. The explanation of the difference is still not clear; one suggestion is that the large IgM molecules are able to reach between two cells and bring them closer together, whereas the small IgG are much less effective. It will be recalled that the valency of IgG is two while that of IgM is five or ten (see p. 145). These incomplete antibodies can prevent the agglutinating action of complete antibodies, and are an example of a blocking antibody (see p. 148); in fact, incomplete anti-Rh was first discovered by this blocking effect.

Rhesus Grouping

Powerful anti-D sera are obtained from women who have already been sensitised during previous pregnancies. A complete anti-D serum is particularly desirable, as it can be used with saline-suspended cells, but often an incomplete serum has to suffice.

A small drop of 5 per cent red-cell suspension in saline is added to an equal quantity of complete anti-D serum in a serological tube, and the mixture is incubated at 37°C for one hour, after which the presence or absence of agglutination is noted. If an incomplete anti-D serum is used, a drop of 30 per cent bovine albumin is added to the tube, and the test is carried out as above. Agglutination indicates that the cells

are Rh-positive. The Coombs technique is unnecessary for Rh grouping, unless the antigen D^u is being investigated.*

Rhesus grouping is also performed on a slide by mixing one drop of a 50 per cent suspension of red cells in serum with one drop of incomplete anti-D serum. The test is read for agglutination in 2 minutes, and the result should agree with that obtained by the tube method outlined above. In the negative control the anti-D is replaced by a drop of albumin.

The all-important antibody is anti-D. It may be accompanied by anti-C or anti-E. It is much rarer to encounter anti-C or anti-E alone. Since anti-c or anti-e are formed by Rh-positive subjects (*CDe/CDe* or *cDE/cDE*), these antibodies are not accompanied by anti-D.

INDICATIONS FOR BLOOD TRANSFUSION

A sudden reduction of blood volume after haemorrhage. Not only is *whole blood transfusion* mandatory after severe haermorrhage, but it is also often used during major operative procedures. The most spectacular example is the use of large quantities of blood in the elaborate extracorporeal circulations set up during open-heart surgery.

An inadequate concentration of circulating haemoglobin which cannot be relieved by specific therapy, e.g. vitamin B$_{12}$ or iron. All severe anaemias are potentially eligible for *packed red-cell transfusion*, but it should be a rare state of affairs for the megaloblastic or iron-deficiency types to require it. A special circumstance may, of course, necessitate transfusion during a severe anaemia, e.g. labour or a surgical operation. Wintrobe rightly castigates the demand of some surgeons, that the haemoglobin concentration be "normal" prior to surgery, as a superstition.[5] Often the patient has adjusted himself to his new haemoglobin level, and a transfusion merely disturbs the equilibrium for the time being. Once symptoms of anaemia have developed (these usually start at a Hb concentration of about 8 g per 100 ml), a transfusion is certainly justified. Transfusions are not free from risk, and the more anaemic the patient, the more carefully should transfusion be performed.

In acute haemolytic anaemia transfusions may be lifesaving while the effect of adrenal steroids or splenectomy is awaited. Transfusions should be used sparingly in the autoimmune haemolytic anaemias. In erythroblastosis fetalis *exchange transfusion* is often imperative to prevent a rise in the plasma level of unconjugated bilirubin by removing cells which have been damaged by antibody. In addition, the anaemia can be corrected (see also p. 634).

In aplastic anaemia transfusions may tide the patient over

---

* The antiglobulin test is in fact more complex than is described above. The reagent commonly used contains antibodies of two separate specificities: anti-human IgG and anti-human C3, C3 being a β_1-globulin and the third component of complement (also called β_1C). The anti-IgG agglutinates red cells coated with IgG antibody; the reaction may be inhibited by free IgG in the solution. Certain incomplete antibodies, commonly IgM, fix complement which is thereby attached to the red cells. Such cells are agglutinated by the anti-β_1-globulin component of Coombs's reagent. This reaction is inhibited by free complement but not by IgG.

* Phenotype cD^ue masquerades as cde, and the antigen D^u may be missed in the albumin test, especially if the anti-D is not very strong. The phenotype is not uncommon in Negroes, and is of importance when Rh-negative donors are being selected. Obviously a D^u donor is Rh-positive.

for a long time in the hope that recovery will ultimately ensue, and there is also a place for them in the leukaemias. The anaemia of chronic renal failure may be relieved in the same way, but invariably the haemoglobin soon falls to its previous low level.

Blood Component Therapy

When whole blood has been lost, it is logical to replace it by whole blood. If, however, the circulating blood is lacking certain components, it is logical to supply these components only. Many are now available from transfusion centres.

Packed red cells. Packed red cells, prepared by removing about 85 per cent of the plasma, are ideal for use in correcting anaemia, especially when there is a danger of circulatory overload (p. 634). In addition, the plasma is available for the preparation of other components.

Platelet-fresh whole blood, platelet-rich plasma, and platelet concentrates. These are useful in thrombocytopenia; a temporary improvement in the platelet count sufficient to arrest bleeding may be achieved. Although intact platelets are readily detectable in stored blood, their viability after transfusion is much impaired. The normal life-span is 8–11 days, but after storage for as little as a day the viability is greatly reduced. Hence platelet transfusions should be given within a few hours of collecting the blood. Platelet transfusions are generally ineffective in patients with severe infections, a large spleen, or with idiopathic thrombocytopenia.

Leucocytes. The transfusion of very large numbers of fresh white cells (e.g. using leukaemic blood) can raise the white-cell count, but the transfused cells have a very short life and the procedure is practical only in special centres.

Fresh frozen plasma. This is prepared by removing plasma from fresh blood and freezing it at −20°C to preserve labile coagulation factors. It is used in the treatment of Christmas disease and also in other bleeding conditions due to proven coagulation defects. Fresh frozen plasma must be transfused as quickly as possible after thawing, and cannot be refrozen. When fresh frozen plasma is thawed at 4°C the Factor VIII precipitates as a cryoglobulin. Such *cryoprecipitates* are the replacement of choice in haemophilia; one unit of cryoprecipitate raises the Factor VIII level of the average adult by 2 per cent.

Other plasma fractions. *Albumin.* This is available for the treatment of haemoconcentration, e.g. following burns, acute pancreatitis, and intestinal obstruction. Supplies are limited, and albumin is of no value in treating the hypoalbuminaemia of chronic renal disease.

Fibrinogen. One gram vials are available, and the usual adult dose is 4–8 g. It is of value in hypofibrinogenaemia, but there is a great risk of virus hepatitis.

γ-Globulin. This is useful in the prophylaxis or attenuation of some virus diseases and in the treatment of agammaglobulinaemia.

Rh(D) immune globulin (human). This is used in the pre-

vention of Rh sensitisation of Rh-negative women after the delivery of a Rh-positive baby or fetus (see p. 594).

THE STORAGE OF BLOOD[6]

Blood is collected aseptically from donors, and is stored in glass bottles or plastic bags. These latter have the advantage of lightness, flexibility, and complete air-tightness. Furthermore, it is possible to give the patient blood under pressure merely by squeezing the bag, without any danger of air embolism.

The anticoagulant usually employed is "ACD", a mixture of citric *a*cid, trisodium *c*itrate, and *d*extrose. Dextrose appears to decrease the rate of hydrolysis of ester phosphate during storage. Acidity also increases the preserving power of the anticoagulant. For platelet transfusions an acidified ACD (ACD-A) is used because it minimises platelet clumping and prolongs their survival.

Stored red cells have an increased affinity for oxygen, and are less ready to release oxygen than are fresh cells. This affinity for oxygen increases with the age of the banked blood. A number of organic phosphate esters, ATP, ADP, and especially 2:3 *diphosphoglycerate (DPG)*, lower this oxygen affinity, particularly at a low oxygen pressure (see p. 585). It has been found that the concentration of 2:3 diphosphoglycerate in the red cells declines on storage, and this is probably the reason for their increased affinity for oxygen. It is useless adding these phosphates to the extracellular medium as they cannot enter the cells, but the effect can be arrested and reversed by adding nucleosides, such as inosine and adenosine. It may be that these are broken down to purine bases and ribose-l-phosphate, which is then converted to 2:3 diphosphoglycerate. Some blood banks add inosine weekly to banked blood to prevent this oxygen-binding effect.[7, 8]

Another anticoagulant solution containing citrate, phosphate, and dextrose (CPD) is less acid than ACD, and the preservation of red-cell DPG is better. It is steadily replacing ACD, particularly when the blood is to be stored.

Blood should be kept stored at a temperature of about 4°C. It has been found that at temperatures above 10°C there is a rapid deterioration of the red cells. On the other hand, slow freezing is to be avoided at all costs. Much of the damage inflicted is due to the residual hypertonic fluid. Once thawing occurs, there is haemolysis when the cells are exposed once more to the isotonic solution. Much research has been done on blood which is frozen very rapidly in liquid nitrogen, and thawed equally rapidly. It has been found that the red cells survive slow freezing only when glycerol is added to the anticoagulant mixture. At a temperature of −50°C there may be no impairment in survival rate even after a year's storage.

The post-transfusion survival of red cells in blood stored at 4°C for various periods, using ACD as the anticoagulant, has been investigated. After 14 days' storage from 6 to 10 per cent of the red cells are destroyed within 24 hours of trans-fusion, but the remainder survive almost as well as do fresh cells. After 28 days' storage there is a 30 per-cent destruction within 24 hours, and the remainder show a considerably more rapid rate of disappearance than normal. It is advisable not to use blood stored longer than 21 days.

Components of a unit of blood. One unit (pint) of whole blood contains approximately 450 ml of blood and 67·5 ml of ACD. The number of red cells is such that the transfusion of one unit should raise the haemoglobin concentration of the average adult by approximately 1 g per 100 ml. At 21 days' storage, the maximum storage time, 70–80 per cent of red cells survive following transfusion. As noted previously, the granulocytes are not viable in stored blood, and in fresh blood there are too few to be effective. White-cell trans-fusions are available in specialised centres only. Platelets are viable only if the blood is less than 24 hours old.

Each unit contains approximately 10 g albumin, 2 g γ-globulin, and 0·7 g fibrinogen. These are relatively stable when stored at 4°C. Prothrombin and Factors VII, IX, and X are also stable. Factors V and VIII are not stable at 4°C, but are stable in fresh frozen plasma.

PREPARATIONS FOR BLOOD TRANSFUSION

Routinely the entire blood grouping and cross-matching procedure takes at least two hours, even if no difficulties are encountered.

Blood grouping. The patient's red cells are tested with anti-A, anti-B, and anti-A plus-B (group O) sera as described. The serum is tested for the presence of the expected alloag-glutinins.

The red cells are tested with anti-Rh (D) by two methods (p. 630).

Antibody screening. *Donor*. Blood issued by trans-fusion services has been screened for the presence of irregular antibodies (e.g., anti-K, anti-c) in the donor's plasma.

Recipient. Trouble due to antibodies can usually be met in advance of cross-matching tests by "screening" the sera of patients likely to require transfusion. Many laboratories use a "pool" of antigens (prepared by mixing the red cells of two or three selected donors) to test the patient's serum for irregular antibodies. A preliminary screening test is parti-cularly helpful in patients anticipating cardiac surgery. Irregular antibodies are then identified by further tests, which may require several hours or days to complete.

Cross-matching of blood. Once the ABO and Rhesus blood groups of donor and recipient are known, it is neces-sary to proceed with a cross-matching of the two specimens of blood before a transfusion can be performed. It is always best to transfuse recipients with blood of their own group insofar as this is possible. The important components to be tested are the donor's red cells and the recipient's serum. The donor's serum is much less important, because any anti-bodies it may contain should be so diluted by the recipient's

plasma as to become ineffectual. Cross-matching is always necessary even if the blood groups of donor and recipient are identical, because (*a*) there may be an error in sample identification, and (b) the recipient's serum may contain antibodies other than anti-A, anti-B, and anti-D.

Group-O donors were often referred to as "universal donors", and there was a temptation to administer uncross-matched group-O Rh-negative blood indiscriminately in times of emergency. While this practice may be absolutely justified by a particular event in which the recipient would have died of exsanguination had he been kept waiting until a proper cross-matching had been performed, it must be realised that the casual use of group-O blood is not free from risk. Occasionally severe haemolytic reactions follow, and these are due to high-titre immune antibodies (usually anti-A) in the donor's plasma reacting with the recipient's red cells, despite the very considerable diluting effect of the recipient's plasma. Even the administration of uncross-matched Rh-negative blood to Rh-positive recipients is not entirely innocuous. Antibodies against Rh-negative cells are well recognised, e.g. anti-c, and severe reactions have been produced by them. Preliminary cross-matching would expose this danger. In practice the use of uncross-matched group-O blood is justifiable *only* for emergency transfusions, e.g., following trauma. In all other cases there should be sufficient time to select donor blood of the same ABO and Rh groups as those of the recipient, and to perform a 15-minute cross-matching test.

The Technique of Cross-Matching

The aim is to demonstrate antibodies in the *recipient's serum* against the *donor's red cells*. These antibodies may be complete IgM or incomplete IgG, therefore two procedures must be carried out:

(a) Agglutination test. Equal volumes of a 2 per-cent saline suspension of donor cells and recipient serum are mixed and left at room temperature for 1 hour. The sedi-mented cells are then examined for agglutinates. This test detects saline agglutinins such as anti-P_1; it also provides a further check that group A blood is not being matched for a group O recipient.

As with ABO grouping, difficulty may be encountered because of pseudoagglutination and autoagglutination. The former is seen in patients with multiple myeloma and macroglobulinaemia, and can hardly be distinguished from true agglutination by microscopy. Dilution with saline breaks up the clumps to some extent. Autoagglutination due to cold agglutinins is prevented by performing the test at 37°C.

(b) Indirect antiglobulin test. Six drops of the patient's serum are mixed with two drops of a 2 per cent suspension of the donor's cells. After incubation at 37°C for 30–60 minutes, the cells are washed three times in large volumes of saline. A drop of antiglobulin serum is added to the final cell button, and the mixture is lightly centrifuged. Agglutination occurs if the cells are "coated" with globulin (antibody). The antiglobulin should contain anti-β_1-globulin as well as anti-γ-globulin in order to react with the complement bound by some antibodies e.g., anti-Le^a, anti-Jk^a (see footnote p. 630). This is the indirect Coombs test, and when properly performed will detect incomplete antibodies of all blood-group systems. Some examples of antibodies of the Duffy and Kidd systems cannot be detected directly as agglutinins in saline or albumin, and are only revealed by the Coombs test. Lewis antibodies may be missed unless fresh serum has been added during the sensitising stage so as to provide complement.

In general, cells which react with the patient's serum *in vitro* at 37°C do not survive well after transfusion. However, when there is doubt about the interpretation of serological tests, a direct measurement of red-cell compatibility can be made by following the survival of 1 ml of the prospective donor's chromium-labelled (^{51}Cr) cells in the patient.

Patients with acquired haemolytic anaemia are a special problem, since the serum may contain a mixture of alloantibodies and autoantibodies. In these and other difficult cases, a sample of the patient's blood should be sent to a Transfusion Centre or Reference Laboratory for further investigation.

THE ADVERSE EFFECTS OF BLOOD TRANSFUSION[9]

These can be classified into those which occur immediately and those which are delayed.

Immediate Reactions

Immediate simple febrile reactions. These are quite common and occur either during or shortly after a transfusion. There are rigors and fever with nausea and vomiting. They may be due to a variety of causes. Most often they can be attributed to the presence of white-cell antibodies formed by the recipient as a result of previous transfusions or pregnancies. Febrile reactions may be quite severe but usually last only a few hours. Nevertheless, although not dangerous they must be investigated, since fever is also a component of the haemolytic reaction (see below). Aspirin will usually alleviate the symptoms, but antihistamine drugs are not effective. If febrile reactions are troublesome in patients who require further transfusions, they may usually be avoided by giving blood from which the white cells have been removed ("buffy-coat poor" blood).

Febrile reactions may also be due to the presence of Gram-negative endotoxin in either the transfusion fluid or the apparatus. Modern disposable apparatus and properly prepared fluids have largely eliminated this complication.

Allergic reactions. Urticarial reactions are usually due to sensitising antibodies in the recipient interacting with an exogenous antigen, e.g. milk or egg protein, in the plasma of the donor. Reactions are therefore most common in patients who suffer from atopic diseases such as asthma or hay-fever.

G.P.—21*

The development of an urticarial reaction is comparatively common; it is usually harmless, and is easily controlled by oral or parenteral antihistamine drugs. Very rarely the reaction has features of generalised anaphylaxis, and can be fatal.

Immediate-type hypersensitivity reactions occur when the transfused plasma (or blood product) contains plasma proteins with antigenic determinants which are lacking in the patient's own plasma proteins and to which he has previously been exposed. Severe anaphylactic reactions can occur due to *anti-IgA* formed as a result of previous transfusion in subjects who either lack IgA or who belong to a different IgA subclass. Similarly, reactions are occasionally seen following the injection of immunoglobulin in patients with agammaglobulinaemia.

Allergic reactions may also occur as a result of the passive transfer of a hypersensitive state from the donor to the recipient. A reaction develops if the recipient happens to come into contact with the relevant antigen. Either immunoglobulin or lymphocytic antibody can be transferred, and donors with a striking history of hypersensitivity should not be accepted.

Haemolytic transfusion reactions. These are usually due to the rapid destruction of donor red cells by antibodies in the recipient's plasma, and are generally the result of transfusion of ABO incompatible blood, for example group A red cells in a group O recipient. This nearly always occurs as a result of an error in the identification of the patient, a specimen, or the unit of blood, rather than a technical failure to detect incompatibility.

The patient, usually soon after the transfusion has begun, complains of a sensation of heat and pain along the transfused vein, and this is followed by facial flushing, rigors, fever, severe pain in the loins, and a feeling of constriction in the chest. Hypotension and shock may follow and terminate in death. In severe cases there is intravascular haemolysis of red cells with haemoglobinaemia, haemoglobinuria, lowering of the haptoglobin level, and the appearance of methaemalbumin in the plasma. Jaundice takes several hours to develop. Oliguria may develop and be followed by acute renal failure. There is little doubt that these dramatic symptoms are due to the substances released as a result of an antigen–antibody reaction, because a similar amount of haemolysed compatible blood does not have such severe effects. Activation of complement probably plays an important part.

The most serious effect is progressive oliguria, which is due to intense renal vasoconstriction. As mentioned on p. 595, the presence of much free haemoglobin in the circulation does cause a degree of interference with the renal blood flow, but acting on its own it is inadequate to produce much damage. In this type of intravascular haemolysis there are the two additional factors of liberated vasoconstrictor substances and above all the primary condition that necessitated transfusion in the first place.

After incompatible transfusion there is often leucopenia

and thrombocytopenia. The lysis of red cells leads to the liberation of clotting substances which cause intravascular fibrin formation, thus leading to a defibrination syndrome with secondary fibrinolysis (p. 622). The incoagulability of the blood causes a generalised bleeding tendency. In anaesthetised patients, whose subjective responses have been abolished, this bleeding tendency is a very important indication of incompatibility. The other suspicious finding is persistent hypotension despite the transfusion.

With other antibodies, especially those of the Rhesus system, red-cell destruction is usually slower and less dramatic. It is nearly always extravascular, occurring in the RE system, especially the spleen (p. 594). Symptoms are usually milder in degree, although haemoglobinaemia may occur with a severe degree of cellular destruction. Renal failure does not occur after extravascular haemolysis.

In the mildest incompatibility reactions there are no obvious symptoms or signs. The anaemia is merely not improved as much as would be hoped, so that another transfusion has to be administered sooner than expected.

Haemolysis also results from transfusion of blood rendered non-viable by faulty storage (freezing or heating), outdating, or bacterial contamination.

Circulatory overload. Congestive heart failure and pulmonary oedema may be precipitated by the excessive or too rapid administration of blood, plasma, or other intravenous fluids, particularly in patients with severe anaemia or pre-existing heart disease.

In susceptible patients it is wise to limit transfusion to two units of packed cells each 24 hours, each unit taking four hours (never more) to transfuse. The patient must be examined frequently throughout the transfusion for evidence of elevated jugular venous pressure and pulmonary oedema. Exchange transfusion or intraperitoneal injection are alternative approaches.

Intraperitoneal injection of blood. Intraperitoneal blood is absorbed by the lymphatics in the diaphragm and travels thence *via* the lymph ducts to the blood. The method is useful in children and in patients with very severe anaemia in whom intravenous transfusion is dangerous. In erythroblastosis fetalis intraperitoneal blood transfusions have been given to the fetus *in utero* in order to correct the anaemia which is the cause of the early fetal death (hydrops fetalis).

Bacterial contamination of blood is due to accidental introduction of organisms during collection or storage. The dangerous ones are cold-growing Gram-negative bacilli of the *Pseudomonas* genus and also certain coliform organisms. After a brief latent period there is profound shock associated with fever and abdominal pain. Death may ensue within a few hours (see p. 425). As a general rule, *a unit of blood should be given within four hours*, for prolonged storage at room temperature encourages the growth of contaminating bacteria.

Biochemical upsets following massive transfusions. [6] With storage there is an increased amount of potassium in the plasma and a decreased amount in the red cells. It sometimes happens that massive transfusions, e.g. exchange transfusions in infants, may be accompanied by transient hyperkalaemia of sufficient severity to produce ECG changes and sudden death. Another danger of this type of transfusion is citrate intoxication, which produces the effects of hypocalcaemia. It is probable that citrate intoxication is not due entirely to hypocalcaemia, because transfused hypocalcaemic blood does not have the same effect as citrate. Nevertheless, the effects are reversed by calcium salts. The actions of hyperkalaemia and citrate intoxication tend to potentiate one another.

The plasma of stored blood has an increased content of ammonia, which may be dangerous in patients with liver failure. [6] The content of organic acids also rises, and the pH of the plasma falls.

Generalised bleeding tendency. *Thrombocytopenia* is an occasional complication of rapidly repeated large transfusions, and it can result in a serious haemorrhagic state. In some cases platelet antibodies are formed against incompatible transfused platelets, and it seems that the antibodies can also damage the recipient's own platelets. Occasionally potent anti-platelet antibodies in the donor's plasma may be found. The generalised bleeding tendency which results from hypofibrinogenaemia has been described above.

Air embolism. The introduction of air through ill-fitting tubing, especially when blood is introduced under pressure, may result in air embolism; the use of plastic bags has virtually eliminated this danger. In terms of experimental work on animals, it would seem that a considerable amount of air (about 200 ml) should be tolerated by man, but there is clinical evidence that as little as 40 ml can have serious results, particularly in severely ill patients. [10]

Delayed Reactions

Sensitisation. The transfusion of red cells, white cells, or platelets carrying antigens not present on the recipient's cells may stimulate the production of alloantibodies directed against the foreign antigen. These alloantibodies may complicate future transfusions or pregnancies. Sensitisation to plasma protein antigens, particularly IgA, has already been noted (pp. 144 and 633).

Delayed haemolytic transfusion reactions. In patients who have become sensitised through transfusion or pregnancy, the titre of the alloantibody may with time fall to such a low level as to be undetectable. During later transfusions blood may be given which appears to be compatible, but which re-stimulates antibody production. The antibody then causes sudden destruction of the transfused cells, usually within 3–7 days following transfusion.

A delayed haemolytic reaction should be suspected when jaundice appears some days after transfusion, or when the haemoglobin concentration fails to rise by the expected amount (p. 632) or drops unexpectedly. Often the irregular antibody is suspected only when further blood is cross-matched, or when the patient's direct antiglobulin (Coombs) test is found to be positive.

Infection introduced from the donor. Syphilis, malaria, brucellosis, and, in tropical Africa and South America, trypanosomiasis may be transmitted by transfusion. The most important hazard, however, is hepatitis; the agents of both the serum (long incubation period) and infective (short incubation period) types may be the cause.

Serum hepatitis is by far the more important, and the presence of the infective agent is related to the presence of Australia antigen.

Australia antigen. This antigen, now more commonly called *hepatitis associated antigen (HAA)* or *Hepatitis B antigen (HBag)*, can be detected by a variety of methods involving the use of serum known to contain high-titre antibody. Immunodiffusion, counter-immunoeletro-phoresis* (immunoelectro-osmophoresis), inhibition of haemagglutination, complement fixation, radio-immunoassay, and electron microscopy have all been used. These vary in sensitivity and ease of performance. At the present time counter-immunoelectrophoresis is commonly used to screen all blood donors. Radio-immunoassay is, however, approximately a hundred times more sensitive, and is being introduced for routine testing of blood donors by the American Red Cross. The incidence of HAA-positivity varies from one community to another and also with the sensitivity of the method used to detect the antigen. Thus the incidence is 0·063 per cent in North Alberta and 0·484 per cent in West Quebec. It is high in the inmates of institutions, particularly prisons (0·903 per cent), and in patients with lepromatous leprosy, Down's syndrome, and immunological deficiency states, patients on renal haemodialysis, those who have had multiple transfusions, and people who have had serum hepatitis. The incidence of antigen is approximately 0·1 per cent of routine blood donors in Britain and the USA, but with professional donors the incidence is ten times higher. It has been estimated that about 50 per cent of people who receive HAA-positive blood develop hepatitis. If the sensitivity of the test employed is known, the expected incidence of hepatitis can be calculated. At present about one in four carriers are detected, and the incidence of hepatitis is about 0·15 per cent following the transfusion from a single donor assuming that HAA positive donors are excluded. The figures quoted are from Mollison (1972) and Moore *et al.* (1972). (see also pp. 290-291.)

Another complication that appears to be infective in nature is the *post-perfusion*, or *post-transfusion, syndrome*. It develops 3 to 5 weeks after the transfusion of fresh blood, often in large amounts as for open-heart surgery, and its

* When placed in an electric field, antigen having a negative charge migrates towards the anode. Antibody under the influence of endosmotic flow migrates towards the cathode. By placing the antigen and antibody in separate wells, a current is passed in such a direction that the antigen and antibody flow towards each other and interact to produce a precipitate. The method is faster and more sensitive than simple double diffusion.

main features are fever, splenomegaly, and atypical lymphocytes in the blood. The condition is a variety of infectious mononucleosis, but the Paul-Bunnell reaction is negative. Some cases are associated with cytomegalovirus infection.[11]

Multiple microembolism. Blood and transfusion fluids have been found to contain particulate matter—particles of rubber bungs, glass particles, and cellulose fibres as well as debris consisting of aggregated platelets and white cells. These may cause significant pulmonary microembolism in a seriously ill patient.[12] Another unknown factor is the importance of plasticisers (usually phthalate derivitives) which are leached by blood from the plastic of the bag and tubing.[13]

Transfusional haemosiderosis. This is a hazard of repeated transfusions given over many years for a chronic condition like aplastic anaemia. The iron deposited in the tissues is derived not only from the blood, but also from the small bowel (see p. 563).

Thrombophlebitis.[14] This is due to the needle or cannula of the infusion set damaging the vein wall. Factors which influence the development of this complication are the period of transfusion (it is progressively more frequent after 12 hours' infusion), the tubing used (rubber is more damaging than plastic tubing), and the administration of autoclaved glucose solutions, which are strongly acid. The practice of giving glucose through a set previously used for blood is also said to predispose to thrombophlebitis, perhaps because the blood haemolyses in contact with the glucose solution.

Indwelling plastic catheters left *in situ* for over 48 hours are frequently contaminated, and can lead to *septic thrombophlebitis* and fatal septicaemia. Indwelling catheters must therefore be changed, ideally every 8 hours.

Graft-versus-host reaction. This rare complication occurs when viable white cells are transfused into an immunologically deficient host (see pp. 172 and 197).

THE HAEMATOLOGICAL HAZARDS OF EXTRACORPOREAL CIRCULATIONS[15]

Extracorporeal circulations maintain an artificially-perfused flow of blood through the tissues while the cardiac action is suspended during open-heart surgery. The underlying principle is that blood, rendered incoagulable with heparin and passed through an oxygenator, is pumped into a large artery (usually the femoral), perfused through the tissues, and then returned to the circuit *via* the venae cavae.

Apart from such immediate mechanical hazards as leakage of blood and inadequate perfusion leading to tissue hypoxia and subsequent metabolic acidosis, a serious, though fortunately rather infrequent, complication is severe postoperative bleeding. The main factors involved are (*a*) the presence of residual heparin in the circulation, (*b*) an early activation of clotting leading to the defibrination syndrome with an activation of the fibrinolytic system, and (*c*) thrombocytopenia, which is probably due to a sequestration of platelets in the tissues and their use in badly-damaged areas; in addition some platelet clumps may be removed by the filters or else become adherent to the oxygenator screen. The first two factors appear to be more relevant to the bleeding tendency than does the platelet deficiency. Another possibility is that some patients have a minor degree of a specific clotting defect, e.g. haemophilia, Christmas disease, or von Willebrand's disease, and under the stress of extracorporeal circulation this is made overt. Only specific assay systems would reveal this defect pre-operatively, whereas routine screening would miss it (see also p. 38). Bleeding may occasionally be due to extensive vascular damage caused by hypoxia or sludging.

Another hazard is extensive mechanical haemolysis during perfusion; in practice this does not seem to cause much harm.

PRECAUTIONS TO BE TAKEN BEFORE AND DURING BLOOD TRANSFUSION

(1) The donor must be carefully selected. A history of malaria, syphilis, or jaundice should exclude a person as a donor.

(2) Thorough grouping and cross-matching of donor and recipient bloods must be carried out. Whenever possible the recipient should be given blood of his own ABO and Rh group. Group-O blood cannot be considered universally suitable.

(3) The container must be correctly and distinctly labelled, so that there is no chance of the recipient being given the wrong blood.

(4) The blood should be kept at 4°C, and not used for transfusion after 3 weeks' storage.

(5) Obviously haemolysed blood should not be used.

(6) If there is any question of contamination, a Gram stain of the blood should be performed before it is administered. Packed red cells should not be used later than 24 hours after removing the plasma from the whole blood, unless the manoeuvre has been performed at a transfusion centre under aseptic conditions.

(7) The recipient should be observed so that manifestations of incompatibility, overloading, and allergy can be detected and treated as soon as possible. If there is any question of incompatibility, the transfusion must be stopped at once. The next specimen of urine passed should be examined for free haemoglobin, and the patient's plasma for haemoglobin, methaemalbumin, and bilirubin. If the evidence points to an incompatibility reaction, the cross-matching should be repeated. If there is no obvious error, the help of the transfusion centre must be sought. Meanwhile some of the blood should be cultured to rule out the possibility of contamination.

GENERAL READING

DACIE, J. V. and LEWIS, S. M. (1968). *Practical Haematology*, 4th edn, 568 pp. London: Churchill.
GIBLETT, E. R. (1969). *Genetic Markers in Human Blood*, 629 pp. Oxford: Blackwell.
MOLLISON, P. L. (1972). *Blood Transfusion in Clinical Medicine*, 5th edn, 830 pp. Oxford: Blackwell.
MOORE, B. P. L., HUMPHREYS, P. and LOVETT-MOSELEY, C. A. (1972). *Serological and Immunological Methods, Technical Manual of the Canadian Red Cross Blood Transfusion Service*, 7th edn, 450 pp. Toronto: Canadian Red Cross Society.
RACE, R. R. and SANGER, R. (1968). *Blood Groups in Man*, 5th edn, 599 pp. Oxford: Blackwell.

REFERENCES

1. MARCUS, D. M. (1969). *New England Journal of Medicine*, **280**, 994.
2. SPRINGER, G. F., HORTON, R. E. and FORBES, M. (1959). *Journal of Experimental Medicine*, **110**, 221.
3. SPRINGER, G. F., WILLIAMSON, P. and BRANDES, W. C. (1961). *Journal of Experimental Medicine*, **113**, 1077
4. ROSENFIELD, R. E. *et al.* (1962). *Transfusion (Philadelphia)*, **2**, 287.
5. WINTROBE, M. M. (1967). *Clinical Hematology*, 6th edn, p. 385. Philadelphia: Lea & Febiger.
6. Leading Article (1962). *Lancet*, i, 955.
7. Leading Article (1969). *Lancet*, ii, 784.
8. Leading Article (1970). *Lancet*, ii, 920.
9. SELDON, T. H. (1961). *Anesthesiology*, **22**, 810.
10. DURANT, T. M. *et al.* (1954). *American Journal of Medical Science*, **227**, 509.
11. Leading Article (1969). *Lancet*, ii, 526.
12. McNAMARA, J. J., MOLOT, M. D. and STREMPLE, J. F. (1970). *Annals of Surgery*, **172**, 334.
13. Leading Article (1973). *Lancet*, i, 28.
14. Medical Research Council Report (1957). *Lancet*, i, 595.
15. Various Authors (1963). *Journal of Clinical Pathology*, **16**, 545–572.

Appendix 1. The Principles of Disinfection

Sterilisation is a process whereby all living organisms, including spores, are destroyed. It is to be contrasted with **disinfection**, a process which destroys only the vegetative forms of organisms, but which leaves intact any spores that may be present. In practice it often suffices, because spore-bearing organisms are often not an important hazard. For example, the skin could never be sterilised without its own destruction, but it can be satisfactorily disinfected with an iodine solution. The terms "germicide", "antiseptic", and "disinfectant" refer to chemical agents which kill organisms or prevent their growth. Though there are subtle theoretical differences in the meanings of these three words, in practice the term *disinfectant* can be used quite conveniently to describe any chemical substance with either a bactericidal or a bacteriostatic action.

Asepsis is the technique employed in the treatment of patients, whereby infective agents are prevented from gaining access to uninfected tissues. Aseptic techniques in surgery include not only the sterilisation of all articles coming into contact with the patient and the disinfection of his own skin, but also a painstaking elimination of all sources of cross-infection in the hospital environment (see Chapter 19).

There are two methods of disinfection, physical and chemical. Of these, the physical ones are by far the more important, as they alone can be relied on to ensure the sterilisation of articles used in the treatment of patients.

PHYSICAL METHODS OF DISINFECTION

The most important physical agent is heat which may be either dry or moist.

Dry Heat

The surest form of heat sterilisation is incineration, as is practised by the bacteriologist when flaming his wire-loop.

For the sterilisation of instruments a hot-air oven is used. Hot-air is an inefficient sterilising agent because it is a poor conductor of heat and it penetrates feebly. It is therefore necessary that the oven be fitted with fans to circulate the air through the chamber around the assembled load. A temperature of 160°C will sterilise the contents after one hour. Such a high temperature damages fabrics and melts rubber, and therefore hot-air sterilisation is used only for:

Glassware, especially syringes, in which moisture is a nuisance.

Oily fluids, which are impenetrable to steam.

Powders, which would cake in the presence of moisture. Metallic objects may be sterilised in the hot-air oven, but are alternatively autoclaved. Scalpels are said to retain their sharpness better in the oven than in the autoclave.

Moist Heat

Moist heat is a much more valuable sterilising agent than is dry heat because it is effective at a lower temperature for a shorter period of time. For less ambitious disinfection moist heat is also useful.

Pasteurisation. Milk is pasteurised by heating at 63°C for 30 minutes ("holder" process) or at 72°C for 20 seconds ("flash" process). The pasteurisation of delicate instruments, like cystoscopes, is now a well-established procedure. All pathogenic vegetative organisms should be destroyed by immersing the instrument in a tank of water at about 75°C for a few minutes. Spores survive, but they are of no importance in causing urinary-tract infections.

Boiling. An advantage of boiling over pasteurisation is that it is efficacious in destroying the agents of hepatitis. These are very resistant to heat, but are said to be killed after 10 minutes' boiling at 100°C. Boiling will not destroy spores.

In consulting-room practice syringes and other instruments are disinfected quite satisfactorily by boiling. Admittedly there is a hazard of anaerobic wound infection, but it is not a very real danger in these circumstances. In operating theatres, however, such a risk should never be tolerated. In this respect the ward "sterilisers" are really only "boilers". They do not sterilise. Indeed, pathogenic clostridia have on occasion been isolated from them.

The addition of 2 per cent sodium carbonate is said to impart sterilising qualities to boiling water. As this salt crystallises out on the instruments, it must be removed before they are used.

Tyndallisation. This is the steaming of a solution for 20 minutes on three successive days. After the first steaming only spores are left behind. These germinate in the medium, and are destroyed by the next steaming. Any that survive should be killed after the third steaming. Tyndallisation is, in fact, a true sterilising process, but is applicable only to media in which the spores can germinate and grow as vegetative organisms. It fails when applied to drugs, suture material, and instruments.

Steaming Under Pressure (Autoclaving)

This is the most important method of sterilisation at our disposal, and it is necessary to understand the principles involved. Because water boils when its vapour pressure is equal to that of the surrounding atmosphere, it follows that the boiling point of water can be increased by raising the atmospheric pressure. At normal (sea-level) atmospheric pressure (760 mm Hg or 14·7 lb per square inch) water boils at 100°C, and this pressure is referred to as "zero" on the pressure gauge. If the pressure in increased by 10 lb per square inch, the water boils at 115°C, and if the pressure is 15 lb per square inch, the boiling point rises to 121°C. If material is held under pure steam at a temperature of 121°C for 20 minutes, sterilisation can be guaranteed (in fact, 15 minutes is enough). At 126°C, 10 minutes suffices, and at 134°C sterilisation is complete within 3 minutes.

The great superiority of steam over hot air as a steriliser is due to the following factors:

(*a*) Moist heat kills by its effect in denaturing and coagulating enzymes and proteins, whereas dry heat acts by virtue of a destructive oxidation of cell constituents. Moist heat kills more rapidly and at a far lower temperature than dry heat.

(*b*) As steam condenses, it liberates a wealth of latent heat to the surface. The latent heat of vaporisation of water is 540 calories per gram, and one ml of water vaporises to produce 1 700 ml of steam at 100°C. It is obvious that when steam condenses, not only is a large amount of heat emitted, but there is also a great contraction in its volume. This produces a negative pressure, and brings more steam to the same site. Very soon the temperature of the surface is raised to that of the surrounding steam. Therefore steam acts much more quickly in heating exposed articles than does hot air. A simple proof of this is afforded by placing a finger in a jet of steam from a kettle, and comparing the effect with that produced by the atmosphere of a hot oven!

(*c*) Finally steam penetrates much better than does hot air. This is due in part to its density being only half that of air, and in part to the negative pressure, as already described. Penetration is, of course, of importance only with respect to porous articles.

The all-important factor is the quality of the steam. It must be (*a*) *dry*, i.e. it must not carry suspended droplets of water, because water soaks porous surfaces, thereby interfering with the removal of air and the final drying of the load, (*b*) *close to its point of condensation*, because if it is superheated it does not condense well, its latent heat is not emitted, and its penetrating power vitiated. In fact, superheated steam behaves exactly like hot air and damages fabrics, and (*c*) *free from air*, because the temperature at any pressure is lower when air is mixed with the steam. Air also hinders the penetration of steam, and by virtue of its greater density forms a separate cooler layer at the bottom of the autoclave, thus preventing the steam reaching the articles there.

The autoclave. A steriliser that contains steam under pressure is called an *autoclave*. The simplest type, which still has some use in small laboratories, contains its own water which is boiled under pressure like a domestic pressure-cooker. The steam produced expels the residual air. This type of instrument is quite unsuitable for hospital purposes because of its small size and the inadequacy of air expulsion.

All modern sterilising units are equipped with capacious autoclaves which consist of large, steam-jacketed, metal cylinders fastened by bolted swing-doors. The steam enters the roof of the cabinet from a central supply, from which it emerges under considerable pressure (about 60 lb per square inch). Before entering the autoclave the pressure is reduced to about 20 lb per square inch. This in itself removes excess water from the steam. Some of the steam enters the jacket directly, so that the side walls of the autoclave are heated independently of the steam in the chamber itself. This prevents the loss of heat from the chamber with consequent condensation of water on its walls.

As steam is lighter than air, the air is displaced downwards and is expelled together with the condensed steam through an outlet in the floor of the cabinet. A thermostatic valve, called the *balanced pressure steam trap*, or *near-to-steam trap*, is present in the outlet channel, and controls the discharge through it. At a definite temperature, usually 121°C, it expands sufficiently to occlude the outlet. A thermometer is situated just above this steam trap, which is the coolest part of the autoclave.

This steriliser is called the *downward displacement autoclave*, because air is displaced downwards by the emerging steam. In up-to-date autoclaves there is also fitted a vacuum pump which removes as much air as possible before the steam is admitted. High-vacuum, downward displacement autoclaves are very efficient because the air is removed so expeditiously that the required temperature is reached very rapidly.

In this respect the new *high-vacuum, high-pressure autoclaves* are worthy of mention. In them a very high preliminary vacuum (below 20 mm Hg absolute) is first produced, and then steam at a pressure of 30 lb per square inch introduced. A temperature of about 134°C is attained, and sterilisation is complete within 3 minutes. Unfortunately these instruments are complicated to work and require constant overhauling.

Another variant of the autoclave technique is the use of steam at low pressure and low temperature, e.g. 80°C–90°C. This is useful for such articles as blankets and endoscopes which are damaged by high temperatures. Used alone, the destruction of spores cannot be guaranteed, but if formaldehyde is added to the steam sterility is assured.

In order to operate an autoclave, the following procedures are carried out:

1. The articles are placed in the cabinet and the doors are bolted.

2. A vacuum of about 12 mm Hg absolute is applied in order to evacuate as much air as possible.

3. Steam is then admitted at a pressure of about 15 lb per square inch, and when the thermometer registers the required temperature, say 121°C, sterilisation will have commenced.

4. Sterilisation is continued for the required time, say 20 minutes, and then the steam is turned off.

5. If the articles comprise bottles of fluid, they can simply be left to cool. The steam gradually dissipates, and cooling follows. If the material is porous, it must be quite dry before it is removed from the cabinet, because organisms penetrate moist wrappings with great ease. This drying is carried out by re-applying a vacuum to evacuate the steam, and then by introducing dry, filtered air into the cabinet. This air comes from the outside and it is sterilised by being drawn (by the negative pressure) through an inlet-pipe which is provided with two filters. The drying should continue for about 15 minutes. This air is warmed by its contact with the sides of the autoclave, which are directly heated by the residual steam in the surrounding jacket.

The autoclave is used in the sterilisation of most surgical equipment, e.g. dressings, theatre apparel, rubber material (including gloves), and metal instruments. It is also used in the sterilisation of water, glucose solutions, and saline solutions used parenterally. Some media used in microbiology are similarly treated.

Failures in sterilisation may be due to any of the following factors:

Packing the load. If dressings or theatre garments are to be autoclaved, they must be arranged so loosely that the steam can circulate intimately around them. If they are assembled in metal drums, the vents of these should be orientated to the direction of downward flow of the steam. The vents should be closed expeditiously after autoclaving to prevent subsequent re-contamination. Cardboard boxes are unsuitable when closed, as air cannot be removed from them by downward displacement. Paper packs are very satisfactory. It is recommended that linen be lightly dampened, because if it is dry, it may absorb so much water that the steam becomes superheated.

Defects in the autoclave. Fortunately, old-fashioned autoclaves, e.g. with steam entering *via* the floor, without steam-trap or attached thermometer, or with no drying facilities, have virtually disappeared from hospitals, being replaced by new, efficient instruments. Nevertheless, the perfect autoclave has still not appeared. The snag is the presence of air mixed with the steam; none of the modifications has yet eliminated this nuisance. It may leak in through the door seal or the valves, or it may enter with the steam supply. The door seals and valves must be carefully overhauled, and efficient air pumps must be employed. Various preliminary manoeuvres have been suggested to eliminate as much air as possible, e.g. a double pre-vacuum with steam introduced between each phase, or a continuous influx of steam during the pre-vacuum phase, but none is completely effective.

Defects in the steam. Over-saturated and superheated steam have already been discussed. If the jacket is too warm, the steam inside the cabinet will become superheated.

Faulty operation of the autoclave. It is regrettable that in many hospitals the operation of the autoclave is left to completely untrained staff like porters, who have other duties to perform. Until a fully-trained staff is employed, no expenditure on modern equipment will ensure safety. The responsibility for efficient sterilisation must remain now as always with those who use the finished product, namely the surgeons themselves.

Tests of Efficiency for Heat Sterilisation

The thermocouple. This is by far the most reliable gauge of efficiency, and proper thermometric testing is essential before a new steriliser is put into commission. One recording is taken from a thermocouple placed inside a test pack of towels and another from one in the chamber drain. Comparison between the two recordings gives a good guide to the speed at which steam penetrates the load.

Browne's tubes. These are ampoules that contain a patent chemical indicator which changes from red through amber to green at a specific temperature. Various types are available for use in autoclaves and hot air ovens, each changing colour at a specific temperature.

Autoclave tape. This is a tape printed with a sensitive ink that undergoes a colour change at a specific temperature. It forms the basis of the *Bowie–Dick test* for high-vacuum autoclaves. In the middle of a test pack of towels there is placed a square of paper on to which has been stuck two strips of a specified autoclave tape (3M brand No. 1222) in the shape of a St. Andrew's Cross (diagonally). A temperature of 134–137°C is applied for $3\frac{1}{2}$ minutes. There should be a uniform development of bars throughout the length of the strips. This indicates that the steam has passed freely and rapidly to the centre of the load.

Spores of a non-pathogenic organism. The aerobic spore-bearer *Bacillus stearothermophilus* is used; its spores are killed at 121°C after 20 minutes. Test samples are put through the autoclave and an attempt is subsequently made to culture them. Unfortunately growth is often slow, so that when a positive culture is obtained the load has probably already been used. The method is therefore of little value for routine use, but it still has a place in the testing of new equipment. A similar type of test can be used for ethylene-oxide sterilisation.

Other Physical Methods

Light. If a spectrum is thrown out on to an inoculated plate, it can be shown that most of the bactericidal activity resides in the ultraviolet band. Unfortunately ultraviolet light cannot penetrate to any extent. It can be used to disinfect surfaces. As an air disinfectant it is useful in virological laboratories, but it is unreliable in the presence of large particles of dust. These must first be filtered off, e.g. by electrostatic precipitation.

Ionising radiation. Both γ-rays and β-particles are used. This is a good method of sterilisation, for penetration is satisfactory and closed packs can be used. It is still outside the realm of hospital sterilisation, but is employed with increasing frequency commercially for plastic syringes, tubing, and blood transfusion equipment. These are disposable and should be discarded after use. This is not wasteful, because the expense of repeated cleaning and sterilising is obviated.

Filtration is used by microbiologists to sterilise fluids containing sera and amino acids, which would be denatured by heating. The most commonly-used filters are made either of asbestos discs, e.g. Seitz filters, or of finely-ground glass, fused sufficiently to make the small particles adhere (sintered-glass filters). Filtration is also used in the sterilisation of air in operating theatres. For this purpose disposable fabric and oiled mesh are the most satisfactory.

CHEMICAL DISINFECTANTS

A vast number of these have been tried, but mention will be made only of those in current use. A satisfactory agent should have the following qualities:

(*a*) It should be active against a wide range of organisms and spores. Only a few chemical agents are true sterilisers.

(*b*) It should have a rapid action.

(*c*) It should not be vitiated by organic matter like blood, pus, and faeces. In practice most of these agents combine indifferently with organisms and organic matter, and this impairs their disinfectant powers.

(*d*) It should not be toxic, irritating, or induce hypersensitivity.

Inorganic Disinfectants

Of these the most useful are the *halogens*. They have a rapid action against both vegetative organisms and spores, i.e they are true sterilisers. A grave disadvantage is the ease whereby their action is annulled by foreign organic matter. The halogens of greatest use are iodine and chlorine.

The most important **iodine** disinfectant is the tincture (Weak Iodine Solution, BP), which contains 25 per cent iodine and 2·5 per cent potassium iodide in approximately 90 per cent ethanol. It is the best skin disinfectant, but is irritating to raw areas and may induce an allergic contact dermatitis. More recent additions are the *iodophors*, which are solutions of iodine in non-ionic detergents. The iodine is complexed with surface-active agents, e.g. polyvinyl-pyrrolidone-iodine (povidone-iodine). They are less irritating and stain less than does the tincture, but their activity is equivalent to the available, as compared with the bound, iodine content. As skin disinfectants they are inferior to the tincture. They have also been used on floors with a mop, and are quite effective in disinfecting fomites.

Chlorine is used as sodium hypochlorite, chloramine, and eusol (Solution of Chlorinated Lime with Boric Acid, BPC). Chlorine is used extensively for the sterilisation of water, and the hypochlorite is excellent for disinfecting fomites. It can also be used to irrigate wounds.

The other inorganic disinfectants include the *salts of heavy metals* like mercury and silver, and *oxidising agents* like potassium permanganate and hydrogen peroxide. These are inferior to the halogens being slower in action, less bactericidal, and often more toxic.

Organic Disinfectants

Alcohols. It is interesting that, whereas pure ethanol is useless as a disinfectant, *70 per cent ethanol* is quite effective against vegetative organisms, but not spores. A 50–70 per cent solution of *isopropyl alcohol* is particularly useful as a skin disinfectant.

Aldehydes. *Commercial formalin*, a 37–41 per cent solution of formaldehyde gas in water, is a powerful disinfectant and a true steriliser. Its action is rather slow, and it penetrates organic matter slowly. Obvious disadvantages are its irritating odour and a tendency to produce sensitisation due to a residue of paraformaldehyde. Amongst other aldehydes, *glutaraldehyde* deserves special mention. As a 25 per cent aqueous solution diluted to 2 per cent with sodium bicarbonate solution it is of use as a steriliser for instruments that cannot be autoclaved. It is not volatile, and is less irritant and more rapidly sterilising than formalin.

Phenols. Phenol itself is a fairly efficient disinfectant, though neither it nor any of its many derivatives are true sterilisers. A great advantage of these substances is their continued activity in the presence of organic matter, which makes them admirable for the disinfection of faeces. Phenol itself is far too toxic and expensive to be used as a disinfectant, but closely-related substances, the cresols, are extensively used in routine hospital practice. *Lysol* is a solution of cresols in soap, and "Sudol" is a rather similar preparation. They are relatively cheap, and are somewhat less poisonous than pure phenol. They too are active in the presence of organic matter. Their disadvantages are the objectionable odour and irritant effect on the skin.

Another class of phenolic disinfectants is *chloroxylenol* and its compounds, of which "Dettol" is the best known. These are much less irritating and toxic than the others, but their efficiency is also less. They are inactivated by foreign organic matter. Probably the attached halogen group is responsible for this drawback.

More recently two phenolic derivatives of great importance have been introduced, chlorhexidine and hexachlorophane. *Chlorhexidine*, better known in Britain as "Hibitane", is an extremely powerful disinfectant against most vegetative organisms, especially Gram-positive ones, but not spores. It is of low toxicity. The parent substance is an odourless, white crystalline powder. It can be incorporated into watery or alcoholic solutions, and it provides an admirable disinfectant for the skin. It has been used as a bladder irrigant during cystoscopy. Incorporated in a cream it is often used in obstetrics, and it has also been employed to reduce the staphylococcal population of the hands of nurses.

Hexachlorophane (in the United States Pharmacopoeia it

is called hexachlorophene) is a whitish crystalline powder which often has a faint phenolic odour. Unlike chlorhexidine it is very insoluble in water and even in alcohol, but it can be incorporated into soap. A 1 per cent hexachlorophane soap is powerfully destructive to Gram-positive organisms but much less so to Gram-negative ones, so that *Pseudomonas pyocyanea* has been cultured from a stock bottle of 3 per cent hexachlorophane. Its use on several consecutive occasions cuts down the staphylococcal population of the skin quite remarkably, an effect due in some measure to its capacity to remain on the skin. It is a very useful tool both in the pre-operative toilet of a patient and in cutting down the residual staphylococcal flora on the hands of nursing attendants. A preparation of hexachlorophane mixed with a detergent is available as "pHisoHex".

Rats given hexachlorophane orally may develop cerebral lesions resembling the rare "spongy degeneration" found in infants. Although there is no evidence that this condition is due to hexachlorophane, it has been found that infants treated with the disinfectant (to reduce staphylococcal infection) sometimes have high blood levels of it. Certainly such infants should be thoroughly rinsed to diminish parenteral absorption of the disinfectant. Another hazard is the development of Gram-negative infections, unresponsive to hexachlorophane, in these infants. Because of the misgivings over the value of hexachlorophane and the possibility of its having toxic effects, this compound has been removed from many non-prescription medications.

Cationic surface-active agents. These dissociate in aqueous solution into a large, complex cation which is responsible for the surface activity, and a smaller inactive anion. The cation usually contains a pentavalent nitrogen atom which is often present as a quaternary ammonium group, and so these types of disinfectants are usually referred to as *quaternary ammonium compounds*. They have the usual emulsifying and detergent properties associated with surface-active agents, but in addition they are moderately bactericidal. The one that is best known and most widely used is *cetrimide*; this is a mixture of dodecyl-, tetradecyl-, and hexadecyl-trimethylammonium bromides, and is also known as "CTAB" or "Cetavlon". These compounds are colourless, odourless, non-irritating, and non-toxic in bactericidal doses. They do not act well in acid solutions, and are incompatible with soap, which is an anionic surface-active agent. They are moderately effective against Gram-positive organisms, but often less so than would appear at first sight. Their surface activity produces a delusive absence of organisms in a fluid medium; in fact many bacteria will be found adhering to free surfaces, e.g. the sides of the container. Against Gram-negative organisms this group of disinfectants is particularly ineffectual. Indeed, *Pseudomonas* organisms survive in bottles containing these compounds, after being introduced into them from bark corks used as stoppers. A particular danger with these agents is that they are adsorbed by fabrics. Hence if swabs are repeatedly dipped or soaked in

a solution of cetrimide, the active agent is removed and virtually all that remains is a bottle of contaminated water.

While these agents can be used as preliminary detergents in the pre-operative toilet of skin, they should not be relied on for disinfection.

Dyes. The *aniline dyes* are quite effective against Gram-positive organisms, particularly staphylococci, but their staining properties are a great nuisance.

The *acridine compounds* ("flavines") have a similar action against Gram-positive organisms, and they can be used in the treatment of wounds. In practice they have been superseded by chlorhexidine, which is more effective, faster, and has a wider range of activity.

GASEOUS DISINFECTANTS

Formalin vapour. The sterilising power of formaldehyde has already been noted. Cold formaldehyde does not penetrate well and is adsorbed by fabrics, but hot formaldehyde is much more useful, as it penetrates fabrics with greater ease. Since 3–4 per cent of people are sensitive to paraformaldehyde, formolisation cannot be regarded as a satisfactory commercial undertaking.

Ethylene oxide. This is a colourless fluid which boils at 12°C. It is a powerful steriliser, and has many advantages. Unlike formalin it *penetrates extremely well*, even going through plastics. It can be *used at a low temperature, leaves no residue, is a deodoriser*, and *is comparatively non-toxic*. It must be used at a relative humidity of 40–50 per cent, and unfortunately it is explosive and inflammable. This hazard is averted if it is used as a 10 per cent mixture with CO_2 or an inert gas. At 20–25°C sterilisation takes 18 hours, but if the temperature is raised to 50–60°C the period is reduced to 4 hours. Useful as this method is, it will not supplant the autoclave, which is more predictable in its effects and can be tested much more accurately. Ethylene oxide finds its main use as an alternative to ionising radiations in the sterilisation of plastics commercially, and in the sterilisation of heart-lung machines and similar apparatus in special hospitals.

PRACTICAL STERILISATION

The present tendency in hospitals is to use pre-sterilised, disposable equipment whenever possible, e.g. rubber gloves, scalpel blades, needles, syringes, biopsy punches, haemodialysis equipment, etc. Nevertheless, there are occasions when sterilisation must be performed on the spot, and it is useful to consider the disinfection of a few articles in common hospital use.

Dressings, theatre apparel, and gloves, should all be autoclaved. Provided the autoclave is working properly, there is no reason why gloves should perish in it. Destruction is due to oxidation, and if the air is completely expelled this cannot happen.

Surgical instruments. These too are best autoclaved.

Some surgeons object to the heating of sharp-edged instruments because of the alleged blunting that follows. This is due to oxidation, and should not occur in a properly functioning autoclave.

Chemical sterilisers may also be used. They usually contain formaldehyde as a disinfectant, and they must be non-rusting. A large number of these exist, and they usually contain formalin, phenol, and borax. In fact none of them is reliable, so they should be discarded. It is doubtful whether any of them will kill the spores of *Cl. tetani*.

Catheters. Rubber and plastic catheters can be boiled (spore-bearing organisms do not cause urinary-tract infections). Silk-web (gum-elastic) catheters are most difficult to sterilise. The usual method is suspension in formalin vapour, but this is quite inefficient, and in addition does not penetrate properly. If they are immersed in glutaraldehyde or mercuric chloride solutions, they will certainly be disinfected, but the agents have then to be removed prior to the use of the catheter. This is very difficult without an elaborate rinsing of the lumen. More recently 0·2 per cent chlorhexidine solution has been tried. Ethylene oxide vapour is another possibility. In fact no method is really satisfactory, and we must hope that disposable catheters, which are sterilised commercially by γ-radiation, will soon be available in bulk.

Cystoscopes and other endoscopes. The lens of these instruments is embedded in a cement which may be softened by heat. Pasteurisation at 75°C is usually innocuous to the instrument. A 0·5 per cent solution of chlorhexidine in 75 per cent ethanol has been used, but *Ps. pyocyanea* has been reported in it. A 0·02 per cent chlorhexidine solution combined with 0·05 per cent mercuric oxycyanide is said to be efficacious, and so is glutaraldehyde. The use of subatmospheric steam, preferably with added formaldehyde vapour, at 80°C appears to be the most effective method of sterilising cystoscopes (see p. 638). There are some cystoscopes on the market that can be boiled.

Polythene tubing. Heat causes softening; ionising radiation or ethylene oxide are the best sterilisers.

Anaesthetic face-masks. The mask with its rubber tubing is best disinfected by pasteurisation in water at about 70°C for a few minutes. Chemical disinfectants may damage the skin of the face of the next patient.

Suture material. Catgut is now prepared under licence by a special patent process in order to prevent the possibility of surgical tetanus. If it is rendered unsterile, it can be resterilised by immersion in Lugol's iodine solution for one week. All other suture materials can be autoclaved. The heat causes shrinkage, so the spools should be loosely wound.

Syringes. Plastic disposable syringes are commonly used, but if not available, the all-glass type should be acquired. If the nozzle and shoulder is of metal, it should be attached to the glass body by a cement that can withstand a high temperature. If the cement is of poor quality, the syringe will have to be boiled. In practice it is best to discard all such syringes. Autoclaving is not as satisfactory as dry heat in a hot-air oven, because the steam has to penetrate right through the syringe for sterilisation to be complete. This is impossible if a lubricated plunger is placed in position beforehand. In any case some moisture is bound to remain. This will cause haemolysis if the syringe is used to collect blood for diagnostic purposes.

Fomites. Urinals are best disinfected with a hypochlorite solution, and baths can also be treated with hypochlorite and a detergent. Bedpans should be disinfected with a 2 per cent lysol or 1 per cent "Sudol" solution. Alternatively, an automatic washer-disinfector can be employed. It first flushes the pan, and then exposes it to a jet of steam. This is particularly pleasant from the nurses' point of view. Bowls should be autoclaved. Hospital thermometers are best disinfected in 70 per cent ethanol, preferably with 1 per cent iodine added.

Blankets and other bedclothes. The disinfection of woollen blankets is very difficult. Boiling damages the fabric, and it should not be performed more than a few times a year. Hot formalin vapour, or better still ethylene oxide, is one possibility. The use of a quaternary ammonium compound after laundering at a low temperature is another. "Cirrasol OD", which is cetyl trimethylammonium bromide, is recommended. It is aesthetically objectionable that a new patient should have to use blankets left over from a previous one. It is to be hoped that soon a fabric like cotton will be in general use for the manufacture of blankets. Then each patient can receive clean, boiled blankets when he is admitted to the hospital (see p. 240).

Pillows and mattresses should be made of latex-foam rubber, in which case they can be sterilised by autoclaving, or else merely disinfected on the surface with a hypochlorite solution. If they are made of horse hair or feathers, the same difficulty arises as with blankets. Gaseous sterilisation with ethylene oxide or hot formalin vapour will have to be used.

Rooms. A contaminated room should be disinfected with hot formalin vapour. A less drastic procedure is a washing of all surfaces, including furniture, with a detergent solution and hypochlorite.

Disinfection of skin. As already mentioned, there is no effective method of skin sterilisation. An excellent agent for the pre-operative treatment of skin is tincture of iodine; a patch test should be performed before the operation to detect the hypersensitive patient. Dilute (70 per cent) ethanol on its own is not bad, but cetrimide cannot be relied on. Another good skin disinfectant is 0·5 per cent chlorhexidine in 70 per cent ethanol, but povidone-iodine containing 1 per cent available iodine is better. For surgical personnel an alcoholised chlorhexidine solution is valuable. The continual use of hexachlorophane liquid soap, preferably containing a phenolic preservative chlorocresol (0·3 per cent), is slightly less effective.

The ritual of applying an antiseptic to the skin for a few seconds before taking a blood sample or giving an injection, although commonly practised, is probably of little value, and its omission does not result in local infection. When complete asepsis is required, as with intra-articular or intrathecal manipulations, a thorough skin preparation is necessary.

After attending an infected patient, the hands should be thoroughly scrubbed, and then immersed in an alcohol or hypochlorite solution.

In many up-to-date hospitals the sterilisation of instruments is carried out in a single **central sterile supply department**, which is supervised by the hospital microbiologist. The danger of inadequately sterilised articles is greatly lessened. The nurses' time is saved, and there is little likelihood of instruments being sterilised for too short a period because of impatience or negligence on the part of the staff. The increase in staff that such a department demands is more than offset by the increased efficiency and safety of the finished product.

The maintenance of hospital sterilisation is now a speciality in its own right, and it is just that special regard should be paid to it. The advantages that it brings are much more substantial than those of many other procedures that are carried out in modern hospitals!

REFERENCES

For further information the following sources are recommended:
WILSON, G. S. and MILES, A. A. (1964). In Topley and Wilson's *Principles of Bacteriology and Immunity*, 5th edn, pp. 127–172. London: Arnold. This gives a good account of the principles of disinfection with special regard to chemical agents.
DUGUID, J. P. (1965). In *Medical Microbiology*, 11th edn, pp. 679–721. Edited by Cruickshank, R. Edinburgh: Livingstone. This contains a detailed description of the autoclave.
WILLIAMS, R. E. O., BLOWERS, R., GARROD, L. P. and SHOOTER, R. A. (1966). In *Hospital Infection*, 2nd edn, pp. 291–346. London: Lloyd-Luke. An excellent practical account of hospital disinfection.
KELSEY, J. C. (1964 and 1968). In *Recent Advances in Clinical Pathology*, Series IV, pp. 57–68, and Series V, pp. 101–111. Edited by Duke, S. C. London: Churchill. This provides an addendum about current views on sterilisation.

Appendix 2. The Principles of Bacteriological Diagnosis

THE GENERAL PROPERTIES OF BACTERIA

CONSTITUTION

Although bacteria are generally unicellular, they are often found attached one to another in the form of clusters, chains, or, in the higher *Actinomyces* organisms, an elaborate mass of filaments.

Bacteria vary in size: staphylococci and streptococci are 0·75–1·25 μm in diameter, while one of the largest bacilli, *Bacillus anthracis*, is 1–1·25 μm thick and 3–8 μm long. *Haemophilus influenzae* is a very small bacterium, measuring 0·2–0·4 μm $\times$ 0·7–1·5 μm.

The bacterial body is contained in a rigid cell wall 10–25 nm thick, which encloses a thin cytoplasmic membrane 5–10 nm thick, composed of lipoprotein. On electron microscopy the bacterial cytoplasm is homogeneous and granular. This granularity is due to innumerable ribosomes which contain RNA and manufacture the bacterial proteins and enzymes. There is no endoplasmic reticulum and no mitochondria. The enzymes are present in the cytoplasmic membrane.

The bacterial DNA is contained in the nuclear body. This has no nuclear membrane, nucleolus, or separate chromosomes. It appears that all the bacterial genes are contained by a single linkage group, or chromosome. It is probably a long fibre folded on itself in the form of a skein. There is usually only one nuclear body in each bacterium, but as its division precedes that of the bacterial cell, there is often the suggestion of two, four, or even more.

Bacteria divide by simple binary fission which involves the nuclear body also. There is no evidence of mitosis. The cell divides into two by constriction with or without primary septation. A few groups exhibit sexual conjugation.

ASSOCIATED STRUCTURES

Intracellular granules. Many organisms contain granular aggregations of metabolic substances in their cytoplasm, e.g. volutin, lipid, and starch. *Volutin granules* are particularly important. They stain metachromatically with toluidine blue, turning a violet colour. The nature of volutin granules is obscure; they are said to contain polymerised inorganic polyphosphate which may act as a reserve of energy for cell metabolism. They are of importance in the identification of *Corynebacterium diphtheriae*.

Capsules. A capsule is a gelatinous layer 0·2 μm or more in width which covers the wall of a bacterium. It is usually composed of polysaccharide, but sometimes it is of polypeptide or protein nature. Capsules are of the greatest importance in contributing to the virulence of an organism, and are also of use in typing procedures; both these features are, of course, due to the specific antigens or haptens contained in them. Important capsulated bacteria are the pneumococcus, *Clostridium welchii*, *B. anthracis*, and *Klebsiella pneumoniae*.

Flagella. These are filamentous appendages which act as organs of locomotion, and are possessed by all motile bacteria except spirochaetes, whose motility is apparently a function of the bacterial body itself. Flagella originate in the cytoplasm, and protrude through the cell wall. They contain a protein called *flagellin*, which is related to *myosin*, the contractile protein of muscle.

Fimbriae. These too are filamentous appendages. They are shorter and thinner than flagella, and have nothing to do with locomotion, since they are found in non-motile organisms. It is possible that they act as organs of adhesion to free surfaces.

Spores. A spore is a highly resistant resting phase of a bacterium. It is formed within the body of the organism, i.e it is an endospore, and eventually the whole organism is converted into a single, thick-walled mass which is round or oval in shape, and highly refractile.

Sporulation in bacteria is not a process of multiplication; it is merely a method of survival during unfavourable circumstances, e.g. starvation, desiccation, extremes of temperature, and unsuitable atmospheric conditions. It incorporates some of the chromatin material as well as the bacterial cytoplasm. Spores are characteristic of only a few genera, e.g. *Bacillus* and *Clostridium*. They appear either subterminally, terminally, or equatorially in relation to the bacterial body, and eventually the remainder of the organism disintegrates. The free spore survives, and germinates when conditions are propitious.

L-forms. These are degenerate bacterial variants, first described in the Lister Institute, London (hence the letter L), which are seen in connexion with cocci, bacilli, and vibrios. They lack a rigid cell wall and therefore vary greatly in size and shape—the largest are 10–20 μm and the smallest only 0·1 μm long. They are resistant to the action of penicillin regardless of the sensitivity of the parent organism. L-forms can be isolated from patients with bacterial infections especially if on penicillin or cephalosporin treatment, and can also be induced in culture by drugs, lysozyme, nutritional deficiency, or the action of amboceptor and complement. A variant of L-form obtained from Gram-positive organisms by the action of penicillin or lysozyme is called the *protoplast*. It contains no cell wall, and differs from the usual L-forms in that it can survive only in a hypertonic environment and usually fails to grow in artificial media. Similar spherical variants of Gram-negative organisms have a cell wall which is defective due to the absence of a strengthening muco-protein. These are called *spheroplasts*. Protoplasts and sphero-plasts are laboratory artefacts. L-forms, unlike protoplasts and spheroplasts, can multiply on hypertonic medium, on which characteristic tiny "fried-egg" colonies are produced.

Some L-forms revert to the normal bacterial form especi-ally if the inducing agent, e.g. penicillin, is removed. Others however, are stable and do not revert. These resemble mycoplasma in appearance, but tend to be somewhat larger. They are said to be non-pathogenic to animals, and their relationship to disease is not known (see p. 92).

DEMONSTRATION OF BACTERIA

Unstained preparations are of limited value. The general shape and motility can be ascertained in fluid preparations viewed between a glass slide and a cover-slip. Some organisms, e.g. the spirochaetes, are so slender and feebly refractible that only dark-ground illumination can reveal their presence.

Staining. *Organisms can be made visible with simple stains* like methylene blue and basic fuchsin.

The Gram technique is of greater value, because it helps to distinguish between different groups of organisms. It is described later on. A Gram-positive organism resists decolorisation by alcohol or acetone after it has been stained with a pararosaniline dye, e.g. crystal violet or methyl violet, and then treated with an iodine solution. A Gram-negative organism is decolorised, and takes up the red counter-stain.

This difference in Gram-staining is fundamental, and is reflected in basic differences in the reaction of the organism to antibiotics and disinfectants. Its mechanism is uncertain. It is established that Gram-positivity depends on the in-tegrity of the cellular structure and the presence in the cell of a specific magnesium ribonucleate-protein complex. If the magnesium ribonucleate is removed, a Gram-positive organism becomes Gram-negative. What part the cell wall plays in aiding (or preventing) decolorisation is unknown; it is possible that the wall of a Gram-positive organism is less permeable to the decoloriser than that of a Gram-negative organism.

Flagella and capsules can be demonstrated only by special techniques,* and fimbriae are revealed by means of

---

* *Capsules* are best demonstrated by "negative" or "relief" staining, in which a smear of the organisms is stained with India ink. The unstained capsular areas contrast with the refractile organism and the diffusely stained background.

Flagella are so thin that they can be made visible with the light microscope only after a thick layer of stain has been deposited on them. A mixture of basic fuchsin and tannic acid is efficacious.

the electron microscope. Spores appear as clear spaces within Gram-stained organisms; they do not take up the stain, no doubt because of their thick walls.

Ziehl-Neelsen staining. This is also described later on. It depends on the fact that a few organisms, notably the genus *Mycobacterium*, are particularly rich in lipids. These not only prevent the entry of the usual stains, but also retain any concentrated stain that may have been forced into them by the process of heating. Even strong acid will then not de-colorise these organisms. If the lipids are extracted with fat solvents, this *acid-fastness* is lost.

SHAPE

The following shapes are recognised:

Cocci—spherical (or nearly spherical) cells, e.g. *Staphy-lococcus pyogenes*.

Bacilli—straight and rod-shaped cells, e.g. *Escherichia coli*.

Vibrios—curved and rod-shaped cells—"comma-shaped", e.g. *Vibrio cholerae*.

Spirilla—spirally-twisted rods which are not capable of bending, e.g. *Spirillum minus*.

Spirochaetes—these resemble spirilla, but have an intrinsic bending motion, e.g. *Treponema pallidum*.

Actinomycetes—simple branching filaments aggregated into compact colonies, e.g. *Actinomyces bovis*.

NUTRITIONAL DEMANDS

Nearly all bacteria can grow on artificial cell-free media (*Myco. leprae* and *Tr. pallidum* are exceptions). The nutri-tional requirements are:

(*a*) A source of energy for such metabolic processes as growth and motility.

(*b*) A source of carbon, nitrogen, various inorganic salts, e.g. sulphates and phosphates of sodium, potassium, calcium, and iron, and finally certain *accessory growth factors*. These are "bacterial vitamins", and are necessary for the synthesis of essential metabolites in certain organisms.

Some non-parasitic bacteria are able to utilise CO_2 as a source of carbon, while energy is obtained from the oxidation of inorganic chemicals or directly from sunlight. Most bacteria, however, including all the parasitic ones, require organic nutrients such as carbohydrate, amino acids, and lipids. Some, e.g. *Esch. coli*, are able to synthesise their own amino acids from a source of inorganic nitrogen such as nitrates or ammonium salts.

Most of the pathogens are very exacting in their demands, and require a wide range of amino acids, e.g. tryptophane, methionine, and histidine, and growth factors, e.g. purines and pyrimidines, for nucleic-acid synthesis, and most of the vitamin-B group as precursors for the formation of co-enzymes.

In addition, bacteria vary widely in their oxygen require-ments. Obligatory anaerobes cannot tolerate the presence of oxygen, perhaps because they are damaged by the peroxides they produce. Normally these are destroyed by the enzyme catalase, but anaerobes are lacking in it.

GROWTH PHASES

When bacteria are inoculated into a sterile fluid culture medium and serial counts are performed on viable organisms, the following four phases of multiplication are noted:

Lag phase, which lasts about two hours. There is no change in number, though the size of the bacteria increases.

Logarithmic phase, which lasts up to eight hours in optimal conditions. There is a regular, maximal proliferation of bacteria increasing in geometrical progression per unit time.

Stationary phase, which lasts for several hours to a few days. There is no increase in numbers, as the death rate is as great as that of reproduction.

Phase of decline, which is completed from a few days to some months. The viable count gradually diminishes until the culture becomes sterile once more. The cause of the decline is presumably a combination of exhaustion of nutriment and an accumulation of toxic waste matter.

THE DIAGNOSIS OF INFECTIVE DISEASE

This is based on three postulates originally laid down by Koch (*Koch's postulates*).

1. *The organism should be found in the lesion in a quantity adequate to account for its effects.* In toxic bacterial infections, e.g. due to *C. diphtheriae* and *Cl. tetani*, the remote effects are due to exotoxins, and the organism is present only in the local lesion. Organisms that act by hypersensitivity, e.g. *Myco. tuberculosis* and *Tr. pallidum*, are sometimes very scanty in the lesions they produce, e.g. gummata. On the other hand, carriers may transmit pathogenic organisms in the absence of overt pathological lesions.

2. *The organism from the lesion should be cultivated in a pure state on an artificial medium.* Most bacteria fulfil this requirement; *Myco. leprae* and *Tr. pallidum* are exceptions. The cultivation of viruses requires living cells (see Chapter 22).

3. *The organism grown in artificial culture should be capable of producing a similar lesion in another member of the species.* Theoretically this would entail human transference, which is impracticable except in volunteers. Animal inoculation is used instead of this. As regards viruses the second and third postulates often merge, because the animal provides the living cells necessary for viral growth. On the whole, animal inoculation does not play an important part in routine bacteriological diagnosis; tuberculosis is an exception. Other bacterial infections in which animal inoculation is necessary for diagnosis are diphtheria, anthrax, plague, glanders, and leptospiral jaundice.

A fourth postulate was added after Koch's time: *the presence in the circulation of antibodies against the organism in the later stages of the illness and during convalescence.*

It therefore follows that in routine bacteriological diagnosis the organism should be isolated from the pathological material:

(*a*) by demonstrating it directly using Gram's or Ziehl-Neelsen's stains.

(*b*) by culturing it on suitable media. Animal inoculation is seldom necessary.

If the organism is scanty, e.g. in the blood, it may be demonstrable only by culture methods. Direct examination is seldom successful.

PRACTICAL BACTERIOLOGY

COLLECTION OF SPECIMENS

Pus. This may be taken on a swab, which should then be tightly inserted into a test-tube, so that it does not undergo desiccation. Large amounts of pus are conveniently collected in screw-capped universal containers.

Exudates, e.g. pleural fluid, are collected in universal containers. If a cytological examination is required, an anticoagulant, e.g. potassium oxalate, should be added.

Urine. In both sexes a midstream specimen should be taken. Catheterisation should be avoided (see p. 237). The urine is collected in a universal container.

Sputum and faeces are collected in waxed or plastic cartons which are burnt and destroyed after use.

In the collection of specimens care must be taken to avoid (*a*) desiccation; (*b*) contamination of the specimen; (*c*) infection of personnel handling the material.

THE STAINING OF BACTERIA

The pus or exudate is transferred on to a clean slide, and a film is made. After drying, it is fixed on to the slide by passing it rapidly through a flame. Staining is then carried out:

Gram's stain. (i) 0·5 per cent methyl violet for about 1 minute.

(ii) Wash off with Lugol's or Gram iodine, and apply more iodine solution for about 2 minutes.

(iii) Decolorise with ethanol until the stain ceases to come out of the preparation.

(iv) Wash with water, and counter-stain with 0·1 per cent neutral red for about 2 minutes.

Gram-positive organisms, e.g. staphylococci, streptococci, pneumococci, clostridia, anthrax bacilli, diphtheria bacilli, actinomyces, and fungi, stain blue, whereas *Gram-negative organisms*, e.g. *Neisseria* organisms and intestinal bacilli of the coli-typhoid type, stain red. The nuclei of pus cells are also Gram-negative.

Ziehl-Neelsen stain. This is reserved for *Mycobacteria*, the waxy content of which is impermeable to Gram's stain.

(i) Flood strong carbol fuchsin on to the slide, and keep it steaming for 5 minutes.

(ii) Wash with water, and then apply 20 per cent sulphuric acid. This is washed off after about a minute, and reapplied several times until no more stain comes out of the preparation.

(iii) Wash with water, and apply absolute ethanol for 2 minutes.*

(iv) Wash with water, and counter-stain with 1 per cent methylene blue or malachite green for about 20 seconds.

Acid-fast material stains red; everything else is blue or green. *Myco. leprae* is less acid fast than *Myco. tuberculosis*, and the preparation should be decolorised with 5 per cent sulphuric acid. Some *Nocardia* species are also acid fast, and so are the granules of lipofuscin.

THE CULTIVATION OF BACTERIA

Culture media are divided into 2 classes, fluid and solid:

Fluid media. The basic medium is called *nutrient broth*, which is a mixture of meat extract (Lab-Lemco), commercial bacteriological peptone (a mixture of peptones, amino acids, vitamins, and salts, obtained from the enzymatic breakdown of lean meat and other protein material), sodium chloride, and water.

Some laboratories make up their own broth by extracting lean beef or ox heart muscle in watery solution and then adding peptone and salt (*infusion broth*), or by digesting the meat with trypsin (*digest broth*), in which case peptone does not need to be added. A special fluid medium is *Robertson's meat medium*, which is useful for culturing anaerobes (see Chapter 18).

Fluid media are useful for promoting the growth of bacteria when these are scanty, but they have two disadvantages:

(i) They are of little value in identifying individual organisms.

(ii) They are of no use in separating mixtures of organisms.

Solid media. The usual solidifying element in solid media is agar, a polysaccharide substance derived from certain seaweeds, and the basic solid medium is *nutrient agar*. This consists of nutrient both solidified by the addition of agar (1·2–2 per cent depending on the type). It forms a gel, stable at temperatures well above 37°C.

Nutrient agar can support the growth of some organisms, e.g. staphylococci, but others, like streptococci and *Neisseria* organisms, require the presence of blood or serum products. This is described as *enrichment* of a medium. Although nutrient agar melts at about 95°C, it remains fluid on subsequent cooling down to a temperature as low as 40°C. Therefore blood or serum can be incorporated into molten nutrient agar at about 45°C, at which temperature there is no denaturation of its proteins.

Solid media are usually distributed in flat glass or plastic plates called Petri dishes. They may also be placed in small bottles, universal containers, or test-tubes. The molten medium is allowed to solidify while the container is tilted at an angle. This is a "slope" culture medium.

Blood agar. This consists of 5–10 per cent horse blood in nutrient agar. It is the standard solid medium used in bacteriological laboratories.

Serum agar. This consists of 10 per cent animal serum in nutrient agar. It is useful for the cultivation of gonococci and meningococci, and for demonstrating the volutin granules of *C. diphtheriae*.

Chocolate agar. This is blood agar which is heated to boiling point for about a minute. The breakdown products of haemoglobin, especially haematin ("X Factor"), are useful for the growth of *H. influenzae*.

Solid media enable individual bacteria to grow into discrete, recognisable colonies, and are essential for the identification of organisms. If there are few bacteria in a specimen, it is wise to start with a fluid medium and then to subculture some of this on to a solid medium.

Selective media. If certain substances are added to a fluid or solid medium, they may promote the growth of a particular type of bacterium while inhibiting that of all other organisms. The following selective media are commonly used:

MacConkey's medium. This consists of a peptone solution solidified with agar, to which is added a bile salt (sodium taurocholate), lactose, and a neutral-red indicator. The bile salt inhibits most organisms, but promotes the growth of the Gram-negative intestinal group. *Esch. coli* ferments lactose, and turns the indicator pink (see Chapter 17).

Deoxycholate-citrate-agar. This works on the same principle as MacConkey's medium, but sodium deoxycholate is used instead of sodium taurocholate, and sodium citrate, sodium thiosulphate, and ferric ammonium citrate are included. These salts inhibit the growth of *Esch. coli* while promoting that of *Salmonella* and *Shigella* organisms. This medium is used for the bacteriological examination of faeces, because even in the presence of a typhoid or dysentery infection there is such a predominance of *Esch. coli* that a MacConkey plate would be overgrown with this organism at the expense of all others.

Tetrathionate broth and selenite-F enrichment medium. These two fluid media contain sodium tetrathionate and sodium selenite respectively. These salts are particularly inhibitory to coliform organisms, while allowing *Salmonella* organisms to grow freely. If faeces contain scanty numbers of these organisms, it is best to culture them initially in these selective fluid media, and then to subculture them a day later on to deoxycholate-citrate-agar.

Potassium tellurite media. A considerable number of media containing this salt are in use for the selective growth and identification of *C. diphtheriae*. They inhibit the growth of most of the other organisms found in the throat.

Sodium chloride is useful for the selective cultivation of staphylococci. It is conveniently incorporated into Robertson's meat medium in a 10 per cent concentration.

Sabouraud's medium. This simple medium contains only glucose and peptone as its nutrients, and the low pH and high sugar content make it selective for fungi as against

---

* 3 per cent HCl in 95 per cent ethanol may be substituted for (ii) and (iii).

bacterial contaminants. Antibacterial agents, usually chloramphenicol and cycloheximide, are often added.

Temperature. Nearly all pathogenic organisms grow best at body temperature (37°C). *Myco. ulcerans* and *Myco. balnei* are exceptions, growing best at 31–33°C. Rhinoviruses also need a temperature of 33°C, while some pathogenic fungi grow at room temperature.

Atmospheric conditions. Most organisms flourish well in air, but a few are strict anaerobes (e.g. clostridia). If their presence is suspected, the medium must be incubated in a *McIntosh and Fildes anaerobic jar*. Alternatively, Robertson's meat medium can be used. Gonococci demand an atmosphere containing 5 per cent CO_2, and *Brucella abortus* one of 10 per cent CO_2.

EXAMINATION OF INDIVIDUAL SPECIMENS

PUS

The usual organisms to be expected in pus are:
Pyogenic cocci, i.e. staphylococci and streptococci.
Gram-negative intestinal bacilli.
Clostridial organisms in infected wounds. These organisms seldom occur alone, but are found together with the others.
Myco. tuberculosis and *Actino. israeli* in chronic lesions.

Smear and Gram-stain. In true pus there are numerous pus cells and usually groups of causative organisms among them. If there is only amorphous debris, it is suggestive of tuberculosis.

Culture on blood agar aerobically and anaerobically. Anaerobic culture is essential in all pus from infected wounds, and some of the material must also be inoculated into Robertson's meat medium in case the anaerobic technique is faulty. The meat medium can be subcultured on to blood-agar the next day. In pus from abdominal wounds MacConkey's medium may be used in addition to blood agar because of the probability of infection with Gram-negative intestinal bacilli.

After 24 hours the plates are examined. Staphylococci are coagulase tested, and β-haemolytic streptococci may be Lancefield grouped (see Chapter 17). The Gram-negative intestinal group may need further investigation. If clostridia are isolated, a Nagler test (see Chapter 18) is worth performing. Antibiotic sensitivities are carried out on all pathogenic organisms.

If *tuberculosis* is suspected, a Ziehl-Neelsen stain should be done on the pus (it is usually negative), and some of the material should be inoculated on to Löwenstein-Jensen medium, and some injected into a guinea-pig (see Chapter 20). Six weeks may elapse before a positive result is forthcoming.

If *actinomycosis* is suspected, the pathognomonic sulphur granules must be isolated by shaking up the pus in sterile water. The granules sink rapidly to the bottom, and are easily removed by suction with a Pasteur pipette. They are then crushed between two slides and stained. Some are inoculated on to blood agar and incubated anaerobically (see Chapter 20).

URINE

The usual infecting organisms are:

(*a*) Gram-negative intestinal bacilli.
(*b*) *Strept. faecalis.*
(*c*) *Myco. tuberculosis*, an important cause of "sterile" pyuria.

Centrifuge some of the urine at about 2 000 revolutions per minute for 5–10 minutes, and examine a drop of the unstained deposit under the low power of a microscope at once. The presence of white cells ("pus cells"), red cells, and casts is to be noted. Sometimes motile organisms can be seen among the cells. Gram-staining is not necessary as a routine measure.

More than one white cell per high power field is abnormal, **and then the urine should be cultured on blood agar.** Anaerobic culture is not necessary. MacConkey's medium can also be used.

Nowadays in the investigation of chronic pyelonephritis more precise quantitative tests are done, because a bacterial growth may be merely an expression of contamination by bacteria resident in the urethra. The most important is a *bacterial count*; contamination does not produce a count of more than 10 000 bacteria per ml. Urinary-tract infections are associated with counts above 100 000 per ml, because the bacteria multiply in the urine.

Another test of some value is the *white-cell excretion rate*; if above 200 000 cells per hour it is probably abnormal. Unfortunately it is difficult to distinguish between leucocytes and epithelial cells, but it is less crude than the centrifugation method.

In the investigation of *tuberculosis* it is best to collect three consecutive early-morning specimens of urine, centrifuge them, and stain and culture the sediments.

PLEURAL AND PERITONEAL EXUDATES

The infecting organisms may be pyogenic cocci, e.g. pneumococci, or else *Myco. tuberculosis*.

Smear and Gram-stain of centrifuged deposit.

Culture on to blood agar. It is advisable to culture some of the specimen in nutrient broth, because organisms tend to be scanty in exudates. The broth is subcultured on to blood agar the next day.

If *tuberculosis* is suspected, it is useful to examine the cells in some detail. A tuberculous effusion contains a large number of lymphocytes. The sediment is then stained and cultured.

CEREBRO-SPINAL FLUID

The common infecting organisms are (*a*) meningococci, (*b*) pneumococci, (*c*) *H. influenzae*, (*d*) *Myco. tuberculosis*. The first three produce a frankly purulent fluid, whereas in tuberculous meningitis the fluid is clear and colourless. A "spider-web clot" tends to form as the fluid sediments in the universal container. The fluid must also be examined cytologically and chemically.

Cell count. This is normally not more than 3 lymphocytes per μl.

Biochemistry. The normal range is:

Glucose	60–90 mg per 100 ml
Protein	15–40 mg per 100 ml
Chloride	120–127 m.Eq per litre.

The protein content is raised in all types of meningitis (including virus ones). Both sugar and chloride levels are reduced in all types of bacterial meningitis especially the tuberculous variety.

Smear and Gram-stain of centrifuged deposit. In tuberculous cases some of the spider-web clot is spread on to a slide and stained by the Ziehl-Neelsen method.

Culture on to blood agar; serum agar is useful for meningococci, and chocolate agar for *H. influenzae*. If tuberculosis is suspected, the sediment is carefully collected and cultured.

The term *aseptic meningitis* is applied to clinical conditions of meningitis in which the cerebro-spinal fluid contains an excess of cells (mostly lymphocytes) and protein, but is bacteriologically sterile. It is usually caused by viruses, e.g. (*a*) enteroviruses including polioviruses, (*b*) lymphocytic choriomeningitis virus, (*c*) arboviruses, (*d*) herpes-simplex virus, (*e*) occasionally as a complication of zoster, vaccinia, mumps (which causes a definite encephalitis), measles, influenza, and chickenpox.

BLOOD CULTURE

The important organisms are *Strept. viridans* in subacute infective endocarditis; *Salmonella typhi* and *S. paratyphi A, B, and C*; *Staph. pyogenes* and *Strept. pyogenes*; Gram-negative pyogenic intestinal bacilli; *Brucella* organisms.

About 5–10 ml of blood is collected aseptically from a forearm vein, and is cultured in 50–100 ml of nutrient or digest broth. A large amount of blood is needed, because organisms are usually very scanty even in pronounced septicaemias. A large amount of medium is used in order to dilute natural bactericidal and bacteriostatic substances present in the blood. Trypsin or "Liquoid" (sodium poly-anetholesulphonate) is often incorporated into the broth to annul any such bactericidal activity. In cases of suspected typhoid fever some of the blood should be inoculated into broth containing 0·5 per cent sodium taurocholate. Penicillinase may be added if the patient has been treated with penicillin.

Occasionally subacute infective endocarditis is caused by an anaerobic streptococcus; it is therefore advisable to inoculate some of the blood anaerobically in Robertson's meat medium. *Coxiella burneti* is another cause of endocarditis.

The broth is incubated for 24 hours, and then films of it are made and stained with Gram's stain. Some of it is sub-cultured on to blood agar (and MacConkey's medium, if typhoid fever is likely). This procedure is repeated for 4 consecutive days and after the first and second weeks. After 14 days the culture may be discarded except if brucellosis is suspected, when at least 3 weeks should elapse before a negative result is reported. For *Br. arbortus* the blood-culture must be incubated in an atmosphere of 10 per cent CO_2.

Under unusual circumstances, as following open-heart surgery or in patients on immunosuppressive therapy, endocarditis may be caused by almost any organism, including some like *Staph. albus* that are generally considered to be non-pathogenic, and also fungi. The repeated culture of an organism from the blood-stream should not be lightly dismissed as due to contamination.

SPUTUM

This contains a large number of organisms, e.g. staphylococci, streptococci, pneumococci, Gram-negative intestinal bacilli, and *H. influenzae*. These are isolated quite easily by aerobic culture on blood agar. Colonies of *H. influenzae* tend to aggregate around staphylococcal colonies, a feature called *satellitism*. This is because staphylococci synthesise a factor (the "V factor") which is essential for the growth of *H. influenzae*.

The most important bacterium to be sought in sputum is *Myco. tuberculosis*. When present it should be easily detectable on direct examination. A purulent portion is selected and stained by the Ziehl-Neelsen technique, or else fluorescence microscopy can be used after staining with auramine. In this case the auramine is simply substituted for strong carbol fuchsin. Under the fluorescence microscope the organisms are yellow and luminous against a black background.

In culturing for *Myco. tuberculosis* the sputum must first be homogenised in alkaline or acid solutions, which destroy other organisms while leaving the tubercle bacilli intact. Guinea-pig inoculation should not often be required; direct examination confirmed by Löwenstein-Jensen culture is generally adequate and indeed essential if atypical mycobacteria are to be identified. Culture is important to assess the sensitivity of the organism to antituberculous agents.

FAECES

The important pathogenic bacteria in faeces are the *Salmonella* and *Shigella* species. Enteropathogenic *Esch. coli* may cause epidemics of infantile diarrhoea.

Organism	Lactose	Glucose	Mannitol	Saccharose
SALMONELLA TYPHI	Nil	Acid only	Acid only	Nil
SALMONELLA TYPHIMURIUM	Nil	Acid and gas	Acid and gas	Nil
SHIGELLA SONNEI	Delayed acid only	Acid only	Acid only	Delayed acid only
SHIGELLA SHIGAE	Nil	Acid only	Nil	Nil

Emulsify a suspicious portion of the faeces with saline, and examine it microscopically (unstained). The presence of pus cells suggests a bacillary type of dysentery, but ulcerative colitis and carcinoma of the colon may produce a similar appearance. The presence of amoebae, cysts, and parasitic ova is also noted.

Some of the faeces are inoculated directly on to deoxycholate-citrate-agar, and some into the tetrathionate and selenite-F enrichment media.

The next day colourless colonies are sought on the solid medium, and at the same time the fluid enrichment media are subcultured on to deoxycholate-citrate-agar. They are examined the next day.

Colourless colonies are picked off and subcultured in peptone water.

About 6 hours later the peptone water is subcultured into other peptone waters containing various sugars (e.g. lactose, glucose, mannitol, and saccharose) and a pH indicator. Into the fluid medium there is placed a small inverted tube called a *Durham fermentation tube*. Within 24 hours the organism will have formed acid (with or without gas, which accumulates in the Durham tube) with some, all, or none of the sugars. The above table gives an indication of how the fermentation reactions help in the identification of these organisms.

Other tests of value are indole formation in peptone water (in some *Shigella* species) and urea decomposition to ammonia (which excludes *Proteus* organisms).

Finally, identification is performed by means of agglutination reactions, using specific antisera prepared from rabbits immunised against these organisms.

For enteropathogenic *Esch. coli*, MacConkey's medium is used. It is impossible to distinguish between enteropathogenic and non-enteropathogenic strains by their colonial appearance. All that can be done is to pick off a number of colonies from the plate and perform agglutination tests using specific antisera obtained by immunising rabbits against known enteropathogenic strains.

THROAT SWAB. Important organisms to be sought are *Strept. pyogenes* and *C. diphtheriae*.

Smear and Gram-stain is useful for demonstrating *Borrelia vincenti*, *Fusobacterium fusiforme*, and *Candida albicans*.

Culture. (i) Blood agar for streptococci and *Candida albicans*.

(ii) Serum agar is excellent for stimulating the development of volutin granules in *C. diphtheriae*.

(iii) Tellurite selective media of the solid type not only favour the growth of *C. diphtheriae*, but also show colonial differences between the three types of the organism—gravis, intermedius, and mitis.

If suspicious colonies appear on the tellurite plate, sugar reactions (using serum-water) are carried out to differentiate between harmless diphtheroid organisms and diphtheria bacilli, which ferment glucose but not sucrose.

Finally, pathogenicity tests are performed on guinea-pigs.

REFERENCES

For further information the following sources are recommended:

WILSON, G. S. and MILES, A. A. (1964). In Topley and Wilson's *Principles of Bacteriology and Immunity*, 5th edn, pp. 16–126. London: Arnold. This constitutes a comprehensive study of bacterial morphology, metabolism and growth.

DUGUID, J. P., HAYWARD, N. J. and COLLEY, J. G. (1965). In *Medical Microbiology*, 11th edn, pp. 642–678, 722–809. Edited by Cruickshank, R. Edinburgh: Livingstone. These three chapters give good accounts of staining procedures and culture media used in bacteriology.

DAVIS, B. D., DULBECCO, R., EISEN, H. N., GINSBERG, H. S. and WOOD, W. B. (1967). *Microbiology*, 1464 pp. New York: Harper and Row.

Appendix 3.   The Physics of Ionising Radiation

One pictures an atom as composed of a central nucleus surrounded by a cloud of orbiting *electrons*. Practically all the mass of the atom resides in its nucleus, which (with the exception of hydrogen) consists of a densely-packed assembly of *protons* and *neutrons*. These two particles are of equal mass ($1 \cdot 66 \times 10^{-24}$ g), the proton having a unit positive electrical charge and the neutron having none. An electron has a unit negative charge, but its mass is only about $1/2\,000$ of that of a proton or neutron.

The so-called *atomic number* Z of an element is defined as the number of protons in the nucleus. With the atom in its normal state there is an equal number of orbiting electrons, so that as a whole the atom is electrically neutral. The chemical nature of an element is decided by the number Z. Thus an atom of atomic number Z has Z protons and Z electrons. The *mass number* is the total number of protons and neutrons present in the nucleus.

Hydrogen (Z = 1, the lightest atom) is exceptional, in that in its most common form there are no neutrons in its nucleus but only a single proton, and there is but one orbiting electron. It therefore has the simplest possible atomic structure. It can also exist in two further forms, or *isotopes*.* Chemically these are identical, but they differ in those physical properties which are related to mass.

Hydrogen atom	Deuterium atom	Tritium atom
Atomic Number 1	Atomic Number 1	Atomic Number 1
Mass Number 1	Mass Number 2	Mass Number 3

Figure 111.1

Atoms of higher atomic number have their electrons arranged in definite orbits, or shells, each of which can contain only a precise maximum number of electrons. Thus, the inner shell (K) can contain only two, as in helium.

The chemical stability of an atom depends upon the number of electrons in its outer shell. With the first shell two electrons give stability. The helium atom is stable, while

* Many elements exist in nature as a mixture of isotopes each with the same atomic number Z, but with different mass numbers. The average of the mass numbers is the atomic weight. Thus, chlorine exists as a mixture of $^{35}_{17}$Cl and $^{37}_{17}$Cl in the proportion of almost exactly three to one, so that its atomic weight is $35 \cdot 5$.

hydrogen is not: the latter in fact usually exists as a molecule of two atoms, the one sharing its electron with the other. Oxygen (atomic number 8) has two electrons in its inner but 6 in its outer shell (maximum number in this shell is 8). With

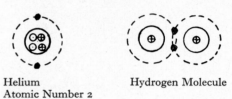

Helium
Atomic Number 2
Mass Number 4

Hydrogen Molecule

Figure 111.2
Both the helium atom and the hydrogen molecule are stable.

the exception of hydrogen and helium, atoms are most stable when their outer shells contain 8 electrons, and they can attain this configuration in two ways. Firstly, one atom may donate an electron to another. As an example, $^{23}_{11}$Na and $^{35}_{17}$Cl (sodium and chlorine) combine as follows:

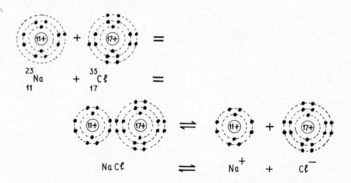

Figure 111.3
The atom of sodium is unstable because it has one electron in its outer shell. Likewise the chlorine atom is unstable due to its seven outer electrons. By donating an electron stable sodium chloride is formed. In solution this molecule may split to produce two charged and stable ions.

The sodium, by donating an electron, and chlorine, by acquiring an electron, both attain a stable configuration to form a molecule of sodium chloride. In solution they may exist as stable charged ions. The chemical properties of these ions, depending upon the number of electrons, are, of course, very different from those of the parent atoms. A second method of attaining stability is by way of a covalent linkage:

in this, electrons are shared, not donated. For instance, water is:

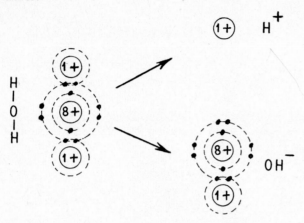

Figure 111.4

This molecule can be dissociated to form the two stable but charged ions: H^+, the positive hydrogen ion, and OH^-, the negative hydroxyl ion. It should be noted that the ions so far described in aqueous solution are stable, and facilitate the conduction of an electric current. The ions produced by the radiations to be described are of a different type, but nevertheless also increase electrical conductivity, e.g. in a gas.

Nature of Ionising Radiations

Certain naturally-occurring elements, like radium, continually emit radiations which may be of one or more of three types:

1. α-"rays". These are, in fact, helium nuclei with mass of 4 and two positive charges.
2. β-"rays", which are electrons of negligible mass, but with one negative charge.
3. γ-"rays". Electromagnetic waves of short wavelength, generally similar to x-rays.

X-rays. Electrons are emitted when a wire is heated, but normally do not escape because of their charge. As they have a negative charge, they can be drawn away by applying a strong electric field provided by a positive charge. This must be done in a vacuum, because they are readily stopped by any matter in their path.

These streams of electrons are in fact similar to the naturally-occurring β-rays. Their energy is dependent upon the voltage applied. It is measured in electron volts, and with electrons is numerically equal to the voltage used to accelerate them. If the electrons hit a "target", much of their energy is transformed into heat, the remainder appearing as electromagnetic radiations (x-rays) of varying wavelengths. The shortest wavelength of the spectrum produced in this way is dependent upon the energy of the electrons. When 20 kV is used in an x-ray tube, the rays have a long wavelength and relatively poor penetrating power ("soft"). For

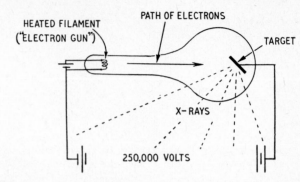

Figure 111.5
Diagrammatic representation of an x-ray tube. The filament is heated by a small electric current which can be varied. The emitted electrons are drawn to the target (anode) where they are stopped, and their energy converted into heat and x-radiation. A cooling mechanism is therefore required to dissipate the heat, while a suitable lead shield allows the x-rays to pass through only one controlled gap. The tube current (i.e. the electron stream between cathode and target) determines the quantity of x-rays generated. It is measured in milliamperes, mA, and is itself related to the temperature of the filament. The energy (i.e. wavelength) of the x-rays is related to the kilovoltage applied, and in the above diagram 250 kV is shown.

many years machines with a "harder" ray generated at about 250 kV were used. Nowadays x-rays generated at several million volts can be produced, and are commonly used in the treatment of cancer. The naturally-emitted γ-rays do not differ from these high energy x-rays. Thus the rays from ^{60}Co are the same as the hardest x-rays generated at about 1·2 MeV.*

Streams of electrons, protons, neutrons, and the charged nuclei of heavier atoms can be generated in various ways, and are being used in radiotherapy.

Changes Induced in Matter by the Passage of Ionising Radiation

The changes that occur have been studied mostly in gases, and it is assumed that liquids and solids behave in a similar manner.

β-Particles. Because of their charge and negligible mass they are rapidly slowed down, giving up their energy to atoms through which they pass. Electrons at 2 MeV have a maximum range of about 1 cm in water.

α-Particles. These have a double positive charge and a mass of 4. Because of their high charge and relatively low velocity, they have little penetrating power.

Protons. With mass of 1 and charge of +1 they are intermediate between γ-rays and β-particles in their power of penetration.

Neutrons. These particles with no charge and a mass of 1 can readily penetrate tissue, and are impeded only when they collide with atomic nuclei. With fast neutrons a proton is

*The maximum energy of such x-rays is 1·2 MeV (million electron-volts). ^{60}Co emits 2 γ-rays of energy 1·17 and 1·33 MeV.

knocked out of the nucleus, and the effects are due to this released particle. With slow neutrons no proton is ejected, but the nucleus traps the neutron. In this way the atom increases its mass number by one, and frequently the isotope so formed is radioactive. It may then emit either β- or γ-rays or both, and (rarely) α-particles. Neutron-induced radio-activity is used in atomic reactors for manufacturing isotopes, and is one of the sources of the radioactivity following nuclear explosions. Electromagnetic radiation and β-particles of very high energy, e.g. over 8 MeV, may also induce radioactivity.

Gamma and X-rays. These electromagnetic radiations have great penetrating power; the shorter the wavelength, the greater their penetration. It should be noted that the particulate radiations have a definite range in matter: electromagnetic radiations, on the other hand, are merely reduced in quantity. Thus, a particular thickness of a material (the *half-value thickness*) will reduce the intensity by half, a further thickness by another half, etc. When they traverse matter, they give up quanta of energy which cause atoms to emit high-energy electrons. In this way a positive ion is formed. The electrons then behave like β-particles, causing other atoms to eject further electrons. These slower electrons are more readily deflected, and finally are caught in the orbit of some atom to produce a negative ion. For each electron ejected an ion pair is formed, and the *density of this ionisation* varies with the different radiations. The density of ionisation for charged particles is directly proportional to the square of their charge and inversely proportional to their velocity. Electrons and protons of equal velocity produce the same ion density, but as they slow down, the density increases. α-particles, on the other hand, with their double charge and slow velocity, produce dense ionisation. Gamma and x-rays of high energy (short wavelengths) produce fewer ionisations than do low-energy rays.

Ion Formation

The ions formed by radiation are not the same as those of salts in solution, e.g. Na^+, Cl^-, OH^-, etc. If a molecule of water ejects an electron, the ion H_2O^+ is formed:

$$H_2O \rightarrow H_2O^+ + e$$

The electron may be captured by another molecule of water

$$H_2O + e \rightarrow H_2O^-$$

These charged ions are unstable and decompose immediately:

$$H_2O^+ \rightarrow H^+ + OH^{\cdot}$$
$$H_2O^- \rightarrow H^{\cdot} + OH^-$$

The radicals $OH^{\cdot}$ and $H^{\cdot}$, although electrically neutral, are highly unstable and reactive, because they have an odd number of outer orbiting electrons.

Although there can be little doubt that when aqueous solutions are irradiated, the hydroxyl radical $OH^{\cdot}$ is formed,

because oxidative reactions predominate, there is some doubt about the $H^{\cdot}$ radical (or hydrogen atom). It has been suggested that H_2O^- breaks down as follows:

$$H_2O^- + H_2O \rightarrow H_2 + OH^{\cdot} + OH^-$$

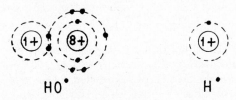

Figure 111.6
Ionising radiations lead to the formation of the free radicals $OH^{\cdot}$ and $H^{\cdot}$ (the hydrogen atom). Although electrically neutral these radicals are highly unstable because of the seven outer electrons in the case of the $OH^{\cdot}$ radical and the odd electron in the hydrogen atom. By convention a dot is placed after these radicals to distinguish them from the charged ions OH^- and H^+.

In the presence of oxygen further powerfully oxidising radicals are formed:

$$H_2O + O_2 \xrightarrow[\text{radiation}]{\text{ionising}} OH^{\cdot} + HO$$
$$H^{\cdot} + O_2 \rightarrow HO_2^{\cdot}$$
$$HO_2^{\cdot} + HO_2^{\cdot} = H_2O_2 + O_2$$

Oxidising compounds are certainly formed; many of them are in a very active state as free radicals, and have an existence of only a small fraction of a second.

Although most work has been directed to the effects of radiation on water, other substances are also changed. In addition to the formation of free radicals, some molecules are "excited" by a change in the energies of their electrons. Much has yet to be learned even about the changes occurring in simple solutions on irradiation.

Radioactive Elements

Some elements, like radium, are not stable, but show a continuous loss of energy and mass due to the emission of radiations of some kind. Alpha, beta, or gamma radiations are given off either singly or in combination, each radioactive element having its own characteristic properties. The energy of each radiation also varies from one element to another. For instance, tritium, ^3_1H, emits β-particles of 0·018 MeV, while $^{131}_{53}I$ emits β-particles (0·605 MeV) and γ-rays of two separate energies.

The activity of any portion of a radioactive material is measured by the number of atoms which disintegrate each second. In 1 gram of radium there are $3·7 \times 10^{10}$ disintegrations every second, and this is arbitrarily taken to be one unit —the Curie. *One Curie* is thus that amount of any element which produces $3·7 \times 10^{10}$ disintegrations per second. The actual weight of material will vary from micrograms to tons, depending upon the speed at which the element decays.

Measurement of Radiations

The Roentgen. Since the radiations produce ion pairs in air, a convenient unit of measurement is dependent upon this ionisation, which can be measured by a change in the electrical conductivity of air. *One Roentgen* (r) may be described as that amount of radiation, which under specified conditions produces in 1 ml of air at NTP, 1 ESU* of electricity of either charge.

The effect of radiation is dependent upon the energy actually absorbed by the substance radiated. A more logical unit of measurement is, therefore, dependent upon energy absorbed. *One Rad* is a dose which equals an absorption of 100 ergs per gram of substance irradiated.

When 1 gram of water or soft tissue is exposed to a dose of 1 r of x-radiation, the absorbed dose is almost equal to 1 rad. When, however, other radiations are used, e.g. neutrons, or when bone is irradiated, much more energy is absorbed.

Another unit which has been suggested is the *rep* (*Roentgen equivalent physical*), which is that quantity of radiation which releases the same amount of energy in water as 1 r of x-rays. The unit is now obsolete.

* Electrostatic Unit.

In radiobiology it is the effect on cells which is important. Even with an equal amount of energy absorption, the different radiations produce different biological effects. The *relative biological efficiency* (*RBE*) is a measure of this. Thus the RBE for neutrons compared with x-rays is about 10, when considering the lethal effect on the mouse. This means that if 500 rad of x-rays causes death, then 50 rad of neutrons produces the same effect.

An alternative method of expressing this is to use the *rem* (*Roentgen equivalent man*). The dose in rems = Rads × RBE. Thus in the above example 500 rem of x-rays (500 rad × RBE, i.e. 500 × 1) produces the same effect as 500 rem of neutrons (50 rad × RBE, i.e. 50 × 10).

When considering other biological effects, e.g. chromosomal damage, the RBE is different. In general the RBE is greatest for those radiations which produce the densest ionisation. It should be noted that the RBE is merely a method of comparing the ability of one type of radiation with another to produce a particular biological effect. It is not an absolute figure.

General Reading. See Chapter 31.

Index

Main references are indicated by bold numerals.
Illustrations are referred to by italic numerals.